Stedman's

EQUIPMENT
WORDS

THIRD EDITION

Edited by
Catherine S. Baxter

Stedman's

EQUIPMENT
WORDS

THIRD EDITION

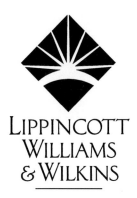

LIPPINCOTT
WILLIAMS
& WILKINS

Series Editor: Beverly J. Wolpert
Editor: Catherine S. Baxter
Associate Managing Editor: Trista A. DiPaula
Associate Managing Editor: William A. Howard
Production Manager: Julie K. Stegman
Production Coordinator: Kevin Iarossi
Typesetter: Peirce Graphic Services, Inc.
Printer & Binder: Data Reproductions Corp.

Copyright © 2001 Lippincott Williams & Wilkins
530 Walnut Street
Philadelphia, Pennsylvania 19106-3620

Printed in the United States of America

Third Edition, 2001

Library of Congress Cataloging-in-Publication Data

01

2 3 4 5 6 7 8 9 10

Stedman's equipment words.— 3rd ed.
    p. ; cm.
    Edited by Catherine S. Baxter.
    Rev. ed. of: Stedman's medical & surgical equipment words. 2nd ed. c1996
    ISBN 0-7817-2703-0
       1. Medical insruments and apparatus—Terminology. 2. Medical technology—
Terminology. I. Title: Equipment words. II. Baxter, Catherine S. III. Stedman,
Thomas Lathrop, 1853-1938. IV. Stedman's medical & surgical equipment words.
       [DNLM: 1. Equipment and Supplies—Terminology—English. W 15 S8112 2001]
R123 .S698 2001
610'.14—dc21
                                              00-052015

Contents

Acknowledgments

An important part of our editorial process is the involvement of medical transcriptionists—as advisors, reviewers, and editors.

We extend special thanks to Catherine S. Baxter for once again undertaking the planning, editing, and researching for yet another edition of *Stedman's Equipment Words*. We also extend special thanks to Jeanne Bock, CSR, MT, for researching and resolving many difficult content questions and editing the manuscript; to Natasha Brown and Patricia L. White, CMT, for editing the manuscript; and to Martha Richards, RRA, for reviewing the previous edition.

Thanks also to our Editorial Advisory Board, including Kay Deering; Carrie Donathan, CMT; Kathryn Mason, CMT; and Peg Nelson, CMT. These individuals served as editors and advisors, in some cases contributing new equipment terms and the benefits of their medical transcription experience to assist in the development of this new edition, and in others, editing the manuscript and appendix sections at different stages. Ellen Atwood; Bonnie Bakal, CMT, CPRS; Shemah Fletcher; Sandy Kovacs, CMT; Robin Koza; and Tina Whitecotton, CMT, spent hours collecting new equipment terms for this new edition. Helen Littrell, CMT, performed the final prepublication format review. Barb Ferretti played an integral role in the process by reviewing the content files for format, updating the database, and providing a final quality check.

As with all our *Stedman's* word references, this resource incorporates the suggestions and expertise of our many contacts in the medical transcriptionist community. Thanks to all of our advisory board participants, reviewers, and editors; AAMT meeting attendees; and others who have written us with requests and comments—keep talking, and we'll keep listening.

Editor's Preface

Stedman's Equipment Words, Third Edition, is "in the can," as someone in the movie industry might comment. Now, it's time to write the preface, that which comes before and introduces the body of the text. After nearly 10 months of blood, sweat, tears, and a database crash, this third edition is truly our best effort yet to provide a comprehensive reference for medical and surgical equipment words and phrases.

The target audience really hasn't changed over the years. We strive to provide accurate, up-to-the-minute information to medical transcriptionists, medical editors, medical translators and interpreters, and anyone who is in the business of using the medical language.

What had really just begun to impact the healthcare industry in 1996 has now become the capstone, the keyword, the motivating force behind most everything we read, namely the Internet, the ".com's," the *www.anythingyoueverwantedtoknow.com,* the ASP (application service provider) model for medical transcription, Internet transmission of voice and text, cyberspace MTs...all very *techie.*

However, the main task of any medical language specialist did not change as we stepped across the precipice into the new millennium. That task is to document and interpret accurately the healthcare data presented to us for the purpose of supporting patient care.

Likewise, what also has not changed is the commitment of Lippincott Williams & Wilkins to provide reference materials of unsurpassed excellence to those of us still pounding the keyboards to make our vitally important contribution to patient care.

Once again, as with the second edition, we were faced with how to add thousands of new terms to a book already testing the limits of its bindings. We started with a detailed review of the second edition, followed by a heavy hand with a red pen, deleting redundant terms and combining similar terms. Every effort was made to remove single-word terms; every term was assigned to a main entry or category to facilitate quick reference checks.

Through the effort of many contributors and our editorial advisory board members, we were able to complete this third edition on time and with confidence that we have prepared the best, most comprehensive reference for medical and surgical equipment words and phrases ever produced!

On a personal note, I'd like to comment on a sentence that I wrote in the Preface for the first edition back in 1993, "Once a medical transcriptionist, always a medical transcriptionist, regardless of what other path I might take in the future."

I've come full circle…again! After being the executive director of the Medical Transcription Industry Alliance (MTIA), I became a consultant and worked for healthcare organizations from Washington to Minnesota to Maine. But, once again, I've returned to my roots in Texas, where I manage the daily operations of the Houston office of the world's largest medical transcription company, MedQuist Inc. I still love to be challenged by a member of my QA Team to come "listen and fill in the blanks." And, I feel comfortably fulfilled when I can pick up one of the Stedman's reference books and point to the answer to that blank. It makes all the work worthwhile and meaningful to me and, hopefully, to all of you who use our references.

Many special thanks go to two people at Lippincott Williams & Wilkins, one newbie and one who has been around since the first edition of this reference. The newbie is the series editor, Beverly Wolpert, and the veteran is my dear friend, Maureen Barlow Pugh, who left that job and the publishing world for an equally daunting position as a full-time mom to Caroline.

Another person who deserves a huge bundle of thanks has worked with me from afar for many years. In fact, we rarely see or talk to each other, but Barb Ferretti is the greatest! Barb is the online editor who translates my red pen notes, lines, and arrows from the hard copy pages to the database that ultimately generates the next edition of this reference.

As the third edition begins the printing process, let the fourth edition begin!

Catherine S. Baxter

Publisher's Preface

When we first published *Stedman's Medical Equipment* Words in 1993 and again with our second edition in 1996, there were no other comprehensive, up-to-date, affordable references that provided listings of generic, trade, and eponymic medical and surgical equipment terms. The same is the case today. The popularity of this reference continues to surge as equipment terminology continues to grow. But now there are even more reasons that this reference is essential. Increasingly, risk management initiatives within healthcare institutions and insurance companies are requiring precise equipment names in medical records to link specific equipment to injury and malpractice claims. Other new requirements amplify the importance of accurately using medical equipment terminology, including the mandate of the Joint Commission on Accreditation of Healthcare Organizations that operative reports specify complete names and model numbers for CT and MRI equipment.

Like the previous two editions, this third edition of the newly titled *Stedman's Equipment Words* is the product of hard work, determination, persistence, and expertise. We started with the equipment terms in the second edition and used database technology to add medical and surgical equipment terms gathered from medical specialty journals, trusted internet sources, manufacturers' printed information and websites, and our other published word books.

To make room for the thousands of terms we added to this third edition, we needed to consolidate some terms listed in the second edition. Our goal, however, was to make way for new terms without taking away any useful information. We therefore retired only those terms that were essentially less descriptive versions of other terms that we retained.

This compilation of more than 100,000 entries, fully cross-indexed for quick access, was built from a base vocabulary of more than 50,000 medical words, phrases, abbreviations, and acronyms. The extensive A to Z list was developed from the database of *Stedman's Medical Dictionary, 27th Edition,* our other word books, and terminology in the current medical literature, including internet sources. For quick reference, a list of top equipment manufacturers and their websites appears as an appendix section at the back of this book.

We at Lippincott Williams & Wilkins strive to provide you with the most up-to-date and accurate word references available. Your use of this word book will prompt new editions, which we will publish as often as updates and revisions justify. We welcome your suggestions for improvements, changes, corrections, and additions—whatever will make this *Stedman's* product more useful to you. Please complete the postpaid card at the back of this book, and send your recommendations care of "Stedman's" at Lippincott Williams & Wilkins.

Explanatory Notes

Medical transcription is an art as well as a science. Both are needed to correctly interpret the dictation of a physician, whose language is a product of education, training, and experience. This variety in medical language means that there are several acceptable ways to express certain terms, including jargon. *Stedman's Equipment Words, Third Edition* provides variant spellings and phrasings for many terms. These elements, in addition to complete cross-indexing, make *Stedman's Equipment Words, Third Edition* a valuable resource for determining the validity of terms as they are encountered.

Alphabetical Organization

Alphabetization of main entries is letter by letter as spelled, ignoring punctuation, spaces, prefixed numbers, or other characters. Greeks are spelled out and placed in alphabetical order. For example:

acid-fast staining method
acid formaldehyde hematin
acid hematin
alpha-acid glycoprotein

In subentry alphabetization, the abbreviated singular form or the spelled-out plural form of the noun main entry word is ignored.

Format and Style

All main entries are in **boldface** to expedite locating a sought-after term, to enhance distinction between main entries and subentries, and to relieve the textual density of the pages.

Irregular plurals and variant spellings are shown on the same line as the singular or preferred form of the word. For example:

scolex, pl. scoleces
curette, curet

Hyphenation

As a rule of style, multiple eponyms (e.g., Mears-Rubash approach) are hyphenated. Also, hyphens have been added between a manufacturer and one or more eponyms (e.g., Vital-Metzenbaum dissecting scissors).

Please note that in many cases, hyphenation is a question of style, not of accuracy, and thus is a matter of choice.

Possessives

Possessive forms have been dropped in this reference for the sake of consistency and conformance with the guidelines of the American Association for Medical Transcription (AAMT), the American Medical Association (AMA), and other groups. Please note, however, that in many cases, retaining the possessive, like hyphenating, is a question of style, not of accuracy, and thus is also a matter of choice. To form the possessive of a word, simply add the apostrophe or apostrophe "s" to the end of the word.

Cross-indexing

The word list is in an index-like main entry-subentry format that contains two combined alphabetical listings:

(1) A *noun* main entry-subentry organization, which is typical of the A–Z section of medical dictionaries like *Stedman's:*

blade
　　Aggressor meniscal b.
　　Baxter disposable b.
　　bent blunt b.
　　carbolized knife b.

clamp
　　Abadie enterostomy c.
　　Adair breast c.
　　Berkeley-Bonney vaginal c.
　　Berke ptosis c.

(2) An *adjective* main entry-subentry organization, which lists words and phrases as you hear them. The main entries are the adjectives or modifiers in a multiword term. The subentries are the nouns around which the terms are constructed and to which the adjectives or modifiers pertain:

Acucise
　　A. balloon
　　A. uretral cutting cautery

chromic
　　c. blue dyed suture
　　c. catgut suture

This format provides the user with more than one way to locate and identify a multiword term. For example:

catheter
Glidewire c.

balloon
Fogarty b.
Garren b.
hydrostatic b.

Glidewire
G. catheter

Fogarty
F. balloon
F. biliary probe
F. irrigation catheter

It also allows the user to see together all terms that contain a particular descriptor, as well as all types, kinds, or variations of a noun entity. For example:

Biograft
Dakin B.
Meadox Dardik B.

collar
Belmont c.
c. brace

Wherever possible, abbreviations are separately defined and cross-referenced. For example:

CFD
color-flow Doppler

color-flow
c.-.f. Doppler (CFD)

Doppler

color-flow D. (CFD)

References

In addition to the manufacturers' literature we gather at various medical meetings, scientific reports from hospitals, and the lists of our MT Editorial Advisory Board members (from their daily transcription work), we used the following sources for new words for *Stedman's Equipment Words, Third Edition:*

Books

Brooks Tighe SM. Instrumentation for the Operating Room: A Photographic Manual, 5th Edition. St. Louis: Mosby, 1999.

Forbis P, Bartolucci SL. Stedman's Medical Eponyms. Baltimore: Lippincott Williams & Wilkins, 1998.

Lance LL. Quick Look Drug Book. Baltimore: Lippincott Williams & Wilkins, 2000.

The Medical Device Register. Montvale, NJ: Medical Economics, 2000.

The Merck Manual, 16th Edition. Rahway, NJ: Merck Research Laboratories, 1992.

Pyle V. Current Medical Terminology, 7th Edition. Modesto: Health Professions Instiitute, 1998.

Stedman's Abbreviations, Acronyms & Symbols, 2nd Edition. Lippincott Williams & Wilkins, 1999.

Stedman's Alternative Medicine Words. Baltimore: Lippincott Williams & Wilkins, 2000.

Stedman's Cardiology & Pulmonary Words, 2nd Edition. Baltimore: Lippincott Williams & Wilkins, 1997.

Stedman's Dermatology & Immunology Words. Baltimore: Lippincott Williams & Wilkins, 1997.

Stedman's GI & GU Words, 2nd Edition. Baltimore: Lippincott Williams & Wilkins, 1996.

Stedman's Medical Dictionary, 27th Edition. Baltimore: Lippincott Williams & Wilkins, 2000.

Stedman's Oncology Words, 3rd Edition. Baltimore: Lippincott Williams & Wilkins, 2000.

Stedman's Ophthalmology Words, 2nd Edition. Baltimore: Lippincott Williams & Wilkins, 2000.

Stedman's Orthopaedic & Rehab Words, 3rd Edition. Baltimore: Lippincott Williams & Wilkins, 1999.

Stedman's Pathology & Lab Medicine Words, 2nd Edition. Baltimore: Lippincott Williams & Wilkins, 1998.

Stedman's Plastic Surgery/ENT/Dentistry Words. Baltimore: Lippincott Williams & Wilkins, 1999.

Stedman's Psychiatry/Neurology/Neurosurgery Words, 2nd Edition. Baltimore: Lippincott Williams & Wilkins, 1999.

Stedman's Radiology Words, 3rd Edition. Baltimore: Lippincott Williams & Wilkins, 2000.

Stedman's Surgery Words. Baltimore: Lippincott Williams & Wilkins, 1998.

Stedman's WordWatcher, 1995–1997. Baltimore: Lippincott Williams & Wilkins, 1998.

Tessier C. The AAMT Book of Style. Modesto: AAMT, 1995.

Tessier C. The Surgical Word Book, 2nd Edition. Philadelphia: Saunders, 199.

Wells MP, Bradley M. Surgical Instruments, 2nd Edition. Philadelphia: Saunders, 1998.

Journals

ACSM's Health & Fitness. American Journal of Audiology. Rockville, MD: American Speech-Language-Hearing Association, 1997–2000.

Alternative Therapies in Health and Medicine. Aliso Viejo, CA: Innovision Communications, 1998–2000.

The American Journal of Cardiology. Belle Mead, NJ: Excerpta Medica, 1996–2000.

The American Journal of Clinical Pathology. Chicago: American Society of Clinical Pathologists, 1997–2000.

The American Journal of Gastroenterology. New York: Elsevier, 1996–2000.

The American Journal of Obstetrics and Gynecology. St. Louis: Mosby, 1999–2000.

The American Journal of Ophthalmology. Baltimore: Lippincott Williams & Wilkins, 1996–2000.

The American Journal of Surgical Pathology. Philadelphia: Lippincott Williams & Wilkins, 1996–2000.

Annals of Surgical Oncology. Philadelphia: Lippincott Williams & Wilkins, 1998–2000.

Applied Radiology. Ocean, NJ: Anderson Publishing, 1998–2000.

Archives of Otolaryngology—Head & Neck Surgery. Chicago: American Medical Association, 1997–2000.

Arteriosclerosis, Thrombosis, and Vascular Biology. Philadelphia: Lippincott Williams & Wilkins, 1998–2000.

AUA News. Baltimore: Lippincott Williams & Wilkins, 1996–2000.

CA-A Cancer Journal for Clinicians, Atlanta: American Cancer Society. 1996–2000.

Cancer. New York: John Wiley & Sons, 1996–2000.

Cardiology in Review. Baltimore: Lippincott Williams & Wilkins, 1996–2000.

Chiropractic Products. Los Angeles: Novicom, 1996–2000.

Circulation. Philadelphia: Lippincott Williams & Wilkins, 1998–2000.

Circulation Research. Philadelphia: Lippincott Williams & Wilkins, 1998–2000.

Clinical Pulmonary Medicine. Baltimore: Lippincott Williams & Wilkins, 1997–2000.

Computer-Aided Surgery. New York: Wiley, 1998–2000.

Contemporary OB/GYN. Montvale, NJ: Medical Economics, 1996–2000.

Cornea. Philadelphia: Lippincott Williams & Wilkins, 1998–2000.

The Endocrinologist. Baltimore: Lippincott Williams & Wilkins, 1997–2000.

Extended Care Product News. Wayne, PA: H M P Communications, 1997–2000.

References

Foot & Ankle International. Seattle: American Orthopaedic Foot & Ankle Society, 1996–2000.

Gastrointestinal Endoscopy. St. Louis: Mosby, 1996–2000.

Hypertension. Philadelphia: Lippincott Williams & Wilkins, 1998–2000.

Implant Dentistry. Philadelphia: Lippincott Williams & Wilkins, 1996–2000.

Infectious Diseases in Clinical Practice. Baltimore: Lippincott Williams & Wilkins, 1996–2000

The Integrative Medicine Consult. Newton, MA: Integrative Medicine Communications, 1998–2000.

Internal Medicine. Montvale, NJ: Medical Economics, 1996–1998.

Journal of Alternative and Complementary Medicine. Larchmont, NY: Mary Ann Liebert, Inc. 1998–2000.

Journal of the American Association for Medical Transcriptionists. Modesto, CA: AAMT, 1996–2000.

Journal of the American College of Cardiology. Philadelphia: Lippincott Williams & Wilkins, 1996–2000.

Journal of the American College of Surgeons. New York: Elsevier, 1996–2000.

Journal of the American Society of Nephrology. Baltimore: Lippincott Williams & Wilkins, 1997–2000.

Journal of Bone and Joint Surgery. Needham, MA: The Journal of Bone and Joint Surgery, Incorporated, 1996–2000.

Journal of Clinical Oncology. Philadelphia: Saunders, 1996–2000.

Journal of Clinical Rheumatology. Baltimore: Lippincott Williams & Wilkins, 1996–2000.

Journal of Foot & Ankle Surgery. Baltimore: H M P Communications, 1997–2000.

Journal of Investigative Medicine. Thorofare: Slack, 1999–2000.

Journal of Oral and Maxillofacial Surgery. Philadelphia: Saunders, 1996–2000.

Journal of the National Cancer Institute. Oxford: Oxford University Press, 1998–2000.

Journal of Neuro-Ophthalmology. Philadelphia: Lippincott Williams & Wilkins, 1998–2000.

Laparoscopic Surgery Update. Hagerstown, MD: Lippincott Williams & Wilkins, 1997–2000.

The Latest Word. Philadelphia: Saunders, 1996–2000.

MT Monthly. Gladstone, MO: Computer Systems Management, 1996–2000.

Neurosurgery. Baltimore: Lippincott Williams & Wilkins, 1996–2000.

O & P Almanac. Alexandria, VA: American Orthotic and Prosthetic Association, 1996–2000.

OB/GYN Clinical Alert. Atlanta: American Health Consultants, 1997–2000.

OB/GYN News. Rockville, MD: International Medical News Group, 1997–2000.

Obstetrical & Gynecological Survey. Philadelphia: Lippincott Williams & Wilkins, 1996–2000.

Obstetrics & Gynecology. New York: Elsevier Science. 1996–2000.

Ophthalmology. Philadelphia: Lippincott Williams & Wilkins, 1996–2000.

Ophthalmology Times. New York: Advanstar Communications, 1997–2000.

Ostomy—Wound Management. Wayne, PA: H M P Communications, 1997–2000.

Otolaryngology—Head and Neck Surgery. St. Louis: Mosby, 1997–2000.

Patient Care. Montvale, NJ: Medical Economics, 1999–2000.

Perspectives on the Medical Transcription Profession. Modesto: Health Professions Institute, 1996–2000.

Physical Therapy Products. Los Angeles: Novicom, 1996–2000.

Plastic and Reconstructive Surgery. Philadelphia: Lippincott Williams & Wilkins/American Society of Plastic Surgeons, 1996–2000.

Plastic Surgery Products. Los Angeles: Novicom, 1996–2000.

Podiatric Products. Los Angeles: Novicom, 1996–2000.

Radiographics. Oak Brook, IL: Radiological Society of North America: 1998–2000.

Radiology. Oak Brook, IL: Radiological Society of North America: 1998–2000.

Retina. Philadelphia: Lippincott Williams & Wilkins, 1998–2000.

Stroke. Philadelphia: Lippincott Williams & Wilkins, 1998–2000.

Websites

http://www.mtdesk.com

http://www.mtdaily.com

http://www.mtmonthly.com

http://www.hpisum.com

http://www.lexi.com/

http://www.health.org/

http://www.parsonstech.com/home/med_list.html

http://www.currentopinion.com/

A1-Askari needle holder
A1, A2 Port multipurpose catheter
A13 Sequel programmable behind-the-ear hearing instrument
A675 Sequel Audio Vision hearing aid
A2008 ABGII hemodialysis machine
AA1 single-chamber pacemaker
Aagesen
    A. disposable rasp
    A. file
AAI
    activating adjusting instrument
Aaron cautery
Abacus Concepts StatView 4.02 statistical analyzer
Abadie
    A. enterostomy clamp
    A. self-retaining retractor
ABaer system
Abanda drape sheet
Abbé condenser
Abbe refractometer
Abbey needle holder
ABBI
    advanced breast biopsy instrumentation
    ABBI system
Abbokinase catheter
Abbott
    A. elevator
    A. infusion pump
    A. LifeCare PCA Plus II infusion system
    A. Lifeshield needleless system
    A. scoop
    A. tube
Abbott-Mayfield forceps
Abbott-Rawson gastrointestinal double-lumen tube
abdominal
    a. aortic counterpulsation device
    a. bandage
    a. binder
    a. brace
    a. left ventricular assist device
    a. patch electrode
    a. ring retractor
    a. scissors
    a. scoop
    a. trocar
    a. vascular retractor
abduction
    a. finger splint
    a. pillow
Abel-Aesculap-Pratt tenaculum
Abelson
    A. adenotome
    A. cricothyrotomy cannula
    A. cricothyrotomy trocar
Aberhart
    A. disposable urinal bag
    A. hemostatic bag
Abernaz strut forceps

aberrometer
    Shack-Hartmann a.
ABG cement-free hip system
Abiomed
    A. biventricular support system
    A. BVAD 5000 cardiac device
ABI PRISM Dye Terminator Cycle Sequencing Ready Reaction Kit
ABL520 blood gas measurement system
Ablaser laser delivery catheter
ablater (var. of ablator)
ablation
    a. catheter
    ThermaChoice thermal balloon a.
ablative device
ablator, ablater
    cautery a.
    Concept a.
    endometrial a.
    Hydro TherAblator a.
    radiofrequency a.
Ablatr temperature control device
Ablaza
    A. aortic wall retractor
    A. patent ductus clamp
Ablaza-Blanco cardiac valve retractor
Ablaza-Morse rib approximator
abortion scoop
Above-Knee Suction Enhancement system
Abradabloc dermabrasion instrument
abrader
    a. bur
    cartilage a.
    cornea a.
    Dingman otoplasty cartilage a.
    Haverhill dermal a.
    Howard corneal a.
    Lieberman a.
    Montague a.
Abraham
    A. contact lens
    A. elevator
    A. iridectomy laser lens
    A. laryngeal cannula
    A. peripheral button iridotomy lens
    A. rectal curette
    A. tonsillar knife
    A. YAG laser lens
Abrams
    A. biopsy needle
    A. pleural biopsy punch
Abrams-Lucas flap heart valve
Abramson
    A. catheter
    A. hook
    A. retractor
    A. sump drain
Abramson-Allis breast clamp
Abramson-Dedo microlaryngoscope
abscess forceps
Abscession fluid drainage catheter
abscission needle

Absolok
> A. endoscopic clip applicator
> A. forceps

Absolute absorbable screw

absorbable
> a. plate
> a. stent

absorber
> Hollister wound exudate a.
> laser fume a.

absorptiometer
> Hologic 1000 QDR dual-energy a.
> Lunar DPX dual-energy a.
> single-energy x-ray a.

A/B switch box

Abuscreen Ontrak

abutment
> CeraOne a.
> Dalla Bona ball and socket a.
> dovetail stress broken a.
> Hex-Lock a.
> IMPAC PDQ a.
> low margin standard a.
> ProTect a.
> Spectra-System a.
> ThreadLoc non-cast-to a.
> tooth-colored a.

AC
> acromioclavicular
> anterior chamber
> AC IOL
> AC lens

ACAT 1 intraaortic balloon pump

accelerator
> alpha particle a.
> Becker a.
> Bevatron a.
> dual-energy linear a.
> electron linear a.
> high-energy bent-beam linear a.
> A. II aspirator
> linear a. (LINAC)
> Mevatron 74 linear a.
> Microtron a.
> Mobetron mobile, self-shielded
>   electron a.
> Philips linear a.
> plasma prothrombin conversion a.
> proserum prothrombin conversion a.
> racetrack Microtron a.
> Siemens Mevatron 74 linear a.
> University of Florida linear a.
> Varian a.

accelerometer
> Caltrac a.
> intracardiac a.
> piezoelectric a.

Accellon Combi cervical biosampler

Accel stopcock

Accent-DG balloon

Ac'cents permanent lash liner

Accents system

Access MV system

accessory
> Auto Glide walker a.

> BabyFace 3-D surface rendering a.
> CUSALap ultrasonic a.
> a. eye implant
> Isola spinal implant system a.
> Wegenke stent exchange a.

Acc ESS Wand

ACCO
> ACCO cotton roll
> ACCO impression material
> ACCO orthodontic appliance

accommodative IOL

Accorde bur

ACCOR dental matrix

accordion
> a. drain
> a. graft
> a. implant

AccuAngle indicator

Accu-Beam suction & irrigation cannula

AccuBrush dental brush

Accucap CO$_2$/O$_2$ monitor

Accucare TENS unit

Accu-Chek
> A.-C. Advantage non-wipe blood
>   glucose monitoring system
> A.-C. Easy glucose monitor
> A.-C. II Freedom blood glucose
>   monitor
> A.-C. II Freedom system
> A.-C. II glucometer
> A.-C. III blood glucose meter
> A.-C. InstantPlus system

Accucom cardiac output monitor

Accucore II biopsy needle

accuDEXA
> a. bone densitometer
> a. bone mineral density assessment
>   system

Accufilm articulating film

Accufix
> A. pacemaker
> A. pacemaker lead

Accu-Flo
> A.-F. button
> A.-F. connector
> A.-F. CSF reservoir
> A.-F. dural film
> A.-F. dural substitute
> A.-F. pressure valve
> A.-F. spring catheter
> A.-F. U-channel stripping cannula
> A.-F. ventricular cannula
> A.-F. ventricular catheter

AccuGel
> A. impression material
> A. lens

Accuguide syringe

Accuject dental needle

**AccuLength arthroplasty measuring
system**

Accu-Line
> A.-L. chamfer resection guide
> A.-L. distal femoral resection
>   instrument
> A.-L. distal femoral resector

A.-L. knee instrumentation
A.-L. patellar instrument
A.-L. surgical marker
A.-L. tibial resector
Acculith pacemaker
AccuMark calibrated infant feeding tube
AccuMax
    A. bed
    A. self-adjusting pressure
      management mattress
AccuMeter
    Aware A.
    ChemTrak A.
    A. cholesterol test system
Accu-Mix
    A.-M. amalgamator
    A.-M. impression material
Accu-o-Matic TENS unit
AccuPoint targeting sphere
AccuPressure heel cup
Accura hydrocephalus shunt
Accurate
    A. catheter
    A. Surgical and Scientific
      Instruments (ASSI)
Accuratome precurved papillotome
Accuray Neurotron 1000 machine
Accurette
    A. endometrial suction curette
    A. microcurette
AccuroX mask
Accurus vitrectomy system
Accusat pulse oximeter
AccuScan CO$_2$ laser scanner
Accuscanner transducer
Accu-Scope
    A.-S. colposcope
    A.-S. microscope
AccuSharp
    A. endoscope
    A. instrument
Accu-Sorb gauze sponge
AccuSpan tissue expander
AccuSway balance measurement system
Accu-Temp cautery
Accutome low-speed diamond saw
Accutorr
    A. A1 blood pressure monitor
    A. bedside monitor
    A. oscillometric device
Accutracker
    A. blood pressure monitor
    A. II
Accuvac smoke evacuation attachment
ACD
    arrhythmia control device
    Res-Q ACD
    ACD resuscitator
ACE
    ACE autografter bone filter
    ACE balloon
    BICAP silver ACE
    ACE bone screw tack
    ACE fixed-wire balloon catheter
    ACE OstseoGenic distractor

Ace
    A. adherent bandage
    A. aerosol cloud enhancer
    A. Brace
    A. halo-cast assembly
    A. halo pelvic girdle
    A. intramedullary femoral nail
      system
    A. longitudinal strips dressing
    A. low-profile MR halo
    A. Mark III halo
    A. pin
    A. spica bandage
    A. Trippi-Wells tong cervical
      traction
    A. Universal tong cervical traction
    A. wire tension assembly
    A. wrap
Ace-Colles half ring
Ace-Fischer
    A.-F. external fixator
    A.-F. frame
Ace-Hershey halo jig
Ace-Hesive dressing
Ace/Normed osteodistractors
acetabular
    a. angle guide
    a. component
    a. endoprosthesis
    a. grater
    a. reconstruction plate
    a. shell guide
    a. skid
ACFS
    anterior cervical plate fixation system
    Dogbone ACFS
achalasia dilator
Achiever
    A. balloon dilatation catheter
    A. balloon dilator
Achilles densitometer
Achilles+ ultrasonometer
Achillotrain
    A. active Achilles tendon support
    Bauerfeind A.
Acier stainless steel suture
AC-IOL
    anterior chamber intraocular lens
Ackerman
    A. clip
    A. lingual bar
    A. needle
Ackrad
    A. balloon-bearing catheter
    A. Bronchitrac "L" suction catheter
    A. Cervicet dilator
    A. esophageal balloon catheter
    A. H/S Elliptosphere catheter
    A. Tampa catheter set
ACL
    ACL drill
    ACL drill guide
    ACL graft knife
Acland
    A. clasp

Acland *(continued)*
    A. clip
    A. microvascular clamp
    A. needle
Acland-Banis arteriotomy set
Acland-Bunke counterpressor
Aclec resin
Acme articulator
ACMI
    ACMI ACN-2 flexible cystonephroscope
    ACMI Alcock catheter
    ACMI antroscope
    ACMI bag
    ACMI biopsy loop electrode
    ACMI Bunts catheter
    ACMI cautery
    ACMI coated Foley catheter
    ACMI cystoscopic tip
    ACMI cystourethroscope
    ACMI duodenoscope
    ACMI Emmett hemostatic catheter
    ACMI endoscope
    ACMI fiberoptic colonoscope
    ACMI fiberoptic esophagoscope
    ACMI fiberoptic proctosigmoidoscope
    ACMI flexible sigmoidoscope
    ACMI gastroscope
    ACMI Marici bronchoscope
    ACMI Martin endoscopic forceps
    ACMI Micro-H hysteroscope
    ACMI microlens Foroblique telescope
    ACMI monopolar electrode
    ACMI operating colonoscope
    ACMI Owens catheter
    ACMI Pezzer drain
    ACMI positive pressure catheter
    ACMI proctoscope
    ACMI resectoscope
    ACMI retrograde electrode
    ACMI severance catheter
    ACMI Thackston catheter
    ACMI Transvaginal Hydro laparoscope
    ACMI ulcer-measuring device
    ACMI ureteral catheter
    ACMI Word Bartholin gland catheter
Acmix Foley catheter
Acoma scanner
acorn
    a. cannula
    A. II nebulizer
    a. reamer
acorn-shaped eye implant
acorn-tipped
    a.-t. bougie
    a.-t. catheter
Acoustascope esophageal stethoscope
acoustic
    a. densitometry
    a. impedance probe

    a. microscope
    a. myograph
    a. otoscope
acoustically transparent cradle
AcQsim CT simulator
Acra-clip system
Acra-Cut Spiral craniotome blade
Acra-gun system
Acro-Flex artificial disk
acromioclavicular (AC)
acromionizer bur
Acrotorque
    A. bur
    A. hand engine
AcryDerm
    A. hydrogel sheet
    A. Strands
    A. Strands absorbent wound dressing
Acry Island border dressing
acrylic
    a. ball eye implant
    a. bar prosthesis
    a. bite block
    a. cap splint
    a. cement
    a. conformer eye implant
    Dentex a.
    Durabase soft rebase a.
    Durahue a.
    Duralay a.
    Dura-Liner a.
    fast-setting a.
    Flexacryl hard rebase a.
    a. graft
    a. implant material
    a. lens
    a. mold
    a. resin dressing
    Setacure denture repair a.
    Splintline a.
    TAB a.
    TMJ a.
    Vita-Gel a.
    a. wafer TMJ splint
Acryl-X orthopaedic cement removal system
AcrySof foldable intraocular lens
ACS
    Advanced Cardiovascular System
    Alcon Closure System
    automated corneal shaper
    ACS Amplatz guidewire
    ACS Anchor Exchange device
    ACS Angioject
    ACS angioplasty catheter
    ACS angioplasty Y connector
    ACS balloon catheter
    ACS Concorde coronary dilatation catheter
    ACS Concorde OTW catheter
    ACS Endura coronary dilation catheter
    ACS exchange guiding catheter
    ACS Gyroscan

ACS Hi-Torque Balance guidewire
ACS Hi-Torque Balance
Middleweight catheter
ACS Indeflator
ACS JL4 French catheter
ACS LIMA guidewire
ACS microglide wire
ACS Monorail perfusion balloon
catheter
ACS Multi-Link Duet coronary
stent
ACS Multi-Link Tristar coronary
stent
ACS needle
ACS OTW Lifestream coronary
dilation catheter
ACS OTW Photon coronary
dilatation catheter
ACS OTW Solaris coronary
dilatation catheter
ACS percutaneous introducer
ACS percutaneous introducer set
ACS RX Comet coronary dilatation
catheter
ACS RX Comet VP catheter
ACS RX Gemini catheter
ACS RX Lifestream catheter
ACS RX multilink stent
ACS RX Rocket catheter
ACS SULP II balloon
ACS Torquemaster catheter
ACS Tourguide II guiding catheter
ACS Tx2000 VP catheter
ACS Viking catheter
ACT
ACT Microcoil
ACT MicroCoil delivery system
Act
Act joint support
Acticoat silver-based burn dressing
Acticon neosphincter
Acti-Fit brief
Actifoam
A. active hemostat
A. collagen sponge
A. hemostat
A. hemostat sponge
Actigraph
Mini-Motionlogger A.
Action
A. Jr. wheelchair
A. OR pad
A. traction system
Actis
A. venous flow controller
A. venous flow device
**activated balloon expandable
intravascular stent**
activating adjusting instrument (AAI)
activator
Andresen a.
Andresen-Haupl a.
Bimler a.
cutout a.
Karwetsky U-bow a.
Klammt elastic open a.

Metzelder modification a.
Nuva-Lite ultraviolet a.
palate-free a.
Pfeiffer-Grobety a.
Schmuth modification a.
Schwarz bow-type a.
Wunderer modification a.
Activa tremor control system
Active
A. Cath catheter
ACTIVE LIFE
A. L. convex one-piece urostomy
pouch with Durahesive skin
barrier
A. L. FLUSHAWAY one-piece
flushable closed-end pouch system
A. L. one-piece drainable pouch
A. L. one-piece opaque stoma cap
A. L. one-piece precut closed-end
pouch
Activent ear tube
Activitrax
A. single-chamber responsive
pacemaker
A. variable-rate pacemaker
activity-guided pacemaker
activity-sensing pacemaker
actocardiotocograph fetal monitor
ACT-one coronary stent
Actros pacemaker
actuator
NYU-Hosmer electric elbow and
prehension a.
Acucair continuous airflow system
Acucare bed
Acucise
A. balloon
A. cutting balloon device
A. RP retrograde endopyelotomy
catheter
A. ureteral cutting cautery
AcuClip endoscopic multiple-clip applier
Acu-Derm
A.-D. IV/TPN dressing
A.-D. wound dressing
Acufex
A. alignment guide
A. arthroscope
A. basket
A. bioabsorbable Suretac suture
A. bioabsorbable suture anchor
A. curved basket forceps
A. drill
A. drill guide
A. Edge
A. handle
A. MosaicPlasty instruments
A. rotary basket forceps
A. rotary punch
A. straight basket forceps
Acufex-Suretac implant
AcuFix anterior cervical plate system
Acuflex
A. impression material
A. intraocular lens implant

acuiometer
visual a.
acuity
visual a.
a. visual projector
Acumaster acupuncture needle
**AcuMatch M Series modular femoral
hip prosthesis**
Acumed suture anchor
AcuNav ultrasound catheter
AcuPressor myotherapy tool
Acuprobe thermometer
acupuncture laser
Acu-Ray x-ray unit
Acuscope microcurrent stimulator
AcuSnare
A. polypectomy device
A. snare
Acuson
A. 128 apparatus
A. color Doppler
A. echocardiographic equipment
A. 128EP imager
A. 128EP scanner
A. linear array transducer
A. 5-MHz linear array
A. ultrasound
A. ultrasound scanner
A. V5M multiplane TEE transducer
A. V5M transesophageal
echocardiographic monitor
A. XP-10, -128 ultrasonoscope
A. 128XP ultrasound system
Acuspot
Sharplan Laser 710 A.
acute
a. ionization detector
a. ventricular assist device (AVAD)
ACUTENS
ACUTENS transcutaneous nerve
stimulator
**Acutome 2000 Reich-Hasson laparoscopic
CO₂ laser coupler**
AcuTouch tissue forceps
AcuTrainer bladder retraining device
Acutrak
A. bone fixation system
A. bone replacement system
A. fusion system
A. screw
Acutrol suture
Acuvue
A. bifocal lens
A. disposable contact lens
A. Etafilcon A lens
ADAC gamma camera
**ADAC/Vertex dual-headed SPECT
camera**
Adair
A. adenotome
A. breast clamp
A. breast tenaculum
A. screw compressor
A. tissue forceps

A. tissue-holding forceps
A. uterine forceps
Adair-Allis tissue forceps
Adair-Veress needle
Adam and Eve rib belt splint
Adams
A. aspirator
A. clasp
A. kidney stone filter
A. modification of Bethune
tourniquet
A. orthodontic clip
A. retractor
A. rib contractor
A. saw
Adams-DeWeese vena cava serrated clip
Adamson retractor
Adante Monorail catheter shaft
Adaptar "no-line" contact lens
adapter, adaptor
Air-Lon a.
Alcock catheter a.
AMSCO Hall a.
Bard-Tuohy-Borst a.
BD a.
Bernaco a.
BioLase laser a.
Bodai a.
Brown-Roberts-Wells ring a.
butterfly a.
catheter a.
Christmas tree a.
chuck a.
circuit a.
C-mount a.
coil machine a.
collet screwdriver a.
Cook plastic Luer-Lok a.
Cooper laser a.
Cordis-Dow shunt a.
Curry hip nail counterbore with
Lloyd a.
E-to-A a.
Foregger-Racine a.
Freestyle CAPD catheter a.
friction-fit a.
Grace plate 4-hole a.
Greenberg Maxi-Vise a.
halo-ring a.
House a.
Hudson a.
Jacobs chuck a.
Kaufman a.
King connector a.
KleenSpec otoscope a.
Lloyd a.
Luer-Lok a.
Luer suction cannula a.
Mayfield skull clamp a.
Medi-Jector a.
Merrimack laser a.
metal a.
Morch swivel a.
Neuroguide suction-irrigation a.
Nickell cystoscope a.

pediatric Racine a.
Peep-Keep II a.
peripheral interface a.
power a.
resectoscope a.
Rosenblum rotating a.
rotating a.
SACH foot a.
SafeTrak epidural catheter a.
Sanders ventilation a.
sheath with side-arm a.
Sheehy-Urban sliding lens a.
Shiley pressure-relief a.
side-arm a.
sleeve a.
Storz catheter a.
suction a.
swivel a.
T-a.
Telestill photo a.
terminal electrode a.
Trinkle chuck a.
tubing a.
Tuohy-Borst a.
UAM Osteon bur a.
Universal T-a.
venous Y-a.
ventilation a.
Venturi ventilation a.
Volk Minus (-) noncontact a.
Volk Plus (+) noncontact a.
Volk retinal scale a.
Volk Ultra Field aspherical lens a.
Volk yellow filter a.
Wullstein chuck a.
Xanar laser a.
Zeiss cine a.

Adapteur
A. multifunctional drill guide
A. power system

Adaptic
A. gauze
A. gauze dressing
A. II dental restorative material
A. nonadhering dressing

adaptometer
Collin 140 color a.
color a.
Feldman a.

adaptor (*var. of* adapter)

Ada scissors

ADC
analog-to-digital converter
ADC Medicut shears

Add-a-Cath catheter

Add-A-Clamp
Hex-Fix A.-A.-C.

Addix needle

Add-On Bucky digital x-ray image acquisition system

ADD side-directed probe

ADD'Stat laser

A-Dec
A.-D. amalgamator
A.-D. handpiece

adenoid
a. curette
a. cutter
a. forceps
a. punch

adenotome
Abelson a.
Adair a.
a. blade
Box a.
Box-DeJager a.
Breitman a.
Cullom-Mueller a.
Daniels a.
direct-vision a.
guillotine a.
Kelly direct-vision a.
LaForce a.
LaForce-Grieshaber a.
LaForce-Stevenson a.
LaForce-Storz a.
Mueller-LaForce a.
Myles guillotine a.
reverse a.
Shambaugh reverse a.
Shulec a.
Sluder a.
St. Clair-Thompson a.
Stevenson-LaForce a.
Storz-LaForce a.
Storz-LaForce-Stevenson a.
V. Mueller-LaForce a.

Aderer alloy

adherent
a. stent
Tuf-Skin tape a.

Ad-Hese-Away dressing

adhesive
a. absorbent dressing
ADTRA composite external fixator ring a.
Aron Alpha a.
autologous fibrin tissue a.
BA bone cement a.
a. band
a. bandage
bioactive bone cement a.
Biobond tissue a.
Biobrane a.
biologic fibrogen a.
Bond-Eze bond a.
bone cement a.
Brown sterile a.
Cel Touch a.
Chewrite denture a.
Coe-Pak paste a.
composite external fixator ring a.
Coverlet a.
Cover-Roll gauze a.
cyanoacrylate tissue a.
Dermabond topical skin a.
fibrin glue a.
fibrin sealant a.
a. flange

adhesive *(continued)*
  gelatin-resorcin-formalin tissue
    glue a.
  HA a.
  hydroxyapatite a.
  Hy-Tape a.
  Implast bone cement a.
  Indermil tissue a.
  Klutch denture a.
  LPPS hydroxyapatite a.
  Mammopatch gel self a.
  MCW cement a.
  MDS a.
  methyl methacrylate cement a.
  Nexacryl tissue a.
  Nu-Hope a.
  Orthomite II a.
  Orthoset radiopaque bone cement a.
  Palacos cement a.
  a. plastic drape
  Plastodent dental impression a.
  Scanpor acrylate a.
  Silastic medical a.
  silicone a.
  Simplex cement a.
  stoma cap microporous a.
  Superglue a.
  Surfit a.
  surgical appliance a.
  Surgical Simplex P radiopaque a.
  a. tape remover
  Tisseel biologic fibrogen a.
  T-Stick a.
  Urihesive expandable a.
  Uro-Bond II brush-on silicone a.
  Zimmer low-viscosity a.
Adjustaback wheelchair backrest system
adjustable
  a. advanced reciprocating gait
    orthosis
  a. breast implant
  a. headrest
  a. leg and ankle repositioning
    mechanism
  a. ostomy appliance belt
  a. pedicle connector
  a. skull traction tongs
  a. thigh antiembolism stockings
    (ATS)
  a. vaginal stent
Adjust-A-Flow colostomy irrigation kit
Adjusta-Rak hanger
Adjusta-Wrist splint
adjuster
  Serdarevic suture a.
Adkins strut
Adler
  A. attic ear punch
  A. bone forceps
  A. punch forceps
  A. tripronged lens error loop
Adler-Kreutz forceps
adnexal forceps
adolescent vaginal speculum

Adolph Gasser camera system
"adoptable" baby cholangioscope
ADR Ultramark 4 ultrasound
Adson
  A. aneurysm needle
  A. angular hook
  A. arterial forceps
  A. aspirating tube
  A. bayonet dressing forceps
  A. bipolar forceps
  A. blunt dissecting hook
  A. bone rongeur
  A. brain clip
  A. brain-exploring cannula
  A. brain forceps
  A. brain hook
  A. brain retractor
  A. brain suction tip
  A. brain suction tube
  A. bur
  A. cerebellar retractor
  A. clamp
  A. clip-applying forceps
  A. conductor
  A. cranial rongeur
  A. dissecting hook
  A. dissector
  A. drainage cannula
  A. dressing forceps
  A. drill guide
  A. dural hook
  A. dural knife
  A. dural needle holder
  A. dural protector
  A. ganglion scissors
  A. Gigli saw
  A. Gigli-saw guide
  A. headrest
  A. head rest
  A. hemostat
  A. hemostatic forceps
  A. hypophyseal forceps
  A. knot tier
  A. laminectomy chisel
  A. microbipolar forceps
  A. microdressing forceps
  A. microforceps
  A. microtissue forceps
  A. monopolar forceps
  A. neurosurgical suction tube
  A. perforating bur
  A. periosteal elevator
  A. pickups
  A. scalp clip
  A. scalp clip-applying forceps
  A. scalp needle
  A. speculum
  A. spiral drill
  A. splanchnic retractor
  A. suture needle
  A. thumb forceps
  A. tissue forceps
  A. tooth forceps
  A. twist drill
Adson-Beckman retractor

Adson-Biemer forceps
Adson-Brown
    A.-B. clamp
    A.-B. forceps
    A.-B. tissue forceps
Adson-Callison tissue forceps
Adson-Love periosteal elevator
Adson-Mixter neurosurgical forceps
Adson-Murphy trocar point needle
Adson-Rogers
    A.-R. cranial bur
    A.-R. perforating drill
Adson-Vital tissue forceps
Adsorba hemoperfusion cartridge
ADTRA composite external fixator ring
  adhesive
adult
    a. laryngoscope
    a. reverse-bevel laryngoscope
    a. sigmoidoscope
Advance
    A. Dynamicaire sleep surface
    A. EX self-adhesive urinary external catheter
    A. Zoneaire sleep surface
advanced
    A. beta 200 otoscope
    a. breast biopsy instrumentation (ABBI)
    A. Cardiovascular System (ACS)
    A. Collection breast pump
    A. Medical Systems fetal monitoring system
    A. NMR Systems scanner
    a. real-time motion analysis (ARTMA)
    A. Surgical suture applier
advancement
    a. forceps
    a. needle
Advancer
    Arrow A.
Advancit guidewire system
Advantage
    A. glucometer
    A. ultrasound
AdvanTeq II TENS unit
Advantim revision knee system
Advantx LC+ cardiovascular imaging system
Advent
    A. Flurofocon contact lens
    A. implant
    A. pachymeter
AdzorbStar
    EndoDynamics A.
AE-7277 Rubenstein LASIK cannula
Aebli
    A. corneal scissors
    A. tenotomy scissors
Aebli-Manson scissors
AEC pacemaker
AED
    automatic external defibrillator
    AED automatic external defibrillator

AEDP
    automated external defibrillator pacemaker
AEGIS sonography management system
AEM
    ambulatory electrogram monitor
    analytical electron microscope
Aequalis humeral head implant
Aequitron
    A. apnea monitor
    A. pacemaker
    A. ventilator
AER+ automatic endoscope reprocessor
AerobiCycle
    Universal A.
AeroChamber
    A. bronchial inhaler
    A. face mask
    A. metered-dose inhaler
    A. pediatric spacer device
AeroEclipse device
Aero-Kromayer lamp
aeroplane splint
Aeroplast dressing
aerosol-barrier pipette tip
Aerosol Cloud Enhancer
AeroSonic personal ultrasonic nebulizer
AeroTech II nebulizer
AERx
    A. diabetes management system
    A. electronic inhaler
    A. pain management system
    A. pulmonary drug delivery system
AES
    antiembolic stockings
    Auger electron spectroscopy
Aesculap
    A. argon ophthalmic laser
    A. drill
    A. excimer laser
    A. forceps
    A. needle holder
    A. skull perforator
    A. traction bow
Aesculap-Meditec excimer laser
Aesculap-Pratt tenaculum
AE-series implantable pronged unipolar electrode
Aesop 2000, 3000 endoscopic stabilizer robot
AFB
    air-fluidized bed
Affinity bed
Affirm VP microbial identification system
Affymetrix GeneChip system
a-fiX cannula seal
AFO
    ankle-foot orthosis
    AFO brace
    Littig strut AFO
    sliding AFO
A-frame
    A.-f. orthosis
aftercataract bur

afterload
    a. applicator
    a. colpostat
afterloader
    Fletcher a.
    Henschke a.
    Nucletron MicroSelectron/LDR
      remote a.
afterloading
    a. catheter
    a. implant
Agarloid impression material
agate burnisher
AGC
    anatomic graduated components
    AGC Biomet total knee system
    AGC dual-pivot resection guide
    AGC Modular Tibial II component
    AGC porous anatomic femoral
      component
    AGC unicondylar knee component
Agee
    A. carpal tunnel release system
    A. endoscope
    A. 4-pin fixation device
    A. WristJack fracture reduction
      system
agent
    Helitene absorbable collagen
      hemostatic a.
    Instat collagen absorbable
      hemostatic a.
    ProBond dentin bonding a.
    Surgicel Nu-Knit absorbable
      hemostatic a.
Agfa
    A. CR system
    A. Medical scanner
    A. PACS system
aggregate
    bone a.
aggregometer
    Alivi a.
Aggressor
    A. meniscal blade
    A. meniscal shaver
Agnew
    A. canaliculus knife
    A. keratome
    A. splint
    A. tattooing needle
agraffe clamp
Agrikola
    A. eye speculum
    A. lacrimal sac retractor
    A. refractor
    A. tattooing needle
Agris-Dingman submammary dissector
Agris rasp
AgX antimicrobial Foley catheter
Ahlquist-Durham embolism clamp
Ahmed glaucoma artificial valve
AI
    AI 5200 diagnostic ultrasound

AI 5200 diagnostic ultrasound
    system
AI 5200 S open color Doppler
    imaging system
AICD
    automatic implantable cardiovascular
    defibrillator
    Cadence AICD
    Guardian AICD
    AICD pacemaker
    AICD plus Tachylog device
    Res-Q AICD
    Ventak Mini II AICD
aid
    air-conduction hearing a.
    Amplitone-3 hearing a.
    Argosy Cameo CIC hearing a.
    Argosy in-the-ear hearing a.
    A675 Sequel Audio Vision
      hearing a.
    Audibel ear a.
    Audicraft VIP-I hearing a.
    Audionics PB Max hearing a.
    Audiotone hearing a.
    Audivisette hearing a.
    Auriculina hearing a.
    Bansaton behind-the-ear hearing a.
    BD Sensability breast self-
      examination a.
    behind-the-ear hearing a.
    bone-anchored hearing a.
    bone-conduction hearing a.
    Canal-Mate hearing a.
    Carex ambulatory a.
    completely-in-the-canal hearing a.
    compression hearing a.
    cryostat frozen sectioning a.
    Crystal Tone I in-the-ear hearing a.
    Dahlberg hearing a.
    Ear-Tronics hearing a.
    Euroton hearing a.
    eyeglass hearing a.
    Fonix hearing a.
    Giller hearing a.
    hearing a.
    in-the-ear hearing a.
    Jade Audio-Starr hearing a.
    linear hearing a.
    Lion hearing a.
    Listening Glass hearing a.
    low-vision a.
    Magnatone hearing a.
    Maico Gamma hearing a.
    MasterCraft hearing a.
    Mecon-I hearing a.
    Metavox hearing a.
    Microson hearing a.
    Nuway in-the-ear hearing a.
    Omnitone hearing a.
    Ortho-Turn transfer a.
    Ovation in-the-ear hearing a.
    Pacific Coast hearing a.
    Panasonic hearing a.
    postauricular hearing a.
    Prescriptor hearing a.

Prisma digital hearing a.
Quantum hearing a.
ReSound CC4 hearing a.
ReSound Digital 2000 hearing a.
Rexton hearing a.
Rionet hearing a.
Sensability Breast Self-
  Examination A.
Senso completely-in-the-canal digital
  hearing a.
Servox electronic speech a.
Servox Inton speech a.
sock a.
SolarEar hearing a.
Starkey hearing a.
Star Optica hearing a.
Tactaid hearing a.
Tactaid I vibrotactile a.
Trilogy I hearing a.
Tru-Canal hearing a.
Turn-Easy transfer a.
Ultra Voice speech a.
Unitron Esteem CIC hearing a.
Widex hearing a.

AID-B pacemaker
AIM
AIM femoral nail system
AIM 7 thermocouple input module
aimer
Arthrotek femoral a.
Puddu tibial a.
Ainslie acrylic splint
Ainsworth
A. arch
A. punch
Air
air
a. aspirator needle
a. bag
a. bed
a. chamber
a. compressor
a. cystotome
a. dermatome
a. drill
a. inflatable vessel occluder clamp
a. injection cannula
a. pillow
a. plethysmograph
A. Plus low-air-loss bed
a. pressure dressing
a. saw
a. splint
A. Supply air purifier
A. Temp Advantage back support
  belt
a. trousers
a. uterine displacer
Air-Back spinal system
air-boot
Jobst postoperative a.-b.
Aircast
A. Air-Stirrup leg brace
A. fracture brace

A. pneumatic brace
A. Swivel-Strap brace
air-conduction hearing aid
air-core magnet
Airdance alternating overlay
air-driven
a.-d. artificial heart
a.-d. saw
Aire-Cuf
A.-C. endotracheal tube
A.-C. tracheostomy tube
AirFlex carpal tunnel splint
AirFlo alternating pressure system
air-flow enclosure
air-fluidized bed (AFB)
airfoam splint
airfuge
Beckman a.
AirGEL ankle brace
airgun retractor
Airis II MRI system
Airkair seat cushion
Airlife
A. cannula
A. Dual Spray MiniSpacer
A. MediSpacer
Airlift balloon retractor
Air-Limb edema control system
AirLITE support pad
Air-Lon
A.-L. adapter
A.-L. decannulation plug
A.-L. inhalation cannula
A.-L. inhalation catheter
A.-L. laryngectomy tube
A.-L. tracheal tube
AIR-O-EASE static air flotation mattress
Air-O-Pad pad
airplane splint
air-powered
a.-p. drill
a.-p. nebulizer
Airprene
A. hinged knee prosthesis
A. hinged knee support
Airshields isolette
Air-Shield-Vickers syringe tip
Airsoft dry replacement mattress
air-spaced electrode
AIR3787 static air mattress overlay
Air-Stirrup ankle brace
Airstrip composite dressing
AIR1517 vacuum-formed static air
  wheelchair cushion
airway
Beck mouth tube a.
Berman intubating pharyngeal a.
binasal pharyngeal a.
Coburg-Connell a.
Combitube a.
Concord/Portex a.
Connell a.
disposable a.
double-lumen gastric laryngeal
  mask a.

airway *(continued)*
    esophageal obturator a.
    Foerger a.
    Guedel a.
    laryngeal mask a.
    LMA-Unique disposable laryngeal mask a.
    Lumbard a.
    Luomanen oral a.
    oral pharyngeal a.
    pharyngeal a.
    Portex nasopharyngeal a.
    Robertazzi nasopharyngeal a.
    rubber a.
    Safar-S a.
AITA modular trauma system
AK-10 dialysis machine
Akahoshi
    A. Nucleus Sustainer
    A. phaco prechopper
A-K diamond knife
Aker lens pusher
Akins valve re-do forceps
Akorn Pak
Akron tilt table
Akros
    A. DFD wheelchair wedge cushion
    A. extended-care mattress
AkroTech mattress
Akton
    A. pad
    A. positioning roll
Akutsu III total artificial heart
AL-1 catheter
Alabama
    A. needle holder
    A. University forceps
Alabama-Green eye needle holder
ALAMO alternating low-air-loss mattress overlay
alar
    a. cinch
    a. protector
    a. retractor
    a. screw
alar-columellar implant
alarm
    Bárány a.
    bedwetting a.
    enuresis a.
    Silent Nite a.
AlaSTAT allergy immunoassay system
A-Lastic module
Albany eye guard
Albarran
    A. bridge
    A. laser
    A. laser cystoscope
    A. lens
    A. urethroscope
Albarran-Reverdin needle
Albee
    A. bone graft calipers
    A. bone saw
    A. drill
    A. orthopaedic fracture table
    A. osteotome
Albert
    A. Grass Heritage digital EEG system
    A. slotted bronchoscope
Albert-Andrews laryngoscope
Albert-Smith pessary
Albin-Bunegin pressure sensor
albumin-coated vascular graft
albuminized woven Dacron tube graft
Alcatel pacemaker
Alcock
    A. bladder syringe
    A. catheter adapter
    A. catheter plug
    A. hemostatic bag
    A. lithotrite
    A. obturator
    A. return-flow hemostatic catheter
Alcock-Timberlake obturator
Alcon
    A. A-OK crescent knife
    A. A-OK phacoemulsification slit knife
    A. A-OK ShortCut knife
    A. aspirator
    A. Closure System (ACS)
    A. crescent blade
    A. cryoextractor
    A. cryophake
    A. cryosurgical unit
    A. CU-15 4-mil needle
    A. cystitome
    A. Digital B 2000 ultrasound
    A. disposable drape
    A. hand cautery
    A. I-knife
    A. indirect ophthalmoscope
    A. intraocular lens
    A. irrigating needle
    A. microsponge
    A. Phaco-Emulsifier phacoemulsification unit
    A. pocket blade
    A. reverse cutting needle
    A. spatula needle
    A. sponge
    A. Surgical instruments
    A. suture
    A. taper-cut needle
    A. taper-point needle
    A. tonometer
    A. vitrectomy probe
    A. vitrector
Alcon-Biophysic Ophthascan
Alden retractor
Alden-Senturia specimen collector
Alderkreutz tissue forceps
Aldrete needle
Aldridge rectus fascia sling
Aleman meniscotomy knife
Aleo meter

Alert
    Sears Wee A.
Alesen tube
Alexa 1000 breast diagnostic system
Alexander
    A. antrostomy punch
    A. approximator
    A. bone chisel
    A. bone lever
    A. costal periosteotome
    A. dressing forceps
    A. elevator
    A. mastoid bone gouge
    A. mastoid chisel
    A. otoplasty knife
    A. perforating osteotome
    A. retractor
    A. rib raspatory
    A. tonsillar needle
    A. tonsil needle
Alexander-Ballen orbital retractor
Alexander-Farabeuf
    A.-F. costal periosteotome
    A.-F. elevator
    A.-F. forceps
Alexander-Matson retractor
Alexander-Reiner ear syringe
alexandrite laser
Alexian
    A. Brothers overhead fracture frame
    A. Hospital retractor
ALEXlazr
    Candela A.
Alfa II electrode
ALF DNA Sequencer II
Alfonso
    A. eyelid speculum
    A. guarded bur
Alfreck retractor
Alfred
    A. Becht temporary crown
    A. M. Large vena cava clamp
    A. snare
Algee impression material
Alger brush
algesimeter
    coiled pressure a.
AlgiDERM
    A. wound dressing
alginate
    a. impression material
    a. wound dressing
AlgiSite alginate wound dressing
Algisorb wound dressing
Algitec impression material
Algo newborn hearing screener
Algosteril alginate dressing
Alice 4 diagnostic sleep system
Alien WildEyes lens
Align
    IV A.
aligner
    Charnley femoral inlay a.
    femoral a.
    Geo-Matt 30-degree body a.

    orthodontic a.
    patellar a.
    tibial a.
alignment catheter
AL II guiding catheter
AliMed
    A. diabetic night splint
    A. Freedom arthritis support
    A. QualCraft wrist support
    A. surgical drape
alimentation catheter
Aliplast custom molded foot orthosis
Alivi aggregometer
Alivium prosthesis cup
alkaline battery cautery
Alkare adhesive remover wipe
Alken set
All Access laser system
Alladin InfantFlow nasal continuous
    positive air pressure
Alldress multilayer wound dressing
Allen
    A. anastomosis clamp
    A. applicator
    A. arm surgery table
    A. cecostomy trocar
    A. ePTFE ocular implant
    A. eye implant
    A. fetal stethoscope
    A. finger trap
    A. intestinal clamp
    A. intestinal forceps
    A. laparoscopic stirrups
    A. orbital implant
    A. preschool card
    A. retractor
    A. root pliers
    A. spherical eye introducer
    A. stereo separator
    A. Supramid implant
    A. traction system
    A. Universal stirrup system
    A. uterine forceps
    A. well leg holder
    A. wire threader
Allen-Barkan
    A.-B. forceps
    A.-B. knife
Allen-Braley
    A.-B. forceps
    A.-B. intraocular lens
    A.-B. lens implant
Allen-Brown prosthesis
Allen-Burian trabeculotome
Allen-Hanbury knife
Allen-headed screwdriver
Allen-Heffernan nasal speculum
Allen-Kocher clamp
Allen-Schiotz plunger retractor tonometer
Allen-Thorpe
    A.-T. goniolens
    A.-T. gonioscopic prism
Allen-type hex key
Allerdyce
    A. approximator

Allerdyce *(continued)*
    A. dissector
    A. elevator
Allergan
    A. Medical Optics (AMO)
Allergan-Humphrey
    A.-H. lensometer
    A.-H. photokeratoscope
Allergan-Simcoe C-loop intraocular lens
Allevyn
    A. adhesive hydrocellular dressing
    A. cavity dressing
    A. foam dressing
    A. hydrophilic polyurethane dressing
    A. Island dressing
    A. tracheostomy dressing
Alliance
    A. integrated inflation system
    A. rehabilitation system
alligator
    a. clip
    a. crimper forceps
    a. cup forceps
    a. ear forceps
    a. MacCarty scissors
    a. nasal forceps
    a. pacing cable
Allingham rectal speculum
All-In-One
    A.-I.-O. laparoscopic electrode
all-in-the-bag intraocular lens
Allis
    A. catheter
    A. delicate tissue forceps
    A. dry dissector
    A. hemostat
    A. intestinal forceps
    A. lung retractor
    A. Micro-Line pediatric forceps
    A. periosteal elevator
    A. thoracic forceps
    A. tissue clamp
Allis-Abramson breast biopsy forceps
Allis-Adair
    A.-A. intestinal forceps
    A.-A. tissue forceps
Allis-Coakley
    A.-C. tonsillar forceps
    A.-C. tonsil-seizing forceps
Allis-Duval forceps
Allis-Ochsner
    A.-O. tissue forceps
    A.-O. tonsillar forceps
Allison
    A. clamp
    A. lung retractor
    A. lung spatula
Allis-Willauer tissue forceps
Allkare protective barrier wipe
AlloDerm
    A. dermal graft
    A. processed tissue graft

allogeneic
    a. lyophilized bone graft implant
      material
    a. material
allograft
    AlloGro freeze-dried bone a.
    a. bone vise
    bovine a.
    decalcified freeze-dried bone a.
    intercalary a.
    napkin ring calcar a.
    osteoarticular a.
    Tutoplast processed a.
AlloGro freeze-dried bone allograft
AlloMatrix
    A. injectable putty
    A. injectable putty bone graft
      substitute
AlloMune system
alloplastic graft material
Allo-Pro hip system
alloy
    Aderer a.
    amalgam a.
    Arjalloy a.
    Ceradelta a.
    Ceramalloy a.
    Cerapall a.
    Cer-Mate a.
    Cer-On R a.
    cobalt-chromium-molybdenum a.
    Co-Cr-Mo a.
    Co-Cr-W-Ni a.
    Coltene a.
    Coronet a.
    Co-Span a.
    Degucast a.
    Degudent a.
    Densilay a.
    Dentsply a.
    E-G a.
    Eligoy metal a.
    Everest a.
    Fulcast a.
    GFH a.
    GM a.
    Hammond a.
    Imperial a.
    Leff a.
    Lumi a.
    Ostalloy 202 a.
    Phase-A-Caps a.
    Phasealloy a.
    Primallor a.
    Remanium a.
    Safco a.
    Shasta a.
    Sierra a.
    Stabilor a.
    Steldent a.
    Summar a.
    Summit a.
    Thriftcast a.
    Tivanium Ti-6A1-4V a.
    Ultracast a.

Vera bond a.
Victory a.
Vitallium a.
Wilgnath a.
Wilkadium a.
Wilkoro a.
Wil-Tex a.
Zimaloy cobalt-chromium-
molybdenum a.
all-PMMA one-piece C-loop intraocular lens
Allport
A. cutting bur
A. gauze packer
A. hook
A. mastoid bayonet retractor
A. mastoid searcher
A. mastoid sound
Allport-Babcock
A.-B. mastoid searcher
A.-B. retractor
Allport-Gifford retractor
All-Purpose
A.-P. Boot (APB)
A.-P. Boot Hi
All-Tronics scanner
Allurion foot prosthesis
Alm
A. clip applier
A. dilator
A. microsurgery retractor
A. self-retaining retractor
Almeida forceps
Alnico Magneprobe magnet
Aloka
A. color Doppler system
A. echocardiograph machine
A. linear ultrasound
A. MP-PN ultrasound probe
A. OB/GYN ultrasound
A. SD, SSD ultrasound system
A. sector ultrasound
A. SSD-720 real-time scanner
A. transducer
A. ultrasound linear scanner
A. ultrasound sector scanner
Alpar intraocular lens implant
Alpern cortex aspirator/hydrodissector
ALPHA
A. ACTIVE pressure-relieving
support surface
alpha
a. cradle
A. fiberoptic pocket otoscope
a. particle accelerator
Alphabed
AlphaCare monitor
alpha-chymotrypsin cannula
alpha-particle emitter
AlphaStar operating room table
Alphatec
A. mini lag-screw system
A. small fragment system
Alpine reusable leg bag with Kraylex odor barrier

ALR cystoresectoscope
already-threaded suture
Alta
A. cancellous screw
A. CFX reconstruction rod
A. channel bone plate
A. condylar buttress plate
A. cortical screw
A. cross-locking screw
A. distal fracture plate
A. femoral bolt
A. femoral intramedullary rod
A. femoral plate
A. humeral rod
A. intramedullary rod
A. lag screw
A. modular trauma system
A. reconstruction rod
A. supracondylar bone plate
A. supracondylar screw
A. tibial rod
A. transverse screw
Altchek vaginal mold
Alter lip retractor
alternative communication device
alternator
film a.
ALTERNS therapeutic seating system
Altertome
Microvasive A.
Altmann needle
Alton
A. Deal pressure infuser
A. Dean blood/fluid warmer
Altona finger extension device
Altra Flux hemodialyzer
ALT ultrasound system
Alukart hemoperfusion cartridge
Alumafoam nasal splint
Alumina cemented total hip prosthesis
aluminum
a. cortex retractor
a. eye shield
a. fence splint
a. finger cot splint
aluminum-bronze wire suture
Aluwax impression wax
ALVAD artificial heart
Alvarado surgical knee holder
Alvarez-Rodriguez cardiac catheter
AlveoSampler
Quintron A.
Alvis
A. fixation forceps
A. foreign body eye curette
A. foreign body spud
Alvis-Lancaster sclerotome
Alway groover
Alyea vas clamp
Alzate catheter
Alzer Model 2001 osmotic minipump
ALZET continuous infusion osmotic pump
Alzheimer lamp

AM
  amperemeter
Amadeus ventilator
amalgam
  a. alloy
  a. burnisher
  a. carrier
  a. carver
  a. condenser
  Paragon a.
  a. plugger
  a. plugger elevator
  a. scraper
amalgamator
  Accu-Mix a.
  A-Dec a.
  Bantex a.
  Capmix a.
  crown a.
  Dentomat a.
  McShirley a.
  Vari-Mix II a.
Amazr catheter
AMBI
  AMBI compression hip screw
  system
  AMBI reamer
Ambicor
  A. inflatable prosthesis
  A. penile prosthesis
Ambler dilator
amblyoscope
  Major a.
  Orthoptic Therapy a.
  Worth a.
Ambrose
  A. eye forceps
  A. suture forceps
Ambu
  A. bag
  A. CardioPump
  A. infant resuscitator
  A. respirator
Ambu-E valve
Ambulator
  A. H1200 healing shoe
ambulatory
  a. electrogram monitor (AEM)
  a. infusion management device
Amcath catheter
AMC needle
AMD artificial urinary sphincter
Amdent ultrasonic scaler
Amdur lid forceps
Amelogen
  A. composite dental restorative
  A. dental implant
Amenabar
  A. capsular forceps
  A. counterpressor
  A. discission hook
  A. iris retractor
  A. lens
  A. lens loop
Amercal intraocular lens

Amercal-Shepard intraocular lens
American
  A. artificial larynx
  A. Catheter Corp. biopsy forceps
  A. circle nephrostomy tube
  A. Endoscopy automatic reprocessor
  A. Endoscopy dilator
  A. Hanks uterine dilator
  A. Heyer-Schulte brain retractor
  A. Heyer-Schulte chin prosthesis
  A. Heyer-Schulte elastomer
  A. Heyer-Schulte-Hinderer malar
  prosthesis
  A. Heyer-Schulte mammary
  prosthesis
  A. Heyer-Schulte-Radovan tissue
  expander prosthesis
  A. Heyer-Schulte rhinoplasty
  prosthesis
  A. Heyer-Schulte-Robertson
  suprapubic trocar
  A. Heyer-Schulte sphere
  A. Heyer-Schulte stent
  A. Heyer-Schulte testicular
  prosthesis
  A. Heyer-Schulte T-tube
  A. Hydron instruments
  A. Lapidus bed
  A. Medical Electronics PinSite
  shield
  A. Medical Optics (AMO) Baron
  lens
  A. Medical Source laparoscope
  A. Medical Systems penile
  prosthesis
  A. Medical Systems urethral
  sphincter
  A. Optical Cardiocare pacemaker
  A. Optical coagulator
  A. Optical ophthalmometer
  A. Optical oximeter
  A. Optical photocoagulator
  A. Optical R-inhibited pacemaker
  A. Shared-CuraCare scanner
  A. silk suture
  A. Sterilizer operating table
  A. umbilical scissors
  A. vascular stapler
  A. wire gauge
Amersham
  A. CDCS A-type needle
  A. J tube
Amerson bone elevator
Ames ventriculoperitoneal shunt
Amfit orthotics
Amico
  A. chisel
  A. drill
Amicon
  A. arteriovenous blood tubing set
  A. D-20 filter
Amicus blood collection separator
Amigo mechanical wheelchair
Amko vaginal speculum
AMK total knee system

A

AML
> AML total hip prosthesis

amnifocal lens

Amnihook amniotic membrane perforator

amnioscope
> Erosa a.
> Saling a.

amniotome
> Baylor a.
> Beacham a.
> Glove-n-Gel a.

AMO
> Allergan Medical Optics
> AMO Advent contact lens
> AMO Array foldable intraocular lens
> AMO HPF 500 pump
> AMO intraocular lens
> AMO lensometer
> AMO phacoemulsification lens-folder forceps
> AMO Phacoflex II foldable intraocular lens
> AMO photokeratoscope
> AMO Prestige advanced cataract extraction system
> AMO refractometer
> AMO scleral implant
> AMO Sensar intraocular lens
> AMO Series 4 phaco handpiece
> AMO vitreous aspiration cutter
> AMO YAG 100 laser

Amoena breast form

Amoils
> A. cryoextractor
> A. cryopencil
> A. cryophake
> A. cryoprobe
> A. cryosurgical unit
> A. iris retractor
> A. probe
> A. refractor

Amoils-Keeler cryo unit

AMO-PhacoFlex lens and inserter

AMO-Prestige phaco system

AmpErase electrocautery

amperemeter (AM)

Amplatz
> A. anchor system
> A. angiography needle
> A. aortography catheter
> A. cardiac catheter
> A. coronary catheter
> A. fascial dilator
> A. femoral catheter
> A. Hi-Flo torque-control catheter
> A. injector
> A. retinal snare
> A. sheath
> A. Super Stiff guidewire
> A. Super Stiff guidewire
> A. torque wire
> A. TractMaster system
> A. tube guide

Amplatzer septal occluder

Amplicor typing kit

amplifier
> Botox injection a.
> Cona-Tone office-use hearing a.
> endocardiographic a.
> gradient a.
> hearing aid a.
> lock-in a.
> power a.
> Servox a.

Amplitone-3 hearing aid

Ampoxen sling

amputation
> a. knife
> a. retractor
> a. saw
> a. screw

amputator
> Smith intraocular capsular a.

AMS
> AMS Ambicore penile prosthesis
> AMS 800 artificial urethral sphincter
> AMS autoclavable laparoscope
> AMS CX penile prosthesis cylinder
> AMS 700CX-series penile prosthesis
> AMS disposable trocar
> AMS Endoview camera
> AMS Hydroflex penile prosthesis
> AMS M-series malleable penile prosthesis
> AMS Ultrex penile prosthesis
> AMS urethral stent

AMSCO
> AMSCO Hall adapter
> AMSCO headholder
> AMSCO hysteroscope
> AMSCO light
> AMSCO Orthairtome drill

Amset anterior locking plate system

Amsler
> A. aqueous transplant needle
> A. chart
> A. grid
> A. scleral marker

Amsoft lens

Amsterdam
> A. biliary stent
> A. ventilator

Amsterdam-type prosthesis

Amtech-Killeen pacemaker

AM-UP-75WET dialyzer

Amussat probe

AN69 membrane dialyzer

anal
> a. dilator
> a. EMG PerryMeter sensor
> a. retractor
> a. speculum

analgesia
> patient-controlled a. (PCA)

analgesic cell therapy implantable device

analgizer
> Penthrane a.

analmoscope
  Pickford-Nicholson a.
Analogic Anatom 2000 mobile CT scanner
analog-to-digital converter (ADC)
analysis
  advanced real-time motion a. (ARTMA)
  Fourier harmonic a.
  multidimensional a.
  Multidimensional Scalogram A.
  Point-of-care a.
  Topcon noncontact morphometric a.
analytical electron microscope (AEM)
analyzer
  Abacus Concepts StatView 4.02 statistical a.
  automated cerebral blood flow a.
  automatic chemical a.
  automatic clinical a.
  AVL 9110 pH a.
  BacT/Alert a.
  Beckman ion-selective a.
  Beckman O_2 a.
  BiliChek bilirubin a.
  blood color a.
  BRACAnalyzer gene a.
  Capnomac infrared a.
  Capnomac multiple gas a.
  Capnomac Ultima gas a.
  CA-6000 spine motion a.
  Cat-a-Kit a.
  Cell Soft 2000 semen a.
  Cell Trak/DMS a.
  Cell Trak/S a.
  Cell Trak 11 semen a.
  ChromaVision digital a.
  COBAS Fara H centrifugal a.
  COBAS Helios differential a.
  Corning 170 blood gas a.
  Coulter Channelyser cell a.
  Coulter STKS hematology a.
  C-Trak a.
  Dow Corning hollow-fiber a.
  Ela Medical Elatec V 3.03A arrhythmia a.
  Electra 1000C coagulation a.
  Enzymun-Test System ES22 a.
  fast Fourier transformation spectrum a.
  Fourier transformation spectrum a.
  Friedmann visual field a.
  Futrex a.
  Gas Check blood a.
  GastrograpH Mark III pH a.
  GDx nerve fiber a.
  GEM-Premier point-of-care blood a.
  halothane a.
  Hamilton-Thorn motility a.
  HemoCue blood glucose a.
  HemoCue blood hemoglobin a.
  Hitachi 704, 717 a.
  Humphrey lens a.
  Humphrey visual field a.
  Immulite Dynamic Duo a.
  immunoturbidimetry a.
  Ionalyzer a.
  i-STAT hand-held a.
  IVEC-10 neurotransmitter a.
  Jayco H2 lactose breath a.
  laser microprobe mass a.
  Leadcare handheld blood lead a.
  Malvern a.
  Marquette Series 8000 Holter a.
  medical gas a.
  Medigraphics 2000 a.
  Menuet Compact primary urodynamic nerve fiber a.
  Microlyzer Gas a.
  miniature centrifugal fast a.
  MiniOX 1A, 1000 oxygen a.
  multichannel a.
  Myograph 2000 neuromuscular function a.
  nerve fiber a.
  New Glucorder a.
  Nova Celltrak 12 hematology a.
  Olympus SP-series image a.
  Opti 1 portable pH/blood gas a.
  Orion model AE 940 ion a.
  Osteomeasure computer-assisted image a.
  oxygen a.
  Pachymetric P55 a.
  Packard Auto-Gamma 5650 a.
  Paradigm ocular blood flow a.
  pulse-height a.
  Puritan Bennett ETCO2 multigas a.
  Radiometer ABL 500 blood gas a.
  reflectance TS-200 spectrum a.
  Reynolds Pathfinder 3 a.
  sequential multiple a.
  Serena Mx apnea recorder/a.
  Serono SR1 FSH a.
  Shimadzu DAR-2400 coronary arteriographic a.
  Siemens Somatom DRH CT a.
  single-channel a.
  Sole Primeur 33D a.
  Sonoclot coagulation a.
  SPART a.
  SRI automated immunoassay a.
  Stride a.
  Synchron CX-series automated a.
  Sysmex NE-8000 CBC a.
  Tanita Professional body composition a.
  thermal energy a.
  Tomey retinal function a.
  ultrasound bone a.
  ULT-Svi calibrated end-tidal gas a.
  Vitalab Flexor clinical chemistry a.
  Vitalab ViVa clinical chemistry a.
  ViVa binocular infrared vision a.
anaphylaxis
  passive cutaneous a.
Anastaflo
  A. intravascular shunt
  A. stent
Anastasia bougie

anastigmatic aural magnifier
Anastomark flexible coronary graft marker
anastomosis
    a. apparatus
    a. clamp
    a. forceps
anastomotic button
anatomic
    a. graduated components (AGC)
    A. hip system
    A. Medullary Locking total hip system
    porous-coated a. (PCA)
    A. Precoat hip prosthesis
Anatomic/Intracone reamer
Ancap braided silk suture
anchor
    Acufex bioabsorbable suture a.
    Acumed suture a.
    Arthrex FASTak suture a.
    a. band
    Bio-Anchor suture a.
    Biologically Quiet suture a.
    Bio-Phase suture a.
    BioROC EZ suture a.
    BioSphere suture a.
    Bio-Statak suture a.
    Bone Bullet suture a.
    Catera suture a.
    a. endosteal implant
    E-Z ROC a.
    FASTak suture a.
    FastIn threaded a.
    Hall sacral a.
    Harpoon suture a.
    a. hook
    A. IIa osseointegrated titanium implant system
    Innovasive Devices ROC XS suture a.
    Isola spinal implant system a.
    Kurer a.
    Lemoine-Searcy a.
    Mainstay urologic soft tissue a.
    mini Bio-Phase suture a.
    Mitek asorbable bone a.
    Mitek Fastin threaded a.
    Mitek GII Easy A.
    Mitek GII suture a.
    Mitek GL a.
    Mitek Knotless a.
    Mitek Ligament a.
    Mitek Micro a.
    Mitek Mini GII a.
    Mitek Mini GLS a.
    Mitek Panalok a.
    Mitek Rotator cuff a.
    Mitek Tacit threaded a.
    A. needle holder
    Ogden soft tissue to bone a.
    PaBA a.
    Panalok absorbable a.
    Panalok RC QuickAnchor Plus suture a.

    A. plate
    Radix a.
    Revo suture a.
    ROC XS suture a.
    a. screw
    Searcy fixation a.
    SmartAnchor-D suture a.
    SmartAnchor-L suture a.
    A. soft tissue biopsy device
    a. splint
    Statak suture a.
    A. sterilizer box
    A. surgical needle
    suture a.
    Tacit threaded a.
    TAG Rod II suture a.
    Therap-Loop door a.
    traction a.
    UltraFix a.
anchored catheter
anchor/fixation
    Searcy a./f.
anchoring peg
Anchorlok system
anchor/Snap-Pak
    Mitek Panalok RC a./S.-P.
ANCOR imaging system
Ancrofil clasp wire
Ancure system
Andersen mercury-weighted tube
Anderson
    A. (Abrams modified) biopsy punch
    A. columellar prosthesis
    A. converse iris scissors
    A. curette
    A. double ball
    A. double-end knife
    A. double-end retractor
    A. elevator
    A. flexible suction tube
    A. nasal strut
    A. splint
    A. suture pusher and double hook
    A. traction bow
Anderson-Adson self-retaining retractor
Anderson-Neivert osteotome
Ando
    A. aortic clamp
    A. motor-driven probe
Andre hook
Andresen
    A. activator
    A. monoblock appliance
    A. removable orthodontic appliance
Andresen-Haupl activator
Andrews
    A. applicator
    A. chisel
    A. comedo extractor
    A. infant laryngoscope
    A. mastoid gouge
    A. rigid chest support holder
    A. spinal frame
    A. spinal surgery table
    A. suction tip

Andrews *(continued)*
    A. tongue depressor
    A. tonsillar forceps
    A. tonsil-seizing forceps
    A. tracheal retractor
Andrews-Hartmann
    A.-H. forceps
    A.-H. rongeur
Andrews-Pynchon
    A.-P. suction tube
    A.-P. tongue depressor
Andries stethoscope
AnEber probe
Anel
    A. lacrimal probe
    A. syringe
anemometer
    hot-wire a.
aneroid chest bellows
anesthesiometer
    Semmes-Weinstein pressure a.
Aneuroplast acrylic material
aneurysm
    a. clamp
    a. clip
    a. clip applier
    a. forceps
    a. neck dissector
    a. needle
aneurysmal
    a. clip
    a. coil
AngeCool RF catheter ablation system
AngeFlex lead
Angeion 2000 ICD generator
AngeLase combined mapping-laser probe
Angelchik antireflux prosthesis
Angell
    A. curette
    A. gauze packer
Angell-James
    A.-J. dissector
    A.-J. hypophysectomy forceps
    A.-J. punch forceps
Angell-Shiley
    A.-S. bioprosthetic heart valve
    A.-S. xenograft prosthetic valve
AngelWings device
Ange-Med Sentinel ICD device
Anger
    A. gamma camera system
    A. scintillation camera
Angestat hemostasis introducer
Angetear tear-away introducer
Angiocath
    A. flexible catheter
    A. PRN catheter
angiocatheter
    Brockenbrough a.
    Corlon a.
    Deseret a.
    Eppendorf a.
    Mikro-Tip a.
    a. with looped polypropylene suture

Angiocor prosthetic valve
Angioflow high-flow catheter
angiogram
    Epistar subtraction a.
    FluoroPlus a.
    helical computed tomographic a.
    indocyanine green a.
    MEDIS off-line quantitative
      coronary a.
    Tagarno 3SD cine projector for a.
angiographic
    a. balloon occlusion catheter
    a. portacaval shunt
angiography
    a. catheter
    a. needle
Angioguard catheter device
Angioject
    ACS A.
AngioJet
    A. rheolytic thrombectomy system
    A. thrombectomy catheter
Angio-Kit catheter
angiolaser
    pulsed a.
Angiomat 6000 contrast delivery system
Angiomedics catheter
AngioOPTIC microcatheter catheter
angiopigtail catheter
angioplasty
    a. balloon
    a. balloon catheter
    a. guiding catheter
    a. sheath
AngioRad radiation system
angioscope
    Baxter a.
    Coronary Imagecath a.
    flexible a.
    Imagecath rapid exchange a.
    Masy a.
    Mitsubishi a.
    Olympus a.
    Optiscope a.
angioscopic valvulotome
Angio-Seal
    A.-S. catheter
    A.-S. hemostasis system
    A.-S. hemostatic puncture closure
      device
AngioStent stent
angiotribe
    Ferguson a.
    a. forceps
    Zweifel a.
AngioVista angiographic system
angle
    a. arch
    a. port pump
    a. splint
Anglebasic E arch appliance
angled
    a. ball-end electrode
    a. balloon catheter
    a. biter

A

a. capsular forceps
a. clip
a. counterpressor
a. DeBakey clamp
a. decompression retractor
a. delivery device
a. discission hook
a. guidewire
a. iris retractor
a. iris spatula
a. left cannula
a. lens loop
a. nucleus removal loop
a. peripheral vascular clamp
a. pigtail catheter
a. pleural tube
a. probe
a. right cannula
a. ring curette
a. scissors
a. stone forceps
a. vein retractor
Angle-Pezzer drain
angle-tip
a.-t. electrode
a.-t. Glidewire
a.-t. guidewire
a.-t. urethral catheter
Angstrom MD implantable single-lead cardioverter-defibrillator
angular
a. elevator
a. knife
a. needle
a. scissors
angulated
a. catheter
a. iris spatula
Anis
A. aspirating cannula
A. ball reverse-curvature capsular polisher
A. capsulotomy forceps
A. corneal forceps
A. corneal scissors
A. corneoscleral forceps
A. disk capsular polisher
A. intraocular lens forceps
A. irrigating vectis
A. microforceps
A. microsurgical tying forceps
A. needle holder
A. staple lens
A. straight corneal forceps
A. tying forceps
Anis-Barraquer needle holder
Ankeney sternal retractor
Ank-L-Aid brace
ankle
a. air stirrup
a. hitch
a. orthosis (AO)
a. rehab pump
a. weight
AnkleCiser exerciser

ankle-foot
a.-f. orthosis (AFO)
a.-f. orthotic
a.-f. orthotic splint
AnkleTough ankle rehabilitation system
Ann Arbor
A. A. phrenic retractor
A. A. towel clamp
ANNE anesthesia infuser
annular
a. detector
a. gouge
annular-array transducer
AnnuloFlex flexible annuloplasty ring
AnnuloFlo
anode
molybdenum a.
rhodium a.
a. tube
tungsten a.
anomaloscope
Kamppeter a.
Nagel a.
Pickford-Nicholson a.
anoscope
Bacon a.
Bensaude a.
Bodenheimer a.
Boehm a.
Brinkerhoff a.
Buie-Hirschman a.
Burnett a.
Disposo-Scope a.
Fansler a.
Fansler-Ives a.
fiberoptic a.
Goldbacher a.
Hirschman a.
Ives a.
Ives-Fansler a.
KleenSpec disposable a.
Muer a.
Munich-Crosstreet a.
Otis a.
Pratt a.
Proscope a.
Pruitt a.
rotating speculum a.
Sims a.
Sklar a.
slotted a.
Smith a.
speculum a.
Welch Allyn a.
anosigmoidoscope
Anprolene sterilizer
Ansaldo AU560 ultrasound
Anspach
A. cranial perforator
A. craniotome
A. diamond dissecting cutter
A. 65K drill
A. 65K instrument system
A. leg holder

antegrade
    a. internal stent
    a. ureteral stent
    a. valvulotome
antegrade/retrograde compression nail
Antense anti-tension device
antepartum monitor
anterior
    a. anodal patch electrode
    a. aspect esophageal sensor
    a. bulbi camera
    a. capsule forceps
    a. cervical plate fixation system
    (ACFS)
    a. chamber (AC)
    a. chamber acrylic implant
    a. chamber intraocular lens (AC
    IOL, AC-IOL)
    a. chamber irrigating cannula
    a. chamber irrigating vectis
    a. chamber irrigator
    a. chamber maintainer
    a. chamber synechia scissors
    a. chamber tube shunt encircling
    band
    a. commissure laryngoscope
    a. commissure microlaryngoscope
    a. cruciate ligament drill guide
    a. crurotomy nipper
    a. distraction instrumentation
    a. footplate pick
    a. internal fixation device
    a. prostatic retractor
    a. quadrilateral triplane frame
    a. resection clamp
    a. segment forceps
anterior-posterior
    a.-p. cutting block
    a.-p. cystoresectoscope
Anthony
    A. aspirating tube
    A. cast boot
    A. elevator
    A. enucleation compressor
    A. gorget
    A. mastoid suction tube
    A. orbital compressor
    A. pillar retractor
    A. quadrisected dilator
    A. suction tube
Anthony-Fisher
    A.-F. antral balloon
    A.-F. forceps
Anthron heparinized catheter
anthropometric total hip
antibiotic-coated stent
antibiotic-loaded
    a.-l. acrylic cement
    a.-l. acrylic cement total joint
    prosthesis
antibiotic removal device
anticavitation drill
anticoagulant
anticoagulator
    argon gas a.

anticomplementary
antiembolic stockings (AES)
antiembolism stockings
antifog tube
antifungal
    Triple Care a.
antimicrobial
    a. catheter
    a. removal device
antimony pH electrode
antirotation guide
antiseptic dressing
antishock suit
antisiphon valve
antitachycardia pacemaker
Antoni-Hook lumbar puncture cannula
antral
    a. balloon
    a. bur
    a. chisel
    a. curette
    a. drain
    a. forceps
    a. gouge
    a. irrigator
    a. perforator
    a. punch
    a. rasp
    a. retractor
    a. sinus cannula
    a. trocar
    a. trocar needle
Antron catheter
antroscope
    ACMI a.
    Nagashima right-angle a.
    Reichert a.
antrum-exploring needle
Anustim electronic neuromuscular
    stimulator
anvil
    Bunnell a.
Anzio catheter
A-O
    A.-O. minus cylinder Phoroptor
    A.-O. plus cylinder Phoroptor
AO
    ankle orthosis
    AO brace
    AO dynamic compression plate
    AO dynamic compression plate
    construct
    AO fixateur interne instrumentation
    AO gouge
    AO guidepin
    AO mandibular system
    AO notched instrumentation
    AO reconstruction plate
    AO rigid fixation
    AO stopped-drill guide
AOA cervical immobilization brace
AOA/CHICK ambulatory halo system
AO/ASIF
    A. orthopaedic implant
    A. titanium craniofacial system

AOO pacemaker
AOR
    A. check traction device
    A. collateral ligament retractor
aortic
    a. aneurysm clamp
    a. aneurysm forceps
    a. arch cannula
    a. balloon pump
    a. bioprosthetic valve
    a. cannula clamp
    a. catheter
    A. Connector system
    a. curette
    a. dilator
    a. direct ellipse cannula
    a. occluder
    a. occlusion clamp
    a. occlusion forceps
    a. perfusion cannula
    a. punch
    a. root perfusion needle
    a. sac
    a. sump tube
    a. tube graft
    a. valve retractor
aortography
    a. catheter
    a. needle
aortopulmonary shunt
APB
    All-Purpose Boot
    APB Hi all purpose boot
APC-3, -4 collimator
A-P cutting block
Apdyne phenol applicator kit
APEX
    APEX 409, 410, 415 ECT digital
    γ camera
Apex
    A. irrigation system
    A. pin
Apexo elevator
Apfelbaum
    A. bipolar forceps
    A. cerebellar retractor
    A. micromirror
APF Moore-type femoral stem
Apgar timer
API
    API osteotome
    API Universal foam chin strap
apicitis curette
apicoaortic
    a. conduit heart valve
    a. shunt heart valve
apicolysis retractor
Aplicap
    Espe Ketac-Bond A.
    Espe Photac-Bond A.
Apligraf
    A. graft
    A. Graftskin
    A. skin graft material
    A. venous ulcer graft material

apnea
    a. alarm mattress
    a. monitor
Apogee
    A. CX 200 echo system
    A. ultrasound device
    A. 800 ultrasound system
Apollo
    A. DXA bone densitometry system
    A. 95E tooth-whitening and curing
      system
    A. hip prosthesis
    A. hip system
    A. knee prosthesis
    A. 3 triple-lumen papillotome
APOPPS, transtibial prosthetic socket
A²-Port
A-Port implantable port
apparatus
    Acuson 128 a.
    anastomosis a.
    aspiration a.
    automatic systematic
      desensitization a.
    Bárány alarm a.
    Bárány noise a.
    Barcroft a.
    Barcroft-Warburg a.
    Belzer a.
    Benedict-Roth a.
    biphase Morris fixation a.
    Brawley suction a.
    Buck convoluted traction a.
    Buck extension a.
    Cappio Laurus a.
    C-arm fluoroscopic a.
    cryosurgical a.
    Davidson pneumothorax a.
    dental a.
    Desault a.
    Deyerle a.
    Doppler a.
    electro-oculogram a.
    extension a.
    eye movement measuring a.
    Fell-O'Dwyer a.
    fixation a.
    FracSure a.
    fracture-banding a.
    Frigitronics nitrous oxide
      cryosurgery a.
    Georgiade visor halo fixation a.
    Gibson-Cooke sweat test a.
    Golgi a.
    Guthrie-Smith a.
    Haldane a.
    halo a.
    Heyns abdominal decompression a.
    Hilal embolization a.
    Hodgen a.
    Holman flushing a.
    Horsley-Clarke stereotactic a.
    ICLH a.
    Jackson-Rees a.
    Jaquet a.

apparatus *(continued)*
    juxtaglomerular a.
    Kanavel a.
    Kandel stereotactic a.
    Killian suspension gallows a.
    Kinetron muscle strengthening a.
    Kirschner traction a.
    Kroner a.
    Küntscher traction a.
    lacrimal a.
    Lewy suspension a.
    Light-Veley a.
    Lynch suspension a.
    Malgaigne a.
    Manifold II slot-blot a.
    Marstock a.
    masticatory a.
    Mayfield-Kees skull fixation a.
    McAtee a.
    McKesson pneumothorax a.
    mechanical joint a.
    mobile electroconvulsive therapy a.
    Morwel silhouette suction a.
    Nakayama anastomosis a.
    Naugh os calcis a.
    Neufeld a.
    optoelectric measuring a.
    OsteoStim a.
    Parham-Martin fracture a.
    Pearson flexed-knee a.
    Philips Angiodiagnostics 96 a.
    Plummer-Vinson a.
    pneumothoracic a.
    portable insulin dosage-regulating a.
    Potain a.
    R&B portable pneumothorax a.
    Reichert stereotaxic brain a.
    Robinson artificial pneumothorax a.
    Roger Anderson a.
    Roughton-Scholander a.
    Ruth-Hedwig pneumothorax a.
    Sandow a.
    Sayre suspension a.
    Scholander a.
    Seldinger a.
    self-contained underwater
      breathing a.
    Semm pneumoperitoneum a.
    Singer portable pneumothorax a.
    Skatron a.
    Spiegel-Wycis human a.
    Stader extraoral a.
    Stryker Constavac closed-wound
      suction a.
    suction a.
    surgical exhaust a.
    suspension a.
    Swenko gastric-cooling a.
    Tallerman a.
    Taylor spinal support a.
    Tobold laryngoscopic a.
    traction a.
    triplanar protractor a.
    Vactro perilimbal suction a.
    vacuum a.
    Van Slyke a.
    Venturi a.
    Volutrol control a.
    von Petz a.
    Wagner a.
    Waldenberg a.
    Wangensteen a.
    Warburg a.
    Watanabe a.
    Wells stereotaxic a.
    Zander a.
    Zavod aneroid pneumothorax a.
    Zund-Burguet a.

Appel-Bercie sheath
appendage clamp
appendectomy retractor
appendiceal retractor
applanation tonometer
applanator
    Johnston LASIK flap a.
applanometer
Applause Super-Hemi wheelchair
Apple
    A. laparoscopic stone grabber
    A. Medical bipolar forceps
    A. trocar
appliance
    ACCO orthodontic a.
    Andresen monoblock a.
    Andresen removable orthodontic a.
    Anglebasic E arch a.
    arch bar facial fracture a.
    Balters a.
    Begg light wire a.
    Bimler a.
    biphasic pin a.
    Bipro orthodontic a.
    Bradford fracture a.
    Brooks a.
    Buck fracture a.
    Case a.
    craniofacial fracture a.
    Crozat removable orthodontic a.
    Denholtz muscle anchorage a.
    dental arch bar facial fracture a.
    Dewald halo spinal a.
    double-band navel a.
    Erich facial fracture a.
    extraoral fracture a.
    Fairdale orthodontic a.
    fixed a.
    FracSure a.
    Fränkel a.
    Gentle Touch colostomy a.
    Gerster fracture a.
    Goldthwait fracture a.
    Graber a.
    Hasund a.
    Hawley a.
    Hibbs fracture a.
    Hyrax a.
    ileostomy a.
    intraoral fracture a.
    Janes fracture a.

Jelenko facial fracture a.
Jewett fracture a.
Jobst a.
Johnson twin-wire a.
Joseph septal fracture a.
Karaya adhesive ileostomy a.
Kesling a.
Latham a.
Level Anchorage a.
light wire a.
mandibular advancement a.
mandibular orthopaedic
  repositioning a.
Margolis a.
Marlen colostomy a.
microstomia prevention a.
Mitek anchor a.
Nu-Comfort colostomy a.
obturator a.
Ormco a.
orthodontic a.
ostomy a.
prosthetic a.
Proxi-Floss cleaning a.
Remedy colostomy a.
Remedy ileostomy a.
ribbon arch a.
Roger Anderson pin fixation a.
SACH orthopaedic a.
Schacht colostomy a.
Seep-Pruf ileostomy a.
soft ankle, cushioned heel
  orthopaedic a.
"stick-and-carrot" a.
Stockfisch a.
surgical a.
TheraSnore oral a.
Unitek a.
Universal a.
vasocillator fracture a.
Whip a.
Whitman fracture a.
Wilson fracture a.
Winter facial fracture a.
wire a.
W. W. Walker a.

applicator
Absolok endoscopic clip a.
afterload a.
Allen a.
Andrews a.
Bárány a.
Barth double-end a.
beta irradiation a.
beta-ray a.
beta therapy eye a.
Bloedorn a.
Brown a.
Brown-Dean cotton a.
Buck ear a.
Buck nasal a.
Burnett a.
Campbell-type Heyman fundus a.
cesium a.
Chaoul a.

Cohen suture a.
colpostat a.
Copalite a.
cotton a.
cotton-tipped a.
Dean a.
Delrin a.
ear a.
Ernst radium a.
Falope-ring a.
Farrior suction a.
Filshie clip minilaparotomy a.
Fletcher-Suit a.
a. forceps
Garney rubber band a.
Gass dye a.
Gifford corneal a.
global force a.
Grafco cotton tip a.
Henschke seed a.
HEX heat a.
Holinger a.
Huzly a.
infrared a.
intracavitary afterloading a.
iontophoretic a.
Ivan laryngeal a.
Ivan nasopharyngeal a.
Jackson laryngeal a.
Jobson-Horne cotton a.
Kevorkian-Younge uterine a.
Kyle a.
laryngeal a.
Lathbury cotton a.
Lejeune cotton a.
Ludwig middle ear a.
Ludwig sinus a.
Mayfield clip a.
Mick seed a.
Mick TP-200 a.
Milex Jel-Jector vaginal a.
minilaparotomy Falope-ring a.
MIRALVA a.
Montrose dressing a.
multifire clip a.
multiload occlusive clip a.
NeuroAvitene a.
Nucletron a.
Playfair uterine caustic a.
Plummer-Vinson radium
  esophageal a.
Pynchon a.
Ralks sinus a.
resorbable thread clip a.
ring a.
Roberts a.
Sawtell laryngeal a.
^{90}Sr-loaded eye a.
Stille laryngeal a.
Storz a.
strontium-90 ophthalmic beta ray a.
Syed-Puthawala-Hedger esophageal a.
tandem a.
Ter-Pogossian cervical radium a.
Turnbull a.

applicator *(continued)*
    Uckermann cotton a.
    Uebe a.
    University of Iowa cotton a.
    Wang a.
    Wolf-Yoon a.
    Yoon-ring a.
Applied
    A. Biosystems 340A nucleic acid extractor
    A. Medical mini ureteroscope
applier
    AcuClip endoscopic multiple-clip a.
    Advanced Surgical suture a.
    Alm clip a.
    aneurysm clip a.
    Autoclip a.
    automatic Hemoclip a.
    Auto Suture Clip-A-Matic clip a.
    bayonet clip a.
    clip a.
    Crockard transoral clip a.
    Endo Clip a.
    Gam-Mer clip a.
    Hamby right-angle clip a.
    Heifitz clip a.
    hemostatic clip a.
    Hulka clip a.
    Kaufman clip a.
    Kees clip a.
    Kerr clip a.
    LDS clip a.
    Ligaclip MCA multiple-clip a.
    Malis clip a.
    Mayfield miniature clip a.
    Mayfield temporary aneurysm clip a.
    McFadden Vari-Angle clip a.
    mini a.
    Mount-Olivecrona clip a.
    Mt. Clemens Hospital clip a.
    Multifire Endo hernia clip a.
    multiloaded clip a.
    Olivecrona clip a.
    pivot clip a.
    Raney scalp clip a.
    Right Clip a.
    Sano clip a.
    Schwartz clip a.
    Scoville clip a.
    Scoville-Drew clip a.
    Spetzler clip a.
    Sugita jaws clip a.
    surgical clip a.
    Vari-Angle McFadden clip a.
    vascular clip a.
    Weck clip a.
    Yasargil clip a.
    Zmurkiewicz clip a.
applipak
    IntraSite gel a.
Appolionio eye lens implant
AP portal
Appose skin stapler

approximation forceps
approximator
    Ablaza-Morse rib a.
    Alexander a.
    Allerdyce a.
    Bailey rib a.
    Biemer a.
    Bruni-Wayne clamp a.
    Brunswick-Mack a.
    Bunke-Schulz clamp a.
    Christoudias a.
    Henderson clamp a.
    hook a.
    Ikuta clamp a.
    Iwashi clamp a.
    Kleinert-Kutz clamp a.
    Lalonde tendon a.
    Leksell sternal a.
    Lemmon sternal a.
    Link a.
    microanastomosis a.
    Microspike a.
    Neuromeet nerve a.
    Neuromeet soft tissue a.
    Nunez sternal a.
    Pilling-Wolvek sternal a.
    pivot microanastomosis a.
    rib a.
    sternal a.
    Tamai clamp a.
    Vari-Angle temporary clip a.
    Wolvek sternal a.
APR
    APR acetabular cup
    APR I femoral stem
    APR total hip system
Aprema III device
A-Probe
    Soft-Touch A.-P.
apron
    Grafco x-ray a.
    Hottentot a.
    lead a.
    perineal surgical a.
Aqua
    A. Spray debridement system
    A. Thermassage
Aqua-Cel heating pad system
Aquacel Hydrofiber wound dressing
Aquaciser underwater treadmill
Aquaflex
    A. contact lens
    A. ultrasound gel pad
Aquaflo hydrogel wound dressing
AquaGaiter treadmill
Aquamatic dressing
AquaMED hydrotherapy device
AquaMotion pool
Aquanex hydrodynamic measurement system
Aquaphor
    A. gauze
    A. gauze dressing
Aquaplast
    A. cast

A

A. mask
A. mold
A. splint
A. tie-down dressing
Aqua-Purator suction device
AquaSens
A. FMS 1000 fluid monitoring
system
**AquaShield reusable orthopaedic cast
cover**
Aquasight lens
**Aquasil Smart Wetting impression
bonding**
Aquasorb
A. Border with Covaderm tape
A. transparent hydrogel dressing
AquaTack hydrocolloid barrier
Aquatrek device
aqueous
a. scintillator
a. transplant needle
a. tube shunt
Aquilion CT scanner
AR-1, AR-2 diagnostic guiding catheter
arachnoid
a. Beaver blade
a. knife
arachnoid-shaped blade
Arani double-loop guiding catheter
Arans pulley passer
Arbuckle-Shea trocar
Arbuckle sinus probe
arc
Leksell a.
shoulder ROM a.
xenon a.
Arc-22 catheter
arch
Ainsworth a.
angle a.
a. bar
a. bar cutter
a. bar facial fracture appliance
Bimler a.
extramedullary alignment a.
FemoStop femoral artery
compression a.
lingual a.
a. rake retractor
Simon expansion a.
a. support
Wilson Bimetric a.
Archer splinter forceps
Archimedean drill
Arch-lok
Swede-O A.-l.
archwire
Jarabak-type a.
Arcitumomab diagnostic imaging system
Arclite light source
Arco
A. atomic pacemaker
A. lithium pacemaker

ArCom
A. compression-molded polyethylene
A. processed polyethylene
arc-quadrant stereotactic system
arcuate skin stapler
Ardee denture liner
Arem-Madden retractor
Arem retractor
Arenberg
A. dural palpator elevator
A. endolymphatic sac knife
Arenberg-Denver inner-ear valve implant
areola circle
ArF excimer laser
Argen dental attachment
Arglaes wound dressing
argon
a. beam coagulator
a. blue laser
a. gas anticoagulator
a. green laser
a. guidewire
a. ion laser
a. laser photocoagulator
a. plasma coagulator
a. pump dye laser
a. vessel dilator
argon-fluoride laser
argon-krypton laser
argon-pumped tunable dye laser
Argosy
A. Cameo CIC hearing aid
A. in-the-ear hearing aid
Argyle
A. anti-reflux valve
A. arterial catheter
A. chest tube
A. CPAP nasal cannula
A. endotracheal tube
A. esophageal stethoscope
A. Medicut R catheter
A. oxygen catheter
A. Penrose tubing
A. Sentinel Seal chest tube
A. silicone Salem sump
A. trocar
A. trocar catheter
A. umbilical vessel catheter
Argyle-Dennis tube
Argyle-Salem sump anti-reflux valve
Argyle-Turkel safety thoracentesis system
Arion
A. implant
A. rod eye prosthesis
Arizona Ankle brace
Arjalloy alloy
Arjo Loop Sling
Arkan sharpening-stone needle
ARK-Juno refractor
Arlt
A. fenestrated lens scoop
A. lens loupe
arm
a. board
a. elevator sling

arm *(continued)*
    flexible a.
    Heidelberg a.
    Huang Universal flexible a.
    Leonard a.
    Leyla flexible a.
    mechanical articulated a.
    MonitorMate monitor a.
    pediatric retractor adjustable a.
    Pinpoint stereotactic a.
    a. retractor
    a. and shoulder immobilizer
    Utah artificial a.
    Wittmoser optical a.
armed bougie
Armstrong
    A. beveled grommet drain tube
    A. beveled grommet myringotomy tube
    A. CPR mask
    A. hand-held pulse oximeter
    A. ventilation tube
    A. V-Vent tube
Army
    A. bone gouge
    A. chisel
    A. osteotome
Army-Navy retractor
Arndorfer
    A. esophageal motility probe
    A. infusion system
    A. pneumohydraulic capillary infusion system
Arnett Lefort implant
Arnett-TMP system
Arnoff external fixation device
Arnold brace
Arnold-Bruening
    A.-B. intracordal injection set
    A.-B. syringe
Arnott
    A. bed
    A. dilator
    A. one-piece all-PMMA intraocular lens
AromaScan aroma analysis device
Aron Alpha adhesive
Aronson
    A. esophageal retractor
    A. lateral sternomastoid retractor
Aronson-Fletcher antrum cannula
A rotating joint
AR+ portable heart monitor
array
    Acuson 5-MHz linear a.
    A. foldable intraocular lens
    a. processor
    A. ultrasound transducer
AR 1000 refractor
Arrequi
    A. KPL laparoscopic knot pusher
    A. laparoscopic knot pusher ligator
arrhythmia
    a. control device (ACD)

    a. mapping system
    A. Net monitor
    A. Research 1200 EPX electrocardiograph
Arrow
    A. Advancer
    A. articulation paper forceps
    A. balloon wedge catheter
    A. Blue FlexTip
    A. FlexTip Plus catheter
    A. PICC
    A. pneumothorax kit
    A. pulmonary artery catheter
    A. QuadPolar electrode catheter
    A. QuickFlash arterial catheter
    A. Raulerson introducer syringe
    A. sheath
    A. true torque wire guide
    A. tube
    A. TwinCath multilumen peripheral catheter
    A. two-lumen hemodialysis catheter
    A. UserGard injection cap system
arrow
    Biofix a.
    Bionics a.
    a. pin clasp
    polylactic acid a.
Arrow-Berman
    A.-B. angiographic balloon
    A.-B. balloon catheter
Arrow-Clarke thoracentesis device
Arrow-Fischell EVAN needle
ArrowFlex
    A. intra-aortic balloon catheter
    A. sheath
ArrowGard
    A. Blue antiseptic-coated catheter
    A. Blue central venous catheter
    A. Blue Line catheter
Arrow-Howes
    A.-H. multilumen catheter
    A.-H. quad-lumen catheter
Arrowsmith
    A. corneal marker
    A. electrode
    A. fixation forceps
Arrowsmith-Clerf pin-closing forceps
Arrow-Trerotola
    A.-T. PTD catheter
    A.-T. rotator drive unit
Arroyo
    A. expressor
    A. forceps
    A. implant
    A. protector
    A. trephine
Arruga
    A. curved capsular forceps
    A. extraction hook
    A. eye expressor
    A. eye holder
    A. eye implant
    A. eye retractor
    A. eye speculum

A

A. eye trephine
A. globe retractor
A. globe speculum
A. lacrimal trephine
A. lens
A. lens expressor
A. needle holder
A. protector
A. surface electrode
Arruga-Gill forceps
Arruga-McCool capsular forceps
Arruga-Moura-Brazil orbital implant
ArtAssist
A. arterial assist device
A. compression dressing
A. wrap
Artec balloon catheter
Artecoll injectable microimplant
arterial
a. cannula
a. clamp
a. embolectomy catheter
a. filter
a. forceps
a. graft prosthesis
a. irrigation catheter
a. line pressure bag
a. needle
a. oscillator endarterectomy
  instrument
a. portography
a. silk suture
arteriograph
CAMAC-300 a.
arteriography needle
arteriotomy scissors
arteriovenous catheter
Arthopor acetabular cup
Arthrex   *Bio-Suture Tak*
A. arthroscope
A. drill guide
A. FASTak suture anchor
A. meniscal dart
A. meniscal dart gun
A. sheathed interference screw
A. tibial tunnel guide
A. zebra pin
ArthroCare
A. multielectrode system
Arthrocare
A. Rubo-Vac device
A. thermal wand
ArthroDistractor distractor
Arthrofile orthopaedic rasp
Arthro-Flo powered irrigation system
Arthro Force
A. F. basket cutting forceps
A. F. hook scissors
arthrogram
cine a.
triple-injection cine a.
ArthroGuide carbon dioxide laser
Arthro-Lok
A.-L. knife

A.-L. system
A.-L. system of Beaver blades
arthrometer
Genucom a.
KT1000, 2000 knee ligament a.
KT1000/s surgical a.
Medmetric KT-1000 knee laxity a.
Robinson pocket a.
Stryker a.
ArthroPlastics ankle instrumentation
arthroplasty
ELP stem for hip a.
Global total shoulder a.
Gustilo-Kyle cementless total hip a.
Stanmore shoulder a.
ArthroProbe
A. laser
SLT Contact A.
Arthroscan video system
arthroscope
Acufex a.
Arthrex a.
Baxter angled a.
Circon a.
Citscope a.
Codman a.
Concept Intravision a.
Downs a.
Dyonics rod lens a.
Eagle straight-ahead a.
examining a.
fiberoptic a.
Flexiscope a.
Hopkins a.
Lumina rod lens a.
4M 30-degree a.
Medical Dynamics 5990 needle a.
O'Connor operating a.
Richard Wolf a.
Sapphire View a.
spinal a.
Storz a.
Stryker a.
Takagi a.
Watanabe a.
Wolf a.
Zimmer a.
arthroscopic
a. ankle holder
a. banana blade
a. leg holder
arthroscopy knife
Arthroscrew arthroscopic suturing device
ArthroSew
A. arthroscopic suturing device
A. suturing system
Arthrotek
A. Ellipticut hand instruments
A. femoral aimer
arthrotome
Hall a.
ArthroWand
CAPS A.
Arthur splinter forceps
articular insert

Articu-Lase
    A.-L. laser
    A.-L. laser mirror
articulated
    a. chin implant
    a. chin prosthesis
    a. external fixator
articulating paper forceps
articulator
    Acme a.
    Balkwell a.
    Bergström a.
    Bonwill a.
    Christensen a.
    Denar a.
    Dentatus a.
    Evans a.
    Galetti a.
    Gariot a.
    Granger a.
    Gysi a.
    Hanau 130-21 a.
    Handy II a.
    hinge a.
    hinged a.
    KSK a.
    Ney a.
    non-arcon a.
    Oliair a.
    Olyco a.
    Olympia a.
    plain-line a.
    semi-adjustable a.
    Steele a.
    Stuart a.
    Walker a.
    Whip-Mix a.
Articul-eze hip ball
artificial
    a. eye
    a. heart
    a. hip joint
    a. joint implant
    a. larynx
    a. lung
    a. pacemaker
    a. sphincter
Arti-holder tweezers
Artilk forceps
Artisan wide-angle vaginal speculum
ARTMA
    advanced real-time motion analysis
    ARTMA virtual patient (AVP)
Artmann
    A. disarticulation chisel
    A. elevator
    A. raspatory
Artoscan
    A. MRI scanner
    A. MRI system
ART transducer
Artus power system
ARUM Colles fixation pin
Arvee model 2400 infant apnea monitor
Arzbacher pill electrode

ARZCO
    A. preamplifier
Arzco
    A. model 7 cardiac stimulator
    A. pacemaker
    A. Tapsul pill electrode
AS
    Auto Suture
AS-800 artificial sphincter
Asahi
    A. blood plasma pump
    A. hollow fiber dialyzer
    A. Plasmaflo plasma separator
    A. pressure controller
ASAP
    ASAP channel cut automated biopsy needle
    ASAP prostate biopsy needle
    ASAP Stacker automated multi-sample biopsy system
A-scan
    Contact A.-s.
    A.-s. scanner
    A.-s. ultrasonogram
Ascension Bird
Ascent
    A. catheter
    A. total knee system
Asch
    A. clamp
    A. nasal splint
    A. septal forceps
    A. septal straightener
    A. septum-straightening forceps
    A. uterine secretion scoop
Ascon instruments
ASDOS umbrella occluder
aseptic saw
Asepto
    A. bulb syringe
    A. suction tube
Ash
    A. catheter
    A. dental forceps
    A. septum-straightening forceps
Ashbell hook
Ashby fluoroscopic foreign body forceps
Asher high-pull facebow
Asherman chest seal
Ashhurst leg splint
Ashley
    A. breast prosthesis
    A. cleft palate elevator
    A. retractor
Ashworth-Blatt implant
ASICO multi-angled diamond knife
ASID Bonz PP infusion pump
ASIF
    ASIF broad dynamic compression bone plate
    ASIF screw pin
    ASIF T plate
    ASIF twist drill
ASIS femoral head locator

Asissto-Seat
    Maddapult A.-S.
ASI uroplasty TCU dilatation catheter
Ask-Upmark kidney
Aslan
    A. endoscopic scissors
    A. 2-mm minilaparoscope
    A. needle holder
ASN
    automatic single-needle monitor
Asnis
    A. guided screw
    A. 2 guided screw
    A. III cannulated screw
    A. pin
Aspect computer
Aspen
    A. cervical thoracic orthosis
    A. CTO
    A. digital ultrasound
    A. digital ultrasound system
    A. echocardiography system
    A. electrocautery
    A. Excaliber ESU
    A. laparoscopic electrode
    A. ultrasound platform
AspenVAC smoke evacuation system
aspheric
    a. cataract lens
    a. viewing lens
aspherical ophthalmoscopic lens
Aspiradeps dissector
aspirating
    a. cannula
    a. curette
    a. dissector
    a. needle
    a. syringe
    a. tube
aspiration
    a. apparatus
    a. biopsy needle
aspiration-tulip device
aspirator
    Accelerator II a.
    Adams a.
    Alcon a.
    Aspirette endocervical a.
    blue-tip a.
    Bovie ultrasound a.
    bronchoscopic a.
    Broyles a.
    Carabelli a.
    Care-e-Vac portable a.
    Carmody a.
    Castroviejo orbital a.
    cataract a.
    Cavi-Pulse cavitation ultrasound
      surgical a.
    Cavitron a.
    Cavitron Ultrasonic Surgical a.
      (CUSA)
    Clerf a.
    Cogsell tip a.
    Cook County Hospital a.

Cooper a.
CUSA Excel ultrasonic a.
DeLee meconium trap a.
DeVilbiss Vacu-Aide a.
Dia pump a.
Dieulafoy a.
Egnell uterine a.
Endo-Assist sponge a.
endocervical a.
endometrial a.
faucet a.
Fibra Sonics phaco a.
Fink cataract a.
Flex-O-Jet a.
Fluvog a.
Frazier suction tip a.
Fritz a.
Frye a.
gallbladder a.
Gesco a.
Gomco uterine a.
Gottschalk middle ear a.
Gradwohl sternal bone marrow a.
GynoSampler endometrial a.
Hahnenkratt a.
Hu-Friedy suction tip a.
Huzly a.
Hydrojette a.
Junior Tompkins portable a.
Kelman a.
Leasure a.
Legacy Series 2000 Cavitron/Kelman
  phaco-emulsifier a.
Lukens a.
LySonix 250 a.
meconium a.
middle ear a.
Monoject bone marrow a.
nasal a.
Nugent soft cataract a.
Penberthy double-action a.
phacoemulsifer-a.
Pilling-Negus clamp-on a.
portable suction a.
Potain a.
Printz a.
red-tip a.
Selector ultrasonic a.
Senoran a.
Sharplan Ultra ultrasonic a.
Sklar-Junior Tompkins a.
soft cataract a.
Sonocut ultrasonic a.
Sonop ultrasonic a.
Sorensen a.
Stat a.
Stedman suction pump a.
suction a.
surgical a.
Taylor a.
Thorek gallbladder a.
Tompkins a.
Ultra ultrasonic a.
Universal a.
uterine a.

aspirator *(continued)*
    Vabra cervical a.
    vacuum a.
    Vent-O-Vac a.
    Walker a.
    yellow-tip a.
aspirator/hydrodissector
    Alpern cortex a.
Aspire continuous imaging system
Aspirette endocervical aspirator
Aspir-Vac probe
Aspisafe nasogastric tube
A-splint dental splint
ASR
    ASR blade
    ASR scalpel
assemble
    sleeve/multiple sidehole
      manometric a.
assembly
    Ace halo-cast a.
    Ace wire tension a.
    Brown-Roberts-Wells arc-ring a.
    dilating catheter-gastrostomy tube a.
    Dosick bellows a.
    emergency oxygen mask a.
    Feild retractable blade a.
    infant nasal cannula a.
    Konigsberg 5-channel solid-state
      catheter a.
    linear array-hydrophone a.
    malleus-footplate a.
    malleus-stapes a.
    Massie nail a.
    Vabra a.
Assess
    A. esophageal testing kit
    A. peak flow meter
ASSI
    Accurate Surgical and Scientific
      Instruments
    ASSI bipolar coagulating forceps
    ASSI breast dissector
    ASSI cannula
    ASSI cranial blade
    ASSI METE-5168 Microspike
      approximator clamp
    ASSI METS-3668 Microspike
      approximator clamp
    ASSI MKCV-2040 Microspike
      approximator clamp
    ASSI MSPK-3678 Microspike
      approximator clamp
    ASSI S&T microsurgical instrument
    ASSI wire pass drill
ASSIST
    Thera-Band ASSIST
assist
    Columbus McKinnon lifting a.
    Elite posterior spring a.
Assistant Free
    A. F. calibrated femoral-tibial
      spreader

    A. F. calibrated femoral tibial
      spreader
    A. F. retractor
    A. F. Stulberg leg positioner
    Suture A. F.
Association for the Study of Internal
  Fixation (ASIF) plate
Assure blood glucose monitoring system
Asta-Cath device
600 Asta frameless air support therapy
Astech peak flow meter
Asthma Check peak flowmeter
Asthmastik
    Bird A.
astigmatic marker
astigmatism
    Staar Toric IOL lens for a.
astigmatome
    Terry a.
Aston
    A. cartilage reduction system
    A. facelift scissors
    A. nasal retractor
    A. submental retractor
Astra pacemaker
AstraZeneca dental cartridge
Astro-Med Albert Grass Heritage digital
  EEG system
Astron
    A. dental resin
    A. investment material
    A. resin
Astropulse cuff
Astro-Trace Universal adapter clip
Asuka PTCA catheter
ASVIP
    atrial-synchronous ventricular-inhibited
      pacemaker
    ASVIP pacemaker
asynchronous
    a. mode pacemaker
    a. ventricular VOO pacemaker
Atad
    A. cervical ripening device
    A. Ripener device
Atakr system
A-T antiembolism stockings
Aten olecranon screw
Athena high frequency mammography
  system
Athens
    A. forceps
    A. suture spreader
atherectomy
    a. catheter
    a. device
atheroblation laser
AtheroCath
    A. Bantam coronary atherectomy
      catheter
    DVI Simpson A.
    A. GTO coronary atherectomy
      catheter
    Simpson coronary A.

Simpson peripheral A.
A. spinning blade catheter
Atkins
    A. esophagoscopic telescope
    A. nasal splint
    A. tonsillar knife
Atkins-Cannard tracheotomy tube
Atkinson
    A. corneal scissors
    A. endoprosthesis
    A. 25-G short curved cystitome
    A. introducer
    A. keratome
    A. prosthesis
    A. retrobulbar needle
    A. sclerotome
    A. single-bevel blunt-tip needle
    A. tip peribulbar needle
    A. tube stent
Atkinson-Walker scissors
Atkins-Tucker
    A.-T. antiembolism stockings
    A.-T. shadow-free laryngoscope
    A.-T. surgical shield
ATL
    ATL duplex scanner
    ATL high definition imaging
    systems
    ATL Mark 600 real-time sector
    scanner
    ATL Neurosector real-time scanner
    ATL real-time ultrasound
    ATL Ultramark-series ultrasound
ATL/ADR Ultramark 4/9 HDI
ultrasound
Atlanta-Scottish Rite hip brace
Atlantic
    A. ileostomy catheter
    A. "O-Dor-Less" Pouches
atlas
    A. 2.0 diagnostic ultrasound system
    A. LP PTCA balloon dilatation
    catheter
    A. orthogonal percussion instrument
    Schaltenbrand-Wahren stereotactic a.
    stereotactic a.
    A. ULP PTCA balloon dilatation
    catheter
Atlas-Storz eye magnet
AtLast blood glucose system
Atlee
    A. bronchus clamp
    A. uterine dilator
Atmolit suction unit
atomic absorbance spectrophotometer
atomizer
    DeVilbiss a.
    Jackson laryngeal a.
    laryngeal a.
    Ono laryngobronchoscope a.
ATO walker
A-Trac atraumatic clamping system
Atrac-II double-balloon catheter
Atrac multipurpose balloon catheter
Atra-Grip clamp

Atraloc needle
Atrauclip hemostatic clip
atraumatic
    a. braided silk suture
    a. chromic suture
    a. curved grasper
    a. intestinal clamp
    a. needle
    a. tissue forceps
    a. visceral forceps
Atraumax peripheral vascular clamp
Atraum with Clotstop drain
atrial
    a. cannula
    a. clamp
    a. demand-inhibited pacemaker
    a. demand-triggered pacemaker
    a. electrode
    a. pacing wire
    a. septal defect single disk closure
    device
    a. septal retractor
    a. synchronous ventricular-inhibited
    pacemaker
    a. tracking pacemaker
    a. triggered ventricular-inhibited
    pacemaker
    a. and ventricular implantable
    cardioverter defibrillator
atrial-synchronous ventricular-inhibited
pacemaker (ASVIP)
Atrial View Ventak implantable
cardioverter-defibrillator
Atricor Cordis pacemaker
Atridox drug delivery system
Atrigel drug delivery system
atrioseptostomy catheter
atrioventricular
    a. junctional pacemaker
    a. sequential demand pacemaker
atrioverter
    Metrix implantable a.
Atri-pace I bipolar flared pacing
catheter
Atrisorb
    A. GTR barrier
Atrium
    A. Blood Recovery System
    A. hemodialysis graft
ATS
    adjustable thigh antiembolism stockings
    ATS 500/1500 tourniquet system
attachment
    Accuvac smoke evacuation a.
    Argen dental a.
    bar clip a.
    bar-sleeve a.
    Bivona tracheostomy tube with
    talk a.
    cerebellar a.
    closed chain exercise a.
    Distaflex dental a.
    Hader dental a.
    Hudson cerebellar a.
    Mayfield-Kees table a.

attachment *(continued)*
MP video endoscopic lens a.
O-ring a.'s
pathometer a.
photo-kerato a.
Planarm Haag Streit a.
PRAFO KAFO a.
Preci-Slot dental a.
Roach ball precision a.
specular a.
Stern dental a.
Strauss dental a.
Tach-EZ dental a.
Tasserit shoulder a.
Thomas splint with Pearson a.
Attenborough total knee prosthesis
Attends
A. beltless undergarment
A. brief with Perma Dry Wings
    contoured incontinence brief
A. pad and guard
A. underpad
attic
a. cannula
a. dissector
a. hook
Atwood
A. bridge remover
A. crown remover
A. loop
A. orthodontic cement
A-type dental implant
Audibel ear aid
Audicraft VIP-I hearing aid
audiometer
AudioScope 3 a.
Békésy a.
Crib-O-Gram neonatal screening a.
GSI 16 a.
Madsen OB822 clinical a.
Maico-MA 20 a.
MA 53 two-channel a.
Pilot a.
Audionics PB Max hearing aid
AudioScope 3 audiometer
Audiotone hearing aid
Audisil silicone ear mold material
auditory tube
Audivisette hearing aid
Aufranc
A. arthroplasty gouge
A. cobra retractor
A. cup
A. dissector
A. femoral neck retractor
A. finishing ball reamer
A. finishing cup reamer
A. hip retractor
A. hook
A. offset reamer
A. periosteal elevator
A. psoas retractor
A. push retractor
A. trochanteric awl

Aufranc-Turner hip prosthesis
Aufricht
A. elevator
A. glabellar rasp
A. nasal rasp
A. nasal retractor
A. scissors
A. septal speculum
Aufricht-Lipsett nasal rasp
auger
A. electron spectroscope (AES)
Hough stapedial footplate a.
a. wire
Auger-electron emitter
Augmen bone-grafting material
augmentative communication device
August automatic gauze packer
Augustine boat nail
Ault intestinal clamp
Aura
A. desktop laser
A. laser system
AuRA cemented total hip system
aural
a. forceps
a. magnifier
a. speculum
Aureomycin
A. gauze dressing
A. suture
auricular
a. appendage catheter
a. appendage clamp
a. appendage forceps
a. prosthesis
Auriculina hearing aid
Aurora
A. dedicated breast MRI system
A. diode-based dental laser system
A. dual-chamber pacemaker
A. MR breast imaging system
A. MR breast imaging system
    scanner
A. pulse generator
Aurovest investment material
Ausculscope carotid bruit detector
Aus-Jena-Gullstrand lens loop
Austin
A. attic dissector
A. awl
A. clip
A. dental knife
A. dental retractor
A. dissection knife
A. duckbill elevator
A. endolymph dispersement shunt
A. excavator
A. footplate elevator
A. forceps
A. measuring gauge
A. middle ear instrument
A. Moore bone reamer
A. Moore corkscrew
A. Moore curved endoprosthesis
A. Moore extractor

A. Moore head
A. Moore hip prosthesis
A. Moore inside-outside calipers
A. Moore mortising chisel
A. Moore-Murphy bone skid
A. Moore pin
A. Moore rasp
A. Moore straight-stem
endoprosthesis
A. needle
A. oval curette
A. pick
A. piston
A. right-angle elevator
A. sickle knife
A. strut calipers

Australian
A. orthodontic wire
A. Special Plus wire

Auth
A. atherectomy catheter
A. knife

Autima II dual-chamber cardiac pacemaker

auto
A. Glide walker accessory
a. injector
A. Ref-keratometer instrument
A. Suture (AS)
A. Suture ABBI system
A. Suture clip
A. Suture Clip-A-Matic clip applier
A. Suture curette
A. Suture endoscopic suction-
irrigation device
A. Suture forceps
A. Suture Multifire Endo GIA 30
stapler
A. Suture Premium CEEA stapler
A. Suture Soft Thoracoport
A. Suture surgical mesh
A. Suture surgical stapler
Tranquility a.

autoanalyzer
Beckman 2 a.
Hitachi 737, 747 a.
Kodak Ektachem a.
technetium H2 a.

Auto-Band Steri-Drape drape
Autoblock safety syringe
autoclave sterilizer
Autoclip
A. applier
Totco A.

Autoclix fingerstick lancet device
Autocon electrosurgical unit
Autocorrelator
AutoCyte Image Analysis system
Autoflex II continuous passive motion unit
autofunduscope
autograft
bone-patellar tendon-bone a.

Autohaler
Maxair A.

autoinfuser
Gish a.

Auto-Injector
Lido-Pen A.-I.

autokeratometer
Canon a. K1

auto-kerato-refractometer
KR-7000P a.-k.-r.

AutoLensmeter
Tomey Trooper A.

Autolet fingerstick device
autoLog autotransfusion system
autologous
a. fibrin tissue adhesive
a. stem

automated
a. angle-encoder system
a. cellular imaging system
a. cerebral blood flow analyzer
a. corneal shaper (ACS)
a. endoscope reprocessor
a. endoscopic system for optimal
positioning surgical robot
a. external defibrillator pacemaker
(AEDP)
a. hemisphere perimeter
a. laser-fluorescence sequencer
a. refractor
a. trephine

automatic
a. catheter
a. chemical analyzer
a. clinical analyzer
a. cranial drill
a. endoscopic reprocessor
a. external defibrillator (AED)
a. gas sequencer
a. Hemoclip applier
a. implantable cardiovascular
defibrillator (AICD)
a. implantable cardioverter-
defibrillator
a. intracardiac defibrillator
a. needle driver
a. ratchet snare
a. screwdriver
a. single-needle monitor (ASN)
a. skin retractor
a. stapling device
a. suction device
a. systematic desensitization
apparatus
a. tourniquet
a. twin syringe injector

Automator computerized distraction device
AutoPap
A. automated screening device
A. 300 QC automatic Pap screener
A. reader

autoperfusion
a. balloon
a. balloon catheter

AutoPilot
MKM A.

autopsy
    a. blade
    a. handle
autoradiographic film
Autoread centrifuge hematology system
Autoref keratometer
autorefractor
    Hoya AR-570 a.
    Nikon Retinomax K-Plus a.
    Retinomax cordless hand-held a.
    Tomey a.
AutoSet portable system
AutoSPECT
Autostainer
    Biotek 1000 A.
Autostat
    A. hemostatic clip
    A. ligating clip
Auto Suture (AS) (*See also* auto)
    AS device
    AS Multifire Endo GIA 30
Autosyringe pump
Autotechnicon
autotitrator
    Radiometer a.
autotome drill
autotopographer
    Tomey a.
Autotransfuser
    Biosurge Synchronous A.
Autovac LF autotransfusion system
Autraugrip tissue forceps
Auvard
    A. Britetrac speculum
    A. clamp
    A. cranioclast
    A. weighted vaginal retractor
    A. weighted vaginal speculum
Auvard-Remine vaginal speculum
Auvard-Zweifel
    A.-Z. basiotribe
    A.-Z. forceps
auxiliary lens
AV
    AV DeClot catheter
    AV fistula needle
    AV Gore-Tex graft
    AV junctional pacemaker
    AV sequential demand pacemaker
    AV synchronous pacemaker
AVAD
    acute ventricular assist device
Avalox skin clip
Avance hearing enhancer
Avanta soft skeletal implant
Avant Gauze nonwoven gauze
Avanti introducer
AVA 3Xi venous access device
AVCO aortic balloon
AVE
    AVE GFX coronary stent
    AVE Micro stent
Avenida dilator
Avenida-Torres dilator
Avenue insertion tool

averager
    multichannel signal a.
Averett total hip endoprosthesis
Avian transport ventilator
Avi lens system
A-V Impulse foot pump
Avina female urethral plug
Avitene
    A. hemostatic material
    A. microfibrillar collagen hemostat
AVIT handpiece
Avius sequential pacemaker
Aviva mammography system
AVL 9110 pH analyzer
AvocetPT rapid prothrombin time meter
AVP
    ARTMA virtual patient
AV-Paceport thermodilution catheter

Aware AccuMeter
awl
    Aufranc trochanteric a.
    Austin a.
    bone a.
    Carroll a.
    Carter-Rowe a.
    curved a.
    DePuy a.
    Ferran a.
    Kelsey-Fry bone a.
    Kirklin sternal a.
    lacrimal a.
    Mark II Kodros radiolucent a.
    Mustarde a.
    Obwegeser a.
    pointed a.
    reamer a.
    reaming a.
    rectangular a.
    rib brad a.
    Rochester a.
    Rush pin reamer a.
    starter a.
    Stedman a.
    sternal perforating a.
    sternum-perforating a.
    Swanson scaphoid a.
    T-handle bone a.
    T-handled a.
    trochanteric a.
    Uniflex distal targeting a.
    Wangensteen a.
    Wilson a.
    wire-passing a.
    Zelicof orthopaedic a.
    Zuelzer a.
Axenfeld nerve loop
Axhausen needle holder
axial
    a. gradiometer
    a. tractor
axillary catheter
Axiom
    A. DG balloon angioplasty catheter
    A. drain

A. knee component
A. modular knee system
Axios pacemaker
Axisonic II ultrasound
axis-traction forceps
Axostim nerve stimulator
Axxcess ureteral catheter
AxyaWeld
A. bone anchor system
A. instrument
Ayers
A. chalazion forceps
A. spatula
Ayerst instruments
Aylesbury cervical spatula
Ayre
A. brush

A. cervical spatula
A. cone knife
A. tube
Ayre-Scott cervical cone knife
Azar
A. corneal scissors
A. cystitome
A. intraocular forceps
A. iris retractor
A. lens forceps
A. lens hook
A. lid speculum
A. Mark II intraocular lens
A. needle holder
A. Tripod eye implant
A. tying forceps
A. utility forceps

B-12 dental curette
BA
    BA bone cement
    BA bone cement adhesive
Babcock
    B. empyema trocar
    B. Endo Grasp
    B. Endo-grasper
    B. intestinal forceps
    B. jointed vein stripper
    B. lung-grasping forceps
    B. needle
    B. plate
    B. raspatory
    B. retractor
    B. stainless steel suture wire
    B. thoracic tissue forceps
    B. thoracic tissue-holding forceps
    B. tissue clamp
Babcock-Beasley forceps
Babcock-Vital
    B.-V. atraumatic forceps
    B.-V. intestinal forceps
    B.-V. tissue forceps
BABE OB ultrasound reporting system
Babinski percussion hammer
baby
    b. Adson brain retractor
    b. Adson forceps
    b. Allis forceps
    b. Balfour retractor
    b. Barraquer needle holder
    b. Bishop clamp
    b. Collin abdominal retractor
    b. Crile forceps
    b. Crile needle holder
    b. Crile-Wood needle holder
    B. Dopplex 3000 antepartum fetal monitor
    b. dressing forceps
    b. hemostatic forceps
    b. Inge bone spreader
    b. Inge laminar spreader
    b. intestinal tissue forceps
    b. Kocher clamp
    b. Lane bone-holding forceps
    b. Metzenbaum scissors
    b. Mikulicz forceps
    b. Miller blade
    b. Miller laryngoscope
    b. Mixter forceps
    b. mosquito forceps
    b. Overholt forceps
    b. pylorus clamp
    b. rib contractor
    b. Roux retractor
    b. Satinsky clamp
    b. scope
    b. Senn-Miller retractor
    b. spur crusher
    b. Tischler biopsy punch
    b. Weitlaner self-retaining retractor

BabyBeat ultrasound instrument
BABYbird
    B. II respirator
    B. II ventilator
BabyFace 3-D surface rendering accessory
Babyflex
    B. heated ventilation system
    B. ventilator
Babytherm IC gel mattress
BacFix system
back
    b. brace
    B. Bubble gravity traction unit
    B. Bull lumbar support cushion
    B. Bull lumbar support system
    b. range-of-motion device
    B. Specialist electric table
    B. Specialist manual table
Backbar device
BackBiter instrument
backbiting
    b. bone punch
    b. forceps
backboard
BackCycler continuous passive motion device
Back-Ease aromatherapy hot/cold pack
Backhaus
    B. cervical knife
    B. dilator
    B. forceps
    B. towel clamp
    B. towel clip
Backhaus-Jones towel clamp
Backhaus-Kocher towel clamp
Backhaus-Roeder forceps
Back-Huggar
    Bodyline B.-H.
    B.-H. lumbar support
    B.-H. lumbar support cushion
backing
    Hahnenkratt b.
Backjoy seat
back, leg and chest dynamometer
Backlund
    B. biopsy needle
    B. stereotactic instrument
Backmann thyroid retractor
BackMaster device
Backnobber II massage tool
backplug
back-stop laser probe
Backstroke
    The B.
BackThing lumbar support
BackTracker
backward-cutting knife
Bacon
    B. anoscope
    B. cranial bone rongeur
    B. cranial forceps

B

Bacon (continued)
B. cranial retractor
B. periosteal raspatory
B. proctoscope
B. shears
BacStop checkvalve
BacT/Alert
B. analyzer
B. automated blood culture system
B. glass bottle
**BACTEC automated blood culture
system**
bacterial filter
Badal stimulus system
Badgley
B. laminectomy retractor
B. plate
Baer
B. bone-cutting forceps
B. bone rongeur
B. rib shears
Baerveldt
B. glaucoma implant
B. glaucoma implant tube
B. seton implant
B. shunt
B. shunt tube
baffle
fabric b.
Gore-Tex b.
Senning intraatrial b.
bag
Aberhart disposable urinal b.
Aberhart hemostatic b.
ACMI b.
air b.
Alcock hemostatic b.
Ambu b.
arterial line pressure b.
Bard Dispoz-A-Bag leg b.
Bardex b.
Barnes b.
B. Bath
bile b.
biohazard b.
Bomgart stomal b.
bowel b.
Brake hemostatic b.
breathing b.
Brodney hemostatic b.
Bunyan b.
Cardiff resuscitation b.
b. catheter
Champetier de Ribes obstetrical b.
CLO Cool B.
Coloplast colostomy b.
Coloplast urine leg b.
colostomy b.
Conveen bedside drainage b.
Conveen deluxe contoured leg b.
coudé b.
Curity leg b.
Davol b.
DeRoyal Surgical grab b.

dialysate b.
Diamed leg b.
Douglas b.
drainage b.
Duval b.
Dynacor leg b.
Emmet hemostatic b.
Endobag specimen b.
EndoMate grab b.
Endopouch Pro specimen-retrieval b.
Endosac specimen b.
Endo-Sock specimen retrieval b.
eXtract specimen b.
exudate disposal b.
Foley-Alcock b.
Foley hemostatic b.
four-point spreader b.
Freedom T-tap leg b.
Frenta enteral feeding b.
Gambro freezing b.
GaSampler Multilaminate B.
gauze tissue b.
GEM nonlatex medical b.
Grafco colostomy b.
Grafco ileostomy b.
Greck ileostomy b.
Hagner hemostatic b.
Hagner urethral b.
Hemofreeze blood b.
hemostatic b.
Hendrickson b.
Heyer-Schulte disposal b.
Heyer-Schulte Pour-Safe exudate b.
Higgins b.
Hofmeister drainage b.
Hollister colostomy b.
Hollister drainage b.
Hollister urostomy b.
Hope resuscitation b.
hydrostatic b.
ice b.
ileostomy b.
Incono b.
infusible pressure infusion b.
Infu-Surg pressure infuser b.
intestinal b.
intracervical b.
isolation b.
Karaya seal ileostomy stomal b.
Lahey b.
Lapides collecting b.
Lapides ileostomy b.
latex b.
Le B.
Lifesaver disposable resuscitator b.
Lyster water b.
Mac-Lee enema b.
manual resuscitation b.
Marlen ileostomy b.
Marlen leg b.
b. and mask
Melmed blood freezing b.
micturition b.
millinery b.
3M limb isolation b.

B

Mosher b.
Nesbit hemostatic b.
night drainage b.
ostomy b.
Owen hemostatic b.
Paul condom b.
Paul hemostatic b.
Pearman transurethral hemostatic b.
pear-shaped fluted b.
Peel Pak b.
Pennine leg b.
Perry ileostomy b.
Petersen rectal b.
Pilcher suprapubic hemostatic b.
Plummer b.
pneumatic b.
Politzer air b.
Ponsky Endo-Sock specimen
  retrieval b.
prostatectomy b.
rebreathing b.
replacement collection b.
Robinson b.
Rusch leg b.
Rutzen ileostomy b.
severance transurethral b.
Shea-Anthony b.
short-tip hemostatic b.
sleeve b.
Soft Guard XL fecal
  incontinence b.
Sones hemostatic b.
sterile isolation b.
stomal b.
suprapubic hemostatic b.
SureGrip breathing b.
Sur-Fit colostomy b.
Sur-Fit urinary drainage b.
Surgi-Flo leg b.
Swenko b.
Tassett vaginal cup b.
Tedlar b.
Teflo-Kapton freezing b.
Thackston retropubic b.
The Deluxe Button B.
three-point spreader b.
Travenol heart b.
Uri-Drain leg b.
urinary leg b.
Urocare latex reusable leg b.
Uro-Safe vinyl disposable leg b.
vaginal b.
Van Hove b.
Versi-Splint carry b.
Vi-Drape bowel b.
Voorhees b.
VPI urinary leg b.
Whitmore b.
Wolf hemostatic b.
Bagby compression plate
BagEasy disposable manual resuscitator
bag-fixated intraocular lens
Baggish hysteroscope
Bagley helical basket
Bagley-Wilmer lens expressor

Bagolini lens
bag-valve-mask (B-V-M)
bag-valve resuscitator
Bahama suture scissors
Bahnson
  B. aortic aneurysm clamp
  B. aortic cannula
  B. appendage clamp
  B. sternal retractor
Bahnson-Brown forceps
Bahn spud
Baikoff lens
Bailey
  B. aortic clamp
  B. aortic valve-cutting forceps
  B. aortic valve rongeur
  B. baby rib contractor
  B. chalazion forceps
  B. dilator
  B. drill
  B. duckbill clamp
  B. foreign body remover
  B. Gigli-saw guide
  B. lacrimal cannula
  B. leukotome
  B. punch
  B. rib approximator
  B. rib spreader
  B. round knife
  B. saw conductor
  B. skull bur
  B. transthoracic catheter
  B. wire saw
Bailey-Cowley clamp
Bailey-Gibbon rib contractor
**Bailey-Glover-O'Neill commissurotomy
  knife**
Bailey-Morse
  B.-M. clamp
  B.-M. mitral knife
Bailey-Williamson obstetrical forceps
Bailliart
  B. goniometer
  B. ophthalmodynamometer
  B. ophthalmoscope
  B. tonometer
bail-lock brace
bailout
  b. autoperfusion balloon catheter
  b. stent
Baim pacing catheter
Baim-Turi
  B.-T. cardiac device
  B.-T. monitoring/pacing catheter
Bainbridge
  B. anastomosis clamp
  B. hemostatic forceps
  B. intestinal clamp
  B. intestinal forceps
  B. resection forceps
  B. thyroid forceps
  B. vessel clamp
Bain circle
Baird
  B. chalazion forceps

Baird (continued)
    B. Electric System 5000 Power
    Plus electrosurgical unit
Bair Hugger
    B. H. fluid-warming device
    B. H. forced-air warmer
    B. H. infant warming device
    B. H. patient heating unit
    B. H. patient warming blanket
    B. H. warmer blanket
    B. H. warming body cover
BAK
    BAK cage
    BAK interbody fusion system
BAK-1 interbody fusion system
BAK/C
    BAK/C cervical interbody fusion
    implant
    BAK/C interbody fusion system
Bakelite
    B. cystoscopy sheath
    B. dental chisel
    B. mallet
    B. retractor
    B. spatula
Baker
    B. continuous flow capillary drain
    B. jejunostomy tube
    B. punch
    B. self-sumping tube
    B. tissue forceps
    B. velum
Bakes
    B. bile duct dilator
    B. probe
Bakes-Pearce dilator
BAK/Proximity interbody fusion implant
Bakst
    B. cardiac scissors
    B. valvulotome
BAK/T interbody fusion system
balance
    b. beam scale
    b. board
    b. bridge
    B. hip prosthesis
    Humphriss binocular b.
    B. Master
    B. Master training and assessment
    system
    b. pad
    b. padding orthosis
balanced traction device
Baldwin butterfly ventilation tube
Balectrode
    B. pacing catheter
    B. pacing probe
Balfour
    B. bladder blade
    B. center blade
    B. center-blade abdominal retractor
    B. clamp
    B. lateral blade
    B. pediatric abdominal retractor
    B. retractor with fenestrated blade

    B. self-retaining retractor
Balkan
    B. bed
    B. femoral splint
    B. fracture frame
Balkwell articulator
ball
    Anderson double b.
    Articul-eze hip b.
    birthing b.
    Body B.
    b. burnisher
    Cajal axonal retraction b.
    cauterizing b.
    B. coagulator
    cold-weld femoral b.
    cotton b.
    B. dissector
    b. electrode
    Electrodes b.
    b. extractor
    b. fastener
    Finger Fitness Spring B.
    B. forceps
    Gertie b.
    Gripp squeeze b.
    gym b.
    Gymnastik b.
    Gymnic b.
    hand exercise b.
    HeavyMed b.
    b. joint block
    Jurgan pin b.
    KBM cotton b.
    Ledraplastic exercise b.
    b. nerve hook
    PhysioGymnic exercise b.
    Physio-Roll VisuaLiser exercise b.
    Pinky b.
    b. poppet
    B. reusable electrode
    Silastic b.
    Slo-Mo b.
    Spondex sponge b.
    squeeze b.
    Stycar graded b.
    Super Pinky b.
    Swiss b.
    Thera-Band exercise b.
    Theragym b.
    therapy b.
    b. tipped scissors
    b. valve prosthesis
    b. wedge
    Wooden Wobble balance b.
Ballade needle
Ballance mastoid spoon
ball-and-cage prosthesis
ball-and-socket ankle prosthesis
Ballantine
    B. clamp
    B. hemilaminectomy retractor
    B. hysterectomy forceps
    B. uterine curette
Ballantine-Drew coagulator

Ballantine-Peterson hysterectomy forceps
Ballen-Alexander
    B.-A. forceps
    B.-A. orbital retractor
ball-end elevator
Ballenger
    B. cartilage knife
    B. chisel
    B. ethmoid curette
    B. follicle electrode
    B. gouge
    B. hysterectomy forceps
    B. mastoid bur
    B. mucosal knife
    B. nasal knife
    B. periosteotome
    B. raspatory
    B. septal elevator
    B. septal knife
    B. sponge forceps
    B. swivel knife
    B. tonsillar forceps
Ballenger-Foerster forceps
Ballenger-Hajek
    B.-H. chisel
    B.-H. elevator
Ballenger-Lillie mastoid bur
Ballenger-Sluder
    B.-S. guillotine
    B.-S. tonsillectome
ballistic energy generator
ballistocardiograph
Ballobes gastric balloon
ball-occluder valve
balloon
    Accent-DG b.
    ACE b.
    ACS SULP II b.
    Acucise b.
    angioplasty b.
    b. angioplasty catheter
    Anthony-Fisher antral b.
    antral b.
    Arrow-Berman angiographic b.
    autoperfusion b.
    AVCO aortic b.
    Ballobes gastric b.
    banana-shaped b.
    Bandit low-profile over-the-wire b.
    Bardex b.
    barium enema retention b.
    barostat b.
    Baxter Intrepid b.
    Baylor cervical b.
    bifoil b.
    b. biliary catheter
    Bilisystem stone-removal b.
    Blue Max high-pressure b.
    Brandt cytology b.
    Brighton epistaxis b.
    catheter b.
    b. catheter sealing device
    centering b.
    compliant b.
    Cook b.

B

    counterpulsation b.
    Cribier-Letac aortic valvuloplasty b.
    cutting b.
    cylindrical b.
    Datascope b.
    delivery b.
    detachable b.
    b. dilatation catheter
    b. dilating catheter
    b. dilator
    b. dissector
    Distaflex b.
    doughnut-shaped b.
    electrode b.
    electro-detachable b.
    Eliminator dilatation b.
    b. embolectomy catheter
    endocapsular b.
    Epistat double b.
    epistaxis b.
    esophageal b.
    Express b.
    extraction b.
    Extractor XL triple-lumen
      retrieval b.
    fixed-wire b.
    b. flotation catheter
    Fogarty b.
    Foley b.
    Force b.
    Fox postnasal b.
    French Swan-Ganz b.
    Garren-Edwards gastric b.
    gastric b.
    Gau gastric b.
    Giesy ureteral dilatation b.
    Grüntzig b.
    Guidant b.
    Hadow b.
    Hartzler Micro II angioplasty b.
    helix b.
    Helmstein b.
    high-compliance latex b.
    Honan b.
    Hunter b.
    Hunter-Sessions b.
    hydrostatic b.
    inflated b.
    Inoue self-guiding b.
    Integra II b.
    intraaortic counterpulsation b.
    intragastric b.
    intraocular b.
    Katzin-Long b.
    Kaye tamponade b.
    kissing b.
    Kontron intra-aortic b.
    laser b.
    latex b.
    Lo-Profile b.
    low-compliance b.
    low-profile angioplasty b.
    LPS b.
    Mansfield b.
    metrizamide-filled b.

balloon *(continued)*
 Micross SL b.
 Microvasive retrieval b.
 Microvasive Rigiflex through-the-
  scope b.
 Microvasive Rigiflex TTS b.
 Monorail Speedy b.
 nasomaxillary b.
 NC Cobra b.
 noncompliant b.
 nondetachable endovascular b.
 nondetachable occlusive b.
 NoProfile b.
 NuMED single b.
 occlusion b.
 occlusive b.
 Olbert b.
 Omega-NV b.
 Omniflex b.
 Omni SST b.
 Origin PDB 1000 b.
 Orion b.
 Owen b.
 Passage exchange b.
 PDB preperitoneal distention b.
 Percival gastric b.
 Percor-Stat intra-aortic b.
 PET b.
  positron emission tomography
  balloon
 Piccolino b.
 pillow-shaped b.
 Pivot b.
 POC b.
 polyethylene terephthalate b.
 polyolefin copolymer b.
 polyvinyl chloride b.
 positron emission tomography b.
  (PET balloon)
 postnasal b.
 Preperitioneal distension b.
 Prime b.
 ProCross Rely b.
 Provocative sensitivity b.
 pulmonary b.
 b. pump
 Quantum TTC biliary b.
 QuickFurl double-lumen b.
 QuickFurl single-lumen b.
 radiofrequency hot b.
 Rashkind b.
 rectal b.
 RediFurl double-lumen b.
 RediFurl single-lumen b.
 retrieval b.
 Riepe-Bard gastric b.
 Rigiflex achalasia b.
 Rigiflex TTS b.
 Rushkin b.
 Schneider-Shiley b.
 Schwarten Microglide LP b.
 Sci-Med Express Monorail b.
 scintigraphic b.
 Seloris b.

 Sengstaken b.
 Sengstaken-Blakemore esophageal b.
 Shadow b.
 Shea-Anthony b.
 Short Speedy b.
 b. shunt
 Simpson epistaxis b.
 sinus b.
 sizing b.
 Slalom b.
 Slider b.
 Slinky b.
 Soft-Wand atraumatic tissue
  manipulator b.
 Soto USCI b.
 Spacemaker II b.
 Spears USCI laser b.
 Stack autoperfusion b.
 Stealth catheter b.
 stone-retrieval b.
 Stretch b.
 b. tamponade
 Taylor gastric b.
 TEGwire b.
 Ten b.
 ThermaChoice uterine b.
 thigh b.
 through-the-scope b.
 Thruflex b.
 transluminal b.
 trefoil Schneider b.
 Triad PET b.
 Tri-Ex radiopaque triple-lumen
  extraction b.
 Tru-Trac high-pressure PTA b.
 Tyshak b.
 ultrasmall-shafted b.
 Ultra-Thin b.
 USCI PET b.
 b. valvuloplasty catheter
 b. wedge pressure catheter
 Wilson-Cook dilating b.
 Wilson-Cook gastric b.
 windowed esophageal b.
 wire-guided hydrostatic b.
 Xomed dual-chamber b.
balloon-centered argon laser
balloon-expandable
 b.-e. flexible coil stent
 b.-e. intravascular stent
 b.-e. metallic stent
balloon-flotation pacing catheter
balloon-imaging catheter
ballooning esophagoscope
Balloon-on-a-Wire cardiac device
balloon-tipped
 b.-t. angiographic catheter
 b.-t. flow-directed catheter
ball-peen splint
ballpit
 multisensory b.
ball-tip
 b.-t. coagulating electrode
 b.-t. nerve hook
ball-tipped seeker

B

ball-type retractor
ball-wedge catheter
Balmer tongue depressor
Balmoral shoe
Balnetar implant
Baloser hysteroscope
Balser hook plate
Balshi packer
Balters appliance
Baltherm thermal dilution catheter
Baltimore
    B. nasal scissors
    B. Therapeutic Equipment work
      stimulator
Bamby clamp
Banaji
    B. cannula
    B. spatula
banana
    b. Beaver blade
    b. catheter
    b. finger extension splint
    B. peel sheath
    b. plug dipolar generator
banana-shaped balloon
band
    adhesive b.
    anchor b.
    anterior chamber tube shunt
      encircling b.
    BB b.
    belly b.
    Can-Do Exercise B.
    coffer b.
    copper b.
    Cosgrove-Edwards annuloplasty b.
    Dentaform b.
    elastic rubber b.
    encircling b.
    ExerBand therapy b.
    exercise b.
    Falope-ring tubal occlusion b.
    Fit-Lastic therapy b.
    Flexi-Ty vessel b.
    fracture b.
    Fränkel head b.
    GelBand arm b.
    Hahnenkratt matrix b.
    Harris b.
    Jobst air b.
    Johnson dental b.
    latex O b.
    Lukens orthodontic b.
    Magill orthodontic b.
    Marlex b.
    Matas vessel b.
    matrix b.
    Mersilene b.
    metal b.
    Ormco preformed b.
    Orthoband traction b.
    orthodontic b.
    Parham b.
    Parham-Martin b.
    Parma b.

    patellar b.
    PD copper b.
    PD SS matrix b.
    Q-b.
    Ray-Tec b.
    Remak b.
    REP Bands exercise b.
    scultetus binder b.
    Silastic b.
    silicone elastomer b.
    Simonart b.
    Storz b.
    T b.
    table b.
    Thera-Band Max b.
    Thera-Band therapy b.
    Tofflemire matrix b.
    tooth b.
    tourniquet b.
    True Blue exercise b.
    T-type matrix b.
    vessel b.
    Vistnes rubber b.
    Watzke b.
    Xercise b.
    Zipper Medical hypoallergenic
      tracheostomy tube neck b.
bandage
    abdominal b.
    Ace adherent b.
    Ace spica b.
    adhesive b.
    Band-Aid b.
    barrel b.
    Barton b.
    Bennell b.
    binocle b.
    binocular b.
    Borsch b.
    Bulkee II gauze b.
    Buller b.
    butterfly b.
    capeline b.
    Cellamin resin plaster-of-Paris b.
    Cellona resin plaster-of-Paris b.
    Champ elastic b.
    circular b.
    ClearSite b.
    Coban b.
    Coflex b.
    cohesive b.
    collodion-treated self-adhesive b.
    Comperm tubular elastic b.
    compression b.
    Comprilan b.
    Conco elastic b.
    Conform stretch b.
    cotton elastic b.
    cotton-wool b.
    Cover-Roll stretch b.
    cravat b.
    crepe b.
    crucial b.
    Curad b.
    demigauntlet b.

bandage *(continued)*
Desault wrist b.
Dressinet netting b.
DuoDERM SCB sustained
  compression b.
DuraCast plaster b.
Dyna-Flex elastic b.
Dyna-Flex Layer Three b.
Dyna-Flex Layer Two b.
E-cotton b.
elastic foam b.
Elastikon b.
Elastomull b.
Elastoplast b.
Esmarch b.
eye b.
Fabco gauze b.
fiberglass b.
figure-of-eight b.
fixation b.
flat eye b.
flexible b.
Flexicon gauze b.
Flexilite conforming elastic b.
FoaMTrac traction b.
four-layer b.
four-tailed b.
Fractura Flex b.
Fricke b.
Galen b.
Garretson b.
gauntlet b.
gauze b.
Gauztape b.
Gauztex b.
Genga b.
Gibney fixation b.
Gibson b.
Guibor Expo flat eye b.
Haftelast self-adhering b.
Hamilton b.
hammock b.
Heliodorus b.
Hermitex b.
Hippocrates b.
Hollister medial adhesive b.
Hueter b.
Hydron burn b.
Hypertie b.
immobilizing b.
Kerlix gauze b.
Kiwisch b.
Kling gauze b.
Kold Wrap cold compression b.
Larrey b.
Lister b.
long-stretch b.
Maisonneuve b.
many-tailed b.
Marlex b.
Martin b.
3M Clean Seals waterproof b.
Medi-Band b.
moleskin b.

monocular b.
Morton b.
MPM b.
oblique b.
Orthoflex elastic plaster b.
Ortho-Trac adhesive skin traction b.
Ortho-Vent b.
Pearlcast polymer plaster b.
perineal b.
plano T-b.
plaster b.
plaster-of-Paris b. (POP bandage)
b. plaster shears
Plast-O-Fit thermoplastic b.
polyurethane b.
POP b.
  plaster-of-Paris bandage
pressure b.
Priessnitz b.
Profore four-layer b.
protective b.
recurrent b.
Ribble b.
Richet b.
Robert Jones b.
roller b.
rubber-reinforced b.
Sayre b.
scarf b.
b. scissors
scultetus b.
Setopress high-compression b.
Seutin b.
short-stretch b.
Shur-Band self-closure elastic b.
Silesian b.
sling-and-swathe b.
Sof-Band bulky b.
Sof-Kling conforming b.
b. soft contact lens
Spandage b.
spica b.
spiral reverse b.
spray b.
starch b.
Stepty P hemostasis b.
Steri-Band b.
Steri-Strips b.
stockinette amputation b.
SurePress high-compression b.
Sureseal cellulose sponge b.
Sureseal pressure b.
Surgiflex b.
suspensory b.
T b. (T)
Telfa 4 x 4 b.
Theden b.
Thera-Boot b.
Thermophore b.
Thillaye b.
thumb Spica b.
triangular b.
Tricodur Epi compression support b.
Tricodur Omos compression
  support b.

Tricodur Talus compression
  support b.
Tru-Support EW b.
Tru-Support SA b.
T-Spica b.
Tubegauz seamless tubular knitted
  cotton b.
TubiFast b.
TubiGrip elastic support b.
Tubipad b.
Tubiton tubular b.
Tuffnell b.
Unna boot b.
Unna-Flex paste b.
Velpeau b.
Webril b.
wet b.
woven elastic b.
Y-b.
zinc oxide b.
BandageGuard half-leg guard
Band-Aid
  B.-A. bandage
  B.-A. brand surgical dressing
Bandeloux bed
bander
Bandit
  B. catheter
  B. low-profile over-the-wire balloon
Band-It tennis elbow strap
band-ligator device
bandpass filter
bandsaw
  microcut b.
  minicut b.
Bane
  B. bone rongeur
  B. hook
  B. mastoid rongeur
  B. rongeur forceps
Bane-Hartmann bone rongeur
Bangerter
  B. angled iris spatula
  B. muscle forceps
Bangs bougie
banjo
  b. curette
  b. splint
  b. tractor
Bankart
  B. rasp
  B. rectal retractor
  B. shoulder prosthesis
  B. shoulder repair set
  B. shoulder retractor
Banks bone graft
Banner
  B. enucleation snare
  B. forceps
  B. snare enucleator
Banno catheter
Bannon-Klein implant
Bansal LASIK forceps
Bansaton behind-the-ear hearing aid

Bantam
  B. Bovie coagulator
  B. irrigation set
  B. wire cutter
  B. wire-cutting scissors
Bantex amalgamator
bar
  Ackerman lingual b.
  arch b.
  Bendick dental arch b.
  Berens prism b.
  Bill b.
  Bookwalter horizontal b.
  Bose b.
  Brookdale b.
  Buck extension b.
  Burns prism b.
  calcaneonavicular b.
  clasp b.
  b. clip attachment
  cross b.
  Denis Browne b.
  dental arch b.
  distraction b.
  b. drill
  Dynamic mesh craniomaxillofacial
    pre-angled connecting b.
  Erich arch malleable b.
  Erich dental arch b.
  Erich-Winter arch b.
  Essig arch b.
  facial fracture appliance dental
    arch b.
  Fillauer b.
  fixed arch b.
  fracture b.
  Gerster traction b.
  Goldman b.
  Goldthwait b.
  grab b.
  Greenberg b.
  Hader implant b.
  Hahnenkratt lingual b.
  hex b.
  intramedullary b.
  Jelenko arch b.
  Jewett b.
  Joseph septal b.
  Kangoo Thera-P b.
  Kazanjian T-b.
  Kennedy b.
  Leyla self-retaining tractor b.
  lingual b.
  Livingston intramedullary b.
  Lockjaw arch b.
  longitudinal spinal b.
  lumbrical b.
  mandibular arch b.
  maxillary arch b.
  Niro arch b.
  occlusal rest b.
  palatal b.
  Passavant b.
  posterior thigh b.
  b. prism

bar (*continued*)
    retainer arch b.
    retention b.
    Roger Anderson fixation b.
    screw alignment b.
    Simonart b.
    skiascopy b.
    spondylitic b.
    spreader b.
    stabilizing b.
    stall b.
    strut b.
    T b.
    tarsal b.
    Thera-P exercise b.
    Tommy hip b.
    Tommy trapeze b.
    traction b.
    trapeze b.
    b. T-tube
    unilateral b.
    unsegmented b.
    valgus b.
    Vistnes applier b.
    Winter arch b.
    Zielke derotator b.
bar-and-shoe orthosis
Bárány
    B. alarm
    B. alarm apparatus
    B. applicator
    B. box
    B. chair
    B. noise apparatus
    B. noise apparatus whistle
    B. speculum
Barbara needle
barbed
    b. broach
    b. epicardial pacing lead
    b. myringotome
    b. plastic washer
    b. Richards staple
    b. snare
    b. stapler
barb-tip lead
Barcroft apparatus
Barcroft-Warburg apparatus
Bard
    B. absorption drape
    B. absorption dressing
    B. adhesive and barrier film remover
    B. AlgiDERM dressing
    B. AlgiDERM rope
    B. alligator cup
    B. Ambulatory PCA device
    B. arterial cannula
    B. automatic reprocessor
    B. balloon-directed pacing catheter
    B. biopsy needle
    B. Biopty cut needle
    B. Biopty gun

B. BladderScan bladder volume instrument
B. button
B. cardiopulmonary support (CPS) system
B. cardiopulmonary support pump
B. catheter strap
B. cervical cannula
B. clamshell septal occluder
B. clamshell septal umbrella
B. closed-end adhesive pouch
B. coil stent
B. Companion papillotome
B. Cunningham incontinence clamp
B. disposable male external catheter
B. Dispoz-A-Bag leg bag
B. drainage adhesive pouch
B. electrode
B. electrophysiology catheter
B. evacuator
B. extension tubing
B. Federal containment device
B. forceps
B. gastrostomy catheter
B. gastrostomy feeding tube
B. guiding catheter
B. helical catheter
B. implant
B. Infus-OR syringe-type infusion pump
B. irrigation sleeve
B. leg bag holder
B. male external catheter
B. Medi-aire
B. Neurostim peripheral nerve stimulator
B. nonsteerable bipolar electrode
B. oval cup
B. PCA pump
B. PDA umbrella
B. PEG tube
B. percutaneous cardiopulmonary support system
B. probe
B. protective barrier film
B. PTFE graft
B. regular one-piece stoma
B. resectoscope
B. rotary atherectomy system
B. security pouch
B. self-adhesive fecal containment device
B. Sequence II Plus incontinent skin care kit
B. soft double-pigtail stent
B. Sperma-Tex preshaped mesh
B. sterile infection control tray
B. sterile red rubber catheter
B. sterilizer
B. tip
B. Touchless intermittent catheter
B. TransAct intraaortic balloon pump
B. universal Foley catheter sterile insertion tray

B. ureteroscopic cytology brush
B. urethral catheter sterile tray
B. urethral dilator
B. urinary sterile collection system
B. Urolase fiber laser system
B. wide leg bag strap
B. x-ray ureteral catheter
B. XT coronary stent
Bardam red rubber catheter
Bardco catheter
Bardeleben
    B. bone-holding forceps
    B. rasp
Bardex
    B. all silicone sterile Foley catheter
    B. bag
    B. balloon
    B. drain
    B. I.C. sterile Foley catheter
    B. Lubricath Foley catheter
    B. Lubricath sterile Foley tray
    B. silicone Foley catheter
    B. stent
Bardex-Bellini drain
Bardex-Foley
    B.-F. balloon catheter
    B.-F. return-flow retention catheter
Bard-Hamm fulgurating electrode
Bardic
    B. cannula
    B. curette
    B. cutdown catheter
    B. translucent catheter
    B. tube
    B. Uro Sheath reusable male
      external catheter
Bardic-Deseret Intracath catheter
Bard-Marlex mesh
Bard-Parker
    B.-P. autopsy blade
    B.-P. dermatome
    B.-P. forceps
    B.-P. handle
    B.-P. keratome
    B.-P. knife
    B.-P. razor
    B.-P. scalpel
    B.-P. surgical blade
    B.-P. trephine
    B.-P. U-Mid/Lo humidifier
Bard-Steigmann-Goff variceal ligation kit
Bard-Tuohy-Borst adapter
Bard-U-Cath self-adhering male external
  catheter
Bareskin knee positioner
Bari-800i system bariatric bed
BariKare
    B. advanced power system
Barikare bed
barium enema retention balloon
barium-impregnated poppet
Barkan
    B. bident retractor
    B. goniolens
    B. gonioscope

B. gonioscopic lens
B. goniotomy knife
B. illuminator
B. infant lens
B. infant lens implant
B. iris forceps
B. light
B. operating lens
B. scissors
Barker
    B. calipers
    B. needle
    B. Vacu-tome
    B. Vacu-tome dermatome
    B. Vacu-tome suction knife
Barlow forceps
Barnard mitral valve prosthesis
Barnes
    B. bag
    B. cervical dilator
    B. common duct dilator
    B. compressor
    B. spirometer
    B. suction tube
    B. vessel scissors
Barnes-Crile hemostatic forceps
Barnes-Dormia stone basket
Barnes-Hill forceps
Barnes-Hind ophthalmic dressing
Barnes-Simpson obstetrical forceps
Barnhill adenoid curette
Barnhill-Jones curette
baromacrometer
Baron
    B. ear knife
    B. ear tube
    B. forceps
    B. intraocular lens
    B. retractor
    B. suction tube
    B. suction tube-cleaning wire
Baron-Frazier suction tube
baroreceptor
    cardiac b.
barospirator
barostat balloon
Barouk
    B. button
    B. button spacer
    B. cannulated bone screw
    B. microscrew
    B. microstaple
    B. spacer
Barr
    B. anal speculum
    B. bolt
    B. crypt hook
    B. fistular probe
    B. pin
    B. rectal fistular hook
    B. rectal probe
    B. rectal speculum
    B. self-retaining rectal retractor
Barracuda flexible cystoscopic hot biopsy
  forceps

B

Barraquer
- B. applanation tonometer
- B. baby needle holder
- B. blade
- B. cannula
- B. ciliary forceps
- B. conjunctival forceps
- B. corneal dissector
- B. corneal forceps
- B. corneal knife
- B. corneal section scissors
- B. corneal trephine
- B. curved holder
- B. cyclodialysis spatula
- B. erysiphake
- B. eye needle holder
- B. eye shield
- B. eye speculum
- B. fixation forceps
- B. hemostatic mosquito forceps
- B. implant
- B. iris scissors
- B. iris spatula
- B. irrigator
- B. irrigator spatula
- B. J-loop intraocular lens
- B. keratoplasty knife
- B. lid retractor
- B. microkeratome
- B. needle
- B. needle carrier
- B. needle holder clamp
- B. operating room tonometer
- B. razor bladebreaker
- B. sable brush
- B. silk suture
- B. solid speculum
- B. sweep
- B. vitreous strand scissors
- B. wire guide
- B. wire speculum

Barraquer-Carriazo microkeratome
Barraquer-Colibri eye speculum
Barraquer-DeWecker iris scissors
Barraquer-Douvas eye speculum
Barraquer-Floyd speculum
Barraquer-Karakashian scissors
Barraquer-Katzin forceps
Barraquer-Krumeich-Swinger
- B.-K.-S. refractor
- B.-K.-S. retractor

Barraquer-Troutman
- B.-T. corneal forceps
- B.-T. needle holder

Barraquer-Vogt needle
Barraquer-von Mandach
- B.-v. M. capsule forceps
- B.-v. M. clot forceps

Barraya tissue forceps
barrel
- b. bandage
- b. cutting bur
- b. dressing
- b. guide
- Opti-Vue plastic b.

Barrett
- B. appendix inverter
- B. flange lens manipulator
- B. hebosteotomy needle
- B. hydrodelineation cannula
- B. hydrogel intraocular lens
- B. intestinal forceps
- B. irrigating lens manipulator
- B. lens forceps
- B. placental forceps
- B. tenacular forceps
- B. uterine knife
- B. uterine tenaculum

Barrett-Adson cerebellum retractor
Barrett-Allen
- B.-A. placental forceps
- B.-A. uterine forceps

Barrett-Murphy intestinal forceps
Barrie-Jones angled crocodile forceps
barrier
- ACTIVE LIFE convex one-piece urostomy pouch with Durahesive skin b.
- Alpine reusable leg bag with Kraylex odor b.
- AquaTack hydrocolloid b.
- Atrisorb GTR b.
- Capset bone graft b.
- DermaMend b.
- Durahesive skin b.
- external urethral b.
- B. gown
- Interceed absorbable adhesion b.
- B. laparoscopy drape
- B. laparoscopy LAVH pack
- B. lower extremity sheet
- Marlen SkinShield adhesive skin b.
- b. membrane
- Nu-Hope adhesive waterproof skin b.
- B. phaco extracapsular pack
- Sil-K OB b.
- space-maintaining b.
- sterile field b.
- TC-7 adhesion b.
- VitaCuff tissue-interface b.

Barron
- B. alligator forceps
- B. disposable trephine
- B. donor corneal punch
- B. epikeratophakia trephine
- B. hemorrhoidal ligator
- B. pump
- B. radial vacuum trephine
- B. retractor

Barron-Hessburg corneal trephine
Barr-Shuford speculum
Barsky
- B. cleft palate raspatory
- B. elevator
- B. forceps
- B. nasal osteotome
- B. nasal rasp
- B. nasal retractor
- B. nasal scissors

B

bar-sleeve attachment
bar-supported overdenture
Bart abdominoperipheral angiography
    unit
Barth
        B. double-end applicator
        B. mastoid curette
Bartholdson-Stenstrom rasp
Bartholin gland catheter
Bartkiewicz two-sided drain
Bartlett fascial stripper
Bartley
        B. anastomosis clamp
        B. partial-occlusion clamp
bar-to-bar clamp
Barton
        B. bandage
        B. blade
        B. double hook
        B. dressing
        B. obstetrical forceps
        B. skull traction tongs
        B. sling
        B. suction
        B. traction device
        B. traction handle
        B. wrench
Barton-Cone tongs
Baruch circumcision scissors
BAS-300 transurethral thermotherapy
    device
basal
        b. block cervical saddle
        b. body thermometer
Baschui pigtail catheter
base
        Brown-Roberts-Wells phantom b.
        fixation b.
        Getz rubber b.
        Lok-Mesh bonding b.
        b. plate
        Plexiglas b.
        Profix nonporous tibial b.
baseball finger splint
base-down prism
Basek chisel
Baseline dynamometer
Basic
        One Touch B.
        B. Sequences ColorCards
Basile hip screw
basin
        catch b.
        urological soaking b.
basiotribe
        Auvard-Zweifel b.
        Tarnier b.
Basis breast pump
Basix pacemaker
basket
        Acufex b.
        Bagley helical b.
        Barnes-Dormia stone b.
        biliary stone b.
        Browne stone b.

Councill stone b.
Dormia biliary stone b.
Dormia gallstone b.
Dormia ureteral stone b.
Duette b.
Eliminator stone extraction b.
Ellik kidney stone b.
endotriptor stone-crushing b.
Ferguson stone b.
b. forceps
gallstone b.
Gemini paired helical wire b.
Glassman b.
Hobbs stone b.
Howard stone b.
instrument b.
InSurg common bile duct (CBD) b.
Johns Hopkins stone b.
Johnson ureteral stone b.
laser lithotriptor b.
Medi-Tech multipurpose b.
Medi-Tech stone b.
Memory b.
Mill-Rose spiral stone b.
Mitchell stone b.
Moss-Harms b.
Olympus stone retrieval b.
parrot-beak b.
Pfister-Schwartz stone b.
Pfister stone b.
Positrap mini-retrieval b.
Pursuer CBD helical b.
b. retriever
Robinson stone b.
rotary b.
Rutner stone b.
Schutte shovel-nose b.
Segura CBD b.
Segura-Dretler stone b.
Segura stone b.
six-wire spiral-tip Segura b.
sphincterotomy b.
sterilizing b.
stone b.
stone-holding b.
stone-retrieval b.
Sur-Catch paired-wire b.
ultrasonic cleaner b.
ureteral stone b.
Vantec stone b.
VPI stone b.
Wilson-Cook stone b.
basket-cutting forceps
basket-punch forceps
basket-style scleral supporter speculum
basket-type crushing forceps
Bassett electrical stimulation device
Basswood splint
bastard suture
basting suture
Bastow raspatory
bat
        Mexican b.
Batchelor plate

Bateman
  B. finger prosthesis
  B. UPF II bipolar endoprosthesis
  B. UPF II bipolar knee system
  B. UPF II shoulder prosthesis
bath
  Bag B.
  b. blanket
  blanket b.
  Charcot b.
  Dickson paraffin b.
  electric cabinet b.
  Finsen b.
  HydraClense sitz b.
  immersion b.
  B. respirator
  sitz b.
  ThermaSplint heating b.
  The Travel B.
Bathlifter
  Leo B.
Baton laser pointer
Batson-Carmody elevator
BAT system
batten graft
battery
  Duracell Activair hearing aid b.
  lithium iodine b.
  Panasonic hearing aid b.
  Renata b.
battery-assisted heart assist device
battery-powered endoscope
batting
  cotton b.
Batt tip
bat-wing catheter
batwing dissector
Batzdorf
  B. cervical wire passer
  B. cervical wire twister
Baudelocque pelvimeter
Bauer
  B. dissecting forceps
  B. hernia belt
  B. kidney pedicle clamp
  B. retractor
  B. sponge forceps
  B. Temno biopsy needle
Bauerfeind
  B. Achillotrain
  B. ankle brace
  B. comprifix knee brace
  B. Malleolic ankle orthosis
  B. silicone heel pad
Baumberger forceps
Baumgarten wire twister
Baumgartner
  B. forceps
  B. needle holder
  B. punch
Baum-Hecht tarsorrhaphy forceps
Baum-Metzenbaum sternal needle holder
Baumrucker
  B. clamp irrigator
  B. electrode

  B. post-TUR irrigation clamp
  B. resectoscope
  B. urinary incontinence clamp
Baumrucker-DeBakey clamp
Baum tonsillar needle holder
Bausch
  B. articulation paper forceps
  B. & Lomb Duoloupe lens loupe
  B. & Lomb manual keratometer
  B. & Lomb Optima lens
  B. & Lomb Surgical L161U lens
  B. & Lomb-Thorpe slit lamp
Bausch-Lomb-Thorpe slit lamp
Bavarian splint
Baxa oral dispenser
Baxter
  B. angioplasty catheter
  B. angioscope
  B. angled arthroscope
  B. CA-210 filter
  B. dilatation catheter
  B. disposable blade
  B. fiberoptic spectrophotometry
    catheter
  B. Flo-Gard 8200 volumetric
    infusion pump
  1550 B. hemodialyzer
  B. Interline IV system
  B. InterLink needle system
  B. INtermate
  B. Intrepid balloon
  B. mechanical valve
  B. mechanical valve prosthesis
  B. PCA pump
  B. personal Von-Loc ice pack
  B. PSN dialyzer
  B. surgical clipper
  B. V. Mueller laparoscopic
    instrumentation
  B. volumetric infusion pump
Baxter-V. Mueller catheter
Bayer/Technicon H1 automated flow
  cytometer
Bay external fixator
Bayless neurosurgical headholder
Baylor
  B. adjustable cross splint
  B. amniotic perforator
  B. amniotome
  B. autologous transfusion system
  B. cardiovascular sump tube
  B. cervical balloon
  B. intracardiac sump tube
  B. metatarsal splint
  B. pelvic traction belt
  B. total artificial heart
Bayne Pap brush
Baynton dressing
bayonet
  b. aneurysm clip
  b. bipolar forceps
  b. clip applier
  b. curette
  b. handle
  b. knife

Lucae b.
b. monopolar forceps
b. needle holder
b. osteotome
b. root tip forceps
b. scissors
b. separator
b. transsphenoidal mirror
bayonet-point wire
bayonet-tip electrode
Bazooka support surface bed
BB
blow bottle
body belt
BB band
BB shot forceps
BCD Plus cardioplegic unit
BCELL-HDM - filtering system
BCI 3301 hand-held pulse oximeter
BCNU-impregnated polymer wafer
BCO₂
Cardiac Stimulator BCO_2
BD
Becton Dickinson
BD adapter
BD bone marrow biopsy needle
BD butterfly swab dressing
BD gun
BD Luer syringe
BD Potain thoracic trocar
BD Safety-Gard needle
BD SafetyGlide shielding
hypodermic needle
BD Sensability breast self-
examination
BD Sensability breast self-
examination aid
BDP pad
BDProbeTec ET system
beach
b. bum rocker-bottom cast sandal
shoe
b. chair positioner
Beacham amniotome
bead
b. bed
carbon particle b.
Chelex b.
Cida-Gel absorbent b.'s
Enzymobead b.
B. ethmoidal forceps
glass b.
hydroxyapatite b.
immunomagnetic b.
magnetic b.
methyl methacrylate b.
packed b.
Percoll b.
Sephadex b.
Septobal b.
beaded
b. cerclage wire
b. guidewire

b. hip pin
b. pin wrench
beaded-tip scissors
beaked
b. cowhorn forceps
b. sheath
Beall
B. bulldog clamp
B. circumflex artery scissors
B. disk heart valve
B. mitral valve
B. mitral valve prosthesis
Beall-Feldman-Cooley sump tube
Beall-Morris ascending aortic clamp
Beall-Surgitool
B.-S. ball-cage prosthetic valve
B.-S. disk prosthetic valve
Beamer
B. injection stent system
B. stent
beam splitter
bean forceps
Bear
B. adult-volume ventilator
B. 1, 2 adult-volume ventilator
B. Cub infant ventilator
B. NUM-1 tidal volume monitor
B. 5 respirator
Beard
B. cystitome
B. eye speculum
B. lid knife
Beardsley
B. aortic dilator
B. cecostomy trocar
B. empyema tube
B. esophageal retractor
B. forceps
B. intestinal clamp
bearing-seating forceps
Beasley-Babcock tissue forceps
Beasytrans transfer device
Beath
B. guidewire
B. needle
B. pin
Beatty
B. pillar retractor
B. tongue depressor
Beaufort seating orthosis
Beaulieu camera
Beaupre
B. ciliary forceps
B. epilation forceps
Beaver
B. Arthro-Lok blade
B. bent blade
B. blade cataract knife
B. blade discission knife
B. blade keratome
B. cataract blade
B. cataract cryoextractor
B. cataract knife
B. curette
B. discission blade

B

Beaver *(continued)*
B. dissector
B. ear knife
B. goniotomy needle knife
B. handle
B. keratome blade
B. lamellar blade
B. limbus blade
B. microblade
B. Microsharp blade
B. miniblade
B. myringotomy blade
B. Ocu-1 curved cystitome
B. Optimum blade
B. phacokeratome blade
B. retractor
B. rhinoplasty blade
B. ring cutter
B. scleral Lundsgaard blade
B. tail-tip electrode
B. tonsillar knife
B. tonsillectomy blade
B. Xstar knife
Beaver-DeBakey blade
Beaver-Lundsgaard blade
Beaver-Okamura blade
beaver-tail
b.-t. burnisher
b.-t. retractor
Beaver-Ziegler blade
Bebax
B. Bootie
B. orthosis
Bechert
B. capsular polisher
B. intraocular lens cannula
B. intraocular lens implant
B. lens-holding forceps
B. nucleus rotator
B. one-piece all-PMMA intraocular
lens
B. spatula
Bechert-Hoffer nucleus rotator
**Bechert-Kratz cannulated nucleus
retractor**
Bechert-McPherson tying forceps
Bechert-Sinskey needle holder
Bechtol prosthesis
Beck
B. abdominal scoop
B. aortic clamp
B. forceps
B. gastrostomy
B. gastrostomy scoop
B. mouth tube airway
B. pericardial raspatory
B. pliers
B. tonsillar knife
B. twisted wire snare loop
B. vascular clamp
B. vessel clamp
Becker
B. accelerator
B. accelerator cannula

B. brace
B. breast prosthesis
B. corneal section spatulated
scissors
B. dissector cannula
B. flat dissector tip
B. goniogram
B. gonioscopic prism
B. Greater dissecting cannula
B. hand prosthesis
B. 655 motion control limiter
B. orthopaedic spinal system
(BOSS)
B. orthopaedic spinal system
orthotic device
B. orthopaedic thermoformable ankle
system
B. probe
B. retractor
B. round dissector tip
B. screwdriver
B. septal scissors
B. skull trephine
B. spatulated corneal section
scissors
B. tissue expander
B. tissue expander prosthesis
B. twist dissector tip
B. vibrating cannula system
Becker-Joseph saw
Becker-Parkin pliers
Becker-Park speculum
Becker-Rojas Sub-Sonic surgical system
Beckerscope binocular microscope
Beckman
B. adenoid curette
B. airfuge
B. 2 autoanalyzer
B. distractor
B. goiter retractor
B. ICS Nephelometer system
B. ion-selective analyzer
B. J5.0 elutriation rotor
B. JE-10X elutriation rotor
B. J-6M centrifuge
B. nasal scissors
B. nasal speculum
B. O_2 analyzer
B. probe
B. self-retaining retractor
B. Silastic bulb
B. stomach electrode
B. thyroid retractor
B. UV spectrophotometer
Beckman-Adson
B.-A. laminectomy blade
B.-A. laminectomy retractor
Beckman-Colver nasal speculum
Beckman-Eaton
B.-E. laminectomy blade
B.-E. laminectomy retractor
Beckman-Weitlaner laminectomy retractor
Beck-Mueller tonsillectome

Beck-Potts
    B.-P. aortic clamp
    B.-P. pulmonic clamp
Beck-Satinsky clamp
Beck-Schenck
    B.-S. tonsillar snare
    B.-S. tonsillectome
Beck-Steffee total ankle prosthesis
Beck-Storz tonsillar snare
Becton Dickinson (BD)   (*See also* BD)
    Becton Dickinson guidewire
    Becton Dickinson Teflon-sheathed
      needle
bed
    AccuMax b.
    Acucare b.
    Affinity b.
    air b.
    air-fluidized b. (AFB)
    Air Plus low-air-loss b.
    American Lapidus b.
    Arnott b.
    Balkan b.
    Bandeloux b.
    Bari-800i system bariatric b.
    Barikare b.
    Bazooka support surface b.
    bead b.
    Betabed b.
    BioDyne II kinetic therapy low-air-
      loss b.
    Biologics Airlift b.
    Biomet b.
    Burke bariatric treatment system
      powered bariatric b.
    Burke plus low-air-loss b.
    Cardiopulmonary Paragon 8500 b.
    Chick-Foster orthopedic b.
    CircOlectric b.
    Clensicair low-air-loss
      hydrotherapy b.
    Clini-Care b.
    Clini.Dyne b.
    Clini.Float b.
    Clinitron air b.
    Clinitron air-fluidized b.
    Duratec nursing home b.
    dynamic b.
    electric b.
    Excel electric hospital b.
    Fisher b.
    Flexicair II low-air-loss therapy
      unit b.
    Flexicair MC3 low-air-loss therapy
      unit b.
    Fluid-Air Plus b.
    Foster b.
    fracture b.
    Gatch b.
    Gelastic b.
    GellyComb b.
    Guthrie-Smith b.
    head of b.
    high-air-loss b.
    high-muscular-resistance b.

    HomeKair b.
    hospital b.
    Hough b.
    Hoverbed b.
    hydrostatic b.
    hyperbaric b.
    IC b.
    Isoflex b.
    Keane Mobility b.
    KinAir III, TC low-air-lossb.
    Klondike b.
    Lapidus b.
    low-air-loss b.
    Lumex shower b.
    Magnum 800 b.
    Magnum bariatric patient system b.
    Medicus b.
    Medline Alpha subacute care b.
    Mega-Air b.
    Mega Tilt and Turn b.
    Ohio b.
    Orthoderm consummate air
      therapy b.
    PediKair pediatric low-air-loss b.
    Plastizote foot b.
    Pneu Care ICU dynamic low-air-
      loss b.
    Pneu Care Pedibed dynamic
      pediatric low-air-loss b.
    Pulmonair 40 b.
    pulsating low-air-loss b.
    Restcue b.
    Roho b.
    rotational dynamic air therapy b.
    Roto Kinetic b.
    Roto-Rest b.
    Sanders oscillating b.
    sawdust b.
    Skytron air-fluidized b.
    Spa B.
    Stress echo b.
    Stryker CircOlectric b.
    Swinger car b.
    TheraPulse pulsating air
      suspension b.
    Tilt and Turn Paragon b.
    TriaDyne b.
    Ultra Dream Ride car b.
    water b.
Bedfont carbon monoxide monitor
Bedge
    B. antireflux mattress
    B. pillow
Bedrossian eye speculum
bedside
    b. air chair
    b. scale
    b. spirometer
    b. sterile drainage collection system
bedwetting alarm
Beebe
    B. hemostatic forceps
    B. lens
    B. lens loop
    B. loupe

B

Beebe *(continued)*
  B. wire-cutting forceps
  B. wire-cutting scissors
Beekhuis-Supramid mentoplasty augmentation implant
Beer
  B. blade
  B. canaliculus knife
  B. cataract knife
  B. ciliary forceps
Beeson cast spreader

Begg
  B. light wire appliance
  B. straight-wire combination bracket
Behavior Assessment System for Children monitor
Behen ear forceps
behind-the-ear (BTE)
  b.-t.-e. hearing aid
  b.-t.-e. listening device
Behrend
  B. cystic duct forceps
  B. periosteal elevator
Beimer-Clip aneurysm clip
Beird eye catheter
Békésy audiometer
Belcher clamp
Belin needle holder
bell
  B. erysiphake
  Gomco circumcision b.
  b. rasp
Bellavar medical support stockings
Bellfield wire retractor
bellied bougie
Bellman retractor
Bellocq
  B. cannula
  B. sound
  B. tube
bellows
  aneroid chest b.
  B. cryoextractor
  B. cryoextractor extractor
  B. cryophake
Bellucci
  B. alligator scissors
  B. cannula
  B. curette
  B. ear forceps
  B. elevator
  B. hook
  B. lancet knife
  B. pick
  B. suction tube
Bellucci-Wullstein retractor
belly band
Belmont collar
Bel-O-Pak suction tube
Belos compression pin
below-knee (BK)
  b.-k. prosthesis

  b.-k. walking cast
  b.-k. walking plaster
Belscope
  B. blade
  B. laryngoscope
Belsey perfusor
belt
  adjustable ostomy appliance b.
  Air Temp Advantage back support b.
  Bauer hernia b.
  Baylor pelvic traction b.
  Bili Button abdominal b.
  Black hernia b.
  body b. (BB)
  Carabelt therapeutic b.
  Coloplast ostomy b.
  compression b.
  Conco abdominal b.
  Cool-Flex A/K suspension b.
  Dover abdominal b.
  gait b.
  Grafco pelvic traction b.
  Grotena abdominal b.
  Grotena lumbar b.
  Hackett sacral b.
  Hackett sacroiliac cinch b.
  Little Ones SUR-FIT pediatric b.
  Loc-Light lumbar support b.
  magnetic support b.
  Marsupial b.
  Meek pelvic traction b.
  MicroTeq portable b.
  pelvic traction b.
  Posey b.
  Pouchkins pediatric ostomy b.
  PowerBelt lower back and abdominal support b.
  Pro-Comelastic abdominal b.
  Reed cast b.
  sacroiliac cinch b.
  safety b.
  Serola sacroiliac b.
  SI-LOC sacroiliac b.
  Soma sacroiliac stabilization b.
  Spine Power pelvic stabilizer b.
  Sports Plus II back b.
  traction b.
  Tri-Flex auxiliary suspension b.
  Universal pelvic traction b.
  waist b.
Belzer apparatus
Belz lacrimal sac rongeur
Bemis
  B. suction cannister
  B. Vac-U-Port
Benaron scalp-rotating forceps
bench
  Invacare vinyl transfer b.
  meditation b.
  Paramount 3-Way press b.
  pelvic b.
  b. scale calorimeter
Benchekroun ileal valve
Bend-A-Boot foot splint

B

Benda finger vise
bender
    Bunnell knuckle b.
    French rod b.
    Gratloch wire b.
    Knuckle B.'s
    plate b.
    rod b.
    Tessier bone b.
Bendick dental arch bar
bending pliers
Bendixen-Kirschner traction bow
Benedict
    B. operating gastroscope
    B. retractor
Benedict-Roth
    B.-R. apparatus
    B.-R. calorimeter
    B.-R. spirometer
Benestent
Beneventi self-retaining retractor
Beneys tonsillar compressor
Bengash needle
Benger probe
Bengolea arterial forceps
Béniqué
    B. catheter
    B. dilator
    B. sound
Benjamin
    B. binocular slimline laryngoscope
    B. pediatric operating laryngoscope
    B. tube
Benjamin-Havas fiberoptic light clip
Benjamin-Lindholm microsuspension
    laryngoscope
Ben-Jet tube
Bennell
    B. bandage
    B. forceps
Bennett
    B. bone elevator
    B. bone lever
    B. bone retractor
    B. Cascade II Servo controlled
        heated humidifier
    B. ciliary forceps
    B. common duct dilator
    B. contour mammography system
    B. epilation forceps
    B. foreign body spud
    B. monitoring spirometer
    B. pressure-cycled ventilator
    B. raspatory
    B. respirator
    B. seal
    B. self-retaining retractor blade
    B. tibial retractor
Benoist penetrometer
Bensaude anoscope
Benson
    B. baby pyloric separator
    B. pyloric clamp
    B. pylorus spreader

bent
    b. blunt blade
    b. blunt needle
    b. malleable retractor
Bentall cardiovascular prosthesis
Bentley
    B. button
    B. Duraflo II
    B. Duraflo II extracorporeal
        perfusion circuit
    B. oxygenator
    B. transducer
Bentson
    B. exchange straight guide wire
    B. floppy-tip guide wire
    B. Glidewire guidewire
Bentson-Hanafee-Wilson catheter
Bentson-type Glidewire guide wire
Benzaquen-Chajchir extraction/reinjection
    system
benzene scintillator
Berbecker
    B. needle
    B. pliers
Berchtold cautery
Berci-Schore choledochoscope-nephroscope
Berci-Ward
    B.-W. laryngonasopharyngoscope
    B.-W. laryngopharyngoscope
Bercovici wire lid speculum
Berens
    B. bident electrode
    B. blade
    B. capsular forceps
    B. cataract knife
    B. common duct scoop
    B. conical eye implant
    B. corneal dissector
    B. corneal transplant forceps
    B. corneal transplant scissors
    B. corneoscleral punch
    B. enucleation compressor
    B. esophageal retractor
    B. eye speculum
    B. glaucoma knife
    B. graft
    B. iridocapsulotomy scissors
    B. iris knife
    B. keratoplasty knife
    B. lens expressor
    B. lens loop
    B. lens loupe
    B. lens scoop
    B. lid everter
    B. lid retractor
    B. marking calipers
    B. mastectomy skin flap retractor
    B. muscle clamp
    B. muscle recession forceps
    B. orbital compressor
    B. orbital implant
    B. partial keratome
    B. prism
    B. prism bar
    B. ptosis forceps

Berens *(continued)*
    B. ptosis knife
    B. punctum dilator
    B. pyramidal eye implant
    B. recession forceps
    B. refractor
    B. scleral hook
    B. sclerotomy knife
    B. spatula
    B. sphere eye implant
    B. sterilizing case
    B. suturing forceps
    B. thyroid retractor
    B. tonometer
Berens-Rosa scleral implant
Berenstein
    B. guiding catheter
    B. occlusion balloon catheter
Berens-Tolman ocular hypertension indicator
Bergen retractor
Berger
    B. biopsy forceps
    B. loop
    B. spur crusher
Bergeret-Reverdin needle
Bergeron pillar forceps
Berges-Reverdin needle
Berget lens loop
Bergh ciliary forceps
Berghmann-Foerster sponge forceps
Bergland-Warshawski phaco/cortex kit
Bergman
    B. mallet
    B. plaster saw
    B. plaster scissors
    B. scalpel
    B. tissue forceps
    B. tracheal retractor
    B. wound retractor
Bergmann Optical laser scanner
Bergström
    B. articulator
    B. needle
Bergström-Stille muscle cannula
Berke
    B. ciliary forceps
    B. clamp
    B. double-end lid everter
    B. ptosis clamp
    B. ptosis forceps
Berkefeld filter
Berke-Jaeger lid plate
Berkeley
    B. Bioengineering bipolar cautery
    B. Bioengineering brass scleral plug
    B. Bioengineering infusion terminal port
    B. Bioengineering mechanized scissors
    B. Bioengineering ocutome
    B. Bioengineering ptosis forceps
    B. Bioengineering stiletto
    B. cannula

    B. clamp
    B. retractor
    B. scarifier
    B. suction cup
    B. suction machine
    B. Vacurette
Berkeley-Bonney
    B.-B. self-retaining abdominal retractor
    B.-B. vaginal clamp
Berkovits-Castellanos hexapolar electrode
Berlin curette
Berlind-Auvard
    B.-A. retractor
    B.-A. vaginal speculum
Berliner
    B. neurological hammer
    B. percussion hammer
Berman
    B. angiographic catheter
    B. aortic clamp
    B. balloon flotation catheter
    B. cardiac catheter
    B. foreign body locator
    B. intubating pharyngeal airway
    B. localizer
    B. magnet
    B. vascular clamp
Bermen-Werner probe
Bernaco adapter
Berna infant abdominal retractor
Bernard uterine forceps
Bernay
    B. sponge
    B. tracheal retractor
    B. uterine gauze packer
Berndt hip ruler
Berne
    B. nasal forceps
    B. nasal rasp
Bernell
    B. grid
    B. tangent screen
Bernhard
    B. clamp
    B. towel forceps
Bernstein
    B. catheter
    B. gastroscope
    B. nasal retractor
Berry
    B. pile clamp
    B. rib raspatory
    B. rotating inlet
    B. sternal needle holder
    B. uterine-elevating forceps
Berry-Lambert periosteal elevator
Bertillon
    B. calipers
    B. cephalometer
Bertin hip retractor
BESP
Best
    B. bite block
    B. common duct stone forceps

B. direct forward-vision telescope
B. gallstone forceps
B. intestinal clamp
beStent
    b. balloon-expandable stent
    b. 2 coronary stent
beta
    b. irradiation applicator
    B. Pile II, III splint strap
    b. therapy eye applicator
Betabed bed
Beta-Cap
    B.-C. closure system for catheters
    B.-C. II catheter closure
Betacel-Biotronik pacemaker
Betaclassic surgical table
Beta-Rail catheter
beta-ray applicator
beta-scintillation counter
Betaseron needle-free delivery system
Bethea sheet holder
Bethune
    B. clamp
    B. lobectomy tourniquet
    B. lung tourniquet
    B. nerve hook
    B. periosteal elevator
    B. phrenic retractor
    B. rib shears
Bethune-Coryllos rib shears
Better Than Another Pair of Hands
  retractor system
Bettman empyema tube
Bettman-Noyes fixation forceps
Beurrier connector
Bevalac system
Bevan
    B. gallbladder forceps
    B. hemostatic forceps
Bevatron accelerator
bevel
    Menghini-type coring b.
beveled
    b. chisel
    b. thin-walled needle
bevel-point Rush pin
Beverly referential valve
Beyer
    B. atticus punch
    B. bone rongeur
    B. endaural rongeur
    B. forceps
    B. laminectomy rongeur
    B. paracentesis needle
    B. pigtail probe
Beyer-Lempert rongeur
Beyer-Stille bone rongeur
BF large core bronchoscope
BFO
    BFO Kit
    BFO orthosis
BGC Matrix dressing
B-H forceps
BHTU microscope

BIAcore system
Biad
    B. camera
    B. SPECT imaging system
Bianchi valve
biangled hook
Bi-Angular shoulder prosthesis
BIAS
    BIAS prosthesis
    BIAS slaphammer
    BIAS total hip system
Bias
    B. stockinette
bias-cut stockinette dressing
bias wrap
Biatin foam dressing
bibeveled cutting instrument
bicanalicular
    b. silicone tube
BICAP, BiCAP
    Bipolar Circumactive Probe
    BICAP bipolar hemostasis probe
    BICAP II cautery
    BICAP monopolar electrode
    BICAP silver ACE
    BICAP unit
Bicarbon Sorin valve
Bicek vaginal retractor
Biceps bipolar coagulator
Bicer-val
    B.-v. mitral heart valve
    B.-v. prosthetic valve
Bickel
    B. intramedullary nail
    B. intramedullary rod
    B. ring
Bickle microsurgical knife
BiCoag bipolar laparoscopic forceps
Bicol collagen sponge
Bicomatic bipolar cable
biconcave
    b. contact lens
    b. washer
Bicon dental implant
bicondylar ankle prosthesis
Bicon-Plus cup
biconvex intraocular lens
Bicoral implant
Bicor catheter
bicortical
    b. superior border screw
bicoudé catheter
bicurved needle
bicycle
    b. dynamometer
    b. ergometer
    MedGraphics CPE 2000
    electronically braked b.
    Monark b.
    Schwinn Air-Dyne b.
    Tredex b.
bicylindrical lens
bident retractor
Bidet toilet insert

B

bidirectional
    b. four-pole Butterworth high-pass digital filter
    b. shunt
Biegelseisen needle
Bielawski heart clamp
Biemer
    B. approximator
    B. vessel clip
Bier
    B. amputation saw
    B. lumbar puncture needle
Bierer ovum forceps
Bierman needle
Biestek thyroid retractor
Bietti
    B. eye implant
    B. lens
bifid
    b. gallbladder retractor
    b. hook
bifocal
    b. demand DVI pacemaker
    executive b.
    b. eye implant
    b. glasses
    b. intracorneal lens
    b. multiplane rectal transducer
bifoil
    b. balloon
    b. balloon catheter
bifurcated
    b. bladeplate
    b. drain extension
    b. J-shaped tined atrial pacing and defibrillation lead
    b. retractor
    b. seamless prosthesis
    b. vascular graft
Bigelow
    B. calvaria clamp
    B. evacuator
    B. forceps
    B. lithotrite
Biggs mammoplasty retractor
Bihrle
    B. dorsal clamp
    B. dorsal clamp-T-C needle holder
bikini
    disposable b.
BiLAP
    B. bipolar cautery
    B. bipolar cautery unit
    B. bipolar laparoscopic probe
bilateral
    b. variable screw placement system
    b. ventricular assist device (BIVAD)
bileaflet tilting-disk prosthetic valve
bile bag
bilevel chisel
bili
    B. Button abdominal belt
    b. light
    b. mask eye shield

biliary
    b. balloon catheter
    b. balloon probe
    b. duct balloon dilator
    b. endoprosthesis
    b. retractor
    b. stent
    b. stone basket
Bilibed phototherapy system
BiliBlanket phototherapy system
BiliBottoms
BiliCheck
    B. battery-powered system
BiliChek bilirubin analyzer
Bililite
bilirubin blanket
bilirubinometer
    transcutaneous b.
    Unistat b.
Bilisystem
    B. ERCP cannula
    B. stone-removal balloon
    B. wire-guided papillotome
bili-Timer
Bill
    B. bar
    B. traction handle forceps
Billeau
    B. ear hook
    B. ear loop
    B. ear wax curette
Billeau-House ear loop
Billingham-Bookwalter rectal fenestrated blade
Billroth
    B. curette
    B. ovarian retractor
    B. tube
    B. uterine tumor forceps
Billroth-Stille retractor
Bilos pin extractor
Bilson fixable-removable cross arch bar splint
Biltzer laryngeal blade
bilumen mammary implant
Bi-Metric
    B.-M. hip prosthesis
    B.-M. Interlok femoral prosthesis
    B.-M. porous primary femoral prosthesis
Bimler
    B. activator
    B. appliance
    B. arch
    B. elastic plate
binasal
    b. cannula
    b. pharyngeal airway
binder
    abdominal b.
    breast b.
    compression b.
    Dale abdominal b.
    Dale surgical b.
    HK b.

Orthomatrix b.
OsteoGraf b.
Texal-Muller chest b.
Binder submalar implant
Bingham knee prosthesis
Bing stylet
Binkhorst
B. collar stud intraocular lens
B. collar stud lens implant
B. eye implant
B. four-loop iris-fixated implant
B. hooked cannula
B. irrigating cannula
B. lens forceps
B. lens implant
B. mustache lens intraocular lens
B. tip
B. two-loop intraocular lens implant
B. two-loop lens
B. two modified J-loops intraocular lens
Binkhorst-Fyodorov lens
Binner
B. diaphanoscope
B. head lamp
binocle bandage
binocular
b. bandage
b. eye dressing
b. fixation forceps
b. indirect ophthalmoscope with SPF
b. loupe
b. shield
binophthalmoscope
binoscope
Bio
B. Core therapeutic mattress
B. Flote
B. Flote air flotation system
B. Gard Plus
B. therapy
BIO101MERmaid kit
bioabsorbable
b. closure device
b. double-spiral stent
b. interference screw
b. staple
bioactive
b. bone cement adhesive
Bio-Anchor suture anchor
bioartificial liver support device
BioBands bracelet
biobarrier membrane
Biobond tissue adhesive
Biobrane
B. adhesive
B. glove
B. glove dressing
B. sheet
Biobrane/HF
B. experimental skin substitute
B. graft material
B. wound dressing

BioCare
B. implant
B. thread
Biocell
B. anatomical reconstructive mammary implant
B. RTV breast implant
B. textured implant
B. textured silicone
B. wrap
bioceramic implant material
Bioceram two-stage series II endosteal dental implant
Bio-Chromatic hand prosthesis
Biocide
Bioclad with pegs reinforced acetabular prosthesis
Bioclusive
B. drape
B. MVP Select transparent dressing
Biocol dressing
biocompatible spacing material
biocompression pneumatic sleeve
Biocon impedance plethysmography cardiac output monitor
Biocor
B. porcine stented aortic valve
B. porcine stented mitral valve
B. prosthetic valve
B. stentless porcine aortic valve
Biocoral graft
BioCore collagen dressing
biodegradable
b. plate
b. polymer scaffold
b. stent
b. surgical tack
Biodel implant
Biodex
B. isokinetic dynamometer
B. isokinetic testing machine
B. Unweighing system
B. XYZ imaging table
BioDIMENSIONAL
B. saline-filled implant
BioDimensional system
BioDivYsio stent
Biodrape dressing
Biodynamic
B. acetabular component
B. molding system
BioDyne
B. II kinetic therapy low-air-loss bed
Bio-Esthetic abutment system
Bio-eye
B.-e. hydroxyapatite ocular implant
biofeedback
B. 5DX device
b. electroencephalograph
b. electromyometer
b. galvanic skin response device
b. instrumentation
Biofil
Trio-Temp X B.

BioFilm
> THINSite with B.

Biofilter cardiovascular hemoconcentrator
Bio-Fit total hip system
Biofix
> B. absorbable rod
> B. absorbable screw
> B. arrow
> B. arrow gun
> B. biodegradable implant
> B. fixation rod
> B. system pin

BIOflex
> B. Magnet Back Support
> B. magnetic brace
> B. penile orthotic

Biofoot orthotic
biofragmentable anastomotic ring
Biofreeze with Ilex
Biogel
> B. orthopaedic surgical gloves
> B. Reveal puncture indication
> system
> B. Sensor surgical glove
> B. surgeons' gloves

BioGen nonporous barrier membrane
Bio-Gide
> B.-G. resorbable barrier membrane

Bioglass
> B. bone substitute material
> low-surface reactive B.
> B. prosthesis

Bio-Glide
> Import vascular access port
> with B.-G.

BioGlide catheter
BioGlue glue
Biograft
> B. bovine heterograft material
> Dakin B.
> Dardik B.
> B. graft
> Meadox Dardik B.

BioGran resorbable synthetic bone graft
Bio-Groove
> B.-G. acetabular prosthesis
> B.-G. hip
> B.-G. Macrobond HA femoral
> prosthesis
> B.-G. stem

Bio-Guard spectrum antimicrobial
  bonded catheter
biohazard bag
BioHorizon
> B. implant
> B. thread

bioimpedance electrocardiograph
bioimplant
> DynaGraft b.

biointerference screw
Bioject jet injector
Biojector 2000 needle-free injection
  management system
Biokinetics pedobarograph
Bio-kinetics reader

BioKnit garment electrode
BioLab modular motility system
BioLase laser adapter
Biolex
> B. impregnated dressing
> B. wound glue

Biolite ventilation tube
Biologically Quiet
> B. Q. interference screw
> B. Q. reconstruction screw
> B. Q. suture anchor

biological tissue valve
BioLogic DT-HT system
biologic fibrogen adhesive
Biologics Airlift bed
Biolox
> B. ball head
> B. ball head prosthesis
> B. ceramic ball head for hip
> replacement

biomagnet
biomagnetometer
> Magnes b.

BioMask
biomaterial
> DualMesh + b.
> DualMesh Plus b.
> Gore-Tex DualMesh Plus b.
> Gore-Tex MycroMesh Plus b.
> MycroMesh + b.
> MycroMesh Plus b.
> polymeric b.

Biomatrix ocular implant
Bio-Medicus
> B.-M. arterial catheter
> B.-M. centrifugal pump
> B.-M. percutaneous cannula set

Bio-Med MVP-10 pediatric ventilator
BioMed TENS unit
BioMedx portable air flotation system
biomembrane
BioMend
> B. collagen membrane
> B. periodontal material

Biomer microsuturing instrument
Biomet
> B. AGC knee component
> B. AGC knee prosthesis
> B. AGC primary and posterior
> stabilized component
> B. ankle arthrodesis nail
> B. Ascent total knee system
> B. bed
> B. Bi-Polar component
> B. button
> B. cement removal hand chisel
> B. custom implant
> B. Finn salvage/oncology knee
> reconstruction system
> B. fracture brace
> B. Genus uniknee system
> B. hip
> B. hip prosthesis
> B. hip stem
> B. MARS acetabular component

B. Maxim revision knee system
B. Maxim total knee system
B. plug
B. Repicci II unicompartment knee component
B. revision acetabular component
B. shoulder component
B. total toe prosthesis
B. Ultra-Drive cement remover
B. Ultra-Drive ultrasonic revision system

Biometer
Ophthasonic Ultrasonic B.

Biometric prosthesis
biometry probe
Biomicroscope
Nikon FS-3 photo slit lamp B.

biomicroscope
high-frequency ultrasound b.
ultrasonic b.

biomicroscopic indirect lens
Bio-Modular
B.-M. humeral rasp
B.-M. shoulder component
B.-M. total shoulder system

Bio-Moore
B.-M. endoprosthesis
B.-M. II instrumentation
B.-M. II provisional neck spacer
B.-M. II stem impactor
B.-M. rasp

Bionicare
B. stimulator
B. 1000 stimulator system

Bionic ear prosthesis
Bionics arrow
Bionit
B. vascular graft
B. vascular prosthesis

Bionix
B. nasal speculum
B. self-reinforced PLLA smart screw

Bio-Optics
B.-O. Bambi cell analysis system
B.-O. Bambi image analysis system
B.-O. camera
B.-O. specular microscope

BIO-OSS
B.-O. freeze-dried demineralized bone
B.-O. maxillofacial bone filler

Biopac gingival retraction cord
BIOPATCH
B. antimicrobial dressing with chlorhexidine gluconate
B. antimicrobial foam wound dressing

Bio-Pen biometric ruler
Biopharm leeches
Bio-Phase suture anchor
Biophysic
B. Medical YAG laser
B. Ophthascan S instrument

Bioplant hard tissue replacement (HTR) synthetic bone
Bioplastique
B. augmentation material
B. injectable microimplant
B. polymer

Bioplate
B. screw fixation system

Bio-Plug
B.-P. canal plug
B.-P. component

Bioplus dispersive electrode
BioPolyMeric
B. femoropopliteal bypass graft
B. vascular graft

Biopore membrane
Bioport collection and transport system
biopotential skin electrode
bioprosthesis
Carpentier-Edwards Perimount RSR pericardial b.
Carpentier-Edwards porcine b.
Freestyle aortic root b.
Hancock M.O. II porcine b.
Mosaic cardiac b.
pericarbon b.
Perimount RSR pericardial b.
PhotoFix alpha pericardial b.
porcine b.
SJM X-Cell cardiac b.
Toronto b.

bioprosthetic
b. heart valve

biopsy
b. cannula
b. gun
b. loop electrode
b. needle
b. probe
b. punch
b. punch forceps
b. specimen forceps
b. suction curette
b. telescope

Biopsys mammotome
bioptic
b. amorphic lens system
b. telescope

bioptome
Bycep PC Jr b.
Caves b.
Caves-Schultz b.
Cordis b.
King cardiac b.
Mansfield b.
Scholten endomyocardial b.
Stanford b.
Stanford-Caves b.

Biopty
B. cut biopsy needle
B. gun

Bio-Pump pump
BioRad Model 5000 Titanium system
Biorate pacemaker

bioresorbable
  b. drug delivery system
  b. implant
BioROC EZ suture anchor
Bio-R-Sorb resorbable poly-L-lactic acid ministaple
biosampler
  Accellon Combi cervical b.
BioScrew
Biosearch
  B. anal biofeedback device
  B. female intermittent urinary catheter
  B. jejunostomy kit
  B. male intermittent urinary catheter
  B. needle
Biosense NOGA catheter-based endocardial mapping system
Bio-sentry telemeter
BioSkin support
BioSorb
  B. endoscopic browlift screw
  B. suture
Biosound
  B. AU (Advanced Ultrasonography) system
  B. 2000 II ultrasound unit
  B. Phase 2 ultrasound system
  B. Surgiscan echocardiograph
  B. wide-angle monoplane ultrasound scanner
Biospal
  B. filter
  B. hemodialyzer
Biospan
  B. anatomical tissue expander
BIOSPAN breast tissue expander
Biospec
  B. MR imaging system
  B. MR imaging system scanner
BioSphere
  B. suture anchor
  B. suture anchor implant
Bio-Statak suture anchor
Biostent
Biostil blood transfusion set
BioStinger
  B. fixation device
  B. fixation system
BioStinger-V bioabsorbable meniscal repair device
Biostop G cement restrictor
Biosurge Synchronous Autotransfuser
Biosyn suture
Biosystems feeding tube Bio-Suture Tak
BioTac (Arthrex)
  B. biopsy cannula
  B. ECG electrode
Biotek 1000 Autostainer
biotelemetry system
Biotens neurostimulator
biothesiometer
  penile b.
Biothotic
  B. foot orthosis

  B. orthotic
  B. orthotic mold
Biotrack coagulation monitor
BioTrainer exercise meter
Biotronik
  B. demand pacemaker
  B. lead
Bio-Vascular prosthetic valve
Bio-Vent implant
Biovert
  B. ceramic implant
  B. implant material
Biovue catheter
BIOWARE software for Biodex isokinetic exercise system
Bio-Wick sock
BI-OX III ear oximeter
BioZ system
BiPAP
  B. Duet LX
  B. unit
biphase Morris fixation apparatus
biphasic
  b. pin
  b. pin appliance
  b. system
bipivotal hinge knee brace
biplanar fixator
biplane
  b. intracavitary probe
  b. sector probe
bipolar
  b. bayonet forceps
  b. cautery
  b. cautery scissors
  B. Circumactive Probe (BICAP, BiCAP)
  b. coagulating forceps
  b. coagulator
  b. coaptation forceps
  b. connection cord
  b. cutting forceps
  b. depth electrode
  b. diathermy adapter clip
  b. diathermy forceps tip
  b. electrocautery
  b. electrocautery forceps
  b. electrosurgical unit
  B. EndoStasis probe
  b. eye forceps
  b. glass electrode
  b. hemostasis probe
  b. hip arthroplasty component
  b. irrigating forceps
  b. irrigating stylet
  b. laparoscopic forceps
  b. long-shaft forceps
  b. myocardial electrode
  b. needle
  b. pacemaker
  b. pacing electrode catheter
  b. suction forceps
  b. temporary pacemaker catheter
  b. transsphenoidal forceps
  b. urological loop

BiPort hemostasis introducer sheath kit
BIPP ribbon gauze
biprong muscle marker
Bipro orthodontic appliance
Bipulse stimulator
BI-RADS breast imaging and reporting data system
Birch
    B. lamp
    B. trocar
Bircher
    B. bone-holding clamp
    B. cartilage clamp
    B. meniscus knife
Bircher-Ganske meniscal cartilage forceps
Birch-Hirschfeld lamp
Bird
    Ascension B.
    B. Asthmastik
    B. low-flow blender
    B. machine
    B. Mark 8 respirator
    B. micronebulizer
    B. MK VIII pressure-cycled ventilator
    B. neonatal CPAP generator
    B. OP cup
    B. pressure-cycled ventilator
    B. 8400STi ventilator
    B. vacuum extractor
birdcage
    b. head coil
    b. resonator
    b. splint
bird's-eye catheter
Birdseye quilted underpad
bird's nest IVC filter
Bireks dissecting forceps
Birkenstock
    B. Blue Footbed arch support
    B. high-flange arch support
Birkett hemostatic forceps
Birkhauser eye testing chart
Birks
    B. Mark II Colibri forceps
    B. Mark II grooved forceps
    B. Mark II hook
    B. Mark II micro cross-action holder
    B. Mark II microneedle-holder forceps
    B. Mark II micro push/pull spatula
    B. Mark II needle holder
    B. Mark II needle-holder forceps
    B. Mark II straight forceps
    B. Mark II suture-tying forceps
    B. Mark II toothed forceps
    B. Mark II trabeculectomy scissors
Birks-Mathelone microforceps
BIRO system
Birtcher
    B. cautery
    B. defibrillator
    B. electrocautery probe
    B. electrode

    B. electrosurgical generator
    B. electrosurgical needle
    B. endoscopic forceps
    B. Hyfrecator
    B. Hyfrecator cautery wire
    B. Hyfrecator coagulator
    B. Hyfrecator electrosurgical unit
    B. laparoscopic coagulator
birth cushion
birthing
    b. ball
    b. chair
BIS
    BIS Sensor
    BIS Sensor Plus
bisected minigraft dilator
Bi-Set catheter
Bishop
    B. antral perforator
    B. bone clamp
    B. mastoid chisel
    B. mastoid gouge
    B. oscillatory bone saw
    B. putty
    B. retractor
    B. sphygmoscope
    B. tendon tucker
    B. tissue forceps
Bishop-Black tendon tucker
Bishop-DeWitt tendon tucker
Bishop-Harman
    B.-H. anterior chamber irrigating cannula
    B.-H. anterior chamber irrigator
    B.-H. bladebreaker
    B.-H. dressing
    B.-H. dressing forceps
    B.-H. foreign body forceps
    B.-H. iris forceps
    B.-H. knife
    B.-H. mules
    B.-H. spud
    B.-H. Superblade
    B.-H. tissue forceps
Bishop-Peter tendon tucker
BiSNARE bipolar polypectomy snare
Bi-Soft lens
bispectral index
bispherical lens
Bisping electrode
bisque-baked prosthesis
bistoury
    b. blade
    Brophy b.
    Converse button-end b.
    Jackson tracheal b.
    Jackson tracheotomic b.
    b. knife
    straight b.
Biswas Silastic vaginal pessary
bit
    cannulated drill b.
    drill guide with drill b.
    Howmedica Microfixation System drill b.

B

bit *(continued)*
    Leibinger Micro System drill b.
    Luhr Microfixation System drill b.
    Storz Microsystems drill b.
    Synthes Microsystem drill b.
bite
    b. biopsy forceps
    b. block
    b. force transducer
    b. protector
    b. stick
biteblock, bite block
    Lell b.
Bi-tec forceps
Bitefork face bow
biteplate
biter
    angled b.
    Stille bone b.
    suction b.
biterminal electrode
Bite wafer denture bite wax
biting
    b. forceps
    b. rongeur
Bitome
    B. bipolar sphincterotome
    B. bipolar system
    B. catheter
Bitpad digitizer
Bitumi monobjective microscope
BIVAD
    bilateral ventricular assist device
    BIVAD bilateral left and right
        ventricular assist device
bivalved
    b. anal speculum
    b. cannula
    b. cast
    b. retractor
bivalve nasal splint implant
biventricular assist device
Bivona
    B. cuff maintenance device
    B. Duckbill voice prosthesis
    B. epistaxis catheter
    B. Fome-Cuf tube
    B. Medical Technologies customized
        tracheostomy tube
    B. sleep apnea tracheostomy tube
    B. tracheostomy tube with talk
        attachment
    B. TTS tracheostomy tube
    B. Ultra Low voice prosthesis
Bivona-Colorado
    B.-C. button
    B.-C. dummy prosthesis
    B.-C. sizing device
    B.-C. template
    B.-C. voice prosthesis
Bi-Wave
    B.-W. mattress overlay
    B.-W. plus mattress replacement
Bizzarri-Guiffrida laryngoscope

Bjerrum
    B. scotometer
    B. screen
Björk
    B. diathermy forceps
    B. prosthesis
    B. rib drill
Björk-Shiley
    B.-S. aortic valve prosthesis
    B.-S. convexoconcave 60-degree
        valve prosthesis
    B.-S. floating disk prosthesis
    B.-S. graft
    B.-S. heart valve holder
    B.-S. heart valve sizer
    B.-S. mitral valve
    B.-S. Monostrut valve
Björk-Stille diathermy forceps
BK
    below-knee
    BK prosthesis
BKS refractive system
black
    B. Beauty ureteral stent
    b. braided nylon suture
    b. braided silk suture
    b. braided suture
    b. hatchet
    B. hernia belt
    b. light lamp
    B. Max mid size knee component
    B. meatal clamp
    B. rasp
    B. retractor
    b. twisted suture
Blackburn
    B. skull traction tractor
    B. trephine
Black-Decker needle
blackened
    b. hemostat
    b. speculum
Blackmon needle
Blackstone anterior cervical plate
black/white occluder
Black-Wylie obstetric dilator
bladder
    b. blade
    b. catheter
    b. dilator
    b. evacuator
    b. flap tube
    gel-filled b.
    b. neck support pessary
    b. pacemaker
    PyMaH nylon balanced b.
    b. replacement urinary pouch
    b. retractor
    b. scan
    b. sound
    b. specimen forceps
BladderManager
    B. portable ultrasonic device
    B. portable ultrasound scanner
    B. ultrasound

bladder-neck support prosthesis
BladderScan
    B. BVI2500 scanner
    B. monitor
    B. ultrasound
blade
    Acra-Cut Spiral craniotome b.
    adenotome b.
    Aggressor meniscal b.
    Alcon crescent b.
    Alcon pocket b.
    arachnoid Beaver b.
    arachnoid-shaped b.
    Arthro-Lok system of Beaver b.'s
    arthroscopic banana b.
    ASR b.
    ASSI cranial b.
    autopsy b.
    baby Miller b.
    Balfour bladder b.
    Balfour center b.
    Balfour lateral b.
    Balfour retractor with
      fenestrated b.'s
    banana Beaver b.
    Bard-Parker autopsy b.
    Bard-Parker surgical b.
    Barraquer b.
    Barton b.
    Baxter disposable b.
    Beaver Arthro-Lok b.
    Beaver bent b.
    Beaver cataract b.
    Beaver-DeBakey b.
    Beaver discission b.
    Beaver keratome b.
    Beaver lamellar b.
    Beaver limbus b.
    Beaver-Lundsgaard b.
    Beaver Microsharp b.
    Beaver myringotomy b.
    Beaver-Okamura b.
    Beaver Optimum b.
    Beaver phacokeratome b.
    Beaver rhinoplasty b.
    Beaver scleral Lundsgaard b.
    Beaver tonsillectomy b.
    Beaver-Ziegler b.
    Beckman-Adson laminectomy b.
    Beckman-Eaton laminectomy b.
    Beer b.
    Belscope b.
    Bennett self-retaining retractor b.
    bent blunt b.
    Berens b.
    Billingham-Bookwalter rectal
      fenestrated b.
    Biltzer laryngeal b.
    bistoury b.
    bladder b.
    Blount bent b.
    Blount V-b.
    bone saw b.
    Bookwalter-Cook anal rectal b.
    Bookwalter-Gelpi point retractor b.

    Bookwalter-Kelly retractor b.
    Bookwalter malleable retractor b.
    Bookwalter-Mayo b.
    Bookwalter-Parks anal sphincter b.
    Bookwalter rectal b.
    Bookwalter retractor b.
    Bookwalter vaginal Deaver b.
    Bovie b.
    Bowen BAS-30 b.
    breakable b.
    broken razor b.
    Brown dermatome b.
    capsulotomy b.
    carbolized knife b.
    carbon steel b.
    Caspar b.
    cast b.
    Castroviejo razor b.
    cataract b.
    cervical biopsy b.
    chisel b.
    chondroplasty Beaver b.
    circular b.
    CLM articulating laryngoscope b.
    Cloward single-tooth retractor b.
    Collin radiopaque sternal b.
    conization instrument b.
    Converse retractor b.
    Cooley-Pontius sternal b.
    CooperVision Surgeon-Plus
      Ultrathin b.
    copper b.
    Cottle nasal knife b.
    crescent b.
    crescentic b.
    Crile b.
    Crockard small-tongue retractor b.
    Curdy b.
    Curdy-Hebra b.
    curved meniscotome b.
    Davidoff b.
    Davis b.
    Davis-Crowe tongue b.
    Dean b.
    Deaver b.
    DeBakey b.
    DeBakey-Beaver b.
    deep spreader b.
    Denis Browne abdominal
      retractor b.
    Denis Browne-Hendren pediatric
      retractor b.
    Denis Browne malleable copper
      retractor b.
    Denis Browne mastoid pediatric
      retractor b.
    Denis Browne pediatric abdominal
      retractor b.
    dermatome b.
    diamond b.
    Dingman mouthgag tongue
      depressor b.
    discission b.
    Dixon b.
    double-angled b.

B

blade *(continued)*
    double-vector b.
    Duotrak b.
    Dyonics arthroscopic b.
    Edge b.
    b. electrode
    electrodermatome sterile b.
    E-Mac laryngoscope b.
    Emir razor b.
    Endo-Assist retractable b.
    b. endosteal implant
    English MacIntosh fiberoptic
      laryngoscope b.
    Epstein hemilaminectomy b.
    expandable b.
    eye b.
    Feather carbon breakable b.
    Field b.
    Flagg stainless steel laryngoscope b.
    folding b.
    Genesis diamond b.
    Gigli-saw b.
    Gill b.
    Gillette Blue B.
    Gill-Hess b.
    Gott-Balfour b.
    Gott-Harrington b.
    Gott-Seeram b.
    Goulian b.
    Grieshaber b.
    GS-9 b.
    GSA-9 b.
    Guedel laryngoscope b.
    Hammond winged retractor b.
    b. handle
    Hebra b.
    hemilaminectomy b.
    Hendren pediatric retractor b.
    Henley retractor b.
    Hibbs spinal retractor b.
    Hopp anterior commissure
      laryngoscope b.
    Horgan center b.
    Hoskins razor fragment b.
    House detachable b.
    House knife b.
    House ophthalmic b.
    Incisor arthroscopic b.
    infant urethrotome b.
    jigsaw b.
    K b.
    Katena double-edged sapphire b.
    K-Blade microsurgical b.
    Keeler retractable b.
    Kellan sutureless incision b.
    keratome b.
    Kjelland b.
    Knapp b.
    b. knife
    knife b.
    LaForce adenotome b.
    lamellar b.
    laminectomy b.
    lancet b.

    Lange b.
    laryngoscope b.
    Leivers b.
    Lemmon b.
    Lieberman Wire Aspirating
      Speculum with V-shape b.'s
    Lite b.
    Lundsgaard b.
    MacIntosh fiberoptic laryngoscope b.
    Magrina-Bookwalter vaginal
      Deaver b.
    malleable b.
    Martin b.
    Martinez corneal trephine b.
    Mastel trifaceted diamond b.
    McPherson-Wheeler b.
    meniscectomy b.
    Merlin arthroscopy b.
    Merlin bendable b.
    Meyerding laminectomy b.
    Meyerding retractor b.
    M4-400 Freedom b.
    Micro-Sharp b.
    microvitreoretinal b.
    Miller fiberoptic laryngoscope b.
    miniature b.
    mini-meniscus b.
    Morse b.
    mouthgag tongue depressor b.
    Mueller tongue b.
    Mullins b.
    Murphy-Balfour center b.
    MVB b.
    MVR b.
    Myocure b.
    myringotomy knife b.
    nasal knife b.
    nasal saw b.
    New Skimmer b.
    notchplasty b.
    Nounton b.
    nubular b.
    ocutome vitreous b.
    ophthalmic b.
    Optimum b.
    Orbit b.
    Orca surgical b.
    Organdi b.
    Otocap myringotomy b.
    Oxiport b.
    Padgett dermatome b.
    panar b.
    Park b.
    Parker-Bard b.
    Paufique b.
    pediatric Hendren retractor b.
    pediatric mastoid retractor b.
    Personna prep b.'s
    Personna surgical b.
    b. plate fixation device
    PowerCut drill b.
    5-prong rake b.
    RAD Airway laryngeal b.
    RADenoid adenoidectomy b.
    RAD40 sinus b.

ramus b.
razor b.
rectangular b.
Reese dermatome b.
replaceable b.
retractor b.
retrograde meniscal b.
Rew-Wyly b.
Rhein 3-D trapezoid diamond b.
ribbon b.
ring retractor b.
ring tongue b.
rosette b.
Rubin b.
Rusch laryngoscope b.
Satterlee bone saw b.
SCA-EX ShortCutter catheter b.
b. scalpel
ScalpelTec keratome slit b.
ScalpelTec wound-enlargement b.
Schanz Scheie b.
Scheie b.
scimitar b.
scleral b.
sclerotome b.
Scoville retractor b.
self-retaining retractor b.
semilunar-tip b.
b. septostomy catheter
serrated b.
Sharpoint spoon b.
Sharpoint V-lance b.
Sharptome crescent b.
shoulder b.
sickle b.
sickle-shaped Beaver b.
side b.
side-cutting b.
Skimmer b.
slimcut b.
slit b.
Sofield retractor b.
spear b.
spinal retractor b.
Sputnik Russian razor b.
stainless steel b.
Stealth DBO diamond b.
sterile electrodermatome b.
sternal retractor b.
Storz disposable b.
straight b.
Stryker b.
Superblade No. 75 b.
Super-Cut b.
surgical saw b.
Surgistar ophthalmic b.
Swann-Morton surgical b.
Swiss b.
Synovator arthroscopic b.
synovectomy b.
tapered b.
Taylor laminectomy b.
Taylor spinal retractor b.
Temperlite saw b.
The Edge coated b.

Thornton arcuate b.
Thornton tri-square b.
three-pronged rake b.
throw-away manual dermatome b.
Tiger b.
tongue retractor b.
Tooke b.
Torpin vectis b.
trephine b.
Tricut b.
tri-radial resector b.
Troutman b.
Tucker-Luikart b.
Turner-Warwick b.
Typhoon cutter b.
Typhoon microdebrider b.
UltraEdge keratome b.
ultra-thin surgical b.
Universal nasal saw b.
urethrotome b.
Vascutech circular b.
vectis b.
V-lance b.
V. Mueller myringotomy b.
Weck-Prep b.
Weinberg b.
Welch Allyn laryngoscope b.
Wheeler b.
winged retractor b.
wire side b.
Wisconsin laryngoscope b.
wood tongue b.
Yu-Holtgrewe malleable b.
Zalkind-Balfour b.
Ziegler b.
Zimmer Gigli-saw b.
bladebreaker
Barraquer razor b.
Bishop-Harman b.
Castroviejo b.
b. holder
I-tech-Castroviejo b.
Jarit b.
b. knife
minirazor b.
razor b.
Swiss b.
Troutman b.
Vari b.
blade-form
b.-f. device
b.-f. implant
bladeplate
bifurcated b.
fixed-angle AO b.
Blade-Safe case
Blade-Vent implant system
Blade-Wilde ear forceps
Blair
B. cleft palate clamp
B. cleft palate elevator
B. cleft palate knife
B. four-prong retractor
B. Gigli-saw guide
B. head drape

Blair *(continued)*
  B. modification of Gellhorn pessary
  B. nasal chisel
  B. palate hook
  B. serrefine
  B. silicone drain
  B. stiletto
  B. talar body fusion blade plate
  B. tibiotalar arthrodesis blade plate
Blair-Brown
  B.-B. graft
  B.-B. implant
  B.-B. needle
  B.-B. needle holder
  B.-B. skin graft knife
  B.-B. vacuum retractor
Blair-Ivy loop
Blajwas-Schwartz-Marcinko irrigation drainage system
Blake
  B. dressing forceps
  B. ear forceps
  B. embolus forceps
  B. gallstone forceps
  B. gingivectomy knife
  B. silicone drain
  B. uterine curette
Blakemore
  B. esophageal tube
  B. nasogastric tube
Blakemore-Sengstaken tube
Blakesley
  B. ethmoid forceps
  B. grasper
  B. lacrimal trephine
  B. laminectomy rongeur
  B. septal bone forceps
  B. septal compression forceps
  B. tongue depressor
  B. uvular retractor
Blakesley-Weil upturned ethmoid forceps
Blakesley-Wilde
  B.-W. ear forceps
  B.-W. nasal forceps
Blalock
  B. forceps
  B. pulmonary artery clamp
  B. shunt
  B. suture
Blalock-Kleinert forceps
Blalock-Niedner pulmonic stenosis clamp
Blalock-Taussig shunt
Blanchard
  B. cryptotome
  B. hemorrhoidal forceps
  B. pile clamp
  B. traction device
  B. traction device blade plate
Blanco
  B. retractor
  B. scissors
  B. valve spreader
Bland
  B. cervical traction forceps

  B. perineal retractor
  B. vulsellum
  B. vulsellum forceps
blank
  implant b.
  Nickelplast b.
blanket
  Bair Hugger patient warming b.
  Bair Hugger warmer b.
  b. bath
  bath b.
  bilirubin b.
  CareDrape b.
  circulating water b.
  cooling b.
  EBI Temptek b.
  Gaymar water-circulating b.
  Hollister Hot/Ice knee b.
  Hot/Ice System III knee b.
  hypothermia b.
  Rowe b.
  b. suture
  thermal space b.
Blasucci
  B. clamp
  B. pigtail ureteral catheter
Blauth knee prosthesis
Blaydes
  B. angled lens forceps
  B. corneal forceps
  B. lens-holding forceps
Bledsoe
  B. adjustable post-op brace
  B. cast brace
  B. knee brace
bleeding needle
Bleier clip
blender
  Bird low-flow b.
Blenderm
  B. surgical tape dressing
  B. tape
blepharochalasis forceps
blepharoplasty clip
blepharostat
  b. clamp
  McNeill-Goldmann b.
  b. ring
  Schachar b.
blind
  b. endosonography probe
  b. loop
  b. medullary nail
Bliskunov implantable femoral distractor
BlisterFilm transparent wound dressing
block
  acrylic bite b.
  anterior-posterior cutting b.
  A-P cutting b.
  ball joint b.
  Best bite b.
  bite b.
  Brightbill corneal cutting b.
  Bunnell b.
  calipers b.

B. cardiac device
Cerrobend trim b.
corneal b.
4-in-1 cutting b.
cutting Delrin b.
cutting Teflon b.
Dembone demineralized cortical
  dental b.
disposable Styrofoam b.
ENT bite b.
ESI bite b.
Ethox bite b.
Fine folding b.
GeneraBloc bite b.
Greco cutting b.
Guilford-Wright cutting b.
hand b.
House-Delrin cutting b.
House Teflon cutting b.
Jackson bite b.
lead b.
Lell bite b.
MaxBloc bite b.
methyl methacrylate b.
Neumann calipers b.
New Orleans corneal cutting b.
OB-10 Comfort bite b.
Omni Bloc bite b.'s
Ora-Gard disposable intraoral bite b.
Oxyguard mouth b.
paraffin b.
pelvic b.
perspex b.
Plexiglas tissue equivalency b.
punch b.
push-up b.
B. right coronary guiding catheter
Shepard calipers b.
Shepard-Kramer calipers b.
shielding b.
shock b.
silicone b.
Southern Eye Bank corneal
  cutting b.
Speed-E-Rim denture bite b.
Stahl calipers b.
Tanne corneal cutting b.
Teflon b.
tibial augmentation b.
tibial cutting b.
Ultima Bloc bite b.
Wright-Guilford cutting b.
blocker
hook b.
MacIntosh b.
Wallach cryosurgical pain b.
Block-Potts intestinal forceps
Bloedorn applicator
Blohmka
B. tonsillar forceps
B. tonsillar hemostat
Blom-Singer
B.-S. esophagoscope
B.-S. indwelling low-pressure voice
  prosthesis

B.-S. tracheoesophageal prosthesis
B.-S. valve
blood
b. agar plate
b. cell separator
b. color analyzer
b. flow imaging
b. glucose reagent strip
b. perfusion monitor
b. pressure cuff
b. pressure recorder
b. pump
b. warmer cuff
blood-contactin catheter
blood-flow probe
bloodless circumcision clamp
Bloodshot WildEyes lens
Bloodwell
B. tissue forceps
B. vascular forceps
Bloodwell-Brown forceps
Bloomberg
B. lens forceps
B. SuperNumb anesthetic ring
B. trabeculotome set
bloomer
KINS pull-on waterproof b.
Bloom programmable stimulator
Blount
B. bent blade
B. blade plate
B. bone spreader
B. brace
B. double-prong retractor
B. epiphyseal staple
B. fracture staple
B. hip retractor
B. knee retractor
B. knife
B. laminar spreader
B. nylon mallet
B. scoliosis osteotome
B. single-prong retractor
B. splint
B. V-blade
Blount-Schmidt-Milwaukee brace
blow bottle (BB)
blow-by ventilator
blower
DeVilbiss powder b.
powder b.
Rica powder b.
SMIC powder b.
B&L pinch gauge
Blucher low-quarter shoe
blue
B. Brand therapy putty
b. Cook sheath
Daimas B.
B. FlexTip catheter
B. Line cuffed endotracheal tube
B. Line orthotic
B. Max balloon catheter
B. Max cannula
B. Max high-pressure balloon

blue *(continued)*
    B. Max triple-lumen catheter
    b. ring pessary
    b. sponge dressing
    b. twisted cotton suture
blue-black monofilament suture
Bluemle pump
blue-tip aspirator
Blum
    B. arterial scissors
    B. forceps
Blumenthal
    B. anterior chamber maintainer
    B. bone rongeur
    B. intraocular lens
    B. irrigating cystitome
    B. uterine dressing forceps
blunt
    b. bullet-tip cannula
    b. dissecting hook
    b. elevator
    b. forceps
    b. hook dissector
    b. iris hook
    b. lacrimal probe
    b. needle
    b. nerve hook
    b. obturator
    b. palpator
    b. rake retractor
    b. suction tube
    b. trocar
blunt-end sialogram needle
blunt-nose hemostat
Bluntport disposable trocar
blunt-ring curette
blunt-tipped obturator
blunt-tip probe
Blythemobile
B-mode handpiece
BMP cabling and plating system
BMSI 5000 electroencephalograph
BMT
**BNA-100-Behring Diagnostics
    immunonephelometer**
board
    arm b., armboard
    balance b.
    cartilage cutting b.
    Competitive Ankle B.
    cutting b.
    Euroglide MKII slide b.
    Fisher tape b.
    Flexisplint arm b.
    full spine b.
    Gabarro b.
    Gibson-Ross b.
    graft b.
    grid maze b.
    Hadfield hand b.
    J b.
    manipulation b.
    memory b.
    papoose b.

    pivoting surgical arm b.
    powder b.
    quad b.
    Rock ankle exercise b.
    rocker b.
    Rock & Roller exercise b.
    Slippery Slider transport b.
    b. splint
    Spri Xercise b.
    Steffensmeier b.
    string drawing b.
    SummaSketch III digitizing b.
    tape b.
    Targa+ image capture b.
    Tegtmeier hand b.
boardlike retractor
Boari button
boat
    b. hook
    b. nail
bobbin
    b. myringotomy tube
bobbin-type laryngectomy button
Bobechko
    B. sliding barrel hook
    B. spreader
Boberg-Ans
    B.-A. intraocular lens
    B.-A. lens implant
Boberg lens
Bock
    B. knee prosthesis
    B. knife
Bodai adapter
Bodenham
    B. dermabrasion cylinder
    B. saw
Bodenham-Blair skin graft knife
Bodenham-Humby skin graft knife
Bodenheimer
    B. anoscope
    B. rectal speculum
Bodenstab tourniquet
BODI
    BODI Dynamic orthosis
    BODI knee extension orthosis
Bodian
    B. discission knife
    B. lacrimal pigtail probe
    B. minilacrimal probe
Bodkin thread holder
Bodnar knee retractor
body
    B. Armor short leg walker
    B. Armor walker cast
    B. Ball
    b. belt (BB)
    B. buddy-body pillow
    Cloward lumbar retractor b.
    b. coil
    Crockard transoral retractor b.
    B. Gard neoprene support
    b. jacket
    B. Logic rehabilitation system

B. Masters MD 510 hi-lo pulley system
b. positioner
B. prop positioning splint
B. Response system
B. Wrap foam positioner
BodyBilt chair
BodyCushion positioner
body-exhaust suit
BodyIce
B. cold pack
B. wrap
Bodyline
B. Back-Huggar
Satalite cushion by B.
B. sleeper mattress overlay
Body-Solid exercise equipment
BodyTable
HiLo B.
TouchAmerica B.
BodyWrap premium overlay
Boebinger tongue depressor
Boehm
B. anoscope
B. drop syringe
B. proctoscope
B. sigmoidoscope
Boehringer
B. Autovac autotransfusion system
B. kit
Boer craniotomy forceps
Boerma obstetrical forceps
Boettcher
B. antral trocar
B. arterial forceps
B. hemostat
B. pulmonary artery clamp
B. pulmonary artery forceps
B. tonsillar artery forceps
B. tonsillar hook
B. tonsillar scissors
Boettcher-Farlow snare
Boettcher-Jennings mouthgag
Boettcher-Schnidt
B.-S. antral trocar
B.-S. forceps
Bogle rongeur
Bograb Universal offset ossicular prosthesis
Böhler
B. exerciser
B. extension bow
B. guideline
B. hip nail
B. iron
B. os calcis clamp
B. pin
B. plaster cast breaker
B. reducing fracture frame
B. rongeur
B. tongs
B. traction bow
B. tractor
B. wire splint

Böhler-Braun
B.-B. fracture frame
B.-B. leg sling
B.-B. splint
Böhler-Knowles hip pin
Böhler-Steinmann pin
Bohlman pin
Bohm dropper sponge
Boies
B. cutting forceps
B. nasal fracture elevator
Boies-Lombard mastoid rongeur
Boiler septal trephine
Boilo retinoscope
Boldrey brace
Bolero lift bath trolley
Bolex
B. cine camera
B. gastrocamera
Boley
B. dental gouge
B. gauge
B. retractor
Bolin wedge filter system
Bollinger knee brace
bolster
b. buddy
Hollister bridge suture b.
knee b.
retention suture b.
roll control b.
b. suture
Telfa b.
tie-over b.
bolt
Alta femoral b.
Barr b.
Camino microventricular b.
cannulated b.
DePuy b.
Fenton tibial b.
Herzenberg b.
hexhead b.
Hubbard b.
Hubbard-Nylok b.
I b.
ICP Camino b.
Norman tibial b.
Nylok b.
Philly b.
Richmond b.
solid hex b.
tibial b.
transfixion b.
trochanteric b.
Webb stove b.
Wilson b.
wire fixation b.
Zimmer tibial b.
Bolton forceps
bolus dressing
Bomgart stomal bag
Bonaccolto
B. cup jaws forceps
B. eye implant

B

Bonaccolto *(continued)*
    B. fragment forceps
    B. jeweler's forceps
    B. magnet
    B. magnet tip forceps
    B. monoplex orbital implant
      material
    B. orbital implant
    B. scleral ring
    B. trephine
    B. utility forceps
Bonaccolto-Flieringa scleral ring
Bonchek-Shiley
    B.-S. cardiac jacket
    B.-S. vein distention system
Bond
    B. arm splint
    B. placental forceps
Bondek
    B. absorbable suture
Bond-Eze bond adhesive
Bondeze resin
bonding
    Aquasil Smart Wetting
      impression b.
    In-Ceram Alumina b.
    In-Ceram Cerestore b.
    In-Ceram Dicor b.
    In-Ceram Empress b.
    In-Ceram Fortress b.
    In-Ceram Optec b.
    In-Ceram Spinell b.
    Poly-Lock b.
bone
    b. abduction instrument
    b. aggregate
    b. awl
    BIO-OSS freeze-dried
      demineralized b.
    Bioplant hard tissue replacement
      (HTR) synthetic b.
    B. Bullet suture anchor
    b. bur
    b. calipers
    b. cement
    b. cement adhesive
    b. chisel
    b. collector
    b. crusher
    b. curette
    b. cutter
    Dembone demineralized human b.
    Dembone freeze dried b.
    demineralized b.
    b. densitometer
    b. elevator
    endochondral b.
    b. extension clamp
    b. femoral plug
    b. file
    b. fixation device
    b. fixation wire
    b. flap fixation plate
    b. gouge

    B. Grafter instrument
    b. guide
    b. hand drill
    b. hole punch
    b. hook
    b. implant material
    B. Injection gun
    Lambone demineralized laminar b.
    Lambone freeze dried b.
    b. lavage
    b. lever
    b. mallet
    b. marrow biopsy needle
    B. Mulch screw
    Osteomin demineralized b.
    Osteomin freeze dried b.
    b. punch forceps
    b. punch rongeur
    b. rasp
    b. reamer
    b. retractor
    b. saw
    b. saw blade
    b. scalpel
    b. screw
    b. screw depth gauge
    b. screw targeter
    b. skid
    b. substitute material
    b. tack system
    Tutoplast b.
    b. wax
    b. wax suture
bone-anchored hearing aid
bone-biting
    b.-b. forceps
    b.-b. rongeur
BoneCollector device
bone-conduction hearing aid
bone-cutting
    b.-c. double-action forceps
    b.-c. rongeur
Bone-Dri femoral surgical wick
bone-graft holder
bone-holding
    b.-h. clamp
    b.-h. forceps
Boneloc cement
bone-measuring calipers
bone-patellar tendon-bone autograft
BonePlast bone void filler
bone-plate
    TiMesh b.-p.
bone-reduction forceps
BoneSource
    B. hydroxyapatite cement
    B. implant
bone-splitting forceps
Bonfiglio bone graft
Bongort
    B. Lifestyles Closed-End Pouches
    B. Max-E-Pouch pouch
    B. one-piece drainable pouch
    B. one-piece ostomy pouch
    B. urinary diversion pouch

Bonn
- B. European suturing forceps
- B. iris forceps
- B. iris hook
- B. iris scissors
- B. microhook
- B. microiris hook
- B. peripheral iridectomy forceps
- B. suturing forceps

Bonnano catheter

Bonnet
- Hydro B.

Bonney
- B. blue ink
- B. cervical dilator
- B. clamp
- B. clip
- B. insufflator
- B. needle
- B. retrograde inflator
- B. tissue forceps
- B. uterine tube

Bonnie balloon catheter

Bonta mastectomy knife

Bonwill articulator

bony endplate

book
- Ishihara test chart b.

Bookler swivel-ball laparoscopic instrument holder

Bookwalter
- B. horizontal bar
- B. malleable retractor blade
- B. rectal blade
- B. retractor blade
- B. retractor ring
- B. ring retractor
- B. segmented ring
- B. vaginal Deaver blade
- B. vaginal retractor ring

Bookwalter-Balfour retractor

Bookwalter-Cook anal rectal blade

Bookwalter-Gelpi point retractor blade

Bookwalter-Goulet retractor

Bookwalter-Harrington retractor

Bookwalter-Hill-Ferguson rectal retractor

Bookwalter-Kelly
- B.-K. retractor
- B.-K. retractor blade

Bookwalter-Magrina vaginal retractor

Bookwalter-Mayo blade

Bookwalter-Parks anal sphincter blade

Bookwalter-St. Mark deep pelvic retractor

boomerang
- b. bladder needle
- b. needle holder

Booster clip

boot
- All-Purpose B. (APB)
- Anthony cast b.
- APB Hi all purpose b.
- b. brace
- Bunny b.
- cast b.

Chukka b.
compression b.
ConvaTec Unna-Flex elastic Unna b.
cradle b.
Cryo/Cuff pressure b.
Darkos b.
derotation b.
Duke b.
external sequential pneumatic compression b.
fracture b.
gelatin compression b.
Gelocast Unna b.
Gibney b.
Heelift suspension b.
hyperbaric b.
IPC b.'s
Jobst b.
Junod b.
L'Nard b.
Lunax B.
Markell brace b.
Moon B.
MPO Active walking Multi Podus b.
O_2 B.
open-heeled Unna b.
pneumatic compression b.
Primer flexible Unna b.
Primer modified Unna b.
quadriceps b.
RIK FootHugger fluid heel b.
rocker b.
Rooke perioperative b.
Scotch b.
sheepskin b.
Slimline cast b.
Spenco b.
TENDERWRAP Unna b.
Unna b.
Unna-Flex elastic Unna b.
Venodyne b.
weight b.
Wilke b.

Bootie
- Bebax B.

Boplant graft

borazone blade cutting machine

Borchard
- B. Gigli-saw guide
- B. wire threader

Borchardt olive-shaped bur

Bores
- B. corneal fixation forceps
- B. incision spreader
- B. radial marker
- B. twist fixation ring
- B. U-shaped forceps

Borge
- B. bile duct clamp
- B. catheter

boron counter

Boros esophagoscope

Borsch
- B. bandage
- B. dressing

Borst side-arm introducer set
Bortone shears
Bortz clamp
Boruchoff forceps
Bosch ERG 500 ergometer
Bose
- B. bar
- B. retractor
- B. tracheostomy hook

Bosher commissurotomy knife
Bosker
- B. TMI Reconstruction system
- B. TMI surgery
- B. transmandibular implant
- B. transmandibular reconstructive surgical system

BosPac cardiopulmonary bypass system
BOSS
- Becker orthopaedic spinal system

Bossi cervical dilator
Bostick staple
Boston
- B. bivalve brace
- B. Children's frame
- B. Dynamics surgical simulator
- B. elbow system
- B. Envision lens
- B. gauze sponge
- B. Lying-In cervical forceps
- B. neurosurgical couch
- B. overlap brace
- B. post-op hip orthosis
- B. Scientific Sonicath imaging catheter
- B. scoliosis brace
- B. soft body jacket
- B. soft corset
- B. stethoscope
- B. trephine

Bosworth
- B. coracoclavicular screw
- B. crown drill
- B. headband
- B. nasal snare
- B. nasal wire speculum
- B. nerve root retractor
- B. osteotomy spline
- B. saw
- B. screwdriver
- B. spline plate
- B. temporary crown
- B. tongue depressor

Bosworth-Joseph nasal saw
Botox injection amplifier
bottle
- BacT/Alert glass b.
- blow b. (BB)
- Castaneda b.
- hot water b.
- McGaw plastic b.
- night drain b.
- Nu-Hope urine collection b.

- Ohio safety trap overflow b.
- PlasmaPlex b.
- urinary night drainage b.
- water b.
- Ziegler wash b.

Bottoms-Up posture system
Botvin
- B. iris forceps
- B. vulsellum forceps

Botvin-Bradford enucleator
Bouchayer grasping forceps
Boucheron ear speculum
Bouchut laryngeal tube
bougie
- acorn-tipped b.
- Anastasia b.
- armed b.
- Bangs b.
- bellied b.
- b. à boule
- bronchoscopic b.
- Buerger dilating b.
- bulbous b.
- Celestin b.
- Chevalier Jackson b.
- conic b.
- cylindrical b.
- dilating b.
- b. dilator
- Dittel dilating urethral b.
- Dourmashkin tunneled b.
- ear b.
- elastic b.
- elbowed b.
- EndoLumina illuminated b.
- esophageal mercury-filled b.
- eustachian b.
- filiform b.
- Fort urethral b.
- Friedman-Otis b. à boule
- fusiform b.
- Gabriel Tucker b.
- Garceau b.
- Gruber b.
- b. guide
- Guyon dilating b.
- Guyon exploratory b.
- Harold Hayes eustachian b.
- Hegar b.
- Holinger-Hurst b.
- Holinger infant b.
- Hurst mercury-filled esophageal b.
- Jackson radiopaque b.
- Jackson steel-stem woven filiform b.
- Jackson tracheal b.
- Klebanoff b.
- LeFort filiform b.
- Maloney tapered mercury-filled esophageal b.
- Maloney-type b.
- mercury b.
- mercury-filled esophageal b.
- mercury-weighted rubber b.
- Miller b.

olive-tipped b.
Otis b. à boule
Phillips urethral whip b.
Plummer modified b.
polyvinyl b.
Ravich b.
retrograde b.
rosary b.
Royalt-Street b.
Rusch b.
Ruschelit urethral b.
Savary-Gilliard Silastic flexible b.
Savary-Gilliard wire-guided b.
spiral-tipped b.
Szuler eustachian b.
through-the-scope b.
Trousseau esophageal b.
Tucker retrograde b.
Urbantschitsch eustachian b.
b. urethrotome
Wales rectal b.
Waltham-Street b.
wax b.
whalebone filiform b.
whip b.
Whistler b.
wire-guided polyvinyl b.
yellow-eyed dilating b.
Bourassa catheter
Bourdon
  B. tube
  B. tube pressure gauge
Bourns
  B. electronic adult respirator
  B. infant respirator
  B. LS104-150 infant ventilator
Bourns-Bear I ventilator
Boutin
  B. optics
  B. thoracoscope
boutonniere splint
Bovie
  B. blade
  B. coagulating forceps
  B. conization electrode
  B. CSV coagulator
  B. electrocautery
  B. electrocautery device
  B. electrocautery unit
  B. electrosurgical unit
  B. grounding pad
  B. holder
  B. liquid conductor
  B. needle
  B. retinal detachment unit
  Ritter B.
  B. suction device
  B. ultrasound aspirator
  underwater B.
  B. wet-field cautery
bovine
  b. allograft
  b. biodegradable collagen
  b. collagen implant
  b. collagen material prosthesis

b. collagen plug device
b. heart valve
b. heterograft
b. pericardial heart valve xenograft
b. pericardial valve
b. pericardium dural graft
b. pericardium strips
Bovino scleral-spreading forceps
Bovin-Stille vaginal speculum
Bovin vaginal speculum
bow
  Aesculap traction b.
  Anderson traction b.
  Bendixen-Kirschner traction b.
  Bitefork face b.
  Böhler extension b.
  Böhler traction b.
  Crego-McCarroll traction b.
  Crutchfield traction b.
  extension b.
  Framer finger extension b.
  Granberry finger traction b.
  Hanau face b.
  harelip traction b.
  Keys-Kirschner traction b.
  Kirschner extension b.
  Kirschner wire traction b.
  lip traction b.
  Logan lip traction b.
  Pease-Thomson traction b.
  Peterson skeletal traction b.
  Schwarz finger extension b.
  Schwarz traction b.
  Steinmann extension b.
  traction b.
Bow & Arrow cannulated drill guide
bowel
  b. bag
  b. forceps
  b. grasper
  b. retractor
Bowen
  B. BAS-30 blade
  B. double-bladed scalpel
  B. gooseneck chisel
  B. gouge
  B. osteotome
  B. periosteal elevator
  B. rasp
  B. resin
  B. suction
  B. suction loose body forceps
  B. suture drill
  B. wire tightener
Bowen-Grover meniscotome
Bower PEG tube
Bowers cannula
bowl
  b. curette
  Latham b.
  rubber spa b.
Bowlby arm splint
bowleg brace
Bowling lens
Bowls septal gouge

Bowman
- B. cataract needle
- B. eye knife
- B. eye speculum
- B. iris needle
- B. iris scissors
- B. lacrimal dilator
- B. lacrimal probe
- B. needle stop
- B. stop needle
- B. strabismus scissors
- B. tube

box
- A/B switch b.
- B. adenotome
- Anchor sterilizer b.
- Bárány b.
- bronchoscopic battery b.
- BTE Bolt B.
- carpal b.
- b. curette
- digital constant-current pacing b.
- Elecath switch b.
- Hogness b.
- mammographic view b.
- Mammo-Lume view b.
- B. osteotome
- steam b.
- sterilizer b.
- switch b.

Box-DeJager adenotome
boxing strip
box-joint forceps
Boxwood mallet
Boyce needle holder
Boyd
- B. bone graft
- B. dissecting scissors
- B. orbital implant
- B. perforator
- B. retractor
- B. tonsillar scissors

Boyden
- B. chamber
- B. chamber assay device

Boyd-Stille tonsillar scissors
Boyes-Goodfellow
- B.-G. hook
- B.-G. hook retractor

Boyes muscle clamp
Boyle-Davis mouthgag
Boyle-Rosin clip
Boyle uterine elevator
Boynton needle holder
Boys-Allis tissue forceps
Boys-Smith laser lens
Bozeman
- B. catheter
- B. clamp
- B. curette
- B. dilator
- B. hook
- B. LR dressing forceps
- B. LR packing forceps
- B. LR uterine-dressing forceps
- B. needle holder
- B. scissors
- B. speculum
- B. suture
- B. uterine-dressing forceps
- B. uterine forceps
- B. uterine-packing forceps

Bozeman-Douglas dressing forceps
Bozeman-Finochietto needle holder
Bozeman-Fritsch catheter
Bozeman-Wertheim needle holder
B-P
- B.-P. surgical handle
- B.-P. transfer forceps

BP Cuff pressure infuser
BPS spinal angiographic catheter
900BQ slit lamp
bra
- Circumpress compression b.
- lead b.
- Woods Surgitek b.

Braasch
- B. bladder specimen forceps
- B. bulb
- B. bulb ureteral catheter
- B. direct catheterization cystoscope
- B. ureteral dilator

Braasch-Kaplan direct vision cystoscope
Braastad costal arch retractor
BRACAnalyzer gene analyzer
Bracco system
brace
- abdominal b.
- Ace B.
- AFO b.
- Aircast Air-Stirrup leg b.
- Aircast fracture b.
- Aircast pneumatic b.
- Aircast Swivel-Strap b.
- AirGEL ankle b.
- Air-Stirrup ankle b.
- Ank-L-Aid b.
- AO b.
- AOA cervical immobilization b.
- Arizona Ankle b.
- Arnold b.
- Atlanta-Scottish Rite hip b.
- back b.
- bail-lock b.
- Bauerfeind ankle b.
- Bauerfeind comprifix knee b.
- Becker b.
- BIOflex magnetic b.
- Biomet fracture b.
- bipivotal hinge knee b.
- Bledsoe adjustable post-op b.
- Bledsoe cast b.
- Bledsoe knee b.
- Blount b.
- Blount-Schmidt-Milwaukee b.
- Boldrey b.
- Bollinger knee b.
- boot b.
- Boston bivalve b.
- Boston overlap b.

Boston scoliosis b.
bowleg b.
Buck knee b.
cage-back b.
Caligamed b.
Callender derotational b.
Camp b.
CAM Walker leg b.
CAM Walker walking b.
Can-Am b.
canvas b.
Capener b.
Carpal Lock wrist b.
CASH b.
cast b.
Castaway leg b.
CDO b.
Centec Propoint knee b.
cervical collar b.
chairback b.
Charleston nighttime bending b.
Charleston scoliosis b.
Chopart b.
Cincinnati ACL b.
clamshell b.
CM-Band 505N b.
CM-Band silicone rubber b.
collar b.
contraflexion b.
Cook walking b.
Cotrel-Dubousset orthopaedic b.
Count'R-Force arch b.
CRM rehab b.
CRS b.
Cruiser hip abduction b.
CTEV b.
C.Ti. b.
Cunningham b.
cutout patellar b.
DACO b.
DarcoGel ankle b.
DePuy fracture b.
derotation b.
DonJoy ALP b.
DonJoy four-point Super Sport
 knee b.
DonJoy Goldpoint knee b.
DonJoy Legend ACL knee b.
double Becker ankle b.
drop-foot b.
Duncan shoulder b.
Easy Lok ankle b.
Easy-On elbow b.
Eclipse Gel ankle b.
Edge knee b.
elastic-hinge knee b.
Elite knee b.
English b.
49er knee b.
Exotec b.
Extreme Select ligament b.
figure-of-eight b.
Fisher b.
Flex Foam b.
flexor hinge hand splint b.

FLOAM ankle stirrup b.
Florida back b.
Florida cervical b.
Florida contraflexion b.
Florida extension b.
Florida hyperextension b.
Florida J-24, J-35, J-45, J-55 b.
Florida post-fusion b.
Florida spinal b.
foot-ankle b.
footdrop b.
Forrester cervical collar b.
four-point cervical b.
functional electronic peroneal b.
functional fracture b.
Futuro wrist b.
gaiter b.
gait lock splint b.
Galveston metacarpal b.
Gauvain b.
Generation II knee b.
Genutrain knee b.
G II Unloader ADJ knee b.
Gillette b.
GLS b.
Goldthwait b.
Guilford b.
halo b.
hand b.
head b.
Hessing b.
high-Knight b.
Hilgenreiner b.
Hi-Top foot/ankle b.
Hudson-Jones knee cage b.
Hudson TLSO b.
hyperextension b.
Ilfeld b.
InCare b.
Industrial Work b.
internal tibial torsion b.
I-Plus humeral b.
ischial weightbearing b.
JACE knee b.
Jewett-Benjamin cervical b.
Jewett contraflexion b.
Jewett hyperextension b.
Jewett post-fusion b.
J-59 Florida b.
Jones b.
Joseph nasal b.
J-55 postfusion b.
Kallassy b.
King cervical b.
Klenzak b.
knee cage b.
knee MD b.
Knight b.
Knight-Taylor b.
Korn Cage knee b.
KS 5 ACL b.
KSO b.
Kuhlman cervical b.
Küntscher-Hudson b.
Kydex b.

brace *(continued)*
kyphosis b.
lace-on b.
LDU b.
leaf-spring b.
LeCocq b.
left long leg b.
leg b.
Lenox Hill Spectralite knee b.
Lerman hinge b.
Liberty CMC thumb b.
LLL b.
Lofstrand b.
long double upright b.
long leg b.
Lorenz b.
Lovitt-Uhler modification of Jewett
   post-fusion b.
LSU reciprocation-gait orthosis b.
Lyman-Smith toe drop b.
Maliniac nasal b.
Masterbrace 3 functional ACL
   knee b.
McClintoch b.
McCollough internal tibial torsion b.
McDavid knee b.
McKee b.
McLight PCL b.
MD b.
Medical Design b.
Metcalf spring drop b.
Miami cervical fracture b.
Miami TLSO scoliosis b.
Milwaukee scoliosis b.
MKS II knee b.
Monarch knee b.
Moon Boot b.
MTA b.
Mueller Ultralite b.
Multi-Lock knee b.
Murphy b.
Nakamura b.
neoprene hinged-knee b.
neoprene Osgood-Schlatter knee b.
neoprene wrist b.
New England scoliosis b.
Nextep knee b.
nonweightbearing b.
Northville b.
OA knee b.
OAsys b.
Omni knee b.
Opiela b.
Oppenheim b.
Orbital shoulder stabilizer b.
Orthomedics b.
Ortho-Mold spinal b.
Orthoplast fracture b.
Ortho Tech performer knee b.
OS-5/Plus 2 knee b.
OsteoArthritic knee b.
Pacesetter knee b.
Palumbo dynamic patellar b.
Palumbo stabilizing knee b.

pantaloon b.
Patten-Bottom-Perthes b.
pediatric PRAFO b.
performer ultralight knee b.
Perlstein b.
Phelps b.
Phemister b.
piano-wire dorsiflexion b.
PMT halo b.
Pneu Knee b.
postoperative flexor tendon
   traction b.
Power Play knee b.
Pro-8 ankle b.
ProShifter ACL sports b.
PTB b.
Push medical b.
Quadrant advanced shoulder b.
QualCare knee b.
Raney flexion jacket b.
range-of-motion b.
ratchet-type b.
Rhino Triangle hip abduction b.
Richie b.
rigid postoperative b.
Rolyan tibial fracture b.
ROM knee b.
Sarmiento b.
SAS II b.
Schanz collar b.
SCOI b.
scoliosis b.
Scottish Rite b.
Seton hip b.
short leg caliper b.
shoulder subluxation inhibitor b.
six-point knee b.
SmartBrace b.
SmartWrap elbow b.
Smedberg b.
snap-lock b.
SOMI b.
   sterno-occipital-mandibular
      immobilizer brace
SOMI Jr. b.
Speed b.
Spinal Technology bivalve TLSO b.
Sports-Caster I, II knee b.
sterno-occipital-mandibular
   immobilizer b. (SOMI brace)
Stille b.
Stimprene electrotherapy b.
stirrup b.
straight walker b.
Strap Lok ankle b.
Stromgren ankle b.
Sully shoulder stabilizer b.
Sure Step b.
Swede-O ankle b.
Swede-O-Universal b.
Swivel-Strap ankle b.
Taylor-Knight b.
Taylor spine b.
telescoping b.
Teufel cervical b.

Teurlings wrist b.
The Richie b.
Thermoskin b.
The Unloader b.
Thomas cervical collar b.
Thomas walking b.
thoracolumbar standing orthosis b.
toedrop b.
Townsend knee b.
Tracker knee b.
Tri-angle shoulder abduction b.
Trinkle b.
turnbuckle ankle b.
turnbuckle knee b.
UCLA functional long leg b.
unilateral calcaneal b.
University of British Columbia b.
ValueWalker b.
Verlow b.
VertaBrace b.
walking b.
Warm Springs b.
weightbearing b.
Wheaton b.
Wilke boot b.
Williams back b.
Women's Tradition b.
Wright Universal b.
Wrist Restore b.
Yale b.
Zinco Hyperex thoracolumbar b.
brace/corset
Hoke lumbar b.
bracelet
BioBands b.
Nussbaum b.
Q-Ray b.
^{89}Sr b.
braceRAP wrap
brachial coronary catheter
BrachyVision brachytherapy planning system
Bracken
B. anterior chamber cannula
B. fixation forceps
B. iris forceps
B. irrigating cannula
B. scleral fixation forceps
Bracken-Forkas corneal forceps
bracket
Begg straight-wire combination b.
Broussard b.
curved-base Lewis b.
Cusp-Lok b.
Hanson speed b.
Lee b.
Lee-Fischer plastic b.
Lewis vertical slot b.
ligatureless b.
metal frame reinforced plastic b.
molar b.
Ormco wire b.
orthodontic b.
plastic b.
Siamese twin b.

single width b.
steel-slotted plastic b.
Steiner b.
torqued slot b.
twin edgewise b.
bracketed splint
Brackett dental probe
Brackmann
B. facial nerve monitor
B. II EMG system
B. suction-irrigator
Braden
B. flushing reservoir
B. scale
Bradford
B. enucleation neurotome
B. fracture appliance
B. fracture frame
B. snare enucleator
B. thyroid forceps
Bradshaw-O'Neill aortic clamp
Brady balanced suspension splint
Bragg-Paul respirator
Brahler ultrasonic dental scaler
braid
carbon fiber lamination b.
braided
b. diagnostic catheter
b. Ethibond suture
b. Mersilene suture
b. Nurolon suture
b. nylon suture
b. occlusion device
b. polyamide suture
b. polyester fiber
b. polyester suture
b. silk suture
b. Spectra UHMWPE surgical cable
b. titanium cable
b. Vicryl suture
b. wire
b. wire suture
brain
b. biopsy cannula
b. biopsy needle
b. clip
b. clip carrier
b. clip forceps
b. depressor
b. dressing forceps
b. Neurolite SPECT scan
b. probe
b. scissors
b. silicone-coated retractor
b. spatula
b. spatula forceps
b. tissue forceps
b. trocar
b. tumor forceps
brain-exploring cannula
BrainLAB VectorVision neuronavigational system
BrainSCAN
B. computer planning system

BrainSCAN *(continued)*
    B. II
    B. Linac radiosurgery system
Braithwaite
    B. clip remover
    B. forceps
    B. nasal chisel
    B. skin graft knife
Brake hemostatic bag
Bralon suture
Brand
    B. passing forceps
    B. shunt-introducing forceps
    B. tendon-holding forceps
    B. tendon passer
    B. tendon-passing forceps
    B. tendon stripper
Brandel cell harvester
Brandt
    B. brassiere
    B. cytology balloon
Brandy
    B. scalp stretcher
    B. scalp stretcher I, II, front
      closure
    B. scalp stretcher I, II, rear closure
Branemark
    B. endosteal implant
    B. implant system
    B. osseointegration implant
Brannock
    B. device shoe sizer
    B. foot measuring device
Bransford-Lewis ureteral dilator
Brant aluminum splint
Brantley-Turner vaginal retractor
Branula cannula
BRAS
brass
    b. mallet
    b. scleral plug
    b. wire
Brasseler Optipost
brassiere
    Brandt b.
    Foerster surgical support b.
brassiere-type dressing
Brauer chisel
Braun
    B. cranioclast
    B. decapitation hook
    B. episiotomy scissors
    B. forceps
    B. frame
    B. graft
    B. implant
    B. ligature carrier
    B. needle
    B. obstetrical hook
    B. speculum
    B. stent
    B. uterine depressor
    B. uterine tenaculum
Braun-Schroeder single-tooth tenaculum

Braun-Stadler
    B.-S. episiotomy scissors
    B.-S. sternal shears
Braunstein fixed calipers
Braunwald-Cutter
    B.-C. ball prosthetic valve
    B.-C. ball valve prosthesis
Braunwald heart valve
Braun-Wangensteen graft
Braun-Yasargil right-angle clip
Brawley
    B. nasal suction tube
    B. refractor
    B. scleral wound retractor
    B. sinus rasp
    B. suction apparatus
Brawner orbital implant
bread knife valvulotome
breakable blade
BreakAway
    B. absorptive wound dressing
breakaway
    b. lap cushion
    b. pin
    b. splice
breaker
    Böhler plaster cast b.
    cast b.
    Jarit-Mason cast b.
    Wölfe-Böhler cast b.
Breakstone lithotriptor
breast
    b. binder
    b. calipers
    b. form
    b. implant
    B. Implant Protector
    b. localization needle
    b. reduction pattern
    b. tenaculum
    B. Vest
    B. Vest EXU-DRY one-piece
      wound dressing
BreastAlert
    B. DTS screening device
Breathe Right nasal strips
breathing
    b. bag
    b. pacemaker
breath-operated inhaler
Brecht feeder
Breck
    B. pin
    B. pin cutter
Bredall amalgam plugger
breeder reactor
Breen retractor
Breeze
    B. infant ventilator
    B. respirator
Breinin suction cup
Breisky
    B. vaginal retractor
    B. vaginal speculum

B

Breisky-Navratil
 B.-N. straight retractor
 B.-N. vaginal speculum
Breisky-Stille speculum
Breitman adenotome
Bremer
 B. AirFlo thoracic stabilization vest
 B. halo
 B. halo cervical traction
 B. halo crown
 B. halo crown system
 B. halo crown traction
 B. halo crown traction set
 B. halo vest
 B. torque-limiting cap
Brems Astigmatism Marker
Brenman camera
Brennen biosynthetic surgical mesh
Brenner
 B. carotid bypass shunt
 B. forceps
 B. rectal probe
Brent pressure earring
brephoplastic graft
Brescia-Cimino shunt
Bresgen
 B. cannula
 B. catheter
 B. frontal sinus probe
Brethables air-permeable underpad
Brett bone graft
Brevir-Kaith epidural catheter
Brewer vaginal speculum
Brewster phrenic retractor
bridge
 Albarran b.
 balance b.
 Burns converting b.
 catheter deflecting b.
 ceramometal implant b.
 B. clamp
 B. deep-surgery forceps
 double b.
 B. hemostatic forceps
 B. hip system
 B. intestinal forceps
 Maryland b.
 one-horn b.
 pediatric b.
 retention suture b.
 Rochette b.
 Short b.
 b. splint
 B. telescope
 three-way b.
 Trestle prostatic b.
 Wappler b.
bridged loop-gap resonator
bridgeless mask
Bridgemaster nasal splint
bridle
 control b.
 b. suture
brief
 Acti-Fit b.

Attends brief with Perma Dry
 Wings contoured incontinence b.
ConQuest male continence system
 supporter b.
Conveen disposable stretch b.
First Quality full fit b.
Harmonie Classic Plus b.
KINS all-in-one cotton b.
MaxiCare adult disposable
 contoured b.
Prevent Plus boys training b.
PrimeTime Plus adult disposable b.
Promise b.
Protection Plus b.
SlimLine disposable b.
Slim and Trim b.
Sofnit 300 fitted b.
Soft & Silent vinyl pull-on b.
Soft & Silent vinyl snap-on b.
Ultra-Fit b.
Brierley nucleus splitter
Briesky
 B. Navritrol retractor
 B. pelvimeter
Briggs
 B. laryngoscope
 B. retractor
 B. transilluminator
Brigham
 B. brain tumor forceps
 B. dressing forceps
 B. thumb tissue forceps
 B. 1x2 teeth forceps
Brightbill corneal cutting block
Brighton epistaxis balloon
Brilliant light-cured resin
Brimfield
 B. cannulated grasping hook
 B. magnetic retriever
Brimms
 B. denture reliner
 B. Quik-Fix denture repair kit
Brinker
 B. hygienic tissue retractor
Brinkerhoff
 B. anoscope
 B. rectal speculum
Brink PeriPyriform implant
Brisman-Nova carotid endarterectomy shunt
Bristol-Myers system
Bristow
 B. lever
 B. periosteal elevator
 B. rasp
Bristow-Bankart
 B.-B. humeral retractor
 B.-B. soft tissue retractor
Brite Lite III light
BriteSmile laser tooth whitening system
Britetrac
 B. fiberoptic instrument
 B. illuminator
 B. speculum

Britt
  B. argon pulsed laser
  B. BL-12 laser
  B. krypton laser
  B. pulsed argon laser
BRK-series transseptal needle
broach
  barbed b.
  Charnley femoral b.
  crescent b.
  endodontic b.
  b. extractor
  femoral b.
  Firtel b.
  glenoid fin b.
  Harris b.
  intramedullary b.
  Koenig metatarsal b.
  metacarpal b.
  metatarsal stem b.
  Monaco b.
  orthopedic b.
  phalangeal b.
  root canal b.
  square-hole b.
  starter b.
  Swanson intramedullary b.
  Swanson metatarsal b.
  tibial b.
broad AO dynamic compression plate
broadbill hemostat with push fork
Brock
  B. auricular clamp
  B. biopsy forceps
  B. cardiac dilator
  B. infundibular punch
  B. mitral valve knife
  B. probe
  B. pulmonary valve knife
  B. valvulotome
Brockenbrough
  B. angiocatheter
  B. cardiac device
  B. curved needle
  B. curved-tip occluder
  B. mapping catheter
  B. modified bipolar catheter
  B. transseptal catheter
  B. transseptal needle
Brockington pile clamp
Brodie
  B. director
  B. fistular probe
Brodmerkel colon decompression set
Brodney
  B. catheter
  B. hemostatic bag
  B. urethrographic cannula
  B. urethrographic clamp
Broggi-Kelman dipstick gauge
broken razor blade
Brombach perimeter
Bromley uterine curette
Brompton Hospital retractor

bronchial
  b. biopsy forceps
  b. catheter
  b. dilator
  b. tube
bronchial-grasping forceps
Bronchitrac L flexible suction catheter
Broncho-Cath
  B.-C. double-lumen endotracheal
  tube
bronchocele
  b. sound
  b. sound raspatory
bronchofiberscope
  Pentax b.
bronchoscope
  ACMI Marici b.
  Albert slotted b.
  BF large core b.
  Broyles b.
  Broyles-Negus b.
  Bruening b.
  Chevalier Jackson b.
  Davis b.
  Doesel-Huzly b.
  double-channel irrigating b.
  Dumon-Harrell b.
  Dumon laser b.
  Emerson b.
  fiberoptic b.
  flexible fiberoptic b.
  Foregger b.
  Foroblique b.
  Fujinon EB-410S b.
  Fujinon flexible b.
  Haslinger b.
  Holinger infant b.
  Holinger-Jackson b.
  Holinger ventilating fiberoptic b.
  hook-on b.
  infant b.
  Jackson costophrenic b.
  Jackson full-lumen b.
  Jackson standard b.
  Jackson staple b.
  Jesberg infant b.
  Kernan-Jackson coagulating b.
  LIFE Imaging System and White
  Light b.
  Marici b.
  Michelson infant b.
  Moersch b.
  Negus b.
  Negus-Broyles b.
  Olympus fiberoptic b.
  open-tube rigid b.
  Overholt-Jackson b.
  Pentax b.
  Pilling b.
  respiration b.
  Riecker respiration b.
  Safar ventilation b.
  Savary b.
  SFB-I right-angled b.
  Shapshay laser b.

single-channel fiberoptic b.
Storz infant b.
Tucker b.
Waterman folding b.
Xanar laser b.
Yankauer b.
bronchoscopic
  b. aspirator
  b. battery box
  b. biopsy forceps
  b. bougie
  b. brush
  b. face shield
  b. magnet
  b. probe
  b. ruler
  b. spectacles
  b. sponge
  b. sponge carrier
  b. telescope
bronchoscopy disposable suction tube
bronchospirometric catheter
bronchus-grasping forceps
Bronkhorst High Tec controller
Bronkometer
Bronner clamp
Bronson
  B. magnet
  B. speculum
  B. ultrasonoscope
Bronson-Magnion
  B.-M. eye magnet
  B.-M. forceps
Bronson-Park speculum
Bronson-Ray pituitary curette
Bronson-Turner foreign body locator
Bronson-Turtz
  B.-T. iris retractor
  B.-T. refractor
  B.-T. speculum
bronze wire suture
Brookdale bar
Brooke Army Hospital splint
Brooker
  B. double-locking unreamed tibial
  nail
  B. wire
Brooker-Wills nail
Brookfield viscometer
Brooks
  B. adenoidal punch
  B. appliance
  B. gallbladder scissors
broomstick cast
Brophy
  B. bistoury
  B. bistoury knife
  B. cleft palate knife
  B. dressing forceps
  B. gag
  B. mouthgag
  B. needle
  B. periosteal elevator
  B. periosteotome

  B. plate
  B. scissors
  B. tenaculum
  B. tenaculum retractor
  B. tissue forceps
  B. tooth elevator
Brophy-Deschamps needle
Broselow
  B. chart
  B. tape
Broselow/Hinkle system
Broussard bracket
Broviac
  B. atrial catheter
  B. hyperalimentation catheter
brow
  b. lift suspension screw
  b. tape
Browlift Bone Bridge system
Brown
  B. air dermatome
  B. applicator
  B. chisel
  B. cleft palate knife
  B. cleft palate needle
  B. dermatome blade
  B. dissecting scissors
  B. ear speculum
  B. electrodermatome
  B. hook
  B. lip clamp
  B. mallet
  B. nasal splint
  B. periosteotome
  B. rasp
  B. saw
  B. and Sharp digital electronic
  calipers
  B. side-grasping forceps
  B. sphenoid cannula
  B. staphylorrhaphy needle
  B. sterile adhesive
  B. thoracic forceps
  B. tissue forceps
  B. tonsillar snare
  B. tonsillectome
  B. tooth elevator
  B. uvular retractor
Brown-Adson
  B.-A. side-grasping forceps
Brown-Bahnson bayonet forceps
Brown-Blair
  B.-B. dermatome
  B.-B. skin graft knife
Brown-Bovari machine
Brown-Buerger
  B.-B. cystoscope
  B.-B. dilator
  B.-B. forceps
Brown-Burr modified Gillies retractor
Brown-Cushing forceps
Brown-Davis mouthgag
Brown-Dean cotton applicator
Brown-Dohlman Silastic corneal implant

Browne
- B. splint
- B. stone basket

Brown-Fillebrown-Whitehead mouthgag
Brown-Joseph saw
Brown-McHardy pneumatic dilator
Brown-Mueller
- B.-M. T-bar fastener
- B.-M. T-fastener set

Brown-Pusey corneal trephine
Brown-Roberts-Wells (BRW)
- B.-R.-W. arc-ring assembly
- B.-R.-W. base ring
- B.-R.-W. computer
- B.-R.-W. floor stand
- B.-R.-W. head frame
- B.-R.-W. headrest
- B.-R.-W. head ring halo
- B.-R.-W. phantom base
- B.-R.-W. ring adapter
- B.-R.-W. stereotactic system

Brown-Sanders fascial needle
Brown-Sharp gauge suture
Brown-Swan forceps
Brown-Whitehead mouthgag
Broyles
- B. anterior commissure laryngoscope
- B. aspirator
- B. bronchoscope
- B. esophageal dilator
- B. esophagoscope
- B. nasopharyngoscope
- B. optical forceps
- B. optical laryngoscope
- B. retrograde cystoscope
- B. telescope
- B. wasp-waist laryngoscope

Broyles-Negus bronchoscope
Bruch mastoid retractor
Bruecke tube
Brueckmann lead hand
Bruel
- B. & Kjaer axial transducer
- B. & Kjaer transvaginal ultrasound probe
- B. & Kjaer ultrasound
- B. & Kjaer 1860 ultrasound machine
- B. & Kjaer ultrasound scanner
- B. & Kjaer 1846 ultrasound system

Bruening
- B. biting tip
- B. bronchoscope
- B. cannula
- B. chisel
- B. cutting-tip forceps
- B. ear snare
- B. electroscope
- B. esophagoscope
- B. esophagoscopy forceps handle
- B. ethmoid exenteration forceps
- B. forceps stylet
- B. intracordal injection set
- B. Japanese anastigmatic aural magnifier
- B. nasal-cutting septal forceps
- B. nasal snare
- B. otoscope set
- B. pneumatic otoscope
- B. pressure syringe
- B. punch
- B. retractor
- B. septal forceps
- B. speculum
- B. tongue depressor
- B. tonsillar snare

Bruening-Arnold intracordal injection set
Bruening-Citelli
- B.-C. forceps
- B.-C. rongeur

Bruening-Storz
- B.-S. anastigmatic aural magnifier
- B.-S. diagnostic head

Bruening-Work diagnostic head
Brughleman needle
Bruker
- B. AMX 300 NMR spectrometer
- B. Biospec system
- B. console
- B. CSI MR system
- B. relaxometer
- B. scanner
- B. S 200 MR system

Brun
- B. bone curette
- B. ear curette
- B. guarded chisel
- B. mastoid curette
- B. plaster shears

Bruner vaginal speculum
Brunetti chisel
Bruni counterpressor
Bruni-Wayne clamp approximator
Brunner
- B. chisel
- B. colon clamp
- B. goiter dissector
- B. intestinal clamp
- B. intestinal forceps
- B. ligature needle
- B. probe
- B. raspatory
- B. retractor
- B. rib shears
- B. sigmoid anastomosis forceps
- B. tissue forceps

Bruns bone curette
Brunschwig
- B. arterial forceps
- B. visceral forceps
- B. visceral retractor

Brunswick-Mack
- B.-M. approximator
- B.-M. bur
- B.-M. chisel
- B.-M. rotating drill

Brunswick serrefine
Brunton otoscope
brush
- AccuBrush dental b.

Alger b.
Ayre b.
Bard ureteroscopic cytology b.
Barraquer sable b.
Bayne Pap b.
b. biopsy kit
bronchoscopic b.
bur b.
Castaneda thrombolytic b.
Cohort bone b.
Combo Cath wire-guided
  cytology b.
contour instrument cleaning b.
Contrangle dermabrasion b.
Cox cytology b.
Cragg thrombolytic b.
cytological b.
cytology b.
denture b.
Diaflex cytology b.
Edwards-Carpentier aortic valve b.
endotracheal tube b.
Endovations disposable cytology b.
Geenan biliary cytology b.
Gill biopsy b.
Glassman b.
Grafco tracheal tube b.
Haidinger b.
Hobbs sheath b.
intramedullary b.
Kurtin planing dermabrasion b.
Kurtin wire b.
manual dermatome b.
Marten hair eye b.
Medscand cytology b.
Medscand endometrial b.
Mill-Rose cytology b.
nylon scrub b.
ophthalmic sable b.
Oral-B soft foam interdental b.
Plak-Vac oral suction b.
polishing b.
polypropylene hand b.
protected bronchoscopic b.
protected specimen microbiology b.
rectal snare stem b.
rotating b.
Rusch cleaning b.
sable b.
scraping b.
scrub b.
Sklar b.
soft scrub b.
stomach b.
Stormby b.
Storz cleaning b.
Thomas b.
tracheal tube b.
Wagner laryngeal b.
Wilson-Cook cytology b.

Bruus scoop
BRW
Brown-Roberts-Wells
BRW stereotactic system

Bryant
B. mitral hook
B. nasal forceps
B. traction
B. tractor
Brymill cryosurgical probe
B-scan
Contact B.-s.
Humphrey B.-s.
B.-s. ultrasonogram
B&S gauge suture
BSS Plus
BTA S-2000 biofeedback system
BTE
behind-the-ear
BTE Assembly Tree
BTE Bolt Box
BTE dynamic lift
BTE listening device
BTE Work Simulator
bubble
b. chamber equipment
gastric b.
Guibor Expo eye b.
b. humidifier
b. jar
b. oxygenator
Bubble-Jet
Puritan B.-J.
buccal
b. cortical plate
b. fat extractor
b. fat extractor tip
Buchbinder
B. Omniflex catheter
B. Thruflex Over-the-Wire catheter
Buch-Gramcko gouge
Buchholz
B. acetabular cup
B. hip prosthesis
Bucholz bipolar cauterizer
Buchwald tongue depressor
Buck
B. bone curette
B. convoluted traction apparatus
B. convoluted traction device
B. ear applicator
B. ear curette
B. ear probe
B. earring curette
B. extension
B. extension apparatus
B. extension bar
B. extension frame
B. extension splint
B. femoral cement restrictor
B. femoral cement restrictor inserter
B. foreign body forceps
B. fracture appliance
B. hook
B. knee brace
B. mastoid curette
B. myringotome
B. myringotomy knife
B. nasal applicator

Buck *(continued)*
> B. neurological hammer
> B. osteotome
> B. percussion hammer
> B. periosteal elevator
> B. plug
> B. traction
> B. traction splint
> B. tractor
> B. Universal convoluted traction unit
> B. wax curette

bucket
> Denis Browne b.
> kick b.
> Lenox b.

Buck-Gramcko bone lever
Buck-House curette
Buckingham
> B. drill
> B. mirror

buckle
> wire-fixation b.

Buckley chisel
Buckstein colonic insufflator
Bucky
> B. diaphragm
> B. digital x-ray device
> B. hand drill
> B. high-contrast imaging
> B. view tray

Bucy
> B. cordotomy knife
> B. laminectomy rongeur
> B. spinal cord retractor
> B. suction tube

Bucy-Frazier
> B.-F. coagulation cannula
> B.-F. suction cannula
> B.-F. suction tube

Bud bur
Budde
> B. halo neurosurgical retractor
> B. halo retractor system
> B. halo ring
> B. halo ring retractor

Budde-Greenberg-Sugita stereotactic head frame
BUD drainage catheter
buddy
> bolster b.
> Ostomy Shadow B.
> b. strap
> Wheelchair B.

Budin
> B. hammertoe splint
> B. toe splint

Buechel-Pappas total ankle prosthesis
Buedding squeegee cortex extractor and polisher
Bueleau empyema trocar
Buerger
> B. dilating bougie
> B. prostatic needle

> B. punch
> B. snare

Buerger-McCarthy
> B.-M. bladder forceps
> B.-M. scissors

Buettner-Parel vitreous cutter
Buffalo
> B. dental cement
> B. ultrasonic scaler

buffing sponge
Bugbee
> B. electrocautery
> B. fulgurating electrode

buggy
> cruiser b.
> Maclaren mobile b.

Buhl spirometer
Buie
> B. biopsy forceps
> B. cannula
> B. fistula probe
> B. fulgurating electrode
> B. pile clamp
> B. rectal forceps
> B. rectal scissors
> B. rectal suction tube
> B. retractor
> B. sigmoidoscope
> B. specimen forceps

Buie-Hirschman
> B.-H. anoscope
> B.-H. pile clamp

Buie-Smith
> B.-S. anal retractor
> B.-S. rectal speculum

Builder Grip hand exerciser
build-up eye implant
Bülau trocar
bulb
> Beckman Silastic b.
> Braasch b.
> dilating b.
> b. dynamometer
> b. grenade
> nystagmus b.
> b. retractor
> self-inflating b.
> Selrodo b.
> b. syringe
> b. and thumb screw valve
> b. ureteral catheter

bulb-operated nebulizer
bulbous
> b. bougie
> b. catheter

bulbous-tip ear syringe
Bulkee
> B. II gauze bandage
> B. super fluff sponge

bulky
> b. compressive dressing
> b. hand dressing
> b. pressure dressing

Bullard intubating laryngoscope

bulldog
- b. clamp
- b. clamp-applying forceps
- b. scissors

Buller
- B. bandage
- B. eye shield

bullet
- b. forceps
- b. probe
- b. tip catheter
- tri-point b.

bullet-shaped cannula
Bullseye femoral guide
Bulnes-Sanchez retractor
Bumgardner dental holder
Bumm
- B. placental curette
- B. uterine curette

bumper
- Cloverleaf internal b.
- dome-shaped internal b.
- PEG b.
- b. wedge

Bumpus specimen forceps
Buncke quartz needle
Bunge
- B. curette
- B. evisceration spoon
- B. exenteration spoon
- B. scissors
- B. ureteral meatotome

Bunim urethral forceps
bunion
- b. dissector
- b. last
- b. shield

Bunke clamp
Bunker
- B. implant
- B. modification of Jackson laryngeal forceps

Bunke-Schulz clamp approximator
Bunnell
- B. active hand splint
- B. anvil
- B. block
- B. bone drill
- B. digital exertion measurer
- B. dissecting probe
- B. dressing
- B. finger extension splint
- B. finger loop
- B. forwarding probe
- B. gutter splint
- B. hand drill
- B. knuckle bender
- B. knuckle-bender splint
- B. outrigger splint
- B. pull-out wire
- B. reverse knuckle bender splint
- B. safety-pin splint
- B. tendon needle
- B. tendon passer
- B. tendon stripper
- B. wire pull-out suture

Bunnell-Howard arthrodesis clamp
Bunnell-Littler dressing
Bunny
- B. boot
- B. Boot foot splint

Bunsen burner
Bunt
- B. catheter
- B. forceps holder
- B. tendon stripper

Bunyan bag
bur, burr
- abrader b.
- Accorde b.
- acromionizer b.
- Acrotorque b.
- Adson b.
- Adson perforating b.
- Adson-Rogers cranial b.
- aftercataract b.
- Alfonso guarded b.
- Allport cutting b.
- antral b.
- Bailey skull b.
- Ballenger-Lillie mastoid b.
- Ballenger mastoid b.
- barrel cutting b.
- bone b.
- Borchardt olive-shaped b.
- Brunswick-Mack b.
- b. brush
- Bud b.
- Burwell corneal b.
- Caparosa cutting b.
- carbide finishing b.
- cataract b.
- Cavanaugh-Israel b.
- Cavanaugh sphenoid b.
- choanal b.
- coarse carbide cone b.
- coarse-olive b.
- Concept Ophtho-b.
- cone b.
- conical b.
- corneal foreign body b.
- countersink b.
- cranial b.
- Cross corneal b.
- crosscut straight fissure b.
- curetting b.
- Cushing cranial b.
- cutting b.
- cylinder b.
- Davidson b.
- decortication b.
- Densco b.
- dental b.
- dentate b.
- denture vulcanite b.
- dermabrasion b.
- D'Errico enlarging b.
- D'Errico perforating b.
- Dialom b.

B

bur *(continued)*
diamond barrel b.
diamond-coated b.
diamond-dust b.
diamond finishing b.
Doyen cylindrical b.
Doyen spherical b.
b. drill
Dyonics arthroplasty b.
end-cutting fissure b.
endodontic b.
enlarging b.
eustachian b.
excavating b.
Farrior b.
Feldman b.
fenestration b.
Ferris Smith-Halle sinus b.
FG diamond b.
fine olive b.
finish b.
finishing b.
Fisch cutting b.
fissure b.
flame b.
flame-tip b.
fluted finishing b.
foreign body b.
Frey-Freer b.
Gam-Mer b.
Gates-Glidden b.
gold b.
Guilford-Wright b.
Hall bone b.
Hall mastoid b.
Hannahan b.
high-speed diamond three-tiered
  depth cutting b.
high-speed diamond wheel b.
high-speed tungsten carbide b.
high-speed two-grit b.
high-torque b.
b. hole cover
b. hole transducer
Hough-Wullstein crurotomy saw b.
House b.
House-Wullstein perforating b.
Hudson brace b.
Hudson conical b.
Hudson cranial b.
Hu-Friedy dental b.
inverted cone b.
Jordan-Day cutting b.
Jordan-Day fenestration b.
Jordan-Day polishing b.
Jordan perforating b.
Kopetzky sinus b.
lacrimal sac b.
large nail spicule b.
Le Blond R diamond dental b.
Lee diamond b.
Lempert diamond-dust polishing b.
Lempert fenestration b.
Light-Veley b.

Lindermann b.
long coarse b.
low-speed Christmas tree
  diamond b.
low-speed tapered carbide b.
Martin b.
Masseran trepan b.
mastoid b.
McKenzie enlarging b.
Micro-Aire b.
M-series b. (M-1, M-2, etc.)
MTM 2 b.
Mueller b.
neurosurgical b.
new happy b.
old smoothie b.
orthopedic b.
Osteon b.
oval cutting b.
Parapost b.
paronychia b.
Patton b.
pear-shaped b.
perforating b.
pilot b.
pineapple b.
plug-finishing b.
pointed cone b.
polishing b.
primary trimming b.
Redi B.
Red Witch b.
rhinoplasty diamond b.
rosehead b.
Rosen b.
Rotablator rotating b.
rotary b.
round cutting b.
round diamond b.
Sachs skull b.
Scheer-Wullstein cutting b.
Shannon b.
Shea b.
short coarse b.
short fine b.
side-cutting Swanson b.
sinus b.
skull b.
slotting b.
small nail spicule b.
Smoothie Junior b.
Somerset b.
sphenoidal b.
spherical b.
spiral fluted tungsten carbide b.
S. S. White J-Notch surgical
  handpiece b.
S. S. White 100 K surgical
  handpiece b.
Starlite Omni-AT b.
Stille b.
Storz corneal b.
straight fissure b.
straight shank b.
Stryker b.

Lightning

Stumer perforating b.
Super-Cut diamond b.
Surgair b.
surgical b.
Surgitome b.
tapered fissure b.
Thomas b.
tungsten carbide b.
Turbo-Jet dental b.
vulcanite b.
Wachsberger b.
wheel b.
Wilkerson choanal b.
wire-passing b.
Worst corneal b.
Wullstein diamond b.
Wullstein high-speed b.
Yazujian cataract b.
Zimmer b.

Buratto
  B. flap forceps
  B. flap protector
  B. irrigating cannula
  B. LASIK forceps
  B. ophthalmic forceps
bur-bearing catheter
Burch
  B. biopsy forceps
  B. eye calipers
  B. fixation pick
  B. hook
  B. ophthalmic pick
  B. tendon tucker
Burch-Greenwood tendon tucker
Burdick
  B. cautery
  B. Eclipse ECG machine
  B. microwave diathermy
    electrosurgical unit
Buretrol device
Burette multiple patient delivery system
Burford
  B. clamp
  B. coarctation forceps
  B. rib retractor
  B. rib spreader
Burford-Finochietto
  B.-F. infant rib spreader
  B.-F. rib retractor
  B.-F. rib spreader
Burford-Lebsche sternal knife
Burgess Vibro-Graver
Burget nasal splint
Burge vagotometer
Burhenne steerable catheter
bur-hole button
Burian-Allen
  B.-A. contact lens
  B.-A. contact lens electrode
Burkard spore trap
Burke
  B. bariatric treatment system
    powered bariatric bed

  B. Plus frameless air support
    therapy
  B. plus low-air-loss bed
Bürker chamber
Burlisher clamp
burner
  Bunsen b.
Burnett
  B. anoscope
  B. applicator
  B. cylinder
  B. mouth positioning device
  B. Pap smear kit
  B. Sani-Spec disposable speculum
Burnham
  B. bandage scissors
  B. biopsy forceps
burnisher
  agate b.
  amalgam b.
  ball b.
  beaver-tail b.
  fishtail b.
  fissure b.
  flat b.
  gold b.
  Nordent b.
  SMIC b.
  straight b.
Burn Jel dressing
Burns
  B. bone forceps
  B. bridge telescope
  B. chisel
  B. converting bridge
  B. prism bar
Burr
  B. butterfly needle
  B. corneal ring
  B. silicone button
burr (*var. of* bur)
Burron Discofix stopcock
burst pacemaker
Burton
  B. laryngoscope
  B. osteotome
Burwell corneal bur
Busch umbilical cord scissors
Buselmeier shunt
B.U.S. Endotron-Lipectron ultrasonic
  scalpel
Busenkell posterior hip retractor
Bushey compression clamp
bushing
  patellar planer b.
  reamer b.
  Uniflex drill b.
Bush intervertebral curette
Buster
  Moss Suction B.
Butcher saw
Butler
  B. bayonet forceps
  B. dental retractor
  B. pillar retractor

B

Butler *(continued)*
    B. stimulator
    B. tonsillar suction tube
Butte dissector
Butterfield cystoscope
Butterfly
    B. cushion
    B. cushion with strap
butterfly
    b. adapter
    b. bandage
    b. catheter
    b. clip
    b. drain
    b. dressing
    b. needle
    b. needle infusion port
butterfly-shaped
    b.-s. monoblock vertebral plate
Butterworth bidirectional four-pole high-pass digital filter
button
    Accu-Flo b.
    anastomotic b.
    Bard b.
    Barouk b.
    Bentley b.
    Biomet b.
    Bivona-Colorado b.
    Boari b.
    bobbin-type laryngectomy b.
    bur-hole b.
    Burr silicone b.
    Charnley suture b.
    Chlumsky b.
    collar b.
    Converse fracture-wiring b.
    coronary artery b.
    Davy surgical b.
    DiaTAP vascular access b.
    Drummond b.
    b. electrode
    Emesay suture b.
    Endo b.
    fixation b.
    gastrostomy b.
    B. gastrostomy device
    Groningen b.
    Helsper laryngectomy b.
    b. hook
    Husen b.
    Jaboulay b.
    Kazanjian tooth b.
    Kistner tracheal b.
    Lardennois b.
    Lee lingual b.
    ligament b.
    b. lip lens manipulator
    Microvasive One Step B.
    Moore tracheostomy b.
    Murphy b.
    Murphy-Johnson anastomosis b.
    Norris b.
    B. One-Step gastrostomy device

    Panje voice b.
    patellar b.
    peritoneal b.
    Perspex b.
    polyethylene collar b.
    polypropylene b.
    pull-out b.
    Reuter bobbin collar b.
    Sheehy collar b.
    Silastic suture b.
    silicone b.
    Smithwick buttonhook b.
    b. spacer
    Spitzy b.
    stoma b.
    Surgitek b.
    suture b.
    Teflon collar b.
    Todd bur hole b.
    tracheal b.
    tracheostomy b.
    Villard b.
    voice b.
buttoned device
button-end knife
buttonhook
    b. nerve retractor
    Smithwick b.
button-tip manipulator
button-type G-tube
buttress
    Omni pretibial b.
    b. pad
    b. plate
    Teflon pledget suture b.
    B. thread screw
buttressed hook
buttress-type plate
butyl cyanoacrylate glue
Buxton uterine clamp
Buyes air-vent suction tube
Buzard Diamond Barraqueratome Microkeratome system
Buzard-Thornton fixation ring
BV2 needle
B-V-M
    bag-valve-mask
BVS pump
BWM spine system
Bx
    Bx Velocity coronary artery stent
Byars mandibular prosthesis
Bycep
    B. biopsy forceps
    B. PC Jr bioptome
Bycroft-Brunswick thyroid retractor
Byford retractor
bypass
    endovascular cardiopulmonary b.
    b. graft catheter
    b. machine
    off-pump coronary artery b.
    b. Speedy balloon catheter
BYR-300 imaging and illumination platform

Byrel
    B. SX pacemaker
    B. SX/Versatrax pacemaker

Byrne expulsive hemorrhage lens

C-2
  C-2 hip system
  C-2 OsteoCap hip prosthesis
C.
  C. B. T. bumper wedge
  C. L. Jackson head-holding forceps
  C. L. Jackson pin-bending
    costophrenic forceps
  C. R. Bard catheter
  C. R. Bard Urolase fiber
CA
  CA membrane hollow-fiber dialyzer
CA-5000 drill-guide isometer
CA-6000 spine motion analyzer
CAAS
  Cardiovascular Angiography Analysis
    System
cabin
  magnetic shielded c.
cabinet
  grid c.
  c. respirator
cable
  alligator pacing c.
  Bicomatic bipolar c.
  braided Spectra UHMWPE
    surgical c.
  braided titanium c.
  chrome-cobalt c.
  coaxial c.
  Dall-Miles c.
  ESI Lite-Pipe fiberoptic c.
  European/German bipolar c.
  fiberoptic light c.
  FlexStrand c.
  Gallie fusion-using c.
  c. graft
  internal fiberoptic c.
  interspinous c.
  Oklahoma City c.
  Old Martin bipolar c.
  OxyLead interconnect c.
  SecureStrand c.
  Songer c.
  Sullivan variable stiffness c.
  c. tie
  titanium c.
  c. wire suture
  world standard Olsen bipolar c.
cable-twister orthosis
Cabot
  C. cannula
  C. leg splint
  C. Medical Corporation diagnostic
    laparoscope
  C. Medical Corporation operating
    laparoscope
  C. Medical Corporation videoscope
  C. nephroscope
  C. Optima laparoscopic Roticulator
  C. trocar
cadaveric knee

caddie
  Cath C.
  SwingAlong walker c.
CADD-Plus intravenous infusion pump
CADD-Prizm pain control system
CADD-TPN
  CADD-TPN ambulatory infusion
    system
  CADD-TPN pump
Cadence
  C. AICD
  C. biphasic ICD
  C. implantable cardioverter-
    defibrillator
  C. tiered therapy defibrillator
    system
  C. TVL nonthoracotomy lead
**Cadet V-115 implantable cardioverter-
  defibrillator**
cadmium
  c. iodide detector
  c. selenide Vidicon video camera
Cadogan-Hough footpedal suction control
Cadwell
  C. 5200A somatosensory evoked
    potential unit
  C. 5200A somatosensory evoked
    potential unit device
Cafet system
Caffinière prosthesis
cage
  BAK c.
  carbon-fiber-composite c.
  carbon-fiber-reinforced c.
  c. catheter device
  fusion c.
  Harm c.
  InterFix titanium threaded spinal
    fusion c.
  lumbar intersomatic fusion
    expandable c.
  Moss c.
  Motech c.
  Novus LC threaded interbody
    fusion c.
  Polaris c.
  protrusio c.
  Pyramesh c.
  Ray threaded fusion c.
  stereolithography c.
  Swedish knee c.
  thoracic c.
  threaded interbody fusion c.
  titanium c.
cage-back brace
caged ball valve prosthesis
Cairns
  C. clamp
  C. dissection forceps
  C. hemostatic forceps
  C. rongeur
  C. scalp retractor

C

Cairns-Dandy hemostasis forceps
Cairpad incontinence pad
Cajal axonal retraction ball
"cake mix" kit
Cal-20 central dialysate preparation unit
Calandruccio
    C. clamp
    C. triangular compression fixation
      device
Calasept medicament delivery system
calcaneal spur cookie orthosis
calcaneonavicular bar
calcar
    c. planer
    c. reamer
    c. replacement femoral prosthesis
    c. replacement stem
    c. trimmer
calcified tissue scissors
Calcipulpe cavity liner
Calcitek
    C. drill
    C. drill system
    C. implant
    C. implant system
    C. retaining screw
    C. spline
Calcitite
    C. bone graft
    C. bone replacement
calcium
    c. alginate swab
    c. phosphate ceramic implant
    c. sodium alginate wound dressing
Calculair spirometer
Calcusplit pneumatic lithotriptor
Calcutript
    C. electrohydraulic lithotriptor
    Karl Storz C.
Caldwell
    C. guide
    C. hanging cast
    C. Spectrum 32
calf compression unit
Calgiswab dressing
Calhoun-Hagler lens needle
Calhoun-Merz needle
Calhoun needle
calibrated
    c. clubfoot splint
    c. depth gauge
    c. grasping tube
    c. pin
    c. probe
    c. V-Lok cuff
calibrator
    Fogarty c.
    screw depth c.
Calibri forceps
caliceal system
California hatchet
Caligamed
    C. ankle orthosis
    C. brace

calipers
    Albee bone graft c.
    Austin Moore inside-outside c.
    Austin strut c.
    Barker c.
    Berens marking c.
    Bertillon c.
    c. block
    bone c.
    bone-measuring c.
    Braunstein fixed c.
    breast c.
    Brown and Sharp digital
      electronic c.
    Burch eye c.
    Castroviejo marking c.
    Castroviejo-Schacher angled c.
    Cone ice-tong c.
    Cottle c.
    digital c.
    EKG c.
    electronic c.
    eye c.
    Fat-O-Meter skinfold c.
    Green eye c.
    Harpenden skinfold c.
    House strut c.
    ice-tong c.
    Jameson eye c.
    John Green c.
    Kapp Surgical Instrument total
      hip c.
    Ladd c.
    Lafayette skinfold c.
    Lange skinfold c.
    Machemer c.
    McGaw skinfold c.
    Mendez degree c.
    middle ear c.
    Mipron digital computer-assisted c.
    Mitutoyo Digimatic c.
    ophthalmic c.
    Osher internal c.
    Paparella rasp c.
    Ruddy stapes c.
    ruler c.
    Sentalloy digital c.
    skinfold c.
    Stahl ophthalmic c.
    Storz c.
    strut c.
    Tenzel c.
    Tesa S.A. hand-held electronic
      digital c.
    Thomas c.
    Thorpe c.
    Thorpe-Castroviejo c.
    tibial c.
    tonsillar c.
    Townley c.
    Vernier c.
    V. Mueller ruler c.
    x-ray c.
Cali-Press graft press
calix tube

Callahan
    C. flange
    C. lacrimal rongeur
    C. lens loop
    C. lens loupe
    C. modification speculum
    C. retractor
    C. scleral fixation forceps
Callender
    C. clip
    C. derotational brace
    C. technique hip prosthesis
Callison-Adson tissue forceps
Calman
    C. carotid clamp
    C. ring clamp
Calnan-Nicoll synthetic joint prosthesis
calomel electrode
calorimeter
    bench scale c.
    Benedict-Roth c.
    Scientec c.
Calot jacket
Caltagirone
    C. chisel
    C. skin graft knife
Caltrac accelerometer
Caluso PEG gastrostomy tube
calvarial clamp
Calve cannula
Calypso Rely catheter
CAM
    controlled ankle motion
    CAM stimulator
    CAM tent
    CAM Walker
    CAM Walker leg brace
    CAM Walker walking brace
cam
    c. blade-tipped catheter
    c.-guided trephine
    C. Lock knee joint
CAMAC-300 arteriograph
Camber axis hinge
Cambridge
    C. acuity card
    C. defibrillator
    C. electrocardiograph
    C. jelly electrode
Cameco syringe pistol aspiration device
camera, pl. **camerae**
    ADAC gamma c.
    ADAC/Vertex dual-headed SPECT c.
    AMS Endoview c.
    Anger scintillation c.
    anterior bulbi c.
    APEX 409, 410, 415 ECT digital γ c.
    Beaulieu c.
    Biad c.
    Bio-Optics c.
    Brenman c.
    cadmium selenide Vidicon video c.
    Canon CF-60U fundus c.

Canon CF-60Z fundus c.
Carl Zeiss Jena Retinophot fundus c.
CeraSPECT c.
charge-coupled device monochrome c.
charge-coupled device video c.
Cidtech c.
cine c.
Circon ACMI MicroDigital-I c.
Circon video c.
Coburn c.
CompuCam digital intraoral c.
CooperVision c.
Cr6-45NMf retinal c.
CTI-Siemens 933/8-12 PET c.
Dental Pro II c.
Digirad gamma c.
DigiScope c.
Dine digital macro c.
Docustar fundus c.
Donaldson fundus c.
DSX Sopha c.
dual-head gamma c.
DyoCam 550 arthroscopic video c.
E.CAM photon emission c.
Elscint dual-detector cardiac c.
Endius spinal c.
endo-c.
Endocam digital c.
EndoVideo-Five endoscopic c.
EndoView c.
Endo zoom lens c.
ETV8 CCD ColorMicro video c.
Eyecor c.
field-of-view c.
four-head c.
Fujica c.
fundus c.
fundus-retinal c.
gamma scintillation c.
Gammatone II gamma c.
Garcia-Ibanez M picture c.
GE Maxicamera gamma c.
Genesys Vertex variable angle gamma c.
GE single-detector SPECT-capable c.
GE Starcam single-crystal tomographic scintillation c.
Haifa c.
hand-held fundus c.
Handy non-mydriatic video fundus c.
Helix c.
Holofax Oxford retroillumination cataract c.
House-Urban-Pentax c.
House-Urban-Stille c.
Icarex 25 Med mirror reflex lens c.
immersible video c.
integral uniformity scintillation c.
Isocon c.
Israel c.
Keeler c.

camera *(continued)*
Kowa angiographic c.
Kowa fundus c.
Kowa hand c.
Kowa-Optimed c.
Kowa PRO II retinal c.
Kowa RC-XV fundus c.
Leicaflex c.
Lester A. Dine c.
Macro-5 c.
MedCam Pro Plus video c.
Medicam c.
MedX c.
Micro-Imager high-resolution digital c.
MLR+ c.
multicrystal gamma c.
multiwire gamma c.
Neitz CT-R cataract c.
Nidek 3Dx stereodisk c.
Nikon microprocessor-controlled c.
Nikon Retinopan fundus c.
Olympus OM-1 endoscopic c.
Olympus OM-1 reflex c.
Olympus operating c.
Olympus OTV-S-series miniature c.
ophthalmoscope c.
Orthicon c.
Pentax Spotmatic c.
Picker c.
pinhole c.
Pixsys FlashPoint c.
Polaroid CB-100 c.
Polavision Land c. for endoscopy
positron scintillation c.
Prism 2000XP gamma c.
radioisotope c.
RC-2 fundus c.
Reflec UV instant c.
Reichert c.
Release-NF c.
Retcam 120 digital c.
Retinopan 45 c.
Reveal MLR+ c.
Reveal single lens reflex c.
Robot Starr II c.
rotating gamma c.
Scheimpflug c.
Schepens binocular indirect c.
Scinticore multicrystal scintillation c.
γ-scintillation c.
Siemens Orbiter gamma c.
single-crystal gamma c.
single-head rotating gamma c.
Skylight gantry-free nuclear medicine gamma c.
slip-ring c.
Sony CCD/RGB DXC-151 color video c.
Sopha Medical gamma c.
SP6 c.
SPECT ADAC/Cirrus single-headed c.

SPECT ADAC/Vertex dual-headed c.
Starcam c.
SteriCam Endoscopic c.
Storz c.
Stryker chip c.
Syn-optics c.
Technicare c.
telecentric fundus c.
TeliCam intraoral c.
three-head c.
time-of-flight positron emission tomographic c.
Topcon 50IA c.
Topcon SL-45 c.
Topcon TRC-50IX ICG-capable fundus c.
Topcon TRC-SS2 stereoscopic fundus c.
Topcon TRC-50VT retinal c.
Topcon TRC-50X retinal c.
Topcon TRV-50VT fundus c.
Trionix c.
Trocam endoscopic c.
Urban microsurgery closed-circuit color TV c.
Urocam video c.
Vertex c.
video display c.
Vision c.
Yashica Dental Eye II c.
Zeiss FF450 fundus c.
Zeiss-Nordenson fundus c.
Zeiss operating c.
Zeiss-Scheimpflug c.

camera-processor
Neuroguide c.-p.

Cameron
C. cautery
C. elevator
C. fracture device
C. omni-angle gastroscope
C. periosteal elevator

Cameron-Haight periosteal elevator

Cameron-Miller
C.-M. electrode
C.-M. type monopolar forceps

Camey reservoir

Camino
C. fiberoptic ICP monitor
C. intracranial catheter
C. intracranial pressure monitoring device
C. intracranial pressure monitoring system
C. intraparenchymal fiberoptic device
C. micromanometer catheter
C. microventricular bolt
C. microventricular bolt catheter
C. OLM intracranial pressure monitoring kit
C. postcraniotomy subdural pressure monitoring kit

C. subdural screw
C. transducer catheter
Cammann stethoscope
Camo disposable dental splint
camouflage prosthesis
Campbell
C. airplane splint
C. arthroplasty gouge
C. graft
C. infant catheter
C. lacrimal sac retractor
C. laminectomy rongeur
C. ligature-carrier forceps
C. miniature urethral sound
C. nerve rongeur
C. nerve root retractor
C. osteotome
C. periosteal elevator
C. refractor
C. self-retaining retractor
C. slit lamp
C. suprapubic cannula
C. suprapubic retractor
C. suprapubic trocar
C. traction splint
C. ureteral forceps
C. ureterotome
C. ventricular needle
Campbell-Boyd tourniquet
Campbell-French sound
Campbell-type Heyman fundus applicator
Camp brace
campimeter
stereo c.
Camp-Sigvaris stockings
CamStar
C. exercise machine
C. power leg press
Canadian
C. chest retractor
C. hip disarticulation prosthesis
C. Ibex quilted underpad
C. knee orthosis
Canad meniscal knife
Canakis
C. beaded hip pin
C. wrench
canal
c. chisel
completely in the c. (CIC)
C. Finder system
c. knife
C. Master drill
c. reamer
canalicular scissors
canaliculus
c. dilator
c. knife
c. probe
Canal-Mate hearing aid
Can-Am brace
cancellous
c. bone screw
c. pin

Candela
C. ALEXlazr
C. laser lithotriptor
C. MDA-200 Lasertripter
C. miniscope
C. MiniScope Plus
C. pulsed dye laser
C. ScleroLaser laser
C. videoimaging system
candle
cesium c.
urethral c.
vaginal c.
c. vaginal cesium implant
Can-Do Exercise Band
candy
c. cane cannula
c. cane cannula style II
candy-cane stirrups
cane
C. bone-holding forceps
Double Duty c.
large-base quad c.
MAFO c.
narrow-base quad c.
offset c.
SBQC c.
single-base c.
small-based quad c.
wide-base quad c.
Canfield
C. facial plastics garment
C. tonsillar knife
cannister, canister
Bemis suction c.
coil c.
Evacupack disposable suction c.
Lipovacutainer c.
reusable Sorensen 2000 cc c.
Sep-T-Vac suction c.
Sorensen reusable c.
Cannon
C. Bio-Flek nasal splint
C. endarterectomy loop
Cannon-Rochester lamina elevator
Cannon-type stripper
Cannu-Flex guidewire
cannula, pl. **cannulae, cannula, cannulas**
Abelson cricothyrotomy c.
Abraham laryngeal c.
Accu-Beam suction & irrigation c.
Accu-Flo U-channel stripping c.
Accu-Flo ventricular c.
acorn c.
Adson brain-exploring c.
Adson drainage c.
AE-7277 Rubenstein LASIK c.
air injection c.
Airlife c.
Air-Lon inhalation c.
alpha-chymotrypsin c.
angled left c.
angled right c.
Anis aspirating c.
anterior chamber irrigating c.

C

cannula *(continued)*
    Antoni-Hook lumbar puncture c.
    antral sinus c.
    aortic arch c.
    aortic direct ellipse c.
    aortic perfusion c.
    Argyle CPAP nasal c.
    Aronson-Fletcher antrum c.
    arterial c.
    aspirating c.
    ASSI c.
    atrial c.
    attic c.
    Bahnson aortic c.
    Bailey lacrimal c.
    Banaji c.
    Bard arterial c.
    Bard cervical c.
    Bardic c.
    Barraquer c.
    Barrett hydrodelineation c.
    Bechert intraocular lens c.
    Becker accelerator c.
    Becker dissector c.
    Becker Greater dissecting c.
    Bellocq c.
    Bellucci c.
    Bergström-Stille muscle c.
    Berkeley c.
    Bilisystem ERCP c.
    binasal c.
    Binkhorst hooked c.
    Binkhorst irrigating c.
    biopsy c.
    BioTac biopsy c.
    Bishop-Harman anterior chamber irrigating c.
    bivalved c.
    Blue Max c.
    blunt bullet-tip c.
    Bowers c.
    Bracken anterior chamber c.
    Bracken irrigating c.
    brain biopsy c.
    brain-exploring c.
    Branula c.
    Bresgen c.
    Brodney urethrographic c.
    Brown sphenoid c.
    Bruening c.
    Bucy-Frazier coagulation c.
    Bucy-Frazier suction c.
    Buie c.
    bullet-shaped c.
    Buratto irrigating c.
    Cabot c.
    Calve c.
    Campbell suprapubic c.
    candy cane c.
    candy cane c. style II
    Cantlie c.
    Carabelli mirror c.
    cardiovascular c.
    Casselberry sphenoid c.

    Castaneda c.
    Castroviejo cyclodialysis c.
    cataract-aspirating c.
    caval c.
    cervical c.
    Charlton c.
    Chilcott venoclysis c.
    Christmas tree c.
    Churchill cardiac suction c.
    Cimochowski cardiac c.
    Circon ACMI c.
    Clagett S-c.
    c. clamp
    clysis c.
    Cntour ERCP c.
    Coakley frontal sinus c.
    coaxial c.
    Cobe small vessel c.
    Cobra+ c.
    Cobra K c.
    Cobra K+ c.
    Codman c.
    Cohen-Eder uterine c.
    Cohen intrauterine c.
    Cohen tubal insufflation c.
    Cohen uterine c.
    Coleman aspiration c.
    Coleman V-dissector infiltration c.
    Colt c.
    Concept c.
    Concorde disposable suction c.
    Cone-Bucy c.
    Cone cerebral c.
    Continental c.
    Cooper chemopallidectomy c.
    Cooper double-lumen c.
    Cope needle introducer c.
    Core Dynamics disposable c.
    coronary artery c.
    coronary perfusion c.
    cortex-aspirating c.
    cortical cleaving hydrodissector c.
    Corydon hydroexpression c.
    cricothyrotomy c.
    curved cricothyrotomy c.
    c. cushion
    cyclodialysis c.
    dacryocystorhinostomy c.
    Day attic c.
    De La Vega vitreous-aspirating c.
    Delima ethmoid c.
    Devonshire-Mack c.
    DeWecker syringe c.
    Dexide disposable c.
    Digiflex c.
    disposable cystotome c.
    DLP aortic root c.
    Dohrmann-Rubin c.
    Dorsey ventricular c.
    double irrigating/aspirating c.
    double-lumen irrigation c.
    Dougherty anterior chamber c.
    Douglas c.
    Dow Corning c.
    Drews irrigating c.

Duke c.
Dulaney antral c.
duodenoscope c.
Dupuis c.
ear c.
egress c.
Eichen irrigating c.
Elecath ECMO c.
Elsberg brain-exploring c.
Elsberg ventricular c.
endometrial c.
Endo-Pool suction c.
Endotrac c.
Entree II c.
Entree Plus c.
ERCP c.
Eriksson muscle biopsy c.
esophagoscopic c.
Ethicon disposable c.
Everett fallopian c.
exploring c.
fallopian c.
Fasanella lacrimal c.
Fazio-Montgomery c.
Feaster K7-5460 hydrodissecting c.
Fein c.
Fem-Flex II femoral cannulae
femoral artery c.
femoral perfusion c.
Fink cul-de-sac c.
Fischer c.
Fisher ventricular c.
Fish infusion c.
flattened irrigating c.
Fletcher-Pierce c.
Flexi-Cath silicone subclavian c.
Floyd loop c.
Fluoro Tip ERCP c.
flute c.
Ford Hospital ventricular c.
Franklin-Silverman biopsy c.
Frazier brain-exploring c.
Frazier suction c.
Frazier ventricular c.
Freeman Blue-Max c.
Freeman positioning c.
frontal sinus c.
Fujita suction c.
Futch antral c.
gallbladder c.
Galt aspirating c.
Gans cyclodialysis c.
Gass cataract-aspirating c.
Gass retinal detachment c.
Gass vitreous-aspirating c.
Genitor mini-intrauterine
  insemination c.
Gesco c.
Ghormley double c.
Gill double I&A c.
Gill double Luer-Lok c.
Gill sinus c.
Gill-Welsh aspirating c.
Gill-Welsh double c.
Gill-Welsh irrigating c.

Gill-Welsh olive-tip c.
Gimbel fountain c.
Girard irrigating c.
Goddio disposable c.
Goldstein anterior chamber c.
Goldstein irrigating c.
Goldstein lacrimal c.
golf tee hollow titanium c.
goniotomy knife c.
Gonzalez specialized dissecting c.
Goodfellow frontal sinus c.
Gott c.
Grafco c.
Gram c.
gravity infusion c.
Gregg c.
Grinfeld c.
Grizzard subretinal c.
Gromley-Russell c.
Grüntzig femoral stiffening c.
c. guard
Guell laser-assisted intrastromal
  keratomileusis (LASIK) c.
guiding c.
Gulani triple function laser-assisted
  intrastromal keratomileusis c.
Gulani triple function LASIK c.
Gundry c.
Hahn c.
Hajek c.
Harvard c.
Hasson balloon uterine elevator c.
Hasson-Eder laparoscopy c.
Hasson open-laparoscopy c.
Hasson stable access c.
Haverfield brain c.
Havlicek spiral c.
Haynes brain c.
Healon injection c.
HeartPort-Endoclamp balloon c.
Heartport Endovenous drainage c.
Hendon venoclysis c.
Hepacon c.
Heyer-Schulte-Fischer ventricular c.
Heyner double c.
high-flow coaxial c.
Hilton self-retaining infusion c.
Hilton sutureless infusion c.
Hirschman hooked c.
Hoen ventricular c.
Hoffer forward-cutting knife c.
Holinger c.
hollow c.
Holman-Mathieu salpingography c.
Hudgins salpingography c.
Hudson All-Clear nasal c.
Hulka uterine c.
Hulten-Stille c.
HUMI c.
Hunt-Reich secondary c.
Huse c.
Hyde "frog" irrigating c.
I&A coaxial c.
iliac-femoral c.
Illouz suction c.

cannula *(continued)*
infiltration c.
inflow c.
infusion c.
infusion/infiltration c.
Ingals antral c.
Ingals flexible silver c.
Ingals rectal injection c.
ingress/egress c.
inhalation c.
injection c.
Interlink threaded lock c.
intraarterial c.
intracardiac c.
Intraducer peritoneal c.
intragastric c.
intraocular lens c.
intrauterine balloon c.
intrauterine balloon-type c.
intrauterine insemination c.
IPAS flexible c.
iris hook c.
irrigating c.
irrigating/aspirating c.
I-tech c.
IUI disposable c.
Jarcho self-retaining uterine c.
Jarit air injection c.
Jarit disposable c.
Jarit lacrimal c.
Jensen-Thomas I&A c.
Jetco spray c.
Johnson double c.
J-shaped I&A c.
Judd c.
Kahn trigger c.
Kahn uterine c.
Kanavel brain-exploring c.
Kara cataract-aspirating c.
Karickhoff double c.
Karmen c.
Katena c.
Katzenstein rectal c.
KDF-2.3 intrauterine insemination c.
Keeler-Keislar lacrimal c.
Keisler lacrimal c.
Kellan hydrodissection c.
Kelman cyclodialysis c.
Kesilar c.
Keyes-Ultzmann-Luer c.
Khouri hydrodissection c.
Kidde uterine c.
Killian antral c.
Killian antrum c.
Killian-Eichen c.
Killian nasal c.
Kleegman c.
Klein curved c.
Knolle anterior chamber irrigating c.
Knolle-Pearce c.
Kos attic c.
Kraff cortex c.
Krause nasal snare c.
Kreutzmann c.

lacrimal irrigating c.
Lamb c.
Landolt c.
LaparoSAC single-use obturator and c.
laparoscopic c.
large antral c.
large-bore c.
laryngeal c.
laser-assisted intrastromal keratomileusis c.
lens c.
Leon cobra c.
Lewicky threaded infusion c.
Lichtwicz antral c.
Lifemed c.
ligature c.
Lillie attic c.
Lindeman self-retaining uterine vacuum c.
Linvatec c.
liquid vitreous-aspirating c.
Littell c.
Litwak c.
Look I&A coaxial c.
Lübke uterine vacuum c.
Luer tracheal c.
Lukens c.
lumen c.
Luongo sphenoid irrigating c.
LV apex c.
Makler c.
Malette-Spencer coronary c.
Malström-Westman c.
Mandelbaum c.
Marlow disposable c.
Maumenee goniotomy c.
maxillary sinus c.
Mayo coronary perfusion c.
Mayo-Ochsner c.
McCain TMJ c.
McCaskey sphenoid c.
McGoon c.
McIntyre anterior chamber c.
McIntyre-Binkhorst irrigating c.
McIntyre coaxial c.
McIntyre lacrimal c.
mediastinal c.
Medicut c.
Medi-Tech flexible stiffening c.
Menghini c.
Mercedes tip c.
metal c.
metal-ball tip c.
metallic tip c.
middle ear suction c.
mirror c.
Mladick concave c.
Mladick convex c.
Moehle c.
Moncrieff anterior chamber irrigating c.
Montgomery tracheal c.
Morris c.
Morwel c.

Mueller coronary perfusion c.
MVS c.
Myerson-Moncrieff c.
Myles sinus c.
nasal snare c.
Neal fallopian c.
Neubauer lancet c.
New York Eye and Ear c.
Nichamin hydrodissection c.
Nichamin laser-assisted intrastromal
   keratomileusis (LASIK)
   irrigating c.
nucleus delivery c.
Oaks double straight c.
O'Gawa cataract-aspirating c.
O'Gawa irrigating c.
O'Gawa two-way I&A c.
olive-tipped c.
Olympus disposable c.
O'Malley-Heintz infusion c.
Osher air-bubble removal c.
Osher lens-vacuuming c.
outflow c.
outlet c.
Pacifico c.
Packo pars plana c.
Padgett-Concorde suction c.
Padgett shark-mouth c.
Park irrigating c.
Paterson laryngeal c.
Patton c.
Pautler infusion c.
Peacekeeper c.
Pearce coaxial I&A c.
Peczon I&A c.
Pemco c.
Pereyra ligature c.
perfusion c.
Pierce attic c.
Pierce coaxial I&A c.
Pinto superficial dissection c.
plastic c.
polyethylene c.
Polystan perfusion c.
portal c.
Portex nylon c.
Portnoy ventricular c.
Post washing c.
Power c.
Pritchard c.
ProForma c.
Pye c.
Pynchon c.
pyramid c.
quad-ported laser-assisted intrastromal
   keratomileusis (LASIK)
   irrigating c.
Rabinov c.
Ramirez Silastic c.
Randolph cyclodialysis c.
Ranfac c.
rectal injection c.
Reddick-Saye c.
reel aspiration c.
Reipen c.

Research Medical straight multiple-
   holed aortic c.
return-flow c.
Rica tracheostomy c.
Rigg c.
Riordan flexible silver c.
Robb antral c.
Robles cutting point c.
Rockey mediastinal c.
Rockey tracheal c.
Rohrschneider c.
Rolf-Jackson c.
Roper alpha-chymotrypsin c.
Rosenberg dissecting c.
Rowsey fixation c.
Rubin fallopian tube c.
Rycroft c.
S-c.
Sachs brain-exploring c.
saphenous vein c.
Sarns aortic arch c.
Sarns soft-flow aortic c.
Sarns two-stage c.
Sarns venous drainage c.
Schanz c.
Scheie anterior chamber c.
Scheie cataract-aspirating c.
Scott attic c.
Scott rubber ventricular c.
Sedan c.
Seletz ventricular c.
self-retaining infusion c.
self-retaining irrigating c.
self-sealing c.
Semm uterine vacuum c.
Sewall antral c.
Shahinian lacrimal c.
shark-mouth c.
Sheets irrigating vectis c.
Shepard incision irrigating c.
Shepard radial keratotomy
   irrigating c.
side-cutting c.
side-port c.
sidewall infusion c.
Silastic coronary artery c.
silicone c.
Silver c.
Silverman-Boeker c.
Simcoe cortex c.
Simcoe double-barreled c.
Simcoe II PC double c.
Simcoe nucleus delivery c.
Simcoe reverse-aperture c.
Simcoe reverse I&A c.
Sims c.
single-lumen c.
sinoscopy c.
sinus antral c.
sinus irrigating c.
Skillern sphenoid c.
Slade c.
Sluijter-Mehta SMK-C10 c.
small-bore c.
smooth c.

C

cannula *(continued)*
soft-tipped c.
soft tissue shaving c.
Solos disposable c.
Soresi c.
Southey c.
SpaceSEAL balloon tip c.
spatula c.
Spencer c.
sphenoidal c.
Spielberg sinus c.
Spizziri-Simcoe c.
stable access c.
Stangel fallopian tube c.
step-down c.
Steriseal disposable c.
Storz disposable c.
Storz needle c.
straightening c.
straight lacrimal c.
Strauss c.
subclavian c.
subretinal fluid c.
sub-Tenon anesthesia c.
suction c.
suprapubic c.
surgical c.
Swets goniotomy c.
Sylva irrigating c.
TAC2 atrial caval c.
Tandem XL triple-lumen ERCP c.
Teflon ERCP c.
Tenner lacrimal c.
Texas c.
thin disposable c.
Thomas I&A c.
three-hole aspiration c.
Thurmond nucleus-irrigating c.
Tibbs arterial c.
Toledo V-dissector c.
Tomey angled c.
Tomey G-bevel c.
Tomey standard c.
Topper c.
Torchia nucleus-aspirating c.
tracheal c.
tracheostomy c.
tracheotomy c.
transseptal c.
Tremble sphenoid c.
Trendelenburg c.
Trevisani c.
TriEye c.
trigeminus c.
trigger c.
Tri-Port sub-Tenon anesthesia c.
Trocan disposable CO_2 trocar
  and c.
Troutman alpha-chymotrypsin c.
trumpet c.
TruPro lacrimal c.
tubal insufflation c.
Tulevech lacrimal c.
Turnbull c.

two-stage Sarns c.
two-way cataract-aspirating c.
Ulanday double c.
Uldall subclavian hemodialysis c.
Ultra-Sil c.
Unitech Toomey c.
Unitri c.
Universal c.
urethral instillation c.
urethrographic c.
USCI c.
U-shaped c.
uterine self-retaining c.
uterine vacuum c.
Vabra c.
vacuum intrauterine c.
vacuum uterine c.
Van Alyea antral c.
Van Alyea frontal sinus c.
Van Alyea sphenoid c.
Vancaillie uterine c.
Vance prostatic aspiration c.
Van Osdel irrigating c.
VC2 atrial caval c.
vein graft c.
Veirs c.
vena caval c.
Venflon c.
venoclysis c.
venous c.
ventricular c.
Veress laparoscopic c.
Veress peritoneum c.
Vidaurri c.
Viking c.
Viscoflow angled c.
Visitec anterior chamber c.
Visitec I&A c.
Vitalcor cardioplegia infusion c.
vitreous-aspirating c.
Von Eichen antral c.
Wallace Flexihub central venous
  pressure c.
washout c.
Webb c.
Webster infusion c.
Weck disposable c.
Weil lacrimal c.
Weiner c.
Weisman c.
Wells Johnson c.
Welsh cortex-stripper c.
Welsh flat olive-tipped double c.
Wergeland double c.
West lacrimal c.
Wisap disposable c.
c. with locking dilator
c. with pre-loaded 0.35-inch
  guidewire
Wolf disposable c.
Wolf drainage c.
Wolf return-flow c.
Ximed disposable c.
Yankauer middle meatus c.

Zinn endoillumination infusion c.
Zylik c.
cannular scissors
cannulated
c. bolt
c. bronchoscopic forceps
c. cancellous lag screw
c. cortical step drill
c. drill bit
c. four-flute reamer
c. nail
c. obturator
C. Plus screw system
c. wire threader
cannulation catheter
cannulatome
Cotton c.
Canon
C. autokeratometer K1
C. automatic keratometer
C. auto refraction keratometer
C. auto refractometer
C. CF-60U fundus camera
C. CF-60Z fundus camera
C. perimeter
C. refractor
C. scanner
Can-Opt
C.-O. dual-lumen ERCP system
C.-O. stand-alone dual lumen ERCP catheter
canted finger hook
Cantlie cannula
Cantor intestinal tube
canvas brace
Canyons irrigation syringe
cap
ACTIVE LIFE one-piece opaque stoma c.
Bremer torque-limiting c.
Carnation corn c.'s
CenterPointLock two-piece ostomy system: stoma c.
Cloward drill guard c.
compliance c.
Dansac Colo F mini c.
Dansac Combi micro c.
Dansac Contour I mini c.
digit c.
Gelfilm c.
Guardian two-piece ostomy system stoma c.
Interlink injection c.
Lehnhardt Universal c.
plastic end c.'s
ProtectaCap c.
Silipos mesh c.
c. splint
SupraCAPS quarter-globe c.
Sur-Fit flange c.
syringe c.
Universal reducer c.
Zang metatarsal c.
Zimmer tibial nail c.
CAP/3SBII angiogram projection system

capacitator
MOS c.
capacitive sensor
capacitor
Caparosa
C. cutting bur
C. wire crimper
Capasee diagnostic ultrasound system
CAPDH probe
capeline bandage
Capello slim-line abduction pillow
Capener
C. brace
C. coil splint
C. finger splint
C. nail
C. nail plate
Capes clamp
Capetown
C. aortic prosthetic valve
C. aortic valve prosthesis
cap-fitted
c.-f. endoscope
c.-f. panendoscope
capillary
c. bed shunt
c. flow dialyzer
C. System slide holder
c. tube
Capintec
C. instant gamma counter
C. nuclear VEST monitor
C. VEST system
Capiox
C. hollow flow oxygenator
C. SX gas and heat exchange oxygenation system
Capiox-E bypass system oxygenator
CAPIS
CAPIS bone plate system
CAPIS compression plate
CAPIS reconstruction plate
capitonnage suture
Caplan
C. angular scissors
C. dorsal scissors
C. nasal scissors
Capmix amalgamator
Capner gouge
Capnocheck
C. capnometer
Capnogard capnograph monitor
capnograph
Nellcor N-2500 c.
Tidal Wave hand-held c.
Capnomac
C. infrared analyzer
C. multiple gas analyzer
C. Ultima gas analyzer
C. Ultima monitor
C. Ultima sidestream spirometer
capnometer
Capnocheck c.
Cardiocap c.
MicroSpan c.

C

Capnostat
C. CO_2 sensor
C. Mainstream carbon dioxide module
capped lead
Cappio
C. Laurus apparatus
C. suture passer
Caprolactam suture
CAPS ArthroWand
Capset bone graft barrier
Capsitome cystitome
Capsuel CPAP manometer
capsular
c. forceps
c. knife
c. polisher
c. scraper
c. scrubber
capsular-style lens
capsule
c. applier system
c. coupeur
Crosby c.
Crosby-Kugler biopsy c.
Crosby-Kugler pediatric c.
dental c.
c. fragment spatula
Heyman-Simon c.
NK dental c.
pH-sensitive radiotelemetry c.
c. polisher
pyxigraphic sampling c.
radioisotope c.
Saf-T-Fit amalgamator c.
Watson c.
capsule-grasping forceps
Capsulform lens
capsulorhexis forceps
capsulotome
Darling c.
capsulotomy
c. blade
c. forceps
c. scissors
CapSure
C. cardiac pacing lead
C. electrode
Captiflex polypectomy snare
Captivator polypectomy snare
caput forceps
Carabelli
C. aspirator
C. cancer cell collector
C. endobronchial tube
C. irrigator
C. lumen finder
C. mirror cannula
Carabelt
C. lower back support
C. therapeutic belt
Carapace face shield
Carasyn hydrogel wound dressing

Carb-Bite
C.-B. needle holder
C.-B. tissue forceps
Carb-Edge scissors
carbide finishing bur
carbide-jaw forceps
CarboFlex odor-control dressing
carbolized knife blade
CarboMedics
C. bileaflet prosthetic heart valve
C. cardiac valve prosthesis
C. "Top-Hat" supra-annular valve
C. valve device
carbon
c. arc lamp
C. Copy HP foot prosthesis
C. Copy II foot prosthesis
C. Copy II lightweight prosthesis
c. dioxide (CO_2) laser
c. dioxide (CO_2) laser scalpel
c. fiber
c. fiber lamination braid
c. fiber-reinforced polyethylene
c. implant
c. Monotube long bone fracture external fixation system
c. particle bead
c. steel blade
carbon-fiber-composite cage
carbon-fiber-reinforced cage
Carboplast
C. II sheeting
C. II sheet orthotic material
Carborundum grinding wheel
Carbo-Seal
C.-S. cardiovascular composite graft
C.-S. graft material
Carbo-Zinc skin barrier material
Carcon stent
card
Allen preschool c.
Cambridge acuity c.
digital acuity c.
ECT time test c.
Guthrie c.
Jaeger acuity c.
memory exercise c.
microendoscopic test c.
Novus Medical image c.
pace c.
pattern matching c.
reduced Snellen c.
Sono-Gram fetal ultrasound image c.
Teller acuity c.
Cardak percutaneous catheter introducer
Carden
C. bronchoscopy tube
C. jetting device
C. laryngoscopy tube
cardiac
C. Assist intraaortic balloon catheter
c. balloon pump
c. baroreceptor
c. infant catheter

c. monitor
c. output recorder
c. pacemaker
C. Pacemaker, Inc.
c. probe
c. retraction clip
c. sling
C. Stimulator BCO_2
c. valve dilator
cardiac-apnea monitor
CardiData Prodigy system
Cardiff resuscitation bag
Cardifix EZ cardiac pacing lead
Cardillo retractor
Cardima Pathfinder microcatheter
cardinal suture
Cardio
C. Tactilaze peripheral angioplasty laser catheter
Cardio3DScope imaging system
CardioBeeper CB-12L monitor
CardioCamera imaging system
Cardiocap
C. capnometer
C. 5-patient monitor
Cardiocare stethoscope
CardioCoil
C. coronary stent
C. self-expanding coronary stent
Cardio-Control pacemaker
Cardio-Cool myocardial protection pouch
Cardio-Cuff
Childs C.-C.
CardioData
C. Mark IV computer
C. MK-3 Holter scanner
CardioDiary
C. heart monitor
cardiodilator
cardioesophageal junction dilator
Cardioflon suture
Cardiofreezer cryosurgical system
CardioGenesis PMR system
cardiograph
Minnesota impedance c.
Cardio-Grip
C.-G. anastomosis clamp
C.-G. aortic clamp
C.-G. bronchus clamp
C.-G. iliac forceps
C.-G. ligature carrier
C.-G. pediatric clamp
C.-G. renal artery clamp
C.-G. tangential occlusion clamp
C.-G. tissue forceps
C.-G. vascular clamp
Cardioguard 4000 electrocardiographic monitor
cardiokymograph (CKG)
Cardiology II stethoscope
Cardiomarker catheter
CardioMatic electrocardiograph
Cardiomed
C. Bodysoft epidural catheter

C. endotracheal ventilation catheter
C. thermodilution catheter
Cardiomemo device
Cardiometrics
C. cardiotomy reservoir
C. Flowire Doppler echo crystal
C. Flow-wire guidewire
cardiomyostimulator
Cardionyl suture
Cardio-Pace Medical Durapulse pacemaker
cardioplegic needle
Cardiopoint cardiac surgery needle
cardiopulmonary
C. Paragon 8500 bed
c. support
c. support system
CardioPump
Ambu C.
Cardioscint nuclear detector
cardioscope
Carlens Universal c.
Siemens BICOR c.
Siemens HICOR c.
c. U system
CardioSeal septal occluder
CardioSearch sensor
Cardioserv defibrillator
cardiospasm dilator
CardioSync cardiac synchronizer
Cardiotach fetal monitor
cardiotachometer
Cardiotest portable electrograph
cardiotomy reservoir
cardiovascular
c. anastomotic clamp
C. Angiography Analysis System (CAAS)
c. bulldog clamp
c. cannula
c. monitor
c. needle holder
c. Prolene suture
c. retractor
c. scissors
c. shunt
c. silk suture
c. stylet
c. tissue forceps
cardioverter
Lown c.
cardioverter-defibrillator
Angstrom MD implantable single-lead c.-d.
Atrial View Ventak implantable c.-d.
automatic implantable c.-d.
Cadence implantable c.-d.
Cadet V-115 implantable c.-d.
Contour LTV135D implantable c.-d.
Contour V-145D implantable c.-d.
CPI PRx implantable c.-d.
CPI Ventak PRx c.-d.
Endotak nonthoracotomy implantable c.-d.

cardioverter-defibrillator *(continued)*
    implantable c.-d. (ICD)
    implantable automatic c.-d.
    Intermedics RES-Q implantable c.-d.
    LT V-105 implantable c.-d.
    Medtronic external c.-d.
    Micron Res-Q implantable c.-d.
    nonthoracotomy lead implantable c.-d.
    PCD Transvene implantable c.-d.
    Powerheart automatic external c.-d.
    programmable c.-d. (PCD)
    Res-Q ACD implantable c.-d.
    Siemens Siecure implantable c.-d.
    Telectronics ATP implantable c.-d.
    tiered-therapy implantable c.-d.
    Transvene nonthoracotomy
      implantable c.-d.
    Ventritex Augstrom MD
      implantable c.-d.
    Ventritex Cadence implantable c.-d.
Cardiovit
    C. AT-10 ECG/spirometry
      combination system
    C. AT-10 monitor
    C. AT-series ECG
    C. spirometer
Cardizem Lyo-Ject
Cardona
    C. corneal prosthesis forceps
    C. corneal prosthesis trephine
    C. fiberoptic diagnostic lens
    C. focalizing fundus lens implant
    C. focalizing goniolens
    C. goniofocalizing implant
    C. keratoprosthesis prosthesis
    C. laser
    C. threading lens forceps
CareDrape blanket
CARE electrode
Care-e-Vac portable aspirator
CareMonitor
    Q-Tel Progressive C.
Carex ambulatory aid
Carey-Coons
    C.-C. biliary endoprosthesis kit
    C.-C. soft stent
Carle analytic gas chromatograph
Carlens
    C. bronchospirometric catheter
    C. curette
    C. double-lumen endotracheal tube
    C. forceps
    C. mediastinoscope
    C. needle
    C. tracheotomy retractor
    C. Universal cardioscope
Carlens-Stille tracheal retractor
Carl Zeiss
    C. Z. instruments
    C. Z. Jena Retinophot fundus
      camera
    C. Z. lens
    C. Z. lensometer

    C. Z. myringotomy tube
    C. Z. tonometer
    C. Z. YAG laser
C-arm
    C.-a. fluoroscope
    C.-a. fluoroscopic apparatus
    C.-a. fluoroscopy unit
    C.-a. image intensifier
    MINI 6000 C.-a.
    C.-a. portable x-ray unit
    Siremobil C.-a.
Carmack ear curette
Carmalt
    C. arterial forceps
    C. clamp
    C. hemostat
    C. hemostatic forceps
    C. hysterectomy forceps
    C. splinter forceps
    C. thoracic forceps
Carman rectal tube
Carmeda BioActive surface
  extracorporeal circuit
Carmel clamp
Carmody
    C. aspirator
    C. perforator drill
    C. thumb tissue forceps
    C. valvulotome
Carmody-Batson elevator
Carmody-Brophy forceps
carmustine wafer
Carnation corn caps
Carol Gerard screw
Carolina
    C. color spectrum CW Doppler
    C. rocker
Caroline finger retractor
Carolon
    C. AFO sock
    C. life support antiembolism
      stockings
carotid
    c. angiogram needle
    c. artery clamp
    c. artery forceps
    c. stent
CarotidCoil stent
carpal
    c. box
    C. Care exerciser
    C. Lock cock-up wrist splint
    C. Lock wrist brace
    c. lunate implant
    c. scaphoid screw
    c. tunnel release system device
    c. tunnel surgery relief kit
Carpel speculum
Carpenter dissector
Carpentier
    C. annuloplasty ring prosthesis
    C. pericardial valve
    C. ring
    C. ring heart valve
    C. stent

Carpentier-Edwards
  C.-E. aortic valve prosthesis
  C.-E. bioprosthetic valve
  C.-E. glutaraldehyde-preserved
    porcine xenograft prosthesis
  C.-E. mitral annuloplasty valve
  C.-E. pericardial valve
  C.-E. Perimount RSR pericardial
    bioprosthesis
  C.-E. Physio annuloplasty ring
  C.-E. porcine bioprosthesis
  C.-E. porcine supra-annular valve
  C.-E. xenograft
Carpentier-Rhone-Poulenc mitral ring
  prosthesis
carposcope
Carpule needle
CarraFilm transparent film dressing
CarraGauze
  C. hydrogel wound dressing pad
  C. packing strips
CarraSmart foam
CarraSorb
  C. H calcium alginate wound
    dressing
  C. M freeze-dried gel wound
    dressing
Carrasyn V viscous hydrogel wound
  dressing
Carrel
  C. clamp
  C. hemostatic forceps
  C. mosquito forceps
  C. patch
  C. suture
  C. tube
Carrel-Girard screw
Carrel-Lindbergh pump
Carriazo-Barraquer microkeratome
Carrie car seat
carrier
  amalgam c.
  Barraquer needle c.
  brain clip c.
  Braun ligature c.
  bronchoscopic sponge c.
  Cardio-Grip ligature c.
  Cave-Rowe ligature c.
  clamp c.
  Converta-Litter c.
  Cooley ligature c.
  cotton c.
  DeBakey ligature c.
  DeBakey-Semb ligature c.
  deep ligature c.
  Deschamps ligature c.
  double-headed stereotactic c.
  ear snare wire c.
  Endo-Assist endoscopic ligature c.
  Endoclose suture c.
  Favaloro ligature c.
  Favaloro-Semb ligature c.
  fiberoptic light c.
  Finochietto clamp c.
  Fitzwater ligature c.

  foil c.
  Fragen c.
  gauze pad c.
  goiter ligature c.
  Goldwasser suture c.
  Jackson sponge c.
  Kilner suture c.
  Kwapis ligature c.
  Lahey ligature c.
  laryngeal sponge c.
  ligature c.
  light c.
  linear in-line ligature c.
  London College foil c.
  Macey tendon c.
  Madden ligature c.
  Mayo goiter ligature c.
  Miya hook ligament c.
  Miya hook ligature c.
  nasal snare wire c.
  proctological cotton c.
  Raz double-prong ligature c.
  Rica cotton c.
  sigmoidoscope light c.
  sponge c.
  Storz cotton c.
  suture c.
  Tauber ligature c.
  tendon c.
  Thermafil plastic c.
  Wangensteen deep ligature c.
  Yasargil ligature c.
  Young ligature c.
Carrion penile prosthesis
Carrion-Small penile implant
Carr lobectomy tourniquet
Carroll
  C. aluminum mallet
  C. awl
  C. bone-holding forceps
  C. bone hook
  C. dressing forceps
  C. finger goniometer
  C. forearm tendon stripper
  C. hook curette
  C. needle
  C. offset hand retractor
  C. osteotome
  C. periosteal elevator
  C. rongeur
  C. self-retaining spring retractor
  C. skin hook
  C. tendon passer
  C. tendon-passing forceps
  C. tendon-pulling forceps
  C. tendon retriever
  C. tissue forceps
Carroll-Adson dural forceps
Carroll-Bennett finger retractor
Carroll-Bunnell drill
Carroll-Legg
  C.-L. osteotome
  C.-L. periosteal elevator
Carroll-Smith-Petersen osteotome

C

Carson
> C. internal/external endopyelotomy stent
> C. Zero Tip balloon dilatation catheter

cart
> Datel endoscopy travel c.
> Harloff c.
> MedGraphics CPX/D metabolic c.
> metabolic c.
> MetroFlex endoscopic c.
> Promedica video c.'s
> resuscitation c.

Cartella eye shield
Carten mitral valve retractor
Carter
> C. clamp
> C. immobilization cushion
> C. intranasal splint
> C. pillow
> C. retractor
> C. septal knife
> C. septal speculum
> C. sphere
> C. spherical eye introducer
> C. submucous curette
> C. submucous elevator
> C. Tubal Assistant surgical instrument

Carter-Glassman resection clamp
Carter-Rowe awl
Carter-Thomason
> C.-T. suture passer
> C.-T. UPLIFT

cartesian reference coordinate system
cartilage
> c. abrader
> c. chisel
> c. clamp
> c. crusher
> c. cutting board
> c. elastic pullover kneecap splint
> c. forceps
> c. guide
> c. implant
> c. knife
> c. scissors

cartilage-holding forceps
Carti-Loid syringe
Cartman lens insertion forceps
Cartmill feeding tube kit
cartridge
> Adsorba hemoperfusion c.
> Alukart hemoperfusion c.
> AstraZeneca dental c.
> Clark hemoperfusion c.
> Diakart hemoperfusion c.
> ELAD c.
> Genotropin two-chamber c.
> Hemocal hemoperfusion c.
> Hemokart hemoperfusion c.
> Heparinase test c.
> serum pregnancy assay c.

Cartwright
> C. heart prosthesis
> C. valve prosthesis

caruncle
> c. clamp
> c. forceps

carver
> amalgam c.
> Cooley wax c.
> C. dental wax
> dental wax c.
> Frahm c.
> G-C wax c.
> Hollenback c.
> modeling c.
> Nordent c.
> SMIC c.

CAS-8000V general angiography positioner
Cascade Up and About system
CASE
> CASE computerized exercise EKG system
> CASE Marquette 16 exercise system

case
> C. appliance
> Berens sterilizing c.
> Blade-Safe c.
> Cloward PLIF c.
> Codman dilator c.
> Contique contact lens c.
> C. enamel cleaver
> Fine corneal carrying c.
> Mazzariello-Caprini stone forceps sterilizing c.
> Port-A-FEESST c.

Casebeer-Lindstrom nomogram
CA-series dialyzer
Casey pelvic clamp
CASH brace
CAS-200 image cytometer
Caspar
> C. alligator forceps
> C. anterior cervical plate
> C. anterior instrumentation
> C. blade
> C. cervical retractor
> C. cervical screw
> C. disk space spreader
> C. distraction pin
> C. distractor
> C. drill
> C. hook
> C. plating
> C. retraction post
> C. rongeur
> C. speculum
> C. trapezoidal plate
> C. vertebral body spreader

Caspari
> C. shuttle
> C. suture punch

CASS
> CASS TrueTaper collimator
> CASS whole-brain mapping system

Casselberry
    C. sphenoid cannula
    C. sphenoid tube
    C. suture punch
cassette
    c. cup collecting device
    Kodak X-Omatic C-1 c.
Cassidy-Brophy dressing forceps
cast
    Aquaplast c.
    below-knee walking c.
    bivalved c.
    c. blade
    Body Armor walker c.
    c. boot
    c. brace
    c. breaker
    broomstick c.
    Caldwell hanging c.
    Cerrobend c.
    Comfort C.
    Cotton-Loader position c.
    dermoplasty c.
    Equilizer short leg walking c.
    Fractura Flex c.
    Freedom Thumb spica c.
    Frejka c.
    C. Gard cast protector
    Gypsona c.
    Hexcelite c.
    hinged c.
    hip spica c.
    c. knife
    LAE c.
    LBE c.
    c. liner
    c. lingual splint
    long above-elbow c.
    long arm navicular c.
    long below-elbow c.
    long leg cylinder c.
    long leg plaster c.
    long leg walking c.
    MaxCast c.
    MBE c.
    medium below-elbow c.
    Minerva c.
    Muenster c.
    Neufeld c.
    Orfizip knee c.
    Orthoplast slipper c.
    c. padding
    petaling the c.
    plaster-of-Paris c.
    pontoon spica c.
    Risser-Cotrel body c.
    Risser localizer scoliosis c.
    Risser turnbuckle c.
    SAE c.
    Sarmiento c.
    SBE c.
    semirigid fiberglass c.
    c. shoe
    short above-elbow c.
    short arm cylinder c.

    short arm navicular c.
    short below-elbow c.
    short leg cylinder c.
    short leg nonwalking c.
    short leg nonweightbearing c.
    short leg plaster c.
    short leg walking c.
    spica c.
    c. spreader
    standard above-elbow c.
    sugar-tong c.
    thumb spica c.
    total contact c.
    Velpeau c.
    walking heel c.
CastAlert device
Castallo
    C. eyelid retractor
    C. eye speculum
    C. refractor
Castanares facelift scissors
Castaneda
    C. anastomosis clamp
    C. bottle
    C. cannula
    C. IMM vascular clamp
    C. infant sternal retractor
    C. partial-occlusion clamp
    C. thrombolytic brush
    C. vascular clamp
    C. vascular forceps
Castaneda-Malecot catheter
Castaneda-Mixter
    C.-M. forceps
    C.-M. thoracic clamp
Castaway
    C. leg brace
    C. leg walker
castbelt
    Posey below-the-knee c.
Castech extremity support
Castelli-Paparella collar button tube
Castens
    C. ascites trocar
    C. hydrocele trocar
Castex rigid dressing
Casteyer prostatic punch
CastGuard guard
Castillo catheter
casting wax sheet
Castle
    C. Daystar surgical television system
    C. surgical light
Castmate plaster bandage dressing
cast-molded PMMA intraocular lens
Castorit investment material
Castro-Martinez keratome
Castroviejo
    C. acrylic eye implant
    C. adjustable retractor
    C. angled keratome
    C. anterior synechia scissors
    C. bladebreaker
    C. blade holder

C

Castroviejo (*continued*)
C. capsular forceps
C. capsule forceps
C. clip-applying forceps
C. compressor
C. cornea-holding forceps
C. corneal dissector
C. corneal scissors with inside stop
C. corneal section scissors
C. corneal transplant marker
C. corneal transplant scissors
C. corneal transplant trephine
C. corneoscleral forceps
C. corneoscleral punch
C. cross-action capsular forceps
C. cyclodialysis cannula
C. cyclodialysis spatula
C. dermatome
C. discission knife
C. double-end lacrimal dilator
C. double-end spatula
C. electrokeratotome
C. electromucotome
C. enucleation snare
C. erysiphake
C. eye speculum
C. eye suture forceps
C. fixation forceps
C. iridocapsulotomy scissors
C. iris scissors
C. keratoplasty scissors
C. lacrimal sac probe
C. lens clamp
C. lens loop
C. lens loupe
C. lens spoon
C. lid forceps
C. lid retractor
C. marking calipers
C. microcorneal scissors
C. mosquito lid clamp
C. needle holder
C. needle holder clamp
C. ophthalmic knife
C. orbital aspirator
C. oscillating razor
C. razor
C. razor blade
C. razor holder
C. refractor
C. scleral fold forceps
C. scleral marker
C. scleral shortening clip
C. sclerotome
C. snare enucleator
C. surface electrode
C. suture forceps
C. suturing forceps
C. synechia scissors
C. synechia spatula
C. tenotomy scissors
C. transplant forceps
C. transplant-grafting forceps
C. twin knife

C. tying forceps
C. vitreous-aspirating needle
C. wide grip handle forceps
Castroviejo-Arruga capsular forceps
Castroviejo-Barraquer needle holder
Castroviejo-Colibri corneal forceps
Castroviejo-Furness cornea-holding forceps
Castroviejo-Galezowski dilator
Castroviejo-Kalt eye needle holder
Castroviejo-McPherson keratectomy scissors
Castroviejo-Schacher angled calipers
Castroviejo-Scheie cyclodiathermy
Castroviejo-Simpson forceps
Castroviejo-Steinhauser mucotome
Castroviejo-Troutman scissors
Castroviejo-Vannas capsulotomy scissors
Castroviejo-Wheeler discission knife
catadioptric lens
Cat-a-Kit
C.-a.-K. analyzer
Catalano
C. capsular forceps
C. corneoscleral forceps
C. dilator
C. intubation set
C. muscle hook
C. needle holder
C. tying forceps
Catalyst machine
Catamaran swim plug
cataract
c. aspirator
c. blade
c. bur
c. knife
c. knife guard
c. mask ring
c. needle
c. pencil
c. probe
c. rotoextractor extractor
c. scissors
c. spoon
cataract-aspirating
c.-a. cannula
c.-a. needle
Catarex cataract removal system
catch basin
Catera suture anchor
Cateye Ergociser
catgut
c. needle
Rica surgical c.
SMIC surgical c.
c. suture
Cath
C. Caddie
CV C.
Freedom C.
MMG Ready C.
Uni-Gard Quik C.
Cathcart orthocentric hip prosthesis
cathematic catheter

catheter
A1, A2 Port multipurpose c.
Abbokinase c.
Ablaser laser delivery c.
ablation c.
Abramson c.
Abscession fluid drainage c.
Accu-Flo spring c.
Accu-Flo ventricular c.
Accurate c.
ACE fixed-wire balloon c.
Achiever balloon dilatation c.
Ackrad balloon-bearing c.
Ackrad Bronchitrac "L" suction c.
Ackrad esophageal balloon c.
Ackrad H/S Elliptosphere c.
ACMI Alcock c.
ACMI Bunts c.
ACMI coated Foley c.
ACMI Emmett hemostatic c.
ACMI Owens c.
ACMI positive pressure c.
ACMI severance c.
ACMI Thackston c.
ACMI ureteral c.
ACMI Word Bartholin gland c.
Acmix Foley c.
acorn-tipped c.
ACS angioplasty c.
ACS balloon c.
ACS Concorde coronary
  dilatation c.
ACS Concorde OTW c.
ACS Endura coronary dilation c.
ACS exchange guiding c.
ACS Hi-Torque Balance
  Middleweight c.
ACS JL4 French c.
ACS Monorail perfusion balloon c.
ACS OTW Lifestream coronary
  dilation c.
ACS OTW Photon coronary
  dilatation c.
ACS OTW Solaris coronary
  dilatation c.
ACS RX Comet coronary
  dilatation c.
ACS RX Comet VP c.
ACS RX Gemini c.
ACS RX Lifestream c.
ACS RX Rocket c.
ACS Torquemaster c.
ACS Tourguide II guiding c.
ACS Tx2000 VP c.
ACS Viking c.
Active Cath c.
Acucise RP retrograde
  endopyelotomy c.
AcuNav ultrasound c.
c. adapter
Add-a-Cath c.
à demeure c.
Advance EX self-adhesive urinary
  external c.
afterloading c.

AgX antimicrobial Foley c.
Air-Lon inhalation c.
AL-1 c.
Alcock return-flow hemostatic c.
alignment c.
AL II guiding c.
alimentation c.
Allis c.
Alvarez-Rodriguez cardiac c.
Alzate c.
Amazr c.
Amcath c.
Amplatz aortography c.
Amplatz cardiac c.
Amplatz coronary c.
Amplatz femoral c.
Amplatz Hi-Flo torque-control c.
anchored c.
Angiocath flexible c.
Angiocath PRN c.
Angioflow high-flow c.
angiographic balloon occlusion c.
angiography c.
AngioJet thrombectomy c.
Angio-Kit c.
Angiomedics c.
AngioOPTIC microcatheter c.
angiopigtail c.
angioplasty balloon c.
angioplasty guiding c.
Angio-Seal c.
angled balloon c.
angled pigtail c.
angle-tip urethral c.
angulated c.
Anthron heparinized c.
antimicrobial c.
Antron c.
Anzio c.
aortic c.
aortography c.
Arani double-loop guiding c.
AR-1, AR-2 diagnostic guiding c.
Arc-22 c.
Argyle arterial c.
Argyle Medicut R c.
Argyle oxygen c.
Argyle trocar c.
Argyle umbilical vessel c.
Arrow balloon wedge c.
Arrow-Berman balloon c.
ArrowFlex intra-aortic balloon c.
Arrow FlexTip Plus c.
ArrowGard Blue antiseptic-coated c.
ArrowGard Blue central venous c.
ArrowGard Blue Line c.
Arrow-Howes multilumen c.
Arrow-Howes quad-lumen c.
Arrow pulmonary artery c.
Arrow QuadPolar electrode c.
Arrow QuickFlash arterial c.
Arrow-Trerotola PTD c.
Arrow TwinCath multilumen
  peripheral c.
Arrow two-lumen hemodialysis c.

C

catheter *(continued)*

Artec balloon c.
arterial embolectomy c.
arterial irrigation c.
arteriovenous c.
Ascent c.
Ash c.
ASI uroplasty TCU dilatation c.
Asuka PTCA c.
atherectomy c.
AtheroCath Bantam coronary
  atherectomy c.
AtheroCath GTO coronary
  atherectomy c.
AtheroCath spinning blade c.
Atlantic ileostomy c.
Atlas LP PTCA balloon
  dilatation c.
Atlas ULP PTCA balloon
  dilatation c.
Atrac-II double-balloon c.
Atrac multipurpose balloon c.
atrioseptostomy c.
Atri-pace I bipolar flared pacing c.
auricular appendage c.
Auth atherectomy c.
automatic c.
autoperfusion balloon c.
AV DeClot c.
AV-Paceport thermodilution c.
axillary c.
Axiom DG balloon angioplasty c.
Axxcess ureteral c.
bag c.
Bailey transthoracic c.
bailout autoperfusion balloon c.
Baim pacing c.
Baim-Turi monitoring/pacing c.
Balectrode pacing c.
c. balloon
balloon angioplasty c.
balloon biliary c.
balloon dilatation c.
balloon dilating c.
balloon embolectomy c.
balloon flotation c.
balloon-flotation pacing c.
balloon-imaging c.
balloon-tipped angiographic c.
balloon-tipped flow-directed c.
balloon valvuloplasty c.
balloon wedge pressure c.
ball-wedge c.
Baltherm thermal dilution c.
banana c.
Bandit c.
Banno c.
Bardam red rubber c.
Bard balloon-directed pacing c.
Bardco c.
Bard disposable male external c.
Bard electrophysiology c.
Bardex all silicone sterile Foley c.
Bardex-Foley balloon c.

Bardex-Foley return-flow retention c.
Bardex I.C. sterile Foley c.
Bardex Lubricath Foley c.
Bardex silicone Foley c.
Bard gastrostomy c.
Bard guiding c.
Bard helical c.
Bardic cutdown c.
Bardic-Deseret Intracath c.
Bardic translucent c.
Bardic Uro Sheath reusable male
  external c.
Bard male external c.
Bard sterile red rubber c.
Bard Touchless intermittent c.
Bard-U-Cath self-adhering male
  external c.
Bard x-ray ureteral c.
Bartholin gland c.
Baschui pigtail c.
bat-wing c.
Baxter angioplasty c.
Baxter dilatation c.
Baxter fiberoptic
  spectrophotometry c.
Baxter-V. Mueller c.
Beird eye c.
Béniqué c.
Bentson-Hanafee-Wilson c.
Berenstein guiding c.
Berenstein occlusion balloon c.
Berman angiographic c.
Berman balloon flotation c.
Berman cardiac c.
Bernstein c.
Beta-Cap closure system for c.'s
Beta-Rail c.
Bicor c.
bicoudé c.
bifoil balloon c.
biliary balloon c.
BioGlide c.
Bio-Guard spectrum antimicrobial
  bonded c.
Bio-Medicus arterial c.
Biosearch female intermittent
  urinary c.
Biosearch male intermittent
  urinary c.
Biovue c.
bipolar pacing electrode c.
bipolar temporary pacemaker c.
bird's-eye c.
Bi-Set c.
Bitome c.
Bivona epistaxis c.
bladder c.
blade septostomy c.
Blasucci pigtail ureteral c.
Block right coronary guiding c.
blood-contactin c.
Blue FlexTip c.
Blue Max balloon c.
Blue Max triple-lumen c.
Bonnano c.

Bonnie balloon c.
Borge c.
Boston Scientific Sonicath
  imaging c.
Bourassa c.
Bozeman c.
Bozeman-Fritsch c.
BPS spinal angiographic c.
Braasch bulb ureteral c.
brachial coronary c.
braided diagnostic c.
Bresgen c.
Brevir-Kaith epidural c.
Brockenbrough mapping c.
Brockenbrough modified bipolar c.
Brockenbrough transseptal c.
Brodney c.
bronchial c.
Bronchitrac L flexible suction c.
bronchospirometric c.
Broviac atrial c.
Broviac hyperalimentation c.
Buchbinder Omniflex c.
Buchbinder Thruflex Over-the-
  Wire c.
BUD drainage c.
bulbous c.
bulb ureteral c.
bullet tip c.
Bunt c.
bur-bearing c.
Burhenne steerable c.
butterfly c.
bypass graft c.
bypass Speedy balloon c.
Calypso Rely c.
cam blade-tipped c.
Camino intracranial c.
Camino micromanometer c.
Camino microventricular bolt c.
Camino transducer c.
Campbell infant c.
cannulation c.
Can-Opt stand-alone dual lumen
  ERCP c.
Cardiac Assist intraaortic balloon c.
cardiac infant c.
Cardiomarker c.
Cardiomed Bodysoft epidural c.
Cardiomed endotracheal
  ventilation c.
Cardiomed thermodilution c.
Cardio Tactilaze peripheral
  angioplasty laser c.
Carlens bronchospirometric c.
Carson Zero Tip balloon
  dilatation c.
Castaneda-Malecot c.
Castillo c.
cathematic c.
Cath-Finder c.
Cath-Guide Closed Suction c.
CathLink 20 c.
Cathlon IV c.
Cathmark suction c.

Caud-a-Kaith epidural c.
caval c.
Cayote OTW balloon c.
CCOmbo c.
cecostomy c.
central venous pressure c.
cephalad c.
Cereblate c.
cerebral c.
C-Flex c.
Chaffin c.
16Ch, 18Ch indwelling silicone c.
Cheetah angioplasty c.
Chemo-Port c.
Cholangiocath c.
cholangiographic c.
cholangiography c.
Cholangiolapcath c.
chorionic villus sampling c.
Chubby balloon c.
Cisco covered needle c.
cisterna magna c.
Clark expanding mesh c.
Clark helix c.
Clark rotating cutter c.
Clay Adams PE-series c.
Clear Advantage latex free c.
Clear Advantage silicone male c.
CliniCath peripherally inserted c.
Clisco covered needle c.
Cloverleaf EP c.
coaxial c.
Cobe-Tenckhoff peritoneal dialysis c.
Cobra over-the-wire balloon c.
Codman-Holter c.
Codman ventricular silicone c.
coil c.
Coil-Cath c.
coil-tipped c.
colon motility c.
combination biliary brush c.
Comfort Cath I, II c.
Conceptus Soft Seal cervical c.
Conceptus Soft Torque uterine c.
Conceptus VS c.
condom c.
conductance c.
cone tip c.
conical c.
conical-tip c.
Constantine flexible metal c.
ConstaVac c.
continuous irrigation c.
Contour balloon dilatation c.
Conveen curved/tapered
  intermittent c.
Conveen female intermittent c.
Conveen Security+self-sealing male
  external c.
Cook arterial c.
Cook Cardiovascular infusion c.
Cook Spectrum c.
Cook TPN c.
Cook yellow pigtail c.
Cool Tip c.

C

catheter *(continued)*

Cope loop nephrostomy c.
Cordis BriteTip guiding c.
Cordis Ducor I, II, III coronary c.
Cordis Ducor pigtail c.
Cordis guiding c.
Cordis Lumelec c.
Cordis Predator balloon c.
Cordis Son-II c.
Cordis Titan balloon dilatation c.
Cordis Trakstar PTCA balloon c.
Cordis TransTaper tip c.
Cordis Webster diagnostic/ablation
  deflectable tip c.
Cordis Webster mapping c.
Corlon c.
coronary angiographic c.
coronary dilatation c.
coronary guiding c.
coronary perfusion c.
coronary seeking c.
coronary sinus thermodilution c.
corset balloon c.
Cotton graduated dilation c.
coudé suction c.
coudé-tip demeure c.
coudé urethral c.
Councill retention c.
Cournand quadpolar c.
Coxeter prostatic c.
C. R. Bard c.
Cribier-Letac c.
CritiCath PA c.
CritiCath thermodilution c.
Critikon balloon temporary
  pacing c.
Critikon balloon thermodilution c.
Critikon balloon wedge pressure c.
Critikon-Berman angiographic
  balloon c.
CrossSail coronary dilation c.
cryoablation c.
CUI c.
Cummings four-wing Malecot
  retention c.
Cummings nephrostomy c.
Cummings-Pezzer c.
cup c.
Curl Cath c.
curved c.
cutdown c.
CVIS intravascular US imaging c.
CVP c.
CVS c.
Cynosar c.
Cystocath c.
Dacron c.
Dakin c.
Damato curved c.
Datascope DL-II percutaneous
  translucent balloon c.
Datascope intra-aortic balloon
  pump c.
Datascope true sheathless c.
Davis c.
Davol sterile red rubber c.
Dearor model c.
decapolar electrode c.
decapolar pacing c.
decompression c.
decompression-feeding c.
decompressive enteroclysis c.
deflectable quadripolar c.
c. deflecting bridge
DeKock two-way bronchial c.
Delcath double-balloon c.
DeLee infant c.
DeLee suction c.
DeLee tracheal c.
Dent sleeve c.
DeOrio intrauterine insemination c.
de Pezzer mushroom-tipped c.
de Pezzer self-retaining c.
Derek-Harwood-Nash c.
Deseret flow-directed
  thermodilution c.
Desilets c.
Desilets-Hoffman c.
Devonshire c.
Devonshire-Mack c.
DeWeese caval c.
Diaflex ureteral dilatation c.
diagnostic ultrasound imaging c.
Dialy-Nate c.
dialysis c.
Diasonics c.
Digiflex high-flow c.
dilating pressure balloon c.
dilation balloon c.
dilator c.
Dispatch infusion c.
disposable c.
distal c.
DLP cardioplegic c.
DLP infant ventricular c.
DLP left atrial pressure
  monitoring c.
dog-leg c.
Doppler coronary c.
Dormia stone basket c.
Dorros brachial internal mammary
  guiding c.
Dorros infusion/probing c.
Dorros probing c.
Dotter caged-balloon c.
Dotter coaxial c.
double-chip micromanometer c.
double-current c.
double-J indwelling c.
double-J stent c.
double-J ureteral c.
double-lumen balloon stone
  extractor c.
double-lumen Broviac c.
double-lumen Hickman c.
double-lumen Hickman-Broviac c.
double-lumen injection c.
double-lumen Silastic c.
double-lumen subclavian c.

double-lumen Swan-Ganz c.
double-thermistor coronary sinus c.
Dover Premium teflon-coated latex Foley c.
Dover 100% silicone Foley c.
Dover teflon-coated latex Foley c.
Dover Texas Catheter Disposable Male C.
Dow Corning ileal pouch c.
Dowd, Dowd II prostatic balloon dilatation c.
drainage c.
Drew-Smythe c.
drill-tip c.
dual-lumen c.
dual-sensor micromanometric high-fidelity c.
Dualtherm dual-thermistor thermodilution c.
Ducor angiographic c.
Ducor balloon c.
Ducor cardiac c.
Ducor-Cordis pigtail c.
Ducor HF c.
duo-decapolar c.
Duo-Flow c.
DURAglide stone removal balloon c.
DVI Simpson AtheroCath c.
Dynacor Foley c.
Dynacor suction c.
Easy Rider neurovascular c.
E-cath c.
echo c.
EchoMark angiographic c.
EchoMark salpingography c.
echo transponder electrode c.
Edge dilatation c.
EDM infusion c.
Edslab cholangiography c.
Edwards diagnostic c.
Ehrlich c.
Eichelter-Schenk vena cava c.
EID percutaneous central venous large-bore c.
elbowed c.
Elecath electrophysiologic stimulation c.
Elecath thermodilution c.
electrode c.
electrohemostasis c.
El Gamal coronary bypass c.
El Gamal guiding c.
Elite guide c.
embolectomy c.
Encapsulon epidural c.
en chemise c.
Endeavor nondetachable silicone balloon c.
end-hole balloon-tipped c.
end-hole fluid-filled c.
end-hole French c.
end-hole pigtail c.
end-hole ureteral c.
EndoCPB c.

endoscopic retrograde cholangiopancreatography c.
EndoSonics balloon dilatation c.
EndoSonics IVUS/balloon dilatation c.
EndoSound endoscopic ultrasound c.
Endotak C lead c.
endotracheal c.
Enhanced Torque guiding c.
Entract dilation and occlusion c.
Envy c.
Eppendorf cardiac c.
EPTFE ventricular shunt c.
ERCP c.
ERCPeel Away c.
Erythroflex hydromer-coated central venous c.
esophageal balloon c.
esophageal manometry c.
esophageal perfusion c.
esophagoscopic c.
eustachian c.
Everett eustachian c.
Everett fallopian c.
Evermed c.
Evert-O-Cath drug delivery c.
Everyday self-adhering urinary external c.
eXamine cholangiography c.
exdwelling ureteral occlusion balloon c.
expandable access c.
Explorer pre-curved diagnostic EP c.
Express over-the-wire balloon c.
Express PTCA c.
Extended Wear self-adhering urinary external c.
external ureteral c.
Extractor three-lumen retrieval balloon c.
ExtraSafe c.
extrusion balloon c.
E-Z Cath c.
FACT-22 c.
FACT coronary balloon angioplasty c.
Falcon coronary c.
Falcon single-operator exchange balloon c.
fallopian c.
FAST balloon c.
FAST balloon flotation c.
FasTracker-18 infusion c.
FAST right heart cardiovascular c.
faucial eustachian c.
female c.
femoral cerebral c.
femoral guiding c.
femoral hemodialysis c.
fenestrated c.
Feth-R-Cath epidural c.
fiberoptic oximeter c.
fiberoptic pressure c.
filiform c.

catheter *(continued)*

filiform-tipped c.
fine-bore c.
Finesse large-lumen guiding c.
flat-blade-tipped c.
Flex-Cath double-lumen intra-aortic balloon c.
Flexguard tip c.
flexible metal c.
Flexi-Cath double-lumen intra-aortic balloon c.
Flexitip c.
Flexxicon Blue dialysis c.
Flexxicon II PC internal jugular c.
floating c.
flotation c.
flow-assisted short-term balloon c.
flow-directed balloon cardiovascular c.
flow-directed balloon-tipped c.
flow-directed thermodilution c.
FloWire Doppler c.
flow-oximetry c.
Flow Rider neurovascular c.
fluid-filled balloon-tipped flow-directed c.
Focus PV c.
Fogarty adherent clot c.
Fogarty arterial embolectomy c.
Fogarty arterial irrigation c.
Fogarty balloon biliary c.
Fogarty-Chin extrusion balloon c.
Fogarty-Chin peripheral dilatation c.
Fogarty dilation c.
Fogarty embolus c.
Fogarty gallstone c.
Fogarty graft thrombectomy c.
Fogarty occlusion c.
Fogarty Thru-Lumen c.
Fogarty venous irrigation c.
Fogarty venous thrombectomy c.
Folatex c.
Foley acorn-bulb c.
Foley-Alcock c.
Foley balloon c.
Foley cone-tip c.
Foley three-way c.
Foltz c.
Foltz-Overton cardiac c.
ForeRunner coronary sinus guiding c.
Formex barium c.
four-eye c.
four-lumen polyvinyl manometric c.
four-wing Malecot retention c.
Franz monophasic action potential c.
Freedom external c.
Freedom Pak Seven c.
Frekatheter vena cava c.
French angiographic c.
French Cope loop nephrostomy c.
French curve out-of-plane c.
French double-lumen c.

French Foley c.
French Gesco c.
French in-plane guiding c.
French JR4 Schneider c.
French MBIH c.
French mushroom-tip c.
French pigtail nephrostomy c.
French red-rubber Robinson c.
French Robinson c.
French SAL c.
French shaft c.
French Silastic Foley c.
French sizing of c.
French Teflon pyeloureteral c.
Friend c.
Friend-Hebert c.
Fritsch c.
Frydman c.
FullFlow c.
Furness c.
fused-tip c.
Gambro c.
Ganz-Edwards coronary infusion c.
Garceau ureteral c.
gastroenterostomy c.
Gauder Silicon PEG c.
Geenan graduated dilation c.
Gensini coronary arteriography c.
Gensini Teflon c.
Gentle-Flo suction c.
Gesco c.
Gibbon urethral c.
Gilbert pediatric balloon c.
Gilbert plug-sealing c.
Gilbert-type Bardex Foley c.
Gizmo c.
Glidecath hydrophilic coated c.
Glidewire c.
Glidex coated Percuflex c.
Glo-Tip ERCP c.
Goeltec c.
Gold Probe bipolar hemostasis c.
Gold Probe electrohemostasis c.
Goodale-Lubin cardiac c.
Gore-Tex peritoneal c.
Gorlin pacing c.
Gould PentaCath thermodilution c.
Gouley whalebone filiform c.
Goutz c.
graduated c.
Graft ACE fixed-wire balloon c.
graft-seeking c.
Graham c.
Greenfield caval c.
Grigor fiberoptic guiding c.
Grollman pigtail c.
Grollman pulmonary artery-seeking c.
Groshong double-lumen c.
Grüntzig arterial balloon c.
Grüntzig balloon angiography c.
Grüntzig-Dilaca c.
Grüntzig G, S dilating c.
Grüntzig steerable c.
Guidant guiding c.

c. guide
Guidefather c.
c. guide holder
c. guidewire
guiding c.
Guyon ureteral c.
H-1 c.
Hagner bag c.
Hakim c.
Hakko Dwellcath c.
Halo c.
Halocath c.
Hamilton-Steward c.
Hanafee c.
Hancock coronary perfusion c.
Hancock embolectomy c.
Hancock fiberoptic c.
Hancock hydrogen detection c.
Hancock luminal electrophysiologic
  recording c.
Hancock thermodilution c.
Hancock wedge-pressure c.
Harris c.
Hartmann eustachian c.
Hartzler ACS coronary dilation c.
Hartzler ACX II c.
Hartzler balloon c.
Hartzler dilatation c.
Hartzler Excel c.
Hartzler LPS dilatation c.
Hartzler Micro-600 c.
Hartzler Micro II c.
Hartzler Micro XT c.
Hartzler RX-14 balloon c.
Hartzler Ultra-Lo-Profile c.
Hatch c.
headhunter visceral angiography c.
HealthShield antimicrobial
  mediastinal wound drainage c.
Heartport Endocoronary Sinus c.
helical PTCA dilatation c.
helical-tip Halo c.
helium-filled balloon c.
Helix PTCA dilatation c.
hemodialysis c.
Hemoject injection c.
hemostatic c.
Hepacon c.
heparin-coated c.
hexapolar c.
Heyer-Schulte c.
Heyer-Schulte-Pudenz cardiac c.
H-H open-end alimentation c.
Hickman-Broviac c.
Hickman indwelling right atrial c.
Hickman tunneled c.
Hidalgo c.
Hieshima coaxial c.
Higgins c.
high-fidelity micromanometric c.
high-flow c.
high-speed rotation dynamic
  angioplasty c.
Hilal modified headhunter c.
His bundle c.

Hi5 Torq Flow c.
Hi-Torque Floppy guide c.
Hobbs dilatation balloon c.
hockey-stick c.
Hohn c.
Hollister external c.
Hollister self-adhesive c.
Holter distal atrial c.
Holter distal peritoneal c.
Holter-Hausner c.
Holter lumboperitoneal c.
Holter ventricular c.
Holt self-retaining c.
hooked c.
Hopkins Percuflex drainage c.
hot-tipped c.
Hryntschak c.
HUI c.
Huibregtse-Katon ERCP c.
Hunter-Sessions vena cava-occluding
  balloon c.
Hurwitt c.
HydraCross TLC PTCA c.
HydroCath central venous c.
Hydrogel-coated PTCA balloon c.
Hydromer grafted c.
hydrostatic balloon c.
Hymes double-lumen c.
hyperalimentation c.
hysterosalpingography c.
IAB c.
940 IAB C.
ICP c.
ICP-T fiberoptic ICP monitoring c.
Illumen-8, -9 guiding c.
ILUS c.
Imager Torque selective c.
imaging-angioplasty balloon c.
Imperson c.
implantable
  cardioverter/defibrillator c.
Impra peritoneal c.
indwelling Foley c.
indwelling subclavian c.
indwelling venous c.
infant female c.
infant male c.
inferior vena cava c.
Infiniti c.
inflatable Foley bag c.
Infusaid c.
Infuse-a-Port c.
InfusaSleeve II c.
Infuse-A-Cath c.
infusion c.
Ingram c.
injection electrode c.
Inmed whistle tip urethral c.
Inoue balloon c.
inside-the-needle c. (INC)
inside-the-needle infusion c.
Intact c.
Integra c.
Intellicath pulmonary artery c.
intercostal c.

C

catheter *(continued)*

Interpret ultrasound c.
interventional c.
Intimax biliary c.
Intimax cholangiography c.
Intimax occlusion c.
Intimax vascular c.
intraaortic balloon c.
intraarterial chemotherapy c.
intracardiac c.
Intracath c.
intracoronary guiding c.
intracoronary perfusion c.
intracranial pressure c.
Intraducer peritoneal c.
intraductal imaging c.
intramedullary c.
Intran intrauterine pressure
  measurement c.
intrapleural c.
Intrasil c.
intraurethral prostatic bridge c.
intrauterine c. (IUC)
intrauterine insemination c.
intrauterine pressure c.
intravascular ultrasound c.
intravenous pacing c.
intravenous ultrasound c.
intraventricular pressure
  monitoring c.
Intrepid balloon c.
Intrepid percutaneous transluminal
  coronary angioplasty c.
Intrepid PTCA c.
introducer c.
c. introducer
irrigating c.
irrigation c.
Itard eustachian c.
ITC radiopaque balloon c.
IUI c.
IV c.
Jackman coronary sinus electrode c.
Jackman orthogonal c.
Jackson-Pratt c.
Jacques c.
Jaeger-Whiteley c.
James lumbar peritoneal c.
Javid c.
Jehle coronary perfusion c.
Jelco intravenous c.
Jelm two-way c.
Jinotti dual-purpose c.
JL c.
JL4, JL5 c.
Jo-Kath c.
Josephson quadripolar c.
Jostra c.
JR c.
JR4, JR5 c.
Judkins coronary c.
Judkins curve LAD c.
Judkins curve LCX c.
Judkins curve STD c.

Judkins guiding c.
Judkins left coronary c.
Judkins left 4 (JL4) c.
Judkins left (JL) c.
Judkins right coronary c.
Judkins right (JR) c.
Judkins torque-control c.
Judkins USCI c.
jugular venous c.
J-Vac c.
Kaminsky c.
Karmen c.
Katon c.
Katzen long balloon dilatation c.
Kaufman c.
KDF-2.3 intrauterine insemination c.
Kearns bag c.
Kensey atherectomy c.
kidney internal stent c.
Kifa green, grey, red, yellow, c.
Kimball c.
King guiding c.
King multipurpose coronary graft c.
kink-resistant peritoneal c.
Kinsey atherectomy c.
Kish urethral c.
Koala intrauterine pressure c.
Konigsberg c.
Kontron balloon c.
Kumpe c.
Lacricath lacrimal duct c.
lacrimal balloon c.
Lahey c.
Landmark midline c.
Lane rectal c.
laparoscopic cholangiography c.
Lapides c.
LAP-13 Ranfac cholangiographic c.
Lapras c.
large-bore c.
large-lumen c.
laser delivery c.
latex c.
Latis c.
Latson multipurpose c.
lavaging c.
L-Cath peripherally inserted
  neonatal c.
Ledor pigtail c.
LeFort male c.
LeFort urethral c.
left coronary c.
left heart c.
left Judkins c.
left ventricular sump c.
c. leg strap
c. leg tube holder
Lehman aortographic c.
Lehman pancreatic manometry c.
Lehman ventriculography c.
lensed fiber-tip laser delivery c.
LeRoy ventricular c.
LeVeen c.
Levin tube c.
Leycom volume conductance c.

Lifecath c.
Lifemed c.
Lifestream coronary dilation c.
Lillehei-Warden c.
Lincoff design of Storz scleral
  buckling balloon c.
Lionheart c.
Lloyd bronchial c.
Lloyd double c.
Lloyd esophagoscopic c.
lobster-tail c.
Lofric disposable urethral c.
long ACE fixed-wire balloon c.
Long Brite Tip guiding c.
Longdwel Teflon c.
Long Skinny over-the-wire
  balloon c.
long-term internal jugular c.
Lo-Profile II balloon c.
Lo-Profile steerable dilatation c.
low-profile balloon-positioning c.
low-speed rotation angioplasty c.
LTX PTCA c.
Lucae eustachian c.
Lumaguide infusion c.
lumbar peritoneal c.
lumbar subarachnoid c.
Lumelec pacing c.
Lunderquist c.
Lynx OTW c.
Magill endotracheal c.
Maglinte c.
magnet-tipped flexible c.
Mahurkar curved extension c.
Mahurkar dual-lumen femoral
  dialysis c.
male c.
Malecot two-wing c.
Malecot four-wing c.
Malecot nephrostomy c.
Malecot reentry c.
Malecot self-retaining urethral c.
Malecot Silastic c.
Malecot suprapubic cystostomy c.
Mallinckrodt angiographic c.
Mallinckrodt vertebral c.
Maloney c.
Manashil sialography c.
Mandelbaum c.
Mani cerebral c.
manometer-tipped c.
manometric c.
Mansfield Atri-Pace 1 c.
Mansfield balloon dilatation c.
Mansfield orthogonal electrode c.
Mansfield Scientific dilatation
  balloon c.
Mansfield-Webster c.
Mansfield-Webster deflectable
  curve c.
mapping c.
mapping/ablation c.
Marathon guiding c.
marker c.

Mark IV Moss decompression-
  feeding c.
Marlin thoracic c.
Marrs intrauterine c.
Maryfield introducer c.
mastoid c.
Max Force balloon dilatation c.
Max Force TTS biliary balloon
  dilatation c.
Maxxum balloon c.
McCarthy c.
McCaskey antral c.
McGoon coronary perfusion c.
McIntosh double-lumen
  hemodialysis c.
McIver nephrostomy c.
Meadox Surgimed c.
measuring-mounting c.
Med-Co flexible c.
Medena continent ileostomy c.
mediastinal c.
Medicut c.
Medina ileostomy c.
MediPort-DL (double-lumen) c.
Medi-Tech arterial dilatation c.
Medi-Tech-Mansfield dilating c.
Medi-Tech occlusion balloon c.
Medi-Tech steerable c.
Medrad angiographic c.
Medtronic balloon c.
Medtronic Transvene 6937
  electrode c.
Memokath c.
memory c.
Menlo Care c.
Mentor coudé c.
Mentor Foley c.
Mentor Self-Cath soft c.
Mentor straight c.
Mentor Tele-Cath ileal conduit
  sampling c.
Mentor-Urosan external c.
Mercier c.
metal ball-tip c.
metallic-tip c.
Metaport c.
Metras bronchial c.
Mewissen infusion c.
Micor c.
microendoscopic optical c.
Micro-Guide c.
micromanometer c.
MicroMewi multiple sidehole
  infusion c.
Microsoftrac c.
Micro-Soft Stream sidehole
  infusion c.
Micross dilatation c.
MicroTip c.
Micro-Transducer c.
MicroVac c.
Microvasive Rigiflex balloon c.
MicroView sheath-based IVUS c.
midstream aortogram c.
Mikaelsson c.

C

catheter *(continued)*

Mikro-Tip micromanometer-tipped c.
Millar Doppler c.
Millar micromonometer c.
Millar MPC-500 c.
Millar pigtail angiographic c.
Millar urodynamic c.
Millenia balloon c.
Millenia percutaneous transluminal
  coronary angioplasty (PTCA) c.
Miller-Abbott c.
Miller septostomy c.
Mills operative peripheral
  angioplasty c.
MiniBard c.
Mini-Profile dilatation c.
Minispace IUI c.
Mirage over-the-wire balloon c.
Missouri c.
Mitsubishi angioscopic c.
Mixtner c.
Molina needle c.
MoniTorr CIP lumbar c.
monofoil c.
Monorail angioplasty c.
Monorail imaging c.
Monorail Piccolino c.
Morris thoracic c.
Moss decompression feeding c.
Moss Suction Buster c.
MP-A-1 c.
MP-A-2 c.
MPR drain c.
MS Classique balloon dilatation c.
MTC Ventcontrol ventricular c.
Mueller c.
Mullins transseptal c.
multi-access c.
multielectrode basket c.
multielectrode impedance c.
multiflanged Portnoy c.
Multiflex c.
multilayer design c.
multilumen manometric c.
Multi-Med triple-lumen infusion c.
multiplex c.
multipolar electrode c.
multipolar impedance c.
multipurpose c.
multisensor c.
Multistim electrode c.
mushroom c.
Mylar c.
Mystic balloon c.
Namic c.
NarrowFlex intra-aortic balloon c.
nasal c.
nasobiliary c.
nasocystic c.
nasopancreatic c.
nasotracheal c.
nasovesicular c.
NBIH c.
NC Bandit c.

NC Big Ranger OTW balloon c.
NDSB occlusion balloon c.
Neal c.
c. needle
needle tip c.
Nélaton urethral c.
Neonatal Y TrachCare c.
Neoplex c.
Neo-Sert umbilical vessel c.
nephrostomy c.
Nestor guiding c.
Neuroguide Visicath viewing c.
Nexus 2 linear ablation c.
Niagara temporary dialysis c.
Nichols-Jehle coronary multihead c.
NIH cardiomarker c.
NIH Image 1.54 c.
NIH left ventriculography c.
NIH marking c.
nondetachable silicone balloon c.
nonflotation c.
nonflow-directed c.
nontraumatizing c.
NoProfile balloon c.
Norfolk intrauterine aspiration c.
Norton flow-directed Swan-Ganz
  thermodilution c.
NovaCath multilumen infusion c.
Nova thermodilution c.
Novoste c.
Numed intracoronary Doppler c.
Nutricath c.
Nycore angiography pigtail c.
occlusion c.
octapolar c.
Odman-Ledin c.
Olbert NoProfile balloon
  dilatation c.
olivary c.
olive-tipped c.
Olympus II PTCA dilatation c.
Olympus PW-1L wash c.
Omni c.
OmniCath atherectomy c.
Omniflex balloon c.
On-Command c.
one-hole angiographic c.
Onik-Cohen percutaneous access c.
Opaca-Garcea ureteral c.
open-ended ureteral c.
Opta 5 c.
Optical c.
Opticath oximeter c.
Opti-Flow permanent dialysis c.
Optiscope c.
Optiva c.
Oracle Focus PTCA c.
Oracle Focus ultrasound imaging c.
Oracle intravascular ultrasound c.
Oracle Megasonics c.
Oracle Micro intravascular
  ultrasound c.
Oracle Micro Plus PTCA c.
Oral-Cath c.
ORC-B Ranfac cholangiographic c.

Oreopoulos-Zellerman c.
over-the-needle infusion c.
over-the-wire PTCA balloon c.
Owatusi double c.
Owen Lo-Profile dilation c.
oximetric c.
oximetry c.
pacemaker c.
Paceport c.
Pacewedge dual-pressure bipolar
  pacing c.
Pacifico c.
pacing c.
Panther c.
Paparella c.
Park blade septostomy c.
partially-implantable c.
P.A.S. Port Fluoro-Free c.
Passage balloon dilation c.
Passport Balloon-on-a-Wire
  dilatation c.
Pathfinder c.
PA Watch position-monitoring c.
pectoral c.
pediatric balloon c.
pediatric Foley c.
pediatric pigtail c.
Pedicath c.
peel-away banana c.
peel-off c.
pennate suction c.
Pennine Nélaton c.
PENSIL catheter Penn State
  Intravascular Lung c.
PentaCath c.
Pentalumen c.
PentaPace QRS c.
PE Plus II balloon dilatation c.
PE Plus II peripheral balloon c.
Per-C-Cath c.
Percor dual-lumen (DL) intra-aortic
  balloon c.
Percor-Stat-DL c.
Percuflex nephrostomy c.
percutaneous central venous c.
percutaneous drainage c.
percutaneous intra-aortic balloon
  counterpulsation c.
percutaneous nephrostomy
  Malecot c.
percutaneous rotational
  thrombectomy c.
percutaneous transhepatic biliary
  drainage c.
percutaneous transhepatic pigtail c.
percutaneous transluminal coronary
  angioplasty c.
perfusion balloon c.
Periflow peripheral balloon
  angioplasty-infusion c.
peripheral atherectomy c.
peripheral long-line c.
peripherally inserted c.
peripherally inserted central c.
  (PICC)

peripherally inserted central
  venous c. (PICVC)
peritoneal dialysis c. (PCD)
peritoneal reflux control c.
permanent silicone c.
PermCath dual-lumen c.
Per-Q-Cath CVP c.
Perry-Foley c.
Perry pediatric Foley latex c.
Personal Catheter 100% silicone
  intermittent c.
Per-Stat-DL c.
pervenous c.
Pezzer mushroom-tipped c.
Pezzer self-retaining urethral c.
Pezzer suprapubic cystostomy c.
Pfeifer c.
Phantom V Plus balloon
  dilatation c.
Pharmaseal c.
Pharmex disposable c.
Phillips urethral c.
Phillips urologic c.
Phoenix Anti-Blok ventricular c.
PIBC c.
Piccolino Monorail c.
Pico-ST II low-profile balloon c.
pigtail c.
Pilcher c.
Pilotip c.
Pinkerton balloon c.
Pipelle endometrial suction c.
Pivot fixed-wire balloon c.
plastic Tiemann c.
Pleur-evac chest c.
pleurx c.
c. plug
pneumatic balloon c.
POC Bandit c.
Polaris LE c.
Polaris steerable diagnostic c.
POLY balloon c.
Poly-Cath c.
polyethylene intravenous c.
Polysil-Foley c.
Polystan venous return c.
PolyTech nonlatex self-adhering
  urinary external c.
polyurethane nasoenteric c.
polyvinyl c.
"pop-on" self-adhering male
  external c.
Port-A-Cath implantable c.
portal c.
Portex chorionic villus sampling c.
Portex-Gibbon c.
Portnoy multiflanged c.
Portnoy ventricular c.
Porto-Vac c.
position-sensing c.
Positrol II Bernstein c.
Positrol USCI c.
Pousson pigtail c.
Predator balloon c.
preformed Cordis c.

C

catheter *(continued)*

preshaped c.
Priestly c.
Prima Laser c.
Pro-Bal protected balloon-tipped c.
probe balloon c.
c. probe ultrasound
probing sheath exchange c.
Procath electrophysiology c.
ProCross Rely over-the-wire
 balloon c.
Profile Plus balloon dilatation c.
Proflex dilatation c.
Pro-Flo XT c.
Prostaprobe c.
prostatic bridge c.
ProSys silicone sterile 2-way, 3-way
 Foley c.
Pruitt-Inahara balloon-tipped
 perfusion c.
Pruitt irrigation c.
Pruitt occlusion c.
PTBD c.
PTCA c.
Pudenz barium cardiac c.
Pudenz-Heyer vascular c.
Pudenz infant cardiac c.
Pudenz peritoneal c.
Pudenz ventricular c.
pulmonary arterial c.
pulmonary artery c.
pulmonary flotation c.
pulmonary triple-lumen c.
pulse spray c.
Pursuit c.
pusher c.
push-pull c.
Putnam evacuator c.
pyeloureteral c.
Q-cath c.
Quadra-Flo infusion c.
quadripolar electrode c.
quadripolar 6-French diagnostic
 electrophysiology c.
quadripolar pacing c.
quadripolar steerable electrode c.
quadripolar steerable
 mapping/ablation c.
Quanticor c.
Quantum Ranger OTW balloon c.
quick c.
QuickFlash arterial c.
Quinton biopsy c.
Quinton central venous c.
Quinton dual-lumen c.
Quinton-Mahurkar dual-lumen
 peritoneal c.
Quinton peritoneal c.
Quinton PermCath c.
Quinton Q-Port c.
Raaf Cath vascular c.
Raaf dual-lumen c.
Racz c.
radial artery c.

Radiofocus Glidewire angiography c.
radiofrequency-generated thermal
 balloon c.
radiopaque calibrated c.
radiopaque ERCP c.
radiopaque silastic c.
railway c.
Raimondi peritoneal c.
Raimondi ventricular c.
Ramirez winged c.
Ranfac cholangiographic c.
Ranger OTW balloon c.
rapid exchange balloon c.
rapid exchange Flowtrack c.
Rashkind septostomy balloon c.
rat-tail c.
RC1, RC2 c.
recessed balloon septostomy c.
rectal c.
Reddick cystic duct
 cholangiogram c.
Reddick-Saye screw c.
RediFurl TaperSeal IAB c.
RediGuard c.
RediGuard IAB c.
red Robinson c.
red rubber c.
reference c.
Reif c.
Reliance urinary control insert c.
Rentrop infusion c.
reperfusion c.
Replogle c.
retention c.
retrograde femoral c.
retrograde occlusion balloon c.
retroperfusion c.
return-flow hemostatic c.
return-flow retention c.
Revivac c.
Reynolds infusion c.
RF Ablatr ablation c.
RF balloon c.
RF Marinr c.
RF Performer c.
rheolytic c.
Rica eustachian c.
right-angle chest c.
right Judkins c.
Rigiflex ABD balloon dilatation c.
Rigiflex biliary balloon dilatation c.
Rigiflex OTW balloon dilatation c.
Rigiflex TTS balloon dilatation c.
RIJ c.
Ring biliary drainage c.
Ring-McLean c.
Ritchie c.
Rivas vascular c.
Robinson urethral c.
Rochester Medical self-adhering
 male external c.
Rochester Medical 100% silicone
 Foley c.
Rockey-Thompson c.
Rodriguez c.

Rodriguez-Alvarez c.
Rolnel c.
Rosch c.
Ross c.
Rotacs motorized c.
Rothene c.
round-tip c.
rove magnetic c.
Royal Flush angiographic flush c.
rubber c.
rubber-shod c.
Rumel c.
Rusch bronchial c.
Rusch coudé c.
Ruschelit c.
Rusch external c.
Rusch-Foley c.
Rutner nephrostomy balloon c.
Rutner wedge c.
RX-014 balloon c.
RX perfusion c.
RX Streak balloon c.
Sable balloon c.
Sacks QuickStick c.
Sacks Single-Step c.
Safe-Dwel Plus c.
Safe-T-Coat heparin-coated
  thermodilution c.
SafTouch c.
Salvage c.
Saratoga sump c.
Sarns wire-reinforced c.
SCA-EX ShortCutter c.
Schneider c.
Schneider-Shiley dilatation c.
Schoonmaker femoral c.
Schoonmaker multipurpose c.
Schrotter c.
Schwarten balloon dilatation c.
Schwarten LP balloon c.
Science-Med balloon c.
Sci-Med angioplasty c.
Sci-Med guiding c.
Scimed rTRA-GC guiding c.
Sci-Med SSC "Skinny" c.
scleral buckling c.
Scoop 1, 2 c.
Scoop transtracheal c.
Security+ self-sealing Urisheath
  external c.
Seidel c.
Seldinger cardiac c.
Selecon coronary angiography c.
Selective-HI c.
Seletz c.
Self-Cath coudé tipped c.
Self-Cath soft c.
Self-Cath straight tipped female c.
Self-Cath straight tipped pediatric c.
Self-Cath straight tipped soft c.
self-guiding c.
self-retaining c.
Sellheim uterine c.
semirigid c.
Semm uterine vacuum c.

Sensation intra-aortic balloon c.
sensing c.
Sentron pigtail angiographic
  micromanometer c.
Sentron pigtail microtip-
  manometer c.
septostomy balloon c.
Seroma-Cath wound drainage c.
serrated c.
SET three-lumen thrombectomy c.
S-G c.
Shadow over-the-wire balloon c.
Shadow-Stripe c.
Shaldon c.
shaver c.
Shaw c.
c. sheath
Sheldon c.
shellac-covered c.
shepherd's hook c.
Sherpa guiding c.
Shiley guiding c.
Shiley-Ionescu c.
Shiley irrigation c.
Shiley MultiPro c.
Shiley soft-tip guiding c.
SHJR4, SHJR4s c.
short-arm Grollman c.
ShortCutter c.
Shulitz c.
side-hole Judkins right, 4-cm
  curved, short c.
side-hole pigtail c.
sidewinder percutaneous intra-aortic
  balloon c.
Siegel-Cohen dilating c.
Silastic Brand sterile Foley c.
Silastic elastomer infusion c.
Silastic ileal reservoir c.
Silastic mushroom c.
Silcath subclavian c.
silicone elastomer infusion c.
silicone epistaxis c.
silicone Robinson c.
silicone rubber Dacron-cuffed c.
Silicore c.
Silitek c.
silk-and-wax c.
Sil-Med c.
silver c.
Simmons 1, 2, 3 c.
Simmons II, III c.
Simmons sidewinder c.
Simplastic c.
Simplus PE/t dilatation c.
Simpson atherectomy c.
Simpson coronary AtheroCath c.
Simpson-Robert ACS dilatation c.
Simpson suction c.
Simpson Ultra Lo-Profile II
  balloon c.
single-lumen balloon stone
  extractor c.
single-lumen infusion c.
single-stage c.

catheter *(continued)*
six-eye c.
Skene c.
Skinny balloon c.
Skinny dilatation c.
Skinny over-the-wire balloon c.
Sleek c.
Slider c.
sliding-rail c.
Slinky balloon c.
Slinky PTCA c.
Slip-Sheen c.
Smart position-sensing c.
SMIC eustachian c.
snare c.
Soehendra dilating c.
Soehendra Universal c.
Soft-Cell permanent dual-lumen c.
SOF-T guiding c.
Softip arteriography c.
Softip diagnostic c.
Softouch Cobra 1, 2 c.
Softouch Headhunter 1 c.
Softouch Multipurpose B2 c.
Softouch Simmons 1, 2 c.
Softouch spinal angiography c.
Softouch UHF cardiac pigtail c.
Softrac-PTA c.
Soft Torque uterine c.
Soft-Vu angiographic c.
Soft-Vu Omni flush c.
solid-state esophageal manometry c.
solid-tip c.
Solo c.
SoloPass c.
Sones Cardio-Marker c.
Sones coronary c.
Sones Hi-Flow c.
Sones Positrol c.
Sones vent c.
Sones woven Dacron c.
Sonicath endoluminal ultrasound c.
Sonicath imaging c.
Sonicath intravascular ultrasound c.
Sorenson thermodilution c.
Soules intrauterine insemination c.
Spectra-Cath STP c.
Spectraprobe-PLS laser
  angioplasty c.
Speedy balloon c.
Spetzler subarachnoid c.
SPI-Argent II peritoneal dialysis c.
spinal c.
SpineCATH intradiscal c.
spiral-tipped c.
split-sheath c.
Spring c.
Sprint c.
Squibb c.
Squire c.
Stack perfusion coronary
  dilatation c.
Stamey Malecot c.
Stamey open-tip ureteral c.

Standard Care sterile urethral c.
standard ERCP c.
standard Lehman c.
Stanford end-hole pigtail c.
Stargate falloposcopy c.
StatLock-Foley c.
St. Bartholomew barium c.
Stealth angioplasty balloon c.
steerable decapolar electrode c.
steerable guidewire c.
steering c.
Steerocath c.
stenting c.
Steri-Cath c.
Stertzer brachial guiding c.
stimulating c.
Stitt c.
Storz bronchial c.
Storz-DeKock two-way bronchial c.
Storz scleral buckling balloon c.
straight flush percutaneous c.
Streamline peripheral c.
StressCath c.
Stretzer bent-tip USCI c.
Stringer tracheal c.
Stripseal c.
styletted tracheobronchial c.
subclavian apheresis c.
subclavian dialysis c.
subclavian hemodialysis c.
subclavian vein access c.
submicroinfusion c.
Sub-4 small-vessel balloon
  dilatation c.
suction c.
Suction Buster c.
Suggs c.
Sugita c.
SULP II balloon c.
sump pump c.
Supercath intravenous c.
Superflow guiding c.
Super-9 guiding c.
Superior suction c.
Super Torque Plus c.
SupraFoley c.
suprapubic c.
SureCath port access c.
Sure Seal Golden Drain c.
Surflo IV c.
surgically implanted hemodialysis c.
Surgimedics cholangiography c.
Surgitek Double-J ureteral c.
Swan-Ganz balloon flotation c.
Swan-Ganz bipolar pacing c.
Swan-Ganz flow-directed c.
Swan-Ganz guidewire TD c.
Swan-Ganz Pacing TD c.
Swan-Ganz pulmonary artery c.
Swan-Ganz thermodilution c.
swan-neck Missouri c.
swan-neck pediatric Coil-Cath c.
Switzerland dilatation c.
TAC atherectomy c.
Tactilaze angioplasty laser c.

Tandem thin-shaft transureteroscopic balloon dilatation c.
tapered c.
tapered-tip hydrophilic-coated push c.
Tauber male urethrographic c.
Taut cholangiographic c.
Taut cystic duct c.
Taut M55, M56, M57 c.
TEC extraction c.
Tefcat intrauterine insemination c.
Teflon ERCP c.
Teflon guiding c.
Teflon injection c.
Teflon needle c.
Teflon-tipped c.
TEGwire balloon dilatation c.
telescoping plugged c.
temporary pacing c.
Tenckhoff 2-cuff c.
Tenckhoff peritoneal c.
Tenckhoff renal dialysis c.
Tennis Racquet angiographic c.
Ten system balloon c.
Terumo SP coaxial c.
Terumo Surflo intravenous c.
Tesio c.
tetrapolar esophageal c.
Texas condom c.
ThermaChoice c.
thermistor thermodilution c.
thermodilution balloon c.
thermodilution pacing c.
thermodilution Swan-Ganz c.
thin-wall introducer c.
Thompson bronchial c.
ThoraCath c.
thoracic c.
three-way Foley c.
three-way irrigating c.
thrombectomy c.
thrombosuction c.
Thruflex PTCA balloon c.
Tiemann coudé c.
Tiemann-Foley c.
Tiemann Neoflex c.
Timberlake c.
tip-deflecting c.
c. tip occluder
Tis-U-Trap endometrial suction c.
Tital balloon c.
Titan-Mega c.
TLC Baxter balloon c.
Tolantins bone marrow infusion c.
Tomac c.
Tomac-Nélaton c.
toposcopic c.
Torcon NB selective angiographic c.
Torktherm torque control c.
Toronto-Western c.
torque-control balloon c.
totally-implantable c.
Tourguide guiding c.
Trabucco double balloon c.
tracer c.

TrachCare multi-access c.
tracheal c.
Tracker infusion c.
Tracker Soft Stream side-hole microinfusion c.
Tracker-18 Unibody c.
Trac Plus c.
Trakstar balloon c.
transcervical tubal access c.
transcutaneous extraction c.
transducer-tipped c.
transfemoral endoaortic occlusion c.
translumbar inferior vena cava c.
transluminal angioplasty c.
transluminal endarterectomy c.
transnasal intraduodenal feeding c.
transoral c.
Transport c.
transseptal c.
transthoracic c.
transtracheal oxygen c.
transurethral c.
transvenous pacemaker c.
Trattner urethrographic c.
trefoil balloon c.
Triguide c.
Trilogy low-profile balloon dilatation c.
triple-lumen Arrow c.
triple-lumen balloon flotation thermistor c.
triple-lumen biliary manometry c.
triple-lumen central c.
triple-lumen manometry c.
triple-thermistor coronary sinus c.
tripolar Damato curve c.
tripolar electrode c.
tripolar w/Damato curve c.
Trocath peritoneal dialysis c.
Troeltsch eustachian c.
True Sheathless c.
T-TAC c.
TTS c.
T-tube c.
tunnelable ventricular ICP c.
Tuohy c.
twist drill c.
two-way c.
Tygon c.
Tyshak balloon valvuloplasty c.
UCAC diagnostic c.
Uldall subclavian hemodialysis c.
Ultraflex self-adhering male external c.
Ultramer c.
c. ultrasound probe
umbilical venous c.
UMI c.
Unicath all-purpose c.
UNI shunt c.
Universal drainage c.
Uniweave c.
Ureflex ureteral c.
Uresil biliary c.

C

catheter *(continued)*

Uresil embolectomy
thrombectomy c.
Uresil irrigation c.
Uresil occlusion balloon c.
ureteral dilatation c.
ureteral occlusion c.
urethral c.
urethrographic c.
Uridome c.
Uridrop c.
urinary c.
Urocare Foley c.
Uro-Cath molded latex male
external c.
Uro-Con Texas style male
external c.
urodynamic c.
Urofoam-1, -2 adhesive foam strip
for male external c.
urological c.
UroMax II high-pressure balloon c.
Uro-San Plus external c.
USCI Bard c.
USCI Finesse guiding c.
USCI guiding c.
USCI Mini-Profile balloon
dilatation c.
USCI Positrol coronary c.
uterine cornual access c.
uterine ostial access c.
Vabra c.
Vacurette c.
vacuum aspiration c.
valve-ended c.
valvuloplasty balloon c.
Van Aman pigtail c.
Van Buren c.
Vance-Kish urethral illuminated c.
Vance percutaneous Malecot
nephrostomy c.
van Sonnenberg gallbladder c.
van Sonnenberg sump c.
van Sonnenberg-Wittich c.
Van Tassel pigtail c.
Vantec occlusion balloon c.
Vantec ureteral balloon dilatation c.
Variflex c.
Vas-Cath Opti-Plast peripheral
angioplasty c.
vascular access c.
Vaso-Cath peritoneal dialysis c.
Vaxcel c.
Vector large-lumen guiding c.
VectorX large-lumen guiding c.
Venaport c.
venous irrigation c.
venous thrombectomy c.
venting c.
Ventra c.
ventricular c.
ventriculography c.
Ventureyra ventricular c.
Verbatim balloon c.

Versaflex steerable c.
vertebrated c.
vessel-sizing c.
Viper PTA c.
Virden rectal c.
Visicath viewing c.
Vision PTCA c.
Visi-Tube c.
Vitalcor venous return c.
Vitatron E c.
Vitax female c.
Vitesse Cos laser c.
Vitesse E-II coronary c.
c. vitrector
Vivonex jejunostomy c.
V. Mueller embolectomy c.
Voda c.
Von Andel biliary dilation c.
VPI nonadhesive condom c.
Vygon Nutricath S c.
c. waist tube holder
Walrus Advancit c.
Walrus Angioflus c.
Walther female c.
Was-Catheter c.
washing c.
Watanabe c.
water-infusion esophageal
manometry c.
water-perfused c.
wave guide c.
Weber rectal c.
Weber winged c.
Webster coronary sinus c.
Webster orthogonal electrode c.
wedge pressure balloon c.
Western external urinary c.
Wexler c.
whalebone filiform c.
whistle-tip Foley c.
whistle-tip ureteral c.
Wholey balloon occlusion c.
Wholey-Edwards c.
Wick c.
Wideband urinary c.
Williams L-R guiding c.
Wilson-Cook fine-needle-aspiration c.
Wilton-Webster coronary sinus
thermodilution c.
Wilton-Webster thermodilution flow
and pacing c.
Winer c.
winged c.
Winston SD c.
wire stylet c.
Wishard ureteral c.
Witzel enterostomy c.
Wolf nephrostomy c.
Woodruff ureteropyelographic c.
Word Bartholin gland c.
woven Dacron c.
woven silk c.
Wurd c.
Xemex pulmonary artery c.

XL-11 Ranfac percutaneous cholangiographic c.
Xpeedior c.
X-Trode electrode c.
Yankauer eustachian c.
Y-trough c.
Zavod bronchospirometry c.
Zimmon c.
Z-Med balloon c.
Zucker cardiac c.
Zucker multipurpose bipolar c.
Zuma coronary guiding c.
Zurich dilatation c.
catheter-based ultrasound probe
catheter-borne sector transducer
catheter-introducing forceps
catheterizing Foroblique telescope
Catheter-Secure tape
catheter-tip micromanometer system
catheter-tipped manometer
Cath-Finder
    C.-F. catheter
    C.-F. catheter tracking system
Cath-Guide Closed Suction catheter
CathLink
    C. 20 catheter
    C. implantable vascular access device
Cath-Lok catheter locking device
Cathlon IV catheter
Cathmark suction catheter
cathode
    c. ray oscilloscope
    c. ray tube (CRT)
Cath-Secure
    C.-S. catheter holder
    C.-S. Dual Tab holder
    C.-S. tape
Cath-Strip catheter fastener
CathTrack catheter locator system
Catlin amputation knife
CatsEye digital camera system
Cat's Paw exerciser
cat's paw retractor
Cattell
    C. forked-type T- tube
    C. gallbladder tube
Caud-a-Kaith epidural catheter
caudal
    c. hook
    c. needle
caulking gun
Cault punch
Causse piston
cauterizer
    Bucholz bipolar c.
cauterizing ball
cautery
    Aaron c.
    c. ablator
    Accu-Temp c.
    ACMI c.
    Acucise ureteral cutting c.
    Alcon hand c.
    alkaline battery c.

Berchtold c.
Berkeley Bioengineering bipolar c.
BICAP II c.
BiLAP bipolar c.
bipolar c.
Birtcher c.
Bovie wet-field c.
Burdick c.
Cameron c.
c. clamp
Codman-Mentor Wet-Field c.
cold (carbon dioxide) c.
Colorado tip c.
Concept disposable c.
Concept hand-held c.
Corrigan c.
cutting c.
Davis-Bovie c.
Denis bipolar c.
disposable c.
Downes c.
electrocautery c.
c. electrode
Eraser c.
Eraser-tip c.
Fine micropoint c.
Geiger c.
Gonin c.
Goodhill c.
hand-control c.
Hildreth ocular c.
c. hook
Hotsy high-temperature c.
Ishihara I-Temp c.
Khosia c.
c. knife electrode
L-shaped c.
Magielski coagulation c.
MegaDyne c.
Mentor Wet-Field c.
Mira c.
monopolar c.
Mueller alkaline battery c.
Mueller Currentrol c.
National c.
needlepoint c.
NeoKnife c.
ocular c.
Op-Temp c.
Paquelin c.
Parker-Heath c.
pencil c.
pencil-tip c.
phacoemulsification c.
Prince eye c.
right-angle bipolar c.
Rommel c.
Rommel-Hildreth c.
Schanz c.
Scheie ophthalmic c.
Schepens eye c.
c. snare
Souttar c.
Statham c.
stepped-down c.

C

cautery *(continued)*
    suction c.
    Todd c.
    unipolar c.
    Valleylab c.
    von Graefe c.
    Wadsworth-Todd eye c.
    Walker c.
    Wappler cold c.
    Wepsic fiberoptic c.
    wet-field c.
    Wills Hospital eye c.
    Ziegler c.

caval
    c. cannula
    c. catheter
    c. occlusion clamp

Cavanaugh-Israel bur
Cavanaugh sphenoid bur
Cavanaugh-Wells tonsillar forceps
Cave
    C. cartilage knife
    C. knee retractor
    C. scaphoid gouge
    C. scaphoid spatula

CaverMap surgical device
cavernospongiosum shunt
Cavernotome C&R
Cave-Rowe ligature carrier
Caves bioptome
Caves-Schultz bioptome
Cavi-Endo
    C.-E. ultrasonic system

Cavi-Jet dental prophylaxis device
Cavi-Pulse cavitation ultrasound surgical aspirator
Cavitec cavity liner
Cavitron
    C. aspirator
    C. cautery unit
    C. dissector
    C. I&A handpiece
    C. I&A system
    C. laser
    C. machine
    C. phacoemulsification unit
    C. Phaco-Emulsifier
    C. scalpel
    C. SPS ultrasonic scaler
    C. Ultrasonic Surgical aspirator (CUSA)

Cavitron-Kelman
    C.-K. I&A system
    C.-K. phacoemulsification machine

Cavoline cavity liner
Cawood nasal splint
Caylor scissors
Cayote OTW balloon catheter
CB
    CB Diode/532 laser
    CB Erbium/2.94 laser
    CB Erbium/2.94 laser system

C-bar web-spacer
CBD 2 choledochoscope

CBI
    CBI stereotactic head holder
    CBI stereotactic ring

C.B.T.
    C.B.T. conductive stretcher pad
    C.B.T. nonconductive stretcher pad
    C.B.T. Siderail bumper pad

CC
    Coulter counter

CCCS
CCD Spirette
CCK femoral stem provisional guide
C-clamp
CCOmbo catheter
CC Rider closed-chain rehabilitation system
CCS endocardial pacing lead
C-D
    C-D hook
    C-D instrumentation
    C-D instrumentation device

CD-5 needle
CD8 AIS CELLector
C-Dak dialyzer
CDH
    CDH Precoat Plus hip prosthesis
    CDH stapler

CDI
    Cotrel-Dubousset instrumentation
    CDI 2000 blood gas monitor
    CDI 2000 blood gas monitoring system

cDNA probe
CDO brace
CDRPan digital x-ray system
CE-24 needle
CE-2 cryostat
Cebotome drill
Cecar electrode
Cecil dressing
cecostomy
    c. catheter
    c. retractor

Cedar anesthesia face rest
CEEA stapler
Ceegraph 128 EEG system
CeeOn heparinized intraocular lens
Cel
    C. Touch adhesive
    C. Touch white indicator powder

Celay
    C. InCeram crown
    C. milling unit
    C. system
    C. Tech light curing resin

Celestin
    C. bougie
    C. endoesophageal prosthesis
    C. endoesophageal tube
    C. endoprosthesis
    C. graduated dilator
    C. graft material
    C. implant
    C. latex rubber tube

celiac clamp

Celita
C. Elite knife
C. Sapphire knife
Cell
C. Analysis system
C. Recovery System
C. Saver 4 cardiopulmonary bypass blood centrifuge and washing equipment
C. Saver Haemolite
C. Saver Haemonetics autotransfusion system
C. Soft 2000 semen analyzer
C. Soft system
C. Trak/DMS analyzer
C. Trak/S analyzer
C. Trak 11 semen analyzer
Cellamin resin plaster-of-Paris bandage
CELLector
CD8 AIS C.
CellFIT acquisition system
Cell-O-Gen
Cellolite
C. material
C. patty
Cellona resin plaster-of-Paris bandage
cellophane dressing
cell-seeded stent
Cell-Track
celltrifuge
CritSpin c.
c. device
celluloid
c. implant
c. implant material
c. linen suture
cellulose
c. acetate device (CA-series dialyzer)
c. surgical sponge
Celluron dental roll
Cell-VU disposable semen analysis chamber
Celsite
C. brachial port
C. implanted port
C. pediatric port
Cemax/Icon scanner
Cemax PACS platform
cement
acrylic c.
antibiotic-loaded acrylic c.
Atwood orthodontic c.
BA bone c.
bone c.
Boneloc c.
BoneSource hydroxyapatite c.
Buck femoral c. restrictor
Buffalo dental c.
c. centralizer
Ceramco dental c.
Ceramlin dental c.
Ceramsave dental c.
Compacement dental c.
composite dental c.
Conclude dental c.

copper phosphate c.
dental c.
DePuy 1 bone c.
dermatome c.
Diaket root canal c.
Duall #88 c.
Durelon dental c.
Eastman dental c.
c. eater
c. eater drill
Endurance bone c.
Epoxylite CBA dental resin c.
Freegenol c.
Fuji dental c.
Gembase dental c.
Gemcem dental c.
Gemcore dental c.
glass ionomer c.
Howmedica Simplex P c.
Implast bone c.
IMProv c.
inorganic dental c.
Ketac Fil c.
Ketac Silver c.
Kirkland c.
low-viscosity bone c.
master c.
modified zinc oxide-eugenol c.
Mynol endodontic c.
Neutrocim dental c.
Nobetec dental c.
Nogenol dental c.
Norian Skeletal Repair System cancellous bone c.
Norian SRS c.
organic dental c.
Orthocomp c.
orthodontic c.
Orthoset c.
Osteobond copolymer bone c.
Palacos radiopaque bone c.
Petralit dental c.
polycarboxylate c.
polymethyl methacrylate bone c.
Pronto c.
prosthetic antibiotic-loaded acrylic c.
resin c.
c. restrictor
c. restrictor inserter
Roth dental c.
Selfast dental c.
Shofu dental c.
silicate c.
Simplex-P bone c.
Skin-Bond skin c.
c. spacer inserter
c. spatula
Sulfix-6 c.
Super-Dent orthodontic c.
SuperEBA c.
Surgical Simplex P radiopaque bone c.
Tempbond dental c.
Temrex dental c.
tooth c.

C

cement *(continued)*
    Torbot c.
    Wacker Sil-Gel 604 silicone c.
    Zimmer bone c.
cemental spike
Cementless
    C. Sportorno hip arthroplasty stem
    C. Sportorno hip arthroplasty stem
      device
cement-removal hand chisel
Cemex system
Cencit
    C. facial scanner
    C. imaging system
    C. surface scanner
Cenflex central monitoring system
Centauri Er:YAG laser system
Centaur trial cup
Centec Propoint knee brace
center-action forceps
centering
    c. balloon
    c. drill
    c. ring
Centermark vascular access device
CenterPointLock
    C. two-piece ostomy system: closed
      mini-pouch
    C. two-piece ostomy system: closed
      pouch
    C. two-piece ostomy system:
      drainable mini-pouch
    C. two-piece ostomy system:
      drainable pouch
    C. two-piece ostomy system: stoma
      cap
    C. two-piece ostomy system: stoma
      irrigator drain
centimeter subtraction ruler
Centimist nebulizer
Centra-Flex lens
central
    c. core wire
    c. retinal lens
    c. terminal electrode
    c. venous pressure catheter
Centralign Precoat hip prosthesis
centralizer
    cement c.
    Integral distal c.
    PMMA c.
Centrax
    C. bipolar endoprosthesis
    C. bipolar system
Centricon-10 filter
Centriflow membrane cone
centrifugal pump
centrifuge
    Beckman J-6M c.
    Eppendorf c.
    Ficoll-Hypaque gradient c.
    MicroMax c.
    Polyprep c.

Centrix
    C. PDQ ligator
    C. syringe
Centronic 200 MGA respiratory mass spectrometer
Centry 2 cps dialysis unit
Centurion
    C. needleless catheter extensions
    C. SorbaView window dressing
Century
    C. bicarbonate dialysis control unit
    C. birthing chair
    C. urodynamics chair
cephalad catheter
cephalic blade forceps
cephalometer
    Bertillon c.
    GX c.
    Plasticeph c.
    Wehmer c.
cephalometric protractor
cephalostat
cephalotribe
    Tarnier c.
Ceprate SC Instrument II
CerAdapt
Ceradelta alloy
Ceramalloy alloy
Ceramco
    C. dental cement
    C. porcelain kit
ceramic
    c. endosteal implant
    c. ossicular prosthesis
    c. vertebral spacer
Ceramion prosthesis
Ceramlin dental cement
ceramometal implant bridge
Ceramsave dental cement
CeraOne
    C. abutment
    C. abutment implant
    C. implant system
Cerapall alloy
CeraSPECT camera
Ceravital incus replacement prosthesis
cerclage
    Howmedica c.
    McDonald c.
    Tylok c.
    c. wire
    c. wire twister
cerebellar
    c. attachment
    c. electrode
    c. retractor
Cereblate catheter
cerebral
    c. angiography needle
    c. catheter
    c. function monitor
    c. retractor
Cerebrograph
cerebrospinal fluid shunt
Cer-Mate alloy

Cer-On R alloy
Cerrobend
    C. cast
    C. trim block
Cerva crane halter
Cervex-Brush
    C.-B. cervical cell collector
    Unimar C.-B.
cervical
    c. AOA halo traction
    c. biopsy blade
    c. biopsy curette
    c. biopsy forceps
    c. block kit
    c. cannula
    c. clamp
    c. collar
    c. collar brace
    c. cone knife
    c. conization electrode
    c. dilator
    c. disk retractor
    c. drill
    c. grasping forceps
    c. hemostatic forceps
    c. immobilization device
    c. mallet
    c. orthosis (CO)
    c. plate
    c. punch
    c. punch forceps
    c. range-of-motion device
    c. range-of-motion instrument
    c. roll
    c. rongeur
    c. saddle
    c. sleep pillow
    c. suture
    c. suture needle
    c. tenaculum
    c. thoracic orthosis
    c. traction forceps
    c. vulsellum
cervical/lumbar hammer
cervicothoracic
    c. jacket
    c. orthosis
Cer-View lateral vaginal retractor
CerviFix system
CerviSoft cytology collection device
Cervitrak device
cesarean forceps
cesium
    c. applicator
    c. candle
    c. cylinder
    c. fluoride scintillation detector
    c. needle
    c. source
cesium-137 wire
CF-200Z Olympus colonoscope
CFC BioScanner system
C-Flex
    C.-F. Amsterdam stent
    C.-F. catheter

    C.-F. supine cervical traction
    C.-F. ureteral stent
CFS
    contoured femoral stem
    CFS hip prosthesis
CF-UM3 echocolonoscope
CFV wrist component
CGI-1 contact lens
CGR biplane angiographic system
Chadwick scissors
Chaffin catheter
Chaffin-Pratt drain
Chailey go-cart
chain saw
chair
    Bárány c.
    bedside air c.
    birthing c.
    BodyBilt c.
    Century birthing c.
    Century urodynamics c.
    Combisit surgeon's c.
    computerized rotary c.
    dynamic integrated stabilization c.
    EasyChair massage c.
    EZ Rider support c.
    fluoroscopic imaging c.
    Gardner c.
    geriatric c.
    Invacare padded shower c.
    invalid c.
    Kaleidoscope c.
    Midmark 413 power female
        procedure c.
    mobile air c.
    OB/GYN c.
    Orthokinetics travel c.
    Pigg-O-Stat x-ray c.
    Pogon c.
    Portal Pro 2 treatment c.
    Portazam portable exam c.
    recliner air c.
    reclining c.
    Seated Hamstring Curl exercise c.
    c. shower
    sit/stand c.
    SPECTurn c.
    STC 900-series travel c.
    Vess c.
chairback brace
Chajchir dissector
chalazion
    c. clamp
    c. curette
    c. forceps
    c. knife
    c. retractor
    c. trephine
Challenger digital applanation tonometer
Chalnot valvulotome
Chamber
    Portable Topical Hyperbaric Oxygen
        Extremity C.
chamber
    air c.

C

chamber *(continued)*
    anterior c. (AC)
    Boyden c.
    Bürker c.
    Cell-VU disposable semen analysis c.
    drill c.
    drip c.
    Finn c.
    Fisher-Paykel MR290 water-feed c.
    flush c.
    hyperbaric c.
    Hyper-Oxy portable hyperbaric c.
    Makler counting c.
    Makler reusable semen analysis c.
    Microcell c.
    moisture c.
    MR 290 humidification c.
    multiwire proportional c.
    parallel-plate flow c.
    plasma clot diffusion c.
    portable topical hyperbaric oxygen extremity c.
    Pudenz flushing c.
    pulp c.
    reentrant well c.
    Sechrist Model 2500E, 3200E, 7200 hyperbaric c.
    Sechrist monoplace hyperbaric c.
    Shandon cytospin c.
    Storm Von Leeuwen c.
    Ussing c.
Chamberlain-Fries atraumatic retractor
Chamberlain tongue depressor
Chamberlen obstetrical forceps
ChamberLift 2000 patient lift system
Chambers
    C. doughnut pessary
    C. intrauterine cup
    C. intrauterine pessary
chamfer
    c. guide
    c. jig
    c. reamer
Chamois
    C. swab
    C. underpad
Champ
    C. cardiac device
    C. elastic bandage
    C. Insulated Propac II
Champetier de Ribes obstetrical bag
Championnière
    C. bone drill
    C. forceps
Champion Power Sox
Champy miniplate rigid fixation system
Chandler
    C. bone elevator
    C. felt collar splint
    C. iris forceps
    C. knee retractor
    C. laminectomy retractor
    C. mallet

    C. spinal-perforating forceps
    C. table
    C. unreamed interlocking tibial nail
    C. V-pacing probe
Chang
    C. bone-cutting forceps
    C. Quick Chop Combo
    C. Quick Chop combo ophthalmic instrument
changer
    film c.
    Littmann galilean magnification c.
    Puck cutfilm c.
    Puck film c.
    Sanchez-Perez automatic film cassette c.
    Schonander film c.
    tracheal tube c.
    tube c.
channel
    c. dissector
    c. retractor
Chan wrist rest
Chaoul
    C. applicator
    C. voltage x-ray tube
Chaput tissue forceps
charcoal filter
Charcot bath
Charcot-Bottcher filament
Chardack-Greatbatch
    C.-G. implantable cardiac pulse generator
    C.-G. pacemaker
Chardack Medtronic pacemaker
Charest head frame
char-free carbon dioxide laser
charge-coupled
    c.-c. device
    c.-c. device monochrome camera
    c.-c. device scanner
    c.-c. device video camera
Charles
    C. anterior segment sleeve
    C. contact lens
    C. flute needle
    C. infusion sleeve
    C. intraocular lens
    C. irrigating lens
    C. vacuuming needle
    C. vitrector with sleeve
Charleston
    C. nighttime bending brace
    C. scoliosis brace
Charlton
    C. antral needle
    C. antral trocar
    C. cannula
Charnley
    C. acetabular cup
    C. acetabular cup prosthesis
    C. acetabular scraper
    C. arthrodesis clamp
    C. bone clamp
    C. bone clasp

C. brace handle
C. cemented hip prosthesis
C. cement restrictor
C. centering drill
C. centering ring
C. compressor
C. cup-trimming scissors
C. deepening reamer
C. device
C. double-ended bone curette
C. drain tube
C. expanding reamer
C. external fixation clamp
C. femoral broach
C. femoral condyle drill
C. femoral condyle radius gauge
C. femoral inlay aligner
C. femoral inlay guillotine
C. femoral lever
C. femoral prosthesis neck punch
C. femoral prosthesis pusher
C. flat-back femoral component
C. foam suture pad
C. gouge
C. hip prosthesis
C. horizontal retractor
C. Howorth ExFlow system
C. implant
C. initial incision retractor
C. knee prosthesis
C. knee retractor
C. narrow stem component
C. offset-bore cup
C. pilot drill
C. pin
C. pin clamp
C. pin retractor
C. rasp
C. saw
C. self-retaining retractor
C. socket gauge
C. standard stem retractor
C. starting drill
C. suction drain
C. suture button
C. suture forceps
C. taper reamer
C. template
C. tibial onlay jig
C. total hip prosthesis
C. towel
C. trochanter file
C. trochanter holder
C. trochanter reamer
C. trochanter wire
C. wire-holding forceps
C. wire passer
C. wire tightener
Charnley-Hastings prosthesis
Charnley-Mueller hip prosthesis
Charnley-Riches arterial forceps
Charnow notched ruler
Charriere
C. amputation saw

C. aseptic metacarpal saw
C. bone saw
chart
Amsler c.
Birkhauser eye testing c.
Broselow c.
contemporary nearpoint c.
cross-Polaroid projection c.
Ferris c.
Hawley c.
Illiterate E c.
Jaeger eye c.
Jaeger reading c.
Konig bar c.
Landolt C acuity c.
Lea Symbol c.
Lebensohn c.
Lighthouse ET-DRS acuity c.
logMAR c.
Mentor B-VAT visual acuity c.
Pelli-Robson letter c.
POMARD anthropomorphic
  measurement reference c.
Regan low-contrast acuity c.
sclerotome pain c.
Snellen c.
Turtle c.
Vistech wall c.
Chaston eye pad
Chatfield-Girdlestone splint
Chatillon dolorimeter
Chattanooga Balance system
Chatzidakis implant
Chauffin-Pratt tube
Chaussier tube
Chavantes-Zamorano neuroendoscope
Chavasse
C. squint hook
C. strabismus hook
Chayes handpiece
Chayet corneal marker
Cheanvechai-Favaloro retractor
Cheatle sterilizing forceps
Checkerboard wheelchair cushion
Check-Flo introducer
checkvalve
BacStop c.
check-valve sheath
cheek retractor
Cheetah angioplasty catheter
cheiroscope
Chelex bead
Chelsea-Eaton anal speculum
ChemoBloc vial venting system
chemonucleolysis table
Chemo-Port
C.-P. catheter
C.-P. perivena catheter system
C.-P. perivena catheter system
  device
**Chemstrip MatchMaker blood glucose
  meter**
ChemTrak AccuMeter
Chen-Smith image coder

C

Cherf
 C. cast stand
 C. leg holder
Chermel
 C. bone chisel
 C. bone gouge
 C. osteotome
Chernov tracheostomy hook
Cheron uterine dressing forceps
cherry
 C. brain probe
 C. drill
 C. forceps
 C. laminectomy self-retaining retractor
 C. osteotome
 C. screw extractor
 C. Secto dissector
 c. sponge
 C. S-shaped brain retractor
 C. S-shape scissors
 C. traction tongs
Cherry-Adson forceps
Cherry-Austin drill
Cherry-Kerrison
 C.-K. forceps
 C.-K. laminectomy rongeur
Cheshire electrosurgical pencil
Cheshire-Poole-Yankauer suction instrument
chessboard implant
chest
 c. dressing
 c. shell
 c. strap
 c. tube
 c. tube stripper
chest-band transmitter
Chester sponge forceps
Chevalier
 C. Jackson bougie
 C. Jackson bronchoesophagoscopy forceps
 C. Jackson bronchoscope
 C. Jackson esophagoscope
 C. Jackson gastroscope
 C. Jackson laryngeal speculum
 C. Jackson laryngoscope
 C. Jackson scissors
 C. Jackson tracheal tube
Chewrite denture adhesive
Cheyne
 C. dissector
 C. periosteal elevator
 C. retractor
Chiba
 C. biopsy needle
 C. eye needle
 C. transhepatic cholangiography needle
Chicco breast pump
Chick
 C. CLT operating frame
 C. CLT operating table
 C. patient transfer device

 C. sterile dressing
 C. surgical light
 C. surgical table
chicken-bill rongeur forceps
Chick-Foster orthopedic bed
Chick-Langren table
Chid breast pump
Chiesi powder inhaler
Chilcott venoclysis cannula
child
 C. clip-applying forceps
 c. esophagoscope
 C. intestinal forceps
 c. rectal dilator
Child-Phillips
 C.-P. forceps
 C.-P. intestinal plication needle
Children's Hospital
 C. H. brain spatula
 C. H. clip
 C. H. dressing forceps
 C. H. hand drill
 C. H. intestinal forceps
 C. H. mallet
 C. H. pediatric retractor
 C. H. screwdriver
child-resistant container
child-restraint device
Childs Cardio-Cuff
Chimani pharyngeal forceps
chin
 c. implant
 c. support
Chinese
 C. fingerstraps traction device
 C. fingertrap suture
 C. twisted silk suture
ChinUpps cervicofacial support
chip
 Dembone demineralized corticocancellous c.'s
Chiroflex C11UB lens
Chiroflow back rest
Chiron
 C. ACS microkeratome
 C. automated corneal shaper
 C. Hansatome
chiropractic
 c. adjusting instrument
 C. Strength Flex-all 454
Chiroslide measuring device
Chirotech x-ray system
chisel
 Adson laminectomy c.
 Alexander bone c.
 Alexander mastoid c.
 Amico c.
 Andrews c.
 antral c.
 Army c.
 Artmann disarticulation c.
 Austin Moore mortising c.
 Bakelite dental c.
 Ballenger c.
 Ballenger-Hajek c.

Basek c.
beveled c.
bilevel c.
Biomet cement removal hand c.
Bishop mastoid c.
c. blade
Blair nasal c.
bone c.
Bowen gooseneck c.
Braithwaite nasal c.
Brauer c.
Brown c.
Bruening c.
Brunetti c.
Brun guarded c.
Brunner c.
Brunswick-Mack c.
Buckley c.
Burns c.
Caltagirone c.
canal c.
cartilage c.
cement-removal hand c.
Chermel bone c.
Cinelli c.
Cinelli-McIndoe c.
Clawicz c.
Clevedent-Gardner c.
Clevedent-Wakefield c.
Cloward-Harman c.
Cloward-Puka c.
Cloward spinal fusion c.
Cobb c.
Compere bone c.
Converse guarded nasal c.
Cooley c.
cornea c.
corneal c.
costotome c.
Cottle antral c.
Cottle crossbar fishtail c.
Cottle curved c.
Cottle fishtail c.
Cottle nasal c.
Councilman c.
Crane bone c.
crossbar fishtail c.
crurotomy c.
curved c.
Dautrey c.
Derlacki c.
Derlacki-Shambaugh c.
D'Errico laminectomy c.
disarticulation c.
dissecting c.
double-guarded c.
double safe-sided c.
Duray-Read c.
Duray-Wood c.
Dworacek-Farrior canal c.
Ecker-Roopenian c.
Eicher tri-fin c.
c. elevator
endaural surgery c.
ethmoidal c.

Farrior-Derlacki c.
Farrior-Dworacek canal c.
Faulkner antral c.
Faulkner-Browne c.
fishtail c.
Fomon nasal c.
footplate c.
fracture c.
Freer bone c.
Freer lacrimal c.
Freer nasal c.
Freer submucous c.
French c.
frontal sinus c.
Gardner bone c.
Gauje curved c.
Goldman guarded c.
gold-paneled c.
gooseneck c.
guarded c.
Hajek septal c.
Halle c.
Harmon c.
Hatch c.
Heermann c.
Henderson bone c.
Hibbs bone c.
hollow c.
Holmes c.
Hough c.
House c.
House-Derlacki c.
Jenkins c.
Jordan-Hermann c.
Joseph c.
Katsch c.
Keyes bone-splitting c.
Kezerian c.
Killian-Claus c.
Killian frontal sinus c.
Killian-Reinhard c.
Kilner c.
Kos c.
Kreischer bone c.
lacrimal sac c.
Lambert-Lowman c.
Lambotte bone c.
laminectomy c.
Lebsche sternal c.
Lexer c.
Lorenz c.
Lowman c.
Lowman-Hoglund c.
Lucas c.
MacAusland c.
Magielski stapes c.
Magnum c.
Mannerfelt c.
Martin cartilage c.
mastoid c.
McIndoe nasal c.
Metzenbaum c.
Meyerding c.
middle ear c.
Miles bone c.

C

chisel *(continued)*
    Moberg c.
    monoangle c.
    Moore hollow c.
    Moore prosthesis-mortising c.
    mortising c.
    Murphy c.
    nasal c.
    Neivert c.
    Nordent bone c.
    Nordent-Ochsenbein periodontic c.
    Obwegeser splitting c.
    Oratek c.
    orthopedic c.
    Partsch bone c.
    Passow c.
    peapod c.
    Pearson c.
    Peck c.
    Pick c.
    pterygoid c.
    Puka c.
    Read c.
    Rica mastoid c.
    Richards c.
    Richards-Hibbs c.
    Rish c.
    Roberts hip dissecting c.
    Rollet c.
    Rubin nasal c.
    Schuknecht c.
    Schwartze c.
    septal c.
    Sewall ethmoidal c.
    Shambaugh-Derlacki c.
    Sheehan nasal c.
    Sheehy-House c.
    Silver c.
    Simmons c.
    single safe-sided c.
    sinus c.
    Skoog nasal c.
    SMIC bone c.
    SMIC mastoid c.
    SMIC sternal c.
    Smillie cartilage c.
    Smillie meniscectomy c.
    Smith-Petersen c.
    spinal fusion c.
    splitting c.
    stapes c.
    Stille bone c.
    submucous c.
    Swedish-pattern c.
    Swiderski nasal c.
    tri-fin c.
    Troutman mastoid c.
    twin-pattern c.
    unibevel c.
    U. S. Army bone c.
    Virchow c.
    vulcanite c.
    Walsh footplate c.
    Ward nasal c.

    West lacrimal c.
    West nasal c.
    White bone c.
    Wilmer c.
    Worth c.
Chitten-Hill retractor
chloramine catgut suture
Chlumsky button
choanal bur
Chocstruct chondral repair system
Cho/Dyonics two-portal endoscope
Choice
    Medi-Jector C.
    C. PT guidewire
Cholangiocath catheter
cholangioclamp
cholangiogram
    T-tube c.
cholangiographic catheter
cholangiography
    c. catheter
    c. clamp
cholangiograsper
    Storz c.
Cholangiolapcath catheter
cholangiopancreatogram
    endoscopic retrograde c. (ERCP)
    magnetic resonance c.
cholangioscope
    "adoptable" baby c.
    Olympus CHF-Q10 c.
    prototype c.
choledochocystonephrofiberscope
    Pentax c.
choledochofiberscope
    Olympus URF-P2
        translaparoscopic c.
choledochoscope
    CBD 2 c.
    fiberoptic c.
    Olympus CHF-P-series c.
    Olympus CHF-series c.
choledochoscope-nephroscope
    Berci-Schore c.-n.
    Storz c.-n.
Cholestech L-D-X office lab system
chondroplasty Beaver blade
chondrotome
    Stryker c.
Chopart
    C. brace
    C. partial foot prosthesis
Cho-Pat
    C.-P. Achilles tendon strap
    C.-P. elbow strap
    C.-P. knee strap
CHOP frame
chopper
    Davidoff ambidextrous nucleus c.
    He Hook c.
    Koch c.
    Nagahara karate c.
    Nagahara phaco c.
    Nichamin quick c.
    Nichamin triple c.

Nichamin vertical c.
Olson phaco c.
Seibel nucleus c.
Shepherd Tomahawk c.
Steinert double-ended claw c.
Sung reverse nucleus c.
chorda tympani pusher
chorionic
c. villus sampler
c. villus sampling catheter
chorionscope
Chorus
C. DDD pacemaker
C. RM rate-responsive dual-chamber pacemaker
Cho two-portal Dyonics endoscope
Choyce
C. intraocular lens forceps
C. lens-inserting forceps
C. Mark intraocular lens
C. Mark VIII eye implant
C. Mark VIII lens
C. MK II keratoprosthesis prosthesis
Choyce-Tennant lens
Christensen articulator
Christie gallbladder retractor
Christmas
C. tree adapter
C. tree cannula
Christopher-Stille forceps
Christoudias
C. approximator
C. fascial closure device
Chromaser dermatology laser
chromated catgut suture
chromatograph
Carle analytic gas c.
column c.
gas c.
high-performance liquid c.
high-pressure liquid c.
ion c.
Quintron Microlyzer 12 c.
solid-phase extraction c.
thin-layer c.
Varian model 3600 gas c.
chromatoptometer
chromatoskiameter
ChromaVision digital analyzer
chrome-cobalt cable
Chromel-Alumel thermocouple
chrome probe with eye
chromic
c. blue dyed suture
c. catgut suture
c. collagen suture
c. gut suture
chromicized catgut suture
chromium-cobalt alloy implant
chromoendoscope
Chromos imager system
ChromoVision video system
chronaximeter

Chronicure
C. protein hydrolysate powder
C. wound dressing
Chronocor IV external pacemaker
Chronos pacemaker
Chrys surgical CO_2 laser
CHS
compression hip screw
CHS supracondylar bone plate
Chubb tonsillar forceps
Chubby balloon catheter
chuck
c. adapter
c. drill
Gam-Mer c.
gold-handled c.
Jacobs snap-lock c.
Jacobs T-handled c.
pin c.
press-button c.
Steinmann pin c.
T-handle Jacob c.
T-handle Zimmer c.
Trinkle c.
Wozniak Sur-Lok c.
Chu foldable lens cutter
Chukka boot
Churchill
C. cardiac suction cannula
C. sucker
Church pediatric scissors
Chuter endovascular device
Chux incontinent dressing
CI
300 CI
Ciaglia
C. Blue Rhino percutaneous tracheostomy introducer set
C. percutaneous tracheostomy introducer
C. percutaneous tracheostomy introducer set
Ciba
C. Soft lens
C. Thin lens
Ciba-Corning 2500 co-oximeter
Cibathin lens
Cibis
C. electrode
C. ski needle
Cibis-Vaiser muscle retractor
CIC
completely in the canal
CIC listening device
Cica-Care silicone gel sheet dressing
Cicherelli
C. bone rongeur
C. forceps
CIDA foam
Cida-Gel absorbent beads
CIDS
continuous insulin delivery system
Cidtech camera
CIF needle
cigarette drain

C

cigar handle basket punch
Cikloid dressing
Cilacalcin double-chambered syringe
Cilco
    C. argon laser
    C. Frigitronics
    C. Frigitronics laser
    C. Hoffer Laseridge
    C. Hoffer Laseridge laser
    C. intraocular lens
    C. krypton laser
    C. Lasertek argon laser
    C. lens forceps
    C. MonoFlex PMMA lens
    C. ophthalmic endoscope
    C. Optiflex intraocular lens
    C. perimeter
    C. posterior chamber intraocular lens
    C. Slant lens
    C. ultrasound unit
    C. viscoelastic
    C. vitrector
    C. YAG laser
Cilco-Simcoe II lens
Cilco-Sonometrics lens
cilia suture forceps
cilium pacemaker
CIMA*flex* 411 foldable silicone lens
Cimino
    C. arteriovenous shunt
    C. dialysis shunt
    C. fistula
Cimino-Brescia arteriovenous fistula
Cimochowski cardiac cannula
cinch
    alar c.
    C. bladder neck suspension anchor system
    Daw C.
    joint c.
Cincinnati ACL brace
cine
    c. arthrogram
    c. camera
    c. CT scanner
    c. gastrocamera
    c. magnetic resonance imaging (cine MRI)
    c. microscope
cine camera
    Bolex c. c.
    House-Urban microsurgery c. c.
    House-Urban UEM-100 c. c.
Cinelli
    C. chisel
    C. osteotome
    C. periosteal elevator
Cinelli-Fomon scissors
Cinelli-McIndoe chisel
Cineloop image review ultrasound system
cine-magnetic resonance imaging
Cine-Microscope

cine MRI
    cine magnetic resonance imaging
CineView Plus Freeland system
Cintor knee prosthesis
Cipro cystitis pack
Circadia dual-chamber rate-adaptive pacemaker
circadian event recorder
Circ-Aid elastic stockings
circle
    areola c.
    Bain c.
    DataVue calibrated reference c.
    c. knife
    pediatric c.
    Randot c.
Circline magnifier
CircOlectric bed
Circon
    C. ACMI cannula
    C. ACMI diagnostic laparoscope
    C. ACMI hysteroscope
    C. ACMI MicroDigital-I camera
    C. ACMI MR-series ureteroscope
    C. ACMI trocar
    C. arthroscope
    C. leg holder
    C. Tripolar forceps
    C. video camera
    C. videohydrothoracoscope
Circon-ACMI
    C.-A. electrohydraulic lithotriptor probe
    C.-A. endoscope
    C.-A. lithotriptor
CircPlus
    C. bandage/wrap system
    C. compression dressing
    C. wrap
circuit
    c. adapter
    Bentley Duraflo II extracorporeal perfusion c.
    Carmeda BioActive surface extracorporeal c.
    Intertech anesthesia breathing c.
    Intertech Mapleson D nonrebreathing c.
    Intertech nonrebreathing modified Jackson-Rees c.
    Jackson-Rees c.
    low-flow c.
    Magill c.
    multipurpose breathing c.
    phototube output c.
    Tygon tubing c.
Circulaire aerosol drug delivery system
Circul'Air shoe system
circular
    c. bandage
    c. blade
    c. cup bronchoscopic biopsy forceps
    c. external fixator
    c. intraluminal stapler
    c. mechanical stapler

c. stapling device
c. suture
circulating water blanket
circulator
  sequential c.
Circulator boot system
Circulon
  C. dressing
  C. System Step 1, 2 venous ulcer kit
  C. wrap
circumcisional
  c. shield
  c. suture
circumcision clamp
circumdential wire
circumductor table
circumferential
  c. dressing
  c. extremity coil
circumflex artery scissors
Circumpress
  C. chin strap
  C. compression bra
  C. facelift dressing
  C. gynecomastia vest
Circumstraint restraint
Cirrus
  C. composite prosthetic foot
  C. foot prosthesis
CIS-2 system
Cisco covered needle catheter
cisterna magna catheter
Citelli
  C. laminectomy punch
  C. punch forceps
  C. sphenoid rongeur
Citelli-Bruening ear forceps
Citelli-Meltzer atticus punch
Citscope arthroscope
Civiale forceps
CKG
  cardiokymograph
CKS knee system
Claes scleral depressor
Clagett
  C. needle
  C. S-cannula
Clairborne clamp
clamp
  Abadie enterostomy c.
  Ablaza patent ductus c.
  Abramson-Allis breast c.
  Acland microvascular c.
  Adair breast c.
  Adson c.
  Adson-Brown c.
  agraffe c.
  Ahlquist-Durham embolism c.
  Alfred M. Large vena cava c.
  Allen anastomosis c.
  Allen intestinal c.
  Allen-Kocher c.
  Allison c.
  Allis tissue c.

Alyea vas c.
anastomosis c.
Ando aortic c.
aneurysm c.
angled DeBakey c.
angled peripheral vascular c.
Ann Arbor towel c.
anterior resection c.
aortic aneurysm c.
aortic cannula c.
aortic occlusion c.
appendage c.
arterial c.
Asch c.
ASSI METE-5168 Microspike approximator c.
ASSI METS-3668 Microspike approximator c.
ASSI MKCV-2040 Microspike approximator c.
ASSI MSPK-3678 Microspike approximator c.
Atlee bronchus c.
Atra-Grip c.
atraumatic intestinal c.
Atraumax peripheral vascular c.
atrial c.
Ault intestinal c.
auricular appendage c.
Auvard c.
Babcock tissue c.
baby Bishop c.
baby Kocher c.
baby pylorus c.
baby Satinsky c.
Backhaus-Jones towel c.
Backhaus-Kocher towel c.
Backhaus towel c.
Bahnson aortic aneurysm c.
Bahnson appendage c.
Bailey aortic c.
Bailey-Cowley c.
Bailey duckbill c.
Bailey-Morse c.
Bainbridge anastomosis c.
Bainbridge intestinal c.
Bainbridge vessel c.
Balfour c.
Ballantine c.
Bamby c.
Bard Cunningham incontinence c.
Barraquer needle holder c.
Bartley anastomosis c.
Bartley partial-occlusion c.
bar-to-bar c.
Bauer kidney pedicle c.
Baumrucker-DeBakey c.
Baumrucker post-TUR irrigation c.
Baumrucker urinary incontinence c.
Beall bulldog c.
Beall-Morris ascending aortic c.
Beardsley intestinal c.
Beck aortic c.
Beck-Potts aortic c.
Beck-Potts pulmonic c.

C

clamp *(continued)*
Beck-Satinsky c.
Beck vascular c.
Beck vessel c.
Belcher c.
Benson pyloric c.
Berens muscle c.
Berke c.
Berkeley c.
Berkeley-Bonney vaginal c.
Berke ptosis c.
Berman aortic c.
Berman vascular c.
Bernhard c.
Berry pile c.
Best intestinal c.
Bethune c.
Bielawski heart c.
Bigelow calvaria c.
Bihrle dorsal c.
Bircher bone-holding c.
Bircher cartilage c.
Bishop bone c.
Black meatal c.
Blair cleft palate c.
Blalock-Niedner pulmonic stenosis c.
Blalock pulmonary artery c.
Blanchard pile c.
Blasucci c.
blepharostat c.
bloodless circumcision c.
Boettcher pulmonary artery c.
Böhler os calcis c.
bone extension c.
bone-holding c.
Bonney c.
Borge bile duct c.
Bortz c.
Boyes muscle c.
Bozeman c.
Bradshaw-O'Neill aortic c.
Bridge c.
Brock auricular c.
Brockington pile c.
Brodney urethrographic c.
Bronner c.
Brown lip c.
Brunner colon c.
Brunner intestinal c.
Buie-Hirschman pile c.
Buie pile c.
bulldog c.
Bunke c.
Bunnell-Howard arthrodesis c.
Burford c.
Burlisher c.
Bushey compression c.
Buxton uterine c.
C-c.
Cairns c.
Calandruccio c.
Calman carotid c.
Calman ring c.
calvarial c.

cannula c.
Capes c.
Cardio-Grip anastomosis c.
Cardio-Grip aortic c.
Cardio-Grip bronchus c.
Cardio-Grip pediatric c.
Cardio-Grip renal artery c.
Cardio-Grip tangential occlusion c.
Cardio-Grip vascular c.
cardiovascular anastomotic c.
cardiovascular bulldog c.
Carmalt c.
Carmel c.
carotid artery c.
Carrel c.
c. carrier
Carter c.
Carter-Glassman resection c.
cartilage c.
caruncle c.
Casey pelvic c.
Castaneda anastomosis c.
Castaneda IMM vascular c.
Castaneda-Mixter thoracic c.
Castaneda partial-occlusion c.
Castaneda vascular c.
Castroviejo lens c.
Castroviejo mosquito lid c.
Castroviejo needle holder c.
cautery c.
caval occlusion c.
celiac c.
cervical c.
chalazion c.
Charnley arthrodesis c.
Charnley bone c.
Charnley external fixation c.
Charnley pin c.
cholangiography c.
circumcision c.
Clairborne c.
Clevis c.
cloth-shod c.
coarctation c.
Codman cartilage c.
Codman towel c.
Collier thoracic c.
Collin umbilical c.
colon c.
colostomy c.
columellar c.
Conger perineal urethrostomy c.
contour block c.
Cooley acutely-curved c.
Cooley anastomosis c.
Cooley aortic aneurysm c.
Cooley aortic cannula c.
Cooley-Baumgarten aortic c.
Cooley-Beck vessel c.
Cooley bronchial c.
Cooley bulldog c.
Cooley carotid c.
Cooley caval occlusion c.
Cooley coarctation c.
Cooley cross-action bulldog c.

Cooley curved cardiovascular c.
Cooley-Derra anastomosis c.
Cooley double-angled c.
Cooley graft c.
Cooley iliac c.
Cooley neonatal vascular c.
Cooley partial-occlusion c.
Cooley patent ductus c.
Cooley pediatric vascular c.
Cooley peripheral vascular c.
Cooley renal artery c.
Cooley-Satinsky c.
Cooley subclavian c.
Cooley tangential pediatric c.
Cooley vena cava c.
Cope crushing c.
Cope-DeMartel c.
Cope modification of a Martel
  intestinal c.
cordotomy c.
Cottle columellar c.
cotton-roll rubber-dam c.
Crafoord aortic c.
Crafoord auricular c.
Crafoord coarctation c.
Crafoord-Sellors auricular c.
Crenshaw caruncle c.
Crile appendiceal c.
Crile crushing c.
Crile-Crutchfield c.
Crile hemostatic c.
Cross c.
cross-action bulldog c.
cross-action towel c.
Cruickshank entropion c.
crushing c.
Crutchfield carotid artery c.
Cunningham urinary incontinence c.
curved-8 c.
curved cardiovascular c.
curved Mayo c.
curved mosquito c.
Cushing c.
cystic duct catheter c.
Dacron graft c.
Daems bronchial c.
D'Allesandro c.
Dandy c.
Daniel colostomy c.
Dardik c.
D'Assumpcão c.
David-Baker lip c.
Davidson muscle c.
Davidson pulmonary vessel c.
Davila atrial c.
Davis aortic aneurysm c.
Dean MacDonald gastric
  resection c.
Deaver c.
DeBakey aortic aneurysm c.
DeBakey aortic exclusion c.
DeBakey arterial c.
DeBakey-Bahnson vascular c.
DeBakey-Bainbridge vascular c.
DeBakey-Beck c.

DeBakey bulldog c.
DeBakey coarctation c.
DeBakey-Crafoord vascular c.
DeBakey cross-action bulldog c.
DeBakey curved peripheral
  vascular c.
DeBakey-Derra anastomosis c.
DeBakey-Harken auricular c.
DeBakey-Howard aortic aneurysm c.
DeBakey-Kay aortic c.
DeBakey-McQuigg-Mixter
  bronchial c.
DeBakey patent ductus c.
DeBakey pediatric c.
DeBakey peripheral vascular c.
DeBakey ring-handled bulldog c.
DeBakey-Satinsky vena cava c.
DeBakey-Semb c.
DeBakey S-shaped peripheral
  vascular c.
DeBakey tangential occlusion c.
DeCourcy goiter c.
DeMartel vascular c.
DeMartel-Wolfson anastomosis c.
DeMartel-Wolfson colon c.
DeMartel-Wolfson intestinal c.
Demel wire c.
Demos tibial artery c.
Dennis anastomotic c.
Dennis intestinal c.
Derra anastomosis c.
Derra aortic c.
Derra vena cava c.
Derra vestibular c.
Desmarres lid c.
Devonshire-Mack c.
DeWeese vena cava c.
Dick bronchus c.
Dick pressure c.
Dieffenbach bulldog c.
Diethrich aortic c.
Diethrich graft c.
Diethrich microcoronary bulldog c.
Diethrich shunt c.
Dingman cartilage c.
disposable muscle biopsy c.
dissecting c.
distraction c.
Dixon-Thomas-Smith intestinal c.
Dobbie-Trout bulldog c.
Doctor Collins fracture c.
Doctor Long c.
Dogliotti-Gugliel mini c.
Dolphin cord c.
Donald c.
double-angled c.
double Softjaw c.
double towel c.
Downing c.
Doyen intestinal c.
Doyen towel c.
drape c.
dreamer c.
duckbill c.
ductus c.

C

clamp *(continued)*
    duodenal c.
    Duval lung c.
    Earle hemorrhoidal c.
    C. Ease device
    Eastman intestinal c.
    Edebohls kidney c.
    Edna towel c.
    Edwards double Softjaw c.
    Edwards single Softjaw c.
    Edwards spring c.
    Efteklar c.
    Eisenstein c.
    endoaortic c.
    English c.
    enterostomy c.
    entropion c.
    Erhardt lid c.
    Ericksson-Stille carotid c.
    Ewald-Hudson c.
    Ewing lid c.
    exclusion c.
    extension bone c.
    extracutaneous vas fixation c.
    Falk c.
    Farabeuf bone c.
    Farabeuf-Lambotte bone-holding c.
    Fauer peritoneal c.
    Favaloro proximal anastomosis c.
    Favorite c.
    feather c.
    Fehland intestinal c.
    Fehland right-angled colon c.
    femoral c.
    Ferguson bone c.
    Ferrier 212 gingival c.
    ferrule c.
    fine-tooth c.
    Finochietto arterial c.
    Finochietto bronchial c.
    Fitzgerald aortic aneurysm c.
    flexible aortic c.
    flexible retractor pressure c.
    flexible retractor sliding c.
    flexible vascular c.
    flow-regulator c.
    Fogarty-Chin c.
    Fogarty Hydragrip c.
    c. forceps
    Ford c.
    Forrester c.
    Foss anterior resection c.
    Foss cardiovascular c.
    Foss intestinal c.
    Frahur cartilage c.
    Frazier-Adson osteoplastic c.
    Frazier-Sachs c.
    Freeman c.
    Friedrich c.
    Friedrich-Petz c.
    Fukushima C-clamp c.
    full-curved c.
    Furness anastomosis c.
    Furness-Clute anastomosis c.
    Furness-Clute duodenal c.
    Furness-McClure-Hinton c.
    gallbladder ring c.
    Gam-Mer aneurysm c.
    Gam-Mer occlusion c.
    Gandy c.
    Gant c.
    Garcia aorta c.
    Garcia aortic c.
    Gardner skull c.
    Garland hysterectomy c.
    Gaskell c.
    gastric c.
    gastroenterostomy c.
    gastrointestinal c.
    Gavin-Miller c.
    Gemini c.
    Gerald c.
    Gerbode patent ductus c.
    Gerster bone c.
    GI c.
    gingival c.
    Gladstone-Putterman transmarginal
      rotation entropion c.
    Glass liver-holding c.
    Glassman-Allis c.
    Glassman bowel atraumatic c.
    Glassman intestinal c.
    Glassman liver-holding c.
    Glassman noncrushing
      gastroenterostomy c.
    Glassman noncrushing
      gastrointestinal c.
    Glover auricular c.
    Glover auricular-appendage c.
    Glover bulldog c.
    Glover coarctation c.
    Glover curved c.
    Glover-DeBakey c.
    Glover patent ductus c.
    Glover spoon-shaped anastomosis c.
    Glover-Stille c.
    Glover vascular c.
    goiter c.
    Goldblatt c.
    Goldstein Microspike
      approximator c.
    Goldvasser c.
    Gomco bell c.
    Gomco bloodless circumcision c.
    Gomco umbilical cord c.
    Goodwin bone c.
    Grafco incontinence c.
    Grafco umbilical cord c.
    graft c.
    Grant aortic aneurysm c.
    grasping c.
    Gray c.
    Greenberg c.
    Green bulldog c.
    Green lid c.
    Green suction tube-holding c.
    Gregory baby profunda c.
    Gregory carotid bulldog c.
    Gregory external c.

Gregory stay suture c.
Gregory vascular miniature c.
Gross coarctation c.
Grover Atra-grip c.
Grover auricular appendage c.
Gusberg hysterectomy c.
Gussenbauer c.
gut c.
Gutgemann auricular appendage c.
Guyon kidney c.
Guyon-Péan vessel c.
Guyon vessel c.
Haberer intestinal c.
half-curved c.
Halifax interlaminar c.
Halsted curved mosquito c.
Halsted straight mosquito c.
handleless c.
Haney c.
Harken auricular c.
Harrah lung c.
Harrington-Carmalt c.
Harrington hook c.
Harrington-Mixter thoracic c.
Hartmann c.
Harvey Stone c.
Hatch c.
Hausmann vascular c.
Haverhill c.
Haverhill-Mack c.
Hayes anterior resection c.
Hayes colon c.
Hayes intestinal c.
Heartport endoaortic c.
Heifitz cerebral aneurysm c.
Heitz-Boyer c.
Hemoclip c.
hemorrhoidal c.
hemostatic c.
Hendren cardiovascular c.
Hendren ductus c.
Hendren megaureter c.
Hendren ureteral c.
Henley subclavian artery c.
Henley vascular c.
Herbert Adams coarctation c.
Herff c.
Herrick kidney c.
Herrick pedicle c.
Hesseltine umbilical cord c.
Hex-Fix Universal swivel c.
Heyer-Schulte Rayport muscle
   biopsy c.
Hibbs c.
hilar c.
Hirschman pile c.
Hirsch mucosal c.
Hoffmann ligament c.
Hoff towel c.
Hohmann c.
c. holder
Hollister c.
Holter pump c.
Hopener c.

Hopkins aortic occlusion c.
Hopkins hysterectomy c.
Howard-DeBakey aortic aneurysm c.
Hudson c.
Hufnagel aortic c.
Hume aortic c.
Humphries aortic aneurysm c.
Humphries reverse-curve aortic c.
Hunt colostomy c.
Hunter-Satinsky c.
Hurson flexible pressure c.
Hurson flexible sliding c.
Hurwitz esophageal c.
Hurwitz intestinal c.
Hymes meatal c.
hysterectomy c.
iliac c.
Iliff c.
incontinence c.
c. insert
interlaminar c.
intestinal anastomosis c.
intestinal occlusion c.
intestinal resection c.
intestinal ring c.
isoelastic rip c.
Ivory rubber dam c.
Jackson bone c.
Jackson bone-extension c.
Jackson bone-holding c.
Jacobs c.
Jacobson bulldog c.
Jacobson microbulldog c.
Jacobson-Potts vessel c.
Jacobson vessel c.
Jahnke anastomosis c.
Jahnke-Cook-Seeley c.
Jako c.
Jameson muscle c.
Jansen c.
Jarit anterior resection c.
Jarit cartilage c.
Jarit intestinal c.
Jarit meniscal c.
Jarvis pile c.
Javid bypass c.
Javid carotid c.
Jesberg laryngectomy c.
Johns Hopkins bulldog c.
Johns Hopkins coarctation c.
Johns Hopkins modified Potts c.
Johnston c.
Jones thoracic c.
Jones towel c.
Joseph septal c.
Judd c.
Judd-Allis c.
Juevenelle c.
Julian-Damian c.
Julian-Fildes c.
Kalt needle holder c.
Kane obstetrical c.
Kane umbilical cord c.
Kantor circumcision c.
Kantrowitz hemostatic c.

C

clamp *(continued)*

Kantrowitz thoracic c.
Kapp-Beck bronchial c.
Kapp-Beck coarctation c.
Kapp-Beck colon c.
Kapp-Beck-Thomson c.
Kapp microarterial c.
Karamar-Mailatt tarsorhaphy c.
Kartchner carotid artery c.
Kaufman kidney c.
Kay aortic anastomosis c.
Kay-Lambert c.
Kelly c.
Kelsey pile c.
Kern bone-holding c.
Kersting colostomy c.
K-Gar umbilical c.
Khan-Jaeger c.
Khodadad c.
kidney pedicle c.
Kiefer c.
Kindt arterial c.
Kindt carotid c.
King c.
Kinsella-Buie lung c.
Kitner c.
Kleinert-Kutz c.
Kleinschmidt appendectomy c.
Klevas c.
Klinikum-Berlin tubing c.
Klintmalm c.
Klute c.
Knutsson penile c.
Knutsson urethrography c.
Kocher intestinal c.
Kolodny c.
Krosnick vesicourethral
  suspension c.
Kutzmann c.
Ladd lid c.
Lahey bronchial c.
Lahey thoracic c.
Lalonde bone c.
Lambert aortic c.
Lambert-Kay aortic c.
Lambert-Kay vascular c.
Lambert-Lowman bone c.
Lambotte bone-holding c.
Lamis patellar c.
c. lamp
Lane bone-holding c.
Lane gastroenterostomy c.
Lane intestinal c.
Lane towel c.
laparoscopic Allis c.
Large vena cava c. (Alfred M.
  Large)
laryngectomy c.
LCC lung compression c.
Leahey c.
Lee bronchus c.
Lee microvascular c.
Lees vascular c.
Lees wedge resection c.

Leland-Jones vascular c.
Lem-Blay circumcision c.
Lewin bone-holding c.
lid c.
Liddle aortic c.
Life-Lok c.
ligament c.
Lillie rectus tendon c.
Lin c.
Lindner anastomosis c.
Linnartz intestinal c.
Linnartz stomach c.
Linton tourniquet c.
lion-head c.
lion-jaw c.
lip c.
Litwak c.
liver-holding c.
Lloyd-Davies c.
lobster-type c.
Locke bone c.
locking c.
Lockwood c.
Longmire-Storm c.
Lorna nonperforating towel c.
Lowman bone-holding c.
Lowman-Gerster bone c.
Lowman-Hoglund c.
Lulu c.
lung exclusion c.
MacDonald gastric c.
Madden intestinal c.
Maingot c.
Malgaigne c.
Malis hinge c.
Marcuse tube c.
marginal c.
Martel intestinal c.
Martin cartilage c.
Martin muscle c.
Mason vascular c.
Masters intestinal c.
Masterson pelvic c.
Masters-Schwartz intestinal c.
Masters-Schwartz liver c.
Mastin muscle c.
Matthew cross-leg c.
Mattox aortic c.
Mayfield aneurysm c.
Mayfield head c.
Mayfield three-pin skull c.
May kidney c.
Mayo-Guyon kidney c.
Mayo-Guyon vessel c.
Mayo kidney c.
Mayo-Lovelace spur crushing c.
Mayo-Robson intestinal c.
Mayo vessel c.
McCleery-Miller intestinal
  anastomosis c.
McCullough hysterectomy c.
McDonald gastric c.
McDougal prostatectomy c.'s
McGuire c.
McKenzie c.

McLean c.
McNealey-Glassman c.
McNealey-Glassman-Mixter c.
McQuigg c.
meatal c.
Meeker gallstone c.
Meeker right-angle c.
megaureter c.
meniscal c.
Michel aortic c.
microarterial c.
microbulldog c.
Microspike approximator c.
microvascular c.
Mikulicz peritoneal c.
Mikulicz-Radecki c.
Miles rectal c.
Millard c.
Millin c.
miniature bulldog c.
Mitchel-Adam c.
Mitchel aortotomy c.
Mixter ligature-carrier c.
Mixter thoracic c.
Mogen circumcision c.
Mohr pinchcock c.
Moorehead lid c.
Moreno gastroenterostomy c.
Moria-France
  dacryocystorhinostomy c.
Morris aortic c.
mosquito hemostatic c.
mosquito lid c.
mouse-tooth c.
Moynihan towel c.
Mueller aortic c.
Mueller bronchial c.
Mueller pediatric c.
Mueller vena cava c.
Muir rectal cautery c.
Mulligan anastomosis c.
multipurpose c.
muscle biopsy c.
mush c.
Myles hemorrhoidal c.
myocardial c.
Nakayama c.
Naraghi-DeCoster reduction c.
needle holder c.
neonatal vascular c.
nephrostomy c.
nerve-approximating c.
Nichols aortic c.
Nicola tendon c.
Niedner anastomosis c.
Niedner pulmonic c.
noncrushing anterior resection c.
noncrushing bowel c.
noncrushing gastroenterostomy c.
noncrushing gastrointestinal c.
noncrushing intestinal c.
noncrushing liver-holding c.
noncrushing vascular c.
nonperforating towel c.
Noon AV fistular c.

Nunez aortic c.
Nunez auricular c.
Nussbaum intestinal c.
occluding c.
Ochsner aortic c.
Ochsner arterial c.
Ochsner thoracic c.
Ockerblad kidney c.
Ockerblad vessel c.
O'Connor lid c.
O'Hanlon intestinal c.
Olivecrona aneurysm c.
Olsen cholangiogram c.
Omed bulldog vascular c.
O'Neill cardiac c.
O'Shaughnessy c.
ossicle-holding c.
osteoplastic flap c.
padded c.
parametrium c.
Parham-Martin bone-holding c.
Parker c.
Parker-Kerr intestinal c.
Parsonnet aortic c.
partial-occlusion c.
Partipilo c.
patellar cement c.
patent ductus c.
Payr gastrointestinal c.
Payr pylorus c.
Payr resection c.
Payr stomach c.
Péan hemostatic c.
Péan hysterectomy c.
Péan intestinal c.
Péan vessel c.
pediatric bulldog c.
pedicle c.
Peers towel c.
pelvic c.
Pemberton sigmoid c.
Pemberton spur-crushing c.
penile c.
Pennington c.
Percy c.
pericortical c.
peripheral vascular c.
peritoneal c.
phalangeal c.
Phaneuf c.
phantom c.
Phillips rectal c.
pile c.
Pilling microanastomosis c.
Pilling pediatric c.
pinchcock c.
pin-to-bar c.
placental c.
Plastibell circumcision c.
point-of-reduction c.
Pomeranz aortic c.
Poppen aortic c.
Poppen-Blalock carotid artery c.
Poppen-Blalock-Salibi carotid c.
post-TUR irrigation c.

clamp *(continued)*
Potts aortic c.
Potts cardiovascular c.
Potts coarctation c.
Potts-DeBakey c.
Potts divisional c.
Potts-Niedner aortic c.
Potts patent ductus c.
Potts pulmonic c.
Potts-Satinsky c.
Potts-Smith aortic c.
Potts-Smith pulmonic c.
Poutasse renal artery c.
Presbyterian Hospital occluding c.
Presbyterian Hospital T-c.
Presbyterian Hospital tubing c.
Preshaw c.
Price muscle c.
Price-Thomas bronchial c.
Prince muscle c.
Pringle c.
Providence Hospital c.
ptosis c.
Pudenz-Heyer c.
pulmonary arterial c.
pulmonary embolism c.
pulmonary nodulectomy c.
pulmonary vessel c.
pulmonic stenosis c.
Putterman levator resection c.
Putterman ptosis c.
pylorus c.
Quick Bend flex c.
Ralks thoracic c.
Ramstedt c.
Ranieri c.
Rankin anastomosis c.
Rankin intestinal c.
Rankin stomach c.
Ranzewski intestinal c.
ratchet c.
Ravich c.
Rayport muscle c.
reamer c.
rectal c.
Redo intestinal c.
Reich-Nechtow arterial c.
Reinhoff swan neck c.
renal artery c.
renal pedicle c.
resection c.
Reul aortic c.
reverse-curve c.
Reynolds dissecting c.
Reynolds resection c.
Reynolds vascular c.
Rhinelander c.
Rica arterial c.
Rica microarterial c.
Rica stem c.
Rica vessel c.
Richards bone c.
right-angle colon c.
ring c.

ring-handled bulldog c.
ring-jawed holding c.
R-N c.
Robin chalazion c.
Rochester hook c.
Rochester-Kocher c.
Rochester-Péan c.
Rochester sigmoid c.
Rockey vascular c.
Roe aortic tourniquet c.
Roeder towel c.
Roosen c.
Roosevelt gastroenterostomy c.
Roosevelt gastrointestinal c.
root rubber dam c.
rubber-dam c.
rubber shod c.
Rubin bronchial c.
Rubio wire-holding c.
Rubovits c.
Rumel myocardial c.
Rumel rubber c.
Rumel thoracic c.
Rush bone c.
Salibi carotid artery c.
Santulli c.
Sarnoff aortic c.
Sarot arterial c.
Sarot bronchus c.
Satinsky anastomosis c.
Satinsky aortic c.
Satinsky pediatric c.
Satinsky vascular c.
Satinsky vena cava c.
Schaedel cross-action towel c.
Schlein c.
Schlesinger c.
Schnidt c.
Schoemaker intestinal c.
Schumacher aortic c.
Schutz c.
Schwartz arterial aneurysm c.
Schwartz bulldog c.
Schwartz intracranial c.
Schwartz vascular c.
Scoville-Lewis c.
screw occlusive c.
Scudder intestinal c.
Scudder stomach c.
Sehrt c.
Seidel bone-holding c.
Sellor c.
Selman c.
Selverstone carotid artery c.
Semb bone-holding c.
Semb bronchus c.
Senning featherweight bulldog c.
Senning-Stille c.
septal c.
serrefine c.
Sheehy ossicle-holding c.
Sheldon c.
shutoff c.
side-biting c.
sidewinder aortic c.

Siegler-Hellman c.
sigmoid anastomosis c.
Silber microvascular c.
Silber vasovasostomy c.
Sims-Maier c.
Singley intestinal c.
Siniscal eyelid c.
skull c.
Slim Fit flex c.
Slocum meniscal c.
slotted nerve c.
SMIC intestinal c.
Smith bone c.
Smith cordotomy c.
Smith marginal c.
Smithwick anastomotic c.
Softjaw c.
Somers uterine c.
Southwick c.
sponge c.
spoon anastomosis c.
spur-crushing c.
S-shaped peripheral vascular c.
S. S. White c.
stainless steel c.
Stallard head c.
Stanton cautery c.
Stayce adjustable c.
Stay-Rite c.
Steinhauser bone c.
Stemp c.
stenosis c.
Stepita meatal c.
Stetten intestinal c.
Stevenson c.
Stille-Crawford coarctation c.
Stille kidney c.
Stille vessel c.
Stimson pedicle c.
Stiwer towel c.
St. Mark c.
Stockman meatal c.
Stockman penile c.
stomach c.
Stone-Holcombe anastomosis c.
Stone-Holcombe intestinal c.
Stone intestinal c.
Stone stomach c.
Stony splenorenal shunt c.
Storey c.
Storz meatal c.
straight mosquito c.
Stratte kidney c.
Strauss meatal c.
Strauss penile c.
Strauss-Valentine penile c.
Strelinger colon c.
St. Vincent tube c.
Subramanian classic miniature
  aortic c.
Subramanian sidewinder aortic c.
Sugarbaker retrocolic c.
Sugita head c.
Sumner c.
SurgiMed c.

Swan aortic c.
swan-neck c.
Swenson ring-jawed holding c.
Swiss bulldog c.
Sztehlo umbilical c.
T c.
tangential occlusion c.
tangential pediatric c.
Tatum meatal c.
Taufic cholangiography c.
Tehl c.
temporalis transfer c.
tension c.
Textor vasectomy c.
Thoma c.
Thompson carotid artery c.
Thomson lung c.
thoracic c.
Thorlakson lower occlusive c.
Thorlakson upper occlusive c.
three-bladed c.
Thumb-Saver introducer c.
tissue occlusion c.
tonsil c.
tonsillar c.
towel c.
Trendelenburg-Crafoord coarctation c.
Treves intestinal c.
trochanter-holding c.
truncus c.
Trusler infant vascular c.
tube-occluding c.
tubing c.
Tucker appendix c.
turkey-claw c.
Tydings tonsillar c.
Tyrrell c.
Ullrich tubing c.
Ulrich bone-holding c.
umbilical cord c.
umbiliclamp c.
Umbilicutter c.
Universal wire c.
upper occlusive c.
ureteral c.
urethrographic cannula c.
urinary incontinence c.
uterine c.
vaginal cuff c.
Valdoni c.
Vanderbilt vessel c.
Varco dissecting c.
Varco gallbladder c.
vas c.
Vasconcelos-Barretto c.
VascuClamp minibulldog vessel c.
VascuClamp vascular c.
vascular graft c.
vasovasostomy c.
Veidenheimer resection c.
vena cava c.
Verbrugge bone c.
Verbrugge bone-holding c.
Verse-Webster c.
vessel c.

clamp *(continued)*
vessel-occluding c.
vestibular c.
Virtus splinter c.
V. Mueller aortic c.
V. Mueller auricular appendage c.
V. Mueller bulldog c.
V. Mueller cross-action bulldog c.
V. Mueller vena cava c.
von Petz intestinal c.
Vorse tube-occluding c.
Vorse-Webster tube-occluding c.
vulsellum c.
Wadsworth lid c.
Walther-Crenshaw meatal c.
Walther kidney pedicle c.
Walther pedicle c.
Walton meniscal c.
Wangensteen anastomosis c.
Wangensteen gastric-crushing
 anastomotic c.
Wangensteen patent ductus c.
Warthen spur-crushing c.
Watts locking c.
Weaver chalazion c.
Weber aortic c.
Weck c.
Weck-Edna nonperforating towel c.
wedge resection c.
Weldon miniature bulldog c.
Wells pedicle c.
Wertheim-Cullen kidney pedicle c.
Wertheim kidney pedicle c.
Wertheim-Reverdin pedicle c.
Wester meniscal c.
West Shur cartilage c.
White c.
Whitver penile c.
Wikström gallbladder c.
Wikström-Stilgust c.
Willett c.
Williams c.
Wilman c.
Wilson c.
Winkelmann circumcision c.
Winston cervical c.
wire-tightening c.
Wirthlin splenorenal shunt c.
Wister vascular c.
Wolfson intestinal c.
Wolfson spur-crushing c.
Wood bulldog c.
Wylie carotid artery c.
Wylie hypogastric c.
Wylie "J" c.
Wylie lumbar bulldog c.
X-c.
Yasargil carotid c.
Yellen circumcision c.
Young renal pedicle c.
Zachary-Cope c.
Zachary-Cope-DeMartel colon c.
Z-clamp c.
Zeppelin c.

Ziegler-Furness c.
Zimmer cartilage c.
Zinnanti c.
Zipser meatal c.
Zipser penile c.
Zutt c.
Zweifel appendectomy c.
Zweifel pressure c.
clamshell
c. brace
c. device
c. prosthesis
C. septal umbrella
Clar head light
Clarion multi-strategy cochlear implant
Clark
C. capsule fragment forceps
C. common duct dilator
C. expanding mesh catheter
C. eye speculum
C. helix catheter
C. hemoperfusion cartridge
C. hemoperfusion system
C. ligator scissor forceps
C. oxygen electrode
C. rotating cutter catheter
C. vein stripper
Clarke-Reich
C.-R. knot pusher
C.-R. ligator
Clarke stereotactic instrument
Clark-Guyton forceps
Clark-Verhoeff capsular forceps
Clarus
C. model 5169 peristaltic pump
C. SpineScope
clasp
Acland c.
Adams c.
arrow pin c.
c. bar
Charnley bone c.
Crozat c.
Damon c.
Duyzings c.
EPI Sport epicondylitis c.
eyelet c.
Hahnenkratt dental c.
c. knife
preformed c.
Roach c.
Sumpter c. spring-lock
Classic II stethoscope
Classix pacemaker
Classon pediatric scissors
Clas von Eichen needle
Claussen fragment stabilizer
Clave needleless system
claw
c. forceps
c. retractor
Clawicz chisel
Clay Adams PE-series catheter
Clayman
C. corneal forceps

C. intraocular guide
C. intraocular lens
C. iris hook
C. lens forceps
C. lens-holding forceps
C. lens implant
C. lens-inserting forceps
C. lid retractor
C. spatula
C. suturing forceps
Clayman-Kelman intraocular lens forceps
Clayman-Knolle irrigating lens loop
Clayman-McPherson tying forceps
Clayman-Troutman corneal scissors
Clayman-Vannas scissors
Clayman-Westcott scissors
Clayton
C. laminectomy shears
C. osteotome
CLC orthotic
Cleanlet lancet
Clean-Wheel disposable neurological pinwheel
clear
C. Advantage latex free catheter
C. Advantage silicone male catheter
C. Image III
c. PVC tube & connector kit
ClearCut
C. 2 electrosurgical handpiece
C. II with smoke eater tube
C. 2 instrument
Clearfix
C. meniscal dart
C. meniscal screw
ClearSite
C. bandage
C. borderless dressing
C. HydroGauze dressing
C. hydrogel absorptive borderline wound dressing
ClearView
C. CO$_2$ laser
C. uterine manipulator
Cleasby
C. iris spatula
C. spatulated needle
cleaver
Case enamel c.
fiber c.
Haefliger c.
Orton enamel c.
cleft
c. palate elevator
c. palate forceps
c. palate needle
c. palate prosthesis
c. palate raspatory
c. palate sharp hook
Clemetson uterine forceps
Clensicair
C. incontinence management system
C. low-air-loss hydrotherapy bed
Clerf
C. aspirator

C. cancer cell collector
C. dilator
C. forceps
C. laryngeal saw
C. laryngectomy tube
C. laryngoscope
C. needle holder
Clerf-Arrowsmith safety pin closer
Clev-Dent excavator
Clevedan positive pressure respirator
Clevedent
C. forceps
C. retractor
Clevedent-Gardner chisel
Clevedent-Lucas curette
Clevedent-Wakefield chisel
Cleveland
C. bone-cutting forceps
C. bone rongeur
C. IMA retractor
Clevis
C. clamp
C. dressing
clicker
compression c.
Click'X
climber
Fitstep II stair c.
Sprint C.
Clinac 600SR stereotactic radiation treatment system
C-line bipolar coagulator
clinical
c. electromagnetic flowmeter
Clinical HandMaster system
Clini-Care
C.-C. bed
C.-C. low-air-loss system
CliniCath
C. peripherally inserted catheter
Clinicel silicon gel-filled cushion
clinic exolever elevator
Clini.Dyne bed
Clini.Float
C. bed
C. flotation therapy bed system
Cliniguard pad
Clinisert mattress
Cliniset infusion set
Clinitemp fever detector
Clinitex Charles endophotocoagulator probe
Clinitron
C. air bed
C. air-fluidized bed
C. Elexis air fluidized therapy unit
C. II air fluidized therapy unit
C. uplift air fluidized therapy unit
clinometer
clip
Ackerman c.
Acland c.
Adams-DeWeese vena cava serrated c.
Adams orthodontic c.

C

clip *(continued)*

Adson brain c.
Adson scalp c.
alligator c.
aneurysm c.
aneurysmal c.
angled c.
c. applier
Astro-Trace Universal adapter c.
Atrauclip hemostatic c.
Austin c.
Autostat hemostatic c.
Autostat ligating c.
Auto Suture c.
Avalox skin c.
Backhaus towel c.
bayonet aneurysm c.
Beimer-Clip aneurysm c.
Benjamin-Havas fiberoptic light c.
Biemer vessel c.
bipolar diathermy adapter c.
Bleier c.
blepharoplasty c.
Bonney c.
Booster c.
Boyle-Rosin c.
brain c.
Braun-Yasargil right-angle c.
butterfly c.
Callender c.
cardiac retraction c.
Castroviejo scleral shortening c.
Children's Hospital c.
Codman c.
Colotzmark c.
cranial aneurysm c.
crankshaft c.
cross-legged c.
curved c.
Cushing c.
Cushing-McKenzie c.
Dandy c.
Delrin plastic scalp c.
Dermaclip c.
DeWeese-Hunter c.
Drake aneurysm c.
Drake fenestrated c.
Drake-Kees c.
Duane U-c.
ear c.
Edslab jaw spring c.
Edwards parallel-jaw spring c.
Elgiloy c.
Elgiloy-Heifitz aneurysm c.
encircling c.
Endo GIA surgical c.
Ethicon c.
Feldstein blepharoplasty c.
fenestrated aneurysm c.
ferromagnetic intracerebral aneurysm c.
Filshie female sterilization c.
Flexi-Seal fecal collector & tail c.
c. force meter

c. forceps
Friedman tantalum c.
gate c.
c. graft
Guilford-Wright c.
Hader bar c.
Halberg c.
Heath c.
Hegenbarth c.
Hegenbarth-Adams c.
Heifitz aneurysm c.
Heifitz-Weck c.
Hem-o-lok polymer ligating c.
hemostasis scalp c.
hemostasis silver c.
hemostatic c.
Herff c.
Hesseltine Umbili C.
holding c.
Horizon surgical ligating and marking c.
House neurovascular c.
Housepian aneurysm c.
Hoxworth c.
Hulka c.
Hulka-Clemens c.
Hylinks c.
inferior vena cava c.
Ingraham-Fowler cranium c.
Ingraham-Fowler tantalum c.
Iwabuchi c.
Janelli c.
jaw spring c.
Kapp c.
Keer aneurysm c.
Khodadad c.
Kifa c.
Koln c.
laparoscopic tie c.
Lapro-Clip ligating c.
LDS c.
lens c.
LeRoy infant scalp c.
LeRoy-Raney scalp c.
Ligaclip surgical c.
L-shaped aneurysm c.
magazine c.
Mayfield CIS-RE aneurysm c.
Mayfield-Kees c.
McDermott c.
McFadden cross-legged c.
McFadden-Kees c.
McFadden Vari-Angle aneurysm c.
McKenzie hemostasis c.
McKenzie silver brain c.
McKenzie V-c.
metal c.
metallic c.
Michel scalp c.
Michel skin c.
Michel suture c.
Michel-Wachtenfeldt c.
microanastomosis c.
microbulldog c.
microvascular c.

Miles skin c.
Miles Teflon c.
Miles vena cava c.
mini-Sugita c.
Moren-Moretz vena cava c.
Moretz c.
Morse towel c.
Mortson V-shaped c.
Moynihan c.
nonferromagnetic c.
nose c.
Olivecrona silver c.
palmar c.
partial-occlusion inferior vena
  cava c.
Paterson long-shank brain c.
Penfield silver c.
Perneczky aneurysm c.
Phynox cobalt alloy c.
pivot aneurysm c.
plastic scalp c.
Poly Surgiclip absorbable c.
Pool-Pfeiffer self-locking c.
primary c.
Raney scalp c.
Raney spring steel c.
c. remover
retractor c.
Rica cross-action towel c.
Rica silver c.
Rica suture c.
right-angle booster c.
ring c.
Samuels-Weck Hemoclip c.
scalp hemostasis c.
Scanlan aneurysm c.
Schaedel c.
Schepens tantalum c.
Schulec silver c.
Schutz c.
Schwartz c.
Schwasser brain c.
Schwasser microclip c.
scleral shortening c.
Scoville c.
Scoville-Lewis aneurysm c.
Secu c.
Selman c.
Seraphim c.
Serature spur c.
silver c.
skin c.
Slimline c.
Smith aneurysm c.
Smithwick silver c.
Sofield retractor c.
Spetzler titanium aneurysm c.
spring c.
sternal c.
Stichs wound c.
straight aneurysm c.
suction tube c.
Sugar aneurysm c.
Sugita aneurysm c.
Sugita cross-legged c.

Sugita-Ikakogyo c.
Sugita side-curved bayonet c.
Sugita temporary straight c.
Sundt booster c.
Sundt cross-legged c.
Sundt encircling c.
Sundt-Kees aneurysm c.
Sundt-Kees booster c.
Sundt-Kees encircling patch c.
Sundt-Kees graft c.
Sundt-Kees Slimline c.
Sundt straddling c.
surgical c.
Surgiclip c.
Surgidev iris c.
Takaro c.
tantalum hemostasis c.
Teflon c.
temporary vascular c.
temporary vessel c.
titanium aneurysm c.
Tomac c.
Totco c.
towel c.
triangular encompassing c.
Tru-clip c.
two-way towel c.
U-c.
Umbili C.
umbilical c.
Uni-Shunt abdominal slip c.
Uni-Shunt cranial anchoring c.
Uni-Shunt right-angle c.
V-c.
Vari-Angle c.
vascular c.
vena cava c.
vessel c.
Vitallium c.
von Petz c.
Wachtenfeldt butterfly c.
Wachtenfeldt suture c.
Wachtenfeldt wound c.
Weck Hemoclip c.
window c.
wing c.
wound c.
Yasargil-Aesculap spring c.
Yasargil cross-legged c.
Zimmer c.
Zmurkiewicz brain c.
clip-applier
  Sundt aneurysm c.-a.
  Yasargil aneurysm c.-a.
clip-applying aneurysm forceps
clip-bending forceps
clip-cutting forceps
clip-introducing forceps
Cliplamp
  Mini C.
Clip-Lite clip-on headlight
clip-on/tie-on occluder
clipper
  Baxter surgical c.
clip-reinforced cotton sling

153

clip-removing
  c.-r. forceps
  c.-r. scissors
ClipTip reusable sensor
Clirans T-series dialyzer
Clisco covered needle catheter
Clitoral therapy device
CLM articulating laryngoscope blade
CLO
  CLO Cool Bag
  CLO Cool Wand
  CLO Recirculating Slim Pack
clock
  Sonic Boom alarm c.
clog
  Hollander c.
  Markell Mobility Health c.'s
C-loop
  C.-l. posterior chamber lens
Cloquet needle
closed
  c. chain exercise attachment
  c. Cotrel-Dubousset hook
  c. iris forceps
  c. Küntscher nail
  c. mini-pouch
  c. suction drain
**closed-circuit television vision
  enhancement system**
closed-loop
  c.-l. device
  c.-l. intraocular lens
closed-suction tube
Close Encounter nut
closer
  Clerf-Arrowsmith safety pin c.
  c. forceps
  safety pin c.
CloseSure procedure kit
closing forceps
closure
  Beta-Cap II catheter c.
  Brandy scalp stretcher I, II,
    front c.
  Brandy scalp stretcher I, II, rear c.
  compression skull cap c.
  DuoLock curved tail c.
  eXit disposable puncture c.
  facial compression finger c.
  facial compression skull cap c.
  hand-sutured c.
  Lowsley retractor with hand-
    sutured c.
  retainer c.
  Steri-Strip skin c.
  Steritapes c.
  Sure-Closure c.
  Sur-Fit/ACTIVE LIFE tail c.
  Sur-Fit irrigation sleeve tail c.
  SutureStrip Plus wound c.
  vacuum-assisted c.
clot forceps
cloth
  Dacron c.
clothesline drain

cloth-shod clamp
Clot Stop drain
Cloutier unconstrained knee prosthesis
cloverleaf
  C. EP catheter
  C. internal bumper
  c. met foot pad
  c. nail
  c. pin
  c. pin extractor
  c. rod
Cloward
  C. anterior fusion kit
  C. blade retractor
  C. bone graft impactor
  C. bone punch
  C. brain retractor
  C. cautery hook
  C. cervical dislocation reducer
  C. cervical drill
  C. cervical drill guard
  C. cervical drill tip
  C. cervical retractor
  C. cervical retractor set
  C. cross-bar handle
  C. curette
  C. depth gauge
  C. double-hinge cervical retractor
    handle
  C. dowel cutter
  C. dowel ejector
  C. dowel handle
  C. dowel impactor
  C. drill guard cap
  C. drill guide
  C. drill shaft
  C. dural hook
  C. dural retractor
  C. hammer
  C. instrument
  C. intervertebral disk rongeur
  C. intervertebral punch
  C. laminectomy rongeur
  C. lumbar retractor body
  C. L-W gauge
  C. nerve root retractor
  C. osteophyte elevator
  C. periosteal elevator
  C. pituitary rongeur
  C. PLIF case
  C. PLIF II kit
  C. posterior lumbar interbody fusion
    kit
  C. self-retaining retractor
  C. single-tooth retractor blade
  C. spanner gauge
  C. spanner wrench
  C. spinal fusion chisel
  C. spinal fusion osteotome
  C. spreader
  C. square punch
  C. surgical saddle
  C. tissue retractor
  C. vertebral spreader

Cloward-Cone
    C.-C. ring curette
Cloward-Cushing vein retractor
Cloward-Dowel punch
Cloward-English
    C.-E. punch
    C.-E. rongeur
Cloward-Harman chisel
Cloward-Harper
    C.-H. cervical punch
    C.-H. laminectomy rongeur
Cloward-Hoen laminectomy retractor
Cloward-Puka chisel
clubfoot splint
Clyburn Colles fracture fixator
Clyman endometrial curette
clysis cannula
CM-Band
    CM-B. 505N brace
    CM-B. silicone rubber brace
CMI/Mityvac cup
CMI/O'Neil cup
CMI vacuum delivery system
C-mount adapter
CMV
    cool mist vaporizer
Cntour ERCP cannula
CO
    cervical orthosis
    CO Sleuth
CO$_2$
    C. cylinder
    C. generator
    C. laser probe
    C. Sharplan laser
CO2SMO monitor
Coach incentive spirometer
Coag-A-Mate
    C.-A.-M. coagulometer
Coag-a-Mate prothrombin device
CoaguChek
    C. portable prothrombin time device
coagulating
    c. electrode
    c. forceps
    c. suction cannula connection cord
    c. suction cannula obturator
coagulation
    c. electrode
    c. forceps
    c. probe
    c. suction tube
coagulation-aspirator tube
coagulator
    American Optical c.
    argon beam c.
    argon plasma c.
    Ball c.
    Ballantine-Drew c.
    Bantam Bovie c.
    Biceps bipolar c.
    bipolar c.
    Birtcher Hyfrecator c.
    Birtcher laparoscopic c.
    Bovie CSV c.

C-line bipolar c.
Codman-Mentor Wet-Field c.
Codman-Shurtleff neo-coagulator c.
cold c.
Concept bipolar c.
Cut-Blot c.
electricator c.
Elektrotom BiCut II c.
Elmed BC 50 M/M digital
    bipolar c.
Erbe Unit argon plasma c.
Evergreen Lasertek c.
Fabry c.
Fukushima monopolar malleable c.
Gam-Mer bipolar c.
Grieshaber microbipolar c.
Hildreth c.
Hyfrecator c.
infrared c.
Jarit bipolar c.
Karl Storz c.
Kirwan bipolar c.
Magielski c.
Makar c.
Malis CMC-II PC bipolar c.
Malis solid state c.
Mentor Wet-Field cordless c.
Meyer-Schwickerath c.
Mira c.
National c.
Polar-Mate bipolar c.
Poppen electrosurgical c.
Redfield IRC 2100 infrared c.
Resnick button bipolar c.
Riddle c.
Ritter c.
Ritter-Bantam Bovie c.
Scanlan bipolar c.
solid-state c.
Storz microsurgical bipolar c.
suction-c.
Tekno c.
Ultroid c.
Walker c.
wet-field c.
xenon arc c.
Zeiss c.
coagulometer
    Coag-A-Mate c.
Coaguloop
    C. resection electrode
Coakley
    C. antral curette
    C. antral trocar
    C. ethmoid curette
    C. frontal sinus cannula
    C. nasal curette
    C. nasal probe
    C. nasal speculum
    C. sinus curette
    C. tenaculum
    C. tonsillar forceps
    C. wash tube
Coakley-Allis tonsillar forceps

coaptation
> c. bipolar forceps
> c. plate
> c. splint

coarctation
> c. clamp
> c. forceps
> c. hook

coarse carbide cone bur
coarse-olive bur
coated
> c. biopsy forceps
> c. polyester suture
> c. Vicryl Rapide suture

coater
> Hummer V Sputter c.
> Polaron sputter c.

coating
> Porocoat c.
> porous c.
> Pro/Pel c.
> Solo catheter with Pro/Pel c.
> Spring catheter with Pro/Pel c.
> Teflon c.

Co-Axa light
coaxial
> c. cable
> c. cannula
> c. catheter
> c. I&A nylon connector
> c. micropuncture introducer set
> c. sheath cut-biopsy needle
> c. snare

Coballoy twist drill
cobalt
> c. blue light
> c. chrome modular head component
> c. megavoltage machine

cobalt-chromium
> c.-c. alloy prosthesis
> c.-c. head
> c.-c. implant

cobalt-chromium-molybdenum
> c.-c.-m. alloy
> c.-c.-m. alloy metal implant

cobalt-chromium-tungsten-nickel alloy
metal implant
Coban
> C. bandage
> C. elastic dressing
> C. wrap

COBAS
> COBAS Fara H centrifugal analyzer
> COBAS Helios differential analyzer

Cobaugh eye forceps
Cobb
> C. bone curette
> C. chisel
> C. osteotome
> C. periosteal elevator
> C. retractor
> C. spinal curette
> C. spinal elevator
> C. spinal gouge
> C. spinal instrument

Cobbett skin graft knife
Cobb-Ragde needle
Cobe
> C. AV fistular needle
> C. AV shunt
> C. blood cell separator
> C. cardiotomy reservoir
> C. 2991 cell processor
> C. CML oxygenator
> C. double blood pump
> C. Optima hollow-fiber membrane oxygenator
> C. small vessel cannula
> C. Spectra apheresis system
> C. staple gun
> C. Trima

Cobe-Stockert
> C.-S. heart lung console
> C.-S. heart-lung machine

Cobe-Tenckhoff peritoneal dialysis
catheter
coblation
> tonsillar c.

Cobra
> C. K+ cannula
> C. K cannula
> C. K+ cannula tip
> C. over-the-wire balloon catheter

Cobra+
> C. cannula
> C. cannula tip

cobra-head
> c.-h. drill
> c.-h. plate
> c.-h. retractor

Coburg-Connell airway
Coburn
> C. anterior chamber intraocular lens implant
> C. camera
> C. equiconvex lens
> C. haptic
> C. I&A system
> C. intraocular lens
> C. lensometer
> C. Mark IX eye implant
> C. Optical Industries-Feaster intraocular lens
> C. refractor
> C. tonometer

Coburn-Rodenstock slit lamp
Coburn-Storz intraocular lens
coccyx
> c. cushion
> C. seat cushion

cochlear implant
cock
> stop c.

Cocke large flap retractor
cock-up
> c.-u. arm splint
> c.-u. wrist support

cocoon
> c. dressing
> c. thread suture

Co-Cr-Mo
 C.-C.-M. alloy
 C.-C.-M. pin
 C.-C.-M. prosthesis
Co-Cr-W-Ni
 C.-C.-W.-N. alloy
 C.-C.-W.-N. alloy implant metal
 C.-C.-W.-N. alloy prosthesis
coder
 Chen-Smith image c.
Codivilla graft
cod liver oil-soaked strips dressing
Codman
 C. Accu-Flow shunt
 C. anterior cervical plating (ACP) system
 C. arthroscope
 C. Bicol sponge
 C. bone gouge
 C. cannula
 C. cartilage clamp
 C. cervical rongeur
 C. clip
 C. cranioblade
 C. cranioclast
 C. cranioplastic material
 C. dilator case
 C. disposable ICP lock
 C. disposable perforator
 C. external drainage system
 C. external drainage ventricular set
 C. fallopian tube forceps
 C. frame
 C. guide
 C. Hakim programmable valve
 C. ICP monitor
 C. ICP monitoring line
 C. IMA kit
 C. intracranial pressure monitor
 C. laminectomy rongeur
 C. lumbar external drain
 C. magnifying loupe
 C. marker
 C. microimpactor
 C. neurological headrest system
 C. osteotome
 C. ovary forceps
 C. Rhoton dissector
 C. scissors
 C. skull perforator guard
 C. spanner
 C. sternal saw
 C. surgical patty
 C. surgical strip
 C. Ti-frame posterior fixation system
 C. towel clamp
 C. vein stripper
 C. ventricular silicone catheter
 C. wire cutter
 C. wire-passing drill
Codman-Holter catheter
Codman-Kerrison laminectomy rongeur
Codman-Leksell laminectomy rongeur
Codman-Medos programmable valve

Codman-Mentor
 C.-M. Wet-Field cautery
 C.-M. Wet-Field coagulator
Codman-Schlesinger cervical laminectomy rongeur
Codman-Shurtleff
 C.-S. cranial drill
 C.-S. neo-coagulator coagulator
Cody
 C. magnetic probe
 C. sacculotomy tack
Coe
 C. impression material
 C. investment material
 C. orthodontic resin
Coe-Comfort tissue conditioner
Coe-Pak
 C.-P. paste adhesive
 C.-P. periodontal dressing
COER-24 delivery system
Coe-Rect denture reliner
Coe-Soft
 C.-S. denture reliner
 C.-S. dressing
coffer band
Coffin
 C. plate
 C. transpalatal wire
Cofield
 C. 2 total shoulder system
Coflex
 C. bandage
 C. wrap
Cogan-Boberg-Ans
 C.-B.-A. lens
 C.-B.-A. lens implant
Cogent
 C. light
 C. LightWear headlight
 C. XL illuminator
Cogsell tip aspirator
CO₂Guard
Cohan-Barraquer microscope
Cohan needle holder
Cohan-Vannas iris scissors
Cohan-Westcott scissors
Cohen
 C. corneal forceps
 C. intrauterine cannula
 C. nasal-dressing forceps
 C. periosteal elevator
 C. retractor
 C. rongeur
 C. sinus rasp
 C. suture applicator
 C. tubal insufflation cannula
 C. uterine cannula
Cohen-Eder uterine cannula
Coherent
 C. 920 argon laser
 C. argon laser photocoagulator
 C. carbon dioxide laser
 C. EPIC laser
 C. 7910 laser
 C. LaserLink slit lamp

C

Coherent *(continued)*
    C. Medical YAG laser
    C. Novus Omni multiwavelength
      laser
    C. photocoagulator
    C. radiation Fluorotron
    C. Selecta 7000 laser
    C. UltraPulse 5000C laser
    C. Versapulse device
cohesive
    c. bandage
    c. dressing
Cohn cardiac stabilizer
Cohney scissors
Cohort
    C. anterior plate system
    C. bone brush
    C. bone screw
    C. spinal impactor
    C. Ti-Spacer
coil
    aneurysmal c.
    birdcage head c.
    body c.
    c. cannister
    c. catheter
    circumferential extremity c.
    collagen-filled interlocking
      detachable c.
    Cook retrievable embolization c.
    crossed c.
    custom-curved c.
    Dacron fiber-coated c.
    detachable c.
    double breast c.
    DuctOcclud c.
    c. electrode
    electro-detachable platinum c.
    embolization c.
    endoanal c.
    endoesophageal MRI c.
    endorectal c.
    endorectal-pelvic phased-array c.
    endoscopic quadrature
      radiofrequency c.
    endovaginal c.
    endovascular c.
    fat-suppressed body c.
    flexible surface c.
    Gianturco occlusion c.
    Gianturco steel c.
    Gianturco-Wallace-Anderson c.
    Gianturco wool-tufted wire c.
    Golay gradient c.
    gradient sheet c.
    Guglielmi detachable c.
    head c.
    helical c.
    Helmholtz double-surface c.
    Hilal c.
    interlocking detachable c.
    intraurethral c.
    Ivalon wire c.
    liver c.

    local gradient c.
    c. machine adapter
    Margulies c.
    Medrad Mrinnervu endorectal colon
      probe c.
    modified birdcage c.
    occlusion c.
    opposed loop-pair quadrature
      magnetic resonance c.
    orthogonal radiofrequency c.
    pelvic phased-array c.
    phased-array torso c.
    planar circular c.
    platinum embolization c.
    posterior neck surface c.
    Prolapse c.
    quadrature cervical spine c.
    quadrature radiofrequency receiver c.
    quadrature T/L surface c.
    radiofrequency c.
    receive-only circular surface c.
    right ventricular c.
    saddle c.
    sensing c.
    shim c.
    shoulder surface c.
    solenoid surface c.
    steel embolization c.
    surface c.
    tantalum balloon-expandable stent
      with helical c.
    three-axis gradient c.
    torso phased-array c.
    transmit-receive c.
    transverse gradient c.
    c. vascular stent
    VORTX vascular occlusion c.
    z-gradient c.
Coil-Cath catheter
coiled
    c. pressure algesimeter
    c. spiral pusher wire
    c. spring
coilette
    FLX flexible treatment c.
coil-tipped catheter
Co₂ject system
Colapinto
    C. sheath
    C. transjugular biopsy set
    C. transjugular needle
Colclough laminectomy rongeur
Colclough-Love-Kerrison laminectomy
  rongeur
cold
    c. beam laser
    c. biopsy forceps
    c. (carbon dioxide) cautery
    c. coagulator
    C. Compress mask
    c. coning knife
    c. cup biopsy forceps
    c. knife hook
    c. pad

c. rolled rod
c. scissors
Coldhot pack
Coldite transilluminator
cold-mist humidifier
cold-weld femoral ball
Cole
    C. duodenal retractor
    C. endotracheal tube
    C. hyperextension fracture frame
    C. orotracheal tube
    C. pediatric tube
    C. polyethylene vein stripper
    C. uncuffed endotracheal tube
Coleman
    C. aspiration cannula
    C. microinfiltration system
    C. retractor
    C. V-dissector infiltration cannula
Coleman-Taylor IOL forceps
Colibri
    C. corneal forceps
    C. eye forceps
    C. mules
Colibri-Pierse forceps
Colibri-Storz corneal forceps
Colin
    C. ambulatory BP monitor
    C. Electronics BP-508 tonometry
      system
    C. STBP-780 stress test blood
      pressure monitor
CollaCote collagen wound dressing
collagen
    c. absorbable suture
    bovine biodegradable c.
    Contigen glutaraldehyde cross-
      linked c.
    c. dressing
    c. hemostatic material
    c. implant
    InterGard knitted c.
    c. membrane
    microfibrillar c.
    c. plug
    c. scaffold
    c. shield
    c. sponge
collagen-filled interlocking detachable coil
collagen-impregnated
    c.-i. Dacron
    c.-i. knitted Dacron velour graft
CollagENT wand
Collagraft
    C. bone graft matrix
    C. bone graft matrix material
Collamer intraocular lens
CollaPlug wound dressing
collapsible tissue retractor
collar
    Belmont c.
    c. brace
    c. button
    cervical c.
    Colpacs c.

cone c.
Cowboy c.
c. dressing
Exo-Static cervical c.
foam c.
Headmaster c.
heated tracheostomy c.
high-humidity tracheostomy c.
Houston halo traction c.
implant c.
Little Ones SUR-FIT flexible wafer,
  white c.
MAC cervical c.
Marlin cervical c.
Miami Acute Care cervical c.
Miami J cervical c.
Minerva c.
Nec Loc cervical c.
Newport c.
Peterson cervical c.
Philadelphia cervical c.
plastic c.
Plastizote cervical c.
Pneu-trac cervical c.
c. prosthesis
2+2 Rehab c.
Schanz c.
c. scissors
Thomas c.
collar-button
    c.-b. iris retractor
    c.-b. tube
collared Press-Fit femoral stem
    implantation
collarless
    c. polished taper
    c. stem
Collastat
    C. OBP microfibrillar collagen
      hemostat
CollaTape
    C. tape
    C. wound dressing
CollectFirst system
collecting tube
collection trap
collector
    Alden-Senturia specimen c.
    bone c.
    Carabelli cancer cell c.
    Cervex-Brush cervical cell c.
    Clerf cancer cell c.
    Conveen drip c.
    Cuputi sputum c.
    Cytobrush Plus cell c.
    Cytopick endocervical and
      uterovaginal cell c.
    Davidson c.
    drainable fecal c.
    Endocell endometrial cell c.
    fetal incontinence c.
    Flexi-Seal fecal c.
    Grass force displacement fluid c.
    Herchenson esophageal cytology c.
    Leukotrap red cell c.

C

collector *(continued)*
    Little Ones Pediatric Urine C.
    Lukens c.
    Medscand Cytobrush Plus cell c.
    Misstique female external urinary c.
    Moffat-Robinson bone pate c.
    Papette cervical c.
    Pilling c.
    Senturia-Alden specimen c.
    Sheehy Pate C.
    stool c.
    Uterobrush endometrial sample c.
    Wallach-Papette disposable cervical cell c.
    Ware cancer cell c.
    wound drainage c.
    Xomed sinus-secretion c.

College
    C. forceps
    C. Park TruStep foot
    C. Park TruStep foot prosthesis
    C. pliers

Collen-Pozzi tenaculum
Coller
    C. arterial forceps
    C. hemostatic forceps

Colles
    C. external fixation frame
    C. needle holder
    C. sling
    C. snare
    C. splint

collet
    c. screwdriver adapter
    tibial c.

Colley
    C. tissue forceps
    C. traction forceps

Collier
    C. hemostatic forceps
    C. needle holder
    C. thoracic clamp

Collier-Crile hemostatic forceps
Collier-DeBakey
    C.-D. hemostat
    C.-D. hemostatic forceps

Collier-Martin hook
collimated
    c. beam handpiece
    c. beam handpiece (CBH-1) for laser surgery

collimator
    APC-3, -4 c.
    CASS TrueTaper c.
    converging c.
    diverging c.
    Eureka c.
    external c.
    fan-beam c.
    c. helmet
    high-resolution multileaf c.
    high-sensitivity c.
    511-keV c.
    Leur-par c.

    long-bore c.
    low-energy c.
    Machlett c.
    medium-energy c.
    Micro-Cast c.
    multileaf c.
    multirod c.
    parallel-hole medium sensitivity c.
    Picker Dyna Mo c.
    pinhole c.
    C. plugging pattern
    slant hole c.
    Sophy high-resolution c.
    StereoGuide c.
    Summit LoDose c.

Collin
    C. abdominal retractor
    C. amputation knife
    C. 140 color adaptometer
    C. dressing forceps
    C. intestinal forceps
    C. lung-grasping forceps
    C. mesher
    C. mucous forceps
    C. osteoclast
    C. ovarian forceps
    C. pelvimeter
    C. pleural dissector
    C. radiopaque sternal blade
    C. raspatory
    C. rib shears
    C. sternal self-retaining retractor
    C. tissue forceps
    C. tongue forceps
    C. tongue-seizing forceps
    C. umbilical clamp
    C. uterine curette
    C. uterine-elevating forceps
    C. vaginal speculum

Collin-Duval-Crile intestinal forceps
Collin-Duval intestinal forceps
Collings
    C. electrosurgery knife
    C. fulguration electrode
    C. knife electrode

Collin-Hartmann retractor
Collin-Pozzi uterine forceps
Collins
    C. bicycle ergometer
    C. Dry spirometer
    C. dynamometer
    C. Eagle I spirometry unit
    C. leg holder
    C. respiratometer
    C. Survey spirometer
    C. SurveyTach pneumotachometer

Collins-Mayo mastoid retractor
Collis
    C. anterior cervical retractor
    C. microforceps
    C. microscissors
    C. mouthgag
    C. posterior lumbar retractor
    C. spirometer

C. TDR instrument
C. Universal laminectomy set
Collis-Maumenee corneal forceps
Collison
    C. body drill
    C. cannulated hand drill
    C. screw
    C. screwdriver
    C. tap drill
Collis-Taylor retractor
collodion dressing
collodion-treated self-adhesive bandage
Collostat sponge
Collyer pelvimeter
Colmascope
colon
    c. clamp
    c. motility catheter
Colonial retractor
colonic insufflator
colonofiberscope
    Olympus CF-series c.
    Olympus CG-P-series c.
colonography
    computed tomographic (CT) c.
colonoscope, coloscope
    ACMI fiberoptic c.
    ACMI operating c.
    CF-200Z Olympus c.
    EVIS 200I c.
    Fujinon EC-series video c.
    magnifying c.
    Olympus CF-HM-series
      magnifying c.
    Olympus CF-MB-series c.
    Olympus CF-PL-series c.
    Olympus CF-P-series c.
    Olympus CF-series c.
    Olympus CF-T-series c.
    Olympus CF-UM3 c.
    Olympus CF-VL-series c.
    Olympus CF-200Z c.
    Olympus CV-series c.
    Olympus EVIS video c.
    Olympus PCF-series pediatric c.
    Pentax FC-series c.
    Pentax VSB-P2900 pediatric c.
    standard c.
    Toshiba TCE-M-series c.
    Welch Allyn video c.
    ZM-1 c.
Colopast Sween sealed dispensing system
Coloplast
    C. colostomy bag
    C. deluxe irrigation kit
    C. dressing
    C. economy irrigation set
    C. hospital irrigation set
    C. irrigation faceplate
    C. one-piece closed pouch with
      filter
    C. one-piece conseal plug
    C. one-piece post-op drainable
      pouch
    C. one-piece small drainable pouch

C. one-piece standard drainable
    pouch
C. ostomy belt
C. stoma cone
C. transparent irrigation sleeve
C. two-piece conseal plug
C. two-piece small drainable pouch
C. two-piece small urostomy pouch
C. two-piece sterile post-op set
C. two-piece stoma cap with filter
C. urine leg bag
C. wafer
color
    c. adaptometer
    C. Bar Schirmer strip
    c. Doppler ultrasound
    C. Power Angio imaging
Colorado
    C. Cycle
    C. electrocautery tip
    C. microdissection needle
    C. MicroNeedle needle electrode
    C. tip cautery
ColorCards
    Basic Sequences C.
    Everyday Objects C.
    Preposition C.
ColorChecker
    Macbeth C.
color-coded therapy putty
color-flow
    c.-f. Doppler
    c.-f. Doppler real-time 2-D blood
      flow imaging
colorimeter
    differential scanning c.
ColorpHast Indicator Strips
Colorscan II
colorvascular Doppler ultrasound
ColorZone tape
coloscope (*var. of* colonoscope)
Coloscreen VPI
colostomy
    c. bag
    c. clamp
    c. rod
    takedown of c.
    Ultra Duet C.
Colotzmark clip
Coloviras-Rumel thoracic forceps
Colpacs
    C. collar
    C. pack
colpomicrohysteroscope
    Hamou c.
colposcope
    Accu-Scope c.
    CooperSurgical overhead c.
    Cryomedics c.
    Frigitronics c.
    Jena c.
    Leisegang c.
    MM-6000 c.
    OpMi c.
    Wallach ZoomStar c.

C

colposcope *(continued)*
  Zeiss c.
  Zoomscope c.
colpostat
  afterload c.
  c. applicator
  dome c.
  FSD c.
  Hejnosz radium c.
  Henschke c.
  Homiak radium c.
  Landon c.
  Regaud radium c.
Colt cannula
Coltene
  C. alloy
  C. direct inlay system
  C. impression material
  C. Magicap
  C. oven
Coltex impression material
Colton empyema tube
Colts cutting needle
Columbia scaler
Columbus
  C. McKinnon Hugger device
  C. McKinnon lifting assist
columellar
  c. clamp
  c. implant
column
  c. chromatograph
  contrast c.
  immunoadsorption c.
  NHS-activated HiTrap affinity c.
  PD-10 disposable Sephadex G-25 c.
  plasmapheresis through a
    Prosorba c.
  Prosorba c.
Colvard pupillometer
Colver
  C. examining hook
  C. retractor hook
  C. tonsillar dissector
  C. tonsillar knife
  C. tonsillar needle
  C. tonsillar pillar-grasping forceps
  C. tonsillar retractor
  C. tonsil-seizing forceps
Colver-Coakley tonsillar forceps
Colver-Dawson tongue depressor
comb
  Cottle periosteal c.
  toe c.
Combi-40 cochlear implant
CombiDerm absorbent cover dressing
Combi Multi-Traction system
combination
  c. biliary brush catheter
  c. cone/tube irrigator kit
  c. cone/tube stoma irrigator drain
  c. gel and inflatable mammary
    prosthesis
  c. needle electrode

combined wire guide bone elevator
Combisit surgeon's chair
Combitrans transducer
Combitube
  C. airway
  C. endotracheal tube
Combo
  C. Cath wire-guided cytology brush
  Chang Quick Chop C.
COMED
  C. footgear
  C. postoperative shoe
  C. postsurgical footgear
comedo extractor
Comfeel
  C. contour dressing
  C. hydrocolloid dressing
  C. Plus pressure relief dressing
  C. powder
  C. Purilon dressing
Comfit
  C. endotracheal tube
  C. endotracheal tube holder
comfort
  C. Ag prosthetic sock
  C. Care bed system
  C. Cast
  C. Cast casting system
  C. Cast stirrup
  c. Cath I or II
  C. Cath I, II catheter
  c. leg bag strap
  C. nylon mattress
  C. Plus cushion
  C. Quilt underpad
  C. Take-Along wheelchair cushion
  C. wrist immobilizer
ComfortCuff blood pressure cuff
comforter
  Thermo hand c.
  Thermo knee c.
Comf-Orthotic
  C.-O. 3/4 length insole
  C.-O. sports replacement insole
Comfortseat
  Flo-Fit C.
ComfortWalk$_2$ prosthetic foot
ComfortWear pouch cover
Comfy
  C. Elbow orthosis
  C. elbow splint
  C. Knee orthosis
  C. walker
Command
  C. hip instrumentation system
  C. PS pacemaker
Commander
  C. angioplasty guidewire
  C. PTCA wire
commissure laryngoscope
committed mode pacemaker
common
  c. bile duct dilator
  c. duct-holding forceps
  c. duct probe

c. duct stone forceps
c. duct stone scoop
c. McPherson forceps
c. pH electrode
CO$_2$mmO$_2$n sensor transcutaneous gas electrode
Commucor A+V Patient monitor
Compacement dental cement
Compac microcentrifuge
compactor
McSpadden c.
Micro-Flow c.
Compafill MH dental restorative material
Compak-200 mini-excimer
Compalay dental restorative material
Compamolar dental restorative material
Companion
C. 2 blood glucose monitor
C. feeding pump
C. 314, 318 nasal CPAP system
C. 2 self blood glucose monitoring device
comparison eyepiece
compass
C. arc-quadrant stereotactic system
C. CT stereotaxic adaptation system
C. frame-based stereotactic system
C. hinge
Mastel diamond c.
C. stereotactic frame
C. stereotactic phantom
Compat
C. enteral feeding pump
C. surgical feeding tube
Compeed Skinprotector dressing
compensating eyepiece
compensator
multivane intensity modulation c.
scattering foil c.
time-gain c.
Compere
C. bone chisel
C. fixation wire
C. threaded pin
Comperm tubular elastic bandage
Competitive Ankle Board
Complement C31 desArg Biotrack RIA system
complete
C. implant
c. upper and lower dentures
completely in the canal (CIC)
completely-in-the-canal
c.-i.-t.-c. hearing aid
c.-i.-t.-c. listening device
Complex Cu3 dressing
compliance cap
compliant balloon
ComPly panty shield
component
acetabular c.
AGC Modular Tibial II c.
AGC porous anatomic femoral c.
AGC unicondylar knee c.

anatomic graduated c.'s (AGC)
Axiom knee c.
Biodynamic acetabular c.
Biomet AGC knee c.
Biomet AGC primary and posterior stabilized c.
Biomet Bi-Polar c.
Biomet MARS acetabular c.
Biomet Repicci II unicompartment knee c.
Biomet revision acetabular c.
Biomet shoulder c.
Bio-Modular shoulder c.
Bio-Plug c.
bipolar hip arthroplasty c.
Black Max mid size knee c.
CFV wrist c.
Charnley flat-back femoral c.
Charnley narrow stem c.
cobalt chrome modular head c.
Definition PM (Pre-Mantle) femoral implant c.
Deyerle c.
Duramer polyethylene c.
Freeman femoral c.
Harris-Galante hip replacement acetabular c.
Harris-Galante I porous-coated acetabular c.
Harris-Galante porous acetabular c.
Harris-Galante porous-coated femoral c.
Healey revision acetabular c.
HGP II acetabular c.
Hoffmann II compact external fixation c.
hybrid fixation of hip replacement c.
Interlok primary femoral c.
Ionguard titanium modular head c.
Isola spinal implant system c.
Judet impactor for acetabular c.
Kirschner Universal self-centering captive-head bipolar c.
Kudo elbow c.
Lubinus acetabular c.
Mallory-Head Interlok primary femoral c.
MARS revision acetabular c.
Meridian ST femoral implant c.
Metasul hip joint c.
monoblock femoral c.
Morse taper lock of modular hip implant c.
NexGen knee c.
OEC Dual-Op barrel/plate c.
Ogee acetabular c.
Omnifit HA femoral c.
Opti-Fix femoral c.
Osteolock HA femoral c.
Osteolock NP acetabular c.
Osteonics Omnifit-HA c.
PCA hip c.
PFC c.
polyethylene liner implant c.

C

component *(continued)*
    Precision Osteolock femoral c.
    Press-Fit condylar c.
    Press-Fit femoral c.
    Profix porous femoral c.
    Pugh barrel c.
    Reliance CM femoral c.
    roof-reinforcement ring hip
      arthroplasty c.
    Rothman Institute porous femoral c.
    Smith & Nephew reflection
      acetabular cup implant c.
    Sofomor-Danek c.
    Springlite G foot c.
    Springlite II foot c.
    supracondylar barrel/plate c.
    Taperloc femoral c.
    Tharies femoral resurfacing c.
    Tharies hip c.
    Ti-BAC acetabular c.
    trial c.
    Tri-Con c.
    Ultima C femoral c.
    Universal radial c.
    Vitallium mesh c.
    Vitalock cluster acetabular c.
    Vitalock solid-back acetabular c.
    Vitalock talon acetabular c.

composite
    C. Cultured Skin
    c. dental cement
    dentin-bonded resin c.
    c. dressing
    DRS c.
    c. external fixator ring adhesive
    Phaseafill dental c.
    c. polymer stent
    Sepramesh biosurgical c.
    c. spring elastic splint

compound
    c. curved rasp
    Dermatex c.
    c. dressing
    Finite dental glazing c.
    Microfil silicone-rubber injection c.
    OCT c.
    Pediplast moldable footcare c.
    c. spectacles
    c. suture

compress
    Cool Tops c.
    Discover cryotherapy c.
    Kold Wrap freezable c.

compressed Ivalon patch graft
compressible acrylic intraocular lens
compression
    c. bandage
    c. belt
    c. binder
    c. boot
    c. clicker
    c. device
    c. dressing
    c. earring

    c. forceps
    c. garment
    c. girdle
    c. hearing aid
    c. hip screw (CHS)
    c. hook
    c. instrumentation posterior construct
    c. paddle
    c. plate
    c. pump
    c. rod
    c. skull cap closure
    c. sleeve shin splint
    c. spring
    c. stockings
    c. U-rod instrumentation

compression-molded PMMA intraocular lens
compressive
    c. internal fixating device
    c. plastic splint

compressor
    Adair screw c.
    air c.
    Anthony enucleation c.
    Anthony orbital c.
    Barnes c.
    Beneys tonsillar c.
    Berens enucleation c.
    Berens orbital c.
    Castroviejo c.
    Charnley c.
    Conn aortic c.
    continuous air c.
    Deschamps c.
    enucleation c.
    external inflatable c.
    Freeway Lite portable aerosol c.
    orbital c.
    Pulmo-Mist c.
    Riahl coronary c.
    screw c.
    Sehrt c.
    shot c.
    tonsillar c.
    tubing c.

Comprifix
    C. active ankle support
    C. ankle splint

Compriform support stockings
Comprilan bandage
Comprol dressing
Compton
    C. suppression spectrometer
    C. suppression system

CompuCam digital intraoral camera
Compu-Neb ultrasonic nebulizer
Compuscan-P pachymeter
computed
    C. Anatomy Corneal Modeling
      System
    c. tomographic (CT) colonography
    c. tomography scan (CT scan)

computer
    Aspect c.

c.-assisted neurosurgical navigational system
Brown-Roberts-Wells c.
CardioData Mark IV c.
Digitrace home c.
Digitron DVI/DSA c.
electromechanical slope c.
Inspiron Instromedix c.
leukocyte automatic recognition c.
on-demand analgesia c.
Sequential Multiple Analyzer C. (SMAC)
Silicon Graphics Indigo 2 c.
thermodilution cardiac output c.

computer-aided
c.-a. fluency establishment trainer
c.-a. sleep system

computer-assisted videokeratoscope
computer-controlled
c.-c. infusion pump
c.-c. neurological stimulation system

computerized
c. bedside transfusion identification system
c. image analysis system
c. isokinetic dynamometer
c. morphometric system
c. pattern generator
c. rotary chair

ComputeRow
Computon microtonometer
Comtesse medical support stockings
Comyns-Berkeley retractor
Cona-Tone office-use hearing amplifier
concave
c. gouge
c. loading socket
c. obturator
c. sheath

concentrator
Keystone Plus oxygenator c.
Millennium oxygen c.
NewLife oxygen c.
SolAiris III oxygen c.
stem cell c.

concentric
c. needle
c. needle electrode

Concentrix Fluidics
Concept
C. ablator
C. ACL/PCL graft passer
C. arthroscopic knife
C. arthroscopy rasp
C. beachchair shoulder positioning system
C. bipolar coagulator
C. bone tunnel plug
C. cannula
C. C-reamer
C. CTS Relief kit
C. curette
C. digit trap
C. disposable cautery

C. hand-held cautery
C. II rowing ergometer
C. Intravision arthroscope
C. mesh grafter dermatome
C. Multi-Liner lining needle
C. nerve stimulator
C. Ophtho-bur
C. 2-pin passer
C. Precise ACL guide system
C. PuddleVac floor suction device
C. rotator cuff repair system
C. self-compressing cannulated screw system
C. shaver
C. Sterling arthroscopy blade system
C. suturing needle
C. tibial guide
C. traction tower
C. video imaging system
C. zone-specific cannula system

Conceptus
C. fallopian tube catheterization system
C. Robust guide wire
C. Soft Seal cervical catheter
C. Soft Torque uterine catheter
C. VS catheter

conchotome
Hartmann nasal c.
Henke-Stille c.
Olivecrona c.
Stille c.
Struyken c.
Watson-Williams c.
Weil-Blakesley c.

Concise
C. compression hip screw
C. resin
C. side plate

Conclude dental cement
Conco
C. abdominal belt
C. elastic bandage

Concorde
C. disposable skin stapler
C. disposable suction cannula

Concord line draw syringe
Concord/Portex airway
condenser
Abbé c.
amalgam c.
Nordent amalgam c.

condensing lens
conditioner
Coe-Comfort tissue c.
Shuttle cardiomuscular c.

condom
c. catheter
c. catheter collecting system
female c.
male c.
c. urinal

conductance catheter

conductive
c. Hydrogel wound dressing
c. V-Lok cuff

conductor
Adson c.
Bailey saw c.
Bovie liquid c.
Davis c.
Gigli saw c.
Kanavel c.
Martel c.
Souttar esophageal c.
Xomed Audiant bone c.

conduit
Rastelli c.

condylar
c. implant
c. lag screw plate
c. neck retractor

condyle rod

cone
c. biopsy needle
C. bone punch
c. bur
Centriflow membrane c.
C. cerebral cannula
c. collar
Coloplast stoma c.
C. guide
hand c.
C. ice-tong calipers
C. laminectomy retractor
McIntyre truncated c.
C. nasal curette
nose c.
Placido 25-ring c.
Posey Palm C.
C. ring curette
C. scalp retractor
C. self-retaining retractor
shielded open-end c.
C. skull punch
C. splint
stacking c.
stoma c.
C. suction biopsy curette
C. suction tube
c. tip catheter
C. ventricular needle
VISI-FLOW stoma c.
C. wire-twisting forceps

Cone-Bucy
C.-B. cannula
C.-B. suction cannula set
C.-B. suction tube

coned heparin tip

Confide HIV test kit

confidence ring

confocal
c. laser scanning ophthalmoscope
c. microscope
c. optics
c. scanning laser ophthalmoscope
c. scanning laser polarimeter

CONFORM
C. II w/heel-ease Nature Sleep pressure pad

Conformant
C. 2 nonadherent transparent wound veil
C. wound dressing

conformer
Fox c.
McGuire c.
Moore-Wilson hyperopic c.
silicone c.
Universal c.

Conform stretch bandage

Conger perineal urethrostomy clamp

conical
c. bur
c. catheter
c. centrifuge tube
c. eye implant
c. inserter tip
c. probe

conical-tip
c.-t. catheter
c.-t. electrode

conic bougie

conization
c. electrode
c. instrument
c. instrument blade

Conjugate export pump

conjunctival
c. fixation forceps
c. scissors
c. spreader

Conley
C. mandibular prosthesis
C. pin
C. tracheal stent

Conmed Aspen Excalibur-Plus electrosurgical unit

Conn
C. aortic compressor
C. pneumatic tourniquet
C. Universal tourniquet

connecting
c. plate
c. tubing

connection
c. cord
internal hex-thread c.
Luer c.

connector
Accu-Flo c.
ACS angioplasty Y c.
adjustable pedicle c.
Beurrier c.
coaxial I&A nylon c.
Denver c.
domino spinal instrumentation c.
drain-to-wall suction c.
dual bypass c.
extension tubing with c.
c. forceps
Holter c.

Humid-Vent Port 1 elbow c.
intrinsic transverse c.
Karl Storz light source c.
Luer c.
Luer-Lok jet ventilator c.
Machida light source c.
McIntyre nylon cannula c.
Olympus light source c.
pedicle c.
Pentax light source c.
plastic c.
Prolene Hernia system c.
Pudenz c.
quick c.
Saf-T-Flo T-tube c.
SidePort AutoControl airway c.
straight c.
tandem c.
Touhy-Borst c.
transverse c.
Tunstal c.
Tuohy-Borst c.
Uni-Gard piggyback c.
Universal c.
venous Y c.
c. with lock washer
Y-port c.

Connell
C. airway
C. breathing tube
C. ether vapor tube
C. suture

Connor
C. straight nonirrigating wand

ConQuest
C. female continence system pressure pad with preattached flange
C. incontinent system
C. male continence system condom catheter with preattached flange
C. male continence system leg bag kit
C. male continence system supporter brief

Conrad-Crosby bone marrow biopsy needle

console
Bruker c.
Cobe-Stockert heart lung c.
Hitachi EUB-515C ultrasound c.
Siemens Satellite CT evaluation c.

constant
c. current stimulator
c. passive-motion machine (CPMM)

Constantine flexible metal catheter

ConstaVac
C. autoreinfusion system
C. catheter

constrained
c. hinged knee prosthesis
c. nonhinged knee prosthesis

constriction ring

construct
AO dynamic compression plate c.

compression instrumentation posterior c.
double-rod c.
Edwards modular system compression c.
Edwards modular system kyphoreduction c.
Edwards modular system neutralization c.
Edwards modular system rod-sleeve c.
Edwards modular system scoliosis c.
Edwards modular system standard sleeve c.
Guiot-Talairach c.
hook-to-screw L4-S1 compression c.
iliosacral and iliac fixation c.
pedicle screw c.
rod-hook c.
screw-to-screw compression c.
segmental compression c.
single-rod c.
tissue-engineered c.
titanium c.
triplane c.
TSRH double-rod c.
TSRH pedicle screw-laminar claw c.
upper cervical spine anterior c.
upper cervical spine posterior c.
Wiltse system double-rod c.
Wiltse system H c.
Wiltse system single-rod c.

Constructa-Foam

contact
C. A-scan
c. bandage lens
C. B-scan
c. B-scan ultrasonography
c. compressive forceps
c. glasses
c. hysteroscope
C. Laser bullet probe
C. Laser chisel probe
C. Laser conical probe
C. Laser convex probe
C. Laser flat probe
C. Laser interstitial probe
C. Laser round probe
C. Laser scalpel
c. lens training mirror
c. low-vacuum lens
c. shell implant
c. shield
C. SPH cups system

contact-layer wound dressing

contact-tip laser system

container
child-resistant c.
cryogenic storage c.
Fenwal cryocyte freezing c.
instrument retrieval c.
Mini-Bag Plus c.
non-child-resistant c.

container (*continued*)
    Perative enteral feeding c.
    Promoe enteral feeding c.
    quartz-glass c.
    Quickbox c.
contemporary nearpoint chart
Contigen
    C. Bard collagen implant
    C. glutaraldehyde cross-linked
    collagen
    C. tube
contiguous spinal fluid reservoir
Contimed
    C. II measuring unit
    C. II pelvic floor muscle monitor
Continental
    C. cannula
    C. needle
continuous
    c. air compressor
    c. bar retainer
    c. clip forceps
    c. insulin delivery system (CIDS)
    c. irrigation catheter
    c. microinfusion device
    c. passive motion device
    c. subcutaneous insulin infusion
    pump
    c. suction tube
continuous-flow
    c.-f. Wolfe resectoscope
continuously perfused probe
continuous-wave
    c.-w. argon laser
    c.-w. arthroscopy pump
    c.-w. diode laser
    c.-w. laser system
continuous-wave, high-frequency Doppler
ultrasound system
Continuum
    C. knee system
    C. knee system implant
Contique contact lens case
contour
    C. back cushion
    C. balloon dilatation catheter
    c. block clamp
    c. defect molding kit
    C. Emboli artificial embolization
    device
    C. Genesis ultrasonic-assisted
    liposuction system
    c. instrument cleaning brush
    C. LTV135D implantable
    cardioverter-defibrillator
    C. MD implantable single-lead
    cardioverter defibrillator
    C. Profile Natural saline breast
    implant
    C. Profile silicone breast implant
    prosthetic buttock c.
    c. scalp retractor
    C. tilting compression
    mammography system

    C. V-145D implantable cardioverter-
    defibrillator
    Ventritex C.
contoured
    c. anterior spinal plate
    c. anterior spinal plate drill guide
    c. femoral stem (CFS)
    c. washer
contour-facilitating instrument
contra-angle head
contractor
    Adams rib c.
    baby rib c.
    Bailey baby rib c.
    Bailey-Gibbon rib c.
    Cooley rib c.
    CraXoord c.
    Effenberger c.
    Finochietto-Burford rib c.
    Finochietto infant rib c.
    Graham rib c.
    Lemmon rib c.
    Medicon c.
    Reinhoff-Finochietto rib c.
    rib c.
    Scanlan-Crafoord c.
    Sellor rib c.
    Stille-Bailey-Senning rib c.
    surgical c.
    Waterman rib c.
contraflexion brace
Contrajet ERCP contrast delivery system
Contrangle dermabrasion brush
contrast column
contrast-enhanced CT
Contraves stand
control
    c. adjustment strap
    c. bridle
    Cadogan-Hough footpedal suction c.
    DryTime for bladder c.
    FlexDial stimulus c.
    Generation II all-in-one-hand c.
    Hough-Cadogan footpedal suction c.
    Hunstad Handle flow c.
    MegaDyne all-in-one hand c.
    PSC pronation/spring c.
    C. Release pop-off needle
    c. wire
controlled
    c. ankle motion (CAM)
    c. drain
controller
    Actis venous flow c.
    Asahi pressure c.
    Bronkhorst High Tec c.
    IMED Gemini PC-2 volumetric c.
    IVAC 831 drip c.
    MAGneedle c.
    mass flow c.
    shoulder c.
    C. Shoulder Orthosis
    voice intensity c.
ControlWire guidewire
Contura medicated dressing

ConvaTec
    C. ostomy pouch
    C. Unna-Flex elastic Unna boot
    C. urostomy pouch
Conve back support
Conveen
    C. bag hanger
    C. bedside drainage bag
    C. curved/tapered intermittent
    catheter
    C. deluxe contoured leg bag
    C. disposable stretch brief
    C. drip collector
    C. female intermittent catheter
    C. leg bag strap
    C. net pant
    C. Security+male external catheter
    & liner
    C. Security+self-sealing male
    external catheter
    C. self-sealing Urisheath
conventional
    c. needle
    c. reform eye implant
    c. shell-type eye implant
    c. silicone elastomer
    c. static scanner
    c. stent
    c. transmission electron microscope
Convergent color Doppler
converging collimator
convergiometer
Converse
    C. alar elevator
    C. blade retractor
    C. button-end bistoury
    C. double-ended alar retractor
    C. fracture-wiring button
    C. guarded nasal chisel
    C. hinged skin hook
    C. nasal knife
    C. nasal retractor
    C. nasal root rongeur
    C. nasal saw
    C. nasal speculum
    C. nasal tip scissors
    C. needle holder
    C. osteotome
    C. periosteal elevator
    C. rasp
    C. raspatory
    C. retractor blade
    C. splint
    C. sweeper curette
Converse-Lange rongeur
Converse-MacKenty periosteal elevator
Converse-Wilmer conjunctival scissors
conversion
    Tilt-In-Space wheelchair c.
Converta-Litter carrier
converter
    analog-to-digital c. (ADC)
    D/A c.
    digital-to-analog c.
    motion-compensating format c.

    real-time format c.
    sequential video c.
    SRR-5 digital-analogue c.
    time-to-pulse height c.
convertible
    c. fin
    Orthoderm c.
    c. telescope
    C. trocar system
    WonderBrace C.
Convertors surgical drape
convex
    c. obturator
    c. probe
    c. rasp
    c. sheath
convexoconcave heart valve
CONVO-GEL cushion
convoluted
    c. foam mattress
    C. mattress pad
    c. wheelchair cushion
convolution mask
Conway
    C. lid retractor
    C. lid speculum
Conzett goniometer
Cook
    C. arterial catheter
    C. balloon
    C. biopsy gun
    C. Cardiovascular infusion catheter
    C. continence cuff
    C. continence ring
    C. County Hospital aspirator
    C. County Hospital tracheal suction
    tube
    C. deflector
    C. drainage pouch set
    C. endomyocardial needle
    C. endoscopic curved needle driver
    C. eye speculum
    C. filter
    C. flexible biopsy forceps
    C. FlexStent stent
    C. helical stone dislodger
    C. intracoronary stent
    C. locking stylet
    C. Longdwel needle
    C. micropuncture introducer
    C. osteotome
    C. pacemaker
    C. Peel-Away introducer
    C. percutaneous entry needle
    C. plastic Luer-Lok adapter
    C. rectal retractor
    C. rectal speculum
    C. retrievable embolization coil
    C. Spectrum catheter
    C. stent positioner
    C. stereotaxic guide
    C. straight guidewire
    C. tissue morcellator
    C. TPN catheter
    C. ureteral stent

Cook *(continued)*
    C. urological trocar
    C. Urosoft stent
    C. walking brace
    C. yellow pigtail catheter
Cook-Amplatz dilator
cookie
    c. cutter
    Gelfoam c.
    metatarsal c.
cool
    C. Comfort cold pack
    c. mist vaporizer (CMV)
    c. pack
    C. Tip catheter
    C. Tops compress
Cool-Aid continuous controlled cold therapy
cooler
    EMI FACT 50 MK III c.
    Hot/Ice cold therapy c.
Cooley
    C. acutely-curved clamp
    C. anastomosis clamp
    C. anastomosis forceps
    C. aortic aneurysm clamp
    C. aortic cannula clamp
    C. aortic forceps
    C. aortic retractor
    C. aortic sump tube
    C. aortic vent needle
    C. arterial occlusion forceps
    C. arteriotomy scissors
    C. atrial valve retractor
    C. auricular appendage forceps
    C. bronchial clamp
    C. bulldog clamp
    C. cardiac tucker
    C. cardiac tunneler
    C. cardiovascular forceps
    C. cardiovascular scissors
    C. cardiovascular suction tube
    C. carotid clamp
    C. carotid retractor
    C. caval occlusion clamp
    C. chisel
    C. coarctation clamp
    C. coarctation forceps
    C. coronary dilator
    C. cross-action bulldog clamp
    C. curved cardiovascular clamp
    C. curved forceps
    C. Dacron prosthesis
    C. double-angled clamp
    C. double-angled jaw forceps
    C. femoral retractor
    C. first-rib shears
    C. graft clamp
    C. graft forceps
    C. graft suction tube
    C. iliac clamp
    C. iliac forceps
    C. intracardiac suction tube
    C. ligature carrier

    C. mitral valve retractor
    C. MPC cardiovascular retractor
    C. neonatal instruments
    C. neonatal scissors
    C. neonatal sternal retractor
    C. neonatal vascular clamp
    C. neonatal vascular forceps
    C. partial-occlusion clamp
    C. patent ductus clamp
    C. patent ductus forceps
    C. pediatric aortic forceps
    C. pediatric dilator
    C. pediatric vascular clamp
    C. peripheral vascular clamp
    C. peripheral vascular forceps
    C. pick
    C. probe-point scissors
    C. renal artery clamp
    C. reverse-cut scissors
    C. rib contractor
    C. rib retractor
    C. rib shears
    C. sternotomy retractor
    C. subclavian clamp
    C. sump suction tube
    C. tangential pediatric clamp
    C. tangential pediatric forceps
    C. tissue forceps
    C. U-sutures
    C. valve dilator
    C. vascular dilator
    C. vascular suction tube
    C. vascular tissue forceps
    C. vena cava clamp
    C. ventricular needle
    C. ventricular sump
    C. Vital microvascular needle holder
    C. wax carver
    C. woven Dacron graft
Cooley-Anthony suction tube
Cooley-Baumgarten
    C.-B. aortic clamp
    C.-B. aortic forceps
    C.-B. wire twister
Cooley-Beck vessel clamp
Cooley-Bloodwell-Cutter valve
Cooley-Bloodwell mitral valve prosthesis
Cooley-Cutter disk prosthetic valve
Cooley-Derra
    C.-D. anastomosis clamp
    C.-D. anastomosis forceps
Cooley-Merz
    C.-M. sternal retractor
    C.-M. sternum retractor
Cooley-Pontius
    C.-P. sternal blade
    C.-P. sternal shears
Cooley-Satinsky clamp
Cool-Flex A/K suspension belt
Coolidge
    C. transformer
    C. tube
cooling
    c. blanket

c. helmet
c. machine
CoolPac hands-free unit
CoolSorb absorbent cold transfer dressing
cool-tip laser
CoolTouch Nd:YAG laser
Cool-vapor vaporizer
Coombs bone biopsy system
Coonrad-Morrey total elbow prosthesis
Coons Super Stiff long-tip guidewire
Cooper
C. argon laser
C. aspirator
C. basal ganglia guide
C. chemopallidectomy cannula
C. chemopallidectomy needle
C. cryoprobe
C. disk cryostat
C. double-lumen cannula
C. endotracheal stylet
C. herniotome
C. implant
C. laser adapter
C. LaserSonics laser
C. ligature needle
C. pallidectomy needle
C. spinal fusion elevator
C. spinal fusion gouge
Cooper-Rand intraoral artificial larynx
CooperSurgical
C. monopolar ELSG LEEP system
C. overhead colposcope
CooperVision
C. argon laser
C. camera
C. Diagnostic Imaging refractor
C. Fragmatome
C. I&A machine
C. I&A unit
C. imaging perimeter
C. irrigating needle
C. irrigation/aspiration handpiece
C. microscope
C. ocutome
C. PMMA-ACL Flex lens
C. refractive surgery photokeratoscope
C. spatulated needle
C. Surgeon-Plus Ultrathin blade
C. ultrasound
C. viscoelastic
C. vitrector
C. YAG laser
CooperVision-Cilco
C.-C. Novaflex anterior chamber intraocular lens
CooperVision-Cilco-Kelman multiflex all-PMMA intraocular lens
Coordinate complete revision knee system
co-oximeter
Ciba-Corning 2500 c.-o.
IL-282 c.-o.
Copalite applicator

Cope
C. crushing clamp
C. double-ended retractor
C. gastrointestinal suture anchor set
C. loop nephrostomy catheter
C. loop nephrostomy tube
C. lung forceps
C. mandrel guidewire
C. modification of a Martel intestinal clamp
C. needle introducer cannula
C. pleural biopsy needle
C. thoracentesis needle
C. wire
Cope-DeMartel clamp
Copeland
C. anterior chamber intraocular lens
C. fetal scalp electrode
C. intraocular lens implant
C. radial loop intraocular lens
C. radial panchamber UV lens
C. streak retinoscope
Cope-Saddekni
C.-S. catheter tip
C.-S. introducer
copolymer
c. ankle-foot orthosis
c. stapler
copper
c. band
c. band-acrylic splint
c. blade
c. bromide laser
c. mallet
c. phosphate cement
c. vapor pulsed laser
Copper-7 intrauterine device
copper-clad steel needle
copper-constantan thermocouple
Coppridge
C. grasping forceps
C. urethral forceps
coquille plano lens
Corail
C. HA-coated stem
C. HA-coated stem hip implant
C. hip system
coral
madreporic c.
coralline
c. hydroxyapatite Goniopora
c. PBHA bone graft
c. porous block hydroxyapatite bone graft
Coratomic
C. implantable pulse generator
C. prosthetic valve
C. R-wave inhibited pacemaker
Corbett
C. bone-cutting forceps
C. bone rongeur
C. foreign body spud
Corboy
C. hemostat
C. needle holder

C

cord
- Biopac gingival retraction c.
- bipolar connection c.
- coagulating suction cannula connection c.
- connection c.
- diathermy c.
- Frazier monopolar cautery c.
- Poppen monopolar cautery c.
- Racestyptine c.
- Sport C.

Cordes
- C. circular punch
- C. esophagoscopy forceps
- C. ethmoidal punch
- C. punch forceps tip
- C. semicircular punch
- C. sphenoidal punch
- C. square punch

Cordes-New
- C.-N. laryngeal punch elevator
- C.-N. laryngeal punch forceps

Cordguard
- C. II
- C. umbilical cord sampler

Cordis
- C. Ancar pacing leads
- C. Atricor pacemaker
- C. bioptome
- C. Bioptone sheath
- C. BriteTip guiding catheter
- C. Chronocor IV pacemaker
- C. Crossflex stent
- C. dilator
- C. Ducor I, II, III coronary catheter
- C. Ducor pigtail catheter
- C. Ectocor pacemaker
- C. endovascular system
- C. fixed-rate pacemaker
- C. Gemini cardiac pacemaker
- C. guiding catheter
- C. Hakim pump
- C. implantable drug reservoir device
- C. injector
- C. lead conversion kit
- C. Lumelec catheter
- C. Multicor pacemaker
- C. multipurpose access port
- C. Omni Stanicor Theta transvenous pacemaker
- C. Predator balloon catheter
- C. radiopaque tantalum stent
- C. Secor implantable pump
- C. Sentron transducer
- C. Sequicor cardiac pacemaker
- C. Son-II catheter
- C. Stabilizer marker wire
- C. Stanicor unipolar ventricular pacemaker
- C. Synchrocor pacemaker
- C. Theta Sequicor DDD pulse generator
- C. Titan balloon dilatation catheter
- C. Trakstar PTCA balloon catheter
- C. TransTaper tip catheter
- C. Ventricor pacemaker
- C. Webster diagnostic/ablation deflectable tip catheter
- C. Webster mapping catheter

Cordis-Dow shunt adapter

Cordis-Hakim
- C.-H. shunt
- C.-H. valve

cordless
- c. dermatome
- c. monocular indirect ophthalmoscope

Cordon Colles fracture splint

Cordostat
- Foley C.

cordotomy
- c. clamp
- c. knife

core
- C. CO_2 insufflation needle
- C. Dynamics disposable cannula
- C. Dynamics disposable trocar
- C. Hibak Rest
- C. Lobak Rest
- C. Max-Relax cushion
- c. reamer
- C. Sitback Rest
- C. Slimrest
- c. trocar

Core-Check tympanic thermometer

Coremetrics fetal apnea monitor

Coretemp deep tissue thermometer

CoreVent Implant system

Corex instrument

Corey
- C. ovum forceps
- C. placental forceps
- C. tenaculum

Corfit System 7000 Series Lumbosacral Support

Cor-Flex
- C.-F. guidewire
- C.-F. wire guide

Corgill bone punch

Corgill-Hartmann forceps

Corgill-Shapleigh ear curette

Corin
- C. hip system
- C. total hip

coring biopsy gun

Corival 400 ergometer

cork
- c., leather, and elastic orthotic

corkscrew
- Austin Moore c.
- c. dural hook
- Filtzer c.

Corlon
- C. angiocatheter
- C. catheter

Cormed ambulatory infusion pump

cornea
- c. abrader
- c. chisel

cornea-holding forceps
corneal
- c. block
- c. chisel
- c. curette
- c. debrider
- c. erysiphake
- c. fascia lata spatula
- c. fixation forceps
- c. foreign body bur
- c. graft spatula
- c. hook
- c. implant
- c. knife
- c. knife dissector
- c. light shield
- c. microscope
- c. monocular loupe
- c. pachymeter
- c. prosthesis forceps
- c. prosthesis trephine
- c. punch
- c. ring
- c. section-enlarging scissors
- c. section spatulated scissors
- C. Shaper microkeratome
- c. spatulated scissors
- c. splinter forceps
- c. spud
- c. suture needle
- c. topography system
- c. transplant centering ring
- c. transplant forceps
- c. transplant marker
- c. transplant scissors
- c. tube
- c. utility forceps

Corneascope nine-ring photokeratoscope
CorneaSparing LTK system
cornea-splitting knife
cornea-suturing forceps
Corneo-Gage PachKnife
corneoscleral
- c. punch
- c. scissors
- c. suturing forceps

corneoscope
- IDI c.

corner
- C. plug
- c. retractor
- C. tampon

Cornet forceps
Corning
- C. 170 blood gas analyzer
- C. implant

Cornish wool dressing
Cornman dissecting knife
Corometrics
- C. Doppler scanner
- C. Gold Quik Connect Spiral electrode tip
- C. maternal/fetal monitor
- C. Medical Systems Inc. fetal monitoring system

- C. Model 900SC in-office mammography machine

Corometrics-Aloka echocardiograph machine
coronal suture
coronary
- c. anastomotic shunt
- c. angiographic catheter
- c. angiography analysis system
- c. artery button
- c. artery cannula
- c. artery forceps
- c. artery probe
- c. artery scissors
- c. dilatation catheter
- c. dilator
- c. endarterectomy spatula
- c. guiding catheter
- C. Imagecath angioscope
- c. perfusion cannula
- c. perfusion catheter
- c. perfusion tip
- c. seeking catheter
- c. sinus thermodilution catheter

Coronet
- C. alloy
- C. magnet

Coroscop C cardiac imaging system
Corpak
- C. enteral Y extension set
- C. weighted-tip, self-lubricating tube

corrected cosmetic contact shell eye implant
Corrigan cautery
corrugated forehead retractor
corset, corsette
- c. balloon catheter
- Boston soft c.
- Daw Industries orthopaedic c.
- lumbar c.
- lumbosacral c.
- Warm 'n Form lumbosacral c.

Corson
- C. myoma forceps
- C. needle
- C. needle electrosurgical probe

Cortac monitoring electrode
cortex
- c. extractor
- c. retractor
- c. screw

cortex-aspirating cannula
Cortexplorer cerebral blood flow monitor
cortical
- c. cleaving hydrodissector
- c. cleaving hydrodissector cannula
- c. electrode
- c. incision coronary dilator
- c. oral plate
- c. pin
- c. screw
- c. step drill

Cortomic pacemaker
corundum ceramic implant material

Corvita
C. endoluminal graft
C. endovascular graft
C. stent
Corwin
C. knife handle
C. tonsillar forceps
C. tonsillar hemostat
C. wire twister
Corydon hydroexpression cannula
Coryllos
C. periosteal elevator
C. retractor
C. rib raspatory
C. rib shears
C. thoracoscope
Coryllos-Bethune rib shears
Coryllos-Doyen periosteal elevator
Coryllos-Moure rib shears
Coryllos-Shoemaker rib shears
Cosgrove
C. mitral valve replacement
C. mitral valve retractor
Cosgrove-Edwards
C.-E. annuloplasty band
C.-E. annuloplasty system
Cosman ICP Tele-Sensor system
Cosman-Nashold spinal stereotaxic guide
Cosman-Roberts-Wells
C.-R.-W. (CRW) stereotactic frame
C.-R.-W. stereotactic ring
C.-R.-W. stereotactic system
cosmetic contact shell implant
Cosmolon closure for splint
Cosmos
C. 283 DDD pacemaker
C. II DDD pacemaker
C. II multiprogrammable dual-chamber cardiac pulse generator
C. pulse-generator pacemaker
Co-Span alloy
costal
c. arch retractor
c. periosteal elevator
c. periosteotome
Costa wire suture scissors
Costen
C. iris needle
C. suction tube
Costenbader
C. incision spreader
C. retractor
Costen-Kerrison rongeur
Coston-Trent
C.-T. cryoretractor
C.-T. iris retractor
costotome
c. chisel
Tudor-Edwards c.
Vehmehren c.
cot
finger c.
Kenwood finger c.
O'Connor rectal finger c.
Profex finger c.

rectal finger c.
rubber finger c.
Cotrel
C. pedicle screw
C. traction
Cotrel-Dubousset
C.-D. closed hook
C.-D. distraction system
C.-D. dynamic transverse traction device
C.-D. hook-rod
C.-D. instrumentation (CDI)
C.-D. orthopaedic brace
C.-D. pediatric rod
C.-D. pedicle screw instrumentation
C.-D. pedicular instrumentation
C.-D. spinal instrumentation
Cottingham punch
Cottle
C. alar elevator
C. alar protector
C. alar retractor
C. angular scissors
C. antral chisel
C. biting forceps
C. bone crusher
C. bone guide
C. bone lever
C. bulldog scissors
C. calipers
C. cartilage guide
C. columellar clamp
C. crossbar chisel osteotome
C. crossbar fishtail chisel
C. curved chisel
C. dorsal scissors
C. double-edged nasal knife
C. double hook
C. dressing scissors
C. fishtail chisel
C. four-prong retractor
C. heavy septal scissors
C. hook retractor
C. insertion forceps
C. knife guide
C. lower lateral forceps
C. mallet
C. nasal chisel
C. nasal elevator
C. nasal hook
C. nasal knife blade
C. nasal rasp
C. nasal retractor
C. nasal scissors
C. nasal speculum
C. needle holder
C. periosteal comb
C. periosteal elevator
C. pillar retractor
C. profilometer
C. pronged retractor
C. protected knife handle
C. rasp
C. septal elevator
C. septal speculum

C. sharp-prong retractor
C. single-blade retractor
C. single-prong tenaculum
C. skin elevator
C. skin hook
C. soft palate retractor
C. spicule sweeper
C. spring scissors
C. suction tube
C. tissue forceps
C. Universal nasal saw
C. upper lateral exposing retractor
C. weighted retractor
Cottle-Arruga cartilage forceps
Cottle-Jansen
C.-J. forceps
C.-J. rongeur
Cottle-Joseph
C.-J. hook
C.-J. retractor
C.-J. saw
Cottle-Kazanjian
C.-K. bone-cutting forceps
C.-K. nasal forceps
Cottle-MacKenty
C.-M. elevator
C.-M. rasp
Cottle-Neivert retractor
Cottle-Walsham
C.-W. septal straightener
C.-W. septum-straightening forceps
Cotton
C. cannulatome
C. cartilage graft
C. graduated dilation catheter
C.-Loader position cast
C. sphincterotome
cotton
c. applicator
c. ball
c. ball sponge
c. batting
c. bolster dressing
c. carrier
c. Deknatel suture
c. elastic bandage
c. elastic dressing
c. nonabsorbable suture
c. pledget
c. pledget dressing
cotton-ball dressing
cotton-covered tourniquet
Cotton-Huibregtse
C.-H. biliary stent set
C.-H. double pigtail stent
Cotton-Leung
C.-L. biliary stent
C.-L. biliary stent set
cottonoid
c. dissector
neurosurgical c.
c. patty
c. pledget
cotton-roll rubber-dam clamp
cotton-tipped applicator

Cottontome
Wilson-Cook ERCP C.
cotton-wadding dressing
cotton-wool bandage
Cottony
C. Dacron
C. Dacron hollow suture
couch
Boston neurosurgical c.
Siemens c.
couching needle
couch-mounted head frame
coudé
c. bag
c. fulgurating electrode
c. suction catheter
c. urethral catheter
coudé-tip
c.-t. demeure catheter
Coulter
C. Channelyser cell analyzer
C. counter (CC)
C. EPICS C-flow flow cytometer
C. EPICS Elite flow cytometer
C. EPICS 700-series flow cytometer
C. EPICS V-flow cytometer
C. MD 16 hemocytometer
C. S-Plus 5 automated red cell counter
C. STKS hematology analyzer
coumarin
c. pulsed dye laser
coumarin-flashlamp-pumped pulsed-dye laser
Coumatrak prothrombin time device
Councill
C. retention catheter
C. stone basket
C. stone dislodger
C. stone scoop
C. ureteral dilator
C. ureteral stone extractor
Councilman chisel
Counsellor
C. plug
C. vaginal mold
counter
beta-scintillation c.
boron c.
Capintec instant gamma c.
Coulter c. (CC)
Coulter S-Plus 5 automated red cell c.
gamma-ray c.
gamma well c.
Geiger c.
Geiger-Müller c.
Gill pressor c.
ionization c.
joule c.
Linson electronic cell c.
LKB/Wallach 1277 automatic gamma c.
LKB/Wallach scintillation c.
pill c.

C

counter *(continued)*
  RackBeta scintillation c.
  scintillation c.
  Sysmex R-1000 reticulocyte c.
  time-based c.
  whole-body c.
  Wizard gamma c.
counterbore
  Lloyd adapter c.
countercurrent heat exchanger
counteroccluder
Counterpoint electromyograph
counterpressor
  Acland-Bunke c.
  Amenabar c.
  angled c.
  Bruni c.
  Gill c.
counterpulsation balloon
counterrotational splint
countersink bur
Count'R-Force arch brace
coupeur
  capsule c.
Coupland
  C. elevator
  C. nasal suction tube
coupler
  Acutome 2000 Reich-Hasson
    laparoscopic CO_2 laser c.
  Ferrier c.
  Precise anastomotic c.
coupling head
Cournand
  C. arterial needle
  C. arteriography needle
  C. cardiac device
  C. quadpolar catheter
Cournand-Grino angiography needle
Cournand-Potts needle
Covaderm
  C. composite wound dressing
  C. Plus tube site dressing
  C. plus V.A.D.
  C. Plus V.A.D. dressing
Coventry stapler
cover
  AquaShield reusable orthopaedic
    cast c.
  Bair Hugger warming body c.
  bur hole c.
  ComfortWear pouch c.
  Dryspell cast c.
  Expo Bubble eye c.
  E-Z Flap burr hole c.
  Hollister replacement filters
    pouch c.
  I.V. House wound c.
  Kold Wrap general use sterile burn
    dressing & emergency wound c.
  Medipore dressing c.
  MIP reusable c.
  Nu-Hope pouch c.
  OxiLink oximetry probe c.

  Pillow perfect zipper c.
  protective mattress c.
  c. screw
  Sheaths ultrasound probe c.
  ShowerSafe waterproof cast and
    bandage c.
  Show'rbag cast and dressing c.
  Silastic bur hole c.
  SofStep wheelchair footplate c.
  Spenco top c.
  Springlite polyolefin BK c.
  Springlite polyurethane AK, BK
    conical c.
  TiMesh burrhole c.
  titanium mini bur hole c.
  Ultra Cover transducer c.
covered
  c. Gianturco stent
  c. Z-stent
Coverlet
  C. adhesive
  C. O.R. adhesive surgical dressing
  C. Strips wound dressing
Cover-Pad dressing
Cover-Roll
  C.-R. adhesive gauze
  C.-R. dressing
  C.-R. gauze adhesive
  C.-R. stretch bandage
Coverslipper
  Jung CV 5000 Robotic C.
Cover-Strip
  C.-S. wound closure strip
Covertell composite secondary dressing
CovRSite dressing
Cowboy collar
cowhorn tooth-extracting forceps
Co-Wrap dressing
Cox
  C. cytology brush
  C. II ocular laser shield
  C. metatarsal spreader
  C. polypectomy snare
Coxeter prostatic catheter
Cox-Uphoff implant
Coyne spoon
Cozean
  C. angled lens forceps
  C. bipolar forceps
  C. implantation forceps
Cozean-McPherson
  C.-M. angled lens forceps
  C.-M. tying forceps
CP2
  CP2 inflatable cold pack
  CP2 Inflat-A-Mask inflatable sinus
    mask
  CP2 Inflat-A-Wrap cold pad
CPAP
  Lightweight and portable Sullivan
    nasal CPAP
  NightBird nasal CPAP
  Revitalizer Soft-Start nasal CPAP
  Tranquility quest CPAP
  CPAP ventilator

CPD Commander combined air/fluid exchange and silicone oil delivery system

CPI

CPI Astra pacemaker
CPI automatic implantable defibrillator
CPI DDD pacemaker
CPI endocardial defibrillation rate-sensing pacing lead
CPI Endotak SQ electrode lead
CPI Endotak transvenous electrode
CPI Maxilith pacemaker
CPI Microthin DI, DII lithium-powered programmable pacemaker
CPI Minilith pacemaker
CPI porous tined-tip bipolar pacing lead
CPI PRx implantable cardioverter-defibrillator
CPI Sentra endocardial lead
CPI Sweet Tip lead
CPI tunneler
CPI Ultra II pacemaker
CPI Ventak AICD device
CPI Ventak PRx cardioverter-defibrillator
CPI Vigor pacemaker
CPI Vista-T pacemaker

CPI90-100 insulin pump
CPI-PRx pulse generator

CPM

CPM device
CPM machine

CPMM

constant passive-motion machine

CPS

CPS modular air cranioclast
CPS unitized air cranioclast

CPT

CPT revision tamp

C-R

C.-R. resin syringe

C&R

Cavernotome C&R

CR-39 nuclear tract detector
Cr6-45NMf retinal camera
Crabtree

C. attic dissector
C. dissector pick

cracker

Ernest nucleus c.
LeVeen plaque c.
Newsom side port nucleus c.
nucleus c.

cradle

acoustically transparent c.
alpha c.
c. arm sling
c. boot
CT scan c.
DG-P pediatric c.
foot c.
Posey bed c.
Spectrum DG-P pediatric c.

Crafoord

C. aortic clamp
C. arterial forceps
C. auricular clamp
C. bronchial forceps
C. coarctation clamp
C. coarctation forceps
C. contractor
C. hemostat
C. lobectomy scissors
C. lung scissors
C. pulmonary forceps
C. retractor
C. thoracic scissors
C. tunneler

Crafoord-Cooley tucker
Crafoord-Sellors

C.-S. auricular clamp
C.-S. hemostatic forceps

Crafoord-Senning heart-lung machine
Cragg

C. Convertible wire
C. endoluminal graft
C. Endopro system
C. FX wire
C. infusion wire
C. stent
C. thrombolytic brush

Craig

C. abduction splint
C. biopsy needle
C. headrest
C. headrest holder
C. nasal-cutting forceps
C. pin
C. scissors
C. septal forceps
C. septum bone-cutting forceps
C. tonsil-seizing forceps
C. vertebral body biopsy instrument set

Craig-Scott orthosis
Craig-Sheehan retractor
Cramer wire splint
Crampton-Tsang percutaneous endoscopic biliary stent set
Crane

C. bone chisel
C. dental pick
C. elevator
C. gouge
C. mallet
C. osteotome

Craniad cup positioner
cranial

c. aneurysm clip
c. bone rongeur
c. bur
c. drill
c. forceps
c. Jacobs hook
c. osteosynthesis system
c. perforator
c. plating system

cranial *(continued)*
   c. retractor
   c. suture
cranioblade
   Codman c.
   Kirwan c.
craniocervical plate
cranioclast
   Auvard c.
   Braun c.
   Codman c.
   CPS modular air c.
   CPS unitized air c.
   Rica c.
   Tarnier c.
   Zweifel-DeLee c.
craniofacial
   c. fracture appliance
   c. instrumentation
CranioFIX device
craniomandibular orthopaedic
  repositioning device
craniomaxillofacial
   c. mesh
   c. plate
   c. plating system
   c. screw
   c. sheet
cranioplastic acrylic cranioplasty material
craniotome
   Anspach c.
   DeMartel c.
   Midas Rex c.
   Verbrugge-Souttar c.
   Williams c.
craniotomy scissors
craniotribe
Craniovac drain
cranium clip-applying forceps
crank
   c. frame retractor
   c. table
crankshaft clip
Crapeau nasal snare
cravat bandage
Crawford
   C. aortic retractor
   C. canaliculus probe
   C. dural elevator
   C. fascial forceps
   C. fascial needle
   C. fascial stripper
   C. head frame
   C. hook
   C. lacrimal set
   C. suture ring
   C. tube
Crawford-Adams acetabular cup
Crawford-Cooley tunneler
Crawford-Knighton forceps
C-reamer
   Concept C.-r.
Credo razor
Creech aortoiliac graft

Creed dissector
Creevy
   C. biopsy forceps
   C. bladder evacuator
   C. calyx stone dislodger
   C. urethral dilator
Crego
   C. periosteal elevator
   C. periosteal retractor
Crego-Gigli saw
Crego-McCarroll traction bow
Cremer-Ikeda
   C.-I. papillotome
   C.-I. sphincterotome
Crenshaw
   C. caruncle clamp
   C. caruncle forceps
crenulated tantalum wire
crepe
   c. bandage
   c. bandage dressing
crescent
   c. blade
   c. broach
   C. graft
   C. memory pillow
   C. plaster knife
   c. snare
crescentic blade
Crescent-Pillo pillow
crib
   c. splint
   TiMesh mandibular c.
Cribier-Letac
   C.-L. aortic valvuloplasty balloon
   C.-L. catheter
Crib-O-Gram neonatal screening
  audiometer
Cricket
   C. disposable skin stapler
   C. pulse oximetry monitor
   C. recording pulse oximeter
   C. stapling device
cricothyrotomy
   c. cannula
   c. trocar tube
Crigler evacuator
Crile
   C. appendiceal clamp
   C. arterial forceps
   C. blade
   C. cleft palate knife
   C. crushing clamp
   C. gall duct forceps
   C. gall hemostat
   C. gasserian ganglion dissector
   C. gasserian ganglion knife
   C. hemostatic clamp
   C. hemostatic forceps
   C. Micro-Line arterial forceps
   C. needle holder
   C. nerve hook
   C. spatula
   C. thyroid double-ended retractor

C. vagotomy stripper
C. wire passer
Crile-Barnes hemostatic forceps
Crile-Crutchfield clamp
Crile-Duval lung-grasping forceps
Crile-Murray needle holder
Crile-Rankin forceps
Crile-Wood needle holder
Crile-Wood-Vital needle holder
crimped
c. Dacron prosthesis
c. toric
crimped-wire prosthesis
crimper
Caparosa wire c.
ENT wire c.
Farrior wire c.
c. forceps
Francis-Gray wire c.
Gruppe wire c.
Juers wire c.
McGee-Caparosa wire c.
McGee-Priest wire c.
McGee wire c.
pin c.
Schuknecht wire c.
Sheer wire c.
washer c.
Wayne U-c.
wire c.
crimping forceps
Crinotene dressing
Cripps obturator
Criss Cross Cradle device
Cristobalite investment material
Critchett eye speculum
Crites laryngeal cotton screw
Critical
C. care mattress
C. Care ventilator
Criticare
C. comprehensive vital sign monitor
C. ETCO$_2$/SpO$_2$ monitor
C. HN-Isocal tube feeding set
C. pulse oximeter
C. sensor probe
C. 507-series noninvasive blood
pressure monitor
CritiCath
C. PA catheter
C. thermodilution catheter
CritiCore monitoring system
Critikon
C. automated blood pressure cuff
C. balloon temporary pacing
catheter
C. balloon thermodilution catheter
C. balloon wedge pressure catheter
C. guidewire
C. oximeter
C. pressure infuser
**Critikon-Berman angiographic balloon
catheter**
CRIT-LINE instrument

CritSpin
C. celltrifuge
CRM
CRM cup
CRM rehab brace
Crockard
C. hard palate retractor
C. ligament grasping forceps
C. microdissector
C. midfacial osteotomy retractor
plate
C. odontoid peg-grasping forceps
C. pharyngeal retractor
C. small-tongue retractor blade
C. sublaminar wire guide
C. suction tube holder
C. transoral clip applier
C. transoral retractor body
crocodile biopsy forceps
Cronin
C. cleft palate elevator
C. mammary implant
C. palate elevator
C. palate knife
C. Silastic mammary prosthesis
Crookes
C. glasses
C. lens
Crookes-Hittorf tube
Crosby
C. biopsy needle
C. capsule
C. knife
Crosby-Kugler
C.-K. biopsy capsule
C.-K. pediatric capsule
cross
c. bar
C. clamp
C. corneal bur
C. needle trocar
C. osteotome
C. scleral trephine
C. Top replacement oxygen sensor
cross-action
c.-a. bulldog clamp
c.-a. capsular forceps
c.-a. towel clamp
crossbar
c. fishtail chisel
cross-bracing
spinal rod c.-b.
Wiltse system c.-b.
crosscut
c. straight fissure bur
crossed coil
Crossen puncturing tenaculum forceps
Crossfire polyethylene material
CrossFlex
C. coil stent
C. LC coronary artery stent
Cross-Jones
C.-J. disk prosthetic valve
C.-J. disk valve prosthesis
cross-legged clip

C

179

crosslink
Edwards modular system rod c.
Galveston fixation with TSRH c.
Texas Scottish Rite Hospital c.
crosslinked poly glaucoma filtration device
cross-Polaroid projection chart
CrossSail coronary dilation catheter
cross-sectional anal sphincter probe
cross-slot screwdriver
cross-talk pacemaker
Crosswire
C. nitinol hydrophilic guidewire
C. PTCA guidewire
crotchless compression garment
Crotti
C. goiter retractor
C. thyroid retractor
Crouch corneal protector
croupette
C. child tent
croup tent
Crowe
C. pilot point
C. pilot point on Steinmann pin
Crowe-Davis
C.-D. mouth gag
C.-D. mouthgag
C.-D. mouth retractor
Crowe-tip pin
Crowley shank
crown
Alfred Becht temporary c.
c. amalgamator
Bosworth temporary c.
Bremer halo c.
Celay InCeram c.
c. drill
c. drill screw
free-standing single c.
Getz c.
Hahnenkratt temporary c.
C. high profile cushion
Kontack temporary c.
C. mattress system
C. needle
PD preformed c.
C. quadtro cushion
C. recliner system
Royal c.
Safco polycarbonate c.
c. saw
c. scissors
stainless steel c.
C. stent
Crown-A-Matic crown and bridge remover
crown-crimping pliers
Crozat
C. clasp
C. orthodontic wire
C. removable orthodontic appliance
CRS
C. brace
C. tibial torsion system

CRS-series alternating overlay with pump
CRT
cathode ray tube
CrTmEr:YAG laser
crucial bandage
cruciate
c. head bone screw
c. ligament guide
c. punch
cruciate-retaining prosthesis
cruciate-sacrificing prosthesis
cruciform
c. anterior spinal hyperextension orthosis
c. head bone screw
c. screwdriver
Cruickshank entropion clamp
cruiser
c. buggy
C. hip abduction brace
Crump-Himmelstein dilator
crumpled aluminum foil
Crump vessel dilator
crural
c. hook
c. nipper forceps
Cruricast dressing
crurotomy
c. chisel
c. saw
crus guide fork
crusher
baby spur c.
Berger spur c.
bone c.
cartilage c.
Cottle bone c.
DeWitt-Stetten colostomy spur c.
Garlock spur c.
Gross spur c.
Lieberman phaco c.
Lowsley stone c.
Mayo-Lovelace spur c.
Mikulicz c.
Ochsner-DeBakey spur c.
Proud fascia c.
Stetten spur c.
ultrasonic stone c.
Warthen spur c.
Wolfson spur c.
Wurth spur c.
crushing clamp
crutch, pl. **crutches**
c. and belt femoral closed nail
EuroCuff forearm c.
Everett c.
c. glasses
Hardy aluminum c.
Kenny c.
Lofstrand c.
Warm Springs c.
crutched stick-type polyurethane endoprosthesis

Crutchfield
  C. bone drill
  C. carotid artery clamp
  C. hand drill
  C. skeletal traction
  C. skeletal traction tongs
  C. skull-tip pin
  C. tongs prosthesis
  C. traction bow
Crutchfield-Raney
  C.-R. drill
  C.-R. skull traction tongs
CRW stereotactic system
CRx valve
Cryer
  C. dental elevator
  C. root elevator
  C. Universal forceps
cryoablation catheter
Cryo-Barrages vitreous implant
Cry-O-Cadet
  Kelman C.-O.-C.
CRYOcare cryoablation system
cryocatheter
  Freezor c.
Cryo/Cuff
  C. ankle dressing
  C. compression dressing
  C. knee compression dressing
    system
  C. pressure boot
Cryocup ice massager
Cryo-Cut microtome
cryoenucleator
  Gallie c.
cryoextractor
  Alcon c.
  Amoils c.
  Beaver cataract c.
  Bellows c.
  Frigitronics Mark II c.
  Keeler c.
  Kelman c.
  Rubinstein c.
  Thomas c.
cryoflex envelope
CryoGenetics CryoPrism
cryogenic
  c. probe
  c. storage container
Cryogun
  Wallach LL100 cryosurgical C.
Cryojet
  Torre C.
Cryolife
  C. homograft
  C. valvular graft
CryoLife-O'Brien valve
cryomagnet
CryoMed 1010A freezer
Cryomedics
  C. colposcope
  C. disposable LLETZ electrode
  C. electrosurgery system

cryopencil
  Amoils c.
  Mira endovitreal c.
cryopexy probe
cryophake
  Alcon c.
  Amoils c.
  Bellows c.
  Keeler c.
  Kelman c.
  Rubinstein c.
cryopreserved homograft valve
CryoPrism
  CryoGenetics C.
cryoprobe
  Amoils c.
  Cooper c.
  cryoptor c.
  DATE c.
  ERBE c.
  Frigitronics c.
  intravitreal c.
  Lee c.
  Linde c.
  MST c.
  Rubinstein c.
  Spembly c.
  Sudarsky c.
  Thomas c.
cryoptor
  c. cryoprobe
  Thomas c.
cryoretractor
  Coston-Trent c.
  Hartstein iris c.
  Thomas c.
CRYO rubber mold
cryostat
  CE-2 c.
  Cooper disk c.
  c. frozen sectioning aid
  Tissue Tek-II c.
Cryostylet
cryosurgical
  c. apparatus
  c. instrument
  c. unit
cryosystem
  Keeler-Amoils ophthalmic c.
cryotherapy probe
cryotome
cryotube
  Nunc c.
CRYO-VAC-A cryostat vacuum system
CryoValve-SG
CryoVein
cryovial
crypt hook
cryptoscope
  Satvioni c.
cryptotome
  Blanchard c.
  Pierce c.

C

crystal
- Cardiometrics Flowire Doppler echo c.
- LZT c.
- piezoelectric c.
- C. Tone I in-the-ear hearing aid

Crystalase
- C. alexandrite DP laser
- C. erbium 2 laser

CrystalEyes endoscopic video system
crystalline lens
Crystar porcelain kit
CS-9000 densitometer
CSC3 cervical support cushion
C-Scan
- TechnoMed C.-S.

CSF
- CSF prosthesis
- CSF reservoir
- CSF shunt-introducing forceps
- CSF T-tube shunt

C-shaped
- C.-s. microplate
- C.-s. plate
- C.-s. resistive magnet

CSI lens
C-sponge
CSV Bovie electrosurgical unit
CT
- contrast-enhanced CT
- CT densitometer
- helical CT
- CT Max 640 scanner
- CT scan
- CT scan cradle
- CT scan gantry
- spiral CT
- Technicare Omega 500 CT
- triphasic spiral CT
- twin-beam CT

CT-10 computerized tonometer
CT1 suture
CTDx electrostimulation system
CTEV brace
CTE:YAG laser
CTI
- CTI cyclotron
- CTI 933/4 ECAT scanner
- CTI infusion pump
- CTI positron emission tomography (PET) scanner

C.Ti. brace
CTI-Siemens 933/8-12 PET camera
CT-MRI-compatible stereotactic head frame system
C-Trak
- C.-T. analyzer
- C.-T. hand-held gamma detector
- C.-T. handheld gamma probe
- C.-T. surgical guidance system

CTS
- CTS gauge
- CTS Gripfit splint
- CTS Relief kit

C-type acupuncture needle

Cu-7 intrauterine device
CU-8 needle
Cubbins
- C. screw
- C. screwdriver

cube
- foam c.
- Gelfoam c.
- c. pessary
- Rancho c.
- Temper Foam c.
- tumbling E c.

Cuchica syringe
Cueva
- C. cranial nerve electrode
- C. cranial nerve electrode monitoring device

cuff
- Astropulse c.
- blood pressure c.
- blood warmer c.
- calibrated V-Lok c.
- ComfortCuff blood pressure c.
- conductive V-Lok c.
- Cook continence c.
- Critikon automated blood pressure c.
- Dacron c.
- Dinamap blood pressure c.
- Ducker-Hayes nerve c.
- c. electrode
- elephant c.
- endotracheal tube c.
- Ethox c.
- Falk vaginal c.
- Finapres finger c.
- finger c.
- First Quality overnight brief with leg c.
- hand c.
- Honan c.
- inflatable tourniquet c.
- inflatable tracheal tube c.
- joint distraction c.
- Kendall endotracheal tube c.
- Kidde tourniquet c.
- C. Link orthopaedic device
- nerve c.
- oscillometric blood pressure c.
- Papercuff disposable blood pressure c.
- pneumatic c.
- Polmedco endotracheal tube c.
- Portex SS endotracheal tube c.
- Portex XL endotracheal tube c.
- pressure c.
- push c.
- Push-Ease Quad c.
- PyMaH pre-gaged c.
- Rusch endotracheal tube c.
- Safe-Cuff blood pressure c.
- Sheridan endotracheal tube c.
- shoulder c.
- sphygmomanometer c.
- Steri-Cuff disposable tourniquet c.

Temp-Kuff blood pressure c.
tourniquet c.
tracheal tube c.
VitaCuff c.
V-Lok disposable blood pressure c.
Watzke c.

cuffed

c. endotracheal tube
c. esophageal endoprosthesis
c. tracheostomy tube

cuff-type inactive electrode

CUI

CUI artificial breast prosthesis
CUI catheter
CUI chin prosthesis
CUI columellar implant
CUI dorsal implant
CUI eye sphere prosthesis
CUI gel mammary prosthesis
CUI joint
CUI malar implant
CUI myringotomy tube
CUI nasal prosthesis
CUI rhinoplasty implant
CUI saline mammary prosthesis
CUI shunt
CUI tendon prosthesis
CUI testicular prosthesis
CUI tissue expander
CUI urological drain

Cuidant system

cuirass

c. jacket
c. respirator
c. ventilator

Cukier nasal forceps

Culbertson canal knife

cul-de-sac

c.-d.-s. irrigating vectis
c.-d.-s. irrigation T-tube

culdoscope

Decker fiberoptic c.

Culler

C. eye forceps
C. fixation forceps
C. iris spatula
C. iris speculum
C. lens spoon
C. rectus muscle hook

Culley ulna splint

Cullom-Mueller adenotome

Cullom septal forceps

Culp biopsy needle

Culpolase laser

CultiSpher-G

culturette

Mini-tip c.

Cummings

C. four-wing Malecot retention
catheter
C. nephrostomy catheter

Cummings-Pezzer catheter

Cun-Meter

Cunningham

C. brace
C. urinary incontinence clamp

Cunningham-Cotton

C.-C. sleeve
C.-C. sleeve coaxial dilator

cup

AccuPressure heel c.
Alivium prosthesis c.
APR acetabular c.
Arthopor acetabular c.
Aufranc c.
Bard alligator c.
Bard oval c.
Berkeley suction c.
Bicon-Plus c.
c. biopsy forceps
Bird OP c.
Breinin suction c.
Buchholz acetabular c.
c. catheter
Centaur trial c.
Chambers intrauterine c.
Charnley acetabular c.
Charnley offset-bore c.
CMI/Mityvac c.
CMI/O'Neil c.
Crawford-Adams acetabular c.
CRM c.
c. curette
dry c.
Dual Geometry HA c.
Duraloc acetabular c.
ear c.
Flo-Trol drinking c.
Galin silicone bleb c.
Gemini c.
Harris-Galante c.
heel c.
HGP II acetabular c.
Instead feminine protection c.
Integrity acetabular c.
Interseal acetabular c.
iodine c.
Kennedy spillproof c.
Laing concentric hip c.
Lord c.
magnetic c.
Malström c.
McBride c.
McGoey-Evans acetabular c.
McKee-Farrar acetabular c.
Mityvac obstetric vacuum
extractor c.
Mityvac Super M c.
MMS low-profile acetabular c.
Mueller-type acetabular c.
multipolar bipolar c.
nasal suction c.
Natural-Lok acetabular c.
New England Baptist acetabular c.
Newhart-Smith c.
O'Connor finger c.
ocular c.
O'Harris-Petruso c.

C

cup *(continued)*
    Omnifit acetabular c.
    ophthalmic c.
    optics c.
    Opti-Fix acetabular c.
    Oves cervical c.
    c. palm manual percussor
    PCA acetabular c.
    c. pessary
    Pierce nasal c.
    Polysorb heel c.
    c. positioner
    prosthetic c.
    c. pusher shaft
    Reflection I, V, and FSO acetabular c.
    Restoration GAP acetabular c.
    Rickham c.
    Riecken PQ premium heel c.
    Rotalok acetabular c.
    Silastic obstetrical vacuum c.
    Silipos silicone wonder c.
    slit-lamp c.
    Smith-Petersen c.
    Soft Touch c.
    Sorbuthane II heel c.
    S-ROM acetabular c.
    stainless steel c.
    Ster-O_2-Mist ultrasonic c.
    suction c.
    Super "M" vacuum extractor c.
    Tender Touch vacuum birthing c.
    Ti-BAC I, II acetabular c.
    Titan hip c.
    trial acetabular c.
    Tri-Lock acetabular c.
    Trilogy acetabular c.
    Tuli heel c.
    University of California Biomechanics Laboratory heel c.
    Veenema-Gusberg prostatic biopsy c.
    Vitallium c.
    wet c.

cup-biting forceps
cupped
    c. curette
    c. forceps
cup-shaped
    c.-s. curette forceps
    c.-s. electrode
    c.-s. inner ear forceps
    c.-s. middle ear forceps
Cuputi sputum collector
Curad
    C. bandage
    C. surgical adhesive dressing
Curaderm hydrocolloid dressing
Curafil
    C. gel wound dressing
    C. hydrogel impregnated gauze
Curafoam
    C. foam wound dressing
    C. island dressing

Curagel
    C. hydrogel island wound dressing
    C. wafer
Curasol sterile wound dressing
Curasorb calcium alginate dressing
Curdy
    C. blade
    C. sclerotome
    C. sclerotome knife
Curdy-Hebra blade
Curet
    Pipet C.
curettage
    Guyon c.
    Gynaspir vacuum c.
curette, curet
    Abraham rectal c.
    Accurette endometrial suction c.
    adenoid c.
    Alvis foreign body eye c.
    Anderson c.
    Angell c.
    angled ring c.
    antral c.
    aortic c.
    apicitis c.
    aspirating c.
    Austin oval c.
    Auto Suture c.
    Ballantine uterine c.
    Ballenger ethmoid c.
    banjo c.
    Bardic c.
    Barnhill adenoid c.
    Barnhill-Jones c.
    Barth mastoid c.
    bayonet c.
    B-12 dental c.
    Beaver c.
    Beckman adenoid c.
    Bellucci c.
    Berlin c.
    Billeau ear wax c.
    Billroth c.
    biopsy suction c.
    Blake uterine c.
    blunt-ring c.
    bone c.
    bowl c.
    box c.
    Bozeman c.
    Bromley uterine c.
    Bronson-Ray pituitary c.
    Brun bone c.
    Brun ear c.
    Brun mastoid c.
    Bruns bone c.
    Buck bone c.
    Buck ear c.
    Buck earring c.
    Buck-House c.
    Buck mastoid c.
    Buck wax c.
    Bumm placental c.
    Bumm uterine c.

Bunge c.
Bush intervertebral c.
Carlens c.
Carmack ear c.
Carroll hook c.
Carter submucous c.
cervical biopsy c.
chalazion c.
Charnley double-ended bone c.
Clevedent-Lucas c.
Cloward c.
Cloward-Cone ring c.
Clyman endometrial c.
Coakley antral c.
Coakley ethmoid c.
Coakley nasal c.
Coakley sinus c.
Cobb bone c.
Cobb spinal c.
Collin uterine c.
Concept c.
Cone nasal c.
Cone ring c.
Cone suction biopsy c.
Converse sweeper c.
Corgill-Shapleigh ear c.
corneal c.
cup c.
cupped c.
cylindrical uterine c.
Daubenspeck bone c.
Daviel chalazion c.
Dawson-Yuhl c.
Dawson-Yuhl-Cone c.
DeLee c.
Dench ear c.
Dench uterine c.
DePuy bone c.
Derlacki ear c.
dermal c.
diagnostic c.
disk c.
disposable vacuum c.
double-ended bone c.
double-ended dental c.
double-ended stapes c.
double-lumen c.
down-biting Epstein c.
Duncan endometrial biopsy c.
Dunning c.
ear c.
embolectomy c.
endaural c.
endocervical biopsy c.
endodontic c.
endometrial c.
endotracheal c.
Epstein down-biting c.
Epstein spinal fusion c.
ethmoidal c.
eye c.
Farrior angulated c.
Farrior ear c.
Faulkner antral c.
Faulkner double-end ring c.

Faulkner ethmoidal c.
Faulkner nasal c.
fenestration c.
Ferguson bone c.
fine c.
fine-angled c.
Fink chalazion c.
flat back c.
c. forceps
foreign body c.
fossa c.
Fowler double-end c.
Fox dermal c.
Franklin-Silverman c.
Freenseen rectal c.
Freimuth ear c.
Frenckner c.
Frenckner-Stille c.
frontal sinus c.
Gam-Mer spinal fusion c.
Garcia-Rock endometrial biopsy c.
Genell biopsy c.
Gifford corneal c.
Gillquist suction c.
Gill-Welsh c.
Goldman c.
Goldstein c.
Goodhill double-end c.
Govons pituitary c.
Gracey c.
Green corneal c.
Greene endocervical c.
Greene placental c.
Greene uterine c.
Gross ear c.
Guilford-Wright c.
Gusberg cervical biopsy c.
Gusberg cervical cone c.
Gusberg endocervical biopsy c.
Halle bone c.
Halle ethmoidal c.
Halle sinus c.
Hannon endometrial c.
Hardy bayonet c.
Hardy hypophysial c.
Hardy modification of Bronson-
   Ray c.
Harrison-Shea c.
Hartmann adenoidal c.
Hatfield bone c.
Hayden tonsillar c.
Heaney endometrial biopsy c.
Heaney uterine c.
Heath chalazion c.
Hebra chalazion c.
Hebra corneal c.
Helix endocervical c.
Helix uterine biopsy c.
Heyner c.
Hibbs bone c.
Hibbs spinal c.
Hibbs-Spratt spinal fusion c.
Hofmeister endometrial biopsy c.
Holden uterine c.
Holtz endometrial c.

C

curette *(continued)*
    hook-type dermal c.
    horizontal ring c.
    Hough c.
    House-Buck c.
    House ear c.
    House-Paparella stapes c.
    House-Saunders middle ear c.
    House-Sheehy knife c.
    House stapes c.
    House tympanoplasty c.
    Houtz endometrial c.
    Howard spinal c.
    Hunter uterine c.
    hypophysial c.
    Ingersoll adenoid c.
    Innomed bone c.
    intervertebral c.
    irrigating uterine c.
    Jacobson c.
    Jansen bone c.
    Jarit reverse adenoid c.
    Jones adenoid c.
    Jordan-Rosen c.
    Juers ear c.
    Kelly c.
    Kelly-Gray uterine c.
    Kerpel bone c.
    Kevorkian endocervical c.
    Kevorkian endometrial c.
    Kevorkian-Younge endocervical
      biopsy c.
    Kevorkian-Younge uterine c.
    Kezerian c.
    Kirkland c.
    Kos c.
    Kraff capsule polisher c.
    Kuhn-Bolger angled c.
    Kushner-Tandatnick endometrial
      biopsy c.
    labyrinth c.
    large bowel c.
    large uterine c.
    Laufe aspirating c.
    Laufe-Novak diagnostic c.
    Laufe-Novak gynecologic c.
    Laufe-Randall gynecologic c.
    Lempert bone c.
    Lempert endaural c.
    Lempert fine c.
    long-handle c.
    loop c.
    Lounsbury placental c.
    Lucas alveolar c.
    Luer bone c.
    Luongo c.
    Lynch c.
    Magnum c.
    Majewski nasal c.
    Malis c.
    Marino rotatable transsphenoidal
      horizontal-ring c.
    Marino rotatable transsphenoidal
      vertical-ring c.

    Marino transsphenoidal c.
    Maroon lip c.
    Martin dermal c.
    Martini bone c.
    mastoid c.
    Mayfield spinal c.
    McCain TMJ c.
    McCaskey antral c.
    McElroy c.
    Meigs endometrial c.
    Meigs uterine c.
    meniscal c.
    Meyerding saw-toothed c.
    Meyhöffer bone c.
    Meyhöffer chalazion c.
    microbone c.
    Microsect c.
    middle ear ring c.
    Middleton adenoid c.
    Milan uterine c.
    Miles antral c.
    Miller c.
    Mi-Mark disposable endocervical c.
    Misdome-Frank c.
    Moe bone c.
    Molt c.
    Mo-Mark c.
    Moorfields c.
    Mosher ethmoid c.
    Moult c.
    Mueller c.
    Munchen endometrial biopsy c.
    Myles antral c.
    nasal c.
    Noland-Budd cervical c.
    Nordent bone c.
    Novak biopsy c.
    Novak-Schoeckaert endometrial c.
    Novak uterine c.
    O'Connor double-edged c.
    optical aspirating c.
    Orban c.
    orthopedic c.
    oval-window c.
    ovum c.
    Paparella angled-ring c.
    Paparella-House c.
    Paparella mastoid c.
    Paparella stapes c.
    periapical c.
    Piffard dermal c.
    Piffard placental c.
    Pipelle-deCornier endometrial c.
    Pipelle endometrial c.
    pituitary c.
    placental c.
    plastic c.
    polyvinyl c.
    Pratt antral c.
    Pratt ethmoid c.
    Pratt nasal c.
    Randall endometrial biopsy c.
    Randall uterine c.
    Rand bayonet ring c.
    Raney spinal fusion c.

Raney stirrup-loop c.
Ray pituitary c.
Read facial c.
Read oral c.
Récamier uterine c.
rectal c.
Reich c.
Reich-Nechtow cervical biopsy c.
Reiner c.
resectoscope c.
retrograde c.
reverse-angle skid c.
reverse-curve adenoid c.
Rheinstaedter flushing c.
Rheinstaedter uterine c.
Rhoton blunt-ring c.
Rhoton horizontal-ring c.
Rhoton loop c.
Rhoton pituitary c.
Rhoton spoon c.
Rhoton vertical ring c.
Rica ear c.
Rica lipoma c.
Rica mastoid c.
Rica uterine c.
Richards bone c.
Richards ethmoid c.
Richards mastoid c.
Ridpath ethmoid c.
right-angle c.
rigid c.
ring bayonet Rand c.
Rock endometrial suction c.
Rosen knife c.
Rosenmüller c.
rotatable transsphenoidal horizontal
  ring c.
rotatable transsphenoidal vertical
  ring c.
ruptured disk c.
salpingeal c.
saw-toothed c.
scarifying c.
Schaefer ethmoid c.
Schaefer mastoid c.
Schede bone c.
Schroeder uterine c.
Schuletz antral c.
Schuletz-Simmons ethmoidal c.
Schwartz endocervical c.
Scoville ruptured disk c.
Semmes c.
serrated c.
Shambaugh adenoidal c.
Shapleigh ear wax c.
Sharman c.
sharp dermal c.
sharp loop c.
Shea c.
Sheehy-House c.
Simon bone c.
Simon cup uterine c.
Simon spinal c.
Simpson antral c.
Sims irrigating uterine c.

sinus c.
Skeele chalazion c.
Skeele corneal c.
Skeele eye c.
skid c.
Skillern sinus c.
SMIC ear c.
SMIC mastoid c.
SMIC pituitary c.
Smith-Petersen c.
soft rubber c.
sonic c.
spinal fusion c.
sponge ear c.
spoon c.
Sprague ear c.
Spratt bone c.
Spratt ear c.
Spratt mastoid c.
stapes c.
St. Clair-Thompson adenoidal c.
stirrup-loop c.
Stiwer c.
Storz resectoscope c.
stout-neck c.
straight ring c.
Strully ruptured-disk c.
Stubbs adenoidal c.
submucous c.
suction tip c.
surgical c.
Sweaper c.
Synthes facial c.
Tabb ear c.
Tamsco c.
Taylor c.
Temens c.
T-handled cup c.
Thomas uterine c.
Thompson adenoid c.
Thorpe c.
tonsillar c.
Townsend endocervical biopsy c.
toxemia c.
Toynbee c.
transsphenoidal c.
Uffenorde bone c.
Ulbrich wart c.
Ultra-Cut Cobb c.
Unimar Pipelle c.
up-angled c.
uterine biopsy c.
uterine irrigating c.
uterine suction c.
uterine vacuum aspirating c.
Vabra suction c.
Vacurette suction c.
vacuum c.
Vakutage c.
vertical ring c.
Visitec capsule polisher c.
V. Mueller mastoid c.
Vogel infant adenoid c.
Volkmann bone c.
Volkmann oval c.

C

curette *(continued)*
>Voller c.
>Walker ring c.
>Walker ruptured-disk c.
>Wallich c.
>Walsh dermal c.
>Walsh hook-type dermal c.
>Walton c.
>wax c.
>Weaver chalazion c.
>Weisman ear c.
>West-Beck spoon c.
>Whiting mastoid c.
>Whitney single-use plastic c.
>Williger bone c.
>Williger ear c.
>Wolf dermal c.
>Wright-Guilford c.
>Wullstein ring c.
>Yankauer ear c.
>Yankauer salpingeal c.
>Yasargil c.
>Younge endometrial c.
>Younge uterine c.
>Zielke c.
>Z-Sampler endometrial suction c.

curetting bur

Curity
>C. ABD pad
>C. cover sponge
>C. disposable laparotomy sponge
>C. dressing
>C. gauze sponge
>C. irrigation tray
>C. leg bag

Curix Capacity Plus film processing system

curl-back shell eye implant

Curl Cath catheter

Curon dressing

Curran knife needle

Curry
>C. cerebral needle
>C. hip nail
>C. hip nail counterbore with Lloyd adapter
>C. walking splint

currycomb instrument

Curschmann trocar

Curtis tissue forceps

curved
>c. array transducer
>c. awl
>c. cardiovascular clamp
>c. catheter
>c. chisel
>c. clip
>c. conventional microscissors
>c. cricothyrotomy cannula
>c. dissecting forceps
>c. electrode
>c. gouge
>c. intraluminal stapler
>c. iris forceps

>c. iris scissors
>c. J-exchange wire
>c. Kelly hemostat
>c. knot-tying forceps
>c. laryngeal mirror
>c. magnifying mirror
>c. Maryland forceps
>c. Mayo clamp
>c. meniscotome blade
>c. microbipolar forceps
>c. micromonopolar forceps
>c. micro-needle holder
>c. mosquito clamp
>c. mosquito hemostat
>c. needle spud
>c. operating scissors
>c. osteotome
>c. retinal probe
>c. suture needle
>c. tenotomy scissors
>c. transjugular needle
>c. turbinate scissors
>c. turbinectomy scissors
>c. tying forceps

curved-8 clamp

curved-base Lewis bracket

curved-on-flat scissors

curved-tip jeweler's bipolar forceps

curved-tipped spatula

curvilinear chin implant

CurvTek
>C. system
>C. TSR bone drill

CUSA
>Cavitron Ultrasonic Surgical aspirator
>CUSA CEM system
>CUSA electrosurgical module
>CUSA Excel ultrasonic aspirator
>CUSA laparoscopic tip
>CUSA system 200 straight autoclavable handpiece

CUSALap
>CUSALap device
>CUSALap ultrasonic accessory
>CUSALap ultrasonic accessory needle

Cusco vaginal speculum

Cushing
>C. aluminum retractor
>C. angled decompression retractor
>C. bayonet forceps
>C. bipolar neurosurgical forceps
>C. bivalve retractor
>C. bone rongeur
>C. brain depressor
>C. brain forceps
>C. brain retractor
>C. clamp
>C. clip
>C. cranial bur
>C. cranial drill
>C. cranial perforator
>C. cranial rongeur forceps
>C. Cushing suture
>C. decompression forceps

C. decompression retractor
C. dressing forceps
C. dural hook
C. dural hook knife
C. flat drill
C. gasserian ganglion hook
C. Gigli-saw guide
C. intervertebral disk rongeur
C. laminectomy rongeur
C. little joker elevator
C. monopolar forceps
C. nerve hook
C. nerve retractor
C. perforator drill
C. periosteal elevator
C. pituitary elevator
C. pituitary rongeur
C. pituitary spoon
C. raspatory
C. saw guide
C. self-retaining retractor
C. spatula spoon
C. S-shaped brain spatula
C. S-shaped retractor
C. staphylorrhaphy elevator
C. straight retractor
C. subtemporal retractor
C. thumb forceps
C. tissue forceps
C. vein retractor
C. ventricular needle
Cushing-Brown tissue forceps
Cushing-Gutsch
   C.-G. dressing forceps
   C.-G. tissue forceps
Cushing-Hopkins periosteal elevator
Cushing-Kocher retractor
Cushing-Landolt transsphenoidal
  speculum
Cushing-McKenzie clip
Cushing-Taylor carbide-jaw forceps
Cushing-Vital tissue forceps
cushion
   Airkair seat c.
   AIR1517 vacuum-formed static air
     wheelchair c.
   Akros DFD wheelchair wedge c.
   Back Bull lumbar support c.
   Back-Huggar lumbar support c.
   birth c.
   breakaway lap c.
   Butterfly c.
   cannula c.
   Carter immobilization c.
   Checkerboard wheelchair c.
   Clinicel silicon gel-filled c.
   coccyx c.
   Coccyx seat c.
   Comfort Plus c.
   Comfort Take-Along wheelchair c.
   Contour back c.
   CONVO-GEL c.
   convoluted wheelchair c.
   Core Max-Relax c.
   Crown high profile c.

Crown quadtro c.
CSC3 cervical support c.
Disc-O-Sit Jr. c.
Dry Flotation wheelchair c.
Easebak lumbar support c.
Easy Up c.
enhancer c.
Ezo denture c.
Flexseat c.
Flo-Fit c.
foam wedge wheelchair c.
gel c.
Gel-Foam Ultra-Wedge c.
Geo-Matt contour c.
Geo-Matt gel c.
Geo-Matt PRT c.
Geo-Matt wheelchair c.
Healthier gel seating c.
heel c.
HeelCare c.
Hudson Hydrofloat c.
hydrofloat c.
invalid c.
ISCH-DISH Plus c.
Jay Rave c.
Jay Triad c.
Jay Xtreme c.
LapTop c.
latex wheelchair c.
MaxiFloat wheelchair c.
Medline gel/foam wheelchair c.
Medline Lap-pal safety c.
Memory II c.
Novex wedged wheelchair c.
OCCI DISH pressure relief head c.
Passavant c.
Pedi-Cushions c.
Pediplast c.
Peri-Comfort seating c.
pommel c.
Posture Curve lumbar c.
Posture Wedge seat c.
Premier pincore latex c.
pressure-relief c.
Prop'r Toes hammer toe c.
Pro Relief gel/foam wheelchair c.
Quadtro c.
Response c.
ring c.
Roho high-profile c.
Roho Pack-It c.
Sacral DISH pressure relief back c.
Samadhi c.
Sat-A-Lite contoured wedge seat c.
scintimammography prone breast c.
Shockmaster heel c.
Sit-Straight wheelchair c.
SkareKare silicon gel-filled c.
Skil-CARE Alarm c.
Snug denture c.
Sof-Care chair c.
Sof-Care Plus c.
Stop-Leak gel flotation c.
Sullivan bubble c.
suture c.

C

cushion *(continued)*
    Temper Foam c.
    Tempur-Med wheelchair c.
    T-Foam c.
    T-Gel c.
    The Corner c.
    The Side Rester c.
    trilaminate c.
    UltraFoam seating c.
    Vac-Lok immobilization c.
    Viscospot heel c.
    Waffle seating c.
    wheelchair c.
    Wool'n Gel seating c.
    Y B Sore c.
cushioned-heel
    solid-ankle, c.-h.
Cushion Grip flatware
Cushman drain
Cusick goniotomy knife
Cusp-Lok
    C.-L. bracket
    C.-L. cuspid traction system
Custodis
    C. implant
    C. sponge
    C. suture
custom
    c. tip
    c. total alloplastic TMJ
      reconstruction prosthesis
custom-contoured implant
CustomCornea wavefront measurement system
custom-curved coil
custom-healing orthotic
Custom Ultrasonic automatic reprocessor
cut
    c. biopsy needle
    c. taper needle
cutaneous
    c. punch
    c. thoracic patch electrode
Cut-Blot coagulator
cutdown catheter
cuticle
    c. nipper
    c. scissors
Cutifilm Plus waterproof wound dressing
Cutinova
    C. alginate dressing
    C. cavity dressing
    C. cavity wound filler
    C. Cavity wound filling material
    C. foam dressing
    C. hydroactive dressing
Cutiplast sterile wound dressing
Cutler
    C. eye implant
    C. forceps
    C. forceps thoracoscope
    C. lens spoon
cutout
    c. activator

    c. patellar brace
    c. table
cutter
    adenoid c.
    AMO vitreous aspiration c.
    Anspach diamond dissecting c.
    C. aortic valve prosthesis
    arch bar c.
    Bantam wire c.
    Beaver ring c.
    bone c.
    Breck pin c.
    Buettner-Parel vitreous c.
    Chu foldable lens c.
    Cloward dowel c.
    Codman wire c.
    cookie c.
    Dedo-Webb c.
    diamond pin c.
    diamond wire c.
    Doret graft c.
    double-action plate c.
    Douvas vitreous c.
    dowel c.
    Dual Geometry c.
    Elmed Bi-Pol c.
    Endopath ELC35 endoscopic
      linear c.
    Endopath ETS-FLEX endoscopic
      articulating linear c.
    Endopath EZ-series endoscopic
      linear c.
    Endopath linear c.
    endoscopic linear c.
    Ethicon endoscopic linear c.
    Expand-O-Graft c.
    fascial c.
    finger ring c.
    flat-end c.
    Gator meniscal c.
    Guilford-Wright wire c.
    guillotine-type c.
    Heath wire c.
    Hefty Bite pin c.
    hollow c.
    Horsley bone c.
    Horsley spine c.
    Hough Teflon c.
    Howmedica Microfixation Sytem
      plate c.
    C. implant
    infusion suction vitreous c.
    Jarit pin c.
    Kalish Duredge wire c.
    Kirschner wire c.
    Kleinert-Kutz bone c.
    Kloti vitreous c.
    Leibinger Micro System plate c.
    Lempert malleus c.
    lens glide c.
    Lindeman bone c.
    Luhr Microfixation System plate c.
    Machemer vitreous c.
    Maguire-Harvey vitreous c.
    malleus c.

SomaSensor d.
SomnoStar apnea testing d.
Sonic Air 1500 d.
Sonoblate ablation d.
Sono-Stat Plus sound d.
Sony Promavica still capture d.
Sorbothane orthotic d.
Spencer incontinence d.
Spenco orthotic d.
Spetzler MacroVac surgical suction d.
Spitz-Holter flushing d.
SplintsRite stabilization d.
SporTX stimulation d.
StairClimber assist d.
stapling d.
Statak soft tissue attachment d.
static topical occlusive hemostatic pressure d.
Stat-Temp II temperature d.
Stellbrink fixation d.
Step d.
stereotaxic d.
Steri-Oss dental implant d.
St. Jude cardiac d.
stoma-measuring d.
Stone clamp-locking d.
Stonetome stone removal d.
Stress-Ray varus-valgus d.
Stretch cardiac d.
STx Saunders lumbar disk d.
subcutaneous peritoneal administration d.
subcutaneous tunneling d.
Sub-Q-Set subcutaneous continuous infusion d.
suction d.
Sukhtian-Hughes fixation d.
Sullivan III nasal continuous positive air pressure d.
superconducting quantum interference d.
Super-9 guiding cardiac d.
Super Pinky d.
SuperQuad assistive d.
Sure-Closure d.
Suretac bioabsorbable shoulder fixation d.
Surgicutt incision d.
Surgiflex WAVE suction-irrigation d.
Surgitron 3000 ultrasound d.
Surgiwand suction/irrigation d.
Sutter-CPM knee d.
Suture Lok d.
Swedish Helparm d.
Swiss Kiss intrastent balloon inflation d.
Symbion cardiac d.
Symbion pneumatic assist d.
SynchroMed drug administration d.
Synergist vacuum erection d.
Tacticon peripheral neuropathy screening d.
Tandem cardiac d.

Tano d.
TaperSeal hemostatic d.
targeted cryoablation d.
Tatum Tee intrauterine d.
Taylor halter d.
Teaser d.
TEC atherectomy d.
TechMate 500 automatic immunostaining d.
Techstar percutaneous closure d.
Techstar suturing closure d.
tedding d.
Tekscan in-shoe monitoring d.
Telectronics Guardian ATP 4210 d.
Telos radiographic stress d.
temperature and galvanic skin response biofeedback d.
Tenderfoot incision-making d.
Tenderlett d.
terminal d.
Texas Scottish Rite Hospital corkscrew d.
Texas Scottish Rite Hospital mini-corkscrew d.
Thera-Band therapy d.
Thera-Putty therapy d.
TheraSnore d.
ThermaStim muscle warming d.
Thermedics cardiac d.
Thermedics HeartMate 10001P left anterior assist d.
Thermedics left ventricular assist d.
Thermex-II transurethral prostate heating d.
Thermo Cardiosystems left ventricular assist d.
The Rope stretching d.
The Rope stretch and traction d.
Thoratec biventricular assist d.
Thoratec cardiac d.
Thoratec right ventricular assist d.
thread-locking d.
Threshold inspiratory muscle trainer d.
Threshold positive expiratory pressure d.
Throat-E-Vac suction d.
Thumper d.
Tibbs semiautomatic suturing d.
tiered-therapy antiarrhythmic d.
titanium fixation d.
Titanium Wedge electrosurgical resection d.
tongue-retaining d.
tooth-borne distraction d.
Trach-Talk d.
traction d.
transcatheter d.
transdermal fentanyl d.
transparent elastic band ligating d.
transpedicularly implanted anterior spinal support d.
d. for transverse traction
Trapper catheter exchange d.
TriggerWheel d.

device *(continued)*
　　Trimedyne Optilase 1000 d.
　　Tru-Area Determination wound
　　　measuring d.
　　tube attachment d.
　　ultrasonic aspirating d.
　　Unilink anastomotic d.
　　Universal joint d.
　　urethral barrier d.
　　Uri-Drain male incontinence d.
　　urine collection d.
　　Urosheath incontinence d.
　　Uterine Explora Curette endometrial
　　　sampling d.
　　UV-Flash ultraviolet germicidal
　　　exchange d.
　　Vacuconstrictor erection d.
　　vacuum-assisted closure d.
　　vacuum constriction d.
　　vacuum entrapment d.
　　vacuum erection d.
　　vacuum extraction d.
　　vacuum tumescence-constrictor d.
　　Valtrac anastomosis d.
　　VAPR coagulation and cautery d.
　　Vasceze vascular access flush d.
　　vascular access d. (VAD)
　　vascular access flush d.
　　vascular hemostatic d.
　　vascular sealing d.
　　VasoSeal vascular hemostasis d.
　　Venodyne pneumatic compressive d.
　　venous access d. (VAD)
　　ventricular assist d. (VAD)
　　Ventritex Cadence d.
　　Venturi aspiration vitrectomy d.
　　Versa-Fx femoral d.
　　Versalok low-back fixation d.
　　VestaBlate system balloon d.
　　Vidal d.
　　Vidal-Ardrey modified Hoffman d.
　　Viking II nerve monitoring d.
　　VitaCuff infection control d.
　　Vitallium d.
　　Vita-Stat automatic d.
　　Voyager Aortic IntraClusion d.
　　Wagner leg-lengthening
　　　distraction d.
　　Wallach Endocell d.
　　Wallach freezer cryosurgical d.
　　Wallach pencil cryosurgical d.
　　Wallstent delivery d.
　　WD2 welding d.
　　wearable cardioverter-defibrillator d.
　　Wedge electrosurgical resection d.
　　Williams cardiac d.
　　wire-guided metal spiral retrieval d.
　　Wizard cardiac d.
　　Wizard disposable inflation d.
　　Wolf Piezolith 2300 lithotripsy d.
　　Wolvek fixation d.
　　Wright Care-TENS d.
　　Xercise tube resistive d.
　　Y-Knot d.

　　Zilkie d.
　　Zipper anti-disconnect d.
　　Z sampler endometrial sampling d.
　　Zucker-Myler cardiac d.
Devices, Ltd. pacemaker
DeVilbiss
　　D. atomizer
　　D. CPAP manometer
　　D. cranial forceps
　　D. cranial rongeur
　　D. eye irrigator
　　D. I&A unit
　　D. Mini-Dop fetal monitor
　　D. OB-Dop fetal monitor
　　D. powder blower
　　D. Pulmo-Aide nebulizer
　　D. skull trephine
　　D. suction pump
　　D. suction tube
　　D. syringe
　　D. Vacu-Aide aspirator
　　D. vaginal speculum
DeVilbiss-Stacy speculum
Devine-Millard-Aufricht retractor
**Devine-Millard-Frazier fiberoptic suction
　tube**
Devon-Pura stent
Devonshire
　　D. catheter
　　D. knife
　　D. needle
　　D. roller
Devonshire-Mack
　　D.-M. cannula
　　D.-M. catheter
　　D.-M. clamp
　　D.-M. stop
Dewald halo spinal appliance
Dewar
　　D. elevator
　　D. flask
DeWecker
　　D. eye implant
　　D. forceps
　　D. iridectomy scissors
　　D. iris scissors
　　D. iris spatula
　　D. syringe cannula
DeWecker-Pritikin iris scissors
DeWeese
　　D. axis traction obstetrical forceps
　　D. caval catheter
　　D. vena cava clamp
DeWeese-Hunter clip
Dewey obstetrical forceps
DeWitt-Stetten colostomy spur crusher
DEXA
　　DEXA densitometer
　　DEXA scan
Dexide
　　D. disposable cannula
　　D. laparoscopic trocar
Dexon
　　D. absorbable synthetic polyglycolic
　　　acid suture

D. II suture
D. Plus suture
D. polyglycolic acid mesh
D. surgically knitted mesh
DextBrush
Dexterity
D. Pneumo Sleeve
D. Protractor
Dextran-70 barrier material
dextrose stick
Deyerle
D. apparatus
D. bone graft plate
D. component
D. drill
D. fixation device
D. pin
D. punch
D. screw
Deyo device
Dey-Pak
3D-flat
-f. Lactosorb plate
D/Flex filter
D-Foam
DFP+/DXP+
MaxiFloat pressure reduction
mattress model DFP+/DXP+
DFS 2 mattress replacement system
DG-P pediatric cradle
DG Softgut suture
DH pressure relief walker
Diab-A-Foot
D.-A.-F. protection system
D.-A.-F. rocker insole
Diab-A-Pad insole
Diab-A-Sheet
Diab-A-Sole insole
Diab-A-Thotics orthotic
diabetic
D. Diagnostic Insole
D. D-Sole foot orthosis
d. orthosis kit
d. pressure relief shoe
d. sock
Diabeticorum dressing
DiabGel hydrogel dressing
diacrylate resin
Diaflex
D. cytology brush
D. dilator
D. grasping forceps
D. retrieval loop
D. ureteral dilatation catheter
diagnostic
d. curette
d. duodenoscope
d. fiberoptic lens
d. hysteroscope
d. tube
d. tympanometer
d. ultrasound imaging catheter
Diakart hemoperfusion cartridge
Diaket root canal cement

dial
Mendez astigmatism d.
Regan-Lancaster d.
dialer
intraocular lens d.
IOL d.
irrigating d.
Spadafora MemoryLens d.
Visitec intraocular lens d.
Dialix dialyzer
dial-lock orthosis
Dialog pacemaker
Dialom bur
dial-type ophthalmodynamometer
Dialy-Nate catheter
Dialys-Aids System
dialysate
d. bag
d. preparation module
d. tubing
dialysis
d. catheter
d. shunt
d. tubing
dialyzer
AM-UP-75WET d.
AN69 membrane d.
Asahi hollow fiber d.
Baxter PSN d.
CA membrane hollow-fiber d.
capillary flow d.
CA-series d.
cellulose acetate device
C-Dak d.
Clirans T-series d.
DAS single pass d.
Dialix d.
Digi-Dyne d.
Eri-Flo d.
Filtryzer d.
Fresenius AG d.
F-series d.
Gambro d.
Gambro-Lundia coil d.
HD Secura d.
Hemoclear d.
HF d.
hollow filter dialyzer
high flux d.
hollow fiber capillary d.
hollow filter d. (HF dialyzer)
Idecap d.
low-flux cuprammonium d.
Nephross d.
parallel flow d.
parallel plate d.
polysulfone d.
Renaflo hollow fiber d.
Renalin d.
Renal systems d.
Renatron d.
Sorbiclear d.
TAF175 d.
Terumo d.
Terumo-Clirans d.

D

dialyzer *(continued)*
    T220L d.
    twin-coil d.
Diamatrix trapezoidal diamond knife
Diamed leg bag
diamond
    d. barrel bur
    D. biomechanical table
    d. blade
    d. blade knife
    d. dermabrader
    d. electrode
    d. finishing bur
    d. fraise
    d. grip needle holder
    d. high-speed air drill
    d. inlay bone graft
    d. instrument
    d. micrometer
    d. nail
    d. phaco knife
    d. pin cutter
    d. pyramid indenter
    d. rasp
    d. saw
    D. SharpPoint needle
    D. valve
    d. wafering saw
    d. wire cutter
diamond-coated bur
diamond-dust bur
diamond-dusted knife
diamond-edge scissors
Diamond-Flex trocar
Diamond-Jaw needle holder
Diamond-Lite
    D.-L. cardiovascular instrument
    D.-L. titanium instruments
diamond-point suture needle
Diamontek knife
diaper
    KINS prefolded flat 100% cotton flannelette d.
    reusable and washable adult pin-style d.
    reusable and washable adult snap d.
    Safe & Dry d.
diaphanoscope
    Binner d.
DiaPhine
    D. corneal trephination device
    D. trephine
diaphragm
    Bucky d.
    d. inserter
    Ortho All-Flex d.
    d. pessary
    Potter-Bucky d.
    Ramses d.
    wide-seal d.
Diapulse
Dia pump aspirator
diary
    Holter d.

Diasensor 1000 sensor
Diasonics
    D. Cardiovue SectOR scanner
    D. catheter
    D. DRF ultrasound unit
    D. Sonotron Vingmed CFM 800 imaging system
    D. Therasonic lithotriptor
    D. transducer
    D. ultrasound
Diastat vascular access graft
diastolic fluttering aortic valve
DIASYS Novacor cardiac device
DiaTAP vascular access button
Diatek 9000 Insta-Temp
diathermal
    d. needle
    d. snare
diathermic
    d. forceps
    d. precut needle
    d. retinal electrode
    d. snare
diathermocoagulator
diathermy
    d. cord
    d. electrode
    d. forceps
    d. knife
    Mira d.
    d. scissors
    d. tip
    underwater d.
    d. unit
    d. wire
Diatube-H
dichroic filter system
dichromate dosimeter
Dick
    D. bronchus clamp
    D. cardiac valve dilator
    D. pressure clamp
Dickinson FACS 400-series flow cytometer
Dickson paraffin bath
DIC tracheostomy tube
die
    pin-deburring d.
    Schuknecht-Paparella wire-bending d.
Dieckmann intraosseous needle
Diederich empyema trocar
Dieffenbach
    D. bulldog clamp
    D. forceps
    D. scalpel
    D. serrefine
    D. tenotome
Dienco flowmeter
Diener forceps
Dieter
    D. malleus forceps
    D. nipper
Dieter-House nipper
Diethrich
    D. aortic clamp

D. circumflex artery scissors
D. coronary artery bypass kit
D. coronary artery scissors
D. coronary artery set
D. graft clamp
D. microcoronary bulldog clamp
D. right-angled hemostatic forceps
D. shunt clamp
D. valve scissors
Diethrich-Hegemann scissors
Diethrich-Jackson femoral graft tunneler
Dieulafoy aspirator
Difco ESP testing system
Difei glasses
differential
d. scanning colorimeter
d. temperature sensor
diffuser
cylindrical d.
diffusion-weighted MR imaging
digestive tube
Digi
D. Grip traction system
D. Sleeve stockinette dressing
Digibind pneumatonometer
Digi-Dyne
D.-D. cardiopulmonary bypass
oxygenator
D.-D. dialyzer
Digiflator digital inflation device
Digi-Flex
D.-F. exercise system
D.-F. finger exerciser
D.-F. hand exerciser
Digiflex
D. cannula
D. high-flow catheter
Digikit finger tourniquet
Digilab
D. perimeter
D. tonometer
Digirad
D. gamma camera
D. 2020 TC imager
digiscope
Direx d.
DigiScope camera
DigiSound
digit
D. Aid splint
d. cap
d. splint
d. tube
d. wrap
digital
d. acuity card
D. Add-On Bucky image acquisition
system
D. Add-On Bucky x-ray device
D. B system
d. calipers
D. Care kit
d. constant-current pacing box
d. edge-detection
D. fundus imager

d. goniometer
d. imaging spectrophotometer
(DISEASE)
D. Inflection Rigidometer
D. OsteoView
d. slide scanner
D. slit-lamp imager
d. subtraction photokeratoscopy
D. Traumex system
d. voltmeter
d. x-ray detector
digital-to-analog
d.-t.-a. converter
DIGIT-grip
D.-g. device
Digitimer pattern reversal stimulator
digitized instrument
digitizer
Bitpad d.
Cyberware 3030RGB d.
Hough-Powell d.
Metrecom d.
optical d.
Pixsys FlashPoint d.
Polhemus 3 d.
Polhemus 3Space d.
Scanmaster D x-ray film d.
Scanmaster DX x-ray film d.
three-dimensional sonic d.
digitizing pad
Digitrace home computer
Digitrapper
D. EGG recorder
D. Mark III sleep monitor
D. Mark II pH monitoring system
D. MKIII
Synthetics dual-channel, solid-
state D.
Digitron
D. dialysis chair scale
D. digital subtraction imaging
system
D. DVI/DSA computer
Dignity
D. easy access pant
D. Plus briefmates beltless
undergarment
D. Plus briefmates guard
D. Plus briefmates pad
D. Plus briefmates stretch mesh
pant
D. Plus liner
D. Plus regular pant
D. Plus underpad
Dilamezinsert
D. device
D. dilator
D. penile prosthesis
Dilapan
D. hygroscopic cervical dilator
D. laminaria
Dilaprobe
D. dilator
Mixter common duct irrigating D.

D

dilating
    d. bougie
    d. bulb
    d. catheter-gastrostomy tube
    assembly
    d. forceps
    d. pressure balloon catheter
    d. probe
dilation balloon catheter
dilation-tracheobronchoscope
    Edens d.-t.
dilator
    achalasia d.
    Achiever balloon d.
    Ackrad Cervicet d.
    Alm d.
    Ambler d.
    American Endoscopy d.
    American Hanks uterine d.
    Amplatz fascial d.
    anal d.
    Anthony quadrisected d.
    aortic d.
    argon vessel d.
    Arnott d.
    Atlee uterine d.
    Avenida d.
    Avenida-Torres d.
    Backhaus d.
    Bailey d.
    Bakes bile duct d.
    Bakes-Pearce d.
    balloon d.
    Bard urethral d.
    Barnes cervical d.
    Barnes common duct d.
    Beardsley aortic d.
    Béniqué d.
    Bennett common duct d.
    Berens punctum d.
    biliary duct balloon d.
    bisected minigraft d.
    Black-Wylie obstetric d.
    bladder d.
    Bonney cervical d.
    Bossi cervical d.
    bougie d.
    Bowman lacrimal d.
    Bozeman d.
    Braasch ureteral d.
    Bransford-Lewis ureteral d.
    Brock cardiac d.
    bronchial d.
    Brown-Buerger d.
    Brown-McHardy pneumatic d.
    Broyles esophageal d.
    canaliculus d.
    cannula with locking d.
    cardiac valve d.
    cardioesophageal junction d.
    cardiospasm d.
    Castroviejo double-end lacrimal d.
    Castroviejo-Galezowski d.
    Catalano d.
    d. catheter

Celestin graduated d.
cervical d.
child rectal d.
Clark common duct d.
Clerf d.
common bile duct d.
Cook-Amplatz d.
Cooley coronary d.
Cooley pediatric d.
Cooley valve d.
Cooley vascular d.
Cordis d.
coronary d.
cortical incision coronary d.
Councill ureteral d.
Creevy urethral d.
Crump-Himmelstein d.
Crump vessel d.
Cunningham-Cotton sleeve coaxial d.
Dagger d.
DeBakey-Cooley valve d.
DeBakey vascular d.
Delaborde tracheal d.
Delaborde-Trousseau tracheal d.
Delclos d.
Denniston d.
Derra cardiac valve d.
de Signeux d.
Desjardins d.
Diaflex d.
Dick cardiac valve d.
Dilamezinsert d.
Dilapan hygroscopic cervical d.
Dilaprobe d.
disposable cervical d.
Dittel uterine d.
Dittman d.
Dittsburg d.
Dotter d.
double-ended d.
Dourmashkin d.
duct d.
Eder-Puestow esophageal d.
Einhorn esophageal d.
Eliminator PET biliary balloon d.
Encapsulon vessel d.
ERCP d.
esophageal balloon d.
esophagospasm d.
expandable cervical d.
expansile d.
Falope-ring d.
Feldbausch d.
Fenton uterine d.
Ferris biliary duct d.
Ferris filiform d.
fixed cervical d.
fluoroscopy-guided balloon d.
French-Hanks uterine d.
French lacrimal d.
French-McRea d.
Frommer d.
frontal sinus d.
Galezowski lacrimal d.
gall duct d.

gallstone d.
Gerbode mitral valvulotomy d.
Gillquist-Oretorp-Stille d.
Glover modification of Brock
  aortic d.
Godelo d.
Gohrbrand cardiac d.
Goodell uterine d.
Gouley d.
graduated Garrett d.
Grüntzig balloon d.
Guggenheim-Gergoiye d.
Guyon d.
Hanks-Bradley uterine d.
Hanks uterine d.
Hayman d.
Hearst d.
Heath punctum d.
Hegar-Goodell d.
Hegar rectal d.
Hegar uterine d.
Henley d.
Henning cardiac d.
Heyner d.
Hiebert vascular d.
high-diameter d.
Hohn vessel d.
Hopkins d.
Hosford double-ended lacrimal d.
House lacrimal d.
Hurst bullet-tip esophageal d.
Hurst-Maloney d.
Hurst mercury-filled d.
Hurst-Tucker pneumatic d.
Hurtig d.
hydrophilic d.
hydrostatic d.
Iglesias d.
implant site d.
incision d.
infant d.
Ivinsco cervical d.
Jackson bronchial d.
Jackson esophageal d.
Jackson-Mosher cardiospasm d.
Jackson-Plummer d.
Jackson tracheal d.
Jackson triangular brass d.
Jackson-Trousseau d.
Jewett uterine d.
Johnston infant d.
Jolly uterine d.
Jones lacrimal canaliculus d.
Jones punctum d.
Jordan wire loop d.
Kahn uterine d.
Kearns bladder d.
Kelly orifice d.
Kelly sphincter d.
Kelly uterine d.
Keuch pupil d.
KeyMed d.
Kleegman d.
Kohlman urethral d.
K-Pratt d.

Krol esophageal d.
Krol-Koski tracheal d.
Kron bile duct d.
Laborde tracheal d.
lacrimal canaliculus d.
laminaria seaweed obstetrical
  cervical d.
Landau d.
laryngeal d.
Laufe cervical d.
Leader-Kohlman d.
LeFort d.
LeMaitre-Bookwalter d.
Lucchese mitral valve d.
Mahoney d.
Mahorner d.
Maloney-Hurst d.
Maloney mercury-filled
  esophageal d.
Maloney tapered-tip d.
mandrin d.
Mantz rectal d.
Marax d.
Marritt d.
McCrea d.
meatal d.
Medi-Tech fascial d.
mercury-filled d.
mercury-weighted d.
metal-olive d.
micrograft d.
Microvasive controlled radial
  expansion esophageal d.
Microvasive Rigiflex balloon d.
Miller d.
minigraft d.
mitral valve d.
Mixter common duct irrigating
  Dilaprobe d.
Moersch cardiospasm d.
Mosher d.
Muldoon lacrimal d.
Murphy common duct d.
myocardial d.
nasal d.
Nettleship canaliculus d.
Nettleship-Wilder lacrimal d.
Nottingham One-Step tapered d.
Nottingham ureteral d.
Olbert balloon d.
olive-tipped d.
Optilume prostate balloon d.
Otis bougie à boule d.
Ottenheimer common duct d.
Outerbridge uterine d.
over-the-endoscope Witzel d.
over-the-guidewire esophageal d.
Palmer uterine d.
Parsonnet d.
Patton esophageal d.
pediatric rectal d.
Percor d.
Pharmaseal disposable cervical d.
Phillips d.
Pilling d.

D

dilator *(continued)*
    Plummer-Vinson esophageal d.
    Plummer water-filled pneumatic
      esophageal d.
    pneumatic balloon d.
    pneumostatic d.
    polyvinyl d.
    Porges Neoflex d.
    Potts expansile d.
    Potts-Riker d.
    Pratt rectal d.
    Pratt uterine d.
    probe d.
    d. probe
    progressive d.'s
    Puestow d.
    punctal d.
    punctum d.
    pupil d.
    pyloric stenosis d.
    quadrisected minigraft d.
    Quantum TTC biliary balloon d.
    Ramstedt pyloric stenosis d.
    Ravich ureteral d.
    rectal d.
    Reich-Nechtow d.
    Richards-Moeller pneumatic air-
      filled d.
    Rider-Moeller cardiac d.
    Rigiflex achalasia balloon· d.
    Rigiflex TTS balloon d.
    Ritter meatal d.
    Rockert d.
    Roland d.
    Rolf punctum d.
    Royal Hospital d.
    Rubbs aortic d.
    Ruedemann lacrimal d.
    Russell hydrostatic d.
    Russell peel-away sheath d.
    Saint Mark d.
    Savary esophageal d.
    Savary-Gilliard esophageal d.
    Savary-Gilliard over-the-wire d.
    Savary tapered thermoplastic d.
    Scanlan vessel d.
    Simpson lacrimal d.
    Simpson uterine d.
    Sims uterine d.
    Sinexon d.
    sinus d.
    Sippy esophageal d.
    Smedberg d.
    Soehendra catheter d.
    sphincter d.
    Spielberg d.
    stapes d.
    Starck d.
    Starlinger uterine d.
    Steele bronchial d.
    Stille uterine d.
    Stucker bile duct d.
    synthetic hygroscopic cervical d.
    Szulc vascular d.

    Taylor pulmonary d.
    Theobald lacrimal d.
    through-the-scope d.
    tracheal d.
    tracheoesophageal puncture d.
    transventricular d.
    Trousseau-Jackson esophageal d.
    Trousseau-Jackson tracheal d.
    Trousseau tracheal d.
    TTS d.
    Tubbs aortic d.
    Tubbs mitral valve d.
    Tubbs two-bladed d.
    Tucker cardiospasm d.
    Turner d.
    two-bladed d.
    ureteral stone d.
    urethral female d.
    urethral male d.
    urethral meatus d.
    uterine d.
    vaginal d.
    valve d.
    Van Buren d.
    Vantec d.
    vascular d.
    vein d.
    vessel d.
    Wales rectal d.
    Walther urethral d.
    Weiss gold d.
    Whylie uterine d.
    Wilder lacrimal d.
    Williams lacrimal d.
    wire-guided oval intracostal d.
    wire loop stapes d.
    Wise d.
    Wylie uterine d.
    Young pediatric rectal d.
    Young vaginal d.
    Ziegler lacrimal d.
    Zipser meatal d.
dilator-sheath system
Dilner-Doughty mouthgag
Di-Main retractor
DIMAQ integrated ultrasound system
Dimension
    D. hip prosthesis
    D. hip system
Dimension-C femoral stem prosthesis
Dimitry
    D. chalazion trephine
    D. dacryocystorhinostomy trephine
    D. erysiphake
Dimitry-Bell erysiphake
Dimitry-Thomas erysiphake
Dinamap
    D. automated blood pressure device
    D. blood pressure cuff
    D. monitor/Oxytrak pulse oximeter
    D. Plus vital signs monitor
    D. 1846SX oscillometric blood
      pressure device
    D. system

D. ultrasound blood pressure manometer

Dine

D. digital macro camera
D. digital scanner

Dingman

D. bone-holding forceps
D. breast dissector
D. cartilage clamp
D. flexible retractor
D. Flexsteel retractor
D. malleable passing needle
D. mouthgag
D. mouthgag frame
D. mouthgag tongue depressor blade
D. oral retraction system
D. osteotome
D. otoabrader
D. otoplasty cartilage abrader
D. periosteal elevator
D. wire passer
D. zygoma elevator
D. zygoma hook retractor
D. zygomatic hook

Dingman-Millard mouthgag
Dingman-Pollock septal displacer
Dingman-Senn retractor
Dintenfass-Chapman ear knife
diode

d. detector
d. endolaser
infrared light-emitting d.
laser d.
light-emitting d. (LED)
Microlase transpupillary d.
d. pumped Nd:YAG laser
Zener d.

DioLite 532 laser system
Diomed surgical diode laser
Dionex BioAutolon 450 Data System amperometric detector
diopsimeter
diopter

d. lens
d. prism

Dioptimum system
dioptrometer, dioptometer
dioptroscope
Dip

Silipos Distal D.

diploscope
Diplos M 5 pacemaker
dipstick

Fyodorov d.
Kelman d.
Knolle d.

direct

d. current generator
d. electrical nerve stimulator
d. forward-vision telescope
d. gonioscopic lens
d. laryngoscope
D. Optical Research Company (DORC)
d. retainer

direct-current bone growth stimulator
directional atherectomy device
Directon resin
director

Brodie d.
Doyen d.
Dr. Quickert d.
Durnin angled d.
grooved d.
D. Guidewire system
Kocher goiter d.
Kocher grooved d.
Koenig grooved d.
Larry rectal d.
Laser Fiber D.
Leksell grooved d.
ligature d.
Ormco ligature d.
Payr grooved d.
plain-end grooved d.
Pratt rectal d.
probe-ended grooved d.
Putti-Platt d.
Quickert grooved d.
Stiwer grooved d.
Toennis d.
ultrasonic flow d.

DirectRay

D. direct-to-digital x-ray capture device

direct-vision

d.-v. adenotome
d.-v. telescope

Direx

D. digiscope
D. Thermex
D. Tripter X-1 lithotriptor

disarticulation chisel
Dischler rectoscopic suction insert
DisCide disinfecting towel
discission

d. blade
d. hook
d. knife
d. needle

Discofix stopcock
disconnect wedge
discoscope

percutaneous d.

Disc-O-Sit Jr. cushion
Discover

D. cryotherapy compress
D. Cryo-Therapy unit

Discovery DDDR pacemaker
Discrene breast form
discriminator

EMI APED amplifier d.
Sweet two-point d.
two-point d.

DISEASE

digital imaging spectrophotometer

disengagement mechanism
Disetronic infuser syringe pump
dish

insemination d.

dish *(continued)*
    Lux culture d.
    panning d.
    Petri d.
    scoop d.
    Uri-Two petri d.
disimpaction forceps
disinfector
    DSD-91 endoscope d.
    dual-scope d. (DSD-91)
    Kestrel d.
disintegrator
    SD-1 stone d.
DisIntek reagent strip
disk
    Acro-Flex artificial d.
    d. curette
    Double-hesive adhesive d.
    Eigon d.
    d. electrode
    d. endoscope
    d. forceps
    HCH d.
    Horico d.
    Krupin eye d.
    Krupin valve with d.
    d. lens intraocular lens
    Lillehei-Kaster pivoting d.
    Molnar d.
    Moore d.
    Moran-Karaya d.
    ortho d.
    d. oxygenator
    Placido da Costa d.
    Placido disk
    planoconvex-shaped d.
    d. rongeur
    TRACHO-FOAM adhesive d.
    video d.
Diskard head halter
Disk-Criminator
    D.-C. instrument
    D.-C. nerve stimulation measuring
      device
diskectomy forceps
Diskhaler
    D. inhaler
diskogram needle
diskographic needle
diskoscope
    percutaneous d.
Diskriminator
    MacKinnon-Dellon D.
Diskus inhaler
dislocator
    Kirby lens d.
dislodger
    Cook helical stone d.
    Councill stone d.
    Creevy calyx stone d.
    Davis loop stone d.
    Dormia ureteral stone d.
    Ellik loop stone d.
    filiform stone d.

    Gibson stone d.
    Howard-Flaherty spiral stone d.
    Howard spiral stone d.
    Jimmy d.
    Johnson stone d.
    Levant stone d.
    Mitchell ureteral stone d.
    Morton stone d.
    Ortved stone d.
    Pfister-Schwartz stone d.
    Porges stone d.
    Robinson stone d.
    spiral stone d.
    stone d.
    Storz stone d.
    Tessier d.
    ureteral basket stone d.
    Wullen stone d.
    Zeiss ureteral stone d.
Dispatch infusion catheter
dispenser
    Baxa oral d.
    DropTainer d.
    Exacta-Med oral d.
    Jet Vac cement d.
    Metron Plus d.
    PressPak d.
Dispenstirs
dispersing
    d. electrode
    d. lens
displacement sensing device
displacer
    air uterine d.
    Dingman-Pollock septal d.
display
    virtual reality head-mounted d.
    virtual retinal d.
disposable
    d. acupuncture needle
    d. airway
    d. aortic rotating punch
    d. aspiration needle
    d. bikini
    d. biopsy needle
    d. cannula tip
    d. catheter
    d. cautery
    d. cervical dilator
    d. coaxial Endostat
    d. cystotome cannula
    d. Doppler-constant thermocouple
      sensor
    d. electrode pad
    d. forceps
    d. head halter
    d. injection needle
    d. intraluminal stapler
    d. iris retractor
    d. laryngoscope
    d. measuring guide
    d. microclamp
    d. muscle biopsy clamp
    d. ocutome
    d. probe

d. scalpel
d. sculptured Endostat
d. sheathed flexible sigmoidoscope
d. Styrofoam block
d. surfaces EMG electrode
d. surgical electrode
d. suturing needle
d. trephine
d. TUR drape
d. vacuum curette
d. Yankauer aspirating tube
d. Yankauer suction tube

disposable-sheath flexible gastroscope
Dispo-sand device
Disposashield
Disposatrode disposable electrode
Dispos-a-trode disposable electrode
Dispos-A-Ture single-use surgical needle
Disposiquet disposable tourniquet
Disposo-Scope anoscope
Disposo-Spec disposable speculum
Dissect

Endo D.

dissecting
d. chisel
d. clamp
d. forceps
d. hook
d. probe
d. scissors

dissection
d. forceps
d. knife
d. probe
d. scissors

dissector
Adson d.
Agris-Dingman submammary d.
Allerdyce d.
Allis dry d.
aneurysm neck d.
Angell-James d.
Aspiradeps d.
aspirating d.
ASSI breast d.
attic d.
Aufranc d.
Austin attic d.
Ball d.
balloon d.
Barraquer corneal d.
batwing d.
Beaver d.
Berens corneal d.
blunt hook d.
Brunner goiter d.
bunion d.
Butte d.
Carpenter d.
Castroviejo corneal d.
Cavitron d.
Chajchir d.
channel d.
Cherry Secto d.
Cheyne d.

Codman Rhoton d.
Collin pleural d.
Colver tonsillar d.
corneal knife d.
cottonoid d.
Crabtree attic d.
Creed d.
Crile gasserian ganglion d.
Davis d.
Desmarres corneal d.
Desmarres eye d.
Dingman breast d.
dolphin-nose monopolar
  electrosurgical d.
double-ended d.
Doyen rib d.
ear d.
Effler double-ended d.
Effler-Groves d.
endarterectomy d.
Endo-Assist cutting d.
Endo Dissect d.
endoscopic d.
facial nerve d.
Fager pituitary d.
Falcao suction d.
Feild suction d.
Fisher tonsillar d.
flap knife d.
Freer dural d.
Freer-Sachs d.
Fukushima d.
Gannetta d.
goiter d.
Gorney d.
Green corneal d.
Haines arachnoid d.
Hajek-Ballenger septal d.
Hamrick suction d.
Hardy pituitary d.
Harris d.
Hartmann tonsillar d.
Heath trephine flap d.
Henke tonsillar d.
Herczel d.
Hitselberger-McElveen neural d.
Holinger laryngeal d.
Hood d.
House d.
House-Crabtree d.
House-Urban vacuum rotary d.
Hunt arachnoid d.
Hurd-Morrison d.
Hurd tonsillar d.
Hurd-Weder tonsillar d.
hydrostatic d.
Inaba and Ezaki d.
Israel tonsillar d.
Jackson-Pratt d.
Jannetta aneurysm neck d.
Jazbi tonsillar d.
Jimmy d.
joker d.
Judet d.
Kffttnerblunt d.

D

dissector *(continued)*

Kennerdell-Maroon d.
Killian d.
King-Hurd tonsillar d.
Kitner blunt d.
Kleinert-Kutz d.
knife d.
d. knife
Kocher goiter d.
Kocher periosteal d.
Kurze d.
Kuttner d.
laminar d.
Lane d.
Lang d.
laryngeal d.
Lemmon intimal d.
Lewin bunion d.
Lewin sesamoidectomy d.
Logan d.
Lopez-Reinke tonsillar d.
Lothrop d.
Lynch blunt d.
Lynch laryngeal d.
Lynch tonsillar d.
MacAusland d.
MacDonald d.
Madden d.
Malis d.
Manhattan Eye & Ear corneal d.
Marino rotatable transsphenoidal round d.
Marino rotatable transsphenoidal spatula d.
Maroon-Jannetta d.
Martinez double-ended corneal d.
Maryland monopolar electrosurgical d.
Mason tonsil suction d.
McCabe facial nerve d.
McCabe flap knife d.
McDonald d.
McElveen-Hitselberger neural d.
McWhinnie tonsillar d.
Meeker monopolar electrosurgical d.
microsurgical d.
Milette-Tyding d.
Miller tonsillar d.
Milligan double-ended d.
Mixter d.
Molt d.
Moorehead d.
Morrison-Hurd tonsillar d.
Mulligan d.
nasal d.
needle d.
Neivert d.
nerve root laminectomy d.
neural d.
neurosurgical d.
Niblitt d.
Oldberg d.
Olivecrona d.
Olivecrona-Stille d.

olive-tipped monopolar electrosurgical d.
Paton corneal d.
peanut d.
Peanut Secto d.
Penfield d.
Pennington septal d.
Pierce submucous d.
pleural d.
Polaris reusable d.
Potts d.
prostatic d.
Raney d.
Reinhoff d.
Resposable Spacemaker surgical balloon d.
Rhode Island Secto d.
Rhoton ball d.
Rhoton round d.
Rhoton spatula d.
Rochester laminar d.
Roger submucous d.
Rosebud d.
Rosen d.
rotary d.
rotatable transsphenoidal round d.
rotatable transsphenoidal spatula d.
round d.
Ruddy d.
Sachs-Freer d.
SaphFinder surgical balloon d.
SAPHtrak balloon d.
Schmieden-Taylor d.
Secto d.
Sens d.
septal d.
sesamoidectomy d.
Sheldon-Pudenz d.
Silverstein arachnoid d.
Silverstein auditory canal d.
Sloan goiter flap d.
Smith tonsillar d.
Smithwick nerve d.
Spacemaker hernia balloon d.
spatula d.
Spetzler d.
sponge d.
spud d.
square-tipped arterial d.
Stallard blunt d.
Stiwer tendon d.
Stolte tonsillar d.
straight monopolar electrosurgical d.
submammary d.
submucous d.
suction d.
suction tonsillar d.
synovial d.
teardrop d.
tissue plane d.
Toennis d.
Toennis-Adson d.
Toledo d.
tonsillar d.
Touma d.

transsphenoidal d.
triangle Secto d.
Troutman corneal d.
Troutman nonincisional lamellar d.
Troutman wave-edge corneal d.
Truszkowski dural d.
ultrasonic d.
umbrella d.
vascular d.
Walker suction tonsillar d.
Wangensteen d.
Watson-Cheyne dry d.
Weder d.
West blunt d.
West hand d.
West plastic d.
Wieder tonsillar d.
Woodson double-ended d.
Wynne-Evans tonsillar d.
Yasargil d.
Yoshida tonsillar d.
Young urological d.
Disstik dissection stick
Distaflex
    D. balloon
    D. dental attachment
Distaflo bypass graft
distal
    d. catheter
    d. femoral cutting guide
    d. locking screw
    d. over-shoulder strap
    d. radioulnar joint prosthesis (DRUJ
      prosthesis)
    d. stimulation generator
    d. targeting device
distending obturator
Disten-U-Flo fluid system
distometer
    Haag-Streit d.
distraction
    d. bar
    d. clamp
    d. device
    d. hook
    d. instrumentation
    d. pin
    d. rod
    d. screw
distractor
    ACE OstseoGenic d.
    ArthroDistractor d.
    Beckman d.
    Bliskunov implantable femoral d.
    Caspar d.
    DeBastiani d.
    femoral d.
    hook d.
    Ilizarov d.
    Kaneda d.
    Kessler metacarpal d.
    Mark II distal femur d.
    Molina mandibular d.
    Monticelli-Spinelli d.
    multidirectional d.

MultiGuide mandibular d.
multiplanar mandibular d.
Orthofix M-100 d.
d. pin
Pinto d.
RED system rigid external d.
turnbuckle d.
distribution transformer
Dittel
    D. dilating urethral bougie
    D. urethral sound
    D. uterine dilator
    D. uterine sound
Dittman dilator
Dittrich plug
Dittsburg dilator
Diva
    D. laparoscopic morcellator
    D. laparoscopic morcellator device
divergent outlet forceps
diverging collimator
diversion stent
diverticuloscope
    Holinger-Benjamin laser d.
Diviplast impression material
Dix
    D. double-ended instrument
    D. eye spud
    D. foreign body spud
    D. gouge
    D. needle
    D. spud probe
Dixey spatula
Dixon
    D. blade
    D. center-blade retractor
    D. collar scissors
    D. flamingo forceps
Dixon-Lovelace hemostatic forceps
Dixon-Thomas-Smith intestinal clamp
Dixon-Thorpe vitreous foreign body
  forceps
DL
    double-lumen
      QuickFurl DL
DLP
    DLP aortic root cannula
    DLP cardiac sling
    DLP cardioplegic catheter
    DLP cardioplegic needle
    DLP infant ventricular catheter
    DLP left atrial pressure monitoring
      catheter
    DLP pericardial sump
DMR2 disposable manual resuscitator
D.M.S.
    HomeKair D.M.S.
DMV II contact lens remover
DN acupuncture needle
Doane knee retractor
Dobbhoff
    D. biliary stent
    D. bipolar coagulation probe
    D. gastrectomy feeding tube
    D. gastric decompression tube

D

Dobbhoff *(continued)*
  D. G/J system
  D. nasogastric feeding tube
  D. PEG tube
Dobbie-Trout bulldog clamp
DOC guidewire extension
Docherty cheek speculum
Dockhorn retractor
docking needle
Docktor
  D. needle
  D. suture
  D. tissue forceps
Doc's ear plug
Doctor
  D. Collins fracture clamp
  D. Long clamp
  D. Plymale lift fracture frame
Docustar fundus camera
Dodd perforator
Dodick
  D. lens-holding forceps
  D. Nucleus Cracker forceps
  D. photolysis probe
Dodrill forceps
Doesel-Huzly
  D.-H. bronchoscope
  D.-H. bronchoscopic tube
Dogbone ACFS
dog chain retractor
dog-leg catheter
Dogliotti-Gugliel mini clamp
Dogliotti valvulotome
Doherty
  D. sphere
  D. spherical eye implant
Dohlman
  D. endoscope
  D. esophagoscope
  D. incus hook
  D. plug
Dohn-Carton brain retractor
Dohrmann-Rubin cannula
Dolan extractor
Dolley raspatory
dolorimeter
  Chatillon d.
dolphin
  D. cord clamp
  D. device
  d. dissecting forceps
  d. grasping forceps
  D. hysteroscopic fluid management
    system
  D. instrument
dolphin-billed grasping forceps
dolphin-nose monopolar electrosurgical
  dissector
dolphin-type atraumatic forceps
dome
  d. colpostat
  d. cylinder
  d. hole plug
  d. plunger

dome-shaped internal bumper
domino spinal instrumentation connector
Donaghy angled suture needle holder
Donahoo marker
Donald
  D. clamp
  D. vulsellum
Donaldson
  D. drain tube
  D. eustachian tube
  D. eye patch
  D. fundus camera
  D. myringotomy tube
  D. ventilation tube
Donberg iris forceps
DonJoy
  D. ALP brace
  D. four-point Super Sport knee
    brace
  D. Goldpoint knee brace
  D. knee splint
  D. Legend ACL knee brace
Donnez endometrial ablation device
Donnheim
  D. implant
  D. lens
donor button forceps
Dontrix
  D. gauge
  D. gouge
Dooley nail
Dopcord recorder
Doplette Doppler blood flow detector
Doppler
  Acuson color D.
  D. apparatus
  D. blood flow monitor
  Carolina color spectrum CW D.
  D. Cavin monitor
  color-flow D.
  D. color jet
  Convergent color D.
  D. coronary catheter
  2D D.
  Dopplette D.
  FetalPulse Plus fetal D.
  D. fetal stethoscope
  D. flow echocardiographic probe
  D. FloWire
  D. four-beam laser probe
  D. guidewire
  Hadeco ES100VX mini D.
  Hadeco intraoperative D.
  Hadeco MiniDop D.
  Haemoson ultrasound D.
  Imexdop CT D.
  Imex Pocket-Dop OB D.
  D. IntraDop
  IntraDop intraoperative D.
  D. laser velocimeter
  MD2 D.
  Medasonics transcranial D.
  Minidop ES-100VX Pocket D.
  Mizuho surgical D.
  Multi Dopplex II D.

Neuroguard transcranial D.
Nicolet Elite obstetrical D.
penile D.
power D.
pulsed D.
D. pulsed ultrasound
pulse wave D.
D. Quantum color flow system
D. scope
Siemens Quantum 2000 Color D.
Smartdop D.
spectral D.
transcranial D.
D. transesophageal color flow
  imaging
Ultrascope obstetrical D.
D. ultrasonic blood flow detector
D. ultrasonic fetal heart monitor
D. ultrasonic flowmeter
D. ultrasonic probe
D. ultrasonography
D. ultrasound flowmeter
D. ultrasound monitor
D. ultrasound stethoscope
Doppler-tipped angioplasty guidewire
Dopplette
D. Doppler
Dopplex
Fetal D.
Doptone
D. fetal monitor
D. fetal pulse detector
D. fetal stethoscope
Doran pattern stimulator ophthalmoscope
DORC
Direct Optical Research Company
DORC backflush instrument
DORC fast freeze cryosurgical
  system
DORC handle
DORC microforceps and
  microscissors
DORC subretinal instrument set
DORC surgical instruments
DORC vitreous shaver
Doret graft cutter
Dorian rib stripper
Doriot handpiece
Dormed cranial electrotherapy stimulator
Dormia
D. biliary stone basket
D. extracorporeal shockwave
  lithotripsy system
D. gallstone basket
D. gallstone lithotriptor
D. noose
D. stone basket catheter
D. ureteral stone basket
D. ureteral stone dislodger
D. waterbath lithotriptor
Dornier
D. compact lithotriptor
D. extracorporeal shock-wave
  lithotriptor
D. HM-series lithotriptor

D. Medilas H holmium:YAG
  endourology laser
D. MPL 9000 gallstone lithotriptor
D. scanner
D. Urotract cysto table
Dorros
D. brachial internal mammary
  guiding catheter
D. infusion/probing catheter
D. probing catheter
dorsal
d. angled scissors
d. columellar implant
d. column stimulator
d. column stimulator implant
d. wrist splint with outrigger
Dorsey
D. bayonet forceps
D. cervical foraminal punch
D. dural separator
D. irrigation tubing
D. needle
D. nerve root retractor
D. screwdriver
D. spatula
D. tongue depressor
D. transorbital leukotome
D. ventricular cannula
Dorsiwedge night splint
Dorton self-retaining retractor
Dosick
D. bellows assembly
D. tunneler
dosimeter
dichromate d.
Gardray d.
LiF thermoluminescence d.
Rosenthal-French nebulization d.
silicone diode d.
single-channel in vivo light d.
thermoluminescent d.
Victoreen d.
dosimetrist radiation beam monitor
Dos Santos lumbar aortography needle
Doss automatic percolator irrigator
dot-plotted probe
Dott
D. mouthgag
D. retractor
Dotter
D. caged-balloon catheter
D. coaxial catheter
D. dilator
Dott-Kilner mouthgag
Doubilet sphincterotome
double
d. balloon device
d. Becker ankle brace
d. breast coil
d. bridge
d. bubble flushing reservoir
d. club elevator
D. Duty cane
D. Duty cane reacher
d. hook

D

227

double *(continued)*
    d. irrigating/aspirating cannula
    d. keyhole loop wire
    d. loop tourniquet
    d. right-angle suture
    d. safe-sided chisel
    d. setup endotracheal tube
    d. Softjaw clamp
    d. spatula
    d. spring ball valve
    d. towel clamp
    d.-velour knitted graft
    d. Zielke instrumentation
double-action
    d.-a. bone-cutting forceps
    d.-a. hump forceps
    d.-a. plate cutter
    d.-a. rongeur
double-angled
    d.-a. blade
    d.-a. blade plate
    d.-a. clamp
double-armed suture
double-articulated
    d.-a. bronchoscopic forceps
    d.-a. forceps tip
double-band navel appliance
double-barreled needle
double-bent Hohmann acetabular retractor
double-bubble isolette
double-cannula tracheostomy tube
double-catheterizing
    d.-c. fin
    d.-c. sheath and obturator
    d.-c. telescope
double-channel
    d.-c. endoscope
    d.-c. irrigating bronchoscope
    d.-c. operating sheath
    d.-c. sphincterotome
    d.-c. videoendoscope
double-chip micromanometer catheter
double-cobra retractor
double-concave rat-tooth forceps
double-crank retractor
double-cuff urinary sphincter
double-cupped forceps
double-current catheter
double-cutting sharp cystitome
double-disk ASD closure device
double-dome reservoir
double-edged sickle knife
double-ended
    d.-e. bone curette
    d.-e. chrome probe
    d.-e. dental curette
    d.-e. dilator
    d.-e. dissector
    d.-e. flap knife
    d.-e. nail
    d.-e. needle forceps
    d.-e. nickelene probe
    d.-e. retractor

    d.-e. root tip dental pick
    d.-e. silver probe
    d.-e. stapes curette
    d.-e. suture forceps
    d.-e. tissue forceps
double-fishhook retractor
double-fixation forceps
double-flanged valve sewing ring
double-focus tube
double-guarded chisel
double-headed
    d.-h. P190 stapling device
    d.-h. stereotactic carrier
Double-hesive adhesive disk
double-H plate
double-hub emulsifying needle
double-immunofluorescence microscopy
double-J
    d.-J dangle stent
    d.-J indwelling catheter
    d.-J indwelling catheter stent
    d.-J silicone internal ureteral catheter stent
    d.-J stent catheter
    d.-J ureteral catheter
    d.-J ureteral stent
double-L spinal rod
double-lumen (DL)
    d.-l. balloon stone extractor catheter
    d.-l. breast implant
    d.-l. Broviac catheter
    d.-l. curette
    d.-l. endobronchial tube
    d.-l. endoprosthesis
    d.-l. gastric laryngeal mask airway
    d.-l. Hickman-Broviac catheter
    d.-l. Hickman catheter
    d.-l. injection catheter
    d.-l. irrigation cannula
    d.-l. needle
    d.-l. Silastic catheter
    d.-l. subclavian catheter
    d.-l. suction irrigation tube
    d.-l. Swan-Ganz catheter
    d.-l. tapered-tip papillotome
double-occlusal splint
double-pigtail
    d.-p. endoprosthesis
    d.-p. prosthesis
    d.-p. stent
double-plate Molteno implant
double-pronged
    d.-p. Cottle hook
    d.-p. Fomon hook
    d.-p. forceps
    d.-p. fork
double-ring frame
double-rod construct
double-running penetrating keratoplasty suture
double-spoon
    d.-s. biopsy forceps
double-stem implant
DoubleStent biliary endoprosthesis

doublet
Wollaston d.
double-tenaculum hook
double-thermistor coronary sinus catheter
double-tipped center-threading needle
double-tooth tenaculum
double-umbrella device
double-vector
d.-v. blade
d.-v. brain spatula
double-walled incubator
double-webbed needle
Doubra lens
Douek-MED Bioglass middle ear device
Dougherty anterior chamber cannula
doughnut
d. headrest
d. magnet
d. pessary
d. tip suction tube
d. transformer
doughnut-shaped balloon
Doughty tongue plate
Douglas
D. antral trocar
D. bag
D. bag spirometer
D. cannula
D. ciliary forceps
D. eye forceps
D. graft
D. measuring plate pelvimeter
D. mucosal speculum
D. nasal scissors
D. nasal snare
D. nasal trocar
D. suture needle
D. tonsillar knife
D. tonsillar snare
Dourmashkin
D. dilator
D. tunneled bougie
Douvas
D. rotoextractor
D. Roto-extractor extractor
D. vitreous cutter
Douvas-Barraquer speculum
Dover
D. abdominal belt
D. midstream urine collection kit
D. Premium teflon-coated latex
Foley catheter
D. 100% silicone Foley catheter
D. teflon-coated latex Foley catheter
D. Texas Catheter Disposable Male
Catheter
dovetail stress broken abutment
Dow
D. Corning antifoam agent dressing
D. Corning cannula
D. Corning external breast form
D. Corning hollow-fiber analyzer
D. Corning ileal pouch catheter
D. Corning implant

Dowd, Dowd II prostatic balloon
dilatation catheter
dowel
d. cutter
d. grip
Thompson d.
threaded cortical d.
Down
D. epiphyseal knife
D. flow generator
D. hand dermatome
down-angle hook
down-biting Epstein curette
down-curved rasp
down-cutting rongeur
Downes
D. cautery
D. nasal speculum
Downing
D. cartilage knife
D. cartilage scalpel
D. clamp
D. II laminectomy retractor
D. stapler
Downs arthroscope
downsized circular laminar hook
Doxen mouthgag
Doyen
D. abdominal scissors
D. bone mallet
D. child abdominal retractor
D. costal elevator
D. costal rasp
D. cylindrical bur
D. cylindrical drill
D. director
D. dissecting scissors
D. electrode
D. gallbladder forceps
D. intestinal clamp
D. intestinal forceps
D. myoma screw
D. needle
D. needle holder
D. periosteal elevator
D. rib dissector
D. rib elevator
D. rib hook
D. rib rasp
D. rib raspatory
D. rib spreader
D. rib stripper
D. spatula
D. spherical bur
D. towel clamp
D. towel forceps
D. tumor screw
D. uterine forceps
D. vaginal retractor
D. vaginal speculum
D. vulsellum forceps
Doyen-Ferguson scissors
Doyen-Jansen mouthgag
Doyle
D. bi-valved airway splint

Doyle *(continued)*
    D. Combo nasal airway splint
    D. ear dressing
    D. II silicone stent
    D. intranasal airway splint
    D. Shark nasal splint
    D. vein stripper
Dozier radiolucent Bennett retractor
DPAP
    DPAP interactive airway
      management system
    DPAP Stealth positive airway
      pressure device
DPX-IQ densitometer
Dr.
    Dr. Bruecke aspirating tube
    Dr. Gibaud thermal health support
    Dr. Joseph's footbrush
    Dr. Kho's CMC Support
    Dr. Quickert director
    Dr. Twiss duodenal tube
    Dr. White trocar
Draeger
    D. forceps
    D. high-vacuum erysiphake
    D. modified keratome
    D. tonometer
Dräger
    D. MTC transducer
    D. respirometer
    D. thermal gel mattress
    D. ventilator
    D. volumeter
dragonhead needle
dragon shaver
Dragstedt
    D. graft
    D. implant
drain
    Abramson sump d.
    accordion d.
    ACMI Pezzer d.
    Angle-Pezzer d.
    antral d.
    Atraum with Clotstop d.
    Axiom d.
    Baker continuous flow capillary d.
    Bardex d.
    Bardex-Bellini d.
    Bartkiewicz two-sided d.
    Blair silicone d.
    Blake silicone d.
    butterfly d.
    CenterPointLock two-piece ostomy
      system: stoma irrigator d.
    Chaffin-Pratt d.
    Charnley suction d.
    cigarette d.
    closed suction d.
    clothesline d.
    Clot Stop d.
    Codman lumbar external d.
    combination cone/tube stoma
      irrigator d.

    controlled d.
    Craniovac d.
    CUI urological d.
    Cushman d.
    dam d.
    Davol suction d.
    Davol sump d.
    Deboisans d.
    de Pezzer d.
    Deseret sump d.
    dual-sump silicone d.
    DuoDERM d.
    ERCP nasobiliary d.
    extraventricular d.
    filtered dual-sump d.
    filtered mediastinal sump d.
    fluted J-Vac d.
    flute-end right-angle d.
    Foley straight d.
    four-wing Malecot d.
    Freyer suprapubic d.
    Glove d.
    Gomco d.
    Guardian two-piece ostomy system:
      stoma irrigator d.
    Guibor lacrimal d.
    Hemaduct wound d.
    Hemovac Hydrocoat d.
    Hendrickson suprapubic d.
    Heyer-Robertson suprapubic d.
    Heyer-Schulte wound d.
    high-capacity silicone d.
    Hollister irrigator d.
    Hysto-vac d.
    intercostal d.
    Jackson-Pratt Gold wound d.
    Jackson-Pratt Hemaduct d.
    Jackson-Pratt round PVC d.
    Jackson-Pratt silicone flat d.
    Jackson-Pratt silicone round d.
    Jackson-Pratt suction d.
    Jackson-Pratt T-tube d.
    J-Vac d.
    Keith d.
    Lahey d.
    large-volume round silicone d.
    latex d.
    Leydig d.
    Malecot two-wing d.
    Malecot four-wing d.
    Mantisol d.
    Marion d.
    mediastinal d.
    mesonephric d.
    Mikulicz d.
    Mikulicz-Radecki d.
    Miller-vac d.
    Monaldi d.
    Morris Silastic thoracic d.
    Mosher d.
    nasobiliary d.
    nasocystic d.
    Nélaton rubber tube d.
    papilla d.
    pencil d.

Penrose sump d.
Pezzer d.
Pharmaseal closed d.
pigtail nephrostomy d.
polyethylene d.
polyvinyl d.
PVC d.
Quad-Lumen d.
quarantine d.
Ragnell d.
Redivac suction d.
Redon d.
Relia-Vac d.
Ritter suprapubic suction d.
Robertson suprapubic d.
rubber d.
rubber-dam d.
Sacks biliary d.
Salem sump d.
Seton d.
Shirley sump wound d.
Silastic thoracic d.
Silastic thyroid d.
silicone hubless flat d.
silicone round d.
silicone sump d.
silicone thoracic d.
Snyder Hemovac silicone sump d.
soft rubber d.
Sof-Wick d.
Sonnenberg sump d. (*var. of* van
    Sonnenberg sump d.)
Sovally suprapubic suction cup d.
spaghetti d.
stab-wound d.
Steri-Vac d.
stoma irrigator d.
Stryker d.
subgaleal d.
suction d.
sump d.
suprapubic suction d.
surgical d.
Surgilav d.
Surgivac d.
T-d.
Taut capillary d.
Teflon nasobiliary d.
The MMG Golden d.
thoracic d.
thyroid d.
tissue d.
TLS suction d.
TLS surgical d.
transnasal pancreaticobiliary d.
transpapillary d.
triple-lumen sump d.
T-tube d.
two-wing Malecot d.
umbilical tape d.
Uni-sump d.
U-tube d.
Vacutainer d.
vacuum d.

van Sonnenberg sump d.,
    Sonnenberg sump d.
Varidyne d.
Vigilon d.
Wangensteen d.
Waterman sump d.
water-seal d.
water-trap d.
whistle-tip d.
Wolf d.
wolffian d.
wound d.
Wylie d.
Y-d.
Yeates d.
Younken double-lumen d.

drainable
    d. fecal collector
drainage
    d. bag
    d. catheter
    Snyder Surgivac d.
    Thoracoseal d.
    Thora-Drain III chest d.
drain-to-wall
    d.-t.-w. suction connector
    d.-t.-w. suction tube
Drake
    D. aneurysm clip
    D. fenestrated clip
    D. tourniquet
    D. uroflowmeter
Drake-Kees clip
Drake-Willard hemodialysis machine
Drake-Willock
    D.-W. automatic delivery system
    D.-W. dialysis machine
Drapanas mesocaval shunt
drape
    3M Vi-d.
    adhesive plastic d.
    Alcon disposable d.
    AliMed surgical d.
    Auto-Band Steri-Drape d.
    Bard absorption d.
    Barrier laparoscopy d.
    Bioclusive d.
    Blair head d.
    d. clamp
    Convertors surgical d.
    disposable TUR d.
    eye d.
    Eye-Pak d.
    fenestrated sterile d.
    foot d.
    Gator d.
    Hough d.
    Incise d.
    Ioban antimicrobial incise d.
    Ioban Steri-d.
    iodophor Steri-d.
    Johnson & Johnson Band-Aid
        sterile d.
    Lingeman 3-in-1 procedure d.
    Lingeman TUR d.

D

drape *(continued)*
    3M d.
    MB&J hip d.
    mini-ophthalmic d.
    3M small aperture Steri-Drape d.
    NeuroDrape surgical d.
    O'Connor d.
    OpMi microscopic d.
    Opraflex incise d.
    OpSite d.
    paper d.
    plastic d.
    procedure d.
    Pro-Ophtha d.
    Qualtex surgical d.
    Richards d.
    Rusch perineal d.
    sewn-in waterproof d.
    small aperture Steri-Drape d.
    split d.
    Steri-Drape d.
    sterile d.
    surgical d.
    Surgikos disposable d.
    Surgi-Site Incise d.
    Thompson d.
    towel d.
    Transelast surgical d.
    transparent d.
    Viadrape d.
    Vi-Drape d.
    Visi-Drape Elite ophthalmic d.
    Visi-Drape Mini Aperture d.
    Visi-Drape Mini Incise d.
    Visiflex d.
    V. Mueller TUR d.
    Zeiss OpMi d.
Drapier needle
draw-over vaporizer
drawsheet
Dream
    D. Pillow
    D. Ride car seat
dreamer clamp
Dremel Moto-tool
DressFlex
    D. orthotic
    D. orthotic device
Dressinet netting bandage
dressing
    Ace-Hesive d.
    Ace longitudinal strips d.
    AcryDerm Strands absorbent
     wound d.
    Acry Island border d.
    acrylic resin d.
    Acticoat silver-based burn d.
    Acu-Derm IV/TPN d.
    Acu-Derm wound d.
    Adaptic gauze d.
    Adaptic nonadhering d.
    Ad-Hese-Away d.
    adhesive absorbent d.
    Aeroplast d.

air pressure d.
Airstrip composite d.
AlgiDERM wound d.
alginate wound d.
AlgiSite alginate wound d.
Algisorb wound d.
Algosteril alginate d.
Alldress multilayer wound d.
Allevyn adhesive hydrocellular d.
Allevyn cavity d.
Allevyn foam d.
Allevyn hydrophilic polyurethane d.
Allevyn Island d.
Allevyn tracheostomy d.
antiseptic d.
Aquacel Hydrofiber wound d.
Aquaflo hydrogel wound d.
Aquamatic d.
Aquaphor gauze d.
Aquaplast tie-down d.
Aquasorb transparent hydrogel d.
Arglaes wound d.
ArtAssist compression d.
Aureomycin gauze d.
Band-Aid brand surgical d.
Bard absorption d.
Bard AlgiDERM d.
Barnes-Hind ophthalmic d.
barrel d.
Barton d.
Baynton d.
BD butterfly swab d.
BGC Matrix d.
bias-cut stockinette d.
Biatin foam d.
binocular eye d.
Biobrane glove d.
Biobrane/HF wound d.
Bioclusive MVP Select
  transparent d.
Biocol d.
BioCore collagen d.
Biodrape d.
Biolex impregnated d.
BIOPATCH antimicrobial foam
  wound d.
Bishop-Harman d.
Blenderm surgical tape d.
BlisterFilm transparent wound d.
blue sponge d.
bolus d.
Borsch d.
brassiere-type d.
BreakAway absorptive wound d.
Breast Vest EXU-DRY one-piece
  wound d.
bulky compressive d.
bulky hand d.
bulky pressure d.
Bunnell d.
Bunnell-Littler d.
Burn Jel d.
butterfly d.
calcium sodium alginate wound d.
Calgiswab d.

Carasyn hydrogel wound d.
CarboFlex odor-control d.
CarraFilm transparent film d.
CarraSorb H calcium alginate
  wound d.
CarraSorb M freeze-dried gel
  wound d.
Carrasyn V viscous hydrogel
  wound d.
Castex rigid d.
Castmate plaster bandage d.
Cecil d.
cellophane d.
Centurion SorbaView window d.
chest d.
Chick sterile d.
Chronicure wound d.
Chux incontinent d.
Cica-Care silicone gel sheet d.
Cikloid d.
CircPlus compression d.
Circulon d.
circumferential d.
Circumpress facelift d.
ClearSite borderless d.
ClearSite HydroGauze d.
ClearSite hydrogel absorptive
  borderline wound d.
Clevis d.
Coban elastic d.
cocoon d.
cod liver oil-soaked strips d.
Coe-Pak periodontal d.
Coe-Soft d.
cohesive d.
CollaCote collagen wound d.
collagen d.
CollaPlug wound d.
collar d.
CollaTape wound d.
collodion d.
Coloplast d.
CombiDerm absorbent cover d.
Comfeel contour d.
Comfeel hydrocolloid d.
Comfeel Plus pressure relief d.
Comfeel Purilon d.
Compeed Skinprotector d.
Complex Cu3 d.
composite d.
compound d.
compression d.
Comprol d.
conductive Hydrogel wound d.
Conformant wound d.
contact-layer wound d.
Contura medicated d.
CoolSorb absorbent cold transfer d.
Cornish wool d.
cotton-ball d.
cotton bolster d.
cotton elastic d.
cotton pledget d.
cotton-wadding d.
Covaderm composite wound d.

Covaderm Plus tube site d.
Covaderm Plus V.A.D. d.
Coverlet O.R. adhesive surgical d.
Coverlet Strips wound d.
Cover-Pad d.
Cover-Roll d.
Covertell composite secondary d.
CovRSite d.
Co-Wrap d.
crepe bandage d.
Crinotene d.
Cruricast d.
Cryo/Cuff ankle d.
Cryo/Cuff compression d.
Curaderm hydrocolloid d.
Curad surgical adhesive d.
Curafil gel wound d.
Curafoam foam wound d.
Curafoam island d.
Curagel hydrogel island wound d.
Curasol sterile wound d.
Curasorb calcium alginate d.
Curity d.
Curon d.
Cutifilm Plus waterproof wound d.
Cutinova alginate d.
Cutinova cavity d.
Cutinova foam d.
Cutinova hydroactive d.
Cutiplast sterile wound d.
Dakin d.
Debrisan d.
Decubi-Care pad d.
demigauntlet d.
DermaCare d.
Dermacea alginate d.
DermaCol hydrocolloid wound d.
DermaFilm d.
Dermagran-B hydrophilic wound d.
Dermagran zinc-saline hydrogel
  wound d.
DermaMend foam wound d.
DermaNet contact-layer wound d.
DermaSite transparent film d.
DermaSORB hydrocolloid/alginate
  wound d.
DermAssist gel/gauze d.
DermAssist glycerin hydrogel d.
DermAssist hydrocolloid d.
DermAssist transparent site d.
DermaStat calcium alginate
  wound d.
Dermgran hydrogel wound d.
Dermicel d.
Dermophase d.
Desault d.
Diabeticorum d.
DiabGel hydrogel d.
Digi Sleeve stockinette d.
Dow Corning antifoam agent d.
Doyle ear d.
Drilac surgical d.
Dri-Site d.
dry-and-occlusive d.
dry pressure d.

D

dressing *(continued)*
    dry sterile d.
    dry textile d.
    DuoDERM CGF gel d.
    DuoDERM hydrocolloid d.
    Dyna-Flex compression d.
    Eakin cohesive seal d.
    Elastikon wristlet d.
    Elasto d.
    Elasto-Gel hydrogel wound d.
    Elastomull d.
    Elastoplast d.
    Elastopore d.
    Elta Dermal hydrogel d.
    Enviclusive semi-occlusive adhesive
      film d.
    Envinet gauze d.
    Epigard d.
    Epi-Lock d.
    Episeal wound d.
    Esmarch roll d.
    ethylene oxide d.
    Expo Bubble d.
    Expo eye d.
    ExuDerm RCD hydrocolloid d.
    Exu-Dry absorptive d.
    eye pad d.
    EZ-Derm porcine biosynthetic
      wound d.
    Fabco gauze d.
    Fastrak traction strip d.
    felt d.
    Ferris polyostomy wound d.
    Fibracol collagen alginate wound d.
    figure-of-eight d.
    filiform d.
    film wound d.
    fine-mesh d.
    finger cot d.
    fixed d.
    Flex-Aid knuckle d.
    FlexDerm wound d.
    Flexfilm wound d.
    Flex foam d.
    FlexiGel gel sheet d.
    Flexigrid d.
    Flexinet d.
    Flexzan Extra d.
    Flexzan topical wound d.
    fluff d.
    fluffed gauze d.
    fluffy compression d.
    foam wound d.
    Foille d.
    d. forceps
    four-tailed d.
    Fowler d.
    Fricke scrotal d.
    Fuller rectal d.
    Furacin gauze d.
    FyBron calcium alginate d.
    Galen d.
    Gamgee d.
    Garretson d.

    gauze stent d.
    Gauztex d.
    Gelfilm d.
    Geliperm gel d.
    Gelocast d.
    Gel-Syte wound d.
    gel wound d.
    Gentell foam wound d.
    Gentell hydrogel d.
    Gentell isotonic saline wet d.
    Gibney d.
    Gibson d.
    Gio-occlusive d.
    Glasscock ear d.
    GraftCyte moist wound d.
    Griffin bandage lens d.
    Gypsona plaster d.
    hammock d.
    Harman eye d.
    Harrison interlocked mesh d.
    Hexcel cast d.
    hip spica d.
    hour-glass d.
    Hueter perineal d.
    hyCare G hydrogel d.
    hyCure collagen hemostatic
      wound d.
    Hydragran absorption d.
    Hydrasorb foam wound d.
    hydroactive d.
    hydrocolloid occlusive d.
    Hydrocol sacral wound d.
    HydroDerm transparent d.
    hydrofiber d.
    Hydrogel wound d.
    hydrophilic polyurethane foam d.
    HyFil hydrogel d.
    Hypergel hydrogel wound d.
    Hysorb wound d.
    Iamin hydrating gel wound d.
    impermeable d.
    impregnated d.
    Inerpan flexible burn d.
    InteguDerm d.
    IntraSite gel wound d.
    Iodoflex absorptive d.
    Iodosorb absorptive d.
    IPOP cast d.
    Ivalon d.
    jacket-type chest d.
    jelly d.
    Jelonet d.
    Jobst mammary support d.
    Jobst UlcerCare d.
    Johnson & Johnson d.
    Jones d.
    Kalginate calcium alginate wound d.
    Kaltostat Fortex d.
    Kaltostat wound packing d.
    Karaya d.
    Kelikian foot d.
    Kerlix d.
    Kirkland cement d.
    Kling adhesive d.
    Kling gauze d.

Koagamin d.
Koch-Mason d.
Kollagen d.
Koylon foam rubber d.
Larrey d.
Lipisorb d.
Lister d.
Lubafax d.
Lukens bone wax d.
LYOfoam A water resistant d.
LYOfoam C d.
LYOfoam T d.
mammary support d.
Manchu cotton d.
many-tailed d.
Martin rubber d.
mastoid d.
Maxorb alginate wound d.
mechanic's waste d.
Medical Resources hydrophilic
    wound d.
Medici aerosol adhesive tape
    remover d.
Medifil collagen hemostatic
    wound d.
Medipore Dress-it d.
Medi-Rip d.
Mediskin porcine biological
    wound d.
Medline Derma-Gel d.
Mepiform self-adherent silicone d.
Mepilex foam d.
Mepitel contact-layer wound d.
Mepitel nonadherent silicone d.
Mepore absorptive d.
Merogel d.
Mersilene mesh d.
Merthiolate d.
Mesalt sodium chloride-
    impregnated d.
Metaline d.
Microdon d.
Microfoam d.
Micropore surgical tape d.
Mills d.
Mitraflex sterile spyrosorbent
    multilayer wound d.
Mitrathane wound d.
3M Microdon d.
modified Robert Jones d.
moistened fine mesh gauze d.
moist interactive d.
moisture-retentive d.
moleskin traction hitch d.
monocular eye d.
Montgomery strap d.
Mother Jones d.
moustache d.
MPM conductive hydrogel d.
MPM GelPad d.
MPM hydrogel d.
MPM multilayer d.
3M SoftCloth adhesive wound d.
3M Tegaderm HP high MVTR
    transparent d.

3M Tegasorb hydrocolloid d.
Multidex maltodextrin wound d.
MultiPad absorptive d.
muslin d.
mustache d.
nasal-tip d.
NDM adhesive wound d.
NeoDerm d.
neoprene d.
nonadhering d.
nonadhesive d.
nonocclusive d.
Normlgel protective wound d.
N-Terface contact-layer wound d.
Nu-Derm foam island d.
Nu Gauze d.
Nu-Gel clear hydrogel wound d.
NutraCol hydrocolloid wound d.
NutraDress zinc-saline d.
NutraFil hydrophilic B d.
NutraGauze hydrophilic wound d.
NutraStat calcium alginate wound d.
NutraVue hydrogel d.
Nu-wrap roll d.
Oasis wound d.
occlusive collodion d.
occlusive moisture-retentive d.
occlusive semipermeable d.
O'Donoghue d.
odor absorbent d.
oiled silk d.
Omiderm transparent adhesive
    film d.
Opraflex d.
OpSite Flexifix transparent film d.
OpSite Flexigrid d.
OpSite occlusive d.
OpSite PLUS d.
OpSite wound d.
Orthoflex d.
Orthoplast d.
OsmoCyte island wound care d.
OsmoCyte PCA pillow wound d.
Ostic plaster d.
Owen cloth d.
Owen gauze d.
Owen nonadherent surgical d.
Oxycel d.
oxyquinoline d.
PanoGauze d.
Panoplex hydrogel wound d.
Paracine d.
paraffin d.
patch d.
peacock d.
PEG self-adhesive elastic d.
Peries medicated hygienic wipe d.
petrolatum gauze d.
Piedmont all-cotton elastic d.
Pillo Pro d.
pink d.
plaster-of-Paris d.
plaster pants d.
plastic d.
pledget d.

D

dressing *(continued)*
Polyderm foam wound d.
PolyFlex traction d.
PolyMem adhesive surgical wound d.
PolyMem foam wound d.
Polyskin II d.
PolyTrach d.
PolyWic d.
Pope halo d.
postauricular ear d.
postnasal d.
Preptic d.
Presso-Elastic d.
Pressoplast compression d.
Presso-Superior d.
pressure patch d.
Priessnitz d.
Primaderm foam d.
Primapore tape and gauze wound d.
Primer compression d.
Pro-Clude transparent wound d.
ProCyte transparent adhesive film d.
proflavin wool d.
Profore four-layer wound d.
Pro-Ophtha d.
propylene d.
protective d.
pulped muscle d.
Quadro d.
Queen Anne d.
Qwik-Clean d.
Ray-Tec d.
Red Cross adhesive d.
Release non-adhering d.
RepliCare Thin hydrocolloid d.
Repliderm d.
Reston foam wound d.
Reston hydrocolloid d.
Restore alginate wound d.
Restore CalciCare d.
Restore Cx wound care d.
Restore extra-thin d.
Restore hydrocolloid d.
Restore hydrogel d.
Restore Plus wound care d.
Rezifilm d.
Reziplast spray-on d.
Rhino Rocket d.
Ribble d.
ribbon gauze d.
Richet d.
Robert Jones bulky soft compressive d.
Rochester d.
roller d.
Rondic sponge d.
Rose bed d.
Royl-Derm wound hydrogel nonadherent d.
rubber Scan spray d.
Saf-Gel hydrogel d.
saline d.
saline-saturated wool d.

Sayre d.
Scan spray d.
scarlet red gauze d.
d. scissors
scrotal d.
scultetus binder d.
SeaSorb alginate wound d.
Sellotape tie-over d.
Selofix d.
Selopor d.
semicompressive d.
semiocclusive moisture-retentive d.
semipermeable membrane d.
semipressure d.
Septisol soap d.
Septopack periodontal d.
Setopress d.
Shah aural d.
Shantz d.
sheepskin d.
sheet-wadding d.
SignaDress hydrocolloid d.
Silastic foam d.
Silastic gel d.
silicone d.
Silon wound d.
Siloskin d.
Silverstein d.
SiteGuard transparent d.
Skin-Prep protective d.
SkinTegrity hydrogel d.
SkinTemp biosynthetic collagen d.
sling d.
Snugs d.
Sof-Foam d.
Sof-Rol d.
SofSorb absorptive d.
SoftCloth absorptive d.
Sof-Wick d.
SoloSite hydrogel d.
Sommers compression d.
SorbaView composite wound d.
Sorbex Thin hydrocolloid d.
Sorb-It II d.
Sorbsan alginate d.
Sorbsan gel block topical wound d.
spica d.
Spray Band d.
Spyrogel hydrogel wound d.
squares of d.
starch-based copolymer d.
Sta-Tite gauze d.
stent d.
Stericare copolymer absorbent d.
Stericare hydrogel gauze d.
sterile adhesive bubble d.
sterile compression d.
sterile dry d.
Steri-Pad d.
d. stick
Stimson d.
stockinette d.
StrataSorb composite wound d.
Stretch Net wound d.
Styrofoam d.

subclavian Tegaderm d.
super-absorptive polymer d.
Superflex elastic d.
SuperSkin thin film d.
Super-Trac adhesive traction d.
SurePress compression d.
SureSite transparent adhesive
  film d.
Surfasoft d.
surgical d.
Surgicel gauze d.
Surgicel Nu-Knit d.
Surgifix d.
Surgiflex d.
Surgilast tubular elastic d.
Surgi-Pad combined d.
Surgitube d.
suspensory d.
Sween-A-Peel wound d.
Synthaderm occlusive wound d.
tap water wet d.
T-bandage d.
T-binder pressure d.
Tegaderm semipermeable
  occlusive d.
Tegagel hydrogel d.
Tegagen HG, HI alginate wound d.
Tegapore contact-layer wound d.
Tegasorb occlusive d.
Tegasorb ulcer d.
Telfa Clear nonadherent wound d.
Telfa gauze d.
Telfa island d.
Telfamax ultra absorbent d.
Telfa plastic film d.
Telfa Plus barrier island d.
Telfa Xtra absorbent island d.
Tenoplast elastic adhesive d.
Tensor elastic d.
Tes Tape d.
Thera-Boot compression d.
TheraSkin wound d.
Thillaye d.
thin film d.
THINSite topical wound d.
Tielle hydropolymer d.
tie-over Sellotape d.
Tomac foam rubber traction d.
Tomac knitted rubber elastic d.
Transeal transparent wound d.
TransiGel woven gauze d.
Transorbent topical wound d.
Transorb wound d.
transparent adhesive film d.
Transpore surgical tape d.
Triad hydrophilic wound d.
triangular d.
tube d.
Tube-Lok tracheotomy d.
Tubex gauze d.
TubiGrip d.
tubular d.
tulle gras d.
twill d.
ulcer d.

Ultec Pro alginate hydrocolloid d.
Ultex Thin extra thin
  hydrocolloid d.
Ultrafera wound d.
Uniflex d.
Unna boot d.
Unna-Flex compression d.
Unna-Flex Plus d.
upper body d.
Usher Marlex mesh d.
vacuum assisted closure d.
vapor-permeable d.
Varick elastic d.
Vari/Moist wound d.
Vaseline gauze d.
Vaseline wick d.
Veingard d.
Velcro fastener d.
Velpeau sling d.
Veni-Gard stabilization d.
Ventex d.
Ventifoam traction d.
Viasorb occlusive film d.
Victorian collar d.
Vi-Drape d.
VigiFoam d.
Vigilon gel d.
Vigilon primary wound d.
Vioform gauze d.
Viscopaste PB7 gauze d.
VitaCuff d.
Wangensteen d.
water d.
Watson-Jones d.
Webril d.
Weck-cel d.
wet d.
wet-to-dry d.
whisk-packets d.
wick d.
wood roll d.
wound d.
Woun'Dres natural collagen hydrogel
  wound d.
WoundSpan Bridge II d.
wraparound d.
Xeroflo d.
Xeroform d.
Y-bandage d.
Yield nonadherent gauze d.
Zephyr rubber elastic d.
Zim-Flux d.
Zimocel d.
Zipzoc stocking compression d.
Zobec sponge d.
Zonas porous adhesive tape d.
Zoroc resin plaster d.

Drews

D. capsular polisher
D. cataract needle
D. ciliary forceps
D. cystitome
D. inclined prism
D. intraocular forceps
D. iris retractor

D

Drews *(continued)*
    D. irrigating cannula
    D. lavage needle
    D. lens
Drews-Knolle reverse irrigating vectis
Drew-Smythe catheter
Drews-Rosenbaum iris retractor
Drews-Sato
    D.-S. capsular fragment spatula
    D.-S. suture-pickup hook
    D.-S. suture-pickup spatula
    D.-S. tying forceps
Dreyfus prosthesis forceps
Driessen hinged plate
Dri-flo underpad
Drilac surgical dressing
drill
    ACL d.
    Acufex d.
    Adson-Rogers perforating d.
    Adson spiral d.
    Adson twist d.
    Aesculap d.
    air d.
    air-powered d.
    Albee d.
    Amico d.
    AMSCO Orthairtome d.
    Anspach 65K d.
    anticavitation d.
    Archimedean d.
    ASIF twist d.
    ASSI wire pass d.
    automatic cranial d.
    autotome d.
    Bailey d.
    bar d.
    Björk rib d.
    bone hand d.
    Bosworth crown d.
    Bowen suture d.
    Brunswick-Mack rotating d.
    Buckingham d.
    Bucky hand d.
    Bunnell bone d.
    Bunnell hand d.
    bur d.
    Calcitek d.
    Canal Master d.
    cannulated cortical step d.
    Carmody perforator d.
    Carroll-Bunnell d.
    Caspar d.
    Cebotome d.
    cement eater d.
    centering d.
    cervical d.
    d. chamber
    Championnière bone d.
    Charnley centering d.
    Charnley femoral condyle d.
    Charnley pilot d.
    Charnley starting d.
    Cherry d.

    Cherry-Austin d.
    Children's Hospital hand d.
    chuck d.
    Cloward cervical d.
    Coballoy twist d.
    cobra-head d.
    Codman-Shurtleff cranial d.
    Codman wire-passing d.
    Collison body d.
    Collison cannulated hand d.
    Collison tap d.
    cortical step d.
    cranial d.
    crown d.
    Crutchfield bone d.
    Crutchfield hand d.
    Crutchfield-Raney d.
    CurvTek TSR bone d.
    Cushing cranial d.
    Cushing flat d.
    Cushing perforator d.
    dental d.
    depth check d.
    DePuy d.
    D'Errico perforating d.
    Deyerle d.
    diamond high-speed air d.
    Doyen cylindrical d.
    driver nail d.
    Elan d.
    Elan-E power d.
    electric d.
    extractor nail d.
    fingernail d.
    Fisch d.
    flat d.
    Galt hand d.
    Gates-Glidden d.
    glenoid d.
    Gray bone d.
    Grosse-Kempf bone d.
    d. guard
    d. guide
    d. guide forceps
    d. guide with drill bit
    Hall air d.
    Hall-Dundar d.
    Hall Micro-Aire d.
    Hall Neurairtome d.
    Hall Orthairtome d.
    Hall power d.
    Hall step-down d.
    Hall Surgairtome II d.
    Hall surgical d.
    Hall Versipower d.
    Hamby twist d.
    hand d.
    Harold Crowe d.
    Harris-Smith anterior interbody d.
    Hewson d.
    high-speed d.
    Hudson bone d.
    Hudson cranial d.
    initiator d.
    intramedullary d.

Jacobs chuck d.
Jordan-Day d.
Kerr electro-torque d.
Kerr hand d.
Kirschner bone d.
Kirschner wire d.
Kodex d.
Küntscher d.
Lentulo spiral d.
Light-Veley cranial d.
Loth-Kirschner d.
Luck bone d.
Lusskin bone d.
Macewen d.
Magnuson twist d.
Mathews hand d.
Mathews load d.
McKenzie bone d.
McKenzie cranial d.
McKenzie perforating twist d.
Michelson-Sequoia air d.
Micro-Aire d.
MicroMax speed d.
Midas Rex d.
mini-Stryker power d.
Minos air d.
Mira d.
Modny d.
Moore bone d.
nail d.
Neil-Moore perforator d.
Neurairtome d.
nipper nail d.
Orthairtome II d.
orthopedic Universal d.
OsseoCare d.
Osseodent surgical d.
Osteon d.
ototome otological d.
Patrick d.
Pease bone d.
pencil-tip d.
pencil-tipped d.
penetrating d.
Penn finger d.
perforating twist d.
perforator d.
pilot d.
pistol-grip hand d.
d. point
Portmann d.
Posi-Stop d.
power d.
Powerforma surgical d.
pronator d.
Rainbow d.
Ralks bone d.
Ralks fingernail d.
Raney bone d.
Raney cranial d.
Raney perforator d.
retention d.
rib d.
Rica bone d.
Richards-Lovejoy bone d.

Richards pistol-grip d.
Richmond subarachnoid twist d.
Richter bone d.
right-angle d.
Romano curved surgical d.
root canal d.
scissors nail d.
Shea ear d.
Sherman-Stille d.
Skeeter otologic d.
Sklar bone d.
skull traction d.
Smedberg hand d.
Smedberg twist d.
SMIC sternal d.
Smith d.
spiral d.
Spirec d.
step d.
step-down d.
Stille bone d.
Stille cranial d.
Stille hand d.
Stille-Sherman bone d.
Stiwer hand d.
d. stop cylinder
Stryker d.
Surgairtome air d.
surgical-orthopaedic d.
suture hole d.
Synthes d.
tap d.
Thornwald antral d.
Toti trephine d.
Treace stapes d.
trephine d.
Trinkle bone d.
Trinkle Super-Cut twist d.
Trowbridge-Campau bone d.
Trowbridge triple-speed d.
twist d.
Ullrich drill guard d.
Uniflex calibrated step d.
union broach retention d.
Universal two-speed hand d.
Vitallium d.
Warren-Mack rotating d.
wire d.
Wolferman d.
Wullstein d.
Xoman d.
Zimalate twist d.
Zimmer hand d.
Zimmer-Kirschner hand d.
Zimmer Universal d.

drill-tip catheter
drill-tipped guidewire
D-ring strap
Drinker tank respirator
drip chamber
Dri-Site dressing
driver
    automatic needle d.
    Cook endoscopic curved needle d.
    Eby band d.

D

driver *(continued)*
femoral head d.
Flatt d.
graft d.
Hall d.
Haney needle d.
Harrington hook d.
Jewett d.
Ken d.
Küntscher nail d.
K wire d.
laparoscopic needle d.
Laurus needle d.
Linvatec d.
Lloyd nail d.
MAGneedle d.
Massie d.
Maxi-Driver d.
McNutt d.
McReynolds d.
Micro Series wire d.
Milewski d.
Moore d.
Moore-Blount d.
d. nail drill
needle d.
Neufeld d.
Nystroem nail d.
Nystroem-Stille d.
orthodontic band d.
ParaMax angled d.
Pereyra needle d.
polyethylene-faced d.
prostatic d.
Pugh d.
Put-In d.
Rush d.
Schneider nail d.
Sharbaro d.
surgical pin d.
Sven Johansson d.
Szabo-Berci needle d.
Teflon-coated d.
tibial d.
trial d.
UAM universal fixation d.
wire d.
Zimmer Orthair ream d.
driver-bender-extractor
Rush d.-b.-e.
driver-extractor
Sage d.-e.
Schneider d.-e.
Dromos pacemaker
Drompp meniscotome
drop-entry (closed body) hook
drop-foot
d.-f. brace
d.-f. redression stockings
d.-f. splint
DropTainer dispenser
DRS composite

drug
d. infusion pump
d. infusion sleeve
drug-coated stent
DRUJ prosthesis
drum
d. dermatome
d. elevator knife
d. probe
d. scraper
Drummond
D. button
D. hook
D. hook holder
D. wire
dry
d. cup
D. Flotation wheelchair cushion
Peri-Strips D.
d. pressure dressing
d. sterile dressing
d. sterile fluff
d. sterile gauze
d. textile dressing
d. textile gauze
dry-and-occlusive dressing
dry-powder inhaler
Drysdale nucleus manipulator
Dryspell cast cover
Drystar dry imager
Dry-Therm sterilizer
DryTime for bladder control
DryView laser imaging system
DS-10 mobile dilator storage tray
DS-9 needle
DSD-91 endoscope disinfector
D-shaped implant
DSIS orthotic
D-Soles
D.-S. foot sole
D.-S. insole
D.-S. orthotic
DSP
DSP Micro Diamond-Point
microsurgery instruments
DSP Micro Diamond-Point
microsurgery set
DSX Sopha camera
D syringe
D-Tach removable needle
DU4072 Static air mattress overlay
Dua antireflux valve
dual
d. bypass connector
d. coil transvenous lead
d. distal-lighted laryngoscope
D. Geometry cutter
D. Geometry HA cup
d. lookup table
d. nerve root suction retractor
d. octapolar lead
d. quadrapolar lead
D. Quattrode spinal cord stimulation
system

D. Range Limiter system
d. square-ended Harrington rod

dual-chamber
d.-c. AV sequential pacemaker
d.-c. flushing valve
d.-c. ICD
d.-c. Medtronic.Kappa pacemaker

dual-compartment gel-inflatable mammary implant

dual-energy
d.-e. linear accelerator
d.-e. x-ray absorptiometry densitometer

Dualer
D. Plus
D. Plus system

dual-head gamma camera
Dualine digital hearing instrument
Duall #88 cement
dual-lead electrode
dual-lock total hip prosthesis
dual-lumen
d.-l. catheter
d.-l. papillotome
d.-l. sump nasogastric tube

DualMesh
D. + biomaterial
D. hernia mesh
D. material
D. Plus biomaterial

Dualoop
dual-pass pacemaker
dual-photon
d.-p. densitometer
d.-p. electrospinal orthosis

Dualplace
Sigma II D.

Dual-Port system
dual-scope disinfector (DSD-91)
dual-sensing, dual-pacing, dual-mode pacemaker (DDD pacemaker)
dual-sensor micromanometric high-fidelity catheter
DualStim TENS unit
dual-sump silicone drain
Dualtherm dual-thermistor thermodilution catheter
Duane
D. retractor
D. U-clip

Dubois decapitation scissors
Dubost valvulotome
Dubroff radial loop intraocular lens
Duchenne trocar
duckbill
d. clamp
d. elevator
d. forceps
d. rongeur
d. speculum
d. voice prosthesis

duck-billed anodized spatula
Ducker-Hayes nerve cuff
Duckey nipple

Ducor
D. angiographic catheter
D. balloon catheter
D. cardiac catheter
D. HF catheter
D. tip

Ducor-Cordis pigtail catheter
duct
d. dilator
d. scoop

DuctOcclud coil
ductus clamp
Dudley
D. rectal hook
D. tenaculum hook

Dudley-Smith rectal speculum
Duehr-Allen eye implant
Duet
D. coronary stent
D. glucose control monitor

Duett
D. arterial closure device
D. vascular sealing device

Duette
D. basket
D. double lumen ERCP instrument

Duff debridement needle
Duffield cardiovascular scissors
Duggan rongeur
Duguet siphon
Duguid curved forceps
Dührssen tampon
Dujovny microsuction dissection set
Duke
D. boot
D. cannula
D. trocar
D. tube

Duke-Elder lamp
Dulaney
D. antral cannula
D. intraocular implant lens
D. LASIK marker

dull
d. retractor
d. rotation forceps

dull-pointed forceps
dull-pronged retractor
Dulox suture
Dumas pessary
Dumbach
D. mandibular reconstruction system
D. mini mesh
D. regular mesh
D. titanium mesh

dumbbell needle
dummy
d. source
d. spacer

Dumon
D. laser bronchoscope
D. silicone stent
D. tracheobronchial stent

D

Dumon-Gilliard
  D.-G. endoprosthesis system
  D.-G. prosthesis introducer
Dumon-Harrell bronchoscope
Dumont
  D. dissecting forceps
  D. jeweler's forceps
  D. retractor
  D. Swiss dissecting forceps
  D. thoracic scissors
  D. tweezers
Dumontpallier pessary
Duncan
  D. dural film
  D. endometrial biopsy curette
  D. loop
  D. shoulder brace
Dundas-Grant tube
Dunhill forceps
Dunlap cold compression wrap system
Dunlop
  D. elbow traction
  D. sleeve
  D. thrombus stripper
  D. tractor
Dunn
  D. depressor
  D. fracture device
Dunning
  D. curette
  D. elevator
Duo-Cline contoured bed wedge
Duocondylar knee prosthesis
duo-decapolar catheter
duodenal
  d. clamp
  d. pin
  d. retractor
duodenofiberscope
  Olympus d.
  Pentax FD-series d.
duodenoscope
  ACMI d.
  d. cannula
  diagnostic d.
  Fujinon ED-series d.
  Fujinon FD-series d.
  GF-UM3 d.
  JF-200 d.
  JF-IT20 d.
  JF-1T Olympus adult d.
  JF-V10 d.
  large-channel therapeutic d.
  Machida fiber-d.
  Olympus EW-series fiberoptic d.
  Olympus GIF-series d.
  Olympus JF-series video d.
  Olympus JF-V-series video d.
  Olympus JT-series video d.
  Olympus PJF-series pediatric d.
  Olympus video d.
  Pentax d.
  side-viewing d.
  standard d.

  therapeutic side-viewing d.
  video d.
DuoDERM
  D. CGF gel dressing
  D. drain
  D. hydrocolloid dressing
  D. SCB sustained compression
    bandage
Duo-Drive cortical screw
Duo-Flow catheter
Duo-Klex artificial kidney
DuoLock curved tail closure
Duo-Lock hip prosthesis
Duoloid impression system
Duoloupe lens loupe
Duo-Patellar knee prosthesis
Duostat rotating hemostatic valve
Duotrak blade
Duovisc viscoelastic system
DUPEL iontophoretic drug delivery
  system
Duplay
  D. nasal speculum
  D. tenaculum forceps
  D. uterine tenaculum
Duplay-Lynch nasal speculum
duplex ultrasound
Duplicone silicone dental impression
  material
DuPont
  D. Cronex x-ray film
  D. distal humeral plate
  D. distal humeral plate system
  D. rare earth imaging system
  D. scanner
Dupuis cannula
Dupuy-Dutemps needle
Dupuytren
  D. knife
  D. splint
  D. suture
  D. tourniquet
Dupuy-Weiss tonsillar needle
Dura
  Tutoplast D.
Durabase soft rebase acrylic
durable medical equipment
DuraCast plaster bandage
Duracell Activair hearing aid battery
Duracep biopsy forceps
Duracon
  D. knee implant
  D. prosthesis
  D. PS total knee system
Durafill dental restorative material
Duraflow heart valve
Duragel lens
DuraGen
  D. absorbable dural graft matrix
  D. neurosurgical device
DURAglide stone removal balloon
  catheter
Dura-Guard patch

Durahesive
    D. skin barrier
    D. Wafer pouch
Durahue acrylic
Dura-II
    D.-II concealable penile implant
    D.-II positionable penile prosthesis
Dura-Kold reusable compression ice wrap
dural
    d. elevator
    d. forceps
    d. hook
    d. implant
    d. needle
    d. protector
    d. scissors
    d. separator
    d. substitute
    d. suction retractor
Duralay acrylic
Duraleve custom molded foot orthotic
Dura-Liner acrylic
DuraLite
    D. handle
Duralite tube
Durallium implant
Duraloc
    D. acetabular cup
    D. acetabular cup system
Duralon-UV nylon membrane
Duramer polyethylene component
Duran annuloplasty ring
Dura-Neb
    D.-N. 2000 portable nebulizer
    D.-N. portable nebulizer pump
Durapatite
    D. bone replacement material
    D. implant
DuraPhase
    D. inflatable penile prosthesis
    D. semirigid penile prosthesis
Durapulse pacemaker
Durascope endoscope
Dur-A-Sil
    D.-A.-S. ear impression material
    D.-A.-S. silicone impression system
Durasoft
    D. 2 contact lens
    D. toric lens
Dura-Soft soft-compression reusable ice or heat wrap
Dura-Stick adhesive electrode
Durasul
    D. large diameter head system
    D. polyethylene, high wear resistant acetabular insert
Duratec nursing home bed
Durathane cardiac device
Dura-T lens
Duraval Hook & Loop strap material
Duray-Read
    D.-R. gouge
Duray-Read chisel
Duray-Wood chisel

Duredge knife
Duredge-Paufique knife
Durelon dental cement
Duret system
Durette
    D. dental shield
    D. external laser shield
Durham
    D. needle
    D. tracheostomy tube
    D. tracheotomy trocar
Durkan CTS gauge
Durnin angled director
Duromedics
    D. bileaflet mitral valve
    D. valve prosthesis
Duros leuprolide implant
Durotip scissors
Durrani dorsal vein complex ligation needle
Duryea retractor
Dutchman's roll
Dutch pessary
Duthie reamer
duToit
    d. shoulder staple
    d. stapler
Duval
    D. bag
    D. disposable dermatome
    D. intestinal forceps
    D. lung clamp
    D. lung-grasping forceps
    D. lung tissue forceps
Duval-Allis forceps
Duval-Collin intestinal forceps
Duval-Coryllos rib shears
Duval-Crile
    D.-C. intestinal forceps
    D.-C. lung forceps
    D.-C. lung-grasping forceps
    D.-C. tissue forceps
Duval-Simon portable dermatome
Duval-Vital intestinal forceps
DuVries needle
DUX system
Duyzings clasp
DVI
    DVI pacemaker
    DVI Simpson AtheroCath
    DVI Simpson AtheroCath catheter
Dworacek-Farrior canal chisel
Dwyer
    D. device
    D. instrument
    D. instrumentation
    D. spinal mechanical stapler
    D. spinal screw
Dwyer-Hall plate
DXA
    DXA densitometer
Dybex TENS unit
Dycem roll matting
Dycor prosthetic foot

D

dye
    d. cuvette
    d. yellow laser
¹⁶⁶Dy generator
Dymer
    D. excimer delivery probe
    D. excimer delivery system
DynaBite biopsy forceps
Dynabond resin
Dyna-Care pressure pad system
Dynacor
    D. ear syringe
    D. enema cleansing kit
    D. Foley catheter
    D. leg bag
    D. suction catheter
    D. ulcer syringe
    D. vaginal irrigator set
    D. vaginal speculum
DynaDisc exercise equipment
DYNAfabric material
Dynafill graft biomedium mineralized bone matrix
DynaFix external fixation system
Dyna-Flex
    D.-F. compression dressing
    D.-F. elastic bandage
    D.-F. Layer One padding
    D.-F. Layer Three bandage
    D.-F. Layer Two bandage
    D.-F. multilayer compression system
    D.-F. wrap
DynaFlex
    D. Gyro exerciser
    D. penile implant
    D. penile prosthesis
DynaGraft
    D. bioimplant
    D. putty
Dynagrip blade handle
DynaGuard
    D. APM alternating pressure mattress
    D. LAL low-air-loss pressure management system
DynaHeat hot pack
DynaLator ultrasound unit
DynaLEAP balloon material
Dyna-Lok plating system
Dynalyzer equipment
dynamic
    d. axial fixator
    d. bed
    D. Bridging plate
    d. compression plate
    d. compression plate instrumentation
    d. condylar screw
    d. contrast-enhanced magnetic resonance imaging
    d. contrast-enhanced MRI
    D. cooling device
    D. digit extensor tube
    D. elbow orthosis
    D. foot stabilizer
    d. hip screw

    d. integrated stabilization chair
    D. knee orthosis
    D. mesh craniomaxillofacial pre-angled connecting bar
    D. optical breast imaging system
    D. orthotic cranioplasty device
    d. penile prosthesis
    D. Spacial Reconstructor scanner
    d. splint
    D. transverse traction device
    D. wrist orthosis
    D. Y stent
Dynamite mattress system
dynamometer
    back, leg and chest d.
    Baseline d.
    bicycle d.
    Biodex isokinetic d.
    bulb d.
    Collins d.
    computerized isokinetic d.
    Cybex II isokinetic d.
    electromechanical d.
    handheld d.
    Harpenden handgrip d.
    hydraulic hand d.
    Isobex d.
    Jamar hydraulic hand d.
    Lido Multi Joint II isokinetic d.
    Micro FET isometric force d.
    orthopedic d.
    Padgett hydraulic hand d.
    Smedley d.
    Spark handheld d.
DynaPak electrode kit
Dynaphor iontophoresis
DynaPulse 5000A ambulatory blood pressure monitor
Dynarad portable imaging system
Dynasplint
    D. knee extension unit
    D. shoulder system
DynaSurg electric handpiece
DynaTorq wrench
Dynatrak handpiece
Dynatron
    D. 50, 125, 525 electrotherapy
    D. Mini 2000 electrotherapy
    D. TX 900 electrotherapy
    D. 150 ultrasound
Dynatronics
    D. Model 1620 laser
DynaVox 2 communication device
DynaWell medical compression device
DynaWraps wrap
DyoBrite
    D. illuminator
    D. Xenon light source
DyoCam 550 arthroscopic video camera
Dyonics
    D. arthroplasty bur
    D. arthroscopic blade
    D. arthroscopic instrument
    D. basket forceps

D. Dyosite office arthroscopy system
D. full-radius resector
D. IntelliJet fluid management system
D. meniscotome
D. needle
D. PS3500 drive system
D. rod lens arthroscope

D. rod lens laparoscope
D. suction punch
D. syringe injector
DyoPneumatic insufflator
DyoVac suction punch
dysprosium-holmium (^{166}Dy-166Ho) in vivo generator
Dystrophile exercise unit

D

E

E Clips prescription computer lens
E wildcat orthodontic wire

E.

E. Benson Hood Laboratories
  esophageal tube
E. Benson Hood Laboratories
  salivary bypass tube

e10 electrosurgery system
E-2 foot prosthesis
Eagle

E. II survey spirometer
E. straight-ahead arthroscope

EaglePlug tapered-shaft punctum plug
EAGLE system
EagleVision Freeman punctum plug
Eakin cohesive seal dressing
E-A-R

E.-A.-R. Hi-Fi earplugs
E.-A.-R. LINK eartips
E.-A.-R. TONE earphones

ear

e. applicator
e. bougie
e. cannula
e. clip
e. cup
e. curette
e. dissector
e. forceps with suction
e. furuncle knife
e. hook
e. knife handle
e. loop
e. magnet
e. oximeter
e. pinna prosthesis
e. piston prosthesis
e. polyp forceps
e. polyp snare
e. probe
e. punch forceps
e. rasp
e. scissors
e. snare wire
e. snare wire carrier
e. speculum
e. spoon
e. syringe

EarCheck

E. monitor
E. Pro instrument

earclip

Satlite pulse oximeter with e.

ear-dressing forceps
ear-grasping forceps
Earle

E. hemorrhoidal clamp
E. rectal probe

Early Fit night splint

earphone

E-A-R TONE e.'s
intrameatal e.

EarPlanes silicone earplugs
earplugs

E-A-R Hi-Fi e.
EarPlanes silicone e.

earring

Brent pressure e.
compression e.
Glori pressure e.'s
pressure e.
pressure-producing e.

Earscope otoscope
eartips

E-A-R LINK e.

Ear-Tronics hearing aid
Easebak lumbar support cushion
Easi-Breathe inhaler
Easi-Lav gastric lavage
East-Grinstead

E.-G. needle
E.-G. scissors

Eastman

E. cystic duct forceps
E. dental cement
E. intestinal clamp
E. Kodak scanner
E. suction tube
E. vaginal retractor

Easton cock-up splint
East-West soft tissue retractor
Easy

E. Access foot splint
E. Analysis system
E. Introduction system
E. Lok ankle brace
E. Pivot patient lift
E. Rider neurovascular catheter
E. Sleeve
E. Up cushion

Easycath

MMG E.

EasyChair massage chair
**EasyGuide Neuro image-guided surgery
  system**
Easy-On elbow brace
EasyStep pressure relief walker
EASYTRAK coronary venous lead
eater

cement e.

Eaton

E. nasal speculum
E. trapezium finger joint
  replacement prosthesis

Eber

E. holder
E. needle-holder forceps

EBI

EBI bone healing system
EBI external fixator

E

EBI *(continued)*
>   EBI SPF-2 implantable bone
>   stimulator
>   EBI Temptek blanket

Eby
>   E. band driver
>   E. band setter

EC-5000 excimer laser
E.CAM
>   E.CAM dual-head emission imaging
>   system
>   E.CAM photon emission camera

E-cath catheter
eccentric
>   e. drill guide
>   e. dynamic compression plate
>   e. dynamic compression plating
>   E. Isotac tibial guide
>   E. locked rib shears
>   e. monocuspid tilting-disk prosthetic
>   valve
>   E. "Y" adjustable finger retractor

Eccocee
>   E. ultrasound
>   E. ultrasound system

EccoVision
>   E. acoustic pharyngometer
>   E. acoustic rhinometry system

ECG
>   Cardiovit AT-series ECG
>   KoKo Rhythm PC-Based ECG
>   Micro-Tracer portable ECG
>   MSC-2001 ECG
>   ECG triggering unit

ECG*stat*
>   PalmVue E.

Echlin
>   E. duckbill rongeur
>   E. laminectomy rongeur
>   E. rongeur forceps

echo
>   e. catheter
>   e. probe
>   e. transponder electrode catheter

echocardiograph
>   Biosound Surgiscan e.
>   Siemens Sonoline SL-2 e.
>   Ultramark 9 e.

echocardiographic probe
ECHOCHECK
Echo-Coat ultrasound biopsy needle
echocolonoscope
>   CF-UM3 e.
>   Olympus CF-UM3 flexible e.

echoduodenoscope
>   Olympus XJF-UM20 e.

echoendoscope
>   GF-UM30P linear-oriented radial
>   scanning e.
>   linear-type e.
>   mechanical longitudinal/sector
>   scanning e.
>   oblique-viewing e.
>   Olympus CF-UM-series e.

>   Olympus GF-series e.
>   Olympus GF-UM-series e.
>   Olympus GIF-EUM-series e.
>   Olympus GIF-series e.
>   Olympus GIF-1T10 e.
>   Olympus JF-UM20 e.
>   Olympus UM-series e.
>   Olympus VU-M-series e.
>   Olympus VU-series e.
>   Olympus XIF-series e.
>   Olympus XIF-UM-series e.
>   Pentax FG-36UX linear scanning e.
>   radial sector scanning e.

EchoEye ultrasound
EchoFlow blood velocity meter system
echogastroscope
echogenic needle
Echols retractor
EchoMark
>   E. angiographic catheter
>   E. salpingography catheter

echoplanar magnetic resonance imaging
echoprobe
>   Olympus XMP-U2 catheter e.

EchoScan
>   Nidek E.

echoscanner
Echosight
>   E. Jansen-Anderson intrauterine
>   catheter set
>   E. Patton coaxial catheter set

Echotip
>   E. Baker amniocentesis set
>   E. Dominion needle set
>   E. Kato-Asch needle set

Echovar Doppler system
Echowarm gel warmer
ECI automatic reprocessor
Eckardt
>   E. Heme-Stopper instrument
>   E. temporary keratoprosthesis

Ecker-Kazanjian forceps
Ecker-Roopenian chisel
Eckhoff forceps
Eclipse
>   E. Gel ankle brace
>   E. Gel elbow strap
>   E. holmium laser
>   E. infusion system
>   E. TENS unit
>   E. TMR laser

ECMO
>   extracorporeal membrane oxygenator
>   ECMO pump

EcoCheck oxygen monitor
Econo-Float Water flotation mattress
Econolith device
Econo-Strap
Econo 90 traction unit
Eco-Oxymax
E-cotton bandage
ECT
>   ECT internal fracture fixation
>   ECT pacemaker
>   ECT time test card

Ectocor pacemaker
ectopic
    e. atrial pacemaker
ECTRA carpal tunnel instruments
EDAP LT.1 lithotriptor
EDCS pain management device
Eddey parotid retractor
Edebohls kidney clamp
Edelstein scissors
edema sock
Edens dilation-tracheobronchoscope
EdenTec 2000W in-home
  cardiorespiratory monitor
Edentrace sleep system
Eder
    E. cord blood collection device
    E. esophagoscope
    E. forceps
    E. gastroscope
    E. insufflator
    E. laparoscope
    E. sigmoidoscope
Eder-Bernstein gastroscope
Eder-Chamberlin gastroscope
Eder-Cohn endoscope
Eder-Hufford
    E.-H. esophagoscope
    E.-H. gastroscope
Eder-Palmer
    E.-P. gastroscope
    E.-P. semiflexible fiberoptic
      endoscope
Eder-Puestow
    E.-P. esophageal dilator
    E.-P. guidewire
    E.-P. metal olive
EDGE
    E. coated needle electrode
Edge
    Acufex E.
    E. blade
    E. dilatation catheter
    E. III hydrogel contact lens
    E. knee brace
EdgeAhead
    E. crescent knife
    E. phaco slit knife
edge-detection
    digital e.-d.
EDG system
Edinburgh
    E. brain retractor
    E. suture
Edison fluoroscope
Edmark mitral valve
EDM infusion catheter
Edmonton extension tongs
Edna
    E. towel clamp
    E. towel forceps
Edslab
    E. cholangiography catheter
    E. jaw spring clip
    E. pressure gauge

EDTA-Vacutainer tube
Edwards
    E. diagnostic catheter
    E. D-L modular fixator
    E. double Softjaw clamp
    E. instrumentation
    E. modular system
    E. modular system compression
      construct
    E. modular system kyphoreduction
      construct
    E. modular system neutralization
      construct
    E. modular system rod crosslink
    E. modular system rod-sleeve
      construct
    E. modular system sacral fixation
      device
    E. modular system scoliosis
      construct
    E. modular system standard sleeve
      construct
    E. parallel-jaw spring clip
    E. raspatory
    E. rectal hook
    E. sacral screw
    E. seamless heart valve
    E. seamless prosthesis
    E. single Softjaw clamp
    E. spring clamp
    E. Teflon intracardiac implant
    E. Teflon intracardiac patch implant
      material
    E. Teflon intracardiac patch
      prosthesis
    E. Universal rod
    E. woven Teflon aortic bifurcation
      graft
Edwards-Barbaro T-shaped syringeal
  shunt
Edwards-Carpentier aortic valve brush
Edwards-Duromedics bileaflet heart valve
Edwards-Levine
    E.-L. hook
    E.-L. rod
    E.-L. sleeve
Edwards-Tapp arterial graft
Edwards-Verner raspatory
EDXRF spectrometer
EEA
    EEA Auto Suture
    EEA Auto Suture stapler
    EEA disposable loading unit
    EEA stapling device
EEG
    electroencephalograph
    EEG and PSG instrumentation
eel
    e. cobra tip
    e. wire
EF/EX
    MaxiFloat pressure reduction
      mattress model EF/EX
Effapoxy resin

E

Effenberger
    E. contractor
    E. retractor
Effler
    E. double-ended dissector
    E. tack
Effler-Groves
    E.-G. cardiovascular forceps
    E.-G. dissector
    E.-G. hook
Efica CC dynamic air therapy unit
Efos-Lite
Efteklar-Charnley hip prosthesis
Efteklar clamp
E-G alloy
Egemen keyhole suction-control device
eggcrate
    e. foam
    e. mattress
    e. positioner
    e. protector
Eggers
    E. bone plate
    E. contact splint
    E. screw
Eggsercizer resistive hand exerciser
Egnell
    E. breast pump
    E. uterine aspirator
    E. vacuum extractor
egress
    e. cannula
    e. needle
Ehmke
    E. ear prosthesis
    E. platinum Teflon implant
Ehrlich catheter
Eichelter-Schenk vena cava catheter
Eichen irrigating cannula
Eicher
    E. hip prosthesis
    E. rasp
    E. tri-fin chisel
EID percutaneous central venous large-bore catheter
EIE
    EIE 150F operating microscope
    EIE MiniEndo piezoelectric
        ultrasonic unit
Eigon
    E. CardioLoop recorder
    E. disk
Eiken-Kizai hemodialysis blood tubing set
Eindhoven magnet
Einhorn
    E. esophageal dilator
    E. tube
Einthoven string galvanometer
Eiselsberg ligature scissors
Eiselsberg-Mathieu needle holder
Eisenhammer speculum
Eisenstein
    E. clamp
    E. hysterectomy forceps

EJ bone marrow biopsy needle
ejector
    Cloward dowel e.
    Johnson & Johnson saliva e.
EK-19 pad
EKG
    EKG calipers
    Micro-Tracer portable EKG
Eklund breast positioning system
EL2-LS2 flexible video laparoscope
Ela
    E. Chorus DDD pacemaker
    E. Medical Elatec V 3.03A
        arrhythmia analyzer
    E. ventricular pacing lead
ELAD
    extracorporeal liver assist device
    ELAD cartridge
Elan
    E. drill
    E. electrosurgical unit
Elan-E
    E.-E. electronic motor system
    E.-E. power drill
Elastafit tubing kit
Elastalloy
    E. esophageal endoprosthesis
    E. esophageal stent
    E. Ultraflex Strecker nitinol stent
ElastaTrac
    E. home lumbar traction system
    E. home lumbar traction unit
elastic
    e. back strap
    e. bougie
    e. foam bandage
    maxillomandibular e.
    e. O ring
    e. plastic splint
    e. rubber band
    e. silicone membrane
    Spandage e.
    e. stable intramedullary nail
    e. stockings
    e. suspensor
    e. suture
elastic-hinge knee brace
Elastikon
    E. bandage
    E. elastic tape
    E. wristlet dressing
Elast-O-Chain separator
Elasto dressing
Elasto-Gel
    E.-G. hot/cold wrap
    E.-G. hydrogel sheet
    E.-G. hydrogel wound dressing
    E.-G. shoulder therapy wrap
Elasto-gel
    E.-g. cushions/pressure pads
Elasto-Link joint wrap
elastomer
    American Heyer-Schulte e.
    conventional silicone e.

e. shell
silicone e.
elastomeric pump
Elastomull
    E. bandage
    E. dressing
Elastoplast
    E. bandage
    E. dressing
    E. eye occlusor
Elastopore dressing
Elastorc catheter guidewire
Elastylon gloves
elbow
    e. extension splint
    e. flexion splint
    e. hinge
    e. magnet
    e. sleeve
elbowed
    e. bougie
    e. catheter
elbow-wrist-hand orthosis (EWHO)
Eldridge-Green lamp
Elecath
    E. circulatory support device
    E. ECMO cannula
    E. electrophysiologic stimulation catheter
    E. pacemaker
    E. switch box
    E. thermodilution catheter
ElecroLink TENS electrode
Electra 1000C coagulation analyzer
electric
    e. bed
    e. cabinet bath
    e. cardiac pacemaker
    e. dermatome
    e. drill
    e. generator
    e. laryngofissure saw
    e. nerve stimulator
    e. probe
    e. retinoscope
    e. syringe
    e. tissue morcellator
electrical
    e. brain stimulator
    e. implant
    e. resistance detector
    e. sector scanner
electricator
    e. coagulator
    e. electrosurgical unit
    National e.
Electri-Cool
    E.-C. cold therapy system
    E.-C. continuous controlled cold therapy
electroacupuncture device
Electro-Acuscope
    E.-A. scope
    E.-A. stimulator
Electro-Blend epilator

electrocardioanalyzer
electrocardiograph
    Arrhythmia Research 1200 EPX e.
    bioimpedance e.
    Cambridge e.
    CardioMatic e.
    MAC-VU e.
    Marquette e.
    Megarcart e.
    Mingograf 62 6-channel e.
    signal-averaged e.
electrocardiographic transtelephonic monitor
electrocardioscanner
electrocautery
    AmpErase e.
    Aspen e.
    bipolar e.
    Bovie e.
    Bugbee e.
    e. cautery
    Endo Clip monopolar e.
    Fine micropoint e.
    Geiger e.
    Hildreth e.
    Mentor Wet-Field e.
    Mira e.
    monopolar e.
    Mueller e.
    needlepoint e.
    Neomed e.
    ophthalmic e.
    Op-Temp disposable e.
    Parker-Heath e.
    Prince e.
    Rommel e.
    Rommel-Hildreth e.
    Schanz e.
    Scheie e.
    Todd e.
    Valleylab e.
    von Graefe e.
    Wadsworth-Todd e.
    wet-field e.
    Ziegler e.
electrochemical detector
electrocoagulating biopsy forceps
electrocoagulator
electrode
    abdominal patch e.
    ACMI biopsy loop e.
    ACMI monopolar e.
    ACMI retrograde e.
    AE-series implantable pronged unipolar e.
    air-spaced e.
    Alfa II e.
    All-In-One laparoscopic e.
    angled ball-end e.
    angle-tip e.
    anterior anodal patch e.
    antimony pH e.
    Arrowsmith e.
    Arruga surface e.
    Arzbacher pill e.

E

electrode *(continued)*
Arzco Tapsul pill e.
Aspen laparoscopic e.
atrial e.
ball e.
Ballenger follicle e.
e. balloon
Ball reusable e.
ball-tip coagulating e.
Bard e.
Bard-Hamm fulgurating e.
Bard nonsteerable bipolar e.
Baumrucker e.
bayonet-tip e.
Beaver tail-tip e.
Beckman stomach e.
Berens bident e.
Berkovits-Castellanos hexapolar e.
BICAP monopolar e.
BioKnit garment e.
Bioplus dispersive e.
biopotential skin e.
biopsy loop e.
BioTac ECG e.
bipolar depth e.
bipolar glass e.
bipolar myocardial e.
Birtcher e.
Bisping e.
biterminal e.
blade e.
Bovie conization e.
Bugbee fulgurating e.
Buie fulgurating e.
Burian-Allen contact lens e.
button e.
calomel e.
Cambridge jelly e.
Cameron-Miller e.
CapSure e.
CARE e.
Castroviejo surface e.
e. catheter
cautery e.
cautery knife e.
Cecar e.
central terminal e.
cerebellar e.
cervical conization e.
Cibis e.
Clark oxygen e.
coagulating e.
coagulation e.
Coaguloop resection e.
coil e.
Collings fulguration e.
Collings knife e.
Colorado MicroNeedle needle e.
combination needle e.
common pH e.
CO_2mmO_2n sensor transcutaneous gas e.
concentric needle e.
conical-tip e.

conization e.
Copeland fetal scalp e.
Cortac monitoring e.
cortical e.
coudé fulgurating e.
CPI Endotak transvenous e.
Cryomedics disposable LLETZ e.
Cueva cranial nerve e.
cuff e.
cuff-type inactive e.
cup-shaped e.
curved e.
cutaneous thoracic patch e.
cutting loop e.
cyclodiathermy e.
cystoscopic fulgurating e.
Darox cutaneous thoracic patch e.
Davis coagulation e.
Delgado e.
depolarizing e.
depth e.
Depthalon monitoring e.
diamond e.
diathermic retinal e.
diathermy e.
disk e.
dispersing e.
disposable surfaces EMG e.
disposable surgical e.
Dispos-a-trode disposable e.
Disposatrode disposable e.
Doyen e.
dual-lead e.
Dura-Stick adhesive e.
EDGE coated needle e.
ElecroLink TENS e.
Electro-Mesh e.
El-Naggar-Nashold right-angled nucleus caudalis DREZ e.
EMG e.
EnGuard PFX lead e.
ENT e.
epicardial sock e.
epidural peg e.
epilation e.
Eppendorf needle e.
equipotential e.
ESA acromioplasty e.
ESA hook e.
ESA Jet Stream ball e.
ESA meniscectomy e.
ESA Smillie e.
esophageal pill e.
EVAP roller e.
Excel Plus e.
exploring e.
external e.
eye diathermy e.
E-Z Clean laparoscopic e.
Fast-Patch disposable defibrillation/electrocardiographic e.
fetal scalp e.
fine-needle e.
fine-wire e.
flat spatula e.

flat-tip e.
flat-wire eye e.
flexible fulgurating e.
flexible radiothermal e.
flexible wire e.
follicle e.
fulgurating e.
Galloway e.
glass pH e.
e. glove
Goetz bipolar e.
Gradle needle e.
Grantham lobotomy e.
Greenwald Control Tip
  cystoscopic e.
Greenwald flexible endoscopic e.
Guyton e.
Haiman tonsillar e.
Hamm fulgurating e.
Hamm resectoscope e.
Hildreth e.
Hubbard e.
Hughes fulguration e.
Hurd bipolar diathermy e.
Hurd turbinate e.
Hymes-Timberlake e.
Iglesias e.
impedance e.
impregnated e.
inactive e.
indifferent e.
Innsbruck e.
intracerebral depth e.
intraluminal reference e.
intrameatal e.
intravascular catheter e.
Iomed Phoresor e.
ion-selective e.
iontophoresis e.
Jewett e.
J-loop e.
J orthogonal e.
Josephson quadpolar mapping e.
Kalk e.
Karaya e.
knife e.
Kontron e.
Kronfeld surface e.
LaCarrere e.
lancet-shaped e.
Lane ureteral meatotomy e.
large-loop e.
large-tip e.
Laserdish e.
Levin thermocouple cordotomy e.
Lifeline e.
Littmann ECG e.
LLETZ/LEEP loop e.
lobotomy e.
localizing e.
loop ball e.
loop-tipped e.
LSI silver self-adhesive
  disposable e.
Lynch e.

Mansfield Polaris e.
McCarthy coagulation e.
McCarthy diathermic knife e.
McCarthy fulgurating e.
McCarthy loop operating e.
McCarthy miniature loop e.
McWhinnie e.
meatotomy e.
Medelec DMG 50 Teflon-coated
  monopolar e.
Medi-Trace e.
Meditrode iontophoresis
  Transvene e.
MegaDyne arthroscopic hook e.
MegaDyne/Fann E-Z clean
  laparoscopic e.
metal e.
microcurrent e.
Microglass pH e.
midgastric e.
midoccipital e.
miniature loop e.
Moersch e.
monopolar temporary e.
multilead e.
multiple-point e.
Multi-Ply reusable e.
multipurpose ball e.
Myerson e.
myocardial e.
Myowire II cardiac e.
Nashold TC e.
National cautery e.
needle e.
Neil-Moore meatotomy e.
Neotrode II neonatal e.
Nesbit e.
neutral e.
New York Hospital e.
Nortech SLED e.
Nyboer esophageal e.
ophthalmic cautery e.
optically transparent e.
Osypka Cereblate e.
pacemaker e.
pacing wire e.
pad e.
e. pad
panendoscope e.
parallel-loop e.
pencil-tipped e.
percutaneous epidural e.
periaqueductal gray e.
PE-series implantable pronged
  unipolar e.
Pisces e.
Pischel e.
platinum blade meatotomy e.
platinum oxygen e.
PMT Cortac cortical e.
PMT Depthalon depth e.
point e.
pointed-tip e.
Polaris e.
polarographic needle e.

electrode *(continued)*
    Polystim e.
    Prizm Electro-Mesh Sock e.
    proctological ball e.
    proctoscopic fulguration e.
    prostatic aluminum e.
    punctate e.
    pyramidal e.
    QuadPolar e.
    Quinton Quik-Prep e.
    Ray rhizotomy e.
    Ray RRE-TM thermistor e.
    recording e.
    reference e.
    reimplanted e.
    REM PolyHesive II patient
      return e.
    renal sympathetic nerve activity
      recording e.
    Re-Ply TENS e.
    Resume e.
    retinal diathermy e.
    retrograde e.
    reusable laparoscopic e.
    Riba electrourethrotome e.
    right-angle e.
    ring e.
    Ringenberg e.
    rod e.
    roller e.
    roller-bar e.
    roller-barrel e.
    round-loop e.
    round-wire e.
    Rychener-Weve e.
    saturated calomel e.
    scalp e.
    scalpel e.
    Schepens surface e.
    screw-in epicardial e.
    screw-in sutureless myocardial e.
    semiflat tip e.
    Severinghaus e.
    sew-on e.
    Shank e.
    Shealy facet rhizotomy e.
    silver bead e.
    single-fiber EMG e.
    single-use e.
    single-wire e.
    Skylark surface e.
    Sluder cautery e.
    Sluder-Mehta e.
    small-loop e.
    Smith endoscopic e.
    e. sock
    Soderstrom-Corson e.
    Soft-EZ reusable e.
    Softrace gel e.
    Somatics monitoring e.
    Spencer probe depth e.
    spiral e.
    stab e.
    stab-in epicardial e.

    Stat-Trace e.
    Stern-McCarthy e.
    steroid eluting e.
    stick-on e.
    Stimitrode e.
    stimulating e.
    St. Mark pudendal e.
    Stockert cardiac pacing e.
    Storz cystoscopic e.
    Storz resectoscope e.
    straight-blade e.
    straight-needle e.
    straight-point e.
    straight-tip e.
    straight-wire e.
    subcutaneous patch e.
    subdural grid e.
    subdural strip e.
    surface e.
    surgical e.
    Surgicraft Copeland fetal scalp e.
    Surgicraft pacemaker e.
    sutured plaque e.
    sutureless pacemaker e.
    Tapcath esophageal e.
    Tapsul pill e.
    temporal e.
    temporary percutaneous SCS e.
    Teq-Trode e.
    terminal e.
    Thymapad stimulus e.
    Timberlake e.
    tined ventricular e.
    tissue desiccation needle e.
    tongue plate e.
    tonsillar e.
    Transvene tripolar e.
    transvenous e.
    trigeminal e.
    tripolar defibrillation coil e.
    turbinate e.
    Turner cystoscopic fulgurating e.
    ultrasonic e.
    Ultra Stim silver e.
    underwater e.
    unipolar glass e.
    ureteral meatotomy e.
    Uroloop e.
    USCI Goetz bipolar e.
    USCI NBIH bipolar e.
    USCI pacing e.
    vaginal aluminum e.
    Valleylab ball e.
    Valleylab loop e.
    VaporTome resection e.
    VaporTrode roller e.
    VPL thalamic e.
    Walker coagulating e.
    Walker ureteral meatotomy e.
    Wappler e.
    Weve e.
    Williams tonsillar e.
    Wilson-Cook coagulation e.
    Wolfe loop e.
    Wolfram needle e.

wraparound inactive e.
Wyler subdural strip e.
Ziegler cautery e.
zinc ball e.
Zuker bipolar pacing e.
Zywiec e.

electrodermatome
Brown e.
Hood e.
Padgett e.
e. sterile blade

Electrodes
E. ball
E. loop
E. needle
E. scalpel

electro-detachable balloon
electro-detachable platinum coil
electrodiaphake
LaCarrere e.

Electrodyne pacemaker
electroejaculator
G&S e.

electroencephalograph (EEG)
biofeedback e.
BMSI 5000 e.
Galileo evoked potential e.
Grass e.
Mingograf e.

electrogoniometer
six-degrees-of-freedom e.

electrograph
Cardiotest portable e.

electrogustometer
Nagashima e.

electrohemostasis catheter
electrohydraulic
e. lithotripsy probe
e. lithotriptor
e. lithotriptor probe

electrokeratotome
Castroviejo e.

Electro-Link joint wrap
electrolysis
electromagnet
spring-mounted e.
structured coil e.

electromagnetic
e. flow meter
e. flowmeter
e. flow probe
e. flow transducer
e. focusing field probe
e. lithotriptor

electromechanical
e. artificial heart
e. dynamometer
e. impactor
e. morcellator
e. slope computer

Electro-Mesh
E.-M. electrode
E.-M. sleeve

electromucotome
Castroviejo e.

Steinhauser e.
Steinhauser-Castroviejo e.

electromyogram (EMG)
e. sensor

electromyograph (EMG)
Counterpoint e.

electromyography
integrated e.

electromyometer
biofeedback e.

electron
e. beam CT scanner
e. capture detector
e. gun
e. linear accelerator
e. microscope
e. microscopy
e. multiplier tube
e. probe x-ray microanalyzer

electronic
e. artificial larynx
e. calipers
e. endoscope
e. goniometer
e. infusion device
e. knife
e. microanalyzer
e. muscle stimulator
e. pacemaker
e. stethoscope
e. summation device
e. voltmeter

electronic-amplified stethoscope
Electronics electrical stimulation device
electronystagmogram (ENG)
Nystar Plus e.

electronystagmograph (ENG)
Elmed-Toennis system e.
Nagashima e.
TAR-200 dual-channel e.

electro-oculogram apparatus
electrooculograph
electroperimeter
Electrorelaxor TENS unit
electroretinogram
electroretinograph
Ganzfeld e.

electroscope
Bruening e.
E. disposable scissors

electroshield
E. cylindrical conductive shield
e. monitoring system
E. reusable sheath

electrostatic generator
Electrosurgery
E. forceps
E. snare

electrosurgical
e. biopsy forceps
e. curved scissors
e. filter
e. generator
e. monopolar spatula probe
e. needle

E

electrosurgical *(continued)*
    e. pencil
    e. scalpel
    e. spatula
    e. unit (ESU)
electrotherapy
    Dynatron 50, 125, 525 e.
    Dynatron Mini 2000 e.
    Dynatron TX 900 e.
    Mettler e.
    e. system
electrotome
    McCarthy infant e.
    McCarthy miniature e.
    McCarthy punctate e.
    Nesbit e.
    Stern-McCarthy e.
    Timberlake obturator e.
Elekta
    E. stereotactic head frame
    E. viewing wand
Elektrotom BiCut II coagulator
Elema pacemaker
Elema-Schonander pacemaker
Elema-Siemens AB pressure transducer
element
    Mira encircling e.
elephant cuff
elevated rim acetabular liner
Elevath pacemaker
elevating forceps
elevator
    Abbott e.
    Abraham e.
    Adson-Love periosteal e.
    Adson periosteal e.
    Alexander e.
    Alexander-Farabeuf e.
    Allerdyce e.
    Allis periosteal e.
    amalgam plugger e.
    Amerson bone e.
    Anderson e.
    angular e.
    Anthony e.
    Apexo e.
    Arenberg dural palpator e.
    Artmann e.
    Ashley cleft palate e.
    Aufranc periosteal e.
    Aufricht e.
    Austin duckbill e.
    Austin footplate e.
    Austin right-angle e.
    ball-end e.
    Ballenger-Hajek e.
    Ballenger septal e.
    Barsky e.
    Batson-Carmody e.
    Behrend periosteal e.
    Bellucci e.
    Bennett bone e.
    Berry-Lambert periosteal e.
    Bethune periosteal e.

Blair cleft palate e.
blunt e.
Boies nasal fracture e.
bone e.
Bowen periosteal e.
Boyle uterine e.
Bristow periosteal e.
Brophy periosteal e.
Brophy tooth e.
Brown tooth e.
Buck periosteal e.
Cameron e.
Cameron-Haight periosteal e.
Cameron periosteal e.
Campbell periosteal e.
Cannon-Rochester lamina e.
Carmody-Batson e.
Carroll-Legg periosteal e.
Carroll periosteal e.
Carter submucous e.
Chandler bone e.
Cheyne periosteal e.
chisel e.
Cinelli periosteal e.
cleft palate e.
clinic exolever e.
Cloward osteophyte e.
Cloward periosteal e.
Cobb periosteal e.
Cobb spinal e.
Cohen periosteal e.
combined wire guide bone e.
Converse alar e.
Converse-MacKenty periosteal e.
Converse periosteal e.
Cooper spinal fusion e.
Cordes-New laryngeal punch e.
Coryllos-Doyen periosteal e.
Coryllos periosteal e.
costal periosteal e.
Cottle alar e.
Cottle-MacKenty e.
Cottle nasal e.
Cottle periosteal e.
Cottle septal e.
Cottle skin e.
Coupland e.
Crane e.
Crawford dural e.
Crego periosteal e.
Cronin cleft palate e.
Cronin palate e.
Cryer dental e.
Cryer root e.
Cushing-Hopkins periosteal e.
Cushing little joker e.
Cushing periosteal e.
Cushing pituitary e.
Cushing staphylorrhaphy e.
Davidson-Mathieu-Alexander
  periosteal e.
Davidson periosteal e.
Davidson-Sauerbruch-Doyen
  periosteal e.
Davis periosteal e.

Dawson-Yuhl-Key e.
Dawson-Yuhl periosteal e.
Dean periosteal e.
Derlacki duckbill e.
dermal e.
D'Errico periosteal e.
Desmarres lid e.
Dewar e.
Dingman periosteal e.
Dingman zygoma e.
double club e.
Doyen costal e.
Doyen periosteal e.
Doyen rib e.
duckbill e.
Dunning e.
dural e.
Ellik e.
endaural e.
Endotrac e.
ESI lighted suction e.
Farabeuf periosteal e.
Farrior-Shambaugh e.
Fay suction e.
Federspiel periosteal e.
Fibre-Lite septal e.
file e.
Fiske periosteal e.
Fomon nostril e.
Fomon periosteal e.
footplate e.
fracture reducing e.
Frazier dural e.
Frazier suction e.
Freer double-end e.
Freer periosteal e.
Freer septal e.
Friedman e.
Friedrich rib e.
Gam-Mer periosteal e.
Gillies zygoma e.
Goldman septal e.
Goodwillie periosteal e.
Gorney septal suction e.
Graham scalene e.
Guilford-Wright drum e.
Guilford-Wright duckbill e.
Haberman suction e.
Hajek e.
Hajek-Ballenger septal e.
Halle septal e.
Hamrick suction e.
Hargis periosteal e.
Harper periosteal e.
Harrington spinal e.
Hatt golf-stick e.
Hayden palate e.
Hedblom costal e.
Henahan e.
Henner endaural e.
Herczel periosteal e.
Herczel raspatory e.
Herczel rib e.
Hibbs chisel e.
Hibbs costal e.

Hibbs periosteal e.
Hoen periosteal e.
Hopkins-Cushing periosteal e.
Horsley e.
Hough spatula e.
House ear e.
House endaural e.
House stapes e.
House Teflon-coated e.
Howorth e.
Hu-Friedy e.
Hulka-Kenwick uterine e.
Hurd septal e.
Iowa University periosteal e.
Jackson perichondrial e.
Jacobson counter-pressure e.
Jannetta angular e.
Jannetta duckbill e.
Jarit periosteal e.
joker e.
Jordan canal e.
Jordan-Rosen e.
Joseph-Killian septal e.
Joseph nasal e.
Joseph periosteal e.
J-periosteal e.
Kahre-Williger periosteal e.
Kartush stimulus dissection e.
Kennerdell-Maroon duckbill e.
Key periosteal e.
Killian septal e.
Kilner e.
Kinsella periosteal e.
Kirmisson periosteal e.
Kleesattel e.
Kleinert-Kutz e.
Kocher periosteal e.
Koenig e.
Kos e.
Krego e.
Ladd e.
Lambotte e.
laminar e.
Lamont e.
Lane periosteal e.
Lange bone e.
Langenbeck periosteal e.
Lee-Cohen septal e.
Lemmon sternal e.
lemon-squeezer obstetrical e.
Lempert heavy e.
Lempert narrow e.
Lempert periosteal e.
Lewin e.
Lewis periosteal e.
Lindholm-Stille e.
Logan periosteal e.
Louisville e.
Love-Adson periosteal e.
Lowis periosteal e.
L-shaped e.
lumbosacral fusion e.
Luongo septal e.
MacDonald periosteal e.
MacKenty-Converse periosteal e.

E

elevator *(continued)*
    MacKenty periosteal e.
    MacKenty septal e.
    Magielski e.
    Malis e.
    Matson-Alexander rib e.
    Matson rib e.
    McClamary e.
    McCollough e.
    McGee canal e.
    McGlamry e.
    McIndoe e.
    Mead periosteal e.
    Melt e.
    MGH periosteal e.
    Miller-Apexo e.
    Miller dental e.
    Molt No. 4 e.
    Molt periosteal e.
    Monks malar e.
    Moore bone e.
    Moorehead e.
    mucosal e.
    Murphy-Lane bone e.
    narrow e.
    Netterville double-ended e.
    Neurological Institute periosteal e.
    Norcross periosteal e.
    Nordent oral surgery e.
    Norrbacka bone e.
    Ohl periosteal e.
    Oldberg e.
    orthopedic e.
    OSI extremity e.
    osteophyte e.
    Overholt periosteal e.
    Pace periosteal e.
    palatorrhaphy e.
    Paparella duckbill e.
    Pennington septal e.
    periosteal e.
    Perkins e.
    Phemister raspatory e.
    Pierce e.
    Polcyn e.
    Pollock-Dingman e.
    Pollock sweetheart periosteal e.
    Pollock zygoma e.
    Poppen periosteal e.
    Potts dental e.
    Presbyterian Hospital
      staphylorrhaphy e.
    Pritchard e.
    Proctor mucosal e.
    Quervain e.
    Ramirez periosteal e.
    Raney periosteal e.
    Ray-Parsons-Sunday
      staphylorrhaphy e.
    Read periosteal e.
    Rhoton e.
    Richards-Cobb spinal e.
    Richardson periosteal e.
    right-angle e.

    Rissler periosteal e.
    Roberts-Gill periosteal e.
    Rochester lamina e.
    Rochester spinal e.
    Roger septal e.
    Rolyan arm e.
    Rosen angular e.
    round-tipped periosteal e.
    Rowe bone e.
    Rubin-Lewis periosteal e.
    Rudderman "Frelevator" fragment e.
    Sabbatsberg septum e.
    Sauerbruch-Frey rib e.
    Sauerbruch rib e.
    Sayre double-end periosteal e.
    Scheer knife e.
    Schuknecht e.
    Scott-McCracken periosteal e.
    Sebileau periosteal e.
    Sédillot periosteal e.
    Seldin e.
    septal e.
    Sewall ethmoidal e.
    Sewall mucoperiosteal e.
    Shambaugh-Derlacki duckbill e.
    Shambaugh narrow e.
    Shea e.
    Silverstein dural e.
    Sisson fracture-reducing e.
    skin e.
    skull e.
    SMIC periosteal e.
    Smith-Petersen e.
    Sokolec e.
    Somer uterine e.
    Soonawalla uterine e.
    Spurling periosteal e.
    stapes e.
    staphylorrhaphy e.
    Steele periosteal e.
    Stille-Langenbeck e.
    Stille periosteal e.
    Stolte-Stille e.
    Story orbital e.
    straight inclined plane e.
    straight periosteal e.
    suction e.
    Sunday staphylorrhaphy e.
    Suraci zygoma hook e.
    Swanson e.
    Tabb ear e.
    Tarlov nerve e.
    Tenzel double-end periosteal e.
    Tessier e.
    T-handle e.
    Tobolsky e.
    Traquair periosteal e.
    Tronzo e.
    Turner cord e.
    Turner periosteal e.
    Urquhart periosteal e.
    uterine e.
    von Langenbeck periosteal e.
    Wadia e.
    Walker submucous e.

Ward periosteal e.
Warwick James e.
Watson-Jones e.
West blunt e.
Willauer-Gibbon periosteal e.
Williger e.
Winter e.
Woodson dental periosteal e.
Wright-Guilford drum e.
Wurzelheber dental e.
zygoma e.

El Gamal
E. G. cardiac device
E. G. coronary bypass catheter
E. G. guiding catheter

Elgiloy
E. clip
E. clip material
E. frame
E. lead-tip pacemaker

Elgiloy-Heifitz aneurysm clip
Elias lid retractor
Eliasoph lid retractor
Eligoy metal alloy
Eliminator
E. biliary stent
E. dilatation balloon
E. nasal biliary catheter set
E. pancreatic stent
E. PET biliary balloon dilator
E. stone extraction basket

Elite
E. dual-chamber rate-responsive
pacemaker
E. Farley retractor
E. Farley retractor for spinal
surgery
E. guide catheter
E. hip system
E. knee brace
E. posterior adjustable stop
E. posterior spring assist
E. System rotating resectoscope

Ellik
E. bladder evacuator
E. elevator
E. kidney stone basket
E. loop stone dislodger
E. meatotome
E. resectoscope
E. sound

Ellik-Shaw obturator
Elliot
E. corneal trephine
E. femoral condyle holder
E. knee plate
E. trephine handle

Elliott
E. blade plate
E. gallbladder forceps
E. hemostatic forceps
E. obstetrical forceps

Ellipse compact spacer
ellipsometer
retinal e.

Ellis
E. buttress plate
E. foreign body needle
E. foreign body spud
E. foreign body spud needle probe
E. foreign body spud probe
E. needle holder

Ellison
E. fixation staple
E. glenoid rim punch

Ellman
E. press-form system
E. rotary scaler

Ellsner gastroscope
Elmar artificial kidney
Elmed
E. BC 50 M/M digital bipolar
coagulator
E. Bi-Pol cutter
E. diagnostic laparoscope
E. hysteroscope
E. operating laparoscope
E. peristaltic irrigation pump

Elmed-Toennis system
electronystagmograph
ELMISKOP 101 electron microscope
Elmore tissue morcellator
El-Naggar-Nashold right-angled nucleus
caudalis DREZ electrode
ELP
ELP femoral prosthesis
ELP stem for hip arthroplasty

Elsberg
E. brain-exploring cannula
E. ventricular cannula

Elschnig
E. capsular forceps
E. cataract knife
E. cataract spoon
E. corneal knife
E. cyclodialysis forceps
E. cyclodialysis spatula
E. extrusion needle
E. eye spoon
E. fixation forceps
E. lens scoop
E. lens spoon
E. lid retractor
E. pterygium knife
E. refractor
E. secondary membrane forceps
E. tissue-grasping forceps
E. trephine

Elschnig-O'Brien
E.-O. fixation forceps
E.-O. tissue-grasping forceps

Elschnig-O'Connor fixation forceps
Elschnig-Weber
E.-W. loop
E.-W. loupe

Elscint
E. dual-detector cardiac camera
E. ESI-3000 ultrasound
E. Excel 905 scanner
E. MR scanner

E

Elscint *(continued)*
    E. Planar device
    E. tomography system
    E. Twin CT scanner
Elsie-Brown otoabrader
Elta
    E. Dermal hydrogel dressing
    E. derma sterile impregnated
      hydrogel gauze pad
eluting stent
E-Mac laryngoscope blade
Embarc bone repair material
embolectomy
    e. catheter
    e. curette
embolization
    e. coil
    Silastic bead e.
Embolyx liquid embolic system
Embosphere microsphere
Embryon GIFT transfer catheter set
embryotome
    obstetrical decapitating e.
Emcee lens
EMED
    EMED insole
    EMED scanner
EMED-SF pedobarograph
Emerald implantation system
Emergence Profile implant system
emergency
    e. infusion device
    e. life support system
    e. oxygen mask assembly
Emerson
    E. bronchoscope
    E. cuirass respirator
    E. postoperative ventilator
    E. pump
    E. vein stripper
**Emerson-Birtheez abdominal
  decompressor**
**Emerson-Segal Medimizer demand
  nebulizer**
Emery lens
Emesay suture button
Emesco handpiece
EMG
    electromyogram
    electromyograph
    EMG electrode
    MyoTRac EMG
    Nicolet Viking Iie EMG
    Nomad-LE EMG
    Nordotrack motion EMG
    EMG stimulator
EMHI galvanic electrode stimulator
EMI
    EMI APED amplifier discriminator
    EMI 9813B photomultiplier
    EMI CT scanner
    EMI FACT 50 MK III cooler
    EMI unit
Emiks heart valve

Emir
    E. razor
    E. razor blade
emission spectrometric detector
emitter
    alpha-particle e.
    Auger-electron e.
    gamma e.
    light e.
Emmet
    E. hemostatic bag
    E. needle
    E. obstetrical forceps
    E. obstetrical retractor
    E. ovarian trocar
    E. tenaculum hook
    E. uterine probe
    E. uterine scissors
Emmet-Gellhorn pessary
Emmet-Murphy needle
Emmett cervical tenaculum
Emory EndoPlastic retractor
Empac-Cavitron I&A unit
EMPI Neuropacer TENS unit
Empire needle
EMS
    EMS 2000 neuromuscular stimulator
EnAbl thermal ablation system
ENAC
    ENAC II
    ENAC ultrasonic instrument system
enamel rod
Encapsulon
    E. epidural catheter
    E. sheath introducer
    E. TFX-Medical bacterial filter
    E. vessel dilator
encased screw
en chemise catheter
encircling
    e. band
    e. clip
enclosure
    air-flow e.
Encore
    E. ceramic hip and knee joint
      replacement systems
    E. microptic powder-free latex
      surgical glove
Encor pacemaker
endarterectomy
    e. dissector
    e. scissors
    e. spatula
endaural
    e. curette
    e. elevator
    e. retractor
    e. speculum
    e. surgery chisel
end-biting
    e.-b. blunt-nosed rongeur
    e.-b. forceps

end-cutting
 e.-c. fissure bur
 e.-c. reamer
Endeavor nondetachable silicone balloon catheter
end-end stapler
Ender
 E. nail
 E. pin
 E. rod
Endermologie
 E. adipose destruction system
 E. noninvasive body contouring device
ENDEX apex sensor
end-fire transrectal probe
End-Flo laparoscopic irrigating system
end-hole
 e.-h. balloon-tipped catheter
 e.-h. fluid-filled catheter
 e.-h. French catheter
 e.-h. pigtail catheter
 e.-h. ureteral catheter
Endius
 E. spinal camera
 E. spinal endoscope
Endless Pool physical therapy pool
Endo
 E. Babcock grasper
 E. Babcock stapler
 E. button
 E. Clip applier
 E. Clip ML/Surgiport System pack
 E. Clip monopolar electrocautery
 E. Dissect
 E. Dissect dissector
 E. GIA stapler
 E. GIA surgical clip
 E. Grasp
 E. Hernia stapler
 E. hinged knee prosthesis
 E. Knot suture
 E. Multi-Mode stimulator
 E. Optics MicroProbe
 E. pants
 E. rotating knee joint prosthesis
 E. Shears
 E. sled prosthesis
 E. Stitch
 E. Stitch instrument
 E. stop
 E. Tip port system
 E. Tip Stortz trocar
 E. zoom lens camera
endoanal
 e. coil
 e. ultrasound
endoaortic clamp
Endo-Assist
 E.-A. cutting dissector
 E.-A. disposable needle holder
 E.-A. endoscopic forceps
 E.-A. endoscopic knot pusher
 E.-A. endoscopic ligature carrier
 E.-A. endoscopic needle holder

 E.-A. retractable blade
 E.-A. retractable scalpel
 E.-A. sponge aspirator
Endo-Avitene
 E.-A. collagen hemostatic material
 E.-A. microfibrillar collagen hemostat
Endo Babcock surgical grasping device
Endobag
 E. laparoscopic specimen retrieval system
 E. specimen bag
Endo-Bender bending device
endobiliary stent
EndoBlade
 LaserSonics E.
endobrachial double-lumen tube
endobronchial tube
Endocam
 E. digital camera
 E. endoscope
 E. video camera system
endocamera
 Olympus e.
 Polaroid instant e.
endocapsular
 e. artificial lens intraocular lens
 e. balloon
endocardial
 e. balloon lead
 e. bipolar pacemaker
 e. cardiac lead
 e. screw
 e. wire
endocardiographic amplifier
EndoCatch
 E. II device
endocavitary
 e. applicator system
 e. probe
Endocavity V33W probe
Endocell
 E. endometrial cell collector
 E. endometrial cell sampler
endocervical
 e. aspirator
 e. biopsy curette
 e. probe
endocervicometer scope
endochondral bone
Endoclose suture carrier
endocoagulator
EndoCoil
 E. biliary stent
 E. esophageal stent
EndoCPB catheter
Endodermologie LPG system
endodiathermy
endodontic
 e. broach
 e. bur
 e. curette
 e. endosteal implant
 e. file
 e. pin

E

endodontic *(continued)*
   e. plugger
   e. reamer
EndoDynamics
   E. AdzorbStar
   E. glutameter
   E. suction polyp trap
endoesophageal
   e. MRI coil
   e. stent
   e. tube
EndoFix absorbable interference screw
Endoflex
   E. endoscopic instrument system
   E. endoscopic retractor
   E. endoscopy instrument
   Nucleotome E.
Endo-Flo irrigator
endograft
   Prograft Exluder bifurcated e.
   Talent bifurcated e.
   Vanguard e.
EndoGrasp device
Endo-grasper
   Babcock E.-g.
Endo-Gripper endodontic handpiece
endo-illuminator
   Grieshaber e.-i.
endo-irrigator
Endo-Lase CO$_2$ laser
endolaser
   diode e.
   e. probe
Endolav
   Meditron EL-100 E.
EndoLift device
EndoLive 3-D stereo video endoscope
Endoloop
   E. chromic ligature suture
     instrument
   E. suture
EndoLumina illuminated bougie
endoluminal stent
endolymphatic shunt tube introducer
endolymphatic-subarachnoid shunt
EndoMate grab bag
EndoMax
   E. advanced laparoscopic instrument
   E. endoscope
   E. endoscopic instrumentation
EndoMed LSS laparoscopy system
endometrial
   e. ablator
   e. aspirator
   e. cannula
   e. curette
   e. polyp forceps
endonerve stripper
EndoNet
   Pentax E.
EndoOctopus
endo-osseous dental implant
endo-otoprobe
   Gherini-Kauffman e.-o.

   HGM E.-o.
   Maloney e.-o.
EndoPaddle
Endopap endometrial sampler
Endopath
   E. disposable surgical trocar
   E. ELC35 endoscopic linear cutter
   E. EMS hernia stapler
   E. endoscopic articulating stapler
   E. ES endoscopic stapler
   E. ETS-FLEX endoscopic
     articulating linear cutter
   E. EZ-RF linear cutter and
     coagulation device
   E. EZ-series endoscopic linear
     cutter
   E. laparoscopic trocar
   E. linear cutter
   E. needle tip electrosurgery probe
   E. Optiview laparoscopic obturator
   E. Optiview system
   E. Stealth stapler
   E. TriStar trocar
   E. Ultra Veress needle
Endopearl
   E. bioabsorbable device
Endo-Pool suction cannula
Endopore
   E. dental implant system
   E. implant
Endo-Port
Endopost
   Kerr E.
Endopouch Pro specimen-retrieval bag
Endo-P-Probe
   E.-P.-P. endorectal probe
endoprosthesis
   acetabular e.
   Atkinson e.
   Austin Moore curved e.
   Austin Moore straight-stem e.
   Averett total hip e.
   Bateman UPF II bipolar e.
   biliary e.
   Bio-Moore e.
   Celestin e.
   Centrax bipolar e.
   crutched stick-type polyurethane e.
   cuffed esophageal e.
   double-lumen e.
   double-pigtail e.
   DoubleStent biliary e.
   Elastalloy esophageal e.
   expandable biliary e.
   expandable metal mesh e.
   femoral e.
   IntraStent DoubleStent biliary e.
   IntraStent DoubleStrut biliary e.
   large-bore bile duct e.
   Leinbach head and neck e.
   Matchett-Brown hip e.
   metatarsophalangeal e.
   nonporous-coated e.
   pancreatic e.
   Passager e.

pigtail e.
plastic e.
Proctor-Livingston e.
Ring-Derlan TM biliary e.
Schneider Wallstent biliary e.
self-expandable stainless steel
  braided e.
self-expanding metallic e.
self-expanding Wallstent e.
smooth e.
Thompson e.
tibial e.
Titan e.
transpapillary endoscopic e.
tumor-replacement e.
Unitrax modular e.
Wallgraft e.
Wallstent biliary e.
Wilson-Cook e.
endoprosthetic flange
**Endoprothetik CSL-Plus cemented-hip
  system**
endorectal
  e. coil
  e. surface-coil MR imaging
endorectal-pelvic phased-array coil
EndoRetract retractor
Endosac specimen bag
Endosample endometrial sampling device
EndoSaph vein harvest system
endo-scissors
  rotating e.-s.
endoscope
  AccuSharp e.
  ACMI e.
  Agee e.
  battery-powered e.
  cap-fitted e.
  Cho/Dyonics two-portal e.
  Cho two-portal Dyonics e.
  Cilco ophthalmic e.
  Circon-ACMI e.
  disk e.
  Dohlman e.
  double-channel e.
  Durascope e.
  Eder-Cohn e.
  Eder-Palmer semiflexible
    fiberoptic e.
  electronic e.
  Endius spinal e.
  Endocam e.
  EndoLive 3-D stereo video e.
  EndoMax e.
  end-viewing e.
  ETB e.
  EUM-series e.
  EVIS EXERA e.
  EVIS "Q" series e.
  FG-series two-channel e.
  fiberoptic e.
  flexible fallopian tube e.
  Foroblique e.
  forward-viewing e.
  French-McCarthy e.

Fujinon EG-FP-series e.
Fujinon EG-series e.
Fujinon EVE-series e.
Fujinon EVG-CT-series e.
Fujinon EVG-FP-series e.
Fujinon EVG-F-series e.
Fujinon EVG-series e.
Fujinon FP-series e.
Fujinon UGI-FP-series video e.
Gaab e.
GIF-HM e.
GIF-N-series fiberoptic pediatric e.
GIF-XP-series e.
GIF-XQ-series e.
Hamou e.
Haslinger e.
Jarit Rotator e.
JFB III e.
J-shaped e.
Karl Storz Calcutript e.
Karl Storz flexible e.
Kelly e.
Kuda e.
large-channel e.
Lowsley-Peterson e.
lung imaging fluorescence e.
Machida flexible e.
magnetic resonance e.
McCarthy e.
Messerklinger e.
MicroLap e.
mother-baby e.
mother-daughter e.
Navigator flexible e.
near-infrared electronic e.
Needlescoper e.
nonrigid e.
oblique-viewing e.
Olympus CF-UM20 ultrasonic e.
Olympus CV-series e.
Olympus EU-series e.
Olympus EUS-series e.
Olympus EVIS Q-series e.
Olympus EVIS-series e.
Olympus forward-viewing e.
Olympus GF-UM-series e.
Olympus GIF-HM-series e.
Olympus GIF-J-series e.
Olympus GIFK-XQ-series e.
Olympus GIF-Q-series e.
Olympus GIF-T-series e.
Olympus GIF-XP-series e.
Olympus GIF-XV-series e.
Olympus JF-T-series e.
Olympus JF-TV-series e.
Olympus JF-V-series e.
Olympus N-series ultrathin e.
Olympus PJF-series pediatric e.
Olympus P-series e.
Olympus Q-series e.
Olympus side-viewing e.
Olympus SIF 100 video push e.
Olympus TJF-series e.
Olympus UM-series e.
Olympus V-series e.

E

endoscope *(continued)*
    Olympus VU-M2 e.
    Olympus XCF-series e.
    Olympus XCF-XK-series e.
    Olympus XK-10 e.
    Olympus XP-series e.
    Olympus XQ-series e.
    Ono loupe for e.
    ophthalmic e.
    oral e.
    Padgett e.
    pediatric e.
    Pentax EC-series video e.
    Pentax EG-series video e.
    Pentax EndoNet digital e.
    Pentax FD-series video e.
    Pentax FG-series ultrasound e.
    Pentax FG-series video e.
    Pentax flexible e.
    Pentax side-viewing e.
    percutaneous spinal e.
    rigid e.
    rigid intranasal e.
    Rockey e.
    Satellite ear e.
    semiflexible e.
    semirigid e.
    Sensatec e.
    side-viewing e.
    Simpson e.
    Sine-U-View nasal e.
    Storz Sine-U-View e.
    stylet-scope e.
    Surgenomic e.
    TJF e.
    TJF-100 Olympus e.
    Toshiba video e.
    transpapillary e.
    TroCam e.
    UGI e.
    velolaryngeal e.
    Visicath e.
    Weerda e.
    Welch Allyn video e.
    Wolf e.
    Zeiss Endolive e.
endoscope/camera
endoscopic
    e. access port
    e. Babcock grasper
    e. band ligator
    e. BICAP probe
    e. biopsy forceps
    e. carpal tunnel release system
    e. color Doppler ultrasonography
    e. dissector
    e. electrode handle
    e. flowprobe
    e. grasping forceps
    e. heat probe
    e. hemoclip device
    e. irrigator
    e. linear cutter
    e. quadrature radiofrequency coil

    e. retrograde cholangiopancreatogram (ERCP)
    e. retrograde cholangiopancreatography catheter
    e. scissors
    e. sewing machine
    e. suture-cutting forceps
    e. telescope
    e. threaded imaging port
    e. ultrasonography
    e. washing pipe
endoscopically deliverable tissue-transfixing device
Endo-Set
    Haag-Streit E.-S.
EndoSheath
    E. endoscopy system
    Slide-On E.
    Vision System E.
EndoShield
    E. mask
    E. mask and goggles
endoskeleton
    stationary ankle flexible e.
Endo-Sock specimen retrieval bag
Endosoft reinforced cuffed tube
EndoSonics
    E. balloon dilatation catheter
    E. IVUS/balloon dilatation catheter
endosonography instrument
endosonoprobe
EndoSound
    E. endoscopic ultrasound
    E. ultrasound probe
endospeculum
    e. forceps
    Kogan e.
endosseous
    e. HA implant
    e. hydroxyapatite implant
Endostapler
EndoStasis probe
Endostat
    E. calibration pod insert
    disposable coaxial E.
    disposable sculptured E.
    E. disposable sterile fiber
    E. fiber stripper
    E. II bipolar/monopolar electrosurgical generator
EndoStitch laparoscopic suturing device
Endo-Suction sinus microstat set
Endotak
    E. C lead catheter
    E. C transvenous lead
    E. C tripolar pacing/sensing/defibrillation lead
    E. DSP lead
    E. lead system
    E. nonthoracotomy implantable cardioverter-defibrillator
    E. Picotip
Endotec spreader
Endotek
    E. machine

E. OM-3 Urodata monitor
E. UDS-1000 monitor
E. urodynamics system
endothelial specular microscope
endothelin-1 platinum-Dacron microcoil
Endo-therapy disposable biopsy forceps
EndoTIP
EndoTIP imaging port
Endotorque
Geenan E.
Endotrac
E. blade system
E. cannula
E. elevator
E. endoscopic carpal tunnel release
system
E. endoscopy instrument
E. obturator
E. probe
E. rasp
E. retractor
endotracheal
e. cardiac output monitor
e. catheter
e. catheter forceps
e. curette
e. tube
e. tube brush
e. tube cuff
e. tube forceps
endotriptor stone-crushing basket
Endotrol endotracheal tube
Endotron-Lipectron ultrasonic scalpel
Endo-Tube nasal jejunal feeding tube
endovaginal
e. coil
e. transducer
endovascular
e. cardiopulmonary bypass
e. coil
e. stent
Endovations disposable cytology brush
EndoVideo-Five endoscopic camera
EndoView camera
Endowel
EndoWrist instruments
EndoZime sponge
endplate
bony e.
end plate
Endur
E. bonding material
E. resin
Endura dressing forceps
Endurance bone cement
EnduraSplint splint
Enduron acetabular liner
end-viewing
e.-v. endoscope
e.-v. gastroscope
end-Z file
Enemette enema cleansing kit
Energy Plus shoe insert
Enertrax pacemaker

Enforcer
CVD Focustent E.
ENG
electronystagmogram
electronystagmograph
Engelmann thigh splint
Engel-May nail
Engel plaster saw
Engen
E. palmar finger orthosis
E. palmar wrist splint
Engh porous metal hip prosthesis
engine
Acrotorque hand e.
e. H-file
Robbins Acrotorque hand e.
Englehardt femoral prosthesis
Englert forceps
English
E. anvil nail nipper
E. brace
E. clamp
E. hospital reflex percussor
E. lock
E. MacIntosh fiberoptic laryngoscope
blade
E. tissue forceps
English-McNab shoulder prosthesis
Engstrom
E. multigas monitor
E. respirator
EnGuard
E. double-lead ICD system
E. pacing and defibrillation lead
system
E. PFX lead electrode
enhanced
e. external counterpulsation unit
E. Torque guiding catheter
EnhanCement
E. gun
enhancement gun
enhancer
Ace aerosol cloud e.
Aerosol Cloud E.
Avance hearing e.
e. cushion
XP Xcelerator ultrasound e.
Enker self-retaining brain retractor
enlarging bur
Enneking rod
Ennis forceps
ensheathing trocar
ENSI syringe
ENT
ENT bite block
ENT electrode
ENT scope
ENT speculum
ENT wire crimper
ENtec surgery system
Entegra prosthesis
Entera-Flo enteral feeding pump
enteroclysis tube
enterolysis tube

E

Enteroport feeding pump
enteroscope
    dedicated push e.
    Goldberg MPC operative e.
    Olympus SIF-M-series video e.
    Olympus SIF-series video e.
    Olympus SIF-SW-series video e.
    Olympus SSIF-series video e.
    Olympus XSIF-series video e.
    Pentax VSB-P-series e.
    SIF10 Olympus e.
    Sonde e.
    video push e.
enterostomy clamp
enterotomy scissors
Enterra therapy
Entos vascular and abdominal intraoperative scanhead
Entract
    E. dilation and occlusion catheter
    E. stent
    E. stone retriever
entrapment
    e. sack
    e. sack introducer
Entrease variable depth punch
Entree
    E. disposable CO_2 insufflation needle
    E. II cannula
    E. II trocar
    E. II trocar and cannula system
    E. Plus cannula
    E. Plus trocar
    E. Plus trocar and cannula system
EnTre guidewire
Entrex
    E. small-joint arthroscopy instrument set
EntriStar
    E. feeding tube
    E. percutaneous endoscopic gastrostomy (PEG) tube
entropion
    e. clamp
    e. forceps
enucleation
    e. compressor
    e. scissors
    e. scoop
    e. spoon
    e. wire snare
enucleator
    Banner snare e.
    Botvin-Bradford e.
    Bradford snare e.
    Castroviejo snare e.
    Foster snare e.
    Hardy bayonet e.
    Hardy microsurgical e.
    Marino rotatable transsphenoidal e.
    Rhoton e.
    rotatable transsphenoidal e.
    snare e.

    transsphenoidal e.
    Young prostatic e.
enuresis alarm
envelope
    e. arm sling
    cryoflex e.
Enviclusive semi-occlusive adhesive film dressing
Envinet gauze dressing
Envisan dextranomer pad
Envision endocavity probe
Envy catheter
Enzymobead bead
Enzymun-Test System ES22 analyzer
EOC goniometer
Epic
    E. laser
    E. ophthalmic 3-in-1 laser system
    E. wheelchair
epicardial
    e. defibrillator patch
    e. Doppler flow sector transducer
    e. lead
    e. pacemaker
    e. retractor
    e. sock electrode
Epicel skin graft material
Epicon mesh
EPICS
    EPICS Elite flow cytometry
    EPICS Profile flow cytometer
Epi-Derm silicone gel sheeting
epidural
    e. peg electrode
EpiE-Z
    E.-Z. Pen
    E.-Z. Pen epinephrine injector
    E.-Z. Pen injection device
    E.-Z. Pen-Jr
EpiFlex heel and elbow protector
Epigard
    E. dressing
    E. synthetic skin
epiglottis retractor
Epi-Grip
EpiLaser
    E. hair removal laser
    E. laser-based hair removal system
epilation
    e. electrode
    e. forceps
    e. needle
epilator
    Electro-Blend e.
    Epilot high-frequency needle-type e.
    high-frequency tweezer-type e.
    Removatron e.
    Super Epitron high-frequency e.
    Thermaderm e.
    Trichodemolus e.
Epilatron hair-removal machine
epilepsy implant
EpiLight hair removal system
Epi-Lock dressing
Epilot high-frequency needle-type epilator

EpiPen injection device
EpiPen-Jr injection device
Epiquick
epiretinal delamination diamond knife
episcleral forceps
Episeal wound dressing
episiotomy scissors
EPI Sport epicondylitis clasp
Epistar subtraction angiogram
Epistat double balloon
epistaxis balloon
Epi-Stay device
epithelial
    e. rete peg
    e. scraper
Epitome scalpel
EpiTouch
    E. Alex laser hair removal system
    E. laser
    E. Ruby SilkLaser
    E. ruby SilkLaser hair removal
    system
Epitrain
    E. active elbow support
    E. elastic elbow support
    E. elbow splint
Epoxylite CBA dental resin cement
Eppendorf
    E. angiocatheter
    E. cardiac catheter
    E. centrifuge
    E. cervical biopsy forceps
    E. needle electrode
    E. punch
    E. tube
Epstein
    E. bone rasp
    E. collar stud acrylic implant
    E. collar stud acrylic lens
    E. down-biting curette
    E. hemilaminectomy blade
    E. intraocular lens
    E. needle
    E. neurological hammer
    E. osteotome
    E. posterior chamber lens
    E. spinal fusion curette
Epstein-Copeland lens
EPTFE
    expanded polytetrafluoroethylene
    EPTFE augmentation membrane
    EPTFE graft prosthesis
    EPTFE implant
    EPTFE sutures
    EPTFE vascular suture
    EPTFE ventricular shunt catheter
Epworth Sleepiness Scale
epX suspension sleeve
Equalizer air walker
Equen
    E. stomach magnet
Equen-Neuffer laryngeal knife
Equilizer short leg walking cast
Equinox EEG neuromonitoring system

equipment
    Acuson echocardiographic e.
    Body-Solid exercise e.
    bubble chamber e.
    Cell Saver 4 cardiopulmonary
    bypass blood centrifuge and
    washing e.
    Cybex back rehabilitation e.
    durable medical e.
    DynaDisc exercise e.
    Dynalyzer e.
    ERCP e.
    Invertrac e.
    LKB/Wallac 1217 Rackbeta e.
    Luxar Silhouette noninvasive body
    appearance e.
    OsseoCare drilling e.
    OsteoStat single-use power
    surgical e.
    Procomp pelvic muscle
    reeducation e.
    static gray scale ultrasound e.
    StereoGuide breast biopsy e.
equipotential electrode
Equisetene suture
ERA resectoscope sheath
eraser
    E. cautery
    hemostatic e.
    Mentor Curved e.
    Mentor Wet-Field e.
    Tano e.
Eraser-tip cautery
ERBE
    E. cryoprobe
Erbe
    E. ICC generator
    E. Unit argon plasma coagulator
erbium
    e. CrystaLase laser
    e. Renaissance laser
erbium:YAG
    e. infrared laser
    e. laser
ERCP
    endoscopic retrograde
    cholangiopancreatogram
    ERCP balloon extractor
    ERCP cannula
    ERCP catheter
    ERCP conventional prosthesis
    ERCP dilator
    ERCP equipment
    ERCP guidewire
    ERCP nasobiliary drain
    ERCP sphincterotome
ERCPeel Away catheter
ErCr:YAG
    ErCr:YAG laser
ErecAid
    E. vacuum
    E. vacuum erection device
    E. vacuum system
Erectek external erection device
erector spinae retractor

E

ERG-Jet disposable contact lens
Ergo
    E. bipolar forceps
    E. Cush back support
    E. irrigation system
    E. microaspirator
    E. style flexion table
Ergociser
    Cateye E.
    E. exercise cycle
Ergoflex Premiere back support
ErgoForm contoured cold pack
Ergolift device
Ergoline bicycle ergometer
ErgoLogic keyboard
ergometer
    bicycle e.
    Bosch ERG 500 e.
    Collins bicycle e.
    Concept II rowing e.
    Corival 400 e.
    Cybex cycle e.
    Ergoline bicycle e.
    Gauthier bicycle e.
    Monark bicycle e.
    pedal-mode e.
    Siemens-Albis bicycle e.
    Siemens-Elema AG bicycle e.
    Tunturi EL400 bicycle e.
Ergos
    E. O_2 dual-chamber rate-responsive pacemaker
    E. work simulator
ErgoTec vitreoretinal instrument system
Erhardt
    E. ear speculum
    E. eyelid forceps
    E. lid clamp
Eric
    E. Lloyd extractor
    E. Lloyd introducer
Erich
    E. arch malleable bar
    E. dental arch bar
    E. facial fracture appliance
    E. facial fracture frame
    E. laryngeal biopsy forceps
    E. maxillary splint
    E. nasal splint
    E. swivel
Erich-Winter arch bar
Ericksson-Stille carotid clamp
Erie system
Eri-Flo dialyzer
Eriksson
    E. guide
    E. knee prosthesis
    E. muscle biopsy cannula
Eriksson-Paparella holder
erisophake (var. of erysiphake)
Erlangen
    E. magnetic colostomy device
    E. papillotome
Erlanger sphygmomanometer
Ermold needle holder

Ernest-McDonald
    E.-M. soft intraocular lens
    E.-M. soft intraocular lens-folding forceps
    E.-M. soft IOL folding forceps
Ernest nucleus cracker
Ernst radium applicator
eroder
    facet e.
Erosa
    E. amnioscope
    E. disposable hypodermic needle
Erosa-Spec vaginal speculum
Eros-CTD clitoral therapy device
ERx Avulsed Tooth kit
Er:YAG laser
erysiphake, erisophake
    Barraquer e.
    Bell e.
    Castroviejo e.
    corneal e.
    Dastoor e.
    Dimitry e.
    Dimitry-Bell e.
    Dimitry-Thomas e.
    Draeger high-vacuum e.
    Esposito e.
    Falcao e.
    Floyd-Grant e.
    Harken e.
    Harrington e.
    Johnson e.
    Johnson-Bell e.
    Kara e.
    L'Esperance e.
    Maumenee e.
    Maumenee-Park e.
    New York e.
    nucleus e.
    Nugent e.
    Nugent-Green-Dimitry e.
    oval cup e.
    Post-Harrington e.
    right-angle e.
    Sakler e.
    Searcy oval cup e.
    Simcoe nucleus e.
    Storz-Bell e.
    Viers e.
    Welsh rubber bulb e.
    Welsh Silastic e.
Erythroflex hydromer-coated central venous catheter
erythrolabe
ESA
    ESA acromioplasty electrode
    ESA hook electrode
    ESA Jet Stream ball electrode
    ESA meniscectomy electrode
    ESA Smillie electrode
Esca Buess + fistula funnel
escape pacemaker
Eschenbach low vision rehabilitation guide
Eschenbach Optik lens

Eschmann endotracheal tube introducer
E-Scope electronic stethoscope
Escort
    E. 300A defibrillator/pacer monitor
    E. balloon stone extractor
Esenbach Highlighter
E-series
    E.-s. bipolar forceps
    E.-s. hip system
    E.-s. needle holder
    E.-s. scissors
ESI
    ESI bite block
    ESI fiberoptic light source
    ESI laryngoscope
    ESI lighted suction elevator
    ESI Lite-Pipe fiberoptic cable
    ESI Lite-Pipe fiberoptic instrument
    ESI Lite-Pipe plastic surgery
      instrument
    ESI long, narrow mammoplasty
      retractor
    ESI sigmoidoscope
ESKA-Buess esophageal tube
ESKA-Jonas silicone-silver penile
  prosthesis
Esmarch
    E. bandage
    E. bandage scissors
    E. plaster knife
    E. plaster shears
    E. probe with Myrtle leaf end
    E. roll dressing
    E. tin bullet probe
    E. tourniquet
    E. tube
EsophaCoil
    E. biliary stent
    E. prosthesis
    E. self-expanding esophageal stent
esophageal
    e. balloon
    e. balloon catheter
    e. balloon dilator
    e. balloon tamponade
    e. detection device
    e. forceps
    e. manometry catheter
    e. mercury-filled bougie
    e. obturator airway
    e. perfusion catheter
    e. pill electrode
    e. retractor
    e. scissors
    e. stethoscope
    e. Strecker stent
    e. temperature probe
Esophageal Z-Stent stent
esophagofiberscope
    Olympus e.
esophagoprobe
    Olympus ultrasonic e.
esophagoscope
    ACMI fiberoptic e.
    ballooning e.

    Blom-Singer e.
    Boros e.
    Broyles e.
    Bruening e.
    Chevalier Jackson e.
    child e.
    Denck e.
    Dohlman e.
    Eder e.
    Eder-Hufford e.
    Eutaw-Hoffman e.
    fiberoptic e.
    Foregger rigid e.
    Foroblique fiberoptic e.
    full-lumen e.
    Haslinger e.
    Holinger infant e.
    Hufford e.
    infant e.
    Jackson e.
    Jasbee e.
    Jesberg oval e.
    Jesberg upper e.
    J-scope e.
    Kalk e.
    Lell e.
    LoPresti fiberoptic e.
    Moersch e.
    Mosher e.
    Moure e.
    Olympus e.
    optical e.
    oval e.
    oval-open e.
    pediatric e.
    Roberts folding e.
    Roberts-Jesberg e.
    Roberts oval e.
    Sam Roberts e.
    Schindler optical e.
    standard full-lumen e.
    Storz operating e.
    Storz optical e.
    Storz pediatric e.
    Tesberg e.
    Tucker e.
    Universal e.
    upper e.
    Yankauer e.
esophagoscopic
    e. cannula
    e. catheter
    e. forceps
esophagospasm dilator
ESP
    ESP radiation reduction examination
      glove
Espe
    E. Ketac-Bond Aplicap
    E. Photac-Bond Aplicap
E-speed intraoral film
Espocan combined spinal/epidural needle
Esposito erysiphake
ESPrit ear level speech processor
Esquire dental sterilizer

E

ESSential shaver system
Esser
    E. graft
    E. implant
    E. prosthesis
Essig arch bar
Essrig
    E. dissecting scissors
    E. tissue forceps
Estecar prosthesis
Esterman scale
esthesiometer
    manual e.
esthetic
    e. CO_2 laser
    e. Taylor mandibular angle implant
Estilux
    E. dental restorative material
    E. ultraviolet system
Estridge ventricular needle
Estring
    E. estradiol vaginal ring
    E. silicone vaginal ring
ESU
    electrosurgical unit
    Aspen Excaliber ESU
    ESU dispersive pad
ESWL
    Modulith SL20 device for ESWL
etafilcon A disposable contact lens
ETB endoscope
Etch-Master
    E.-M. electronic stencil
    E.-M. felt pad
    E.-M. kit
Ethalloy TruTaper cardiovascular needle
ether
    e. guard
    e. screen
Ethibond
    E. polybutilate-coated polyester
      suture
    E. polyester suture
Ethicon
    E. BV-75-3 needle
    E. clip
    E. disposable cannula
    E. disposable trocar
    E. endoscopic linear cutter
    E. Endosurgery circular stapler
    E. Ligaclip
    E. mesh
    E. micropoint suture
    E. Polytef paste prosthesis
    E. Sabreloc suture
    E. silk suture
    E. ST-4 straight taper-point needle
    E. TG Plus needle
    E. TGW needle
Ethicon-Atraloc suture
Ethiflex retention suture
Ethiguard needle
Ethilon nylon suture
Ethi-pack suture

Ethitek's automated protection manometer
ethmoid
    e. punch forceps
ethmoidal
    e. chisel
    e. curette
    e. forceps
    e. punch
ethmoid-Blakesley forceps
ethmoid-cutting forceps
Ethox
    E. bite block
    E. cuff
    E. rectal tube
    E. Surgi-Press pressure infuser
Ethridge hysterectomy forceps
Ethrone
    E. implant
    E. prosthesis
ethyl cyanoacrylate glue
ethylene oxide dressing
E-to-A adapter
ETO Sleuth
ET tube
Etude cystometer uroflowmeter
ETV8 CCD ColorMicro video camera
E-type dental implant
EUB-405
    EUB-405 ultrasound scanner
    EUB-405 ultrasound system
Eucotone monitor
EUE tonsillar snare
EUM-series endoscope
Eureka collimator
Euro-Collins multiorgan perfusion kit
EuroCuff forearm crutch
Euroglide MKII slide board
Euro-Med FNA-21 aspiration needle
European/German bipolar cable
European in-the-bag lens
Euro Precision Technology submicron lathe machine
Eurotech table
Euroton hearing aid
eustachian
    e. bougie
    e. bur
    e. catheter
    e. probe
    e. tube
Eutaw-Hoffman esophagoscope
euthyscope
evacuator
    Bard e.
    Bigelow e.
    bladder e.
    Creevy bladder e.
    Crigler e.
    Dentsply MVS e.
    Ellik bladder e.
    high-volume e.
    Hutch e.
    ice clot e.
    Iglesias e.

Kennedy-Cornwell bladder e.
Laparofan smoke e.
Laufe portable uterine e.
Lavacuator gastric e.
McCarthy bladder e.
McKenna Tide-Ur-Ator e.
oval-window piston e.
Plume-Away e.
Sklar e.
smoke e.
SmokEvac smoke e.
Snyder Hemovac e.
Surgilase ECS.1 smoke e.
Thompson e.
Timberlake e.
Toomey bladder e.
e. tubing
Urovac bladder e.
uterine e.
Evacupack disposable suction cannister
Evans articulator
Evans-Vital tissue forceps
EVAP roller electrode
Evazote
E. cushioning material
E. foam
EVE Fujinon videocolonoscope
Eve-Neivert tonsillar wire
Everclear laryngeal mirror
Everest alloy
Everett
E. crutch
E. eustachian catheter
E. fallopian cannula
E. fallopian catheter
E. forceps
Ever-Flex insole
Evergreen
E. Lasertek coagulator
E. Lasertek laser
Evermed catheter
Evershears
E. bipolar curved scissors
E. bipolar laparoscopic forceps
E. bipolar laparoscopic scissors
E. surgical instrument device
everter, eversor
Berens lid e.
Berke double-end lid e.
lid e.
Luther-Peter lid e.
Pess lid e.
Roveda lid e.
Schachne-Desmarres lid e.
Siniscal-Smith lid e.
Strubel lid e.
Vail lid e.
Walker lid e.
everting mattress suture
Evert-O-Cath drug delivery catheter
Everyday
E. Objects ColorCards
E. self-adhering urinary external
catheter
Eves-Neivert tonsillar snare

Eves tonsillar snare
EVIS
EVIS 140 endoscope reprocessing
system
EVIS EXERA endoscope
EVIS 200I colonoscope
EVIS "Q" series endoscope
evisceration spoon
Evolution
E. hip prosthesis
E. XP scanner
**Evoport auditory evoked potential
system**
Ewald
E. elbow prosthesis
E. gastroscope
E. tissue forceps
E. tube
Ewald-Hensler arthroscopic punch
Ewald-Hudson
E.-H. brain forceps
E.-H. clamp
E.-H. dressing forceps
E.-H. tissue forceps
Ewald-Walker knee implant
EWHO
elbow-wrist-hand orthosis
Ewing
E. capsular forceps
E. eye implant
E. lid clamp
Exacta-Med oral dispenser
ExacTech blood glucose meter
Exact-Fit ATH hip replacement system
**Exact-Touch Saccomanno Pap smear
collection system**
EXAKT
EXAKT cutting/grinding system
EXAKT cutting/grinding unit
Exakta Varex gastrocamera
Exami-Gown gown
examination retractor
eXamine cholangiography catheter
examining
e. arthroscope
e. gastroscope
e. hysteroscope
e. lamp
e. spotlight
e. telescope
Excaliber handpiece
Excalibur introducer
excavating bur
excavator
Austin e.
Clev-Dent e.
dental e.
Farrior oval-window e.
fenestration e.
Henry Schein e.
Hough oval-window e.
Hough-Saunders e.
Hough whirlybird e.
House e.
House-Hough e.

E

excavator *(continued)*
Lempert e.
Merlis obstetrical e.
middle ear e.
Nordent e.
oval-window e.
Paparella-Hough e.
PD e.
Schuknecht whirlybird e.
sinus tympani e.
SMIC e.
stapes e.
whirlybird stapes e.

Excel
E. disposable biopsy forceps
E. electric hospital bed
E. GE electrochemical glucose
monitoring test strip
E. Plus electrode
E. Plus underpad
E. quilted underpad

Excelart short-bore MRI
eXcel-DR
e.-D. disposable/reusable Glasser
laparoscopic needle
e.-D. disposable/reusable instrument
e.-D. pneumothorax needle

Excell
E. polishing point
E. polishing wheel

Exceltech imaging
exchange guidewire
exchanger
countercurrent heat e.
head/moisture e.
heat and moisture e.
HumidFilter heat and moisture e.
hygroscopic heat and moisture e.
moisture e.
Portex ThermoVent heat and
moisture e.

Excilon
E. drain sponge
E. dressing sponge
E. IV sponge

ExciMed UV200 excimer laser
excimer
e. cool laser
e. gas laser
e. ultraviolet laser

exclusion clamp
exdwelling ureteral occlusion balloon
catheter
executive bifocal
exenteration
e. forceps
e. spoon

Exerball kit
ExerBand therapy band
exercise
e. band
E. Sandal
e. treadmill

exerciser
AnkleCiser e.
Böhler e.
Builder Grip hand e.
Carpal Care e.
Cat's Paw e.
Cybex II, II+ isokinetic e.
Danniflex CPM e.
Digi-Flex finger e.
Digi-Flex hand e.
DynaFlex Gyro e.
Eggsercizer resistive hand e.
Exer-Cor e.
ExtendaFLEX e.
FiddleLink hand e.
finger e.
Finger Helper hand e.
Finger Platter hand e.
Flextender Plus hand e.
Grahamizer I e.
Gripp squeeze ball hand e.
hand e.
Hand Helper hand e.
isokinetic Unex III e.
Iso-Quadron e.
JACE shoulder e.
jaw e.
Jux-A-Cisor e.
KineTec clubfoot CPM e.
Knead-A-Ball e.
microcomputer upper limb e.
MiniMedBall hand e.
Morpho e.
Motivator FTR2000 e.
MULE upper limb e.
NordiCare Enabler e.
NordiCare Strider e.
NordicTrack ski e.
NuStep e.
Omni-Flexor wrist e.
Oppociser hand e.
Orthotron e.
pedal e.
Physio-Roll-R-Cise e.
PlyoSled e.
Powerflex CMP e.
Power Pogo stationary e.
Power Web hand e.
Preston Traveler CPM e.
ProStretch e.
Pul-Ez e.
Relax-a-Cizor e.
Resistex expiratory resistance e.
resistive e.
rickshaw rehab e.
rocky boat e.
Rotaflex e.
Roylan ergonomic hand e.
Seated Cable Row e.
Soft Touch hand e.
squeeze e.
strengthening e.
Stronghands hand e.
Stryker CPM e.
Stryker leg e.

Swanson Grip-X hand e.
Thera-Band ASSIST e.
Therabite jaw e.
Thera Cane shoulder e.
Theraflex wrist e.
Ther-A-Hoop e.
Thera-Loop e.
Toronto Medical CPM e.
Tuf Nex neck e.
Tunturi hand e.
Walk-'n-tone e.
Exer-Cor exerciser
Exer-Pedic cycle
Exerstrider machine
Exertools gymball
Exeter
E. intramedullary bone plug
E. ophthalmoscope
EX-FI-RE
E.-F.-R. external fixation device
E.-F.-R. external fixation system
eXit
e. disposable puncture closure
e. disposable puncture closure
device
Exmoor plastics aural grommet
Exo-Bed
E.-B. traction unit
E.-B. tractor
exolever forceps
Exonix
E. ultrasonic surgical system
Exo-Overhead traction unit
exophthalmometer
Hertel e.
Krahn e.
LICO Hertel e.
Luedde e.
Marco prism e.
Naugle orbitometer e.
exoplant
EX-OP operating table
Exo-Static
E.-S. cervical collar
E.-S. overhead tractor
Exotec brace
expandable
e. access catheter
e. biliary endoprosthesis
e. blade
e. breast implant
e. cervical dilator
e. esophageal stent
e. intrahepatic portacaval shunt stent
e. LeMaitre valvulotome
e. metallic stent
e. metal mesh endoprosthesis
e. prosthesis
Expandacell sponge
expanded
e. polytetrafluoroethylene (EPTFE)
e. polytetrafluoroethylene (EPTFE)
implant
e. polytetrafluoroethylene (EPTFE)
suture

e. polytetrafluoroethylene vascular
graft
expander
AccuSpan tissue e.
Becker tissue e.
Biospan anatomical tissue e.
BIOSPAN breast tissue e.
CUI tissue e.
field e.
Graether pupil e.
Hextend plasma volume e.
Integra tissue e.
E. mammary implant material
McGhan tissue e.
Mentor Spectrum contour e.
Mentor tissue e.
Meshgraft skin e.
Ormco orthodontic arch-e.
PMT AccuSpan tissue e.
Radovan tissue e.
rectal e.
Ruiz-Cohen round e.
saline-filled e.
self-inflating tissue e.
slow palatal e.
subperiosteal tissue e.
surgical skin graft e.
tissue e.
T-Span tissue e.
expanding
e. reamer
e. valvotome
Expand-O-Graft cutter
**expansible infrastructure endosteal
implant**
expansile
e. dilator
e. forceps
expansion
E. control WAFFLE mattress pad
e. screw
Expert bone densitometer
Expert-XL densitometer
expiratory valve
expirograph
Godart e.
explorer
E. common bile duct exploration
system
dental e.
Nordent e.
operative e.
E. pre-curved diagnostic EP catheter
SMIC e.
Steri-Probe e.
exploring
e. cannula
e. electrode
e. needle
Expo
E. Bubble dressing
E. Bubble eye cover
E. Bubble eye shield
E. eye dressing
eXpose retractor

E

exposure meter
Express
    E. balloon
    E. over-the-wire balloon catheter
    E. PTCA catheter
expressor
    Arroyo e.
    Arruga eye e.
    Arruga lens e.
    Bagley-Wilmer lens e.
    Berens lens e.
    follicle e.
    Fyodorov lens e.
    Goldmann e.
    Heath follicle e.
    Hess tonsil e.
    Heyner e.
    hook e.
    e. hook
    Hosford meibomian gland e.
    intracapsular lens e.
    iris e.
    Kirby hook e.
    Kirby intracapsular lens e.
    lens e.
    lid e.
    McDonald e.
    Medallion lens e.
    meibomian gland e.
    nucleus e.
    Osher nucleus stab e.
    ring lens e.
    Rizzuti iris e.
    Rizzuti lens e.
    Smith lens e.
    Smith lid e.
    Stahl nucleus e.
    tonsillar e.
    Verhoeff lens e.
    Wilmer-Bagley iris e.
    Wilmer-Bagley lens e.
Exprin DQ1 biopsy instrument
expulsion stent
EXS femoropopliteal bypass graft
Extend
    E. stem
    E. total hip system
ExtendaFLEX exerciser
extended
    e. anatomical high-profile malar
        implant
    e. round needle
    e. sector ultrasonic probe
    E. Wear self-adhering urinary
        external catheter
    E. Wear self-adhering urinary
        external catheter starter kit
    E. Wear self-adhering urinary
        external catheter with removable
        tip
extended-wear
    e.-w. soft contact lens
extender
    Kalish Duredge wire e.
    Küntscher nail e.

rear-tip e.
Rousek e.
Superstabilizer cemented stem e.
Superstabilizer press-fit stem e.
Sven Johansson e.
Taq e.
Extend-It finger splint
extension
    e. apparatus
    bifurcated drain e.
    e. bone clamp
    e. bow
    Buck e.
    Centurion needleless catheter e.'s
    deep brain e.
    DOC guidewire e.
    Hudson cerebellar e.
    Jackson-Pratt bifurcated drain e.
    Linx guidewire e.
    LOC guidewire e.
    NexGen offset stem e.
    Orascoptic loupe e.
    radiolucent operating room table e.
    e. tube
    e. tubing with connector
Extensometer
    Laser E.
exterior pelvic device
external
    e. asynchronous pacemaker
    e. auditory larynx
    e. collimator
    e. counterpressure device
    e. demand pacemaker
    e. electrode
    e. functional neuromuscular
        stimulator
    e. inflatable compressor
    e. monitor
    e. orthosis
    e. sequential pneumatic compression
        boot
    e. spinal skeletal fixator
    e. tachyarrhythmia control device
    e. transthoracic pacemaker
    e. ureteral catheter
    e. urethral barrier
    e. vascular compression device
    e. vein stripper
external-alignment compression jig
external-internal pacemaker
externally-controlled noninvasive
    programmed stimulation pacemaker
externally supported Dacron graft
externofrontal retractor
extracapsular forceps
extracardiac right-to-left shunt
extrachromic suture
extracoronal retainer
extracorporeal
    e. liver assist device (ELAD)
    e. membrane oxygenation system
    e. membrane oxygenator (ECMO)
    e. piezoelectric lithotriptor
    e. pump

e. pump oxygenator
e. shock wave lithotriptor
extracting forceps
extraction
e. atherectomy device
e. balloon
e. forceps
e. generator
e. hook
e. pliers
e. trap
extractor
Andrews comedo e.
Applied Biosystems 340A nucleic acid e.
Austin Moore e.
ball e.
Bellows cryoextractor e.
Bilos pin e.
Bird vacuum e.
broach e.
buccal fat e.
cataract rotoextractor e.
Cherry screw e.
cloverleaf pin e.
comedo e.
cortex e.
Councill ureteral stone e.
deluxe FIN e.
DePuy e.
Dolan e.
Douvas Roto-extractor e.
Egnell vacuum e.
ERCP balloon e.
Eric Lloyd e.
Escort balloon stone e.
femoral trial e.
fetal head e.
fetal vacuum e.
food e.
Gill-Welsh cortex e.
Glassman stone e.
Hallach comedo e.
head e.
e. injector
Intraflex intramedullary pin e.
Jarit comedo e.
Jewett bone e.
Kalish Duredge wire e.
Kobayashi vacuum e.
Krwawicz cataract e.
Küntscher e.
Lewicky cortex e.
Lloyd nail e.
Look cortex e.
Luxator e.
magnetic e.
Malström vacuum e.
Mark II femoral component e.
Mark II tibial component e.
Massie e.
McDermott e.
McNutt e.
McReynolds e.
Mignon cataract e.

Mityvac e.
Moore-Blount e.
Moore hooked e.
Moore nail e.
Moore prosthesis e.
M-type e.
Murless fetal head e.
e. nail drill
Rush e.
Rutner stone e.
Saalfeld comedo e.
Schamberg comedo e.
Schneider e.
Silastic cup e.
Silc e.
Simcoe cortex e.
Smirmaul nucleus e.
Smith-Petersen e.
Snap Lock wire/pin e.
Soehendra stent e.
Southwick screw e.
stem e.
Take-Out e.
T-C ring-handle pin and wire e.
Tender Touch e.
E. three-lumen retrieval balloon catheter
Torpin vectis e.
Trizol RNA e.
Troutman cataract e.
Unna comedo e.
ureteral stone e.
Vantos vacuum e.
Visitec cortex e.
Walton comedo e.
Welsh cortex e.
Wilson-Cook eight-wire basket stone e.
E. XL triple-lumen retrieval balloon
Zimmer e.
eXtract specimen bag
extracutaneous vas fixation clamp
extra-depth shoe
Extrafil breast implant
extrahepatic shunt
extramedullary
e. alignment arch
e. alignment guide
e. tibial alignment jig
extraoral
e. bone-anchored implant
e. fracture appliance
e. sigmoid notch retractor
ExtraSafe
E. butterfly infusion needle
E. catheter
E. phlebotomy device
E. syringe
extra-stiff
e.-s. Amplatz wire
e.-s. guidewire
extra-support guidewire
extraventricular drain
Extreme Select ligament brace

E

extremity
>e. mobilization strap
>e. pump

extruded bar polyethylene

extrusion
>e. balloon catheter
>e. needle

exudate disposal bag

ExuDerm RCD hydrocolloid dressing

Exu-Dry absorptive dressing

eye
>artificial e.
>e. bandage
>e. blade
>e. calipers
>e. curette
>e. diathermy electrode
>e. drape
>e. forceps
>e. knife
>e. knife guard
>e. magnet
>e. movement measuring apparatus
>e. needle holder
>e. occluder
>oval e.
>e. pad
>e. pad dressing
>patch e.
>e. patch
>e. probe
>e. protector
>e. shield
>Snellen reform e.
>e. spear
>e. speculum
>e. spherical implant
>e. stitch scissors
>e. suture scissors

EyeClose
>E. Adhesive strip
>E. external eyelid weight

Eyecor camera

eyed
>e. suture needle

eye-dressing forceps

eye-fixation forceps

eyeFix speculum system

eyeglass hearing aid

eyeless atraumatic suture needle

eyelet clasp

eyelid
>e. forceps
>e. retractor
>e. spacer

EyeMap EH-290 corneal tomography system

Eye-Pak drape

eyepiece
>comparison e.
>compensating e.
>demonstration e.
>huygenian e.
>negative e.
>positive e.
>Ramsden e.
>wide-field e.

EyeSys
>E. 2000 corneal topographic mapping system
>E. videokeratoscope

E-Z
>E-Z arm abduction orthosis
>E-Z Cath catheter
>E-Z Clean cautery tip
>E-Z Clean laparoscopic electrode
>E-Z Flap
>E-Z Flap burr hole cover
>E-Z Flap cranial flap fixation system
>E-Z Flap titanium miniplate system
>E-Z Flex jaw exercising device
>E-Z guide
>E-Z hold adhesive catheter tube holder pad
>E-Z hold adhesive/stretchable strap catheter tube holder
>E-Z Ject injector
>E-Z 'Jector injector
>E-Z Reacher
>E-Z ROC anchor
>E-Z syringe
>E-Z Tac soft-tissue reattachment system

EZ
>EZ-Derm porcine biosynthetic wound dressing
>EZ hand pump
>EZ Lift table
>EZ Rider support chair
>EZ Temp thermometer

EZ.1 multifocal contact lens

EZE-FIT IOL system

Ezeform splint

E-Z-EM
>E-Z-EM BioGun automated biopsy system
>E-Z-EM cut biopsy needle
>E-Z-EM PercuSet amniocentesis tray

E-Z-Guard mouthpiece

Ezo denture cushion

EZ-ON traction belt system

E-Z-On vest

EZRest

EZ-Trac orthopaedic suspension device

EZVue violet haptic intraocular lens

Ezy
>E. Wrap lumbosacral support
>E. Wrap shoulder immobilizer

F2L Multineck femoral stem
Fabco
    F. gauze bandage
    F. gauze dressing
    F. wrap
Fabian screw
fabric
    f. baffle
    f. leg bag strap
Fabry coagulator
face
    f. mask
    f. rest
    f. shield
facebow, face-bow
    Asher high-pull f.
    Kinematic f.
    Kloehn f.
    Ortho-Yomy f.
    Rampton f.
    Rickett f.
    root high-pull f.
facehole
Face-It protective shield
FACE kit
facelift, face-lift
    f. flap marker
    f. retractor
    f. scissors
face-out, whole-body plethysmograph
faceplate
    Coloplast irrigation f.
    Sur-Fit irrigation adapter f.
facet
    f. eroder
    f. rasp
    f. screw system
facial
    f. compression finger closure
    f. compression skull cap closure
    F. Flex therapy
    f. fracture appliance dental arch bar
    f. implant
    f. nerve dissector
    f. nerve knife
    f. nerve stimulator
    f. plastics garment
    f. plastic surgery scissors
    f. support
Facit uterine polyp forceps
FACScan flow cytometer
FACSVantage cell sorter
FACT-22 catheter
FACT coronary balloon angioplasty catheter
Fader Tip ureteral stent
Fager pituitary dissector
Fahey-Compere pin
Fahey pin
Fahrenheit flat bath thermometer
fail-safe device
Fairdale orthodontic appliance

Falcao
    F. erysiphake
    F. fixation forceps
    F. suction dissector
Falcon
    F. coronary catheter
    F. filter
    F. FX8000 DEEP CELL alternating support surface system
    F. lens
    F. plastic flask
    F. single-operator exchange balloon catheter
Falconer rongeur
Falk
    F. appendectomy spoon
    F. clamp
    F. lion-jaw forceps
    F. needle
    F. vaginal cuff
    F. vaginal retractor
fallopian
    f. cannula
    f. catheter
    f. tube forceps
falloposcope endoscopic instrument
Falope-ring
    F.-r. applicator
    F.-r. dilator
    F.-r. tubal occlusion band
Falope tubal sterilization ring
false
    f. neurochemical transmitter
fan
    f. elevator retractor
    f. liver retractor
    Schmitt f.
fan-beam collimator
Fansler
    F. anoscope
    F. proctoscope
    F. rectal speculum
Fansler-Ives anoscope
Fanta speculum
Farabeuf
    F. bone clamp
    F. bone-holding forceps
    F. bone rasp
    F. double-ended retractor
    F. periosteal elevator
    F. raspatory
    F. rugine
    F. saw
Farabeuf-Collin
    F.-C. rasp
    F.-C. raspatory
Farabeuf-Lambotte
    F.-L. bone-holding clamp
    F.-L. bone-holding forceps
    F.-L. raspatory
Faraci punch
Faraci-Skillern sphenoid punch

F

Faraday
    F. shield
    F. shielded resonator
Farah cystoscopic needle
Farkas urethral speculum
Farley Elite spinal retractor
Farlow
    F. tongue depressor
    F. tonsillar snare
Farlow-Boettcher snare
Farmingdale retractor
Farnham nasal-cutting forceps
Faro coolbeam lamp
Farr
    F. self-retaining retractor
    F. spring retractor
    F. wire retractor
Farrington
    F. nasal polyp forceps
    F. septal forceps
Farrior
    F. angulated curette
    F. anterior footplate pick
    F. blunt palpator
    F. bur
    F. ear curette
    F. ear speculum
    F. mushroom raspatory
    F. otoplasty knife
    F. oval speculum
    F. oval-window excavator
    F. oval-window pick
    F. posterior footplate pick
    F. rasp
    F. septal cartilage stripper knife
    F. sickle knife
    F. suction applicator
    F. triangular knife
    F. wire crimper
    F. wire-crimping forceps
Farrior-Derlacki chisel
Farrior-Dworacek canal chisel
Farrior-Joseph bayonet saw
Farrior-McHugh ear knife
Farrior-Shambaugh elevator
Farris tissue forceps
Fary anterior chamber maintainer
Fasanella
    F. double-ended iris retractor
    F. lacrimal cannula
fascia
    f. lata heart valve
    f. lata implant
    f. lata prosthesis
    f. lata stripper
fascial
    f. cutter
    f. needle
    f. press
    f. snare
Fascian human fascia lata
fasciatome
    Lane f.
    Luck f.

    Masson f.
    Moseley f.
Fasplint splint
FAST
    flow-assisted short-term
    FAST balloon catheter
    FAST balloon flotation catheter
    FAST right heart cardiovascular
      catheter
fast
    f. Fourier transformation spectrum
      analyzer
    F. Lanex rare earth screen
**F.A.S.T.1 adult intraosseous infusion
    system**
FASTak
    F. suture anchor
    F. suture anchor system
fast-breeder reactor
Fastcure denture repair material
fastener
    ball f.
    Brown-Mueller T-bar f.
    Cath-Strip catheter f.
    Intrafix tibial f.
    NG strip nasal tube f.
    Percu-Stay catheter f.
    ROC XS suture f.
    SmartPins f.
    UC strip catheter tubing f.
**fast-imaging steady precession sequence
    three-dimensional magnetic resonance
    imaging**
FastIn threaded anchor
Fastlok implantable staple
FastOut device
Fast-Pass
    F.-P. endocardial lead
    F.-P. lead pacemaker
**Fast-Patch disposable
    defibrillation/electrocardiographic
    electrode**
FasTrac
    F. hydrophilic-coated guidewire
    F. introducer
FasTracker-18 infusion catheter
Fastrak traction strip dressing
FastRNA Kit-Green
fast-setting acrylic
fastSTART
    f. EMS neuromuscular stimulator
    f. HVPC pulsed stimulator
**FastTake blood glucose monitoring
    system**
fat
    f. pad retractor
    f. towel
Fat-O-Meter skinfold calipers
fat-suppressed body coil
faucet aspirator
faucial eustachian catheter
Fauer peritoneal clamp
Faught sphygmomanometer
Faulkner
    F. antral chisel

F. antral curette
F. double-end ring curette
F. ethmoidal curette
F. folder
F. nasal curette
F. trocar
Faulkner-Browne chisel
Faure
F. peritoneal forceps
F. uterine biopsy forceps
Fauvel laryngeal forceps
Favaloro
F. atrial retractor
F. coronary scissors
F. ligature carrier
F. proximal anastomosis clamp
F. saphenous vein bypass graft
F. self-retaining sternal retractor
Favaloro-Morse rib spreader
Favaloro-Semb ligature carrier
Favorite clamp
Faxitron x-ray machine
Fay
F. suction elevator
F. suction tube
Fazio-Montgomery cannula
Fazioplast
FCD
fecal containment device
Fearon tracheoscope
Feaster
F. Dualens intraocular lens
F. dual-placement intraocular lens
F. K7-5460 hydrodissecting cannula
F. lens hook
F. lens manipulator
F. radial keratotomy knife
feather
F. carbon breakable blade
f. clamp
f. knife
f. scalpel
feathered extended malar implant
Feather-Lite Pouching System
FeatherTouch
F. CO_2 laser
F. SilkLaser
F. SilkLaser system
fecal
f. containment device (FCD)
f. containment system
f. marker
Fechtner
F. conjunctiva forceps
F. intraocular lens
F. ring forceps
Federspiel
F. cheek retractor
F. needle
F. periosteal elevator
F. scissors
feedback
f. control system
f. system

feeder
Brecht f.
Haberman f.
offset suspension f.
Rancho Los Amigos f.
suspension f.
Tumble Forms f.
feeding
f. gastrostomy
f. tube
f. tube attachment device
feeler
O'Donoghue cartilage f.
Feeln' Sure pant
Fe-Ex orogastric tube magnet
Fehland
F. intestinal clamp
F. intestinal forceps
F. right-angled colon clamp
Fehling TOP ejector punch
Feilchenfeld splinter forceps
Feild
F. retractable blade assembly
F. suction dissector
Feild-Lee biopsy needle
Fein
F. antral trocar
F. cannula
F. needle
Feldbausch dilator
Feldenkrais cylinder
Feldman
F. adaptometer
F. bur
F. lid retractor
F. radial keratotomy marker
Feldstein blepharoplasty clip
Felig insulin pump
Fell-O'Dwyer apparatus
Fell sucker tip
felt
f. dressing
f. pledget
F. shears
Teflon f.
female
f. catheter
f. condom
f. sound
f. urinary pouch
f. washer
Fem-Flex II femoral cannulae
Feminal urinal
Femina vaginal weight
femoral
f. aligner
f. artery cannula
f. broach
f. canal restrictor
f. cerebral catheter
f. clamp
f. distractor
f. endoprosthesis
f. guide pin
f. guiding catheter

F

femoral *(continued)*
    f. head driver
    f. hemodialysis catheter
    f. impactor
    f. intermedullary guide
    f. introducer sheath
    f. neck retractor
    f. notch guide
    f. perfusion cannula
    f. plug
    f. rasp
    f. shaft reamer
    f. stem
    f. trial extractor
femorofemoral crossover prosthesis
FemoStop
    F. femoral artery compression arch
    F. inflatable pneumatic compression
      device
FemSoft urethral insert
FemTone vaginal weight
fence
    Kirklin f.
    f. splint
fenestra implant
fenestrated
    f. aneurysm clip
    f. blade forceps
    f. catheter
    f. compression plate
    f. cup biopsy forceps
    f. ellipsoid spiked open span biopsy
      forceps
    f. Moore-type femoral stem
    f. spiked open span jumbo biopsy
      forceps
    f. sterile drape
    f. tracheostomy tube
fenestration
    f. bur
    f. curette
    f. excavator
    f. hook
fenestrator
    Montgomery tracheal f.
    Rosen f.
fenestrometer
    Guilford-Wright f.
    Paparella f.
    Rosen f.
    Wright-Guilford f.
Fenger
    F. gall duct probe
    F. spiral gallstone probe
Fenlin total shoulder system
Fenton
    F. bulldog vulsellum
    F. tibial bolt
    F. uterine dilator
Fenwal
    F. cryocyte freezing container
    F. CS3000 Plus cell separator
    F. hemapheresis pump
FEP-ringed Gore-Tex vascular graft

Ferciot
    F. tip-toe splint
    F. wire guide
Fergie needle
Ferguson
    F. abdominal scissors
    F. angiotribe
    F. angiotribe forceps
    F. bone clamp
    F. bone curette
    F. bone holder
    F. bone-holding forceps
    F. esophageal probe
    F. gallstone scoop
    F. implant
    F. mouthgag
    F. retractor
    F. round-body needle
    F. stone basket
    F. suction
    F. suture needle
Ferguson-Ackland mouthgag
Ferguson-Brophy mouthgag
Ferguson-Frazier suction tube
Ferguson-Gwathmey mouthgag
Ferguson-Metzenbaum scissors
Ferguson-Moon rectal retractor
Fergus percutaneous introducer kit
Fergusson tubular vaginal speculum
Fermit-N occlusal hole blockage material
Ferno
    F. AquaCiser underwater treadmill
      system
    F. Recline-a-Bath bathing system
Fernstroem bladder retractor
Fernstroem-Stille retractor
Ferran awl
Ferree-Rand perimeter
Ferrier
    F. coupler
    F. 212 gingival clamp
    F. separator
Ferris
    F. biliary duct dilator
    F. chart
    F. colporrhaphy forceps
    F. common duct scoop
    F. disposable bone marrow
      aspiration needle
    F. filiform dilator
    F. polyostomy wound dressing
    F. Robb tonsillar knife
    F. Smith bone-biting forceps
    F. Smith cup rongeur forceps
    F. Smith disk rongeur
    F. Smith fragment forceps
    F. Smith-Gruenwald rongeur
    F. Smith-Halle sinus bur
    F. Smith intervertebral disk rongeur
    F. Smith-Kerrison disk rongeur
    F. Smith-Kerrison forceps
    F. Smith-Kerrison laminectomy
      rongeur
    F. Smith-Kerrison punch
    F. Smith-Lyman periosteotome

F. Smith needle holder
F. Smith orbital retractor
F. Smith pituitary rongeur
F. Smith punch
F. Smith rongeur forceps
F. Smith-Sewall orbital retractor
F. Smith-Sewall refractor
F. Smith-Spurling disk rongeur
F. Smith-Spurling intervertebral disk
  forceps
F. Smith-Takahashi forceps
F. Smith-Takahashi rongeur
F. Smith tissue forceps

Ferrolite crown remover
ferromagnetic
f. intracerebral aneurysm clip
f. monitoring device
ferrule clamp
Ferszt
F. dissecting hook
F. ligature passer
fetal
F. Dopplex
F. Dopplex monitor
f. head extractor
f. heart rate monitor
f. incontinence collector
f. scalp electrode
f. stethoscope
f. vacuum extractor
Fetalert fetal heart rate monitor
FetalPulse
F. Plus fetal Doppler
F. Plus monitor
Fetasonde
F. fetal monitor
F. fetal monitoring system
Feth-R-Cath epidural catheter
fetoscope
Pinard f.
Fett carpal prosthesis
Feuerstein
F. drainage tube
F. split ventilation tube
F&F
filiform and follower
FG diamond bur
FG-series two-channel endoscope
fiber
braided polyester f.
carbon f.
f. cleaver
C. R. Bard Urolase f.
Endostat disposable sterile f.
FiberLase flexible f.
laser f.
Laserscope disposable Endostat f.
f. mallet
Micro Link endoscope f.
micro-thin plastic f.
nonmedullated nerve f.
Pinnacle contact Nd:YAG f.
Prolase f.
SLT FiberTact/Contact laser f.
UltraLine Nd:YAG laser f.

Urolase neodymium:YAG laser f.
Versatome laser f.
fibercolonoscope
Olympus CF-20 f.
fiberendoscope
fibergastroscope
fluorescence f.
fiberglass
f. bandage
f. graft
f. staff
FiberLase
F. beam delivery system
F. flexible fiber
F. laser
Fiberlite microscope
fiber-metal peg
fiberoptic
f. anoscope
f. arthroscope
f. bronchoscope
f. catheter delivery system
f. choledochoscope
f. endoscope
f. esophagoscope
f. gastroscope
f. hysteroscope
f. light cable
f. light carrier
f. lighted mirror
f. light pipe
f. light projector
f. light source
f. loupe
f. microscope
f. otoscope
f. oximeter catheter
f. PCO_2 sensor
f. pick
f. pressure catheter
f. probe
f. proctosigmoidoscope
f. retractor
f. right-angle telescope
f. sheath
f. sigmoidoscope
f. slide laryngoscope
f. suction tube
f. surgical field illuminator
f. vaginal speculum
f. videoendoscope
f. video glasses
fiberscope
Hirschowitz gastroduodenal f.
nasopharyngeal f.
Olympus GIF Q30 f.
Olympus OES f.
Olympus XK-series oblique-viewing
  flexible f.
Pentax f.
side-viewing f.
superfine f.
fiberTome
f. system

F

Fibracol collagen alginate wound dressing
Fibra Sonics phaco aspirator
Fibrel gelatin matrix implant
Fibre-Lite septal elevator
fibrin
    f. film stent
    f. glue
    f. glue adhesive
    f. glue-soaked Gelfoam
    f. sealant adhesive
fibroid hook
fibrotome
    Pelosi f.
fibrous shell
Fichman suture-cutting forceps
Ficoll-Hypaque gradient centrifuge
FiddleLink hand exerciser
fiducial marker
FIDUS probe
field
    F. blade
    f. emission tube
    f. expander
    F. tourniquet
field-effect transistor
field-of-view camera
figure-of-eight
    f.-o.-e. bandage
    f.-o.-e. brace
    f.-o.-e. clavicle strap
    f.-o.-e. dressing
    f.-o.-e. suture
filament
    Charcot-Bottcher f.
    cytokeratin f.
    desmin f.
    Semmes-Weinstein pressure aesthesiometer f.
    f. suture
    f. transformer
    vimentin f.
filamentary keratome
Filcard
    F. temporary removable vena cava filter
    F. vena cava filter
fil D'Arion silicone tube
file
    Aagesen f.
    bone f.
    Charnley trochanter f.
    f. elevator
    endodontic f.
    end-Z f.
    Flexicut f.
    Flex-R-File f.
    Hedstrom f.
    Kerr K-Flex f.
    K-Flexofile f.
    Kleinert-Kutz bone f.
    K root canal f.
    Lightspeed f.
    McXIM f.
    Miller bone f.

    Mity Gates Glidden f.
    Mity Hedström f.
    Mity Turbo File f.
    nickel-titanium f.
    Nordent bone f.
    Onyx-R NiTi f.
    orthopedic bone f.
    ProFile f.
    pulp canal f.
    Putti bone f.
    root canal f.
    Schwed Flexicut f.
    scrub f.
    SMIC bone f.
    SMIC periodontal f.
    S root canal f.
    SureFlex nickel-titanium f.
    surgical f.
    taper hand f.
filiform
    f. bougie
    f. bougie probe
    f. catheter
    f. dressing
    f. and follower (F&F)
    f. guide
    LeFort f.
    Rusch f.
    f. steel needle
    f. stone dislodger
filiform-tipped catheter
Fillauer
    F. bar
    F. dorsiflexion assist ankle joint
    F. endoskeletal alignment system
    F. night splint
    F. PDC ankle joint
    F. prosthesis liner
    F. Scottish Rite orthosis kit
    F. silicone suspension liner
filler
    BIO-OSS maxillofacial bone f.
    BonePlast bone void f.
    Cutinova cavity wound f.
    OsteoSet bone f.
    paste f.
    ProOsteon implant 500 coralline hydroxyapatite bone void f.
    spiral f.
    Springlite toe f.
film
    Accufilm articulating f.
    Accu-Flo dural f.
    f. alternator
    autoradiographic f.
    Bard protective barrier f.
    f. changer
    Dentus x-ray f.
    Duncan dural f.
    DuPont Cronex x-ray f.
    E-speed intraoral f.
    GLP7 f.
    Knuttsen bending f.
    Kodak XAR-5 x-ray f.
    Kodak XRP-1 x-ray f.

MDS Truspot articulating f.
3M No Sting barrier f.
No Sting barrier f.
orthogonal f.
Repel bioresorbable barrier f.
Softopac intraoral f.
soft x-ray f.
vaginal contraceptive f.
f. wound dressing

Filshie
F. clip minilaparotomy applicator
F. female sterilization clip

filter
ACE autografter bone f.
Adams kidney stone f.
Amicon D-20 f.
arterial f.
bacterial f.
bandpass f.
Baxter CA-210 f.
Berkefeld f.
bidirectional four-pole Butterworth high-pass digital f.
Biospal f.
bird's nest IVC f.
Butterworth bidirectional four-pole high-pass digital f.
Centricon-10 f.
charcoal f.
Coloplast one-piece closed pouch with f.
Coloplast two-piece stoma cap with f.
Cook f.
D/Flex f.
electrosurgical f.
Encapsulon TFX-Medical bacterial f.
Falcon f.
Filcard temporary removable vena cava f.
Filcard vena cava f.
flattening f.
fluorescence excitation f.
Fresenius F-40 f.
Gambro FH88H f.
Gene Screen nylon membrane f.
Gianturco-Roehm bird's nest vena cava f.
Greenfield titanium inferior vena cava (IVC) f.
Haag-Streit 900 cobalt blue f.
Hamming-Hahn f.
Hann f.
HEPA f.
heparin arterial f.
high-pass f.
Holter in-line shunt f.
Hospal Biospal f.
Hybond-N-f.
inferior vena cava umbrella f.
inherent f.
Interface arterial blood f.
interference barrier f.
Jostra arterial blood f.
Kalman f.

K-edge f.
Kim-Ray Greenfield antiembolus f.
Kim-Ray Greenfield vena cava f.
K-37 pediatric arterial blood f.
LeukoNet f.
LGM f.
Liposorber cholesterol f.
low-pass f.
f. maintainer
mediastinal sump f.
Medi-Tech IVC f.
Millex GS-series f.
Millex GV-series f.
Millipore ultrafree-CL centrifugal f.
Mobin-Uddin umbrella vena cava f.
f. mold
monomer f.
Nalzene f.
f. needle
neutral density f.
notch f.
Pall Biomedical heat- and moisture-exchanging f.
Pall ELD-96 Set Saver f.
Pall leukocyte removal f.
Pall transfusion f.
f. paper
Percoll f.
Portex bacterial f.
power peak f.
PreVENT Anti-Reflux f.
red-free f.
Re/Flex f.
Renal System HF250 f.
rhodium f.
F. Security closed mini-pouch
shunt f.
Simon nitinol inferior vena cava (IVC) f.
Steriflex-Braun bacterial f.
suprarenal Greenfield f.
Swank high-flow arterial blood f.
Thoreau f.
tunable notch f.
umbrella f.
UV blocking f.
Vena Tech dual vena cava f.
Vena Tech-LGM vena cava f.
wedge f.
Wiener MRI f.
William Harvey arterial blood f.
Wratten 6B f.
Zeta probe nylon f.

filtered
f. dual-sump drain
f. mediastinal sump drain
f. specimen trap

FiltraCheck-UTI
Filtryzer dialyzer
Filtzer
F. corkscrew
F. interbody rasp

fin
convertible f.

F

fin *(continued)*
    double-catheterizing f.
    prosthesis f.
final-cut acetabular reamer
Finapres
    F. blood pressure monitor
    F. Dinamap blood pressure machine
    F. finger cuff
finder
    Carabelli lumen f.
    Damian lumen f.
    Dasco Pro angle f.
    gravity-driven angle f.
    hamate f.
    Hedwig lumen f.
    IMP Femur F.
    lumen f.
    Moore direction f.
    pedicle f.
    Tucker vertebrated lumen f.
Findley folding pessary
fine
    f. arterial forceps
    f. chromic suture
    F. corneal carrying case
    F. crescent fixation ring
    f. curette
    f. dissecting forceps
    F. folding block
    f. intestinal needle
    F. magnetic implant
    F. micropoint cautery
    F. micropoint electrocautery
    f. olive bur
    f. silk suture
    F. suture scissors
    F. suture-tying forceps
    f. tissue forceps
fine-angled curette
fine-bore catheter
Fine-Castroviejo suturing forceps
fine-cup forceps
Fine-Gill corneal knife
fine-line tissue marker
fine-mesh dressing
fine-needle electrode
Finesse
    F. cardiac device
    F. large-lumen guiding catheter
Fine-Thornton scleral fixation ring
fine-tipped
    f.-t. mosquito hemostat
    f.-t. up-and-down-angled bipolar
      forceps
fine-tooth
    f.-t. clamp
    f.-t. forceps
fine-wire
    f.-w. electrode
    f.-w. speculum
finger
    F. Blocking Tree
    f. circumference gauge
    f. clip sensor

    f. cot
    f. cot dressing
    f. cot splint
    f. cuff
    f. exerciser
    f. extension clockspring splint
    F. Fitness Spring Ball
    f. flexion glove
    f. flexion splint
    f. gauze
    f. goniometer
    F. Helper hand exerciser
    f. hook
    f. indicator
    f. joint implant
    f. ladder
    f. loop
    mechanical f.
    F. Phantom pulse oximeter testing
      system
    f. plate
    F. Platter hand exerciser
    f. rake retractor
    f. ring cutter
    f. ring saw
    f. separator
    f. sling
Finger-Hugger splint
fingernail drill
FingerPrint oximeter
fingertrap
    Japanese f.
    MicroDigitrapper-HR f.
    MicroDigitrapper-S f.
    MicroDigitrapper-V f.
    f. suture
finish bur
finisher
    Küntscher f.
finishing bur
Finite dental glazing compound
Fink
    F. biprong marker
    F. cataract aspirator
    F. chalazion curette
    F. cul-de-sac cannula
    F. cul-de-sac irrigator
    F. fixation forceps
    F. lacrimal retractor
    F. laryngoscope
    F. muscle marker
    F. oblique muscle hook
    F. refractor
    F. tendon tucker
    F. tendon-tucker forceps
    F. valve
Fink-Jameson oblique muscle forceps
Fink-Rowland keratome
Fink-Scobie hook
Fink-Weinstein two-way syringe
Finn
    F. chamber
    F. chamber patch test device
    F. knee revision prosthesis
    F. knee revision system

finned pacemaker lead
finned-stem punch
Finney
    F. Flexirod penile prosthesis
    F. mask
    F. penile implant
Finnoff
    F. laryngoscope
    F. sinus transilluminator
Finochietto
    F. arterial clamp
    F. bronchial clamp
    F. clamp carrier
    F. hand retractor
    F. infant rib contractor
    F. infant rib retractor
    F. laminectomy retractor
    F. lobectomy forceps
    F. needle
    F. needle holder
    F. rib spreader
    F. stirrup
    F. thoracic forceps
    F. thoracic scissors
Finochietto-Burford
    F.-B. rib contractor
    F.-B. rib spreader
Finochietto-Geissendorfer rib retractor
Finochietto-Stille rib spreader
Finsen
    F. bath
    F. lamp
    F. retractor
    F. tracheal hook
    F. wound hook
Finsterer
    F. myringotomy split tube
    F. suction tube
FIN system
Firlene eye magnet
Firlit-Sugar intermittent catheter   I-Cath
Firm D-Ring wrist support
FirmFlex
    F. custom orthosis
    F. custom orthotic
FIRST
    F. knee prosthesis
first
    F. Beat ultrasound stethoscope
    F. Quality belted undergarment
    F. Quality full fit brief
    F. Quality high performance and
      nighttime underpad
    F. Quality overnight brief with leg
      cuff
    F. Quality pad insert and pant
    F. Response manual resuscitator
    f. rib shears
    F. Step select low-air overlay
FirstChoice
    F. closed pouch
    F. post-operative drainable pouch
    F. urostomy pouch
FirstQ departure alert system
FirstSave automated external defibrillator

FirstStep
    F. mattress
    F. tibial osteotomy instruments
FirstTemp Genius tympanic thermometer
Firtel broach
Fisch
    F. bone drill irrigator
    F. cutting bur
    F. drill
    F. dural hook
    F. dural retractor
    F. microcrurotomy scissors
Fischer
    F. cannula
    F. modular stereotaxic system
    F. nasal rasp
    F. & Paykel HC100 heated
      humidifier
    F. pneumothoracic needle
    F. tendon stripper
Fischer-Leibinger bur hole-mounted
  fixation device
Fischl dissecting forceps
Fischmann angiotribe forceps
Fish
    F. antral probe
    F. grasping forceps
    F. infusion cannula
    F. inlet
    F. nasal-dressing forceps
    F. sinus probe
Fisher
    F. Accumet pH meter
    F. advancement forceps
    F. bed
    F. brace
    F. capsular forceps
    F. double-ended retractor
    F. eye needle
    F. eye spoon
    F. fenestrated lid retractor
    F. half pin
    F. iris forceps
    F. lid retractor
    F. microcapillary tube reader
    F. spud
    F. tape board
    F. tonsillar dissector
    F. tonsillar knife
    F. tonsillar retractor
    F. ventricular cannula
Fisher-Arlt iris forceps
fisherman's pliers
Fisher-Nugent retractor
Fisher-Paykel
    F.-P. heated humidifier
    F.-P. MR290 water-feed chamber
    F.-P. RD1000 resuscitator
Fisher-plus slide
Fisher-Smith spatula
fishhook
    f. lead
    f. needle
fishtail
    f. burnisher

F

fishtail *(continued)*
    f. chisel
    f. spatula
    f. spatula raspatory
Fiskars scissors
Fiske periosteal elevator
Fisk tractor
Fisons
    F. indirect binocular ophthalmoscope
    F. nebulizer
fissure
    f. bur
    f. burnisher
fistula
    Cimino f.
    Cimino-Brescia arteriovenous f.
    Gore-Tex aortofemoral (AF) f.
    f. hook
    f. needle
    f. probe
    f. scissors
fistulotome
    needle-knife f.
Fitch obturator
Fit-Lastic therapy band
Fitnet joint testing system
Fits-All sling
Fitstep
    F. II stair climber
    Universal F.
fitting
    Luer lock f.
    Shrader f.
Fitz-all fabric leg strap
Fitzgerald
    F. aortic aneurysm clamp
    F. aortic aneurysm forceps
Fitzpatrick suction tube
Fitzwater
    F. ligature carrier
    F. peanut sponge-holding forceps
five-pin staple
five-prong rake blade retractor
Fixateur
    F. Interne fixation system
    F. Interne rod
    F. Interne screw
fixation
    AO rigid f.
    f. apparatus
    f. bandage
    f. base
    f. binocular forceps
    f. button
    f. device
    ECT internal fracture f.
    f. jig
    Kempf internal screw f.
    Kirschner pin f.
    Kirschner wire f.
    LactoSorb resorbable
      craniomaxillofacial f.
    Microplate f.
    Modulock posterior spinal f.

    Obwegeser-Dalpont internal screw f.
    OrthoFrame external f.
    OrthoSorb pin f.
    f. pick
    f. pin
    ReUnite hand f.
    ReUnite VersaTile f.
    f. ring
    f. screw
    Searcy f.
    Seidel intramedullary f.
    SOF'WIRE spinal f.
    Spiessel internal screw f.
    Steinhauser internal screw f.
    Turvy internal screw f.
    f. twist hook
    Wolvek sternal approximation f.
fixation/anchor forceps
fixator
    Ace-Fischer external f.
    articulated external f.
    Bay external f.
    biplanar f.
    circular external f.
    Clyburn Colles fracture f.
    DeBastiani external f.
    dynamic axial f.
    EBI external f.
    Edwards D-L modular f.
    external spinal skeletal f.
    Herbert screw f.
    Hex-Fix monolateral external f.
    hinged articulated f.
    Hoffmann external f.
    HTO f.
    Ilizarov circular external f.
    Ilizarov external ring f.
    Ilizarov hybrid f.
    Kessler external f.
    mini-Hoffmann external f.
    mini-Orthofix f.
    Monofixateur external f.
    Olerud internal f.
    Orthofix monolateral femoral
      external f.
    Oxford f.
    Pennig dynamic wrist f.
    Rezinian spinal f.
    spanning external f.
    Stableloc Colles fracture external f.
    Stuhler-Heise f.
    thin-wire Ilizarov f.
    Thomas f.
    Vermont spinal f.
fixed
    f. appliance
    f. arch bar
    f. bearing knee implant
    f. cervical dilator
    f. dressing
    f. expansion prosthesis
    f. femoral head prosthesis
    f. forceps
    f. mandibular implant
    f. ring retractor

fixed-angle AO bladeplate
fixed-beam portal
fixed-focus scope
fixed-offset guide
fixed-rate
    f.-r. asynchronous atrial pacemaker
    f.-r. asynchronous ventricular
      pacemaker
fixed-wire balloon
Fizeau-Tolansky interferometer
Flagg
    F. laryngoscope
    F. stainless steel laryngoscope blade
flame
    f. bur
    f. ionization detector
    f. photometric detector
flame-tip bur
flamingo antrostomy forceps
Flanagan spinal fusion gouge
flange
    adhesive f.
    Callahan f.
    ConQuest female continence system
      pressure pad with preattached f.
    ConQuest male continence system
      condom catheter with
      preattached f.
    endoprosthetic f.
    Scuderi-Callahan f.
flanged Teflon tube
Flannery ear speculum
flap
    f. demarcator
    E-Z F.
    f. knife
    f. knife dissector
    Leibinger E-Z f.
    peg f.
FlapMaker
    F. disposable microkeratome
    F. microkeratome system
Flared
flared
    f. ABS tip
    F. patch mesh
    f. spinal rod
FlashCast
    Delta-Lite F.
flashlamp
    f. pulsed Nd:YAG laser
    f. pumped pulsed dye laser
FlashPoint optical localizer
Flash portable spirometer
flask
    Dewar f.
    Falcon plastic f.
    tissue culture f.
flat
    f. back curette
    f. bottom reservoir
    f. brain spatula support
    f. burnisher
    f. drill
    f. eye bandage

    f. needle spud
    f. spatula
    f. spatula electrode
    f. spatula needle
    f. tenotomy hook
    f. wire coil stent
flat-bladed nasal speculum
flat-blade-tipped catheter
flat-bottomed Kerrison rongeur
Flateau oval punch
flat-end cutter
flat-panel megavoltage imager
Flatt
    F. driver
    F. finger prosthesis
    F. implant
flattened irrigating cannula
flattening filter
F&L attenuating gloves
flat-tip electrode
flatware
    Cushion Grip f.
    Melaware f.
flat-wire eye electrode
flavine wool mold
Flaxedil suture
Fleischer ring
Fleish No. 2 pneumotachograph
Fleming
    F. afterloading tandem
    F. conization instrument
    F. ovoid
Flents breast comfort pack
Fletcher
    F. afterloader
    F. dressing forceps
    F. sponge forceps
    F. tonsillar knife
Fletcher-Delclos dome cylinder
Fletcher-Pierce cannula
Fletcher-Suit
    F.-S. afterloading tandem
    F.-S. applicator
    F.-S. polyp forceps
    F.-S. tandem and ovoid
Fletcher-Suit-Delclos
    F.-S.-D. system
    F.-S.-D. tandem
Fletcher-Van
    F.-V. Doren sponge-holding forceps
    F.-V. Doren uterine forceps
Fletching femoral hernia implant
  material
Fleurant bladder trocar
FLEX
    F. H/A total ossicular prosthesis
Flex
    F. Foam brace
    F. foam dressing
    F. Foam orthosis
    F. stent
    F. Tip guidewire
Flexacryl hard rebase acrylic
Flex-Aid knuckle dressing
Flexblock

F

Flex-Cath
    F.-C. double-lumen intra-aortic balloon catheter
FlexComp/DSP
Flexcon lens
FlexDerm
    F. hydrogel sheet
    F. wound dressing
FlexDial stimulus control
flexer
    X-TEND-O knee f.
Flex-E-Z wax
Flexfilm wound dressing
Flex-Foot prosthesis
Flexguard tip catheter
Flexguide intubation guide
flexible
    f. angioscope
    f. aortic clamp
    f. arm
    f. arm microretractor
    f. aspiration needle
    f. bandage
    f. biopsy needle
    f. blade osteotome
    f. bronchoscopy simulator
    f. cardiac valve
    f. delivery device
    f. digital implant
    f. Dualens implant
    f. endoscopic overtube
    f. endosonography probe
    f. fallopian tube endoscope
    f. fiberoptic bronchoscope
    f. fluoropolymer
    f. fluoropolymer contact lens
    f. foreign body forceps
    f. forward-viewing panendoscope
    f. fulgurating electrode
    f. gastroscope
    f. guidewire
    f. injection needle
    f. intramedullary nail
    f. laminar bone strip
    f. metal catheter
    f. nasopharyngoscope
    f. Olympus GF-eUM3 device
    f. optical biopsy forceps
    f. pump
    f. radiothermal electrode
    f. reamer
    f. retractor pressure clamp
    f. retractor sliding clamp
    f. rod penile implant
    f. sigmoidoscope
    f. socket
    f. sound
    f. surface coil
    f. surface-coil-type resonator
    f. translimbal iris retractor
    f. ureteroscope
    f. vascular clamp
    f. video laparoscope
    f. wand
    f. wire electrode

flexible-loop
    f.-l. anterior chamber intraocular lens
    f.-l. posterior chamber intraocular lens
flexible, steerable nasolaryngopharyngoscope
flexible-tip Bentsen guidewire
flexible-wire bundle reamer
Flexicair
    F. eclipse low-air-loss therapy unit
    F. II low-air-loss therapy unit bed
    F. MC3 low-air-loss therapy unit bed
Flexi-Cath
    F.-C. double-lumen intra-aortic balloon catheter
    F.-C. silicone subclavian cannula
Flexicon gauze bandage
Flexicut file
Flexi-Flate
    F.-F. I, II penile prosthesis
    F.-F. penile implant
Flexiflo
    F. enteral feeding tube
    F. enteral pump
    F. feeding pump
    F. gastrostomy tube enteral delivery system
    F. Inverta-PEG gastrostomy kit
    F. Inverta-PEG tube
    F. Lap G laparoscopic gastrostomy kit
    F. Lap J laparoscopic jejunostomy kit
    F. over-the-guidewire gastrostomy kit
    F. Sacks-Vine tube
    F. Stomate low-profile gastrostomy tube
    F. suction feeding tube
    F. tap-fill enteral tube
    F. Taptainer tube
    F. tungsten-weighted feeding tube
    F. Versa-PEG tube
FlexiGel
    F. gel sheet dressing
    F. strands
Flexigrid dressing
Flexi-Guard
Flexilite conforming elastic bandage
Flexima
    F. biliary stent
Flexinet dressing
flexion glove
Flexipost
Flexi-Rod
    F.-R. II penile implant
    F.-R. penile prosthesis
Flexiscope arthroscope
Flexi-Seal
    F.-S. fecal collector
    F.-S. fecal collector & tail clip
FlexiSensor sensor

Flexisplint
F. arm board
FlexiSport orthotic
Flexistone impression material
Flexi-Therm
F.-T. diabetic diagnostic insole
F.-T. liquid crystal system
Flexitip catheter
Flexitone suture
Flexi-Trak skin anchoring device
Flexi-Ty vessel band
Flexlens lens
Flexlite
Zelco F.
FlexLite hinged knee support
Flexner-Worst iris claw lens
FlexoFiles
Dentsply F.
Flex-O-Jet aspirator
flexometer
Moeltgen f.
Flexon steel suture
Flexoreamer Batt tip
flexor hinge hand splint brace
Flexo wax
FlexPosure endoscopic retractor
Flex-R-File file
Flex-Rite lumbar support
Flexseat cushion
Flexsteel ribbon retractor
FlexStent stent
FlexStrand cable
Flextender Plus hand exerciser
FlexTip
Arrow Blue F.
F. intervertebral rongeur
FLEX-WRAP self-adherent wrap
Flexxicon
F. Blue dialysis catheter
F. II PC internal jugular catheter
Flexzan
F. Extra dressing
F. topical wound dressing
F. L. Fischer
F. L. F. microsurgical neurectomy
bayonet scissors
F. L. F. modular stereotaxy system
Flieringa
F. fixation ring
F. scleral ring
Flieringa-Kayser fixation ring
Flieringa-LeGrand fixation ring
FlimFax teleradiology system
Flint glass speculum
flip-flap
Mathieu-Horton-Devine f.-f.
Flip-Flop pillow
FLOAM ankle stirrup brace
floating
f. catheter
f. disk heart valve
f. lead
f. table
Flocare 500 feeding pump

Flo-Fit
F.-F. Comfortseat
F.-F. cushion
Flo-Gard pump
FloGUN suction/irrigation control handle
FloMap
F. guidewire
F. velocimeter
floor-standing surgical light
floppy
f. tip guidewire
floppy-tipped guidewire
Flo-Restors backbleeding control device
Florex medical compression stockings
Florida
F. back brace
F. cervical brace
F. contraflexion brace
F. extension brace
F. hyperextension brace
F. J-24, J-35, J-45, J-55 brace
F. post-fusion brace
F. spinal brace
F. urinary pouch
Flo-Stat
F.-S. fluid management system
F.-S. fluid monitor
flotation
f. catheter
f. gel pad
Phoenix Powerloft series I, II
alternating air f.
Flote
Bio F.
Flo-Tech prosthetic socket
Flotem IIe fluid-warming device
Flo-Thru intraluminal shunt
Flo-Trol drinking cup
flow
f. cytometer
f. meter
f. probe
f. regulated suction tube
flow-assisted
f.-a. short-term (FAST)
f.-a. short-term balloon catheter
flow-directed
f.-d. balloon cardiovascular catheter
f.-d. balloon-tipped catheter
f.-d. thermodilution catheter
Flowers
F. Mandibular Glove implant
F. Tear Trough implant
FlowGel barrier material
FlowGun suction-irrigator
FloWire
Doppler F.
F. Doppler catheter
F. Doppler guidewire
flowmeter, flow meter
Asthma Check peak f.
clinical electromagnetic f.
Dantec rotating disk f.
Dantec Urodyn 1000 f.
Dienco f.

F

flowmeter *(continued)*
> Doppler ultrasonic f.
> Doppler ultrasound f.
> electromagnetic f.
> Gould electromagnetic f.
> Heidelberg retinal f.
> infrared laser-Doppler f.
> laser Doppler f.
> Life-Tech f.
> MBF3 infrared laser-Doppler f.
> mini-Wright peak f.
> Model 500F electromagnetic f.
> Narcomatic f.
> Parks bidirectional Doppler f.
> Personal Best peak f.
> Pocketpeak peak f.
> preVent Pneumotach f.
> pulsed Doppler ultrasonic f.
> Statham f.
> transit-time f.
> Transonic f.
> Wright peak f.

flowmetry
> laser Doppler f.
> Periflux 3 laser-Doppler f.

flow-over vaporizer
flow-oximetry catheter
FLOWPLUS therapeutic pneumatic compression system
flowprobe
> endoscopic f.

flow-regulator clamp
Flow Rider neurovascular catheter
flow-sensing spirometer
Flowtron
> F. DVT compression device
> F. DVT external pneumatic compression system
> F. DVT prophylactic deep venous thrombosis unit
> F. DVT pump
> F. Excel DVI prophylaxis system
> F. thigh-high device

FlowWire Doppler guide wire
Floxite mirror light
Floyd
> F. loop cannula
> F. pneumothorax needle

Floyd-Barraquer wire speculum
Floyd-Grant erysiphake
fluff
> f. dressing
> dry sterile f.

fluffed gauze dressing
fluffy compression dressing
fluffy-cuffed tube
Fluftex
> F. gauze roll
> F. gauze rolls and sponge

Flu-Glow strip
Fluhrer
> F. bullet probe
> F. rectal probe

fluid
> f. control trauma pad
> f. warmer

Fluid-Air Plus bed
fluid-filled
> f.-f. balloon-tipped flow-directed catheter
> f.-f. pressure monitoring guidewire

Fluidics
> Concentrix F.

fluorescence
> f. detector
> f. excitation filter
> f. fibergastroscope

fluorescence-activated cell sorter
fluorescence-guided "smart" laser
fluorescent
> f. lamp
> f. optode
> f. probe

Fluorescite syringe
Fluor-i-Strip
FluoroCatcher
fluorodopa positron emission tomographic scan
Fluoro-Free
> P.A.S. Port F.-F.

fluorometer
> CytoFluor II f.
> scanning f.

fluorophotometer
> Fluorotron Master f.
> slit-lamp f.

FluoroPlus
> F. angiogram
> F. Roadmapper
> F. Roadmapper digital fluoroscopy
> F. Roadmapper digital fluoroscopy system

fluoropolymer
> flexible f.

fluoroptic
> f. thermometry probe
> f. thermometry system

FluoroScan
> F. C-arm fluoroscope
> F. C-arm fluoroscopy

fluoroscope
> C-arm f.
> Edison f.
> FluoroScan C-arm f.
> Xi-scan f.

fluoroscopic
> f. foreign body forceps
> f. imaging chair

fluoroscopy
> FluoroPlus Roadmapper digital f.
> FluoroScan C-arm f.

fluoroscopy-guided balloon dilator
Fluoro Tip ERCP cannula
Fluorotome double-lumen sphincterotome
Fluorotron
> Coherent radiation F.
> F. Master fluorophotometer

Fluotec vaporizer

flush chamber
flushing
    f. device
    f. reservoir
    f. valve
Flushmesh strap
flute
    f. cannula
    f. needle
fluted
    f. finishing bur
    f. J-Vac drain
    f. reamer
    f. Sampson nail
    f. stem punch
    f. titanium nail
flute-end right-angle drain
Flutter therapeutic device
Fluvog
    F. aspirator
    F. irrigator
FLX flexible treatment coilette
fly
    Titmus stereo f.
"flying spot" excimer laser system
Flynn
    F. lens loop
    F. scleral depressor
Flynt aortography needle
FMA cardiovascular imaging system
F-MAT screening system
F/M base curve contact lens
FMS Intracell stick
FNA-21 syringe
foam
    CarraSmart f.
    CIDA f.
    f. collar
    f. cube
    f. cube mattress
    DermaMend f.
    eggcrate f.
    Evazote f.
    hi-density f.
    Ivalon f.
    Neoplush f.
    nonadherent f.
    open-celled f.
    Pedilen polyurethane f.
    polyethylene f.
    polyvinyl alcohol f.
    prosthetic f.
    PV f.
    Reston polyurethane f.
    f. ring
    f. rubber vaginal stent
    f. tape
    Temper f.
    tube f.
    f. tubing
    f. wedge wheelchair cushion
    f. wound dressing
FOAMART foot impression system
FoaMTrac traction bandage
FocalSeal-R neurosurgical stent

focused, segmented, ultrasound machine
Focus PV catheter
Foerger airway
Foerster
    F. abdominal retractor
    F. capsulotomy knife
    F. enucleation snare
    F. gallbladder forceps
    F. iris forceps
    F. sponge forceps
    F. sponge-holding forceps
    F. surgical support brassiere
    F. tissue forceps
    F. uterine forceps
Foerster-Ballenger forceps
Foerster-Bauer sponge-holding forceps
Foerster-Mueller forceps
Foerster-Van Doren sponge-holding
    forceps
Fogarty
    F. adherent clot catheter
    F. arterial embolectomy catheter
    F. arterial irrigation catheter
    F. balloon
    F. balloon biliary catheter
    F. biliary balloon probe
    F. bulldog clamp-applying forceps
    F. calibrator
    F. dilation catheter
    F. embolus catheter
    F. gallstone catheter
    F. graft thrombectomy catheter
    F. Hydragrip clamp
    F. insert
    F. occlusion catheter
    F. Thru-Lumen catheter
    F. venous irrigation catheter
    F. venous thrombectomy catheter
Fogarty-Chin
    F.-C. clamp
    F.-C. extrusion balloon catheter
    F.-C. peripheral dilatation catheter
Fogarty-Hydragrip insert
Fogarty-Softjaw insert
fog reduction/elimination device
FOII powder inhaler
foil
    f. carrier
    crumpled aluminum f.
    scattering f.
    f. sheet
    Shimstock occlusion f.
    titanium f.
Foille dressing
Folatex catheter
foldable intraocular lens
folded aluminum ear splint
folder
    Faulkner f.
    intraocular lens f.
fold forceps
folding
    f. blade
    f. forceps

F

folding *(continued)*
>   f. laryngoscope
>   f. lens

fold-over finger splint

Foley
>   F. acorn-bulb catheter
>   F. balloon
>   F. balloon catheter
>   F. cone-tip catheter
>   F. Cordostat
>   F. hemostatic bag
>   F. plate
>   F. straight drain
>   F. three-way catheter
>   F. vas isolation forceps

Foley-Alcock
>   F.-A. bag
>   F.-A. catheter

follicle
>   f. electrode
>   f. expressor

follower
>   filiform and f. (F&F)
>   Le Fort f.
>   Rusch f.

Foltz
>   F. catheter
>   F. flushing reservoir
>   F. needle

Foltz-Overton cardiac catheter

Fome-Cuf
>   F.-C. endotracheal tube
>   F.-C. laser kit
>   F.-C. pediatric tracheostomy tube

Fomon
>   F. angular scissors
>   F. double-edge knife
>   F. facelift scissors
>   F. hook retractor
>   F. lower lateral scissors
>   F. nasal chisel
>   F. nasal hook
>   F. nasal rasp
>   F. nasal retractor
>   F. nostril elevator
>   F. osteotome
>   F. periosteal elevator
>   F. periosteotome
>   F. saber-back scissors
>   F. upper lateral scissors

Fonar
>   F. Quad MRI scanner
>   F. Stand-Up MRI scanner
>   F. system

Fonix
>   F. 6500-CX hearing aid test system
>   F. hearing aid

food extractor

foot
>   Cirrus composite prosthetic f.
>   College Park TruStep f.
>   ComfortWalk$_2$ prosthetic f.
>   f. cradle
>   f. drape

>   f. drop night splint
>   Dycor prosthetic f.
>   f. holder
>   F. Hugger foot support
>   Kingsley Steplite f.
>   F. Levelers custom orthotic
>   F. Levelers orthosis
>   f. magnet
>   f. model
>   multiaxis f.
>   f. orthotic device
>   Otto Bock 1A30 Greissinger Plus f.
>   Otto Bock 1D25 Dynamic Plus f.
>   f. pillow
>   f. rest
>   SACH f.
>   single-axis Syme DYCOR f.
>   f. stabilizer
>   f. stool
>   Sure-Flex III prosthetic f.
>   Syme Dycor prosthetic f.
>   The Beachcomber prosthetic f.
>   Trowbridge TerraRound f.
>   Vari-Flex prosthetic f.
>   f. volumeter
>   F. Waffle positioner

foot-ankle brace

footbrush
>   Dr. Joseph's f.

Footdeck Sport exercising footrest

footdrop
>   f. brace
>   f. stop

Foot-Fitter

footgear
>   COMED f.
>   COMED postsurgical f.

foothugger
>   RIK f.

footplate, foot plate
>   f. chisel
>   f. elevator
>   f. hook
>   f. pick

footrest
>   Footdeck Sport exercising f.

Foot-Station 3-D foot imaging system

foramen-plugging forceps

Forbes
>   F. esophageal speculum
>   F. uterine-dressing forceps

force
>   F. balloon
>   F. 2 CEM generator
>   f. fulcrum retractor
>   F. FX generator
>   F. GSU argon-enhanced electrosurgery system
>   F. GSU laparoscopic handset
>   f. transducer
>   F. wire

forced-air active cooling device

forced displacement transducer

forceps
>   Abbott-Mayfield f.

Abernaz strut f.
abscess f.
Absolok f.
ACMI Martin endoscopic f.
Acufex curved basket f.
Acufex rotary basket f.
Acufex straight basket f.
AcuTouch tissue f.
Adair-Allis tissue f.
Adair tissue f.
Adair tissue-holding f.
Adair uterine f.
adenoid f.
Adler bone f.
Adler-Kreutz f.
Adler punch f.
adnexal f.
Adson arterial f.
Adson bayonet dressing f.
Adson-Biemer f.
Adson bipolar f.
Adson brain f.
Adson-Brown f.
Adson-Brown tissue f.
Adson-Callison tissue f.
Adson clip-applying f.
Adson dressing f.
Adson hemostatic f.
Adson hypophyseal f.
Adson microbipolar f.
Adson microdressing f.
Adson microtissue f.
Adson-Mixter neurosurgical f.
Adson monopolar f.
Adson scalp clip-applying f.
Adson thumb f.
Adson tissue f.
Adson tooth f.
Adson-Vital tissue f.
advancement f.
Aesculap f.
Akins valve re-do f.
Alabama University f.
Alderkreutz tissue f.
Alexander dressing f.
Alexander-Farabeuf f.
Allen-Barkan f.
Allen-Braley f.
Allen intestinal f.
Allen uterine f.
alligator crimper f.
alligator cup f.
alligator ear f.
alligator nasal f.
Allis-Abramson breast biopsy f.
Allis-Adair intestinal f.
Allis-Adair tissue f.
Allis-Coakley tonsillar f.
Allis-Coakley tonsil-seizing f.
Allis delicate tissue f.
Allis-Duval f.
Allis intestinal f.
Allis Micro-Line pediatric f.
Allis-Ochsner tissue f.
Allis-Ochsner tonsillar f.

Allis thoracic f.
Allis-Willauer tissue f.
Almeida f.
Alvis fixation f.
Ambrose eye f.
Ambrose suture f.
Amdur lid f.
Amenabar capsular f.
American Catheter Corp. biopsy f.
AMO phacoemulsification lens-folder f.
anastomosis f.
Andrews-Hartmann f.
Andrews tonsillar f.
Andrews tonsil-seizing f.
aneurysm f.
Angell-James hypophysectomy f.
Angell-James punch f.
angiotribe f.
angled capsular f.
angled stone f.
Anis capsulotomy f.
Anis corneal f.
Anis corneoscleral f.
Anis intraocular lens f.
Anis microsurgical tying f.
Anis straight corneal f.
Anis tying f.
anterior capsule f.
anterior segment f.
Anthony-Fisher f.
antral f.
aortic aneurysm f.
aortic occlusion f.
Apfelbaum bipolar f.
Apple Medical bipolar f.
applicator f.
approximation f.
Archer splinter f.
Arrow articulation paper f.
Arrowsmith-Clerf pin-closing f.
Arrowsmith fixation f.
Arroyo f.
Arruga curved capsular f.
Arruga-Gill f.
Arruga-McCool capsular f.
arterial f.
Arthro Force basket cutting f.
Arthur splinter f.
articulating paper f.
Artilk f.
Asch septal f.
Asch septum-straightening f.
Ashby fluoroscopic foreign body f.
Ash dental f.
Ash septum-straightening f.
ASSI bipolar coagulating f.
Athens f.
atraumatic tissue f.
atraumatic visceral f.
aural f.
auricular appendage f.
Austin f.
Auto Suture f.
Autraugrip tissue f.

F

forceps *(continued)*
Auvard-Zweifel f.
axis-traction f.
Ayers chalazion f.
Azar intraocular f.
Azar lens f.
Azar tying f.
Azar utility f.
Babcock-Beasley f.
Babcock intestinal f.
Babcock lung-grasping f.
Babcock thoracic tissue f.
Babcock thoracic tissue-holding f.
Babcock-Vital atraumatic f.
Babcock-Vital intestinal f.
Babcock-Vital tissue f.
baby Adson f.
baby Allis f.
baby Crile f.
baby dressing f.
baby hemostatic f.
baby intestinal tissue f.
baby Lane bone-holding f.
baby Mikulicz f.
baby Mixter f.
baby mosquito f.
baby Overholt f.
backbiting f.
Backhaus f.
Backhaus-Roeder f.
Bacon cranial f.
Baer bone-cutting f.
Bahnson-Brown f.
Bailey aortic valve-cutting f.
Bailey chalazion f.
Bailey-Williamson obstetrical f.
Bainbridge hemostatic f.
Bainbridge intestinal f.
Bainbridge resection f.
Bainbridge thyroid f.
Baird chalazion f.
Baker tissue f.
Ball f.
Ballantine hysterectomy f.
Ballantine-Peterson hysterectomy f.
Ballen-Alexander f.
Ballenger-Foerster f.
Ballenger hysterectomy f.
Ballenger sponge f.
Ballenger tonsillar f.
Bane rongeur f.
Bangerter muscle f.
Banner f.
Bansal LASIK f.
Bard f.
Bardeleben bone-holding f.
Bard-Parker f.
Barkan iris f.
Barlow f.
Barnes-Crile hemostatic f.
Barnes-Hill f.
Barnes-Simpson obstetrical f.
Baron f.

Barracuda flexible cystoscopic hot biopsy f.
Barraquer ciliary f.
Barraquer conjunctival f.
Barraquer corneal f.
Barraquer fixation f.
Barraquer hemostatic mosquito f.
Barraquer-Katzin f.
Barraquer-Troutman corneal f.
Barraquer-von Mandach capsule f.
Barraquer-von Mandach clot f.
Barraya tissue f.
Barrett-Allen placental f.
Barrett-Allen uterine f.
Barrett intestinal f.
Barrett lens f.
Barrett-Murphy intestinal f.
Barrett placental f.
Barrett tenacular f.
Barrie-Jones angled crocodile f.
Barron alligator f.
Barsky f.
Barton obstetrical f.
basket f.
basket-cutting f.
basket-punch f.
basket-type crushing f.
Bauer dissecting f.
Bauer sponge f.
Baumberger f.
Baumgartner f.
Baum-Hecht tarsorrhaphy f.
Bausch articulation paper f.
bayonet bipolar f.
bayonet monopolar f.
bayonet root tip f.
BB shot f.
Bead ethmoidal f.
beaked cowhorn f.
bean f.
Beardsley f.
bearing-seating f.
Beasley-Babcock tissue f.
Beaupre ciliary f.
Beaupre epilation f.
Bechert lens-holding f.
Bechert-McPherson tying f.
Beck f.
Beebe hemostatic f.
Beebe wire-cutting f.
Beer ciliary f.
Behen ear f.
Behrend cystic duct f.
Bellucci ear f.
Benaron scalp-rotating f.
Bengolea arterial f.
Bennell f.
Bennett ciliary f.
Bennett epilation f.
Berens capsular f.
Berens corneal transplant f.
Berens muscle recession f.
Berens ptosis f.
Berens recession f.
Berens suturing f.

Berger biopsy f.
Bergeron pillar f.
Bergh ciliary f.
Berghmann-Foerster sponge f.
Bergman tissue f.
Berke ciliary f.
Berkeley Bioengineering ptosis f.
Berke ptosis f.
Bernard uterine f.
Berne nasal f.
Bernhard towel f.
Berry uterine-elevating f.
Best common duct stone f.
Best gallstone f.
Bettman-Noyes fixation f.
Bevan gallbladder f.
Bevan hemostatic f.
Beyer f.
B-H f.
BiCoag bipolar laparoscopic f.
Bierer ovum f.
Bigelow f.
Billroth uterine tumor f.
Bill traction handle f.
Binkhorst lens f.
binocular fixation f.
biopsy punch f.
biopsy specimen f.
bipolar bayonet f.
bipolar coagulating f.
bipolar coaptation f.
bipolar cutting f.
bipolar electrocautery f.
bipolar eye f.
bipolar irrigating f.
bipolar laparoscopic f.
bipolar long-shaft f.
bipolar suction f.
bipolar transsphenoidal f.
Bircher-Ganske meniscal cartilage f.
Bireks dissecting f.
Birkett hemostatic f.
Birks Mark II Colibri f.
Birks Mark II grooved f.
Birks Mark II microneedle-holder f.
Birks Mark II needle-holder f.
Birks Mark II straight f.
Birks Mark II suture-tying f.
Birks Mark II toothed f.
Birtcher endoscopic f.
Bishop-Harman dressing f.
Bishop-Harman foreign body f.
Bishop-Harman iris f.
Bishop-Harman tissue f.
Bishop tissue f.
bite biopsy f.
Bi-tec f.
biting f.
Björk diathermy f.
Björk-Stille diathermy f.
bladder specimen f.
Blade-Wilde ear f.
Blake dressing f.
Blake ear f.
Blake embolus f.

Blake gallstone f.
Blakesley ethmoid f.
Blakesley septal bone f.
Blakesley septal compression f.
Blakesley-Weil upturned ethmoid f.
Blakesley-Wilde ear f.
Blakesley-Wilde nasal f.
Blalock f.
Blalock-Kleinert f.
Blanchard hemorrhoidal f.
Bland cervical traction f.
Bland vulsellum f.
Blaydes angled lens f.
Blaydes corneal f.
Blaydes lens-holding f.
blepharochalasis f.
Block-Potts intestinal f.
Blohmka tonsillar f.
Bloodwell-Brown f.
Bloodwell tissue f.
Bloodwell vascular f.
Bloomberg lens f.
Blum f.
Blumenthal uterine dressing f.
blunt f.
Boer craniotomy f.
Boerma obstetrical f.
Boettcher arterial f.
Boettcher pulmonary artery f.
Boettcher-Schnidt f.
Boettcher tonsillar artery f.
Boies cutting f.
Bolton f.
Bonaccolto cup jaws f.
Bonaccolto fragment f.
Bonaccolto jeweler's f.
Bonaccolto magnet tip f.
Bonaccolto utility f.
Bond placental f.
bone-biting f.
bone-cutting double-action f.
bone-holding f.
bone punch f.
bone-reduction f.
bone-splitting f.
Bonn European suturing f.
Bonney tissue f.
Bonn iris f.
Bonn peripheral iridectomy f.
Bonn suturing f.
Bores corneal fixation f.
Bores U-shaped f.
Boruchoff f.
Boston Lying-In cervical f.
Botvin iris f.
Botvin vulsellum f.
Bouchayer grasping f.
Bovie coagulating f.
Bovino scleral-spreading f.
bowel f.
Bowen suction loose body f.
box-joint f.
Boys-Allis tissue f.
Bozeman-Douglas dressing f.
Bozeman LR dressing f.

F

forceps *(continued)*

Bozeman LR packing f.
Bozeman LR uterine-dressing f.
Bozeman uterine f.
Bozeman uterine-dressing f.
Bozeman uterine-packing f.
B-P transfer f.
Braasch bladder specimen f.
Bracken fixation f.
Bracken-Forkas corneal f.
Bracken iris f.
Bracken scleral fixation f.
Bradford thyroid f.
brain clip f.
brain dressing f.
brain spatula f.
brain tissue f.
brain tumor f.
Braithwaite f.
Brand passing f.
Brand shunt-introducing f.
Brand tendon-holding f.
Brand tendon-passing f.
Braun f.
Brenner f.
Bridge deep-surgery f.
Bridge hemostatic f.
Bridge intestinal f.
Brigham brain tumor f.
Brigham dressing f.
Brigham thumb tissue f.
Brigham 1x2 teeth f.
Brock biopsy f.
bronchial biopsy f.
bronchial-grasping f.
bronchoscopic biopsy f.
bronchus-grasping f.
Bronson-Magnion f.
Brophy dressing f.
Brophy tissue f.
Brown-Adson side-grasping f.
Brown-Bahnson bayonet f.
Brown-Buerger f.
Brown-Cushing f.
Brown side-grasping f.
Brown-Swan f.
Brown thoracic f.
Brown tissue f.
Broyles optical f.
Bruening-Citelli f.
Bruening cutting-tip f.
Bruening ethmoid exenteration f.
Bruening nasal-cutting septal f.
Bruening septal f.
Brunner intestinal f.
Brunner sigmoid anastomosis f.
Brunner tissue f.
Brunschwig arterial f.
Brunschwig visceral f.
Bryant nasal f.
Buck foreign body f.
Buerger-McCarthy bladder f.
Buie biopsy f.
Buie rectal f.

Buie specimen f.
bulldog clamp-applying f.
bullet f.
Bumpus specimen f.
Bunim urethral f.
Bunker modification of Jackson
  laryngeal f.
Buratto flap f.
Buratto LASIK f.
Buratto ophthalmic f.
Burch biopsy f.
Burford coarctation f.
Burnham biopsy f.
Burns bone f.
Butler bayonet f.
Bycep biopsy f.
Cairns-Dandy hemostasis f.
Cairns dissection f.
Cairns hemostatic f.
Calibri f.
Callahan scleral fixation f.
Callison-Adson tissue f.
Cameron-Miller type monopolar f.
Campbell ligature-carrier f.
Campbell ureteral f.
Cane bone-holding f.
cannulated bronchoscopic f.
capsular f.
capsule-grasping f.
capsulorhexis f.
capsulotomy f.
caput f.
Carb-Bite tissue f.
carbide-jaw f.
Cardio-Grip iliac f.
Cardio-Grip tissue f.
cardiovascular tissue f.
Cardona corneal prosthesis f.
Cardona threading lens f.
Carlens f.
Carmalt arterial f.
Carmalt hemostatic f.
Carmalt hysterectomy f.
Carmalt splinter f.
Carmalt thoracic f.
Carmody-Brophy f.
Carmody thumb tissue f.
carotid artery f.
Carrel hemostatic f.
Carrel mosquito f.
Carroll-Adson dural f.
Carroll bone-holding f.
Carroll dressing f.
Carroll tendon-passing f.
Carroll tendon-pulling f.
Carroll tissue f.
cartilage f.
cartilage-holding f.
Cartman lens insertion f.
caruncle f.
Caspar alligator f.
Cassidy-Brophy dressing f.
Castaneda-Mixter f.
Castaneda vascular f.
Castroviejo-Arruga capsular f.

Castroviejo capsular f.
Castroviejo capsule f.
Castroviejo clip-applying f.
Castroviejo-Colibri corneal f.
Castroviejo cornea-holding f.
Castroviejo corneoscleral f.
Castroviejo cross-action capsular f.
Castroviejo eye suture f.
Castroviejo fixation f.
Castroviejo-Furness cornea-holding f.
Castroviejo lid f.
Castroviejo scleral fold f.
Castroviejo-Simpson f.
Castroviejo suture f.
Castroviejo suturing f.
Castroviejo transplant f.
Castroviejo transplant-grafting f.
Castroviejo tying f.
Castroviejo wide grip handle f.
Catalano capsular f.
Catalano corneoscleral f.
Catalano tying f.
catheter-introducing f.
Cavanaugh-Wells tonsillar f.
center-action f.
cephalic blade f.
cervical biopsy f.
cervical grasping f.
cervical hemostatic f.
cervical punch f.
cervical traction f.
cesarean f.
chalazion f.
Chamberlen obstetrical f.
Championnière f.
Chandler iris f.
Chandler spinal-perforating f.
Chang bone-cutting f.
Chaput tissue f.
Charnley-Riches arterial f.
Charnley suture f.
Charnley wire-holding f.
Cheatle sterilizing f.
Cheron uterine dressing f.
Cherry f.
Cherry-Adson f.
Cherry-Kerrison f.
Chester sponge f.
Chevalier Jackson
  bronchoesophagoscopy f.
chicken-bill rongeur f.
Child clip-applying f.
Child intestinal f.
Child-Phillips f.
Children's Hospital dressing f.
Children's Hospital intestinal f.
Chimani pharyngeal f.
Choyce intraocular lens f.
Choyce lens-inserting f.
Christopher-Stille f.
Chubb tonsillar f.
Cicherelli f.
Cilco lens f.
cilia suture f.
Circon Tripolar f.

circular cup bronchoscopic biopsy f.
Citelli-Bruening ear f.
Citelli punch f.
Civiale f.
clamp f.
Clark capsule fragment f.
Clark-Guyton f.
Clark ligator scissor f.
Clark-Verhoeff capsular f.
claw f.
Clayman corneal f.
Clayman-Kelman intraocular lens f.
Clayman lens f.
Clayman lens-holding f.
Clayman lens-inserting f.
Clayman-McPherson tying f.
Clayman suturing f.
cleft palate f.
Clemetson uterine f.
Clerf f.
Clevedent f.
Cleveland bone-cutting f.
clip f.
clip-applying aneurysm f.
clip-bending f.
clip-cutting f.
clip-introducing f.
clip-removing f.
C. L. Jackson head-holding f.
C. L. Jackson pin-bending
  costophrenic f.
closed iris f.
closer f.
closing f.
clot f.
coagulating f.
coagulation f.
Coakley-Allis tonsillar f.
Coakley tonsillar f.
coaptation bipolar f.
coarctation f.
coated biopsy f.
Cobaugh eye f.
Codman fallopian tube f.
Codman ovary f.
Cohen corneal f.
Cohen nasal-dressing f.
cold biopsy f.
cold cup biopsy f.
Coleman-Taylor IOL f.
Colibri corneal f.
Colibri eye f.
Colibri-Pierse f.
Colibri-Storz corneal f.
College f.
Coller arterial f.
Coller hemostatic f.
Colley tissue f.
Colley traction f.
Collier-Crile hemostatic f.
Collier-DeBakey hemostatic f.
Collier hemostatic f.
Collin dressing f.
Collin-Duval-Crile intestinal f.
Collin-Duval intestinal f.

F

forceps *(continued)*

Collin intestinal f.
Collin lung-grasping f.
Collin mucous f.
Collin ovarian f.
Collin-Pozzi uterine f.
Collin tissue f.
Collin tongue f.
Collin tongue-seizing f.
Collin uterine-elevating f.
Collis-Maumenee corneal f.
Coloviras-Rumel thoracic f.
Colver-Coakley tonsillar f.
Colver tonsillar pillar-grasping f.
Colver tonsil-seizing f.
common duct-holding f.
common duct stone f.
common McPherson f.
compression f.
Cone wire-twisting f.
conjunctival fixation f.
connector f.
contact compressive f.
continuous clip f.
Cook flexible biopsy f.
Cooley anastomosis f.
Cooley aortic f.
Cooley arterial occlusion f.
Cooley auricular appendage f.
Cooley-Baumgarten aortic f.
Cooley cardiovascular f.
Cooley coarctation f.
Cooley curved f.
Cooley-Derra anastomosis f.
Cooley double-angled jaw f.
Cooley graft f.
Cooley iliac f.
Cooley neonatal vascular f.
Cooley patent ductus f.
Cooley pediatric aortic f.
Cooley peripheral vascular f.
Cooley tangential pediatric f.
Cooley tissue f.
Cooley vascular tissue f.
Cope lung f.
Coppridge grasping f.
Coppridge urethral f.
Corbett bone-cutting f.
Cordes esophagoscopy f.
Cordes-New laryngeal punch f.
Corey ovum f.
Corey placental f.
Corgill-Hartmann f.
cornea-holding f.
corneal fixation f.
corneal prosthesis f.
corneal splinter f.
corneal transplant f.
corneal utility f.
cornea-suturing f.
corneoscleral suturing f.
Cornet f.
coronary artery f.
Corson myoma f.

Corwin tonsillar f.
Cottle-Arruga cartilage f.
Cottle biting f.
Cottle insertion f.
Cottle-Jansen f.
Cottle-Kazanjian bone-cutting f.
Cottle-Kazanjian nasal f.
Cottle lower lateral f.
Cottle tissue f.
Cottle-Walsham septum-
  straightening f.
cowhorn tooth-extracting f.
Cozean angled lens f.
Cozean bipolar f.
Cozean implantation f.
Cozean-McPherson angled lens f.
Cozean-McPherson tying f.
Crafoord arterial f.
Crafoord bronchial f.
Crafoord coarctation f.
Crafoord pulmonary f.
Crafoord-Sellors hemostatic f.
Craig nasal-cutting f.
Craig septal f.
Craig septum bone-cutting f.
Craig tonsil-seizing f.
cranial f.
cranium clip-applying f.
Crawford fascial f.
Crawford-Knighton f.
Creevy biopsy f.
Crenshaw caruncle f.
Crile arterial f.
Crile-Barnes hemostatic f.
Crile-Duval lung-grasping f.
Crile gall duct f.
Crile hemostatic f.
Crile Micro-Line arterial f.
Crile-Rankin f.
crimper f.
crimping f.
Crockard ligament grasping f.
Crockard odontoid peg-grasping f.
crocodile biopsy f.
cross-action capsular f.
Crossen puncturing tenaculum f.
crural nipper f.
Cryer Universal f.
CSF shunt-introducing f.
Cukier nasal f.
Culler eye f.
Culler fixation f.
Cullom septal f.
cup biopsy f.
cup-biting f.
cupped f.
cup-shaped curette f.
cup-shaped inner ear f.
cup-shaped middle ear f.
curette f.
Curtis tissue f.
curved dissecting f.
curved iris f.
curved knot-tying f.
curved Maryland f.

curved microbipolar f.
curved micromonopolar f.
curved-tip jeweler's bipolar f.
curved tying f.
Cushing bayonet f.
Cushing bipolar neurosurgical f.
Cushing brain f.
Cushing-Brown tissue f.
Cushing cranial rongeur f.
Cushing decompression f.
Cushing dressing f.
Cushing-Gutsch dressing f.
Cushing-Gutsch tissue f.
Cushing monopolar f.
Cushing-Taylor carbide-jaw f.
Cushing thumb f.
Cushing tissue f.
Cushing-Vital tissue f.
Cutler f.
cutting f.
cylindrical-object f.
cystic duct f.
cystoscopic f.
Czerny tenaculum f.
Dahlgren-Hudson cranial f.
Dahlgren skill-cutting f.
Daicoff needle-pulling f.
Daicoff vascular f.
Dale femoral-popliteal anastomosis f.
Dallas lens-inserting f.
D'Allesandro serial suture-holding f.
Danberg iris f.
Dan chalazion f.
Dandy arterial f.
Dandy hemostatic f.
Dandy-Kolodny hemostatic f.
Dandy scalp hemostatic f.
Dan-Gradle ciliary f.
Dartigues kidney-elevating f.
Dartigues uterine-elevating f.
Davidson pulmonary vessel f.
Davis bayonet f.
Davis capsular f.
Davis coagulating f.
Davis diathermy f.
Davis monopolar bayonet f.
Davis sterilizing f.
Davis thoracic tissue f.
Davol rongeur f.
Dawson-Yuhl-Kerrison rongeur f.
Dawson-Yuhl-Leksell rongeur f.
Dawson-Yuhl rongeur f.
De Alvarez f.
Dean-Shallcross tonsil-seizing f.
Dean tonsillar f.
DeBakey aortic f.
DeBakey Autraugrip f.
DeBakey-Bainbridge vascular f.
DeBakey-Beck multipurpose f.
DeBakey-Coloviras-Rumel thoracic f.
DeBakey-Cooley cardiovascular f.
DeBakey-Derra anastomosis f.
DeBakey-Diethrich coronary artery f.
DeBakey-Diethrich vascular f.
DeBakey dissecting f.

DeBakey-Kelly hemostatic f.
DeBakey-Liddicoat vascular f.
DeBakey-Mixter thoracic f.
DeBakey-Péan cardiovascular f.
DeBakey-Rankin hemostatic f.
DeBakey-Reynolds anastomosis f.
DeBakey-Rumel thoracic f.
DeBakey-Semb f.
DeBakey tangential occlusion f.
DeBakey thoracic f.
DeBakey tissue f.
DeBakey vascular f.
Decker microsurgical f.
Deddish-Potts intestinal f.
deep-surgery f.
deep-vessel f.
Defourmental f.
De Juan f.
DeLee cervical f.
DeLee cervix-holding f.
DeLee dressing f.
DeLee obstetrical f.
DeLee ovum f.
DeLee shuttle f.
DeLee-Simpson f.
DeLee spoon tissue f.
DeLee uterine f.
DeLee uterine-packing f.
delicate thumb-dressing f.
Delrin locking-handle f.
Demarest septal f.
DeMartel appendix f.
DeMartel scalp flap f.
DeMartel-Wolfson closing f.
DeMartel-Wolfson intestinal-
  holding f.
Demel wire-tightening f.
Demel wire-twisting f.
Dench ear f.
Denis Browne tonsillar f.
Dennen f.
Dennis intestinal f.
dental dressing f.
depilatory dermal f.
Derf f.
DermaCare electrosurgical f.
Derra cardiovascular f.
Derra-Cooley f.
Derra urethral f.
D'Errico bayonet pituitary f.
D'Errico dressing f.
D'Errico hypophyseal f.
D'Errico tissue f.
Desjardins gallstone f.
Desjardins kidney pedicle f.
Desmarres chalazion f.
Desmarres lid f.
DeTakats-McKenzie brain clip-
  applying f.
DeVilbiss cranial f.
DeWecker f.
DeWeese axis traction obstetrical f.
Dewey obstetrical f.
Diaflex grasping f.
diathermic f.

F

forceps *(continued)*
  diathermy f.
  Dieffenbach f.
  Diener f.
  Dieter malleus f.
  Diethrich right-angled hemostatic f.
  dilating f.
  Dingman bone-holding f.
  disimpaction f.
  disk f.
  diskectomy f.
  disposable f.
  dissecting f.
  dissection f.
  divergent outlet f.
  Dixon flamingo f.
  Dixon-Lovelace hemostatic f.
  Dixon-Thorpe vitreous foreign
    body f.
  Docktor tissue f.
  Dodick lens-holding f.
  Dodick Nucleus Cracker f.
  Dodrill f.
  dolphin-billed grasping f.
  dolphin dissecting f.
  dolphin grasping f.
  dolphin-type atraumatic f.
  Donberg iris f.
  donor button f.
  Dorsey bayonet f.
  double-action bone-cutting f.
  double-action hump f.
  double-articulated bronchoscopic f.
  double-concave rat-tooth f.
  double-cupped f.
  double-ended needle f.
  double-ended suture f.
  double-ended tissue f.
  double-fixation f.
  double-pronged f.
  double-spoon biopsy f.
  Douglas ciliary f.
  Douglas eye f.
  Doyen gallbladder f.
  Doyen intestinal f.
  Doyen towel f.
  Doyen uterine f.
  Doyen vulsellum f.
  Draeger f.
  dressing f.
  Drews ciliary f.
  Drews intraocular f.
  Drews-Sato tying f.
  Dreyfus prosthesis f.
  drill guide f.
  duckbill f.
  Duguid curved f.
  dull-pointed f.
  dull rotation f.
  Dumont dissecting f.
  Dumont jeweler's f.
  Dumont Swiss dissecting f.
  Dunhill f.
  Duplay tenaculum f.

  Duracep biopsy f.
  dural f.
  Duval-Allis f.
  Duval-Collin intestinal f.
  Duval-Crile intestinal f.
  Duval-Crile lung f.
  Duval-Crile lung-grasping f.
  Duval-Crile tissue f.
  Duval intestinal f.
  Duval lung-grasping f.
  Duval lung tissue f.
  Duval-Vital intestinal f.
  DynaBite biopsy f.
  Dyonics basket f.
  ear-dressing f.
  ear-grasping f.
  ear polyp f.
  ear punch f.
  Eastman cystic duct f.
  Eber needle-holder f.
  Echlin rongeur f.
  Ecker-Kazanjian f.
  Eckhoff f.
  Eder f.
  Edna towel f.
  Effler-Groves cardiovascular f.
  Eisenstein hysterectomy f.
  electrocoagulating biopsy f.
  Electrosurgery f.
  electrosurgical biopsy f.
  elevating f.
  Elliott gallbladder f.
  Elliott hemostatic f.
  Elliott obstetrical f.
  Elschnig capsular f.
  Elschnig cyclodialysis f.
  Elschnig fixation f.
  Elschnig-O'Brien fixation f.
  Elschnig-O'Brien tissue-grasping f.
  Elschnig-O'Connor fixation f.
  Elschnig secondary membrane f.
  Elschnig tissue-grasping f.
  Emmet obstetrical f.
  end-biting f.
  Endo-Assist endoscopic f.
  endometrial polyp f.
  endoscopic biopsy f.
  endoscopic grasping f.
  endoscopic suture-cutting f.
  endospeculum f.
  Endo-therapy disposable biopsy f.
  endotracheal catheter f.
  endotracheal tube f.
  Endura dressing f.
  Englert f.
  English tissue f.
  Ennis f.
  entropion f.
  epilation f.
  episcleral f.
  Eppendorf cervical biopsy f.
  Ergo bipolar f.
  Erhardt eyelid f.
  Erich laryngeal biopsy f.

Ernest-McDonald soft intraocular lens-folding f.
Ernest-McDonald soft IOL folding f.
E-series bipolar f.
esophageal f.
esophagoscopic f.
Essrig tissue f.
ethmoidal f.
ethmoid-Blakesley f.
ethmoid-cutting f.
ethmoid punch f.
Ethridge hysterectomy f.
Evans-Vital tissue f.
Everett f.
Evershears bipolar laparoscopic f.
Ewald-Hudson brain f.
Ewald-Hudson dressing f.
Ewald-Hudson tissue f.
Ewald tissue f.
Ewing capsular f.
Excel disposable biopsy f.
exenteration f.
exolever f.
expansile f.
extracapsular f.
extracting f.
extraction f.
eye f.
eye-dressing f.
eye-fixation f.
eyelid f.
Facit uterine polyp f.
Falcao fixation f.
Falk lion-jaw f.
fallopian tube f.
Farabeuf bone-holding f.
Farabeuf-Lambotte bone-holding f.
Farnham nasal-cutting f.
Farrington nasal polyp f.
Farrington septal f.
Farrior wire-crimping f.
Farris tissue f.
Faure peritoneal f.
Faure uterine biopsy f.
Fauvel laryngeal f.
Fechtner conjunctiva f.
Fechtner ring f.
Fehland intestinal f.
Feilchenfeld splinter f.
fenestrated blade f.
fenestrated cup biopsy f.
fenestrated ellipsoid spiked open span biopsy f.
fenestrated spiked open span jumbo biopsy f.
Ferguson angiotribe f.
Ferguson bone-holding f.
Ferris colporrhaphy f.
Ferris Smith bone-biting f.
Ferris Smith cup rongeur f.
Ferris Smith fragment f.
Ferris Smith-Kerrison f.
Ferris Smith rongeur f.

Ferris Smith-Spurling intervertebral disk f.
Ferris Smith-Takahashi f.
Ferris Smith tissue f.
Fichman suture-cutting f.
fine arterial f.
Fine-Castroviejo suturing f.
fine-cup f.
fine dissecting f.
Fine suture-tying f.
fine-tipped up-and-down-angled bipolar f.
fine tissue f.
fine-tooth f.
Fink fixation f.
Fink-Jameson oblique muscle f.
Fink tendon-tucker f.
Finochietto lobectomy f.
Finochietto thoracic f.
Fischl dissecting f.
Fischmann angiotribe f.
Fisher advancement f.
Fisher-Arlt iris f.
Fisher capsular f.
Fisher iris f.
Fish grasping f.
Fish nasal-dressing f.
Fitzgerald aortic aneurysm f.
Fitzwater peanut sponge-holding f.
fixation/anchor f.
fixation binocular f.
fixed f.
flamingo antrostomy f.
Fletcher dressing f.
Fletcher sponge f.
Fletcher-Suit polyp f.
Fletcher-Van Doren sponge-holding f.
Fletcher-Van Doren uterine f.
flexible foreign body f.
flexible optical biopsy f.
fluoroscopic foreign body f.
Foerster-Ballenger f.
Foerster-Bauer sponge-holding f.
Foerster gallbladder f.
Foerster iris f.
Foerster-Mueller f.
Foerster sponge f.
Foerster sponge-holding f.
Foerster tissue f.
Foerster uterine f.
Foerster-Van Doren sponge-holding f.
Fogarty bulldog clamp-applying f.
fold f.
folding f.
Foley vas isolation f.
foramen-plugging f.
Forbes uterine-dressing f.
foreign body cystoscopy f.
foreign body eye f.
foreign body-retrieving f.
Förster iris f.
forward-grasping f.
Foss cardiovascular f.

F

forceps *(continued)*

Foss clamp f.
Foster-Ballenger f.
Fox bipolar electrocautery f.
Fox tissue f.
fragment f.
Francis spud chalazion f.
Frangenheim biopsy punch f.
Frangenheim hook f.
Fränkel cutting-tip f.
Fränkel esophagoscopy f.
Fränkel laryngeal f.
Fränkel tampon f.
Frankfeldt grasping f.
Fraser f.
Freer-Gruenwald punch f.
Freer septal f.
French-pattern f.
Fricke arterial f.
Friedman rongeur f.
Fry nasal f.
Fuchs capsular f.
Fuchs capsule f.
Fuchs capsulotomy f.
Fuchs extracapsular f.
Fuchs iris f.
Fujinon biopsy f.
Fulpit tissue f.
Furness cornea-holding f.
Furness polyp f.
Gabriel Tucker f.
galeal f.
gallbladder f.
gall duct f.
gallstone f.
Gambale-Merrill bone-cutting f.
Gam-Mer bone-cutting f.
Gardner bone f.
Gardner hysterectomy f.
Garland hysterectomy f.
Garrigue uterine-dressing f.
Garrison f.
Gaskin fragment f.
gastrointestinal f.
Gauss hemostatic f.
Gavin-Miller colon f.
Gavin-Miller intestinal f.
Gavin-Miller tissue f.
Gaylor uterine biopsy f.
Geissendorfer uterine f.
Gelfilm f.
Gelfoam pressure f.
Gellhorn uterine biopsy f.
Gelpi hysterectomy f.
Gelpi-Lowrie hysterectomy f.
Gemini gall duct f.
Gemini hemostatic f.
Gemini Mixter f.
Gemini thoracic f.
general tissue f.
general wire f.
Gerald bayonet microbipolar
    neurosurgical f.
Gerald brain f.

Gerald dressing f.
Gerald monopolar f.
Gerald straight microbipolar
    neurosurgical f.
Gerald tissue f.
Gerbode cardiovascular tissue f.
GI f.
GIA f.
Gifford fixation f.
Gifford iris f.
Gilbert cystic duct f.
Gildenberg biopsy f.
Gill-Arruga capsular f.
Gill-Chandler iris f.
Gill curved iris f.
Gillespie obstetrical f.
Gill-Fuchs capsular f.
Gill-Hess iris f.
Gillies dissecting f.
Gillies tissue f.
Gill incision-spreading f.
Gill iris f.
Gillquist-Oretorp-Stille f.
Gill-Safar f.
Gill-Welsh capsular f.
Ginsberg tissue f.
giraffe biopsy f.
Girard corneoscleral f.
Glassman-Allis intestinal f.
Glassman-Allis noncrushing common
    duct f.
Glassman-Allis noncrushing
    intestinal f.
Glassman-Allis noncrushing tissue-
    holding f.
Glassman-Babcock f.
Glassman noncrushing pickup f.
Glassman pickup f.
Glenn diverticular f.
Glenner vaginal hysterectomy f.
glenoid-reaming f.
globular object f.
Glover anastomosis f.
Glover coarctation f.
Glover curved f.
Glover infundibular rongeur f.
Glover patent ductus f.
Glover spoon-shaped f.
goiter-seizing f.
goiter vulsellum f.
Gold deep-surgery f.
Gold hemostatic f.
Goldman-Kazanjian nasal f.
Goldmann capsulorrhexis f.
Gomco f.
Goodhill tonsillar f.
Good obstetrical f.
Goodyear-Gruenwald f.
Gordon bead f.
Gordon ciliary f.
Gordon uterine f.
Gordon vulsellum f.
Grabow f.
Gradle ciliary f.
Graefe curved iris f.

Graefe dressing f.
Graefe eye-fixation f.
Graefe straight iris f.
Graefe tissue f.
Graefe tissue-grasping f.
Grafco-Halsted f.
grasping biopsy f.
grasping tripod f.
Gray arterial f.
Gray cystic duct f.
Grayson corneal f.
Grayton corneal f.
Grazer blepharoplasty f.
Green-Armytage hemostatic f.
Green capsular f.
Green chalazion f.
Green fixation f.
Green suction tube f.
Green tissue-grasping f.
Green tube-holding f.
Greenwood bipolar coagulation-
    suction f.
Gregory f.
Greven alligator f.
Grey Turner f.
Grieshaber diamond-coated f.
Grieshaber internal limiting
    membrane f.
Grieshaber iris f.
Grieshaber manipulator f.
Griffiths-Brown f.
grooved tying f.
Gross dressing f.
Gross hyoid-cutting f.
Gross sponge f.
Grotting f.
Gruenwald bayonet-dressing f.
Gruenwald-Bryant nasal f.
Gruenwald-Bryant nasal-cutting f.
Gruenwald dissecting f.
Gruenwald dressing f.
Gruenwald Durogrip f.
Gruenwald ear f.
Gruenwald-Jansen f.
Gruenwald-Love neurosurgical f.
Gruenwald nasal-cutting f.
Gruenwald nasal-dressing f.
Gruenwald tissue f.
Gruppe wire-crimping f.
f. guard
Guggenheim adenoidal f.
guide f.
Guilford-Wright f.
guillotome f.
Guist fixation f.
Gunderson bone f.
Gunderson muscle recession f.
Gunnar-Hey roller f.
Guppe f.
Gusberg uterine f.
Gutgemann auricular appendage f.
Gutglass hemostatic cervical f.
Gutierrez-Najar grasping f.
Guyton-Clark f.
Guyton-Clark fragment f.

Guyton-Noyes fixation f.
Guyton suturing f.
Haberer gastrointestinal f.
Haberer-Gili f.
Hagenbarth clip-applying f.
Haig-Ferguson obstetrical f.
Haig obstetrical f.
Hajek antral punch f.
Hajek-Koffler bone punch f.
Hajek-Koffler sphenoidal f.
Hakler f.
Halberg contact lens f.
Hale obstetrical f.
Halifax placement f.
Hallberg f.
hallux f.
Halsey mosquito f.
Halsted arterial f.
Halsted curved mosquito f.
Halsted hemostatic mosquito f.
Halsted Micro-Line arterial f.
Halsted-Swanson tendon-passing f.
Hamby clip-applying f.
Hamilton deep-surgery f.
hammer f.
Hank-Dennen obstetrical f.
Hannahan f.
Hardy bayonet dressing f.
Hardy bayonet neurosurgical
    bipolar f.
Hardy microbipolar f.
Hardy microsurgical bayonet
    bipolar f.
harelip f.
Harken cardiovascular f.
Harken-Cooley f.
Harman fixation f.
Harms corneal f.
Harms microtying f.
Harms suture-tying f.
Harms-Tubingen tying f.
Harms tying f.
Harms utility f.
Harms vessel f.
Harrington clamp f.
Harrington lung-grasping f.
Harrington-Mayo tissue f.
Harrington-Mixter thoracic f.
Harrington thoracic f.
Harrington vulsellum f.
Harrison bone-holding f.
Harris suture-carrying f.
Hartmann alligator f.
Hartmann-Citelli alligator f.
Hartmann-Citelli ear punch f.
Hartmann-Corgill ear f.
Hartmann ear-dressing f.
Hartmann ear polyp f.
Hartmann-Gruenwald nasal-cutting f.
Hartmann hemostatic mosquito f.
Hartmann-Herzfeld ear f.
Hartmann mosquito hemostatic f.
Hartmann nasal-cutting f.
Hartmann nasal-dressing f.
Hartmann nasal polyp f.

F

forceps *(continued)*

Hartmann-Noyes nasal-dressing f.
Hartmann-Proctor ear f.
Hartmann tonsillar punch f.
Hartmann uterine biopsy f.
Hartmann-Weingärtner ear f.
Hartmann-Wullstein ear f.
Haslinger tip f.
Hasner lid f.
Hasson bullet-tip f.
Hasson grasping f.
Hasson needle-nose f.
Hasson ring f.
Hasson spike-tooth f.
Haugh ear f.
Hawkins cervical biopsy f.
Hawks-Dennen obstetrical f.
Hayes anterior resection f.
Hayes Martin f.
Hayes-Olivecrona f.
Hayton-Williams f.
Healy gastrointestinal f.
Healy intestinal f.
Healy suture-removing f.
Healy uterine biopsy f.
Heaney hysterectomy f.
Heaney-Kantor hysterectomy f.
Heaney-Rezek f.
Heaney-Simon hysterectomy f.
Heaney-Stumf f.
Heaney tissue f.
Heath chalazion f.
Heath clip-removing f.
Heath nasal f.
Hecht fascia lata f.
Heermann alligator f.
Heermann ear f.
Hegenbarth clip-applying f.
Hegenbarth-Michel clip-applying f.
Heidelberg fixation f.
Heifitz cup serrated ring f.
Heiming kidney stone f.
Heiss arterial f.
Heiss hemostatic f.
Heiss vulsellum f.
Heller biopsy f.
Hemoclip-applying f.
hemorrhoidal f.
hemostatic cervical f.
hemostatic clip-applying f.
hemostatic neurosurgical f.
hemostatic tissue f.
hemostatic tonsillar f.
hemostatic tracheal f.
Hendren cardiovascular f.
Hendren pediatric f.
Henke punch f.
Henrotin vulsellum f.
Henry ciliary f.
Herff membrane-puncturing f.
Herget biopsy f.
Hermann bone-holding f.
Herrick kidney f.
Hersh LASIK retreatment f.

Hertel kidney stone f.
Hertel rigid dilator stone f.
Hertel rigid kidney stone f.
Herzfeld ear f.
Herz meniscal tendon f.
Hess-Barraquer iris f.
Hessburg lens-inserting f.
Hess capsular f.
Hess-Gill iris f.
Hess-Horwitz iris f.
Hess iris f.
Hevesy polyp f.
Heyman-Knight nasal dressing f.
Heyman nasal f.
Heyman nasal-cutting f.
Heyner f.
Heywood-Smith dressing f.
Heywood-Smith gallbladder f.
Heywood-Smith sponge-holding f.
Hibbs biting f.
Hibbs bone-cutting f.
Hibbs bone-holding f.
Hildebrandt uterine hemostatic f.
Hildyard nasal f.
Himalaya dressing f.
Hinderer cartilage f.
Hirsch hypophysis punch f.
Hirschman hemorrhoidal f.
Hirschman jeweler's f.
Hirschman lens f.
Hirst-Emmet obstetrical f.
Hirst-Emmet placental f.
Hirst obstetrical f.
Hirst placental f.
Hodge obstetrical f.
Hoen alligator f.
Hoen bayonet f.
Hoen dressing f.
Hoen grasping f.
Hoen hemostatic f.
Hoen scalp f.
Hoen tissue f.
Hoffmann ear punch f.
Hoffmann-Pollock f.
holding f.
Holinger specimen f.
hollow-object f.
Holmes fixation f.
Holth punch f.
Holzbach hysterectomy f.
hook f.
Hopkins aortic f.
Horsley bone-cutting f.
Horsley-Stille bone-cutting f.
Horsley-Stille rib shears f.
Hosemann choledochus f.
Hosford-Hicks transfer f.
Hoskins beaked Colibri f.
Hoskins-Dallas intraocular lens-inserting f.
Hoskins fine straight f.
Hoskins fixation f.
Hoskins-Luntz f.
Hoskins microstraight f.

Hoskins miniaturized micro straight f.
Hoskins-Skeleton fine f.
Hoskins-Skeleton grooved broad-tipped f.
Hoskins straight microiris f.
Hoskins suture f.
host tissue f.
hot biopsy f.
hot flexible f.
Hot Sampler disposable hot biopsy f.
House alligator crimper f.
House alligator grasping f.
House alligator strut f.
House cup f.
House-Dieter eye f.
House ear f.
House Gelfoam pressure f.
House grasping f.
House miniature f.
House oval-cup f.
Housepian clip-applying f.
House pressure f.
House strut f.
House-Wullstein cup ear f.
Houspian clip-applying f.
Howard closing f.
Howard tonsillar f.
Howard tonsil-ligating f.
Howmedica Microfixation System f.
Hoxworth f.
Hoyt deep-surgery f.
Hoytenberger tissue f.
Hoyt hemostatic f.
Hubbard corneoscleral f.
Huber f. handle
Hudson brain f.
Hudson cranial f.
Hudson dressing f.
Hudson rongeur f.
Hudson tissue f.
Hufnagel mitral valve f.
Hulka clip f.
Hulka-Kenwick uterine-elevating f.
Hulka-Kenwick uterine-manipulating f.
Hulka tenaculum f.
hump f.
Hunt angled serrated ring f.
Hunt angled-tip f.
Hunt bipolar f.
Hunt chalazion f.
Hunter splinter f.
Hunt grasping f.
Hunt tumor f.
Hunt vessel f.
Hunt-Yasargil pituitary f.
Hurd bone f.
Hurd bone-cutting f.
Hurdner tissue f.
Hurd septal bone-cutting f.
Hurd septum-cutting f.
Hurteau f.
Hyde double-curved corneal f.

hyoid-cutting f.
hypogastric artery f.
hypophyseal f.
hypophysectomy f.
hysterectomy f.
Ilg capsular f.
Ilg curved micro tying f.
Ilg insertion f.
iliac f.
Iliff blepharochalasis f.
IM Jaws alligator f.
Imperatori laryngeal f.
implant f.
implantation f.
Inamura small incision capsulorrhexis f.
infant biopsy f.
infundibular f.
Ingraham-Fowler clip-applying f.
inlet f.
insertion f.
instrument-grasping f.
insulated bayonet f.
insulated monopolar f.
insulated tissue f.
intervertebral disk f.
intestinal anastomosis f.
intestinal closing f.
intestinal holding f.
intestinal tissue f.
intracapsular lens f.
intraocular irrigating f.
intraocular lens f.
intrathoracic f.
introducing f.
Iowa membrane f.
Iowa-Mengert membrane f.
Iowa State fixation f.
iris bipolar f.
iris tissue f.
Iselin f.
isolation f.
I-tech intraocular foreign body f.
I-tech splinter f.
I-tech tying f.
Jackson alligator grasping f.
Jackson approximation f.
Jackson biopsy f.
Jackson broad staple f.
Jackson button f.
Jackson conventional foreign body f.
Jackson cross-action f.
Jackson cylindrical-object f.
Jackson double-concave rat-tooth f.
Jackson double-prong f.
Jackson down-jaw f.
Jackson dressing f.
Jackson dull-pointed f.
Jackson dull rotation f.
Jackson endoscopic f.
Jackson fenestrated peanut-grasping f.
Jackson flexible upper lobe bronchus f.

F

forceps *(continued)*

Jackson forward-grasping f.
Jackson globular object f.
Jackson head-holding f.
Jackson hemostatic f.
Jackson hollow-object f.
Jackson infant biopsy f.
Jackson laryngeal applicator f.
Jackson laryngeal basket f.
Jackson laryngeal-dressing f.
Jackson laryngeal-grasping f.
Jackson laryngeal punch f.
Jackson laryngeal ring-rotation f.
Jackson laryngofissure f.
Jackson papilloma f.
Jackson pin-bending costophrenic f.
Jackson punch f.
Jackson ring-jaw f.
Jackson ring-rotation f.
Jackson sharp-pointed rotation f.
Jackson side-curved f.
Jackson sister-hook f.
Jackson tendon-seizing f.
Jackson tracheal hemostatic f.
Jackson triangular-punch f.
Jacob capsule fragment f.
Jacobs biopsy f.
Jacobs capsular fragment f.
Jacobson bipolar f.
Jacobson dressing f.
Jacobson hemostatic f.
Jacobson mosquito f.
Jacobs vulsellum f.
Jaffe capsulorhexis f.
Jaffe suturing f.
Jager meniscal f.
Jako laryngeal f.
Jako microlaryngeal cup f.
Jako microlaryngeal grasping f.
Jameson muscle recession f.
Jameson strabismus f.
Jameson tracheal muscle f.
James wound-approximation f.
Jannetta alligator grasping f.
Jannetta bayonet f.
Jannetta microbayonet f.
Jansen bayonet dressing f.
Jansen bayonet ear f.
Jansen bayonet nasal f.
Jansen dissecting f.
Jansen dressing f.
Jansen-Gruenwald f.
Jansen-Middleton nasal-cutting f.
Jansen-Middleton punch f.
Jansen-Middleton septal f.
Jansen-Middleton septotomy f.
Jansen-Middleton septum-cutting f.
Jansen monopolar f.
Jansen-Mueller f.
Jansen nasal-dressing f.
Jansen-Struyken septal f.
Jansen thumb f.
Jarcho tenaculum f.
Jarell f.

Jarit-Allis tissue f.
Jarit brain f.
Jarit-Crafoord f.
Jarit-Dandy f.
Jarit-Liston bone-cutting f.
Jarit microsuture tying f.
Jarit mosquito f.
Jarit sterilizer f.
Jarit tendon-pulling f.
Jarit tube-occluding f.
Jarit wire-pulling f.
Jarvis hemorrhoidal f.
Javerts placental f.
Javerts polyp f.
Jayles f.
Jensen intraocular lens f.
Jensen lens-inserting f.
Jerald f.
Jervey capsular fragment f.
Jervey iris f.
Jesberg grasping f.
jeweler's bipolar f.
jeweler's pickup f.
Johns Hopkins gallbladder f.
Johns Hopkins gall duct f.
Johns Hopkins hemostatic f.
Johns Hopkins occluding f.
Johns Hopkins serrefine f.
Johnson brain tumor f.
Johnson ptosis f.
Johnson thoracic f.
John Weiss f.
Jones hemostatic f.
Jones IMA f.
Jones towel f.
Joplin bone-holding f.
Jordan strut f.
Judd-Allis intestinal f.
Judd-Allis tissue f.
Judd-DeMartel gallbladder f.
Judd strabismus f.
Judd suture f.
Juers crimper f.
Juers-Lempert rongeur f.
Juers lingual f.
jugum f.
Julian-Damian thoracic f.
Julian splenorenal f.
Julian thoracic artery f.
jumbo f.
Jurasz laryngeal f.
Kadesky f.
Kahler bronchial biopsy f.
Kahler bronchoscopic f.
Kahler bronchus-grasping f.
Kahler laryngeal biopsy f.
Kahler polyp f.
Kahn tenaculum f.
Kalman occluding f.
Kalman tube-occluding f.
Kalt capsular f.
Kansas University corneal f.
Kantor f.
Kantrowitz dressing f.
Kantrowitz thoracic f.

Kantrowitz tissue f.
Kapp f.
Kapp-Beck f.
Karl Storz reusable multi-function valve trocar take-apart scissors f.
Karp aortic punch f.
Katena f.
Katzin-Barraquer Colibri f.
Katzin-Barraquer corneal f.
Kaufman ENT f.
Kazanjian bone-cutting f.
Kazanjian-Cottle f.
Kazanjian cutting f.
Kazanjian nasal f.
Kazanjian nasal hump f.
Keeler extended round tip f.
Keeler intraocular foreign body grasping f.
Keen Edge disposable biopsy f.
Kelly arterial f.
Kelly dressing f.
Kelly-Gray uterine f.
Kelly hemostatic f.
Kelly-Murphy f.
Kelly ovum f.
Kelly placental f.
Kelly polypus f.
Kelly-Rankin f.
Kelly tissue f.
Kelly urethral f.
Kelman implantation f.
Kelman intraocular f.
Kelman irrigator f.
Kelman-McPherson corneal f.
Kelman-McPherson microtying f.
Kelman-McPherson suture f.
Kelman-McPherson tissue f.
Kelman-McPherson tying f.
Kennedy vulsellum f.
Kennerdell bayonet f.
Kent f.
keratotomy f.
Kern bone-holding f.
Kern-Lane bone-holding f.
Kerrison f.
Kershner one-step micro capsulorhexis f.
Kevorkian uterine biopsy f.
Kevorkian-Younge cervical biopsy f.
Kevorkian-Younge uterine biopsy f.
Khodadad microclip f.
kidney-elevating f.
kidney pedicle f.
kidney stone f.
Kielland f.
Killian-Jameson f.
Killian septal compression f.
Kinder Design pedo f.
King-Prince muscle f.
King-Prince recession f.
Kingsley grasping f.
King tissue f.
King wound f.
Kirby-Arthus fixation f.
Kirby-Bracken iris f.

Kirby capsular f.
Kirby corneoscleral f.
Kirby eye tissue f.
Kirby fixation f.
Kirby intracapsular lens f.
Kirby iris f.
Kirby lens f.
Kirkpatrick tonsillar f.
Kirschner-Ullrich f.
Kirwan-Adson ophthalmic bipolar f.
Kirwan bipolar electrosurgical f.
Kirwan coaptation ophthalmic bipolar f.
Kirwan iris curved ophthalmic bipolar f.
Kirwan iris straight ophthalmic bipolar f.
Kirwan jeweler's curved ophthalmic bipolar f.
Kirwan jeweler's insulated straight ophthalmic bipolar f.
Kirwan-Nadler-style coaptation ophthalmic bipolar f.
Kirwan-Tenzel ophthalmic bipolar f.
Kitner goiter f.
Kitner thyroid-packing f.
Kjelland-Barton f.
Kjelland-Luikart obstetrical f.
Kjelland obstetrical f.
KleenSpec f.
Kleinert-Kutz bone-cutting f.
Kleinert-Kutz rongeur f.
Kleinert-Kutz tendon f.
Kleinert-Kutz tendon-passing f.
Kleinert-Kutz tendon-retrieving f.
Kleppinger bipolar f.
KLI bipolar f.
KLI monopolar f.
Knapp-Luer trachoma f.
Knapp trachoma f.
Knight nasal-cutting f.
Knight nasal septum-cutting f.
Knighton-Crawford f.
Knight polyp f.
Knight septal f.
Knight septum-cutting f.
Knight-Sluder nasal f.
Knight turbinate f.
Knolle lens implantation f.
Knolle-Shepard lens f.
Knolle-Volker lens-holding f.
knot-holding f.
knotting f.
Koby cataract f.
Kocher arterial f.
Kocher artery f.
Kocher hemostatic f.
Kocher kidney-elevating f.
Kocher Micro-Line intestinal f.
Kocher-Ochsner hemostatic f.
Koeberlé f.
Koenig vascular f.
Koerte gallstone f.
Koffler-Lillie septal f.
Koffler septal f.

F

forceps *(continued)*

Kogan endospeculum f.
Kolb bronchial f.
Kolodny f.
Korte gallstone f.
Kos crimper f.
Kraff intraocular utility f.
Kraff lens-inserting f.
Kraff-Osher lens f.
Kraff suturing f.
Kraff tying f.
Kraff-Utrata capsulorrhexis f.
Kraff-Utrata intraocular utility f.
Kraff-Utrata tear capsulotomy f.
Kramer f.
Kratz lens-inserting f.
Krause biopsy f.
Krause esophagoscopy f.
Krause punch f.
Krause Universal f.
Kremer fixation f.
Kremer two-point fixation f.
Kronfeld micropin f.
Kronfeld suturing f.
Krönlein hemostatic f.
Krukenberg pigment spindle f.
K/S-Allis f.
Kuhne coverglass f.
Kuhnt capsular f.
Kuhnt capsule f.
Kuhnt fixation f.
Kulvin-Kalt iris f.
Kurze microbiopsy f.
Kurze micrograsping f.
Kurze pickup f.
Küstner uterine tenaculum f.
Kwapis interdental f.
Laborde f.
Lahey arterial f.
Lahey-Babcock f.
Lahey dissecting f.
Lahey gall duct f.
Lahey goiter-seizing f.
Lahey goiter vulsellum f.
Lahey hemostatic f.
Lahey lock arterial f.
Lahey-Péan f.
Lahey-Sweet dissecting f.
Lahey thoracic f.
Lahey thyroid tenaculum f.
Lahey thyroid tissue traction f.
Lahey thyroid traction vulsellum f.
Lajeune hemostatic f.
Lalonde delicate hook f.
Lalonde extra fine skin hook f.
Lambert chalazion f.
Lambert-Kay anastomosis f.
Lambotte bone-holding f.
Lambotte fibular f.
Lancaster-O'Connor f.
lancet-shaped biopsy f.
Landers vitrectomy lens f.
Landolt spreading f.
Landon f.

Lane bone-holding f.
Lane gastrointestinal f.
Lane intestinal f.
Lane screw-holding f.
Lane tissue f.
Lange approximation f.
Langenbeck bone-holding f.
Lang iris f.
laparoscopic f.
Laplace f.
large-angled f.
LaRoe undermining f.
Larsen tendon f.
Larsen tendon-holding f.
laryngeal applicator f.
laryngeal basket f.
laryngeal biopsy f.
laryngeal bronchial grasping f.
laryngeal curette f.
laryngeal grasping f.
laryngeal punch f.
laryngeal rotation f.
laryngeal sponging f.
laryngofissure f.
laser microlaryngeal cup f.
laser microlaryngeal grasping f.
laser ovary f.
Laufe-Barton-Kjelland obstetrical f.
Laufe-Barton-Kjelland-Piper
   obstetrical f.
Laufe-Barton obstetrical f.
Laufe divergent outlet f.
Laufe obstetrical f.
Laufe-Piper obstetrical f.
Laufe-Piper uterine polyp f.
Laufe uterine polyp f.
Laufman f.
Laurer f.
Laval advancement f.
Lawrence deep f.
Lawrence hemostatic f.
Lawton f.
Lawton-Schubert biopsy f.
Lawton-Wittner cervical biopsy f.
Lazar microsuction f.
Leader vas isolation f.
Leahey chalazion f.
Leahey marginal chalazion f.
Leahey suture f.
Leasure nasal f.
Leaver sclerotomy f.
Lebsche f.
Lees arterial f.
Lees nontraumatic f.
Lefferts bone-cutting f.
Leibinger Micro System plate-
   holding f.
Leigh capsular f.
Lejeune thoracic f.
Leksell rongeur f.
Leland-Jones f.
Lemmon-Russian f.
Lemoine f.
Lempert rongeur f.
lens implantation f.

lens loop f.
lens-threading f.
Leonard f.
Leo Schwartz sponge-holding f.
Leriche hemostatic f.
Leriche tissue f.
LeRoy clip-applying f.
Lester fixation f.
Lester muscle f.
Levenson tissue f.
Levora fixation f.
Levret f.
Lewin bone-holding f.
Lewin spinal-perforating f.
Lewis septal f.
Lewis tonsillar hemostatic f.
Lewis ureteral stone isolation f.
Lewkowitz lithotomy f.
Lewkowitz ovum f.
Lewkowitz placental f.
Lexer tissue f.
Leyro-Diaz thoracic f.
lid f.
Lieberman-Pollock double corneal f.
Lieberman suturing f.
Lieberman tying f.
Lieb-Guerry f.
ligament-grasping f.
ligamentum flavum f.
ligature f.
ligature-carrying f.
Lillehei valve-grasping f.
Lillie intestinal f.
Lillie-Killian septal f.
Lillie tissue-holding f.
Lindsay-Rea f.
Lindstrom lens-insertion f.
lingual f.
Linnartz f.
Linn-Graefe iris f.
lion f.
lion-jaw bone-holding f.
Lister conjunctival f.
Liston bone-cutting f.
Liston-Key bone-cutting f.
Liston-Key-Horsley f.
Liston-Littauer bone-cutting f.
Liston-Stille bone-cutting f.
lithotomy f.
Litt f.
Littauer bone-cutting f.
Littauer ciliary f.
Littauer ear-dressing f.
Littauer ear polyp f.
Littauer-Liston bone-cutting f.
Littauer nasal-dressing f.
Littauer-West cutting f.
Littlewood tissue f.
Livernois lens-holding f.
Livernois pickup and folding f.
Livingston f.
Llobera fixation f.
Llorente dissecting f.
Lloyd-Davies occlusion f.
lobectomy f.

lobe-grasping f.
lobe-holding f.
Lobell splinter f.
Lobenstein-Tarnier f.
lobster bone-reduction f.
Lockwood-Allis intestinal f.
Lockwood-Allis tissue f.
Lockwood intestinal f.
Lockwood tissue f.
Lombard-Beyer f.
London tissue f.
Long Island College Hospital
  placental f.
long-jaw basket f.
long tissue f.
loop-type snare f.
loop-type stone-crushing f.
loose body suction f.
Lordan chalazion f.
Lore subglottic f.
Lore suction tube-holding f.
Lore suction tube and tip-holding f.
Lothrop ligature f.
Love-Gruenwald alligator f.
Love-Gruenwald pituitary f.
Love-Kerrison rongeur f.
Lovelace bladder f.
Lovelace gallbladder traction f.
Lovelace hemostatic f.
Lovelace lung-grasping f.
Lovelace thyroid-traction
  vulsellum f.
Lovelace tissue f.
Lovelace traction lung f.
Lovelace traction tissue f.
Löw-Beer f.
Löwenberg f.
lower gall duct f.
lower lateral f.
Lowis intervertebral disk f.
Lowman bone-holding f.
low outlet f.
Lowsley grasping f.
Lowsley-Luc f.
Lowsley prostatic f.
Luc f.
Lucae bayonet dressing f.
Lucae bayonet ear f.
Lucae bayonet tissue f.
Lucae dissecting f.
Lucae ear f.
Luc ethmoidal f.
Luc nasal-cutting f.
Luc septal f.
Luc septum-cutting f.
Luer curette f.
Luer hemorrhoidal f.
Luer rongeur f.
Luer-Whiting f.
Luer-Whiting rongeur f.
Luhr Microfixation System plate-
  holding f.
Luikart f.
Luikart-Bill f.
Luikart-Kjelland obstetrical f.

F

forceps *(continued)*

Luikart-McLane obstetrical f.
Luikart-Simpson obstetrical f.
lung-grasping f.
lung tissue f.
Lutz septal f.
Lynch cup-shaped curette f.
Lynch laryngeal f.
Lyon f.
MacCarty f.
MacGregor conjunctival f.
Machemer diamond-dust-coated foreign body f.
Machemer diamond-dusted f.
MacKenty tissue f.
MacQuigg-Mixter f.
Madden f.
Madden-Potts intestinal f.
Madden-Potts tissue f.
Magielski coagulating f.
Magielski-Heermann strut f.
Magielski tonsillar f.
Magielski tonsil-seizing f.
Magill catheter f.
Magill endotracheal f.
Maier dressing f.
Maier polyp f.
Maier sponge f.
Maier uterine f.
Mailler colon f.
Mailler cut-off f.
Mailler intestinal f.
Mailler rectal f.
Maingot hysterectomy f.
Malis angled bayonet f.
Malis bipolar coagulation f.
Malis bipolar cutting f.
Malis bipolar irrigating f.
Malis cup f.
Malis-Jensen bipolar f.
Malis-Jensen microbipolar f.
Malis jeweler bipolar f.
Malis titanium microsurgical f.
malleus f.
mammary-coronary tissue f.
Manche LASIK f.
Manhattan Eye & Ear suturing f.
Mann f.
Manning f.
Mansfield f.
Mantis retrograde f.
March-Barton f.
Marcuse f.
marginal chalazion f.
Markwalder rib f.
Marshik tonsillar f.
Marshik tonsil-seizing f.
Martin bipolar coagulation f.
Martin cartilage f.
Martin meniscal f.
Martin nasopharyngeal f.
Martin nasopharyngeal biopsy f.
Martin thumb f.
Martin tissue f.

Martin uterine tenaculum f.
Maryan biopsy punch f.
Masket f.
Masterson hysterectomy f.
Mastin goiter f.
Mastin muscle f.
Mathieu foreign body f.
Mathieu tongue f.
Mathieu urethral f.
matte black f.
Matthew f.
Maumenee capsular f.
Maumenee-Colibri corneal f.
Maumenee corneal f.
Maumenee cross-action capsular f.
Maumenee straight-action capsular f.
Maumenee Suregrip f.
Maumenee tissue f.
Max Fine tying f.
maxillary disimpaction f.
maxillary fracture f.
Maxum Carr-Locke angled f.
Maxum reusable endoscopic f.
Mayer f.
Mayfield aneurysm f.
Mayo bone-cutting f.
Mayo-Harrington f.
Mayo kidney pedicle f.
Mayo-Ochsner f.
Mayo-Robson gastrointestinal f.
Mayo-Russian gastrointestinal f.
Mayo tissue f.
Mayo ureter isolation f.
Mazzariello-Caprini stone f.
Mazzocco flexible lens f.
McCain TMJ f.
McCarthy-Alcock f.
McCarthy visual hemostatic f.
McClintock placental f.
McClintock uterine f.
McCollough tying f.
McCoy septal f.
McCoy septum-cutting f.
McCullough strabismus f.
McCullough suture-tying f.
McCullough suturing f.
McDonald lens-folding f.
McGannon lens f.
McGee-Paparella wire-crimping f.
McGee-Priest-Paparella f.
McGee-Priest wire f.
McGee-Priest wire-closure f.
McGee wire-closure f.
McGee wire-crimping f.
McGill f.
McGivney hemorrhoidal f.
McGravey tissue f.
McGregor conjunctival f.
McGuire marginal chalazion f.
McHenry tonsillar f.
McIndoe bone-cutting f.
McIndoe dissecting f.
McIndoe dressing f.
McIndoe rongeur f.
McIntosh suture-holding f.

McKay ear f.
McKenzie clip-applying f.
McKerman-Adson f.
McKerman-Potts f.
McKernan f.
McKernan-Adson f.
McKernan-Potts f.
McLane-Luikart obstetrical f.
McLane obstetrical f.
McLane pile f.
McLane-Tucker-Kjelland f.
McLane-Tucker-Luikart f.
McLane-Tucker obstetrical f.
McLean capsular f.
McLean muscle-recession f.
McLean ophthalmic f.
McLearie bone f.
McNealey-Glassman-Mixter f.
McNealy-Glassman-Babcock f.
McPherson angled f.
McPherson bent f.
McPherson-Castroviejo f.
McPherson corneal f.
McPherson irrigating f.
McPherson lens f.
McPherson microbipolar f.
McPherson microcorneal f.
McPherson microiris f.
McPherson microsuture f.
McPherson-Pierse microcorneal f.
McPherson-Pierse microsuturing f.
McPherson straight bipolar f.
McPherson suture-tying f.
McPherson tying iris f.
McQueen vitreous f.
McQuigg f.
McQuigg-Mixter bronchial f.
McWhorter tonsillar f.
Meacham-Scoville f.
meat f.
meat-grasping f.
mechanical finger f.
Medicon-Jackson rectal f.
Medicon-Packer mosquito f.
Medicon wire-twister f.
medium f.
Meeker deep-surgery f.
Meeker gallbladder f.
Meeker hemostatic f.
Meeker intestinal f.
meibomian expressor f.
membrane f.
membrane-puncturing f.
Mendel ligature f.
Mendez multi-purpose LASIK f.
Mengert membrane-puncturing f.
meniscal basket f.
Mentor-Maumenee Suregrip f.
Merlin stone f.
Merriam f.
Merz hysterectomy f.
Metico f.
Metzel-Wittmoser f.
Metzenbaum tonsillar f.
Metzenbaum-Tydings f.

MGH uterine vulsellum f.
Michel clip-applying f.
Michel clip-removing f.
Michel tissue f.
Michigan University intestinal f.
Micrins f.
micro-Allis f.
microarterial f.
microbayonet f.
microbiopsy f.
microbipolar f.
microbronchoscopic grasping f.
microbronchoscopic tissue f.
microclamp f.
microclip f.
micro-Colibri f.
microcorneal f.
microcup pituitary f.
microdissecting f.
microdressing f.
microextractor f.
micro-Halstead arterial f.
micro-jewelers monopolar f.
microlaryngeal grasping f.
Micro-Line arterial f.
microneedle holder f.
microneurosurgical f.
Micro-One dissecting f.
micropin f.
Microsnap hemostatic f.
microsurgical biopsy f.
microsurgical grasping f.
microsurgical tying f.
Microtek cupped f.
microtip bipolar jeweler's f.
microtissue f.
Micro-Two f.
microtying f.
microvascular clamp-applying f.
microvascular tying f.
Microvasive disposable alligator-
  shaped f.
Microvasive radial jaw biopsy f.
midcavity f.
middle ear strut f.
Mighty Bite Zimmon lateral biopsy
  cup f.
Mikulicz peritoneal f.
Mikulicz tonsillar f.
Miles punch biopsy f.
Milex f.
Miller articulating f.
Miller bayonet f.
Miller rectal f.
Millin capsular f.
Millin ligature-guiding f.
Millin prostatectomy f.
Millin T-shaped f.
Mill-Rose RiteBite biopsy f.
Mill-Rose Surebrite biopsy f.
Mills tissue f.
miniature intestinal f.
Mitchell-Diamond biopsy f.
mitral valve-holding f.
Mixter arterial f.

F

forceps *(continued)*

Mixter baby hemostatic f.
Mixter gallbladder f.
Mixter gallstone f.
Mixter-McQuigg f.
Mixter mosquito f.
Mixter-O'Shaughnessy dissecting f.
Mixter-O'Shaughnessy hemostatic f.
Mixter-O'Shaughnessy ligature f.
Mixter-Paul arterial f.
Mixter-Paul hemostatic f.
Mixter pediatric hemostatic f.
Mixter thoracic f.
Moberg f.
Moberg-Stille f.
modified Younge f.
Moehle corneal f.
Moersch bronchoscopic f.
Molt pedicle f.
Monod punch f.
monopolar coagulating f.
monopolar insulated f.
monopolar tissue f.
Montenovesi cranial f.
Moody fixation f.
Moolgaoker f.
Moore lens-inserting f.
Morgenstein blunt f.
Moritz-Schmidt laryngeal f.
Morris f.
Morson f.
Mosher ethmoid punch f.
mosquito hemostatic f.
Mount intervertebral disk f.
Mount-Mayfield aneurysm f.
Mount-Olivecrona f.
mouse-tooth f.
Moynihan intestinal f.
Moynihan kidney pedicle f.
Moynihan-Navratil f.
Moynihan towel f.
MPC coagulation f.
Muck tonsillar f.
mucous f.
Mueller f.
Mueller-Markham patent ductus f.
Muir hemorrhoidal f.
Muldoon meibomian f.
Multibite multiple sample biopsy f.
multipurpose f.
multitoothed cartilage f.
Mundie placental f.
Murless head extractor f.
Murphy-Péan hemostatic f.
Murphy tonsillar f.
Murray f.
muscle f.
Museholdt nasal-dressing f.
Museux-Collins uterine vulsellum f.
Museux tenaculum f.
Museux uterine f.
Museux vulsellum f.
Musial tissue f.
Mustarde f.

Myerson bronchial f.
Myerson laryngeal f.
Myles hemorrhoidal f.
Myles nasal f.
Nadler bipolar coaptation f.
Naegele obstetrical f.
nail-cutting f.
nail-extracting f.
nail-pulling f.
Nakao Ejector biopsy f.
nasal alligator f.
nasal bone f.
nasal cartilage-holding f.
nasal-cutting f.
nasal-dressing f.
nasal hump-cutting f.
nasal insertion f.
nasal lower lateral f.
nasal needle holder f.
nasal-packing f.
nasal polyp f.
nasal septal f.
nasopharyngeal biopsy f.
Natvig wire-twister f.
needle f.
needle-holder f.
Negus-Green f.
Negus tonsillar f.
Nelson lung f.
Nelson-Martin f.
Nelson tissue f.
neonatal vascular f.
nephrolithotomy f.
Neubauer foreign body f.
Neubauer vitreous micro-extractor f.
Neubuser tube-seizing f.
neurosurgical dressing f.
neurosurgical ligature f.
neurosurgical suction f.
neurosurgical tissue f.
neurovascular f.
Neuwirth-Palmer f.
Neville-Barnes f.
Nevins dressing f.
Nevins tissue f.
Nevyas lens f.
New biopsy f.
Newman uterine tenaculum f.
New Orleans Eye & Ear fixation f.
New tissue f.
New York Eye and Ear Hospital fixation f.
Nicola f.
Niedner dissecting f.
NIH mitral valve f.
Niro bone-cutting f.
Niro wire-twister f.
Niro wire-twisting f.
Nisbet eye f.
Nisbet fixation f.
Nissen cystic f.
Nissen gall duct f.
Nissen hassux f.
Noble iris f.
noncrushing common duct f.

noncrushing intestinal f.
noncrushing pickup f.
noncrushing tissue-holding f.
nonfenestrated f.
nonmagnetic dressing f.
nonmagnetic tissue f.
nonperforating towel f.
nonslipping f.
nontoothed f.
nontraumatizing visceral f.
Nordan-Colibri f.
Nordan tying f.
Norris sponge f.
Norwood f.
Noto dressing f.
Noto ovum f.
Noto polypus f.
Noto sponge f.
Novak fixation f.
Noyes ear f.
Noyes nasal f.
Noyes nasal-dressing f.
Nugent fixation f.
Nugent rectus f.
Nugent superior rectus f.
Nugent utility f.
Nugowski f.
Nussbaum intestinal f.
Nyhus-Potts intestinal f.
Nystroem tumor f.
Oberhill obstetrical f.
O'Brien-Elschnig f.
O'Brien fixation f.
O'Brien tissue f.
obstetrical f.
occluding f.
Ochsner arterial f.
Ochsner cartilage f.
Ochsner-Dixon arterial f.
Ochsner hemostatic f.
Ochsner tissue f.
Ochsner tissue/cartilage f.
Ockerblad f.
O'Connor biopsy f.
O'Connor-Elschnig fixation f.
O'Connor eye f.
O'Connor grasping f.
O'Connor iris f.
O'Connor lid f.
O'Connor sponge f.
O'Dell spicule f.
odontoid peg-grasping f.
O'Gawa-Castroviejo tying f.
O'Gawa suture f.
O'Gawa suture-fixation f.
O'Gawa tying f.
Ogura cartilage f.
Ogura tissue f.
O'Hanlon f.
O'Hara f.
Oldberg intervertebral disk f.
Oldberg pituitary rongeur f.
Olivecrona aneurysm f.
Olivecrona clip-applying and
  removing f.

Olivecrona rongeur f.
Olivecrona-Toennis clip-applying f.
Olsen bayonet monopolar f.
Olympus alligator-jaw endoscopic f.
Olympus basket-type endoscopic f.
Olympus Endo-Therapy disposable
  biopsy f.
Olympus FB-series biopsy f.
Olympus FG-series f.
Olympus FS-K-series endoscopic
  suture-cutting f.
Olympus FS-series endoscopic
  suture-cutting f.
Olympus grasping rat-tooth f.
Olympus hot biopsy f.
Olympus magnetic extractor f.
Olympus pelican-type endoscopic f.
Olympus rat-tooth endoscopic f.
Olympus reusable oval cup f.
Olympus shark-tooth endoscopic f.
Olympus tripod-type endoscopic f.
Olympus W-shaped endoscopic f.
Ombrédanne f.
optical biopsy f.
oral f.
Orr gall duct f.
orthopedic f.
O'Shaughnessy arterial f.
Osher bipolar coaptation f.
Osher capsular f.
Osher conjunctival f.
Osher foreign body f.
Osher haptic f.
Osher superior rectus f.
ossicle-holding f.
Ossoff-Karlan laser f.
ostrum punch f.
otologic cup f.
Otto tissue f.
Oughterson f.
outlet f.
oval cup f.
ovary f.
Overholt clip-applying f.
Overholt dissecting f.
Overholt-Geissendörfer arterial f.
Overholt-Mixter dissecting f.
Overstreet polyp f.
ovum f.
Pace-Potts f.
Packer mosquito f.
packing f.
Page tonsillar f.
Palmer biopsy f.
Palmer cutting f.
Palmer-Drapier f.
Palmer grasping f.
Palmer ovarian biopsy f.
Pang biopsy f.
Pang nasopharyngeal f.
Panje-Shagets tracheoesophageal
  fistula f.
papilloma f.
parametrium f.
Parker fixation f.

F

forceps *(continued)*

Parker-Kerr f.
Park lens implantation f.
partial-occlusion f.
Passarelli one-pass capsulorrhexis f.
passing f.
patent ductus f.
Paterson brain clip f.
Paterson laryngeal f.
Paton anterior chamber lens
 implant f.
Paton capsular f.
Paton corneal f.
Paton corneal transplant f.
Paton extra-delicate f.
Paton suturing f.
Paton tying/stitch removal f.
Patterson bronchoscopic f.
Patterson specimen f.
Paufique suturing f.
Paulson infertility microtissue f.
Paulson infertility microtying f.
Pauwels fracture f.
Pavlo-Colibri corneal f.
Payne-Ochsner arterial f.
Payne-Péan arterial f.
Payne-Rankin arterial f.
Payr pylorus f.
Péan arterial f.
Péan hemostatic f.
Péan hysterectomy f.
Péan intestinal f.
Péan sponge f.
peanut-fenestrated f.
peanut-grasping f.
peanut sponge-holding f.
peapod bead-type f.
peapod intervertebral disk f.
pediatric f.
pedicle f.
Peet mosquito f.
Peet splinter f.
pelican biopsy f.
Pelkmann foreign body f.
Pelkmann gallstone f.
Pelkmann sponge f.
Pelkmann uterine f.
pelvic reduction f.
pelvic tissue f.
Pemberton f.
Penfield watchmaker suture f.
Penn-Anderson scleral fixation f.
Pennington hemorrhoidal f.
Pennington hemostatic f.
Pennington tissue f.
Pennington tissue-grasping f.
Percy intestinal f.
Percy tissue f.
Percy-Wolfson gallbladder f.
Perdue tonsillar hemostat f.
Perez-Castro f.
peripheral blood vessel f.
peripheral iridectomy f.
peripheral vascular f.

peritoneal f.
Perman cartilage f.
Perone LASIK flap f.
Perritt fixation f.
Perritt lens f.
Perry f.
Peter-Bishop f.
Peters tissue f.
Peyman-Green vitreous f.
Peyman intraocular f.
Peyman vitreous-grasping f.
Pfau polyp f.
Pfister-Schwartz basket f.
phalangeal f.
Phaneuf arterial f.
Phaneuf hysterectomy f.
Phaneuf peritoneal f.
Phaneuf uterine artery f.
Phaneuf vaginal f.
Phillips fixation f.
Phillips swan neck f.
phimosis f.
Phipps f.
phrenicectomy f.
pickup noncrushing f.
Pierse-Colibri corneal utility f.
Pierse corneal Colibri-type f.
Pierse fixation f.
Pierse-Hoskins f.
Pierse tip f.
Pigott f.
Pike jawed f.
pillar f.
pillar-grasping f.
Pilling f.
Pilling-Liston bone utility f.
pin-bending f.
pinch f.
pin-seating f.
Piper obstetrical f.
Piranha uteroscopic biopsy f.
Pischel micropin f.
Pistofidis cervical biopsy f.
Pitanguy f.
Pitha foreign body f.
Pitha urethral f.
pituitary f.
placement f.
placenta previa f.
plain f.
plastic f.
plate-holding f.
platform f.
pleurectomy f.
Pley capsular f.
Pley extracapsular f.
Plondke uterine f.
point f.
Polaris reusable f.
Polk placental f.
Polk sponge f.
Pollock double corneal f.
polyp f.
polypus f.
Poppen intervertebral disk f.

Porter duodenal f.
Post f.
posterior f.
postnasal sponge f.
Potta coarctation f.
Potter sponge f.
Potter tonsillar f.
Potts bronchial f.
Potts bulldog f.
Potts coarctation f.
Potts fixation f.
Potts intestinal f.
Potts-Nevins dressing f.
Potts patent ductus f.
Potts-Smith bipolar f.
Potts-Smith dressing f.
Potts-Smith monopolar f.
Potts-Smith tissue f.
Potts thumb f.
Poutasse renal artery f.
Pozzi tenaculum f.
Pratt hemostatic f.
Pratt-Smith hemostatic f.
Pratt tissue f.
Pratt T-shaped hemostatic f.
Pratt vulsellum f.
Precisor Direct Bite biopsy f.
Prentiss f.
prepuce f.
Presbyterian Hospital f.
pressure f.
Preston ligamentum flavum f.
Price-Thomas bronchial f.
Primbs suturing f.
Prince advancement f.
Prince muscle f.
Prince trachoma f.
proctological grasping f.
proctological polyp f.
Proctor phrenectomy f.
Proctor phrenicectomy f.
prostatectomy f.
prostatic lobe f.
protological biopsy f.
Proud adenoidectomy f.
Providence Hospital arterial f.
ptosis f.
pulmonary arterial f.
pulmonary vessel f.
punch f.
Puntenney tying f.
Puntowicz arterial f.
pupil spreader/retractor f.
QSA dressing f.
quadripolar cutting f.
Quervain cranial f.
Quevedo conjunctival f.
Quevedo fixation f.
Quevedo suturing f.
Quinones-Neubüser uterine-
    grasping f.
Quinones uterine-grasping f.
Quire foreign body f.
Quire mechanical finger f.
Raaf f.

Raaf-Oldberg intervertebral disk f.
Radial Jaw bladder biopsy f.
Radial Jaw hot biopsy f.
Radial Jaw single-use biopsy f.
Raimondi scalp hemostatic f.
Ralks ear f.
Ralks splinter f.
Ralks wire-cutting f.
Rampley sponge f.
Rand f.
Randall stone f.
Raney rongeur f.
Raney scalp clip-applying f.
Raney straight coagulating f.
Rankin arterial f.
Rankin-Crile f.
Rankin hemostatic f.
Rankow f.
Rapp f.
Rappazzo intraocular foreign
    body f.
Ratliff-Blake gallstone f.
Ratliff-Mayo gallstone f.
rat-tooth f.
Ray kidney stone f.
reach-and-pin f.
Read f.
recession f.
rectal f.
Reese advancement f.
Reese muscle f.
Reich-Nechtow hypogastric artery f.
Reich-Nechtow hysterectomy f.
Reill f.
Reiner-Knight ethmoid-cutting f.
Reinhoff arterial f.
Reisinger lens-extracting f.
renal artery f.
Resano sigmoid f.
resection intestinal f.
retrieval f.
Reul coronary f.
reverse-action hypophysectomy f.
Rezek f.
Rhein capsulorhexis cystitome f.
Rhein fine foldable lens-insertion f.
Rhoton-Adson dressing f.
Rhoton-Adson tissue f.
Rhoton bipolar f.
Rhoton cup f.
Rhoton-Cushing tissue f.
Rhoton dural f.
Rhoton grasping f.
Rhoton microcup f.
Rhoton microdissecting f.
Rhoton microtying f.
Rhoton microvascular f.
Rhoton ring tumor f.
Rhoton-Tew bipolar f.
Rhoton tissue f.
Rhoton transsphenoidal bipolar f.
Rhoton tying f.
Riba-Valeira f.
rib rongeur f.
Rica-Adson f.

F

forceps *(continued)*

Rica clip-applying f.
Rica hemostatic f.
Rich f.
Richards f.
Richards-Andrews f.
Richards tonsillar f.
Riches artery f.
Riches diathermy f.
Richmond f.
Richter f.
Richter-Heath clip-removing f.
ridge f.
Ridley f.
right-angle f.
rigid biopsy f.
rigid kidney stone f.
ring f.
ringed formed f.
Ringenberg stapedectomy f.
ring-rotation f.
ring-tip f.
Ripstein arterial f.
Ripstein tissue f.
Ritch-Krupin-Denver eye valve insertion f.
RiteBite biopsy f.
Ritter f.
Rizzuti double-prong f.
Rizzuti fixation f.
Rizzuti-Furness cornea-holding f.
Rizzuti scleral f.
Rizzuti superior rectus f.
Rizzuti-Verhoeff f.
Robb tonsillar f.
Roberts arterial f.
Roberts bronchial f.
Roberts hemostatic f.
Robertson tonsillar f.
Roberts-Singley dressing f.
Roberts-Singley thumb f.
Robson intestinal f.
Rochester-Carmalt hysterectomy f.
Rochester-Davis f.
Rochester-Ewald tissue f.
Rochester gallstone f.
Rochester-Harrington f.
Rochester-Mixter arterial f.
Rochester-Mixter gall duct f.
Rochester-Müeller f.
Rochester-Ochsner f.
Rochester oral tissue f.
Rochester-Péan hysterectomy f.
Rochester-Rankin arterial f.
Rochester Russian tissue f.
Rochester tissue f.
Rockey f.
Roeder f.
Roeltsch f.
Roger vascular-toothed hysterectomy f.
Rolf jeweler's f.
Rolf utility f.
roller f.

rongeur f.
Ronis cutting f.
Rose disimpaction f.
rotating f.
Roubaix f.
round-handled f.
round punch f.
Rovenstine catheter-introducing f.
Rowe bone-drilling f.
Rowe disimpaction f.
Rowe glenoid-reaming f.
Rowe-Harrison bone-holding f.
Rowe-Killey f.
Rowe maxillary f.
Rowe modified-Harrison f.
Rowland double-action f.
Rowland hump f.
Royce f.
rubber-shod f.
Rudd Clinic hemorrhoidal f.
Ruel f.
Rugby deep-surgery f.
Rugelski arterial f.
Rumel dissecting f.
Rumel lobectomy f.
Rumel thoracic f.
Ruskin bone-cutting f.
Ruskin-Liston bone-cutting f.
Ruskin rongeur f.
Ruskin-Rowland bone-cutting f.
Russell f.
Russell-Davis f.
Russell hysterectomy f.
Russian Péan f.
Russian thumb f.
Russian tissue f.
Russ tumor f.
Russ vascular f.
Rycroft tying f.
Sachs tissue f.
Saenger ovum f.
Saenger placental f.
Sajou laryngeal f.
Sam Roberts bronchial biopsy f.
Samuels hemoclip-applying f.
Sanders-Castroviejo suturing f.
Sanders vasectomy f.
Sandt suture f.
Sandt utility f.
Santy ring-end f.
Saqalain dressing f.
Sarot arterial f.
Sarot intrathoracic f.
Sarot pleurectomy f.
Satellight needle holder f.
Satinsky f.
Satterlee advancement f.
Satterlee muscle f.
Sauerbruch pickup f.
Sauerbruch rib f.
Sauer outer ring f.
Sauer suture f.
Sauer suturing f.
Sawtell arterial f.
Sawtell-Davis f.

Sawtell gallbladder f.
Sawtell tonsillar f.
scalp clip-applying f.
Scanlan laparoscopic f.
Scanzoni f.
Schaaf foreign body f.
Schaefer fixation f.
Schanzioni craniotomy f.
Scharff bipolar f.
Schatz utility f.
Scheer crimper f.
Scheie-Graefe fixation f.
Scheinmann esophagoscopy f.
Scheinmann laryngeal f.
Schepens f.
Schick f.
Schindler peritoneal f.
Schlesinger cervical punch f.
Schlesinger intervertebral disk f.
Schlesinger meniscus-grasping f.
Schlesinger rongeur f.
Schnidt gall duct f.
Schnidt-Rumpler f.
Schnidt thoracic f.
Schnidt tonsillar f.
Schoenberg intestinal f.
Schoenberg uterine f.
Scholten endomyocardial biopsy f.
Schroeder-Braun uterine f.
Schroeder tissue f.
Schroeder uterine vulsellum f.
Schroeder-Van Doren tenaculum f.
Schubert cervical biopsy f.
Schubert uterine biopsy f.
Schumacher biopsy f.
Schutz f.
Schwartz clip-applying f.
Schwartz multipurpose f.
Schwartz obstetrical f.
Schwartz temporary clamp-
 applying f.
Schweigger capsule f.
Schweigger extracapsular f.
Schweizer cervix-holding f.
Schweizer uterine f.
scissors f.
scleral twist-grip f.
sclerectomy punch f.
Scobee-Allis f.
Scott lens-insertion f.
Scoville brain f.
Scoville clip-applying f.
Scoville-Greenwood bayonet
 neurosurgical bipolar f.
Scoville-Hurteau f.
screw-holding f.
Scudder intestinal f.
Scuderi bipolar coagulating f.
Searcy capsular f.
Segond hysterectomy f.
Segond-Landau hysterectomy f.
Segond tumor f.
Seiffert esophagoscopy f.
Seiffert laryngeal f.
Seitzinger tripolar cutting f.

seizing f.
Seletz foramen-plugging f.
self-opening f.
self-retaining bone f.
Selman nonslip tissue f.
Selman peripheral blood vessel f.
Selman tissue f.
Selman vessel f.
Selverstone embolus f.
Selverstone intervertebral disk f.
Selverstone rongeur f.
Semb bone f.
Semb bone-cutting f.
Semb bone-holding f.
Semb dissecting f.
Semb-Ghazi dissecting f.
Semb ligature f.
Semb ligature-carrying f.
Semb rib f.
Semb rongeur f.
Semken bipolar f.
Semken dressing f.
Semken infant f.
Semken microbipolar
 neurosurgical f.
Semken thumb f.
Semken tissue f.
Semmes dural f.
Senning cardiovascular f.
Senturia f.
septal bone f.
septal compression f.
septal ridge f.
septum-cutting f.
septum-straightening f.
sequestrum f.
serrated conjunctival f.
serrefine f.
Sewall brain clip-applying f.
Seyfert f.
Shaaf eye f.
Shaaf foreign body f.
Shallcross cystic duct f.
Shallcross-Dean gall duct f.
Shallcross gallbladder f.
Shallcross nasal f.
Shapshay-Healy laryngeal alligator f.
Shark f.
shark-tooth f.
sharp-pointed f.
Shearer chicken-bill f.
Sheehy ossicle-holding f.
Sheets lens f.
Sheets-McPherson angled f.
Sheets-McPherson tying f.
Sheinmann laryngeal f.
Shepard bipolar f.
Shepard curved intraocular lens f.
Shepard lens f.
Shepard-Reinstein intraocular lens f.
Shepard tying f.
Shields f.
Shoemaker intraocular lens f.
short tooth f.
Shuppe biting f.

F

forceps *(continued)*

Shuster suture f.
Shuster tonsillar f.
Shutt Aggressor f.
Shutt alligator f.
Shutt basket f.
Shutt B-scoop f.
Shutt grasping f.
Shutt Mantis retrograde f.
Shutt Mini-Aggressor f.
Shutt retrograde f.
Shutt shovel-nosed f.
Shutt suction f.
side-biting Stammberger punch f.
side-curved f.
side-cutting basket f.
side-grasping f.
side-lip f.
Siegler biopsy f.
Silcock dissection f.
silicone rod and sleeve f.
silicone sponge f.
Silver endaural f.
Simcoe implantation f.
Simcoe lens-inserting f.
Simcoe nucleus f.
Simcoe posterior chamber f.
Simcoe superior rectus f.
Simons stone-removing f.
Simpson-Braun obstetrical f.
Simpson-Luikart obstetrical f.
Simpson obstetrical f.
Sims-Maier sponge and dressing f.
single-tooth f.
Singley intestinal f.
Singley tissue f.
Singley-Tuttle dressing f.
Singley-Tuttle intestinal f.
Singley-Tuttle tissue f.
Sinskey intraocular lens f.
Sinskey-McPherson f.
Sinskey microtying f.
Sinskey-Wilson foreign body f.
sinus biopsy f.
Sisson f.
sister-hook f.
Skeleton fine f.
Skene tenaculum f.
Skene uterine f.
Skene vulsellum f.
Skillern phimosis f.
Skillman arterial f.
Skillman mosquito f.
Skillman prepuce f.
skin f.
sleeve-spreading f.
sliding capsular f.
Sluder-Ballenger tonsillar punch f.
small cup biopsy f.
Smart chalazion f.
Smart nonslipping chalazion f.
Smellie obstetrical f.
Smith grasping f.

Smith-Leiske cross-action intraocular lens f.
Smith lion-jaw f.
Smith & Nephew Richards bipolar f.
Smith obstetrical f.
Smith-Petersen f.
Smithwick clip-applying f.
Smithwick-Hartmann f.
smooth dressing f.
smooth-tipped jeweler's f.
smooth tissue f.
smooth-tooth f.
Snellen entropion f.
Snyder corneal spring f.
Snyder deep-surgery f.
Somers uterine f.
Songer tonsillar f.
Soonawalla vasectomy f.
Sopher ovum f.
Sourdille f.
Spaleck f.
Sparta micro-iris f.
spatula f.
specimen f.
speculum f.
Spence-Adson f.
Spencer biopsy f.
Spencer chalazion f.
Spence rongeur f.
Spencer plication f.
Spencer-Wells arterial f.
Spencer-Wells chalazion f.
Spero meibomian f.
Spetzler f.
sphenoidal punch f.
spicule f.
spinal-perforating f.
spiral f.
splaytooth f.
splinter f.
splitting f.
sponge f.
sponge-holding f.
spoon f.
spoon-shaped f.
spreading f.
spring-handled f.
Spurling intervertebral disk f.
Spurling-Kerrison rongeur f.
Spurling rongeur f.
Spurling tissue f.
square specimen f.
squeeze-handle f.
Stammberger side-biting punch f.
Stamm bone-cutting f.
standard arterial f.
stapedectomy f.
stapes f.
staple f.
Stark vulsellum f.
Starr fixation f.
Staude-Jackson tenaculum f.
Staude-Moore uterine tenaculum f.
Staude tenaculum f.

Stavis fixation f.
St. Clair f.
St. Clair-Thompson adenoidal f.
St. Clair-Thompson peritonsillar
  abscess f.
Steinmann intestinal f.
Steinmann tendon f.
Stephens soft IOL-inserting f.
sterilizing f.
sternal punch f.
Stern-Castroviejo locking f.
Stern-Castroviejo suturing f.
Stevens fixation f.
Stevens iris f.
Stevenson alligator f.
Stevenson cupped-jaw f.
Stevenson grasping f.
Stevenson microsurgical f.
Stieglitz splinter f.
Stille-Adson f.
Stille-Babcock f.
Stille-Barraya intestinal f.
Stille-Barraya vascular f.
Stille-Björk f.
Stille-Crafoord f.
Stille-Crile f.
Stille gallstone f.
Stille-Halsted f.
Stille-Horsley bone-cutting f.
Stille-Horsley rib f.
Stille kidney f.
Stille-Liston bone f.
Stille-Liston rib-cutting f.
Stille-Luer rongeur f.
Stille rongeur f.
Stille-Russian f.
Stille tissue f.
Stille-Waugh f.
Stiwer biopsy f.
Stiwer bone-holding f.
Stiwer dressing f.
Stiwer sponge f.
Stiwer tissue f.
S&T Lalonde hook f.
St. Martin eye f.
St. Martin suturing f.
Stolte capsulorhexis f.
Stone clamp-applying f.
stone-crushing f.
stone-extraction f.
stone-grasping f.
Stone intestinal f.
Stoneman f.
Stone tissue f.
Storey gall duct f.
Storey-Hillar dissecting f.
Storey thoracic f.
Storz biopsy f.
Storz-Bonn suturing f.
Storz bronchoscopic f.
Storz capsular f.
Storz ciliary f.
Storz corneal f.
Storz curved f.
Storz cystoscopic f.

Storz esophagoscopic f.
Storz grasping biopsy f.
Storz kidney stone f.
Storz Microsystems plate-holding f.
Storz miniature f.
Storz nasopharyngeal biopsy f.
Storz optical biopsy f.
Storz sinus biopsy f.
Storz stone-crushing f.
Storz stone-extraction f.
Storz-Utrata f.
strabismus f.
straight coagulating f.
straight-end cup f.
straight knot-tying f.
straight line bayonet f.
straight Maryland f.
straight microbipolar f.
straight micromonopolar f.
straight single tenaculum f.
straight-tip bipolar f.
straight-tip jeweler's bipolar f.
straight tying f.
Strassburger tissue f.
Strassmann uterine f.
Stratte f.
Streli f.
Strelinger catheter-introducing f.
Stringer catheter-introducing f.
Stringer newborn throat f.
Strow corneal f.
Struempel ear alligator f.
Struempel ear punch f.
Struempel-Voss ethmoidal f.
Struempel-Voss nasal f.
Strully dressing f.
Strully tissue f.
strut f.
Struyken ear f.
Struyken nasal f.
Struyken nasal-cutting f.
Struyken turbinate f.
St. Vincent tube-occluding f.
Styles f.
subglottic f.
suction f.
Suker iris f.
superior rectus f.
SureBite biopsy f.
Sutherland-Grieshaber f.
Sutherland vitreous f.
suture clip f.
suture tag f.
suture-tying platform f.
suturing f.
Swan-Brown arterial f.
Sweet clip-applying f.
Sweet dissecting f.
Sweet ligature f.
Syark vulsellum f.
synovium biopsy f.
Szuler vascular f.
Szultz corneal f.
tack-and-pin f.
Takahashi cutting f.

F

forceps *(continued)*
Takahashi ethmoidal f.
Takahashi iris retractor f.
Takahashi nasal f.
Takahashi neurosurgical f.
Take-apart f.
tampon f.
Tamsco f.
tangential f.
taper-jaw f.
Tarnier axis-traction f.
Tarnier obstetrical f.
Taylor-Cushing dressing f.
Taylor dissecting f.
Taylor tissue f.
Teale tenaculum f.
Teale uterine f.
Teale vulsellum f.
Tekno f.
tenaculum f.
tenaculum-reducing f.
tendon f.
tendon-holding f.
tendon-passing f.
tendon-pulling f.
tendon-retrieving f.
tendon-seizing f.
Tennant-Colibri corneal f.
Tennant intraocular lens f.
Tennant lens f.
Tennant-Maumenee f.
Tennant titanium suturing f.
Tennant-Troutman superior rectus f.
Tennant tying f.
Tenzel bipolar f.
Terson capsular f.
Terson extracapsular f.
Thackray dental f.
Therma Jaw hot urologic f.
The Shark disposable biopsy f.
Theurig sterilizer f.
Thomas fixation f.
Thomas shot compression f.
Thompson hip prosthesis f.
Thoms-Allis intestinal f.
Thoms-Allis tissue f.
Thoms-Gaylor uterine f.
Thoms tissue f.
thoracic artery f.
thoracic tissue f.
Thorek gallbladder f.
Thorek-Mixter gallbladder f.
Thornton episcleral f.
Thornton fixation f.
Thornton intraocular f.
Thorpe-Castroviejo corneal f.
Thorpe-Castroviejo fixation f.
Thorpe-Castroviejo vitreous foreign body f.
Thorpe conjunctival f.
Thorpe corneal f.
Thorpe corneoscleral f.
Thorpe foreign body f.
Thrasher intraocular f.

Thrasher lens implant f.
three-prong grasping f.
throat f.
thumb tissue f.
Thurston-Holland fragment f.
thyroid f.
Tickner tissue f.
Tiemann bullet f.
Tiger Shark f.
Tilley dressing f.
Tilley-Henckel f.
Tischler cervical biopsy punch f.
Tischler-Morgan uterine biopsy f.
tissue f.
tissue-grasping f.
tissue-holding f.
tissue-spreading f.
titanium microsurgical bipolar f.
Tivnen tonsillar f.
Tobey ear f.
Tobold-Fauvel grasping f.
Tobold laryngeal f.
Toennis-Adson f.
Toennis tumor-grasping f.
Tomac f.
tongue f.
tonsil f.
tonsillar abscess f.
tonsillar artery f.
tonsillar hemostatic f.
tonsillar pillar grasping f.
tonsillar punch f.
Tooke corneal f.
Toomey f.
toothed thumb f.
toothed tissue f.
tooth-extracting f.
toothless f.
Torchia capsular f.
Torchia-Colibri f.
Torchia lens implantation f.
Torchia microbipolar f.
Torchia tissue f.
Torchia tying f.
Torres cross-action f.
torsion f.
Tower muscle f.
Townley tissue f.
tracheal f.
trachoma f.
traction f.
transfer f.
transsphenoidal bipolar f.
traumatic grasping f.
triangular punch f.
tripod grasping f.
Troeltsch dressing f.
Troeltsch ear f.
Trotter f.
Trousseau dilating f.
Troutman-Barraquer-Colibri f.
Troutman-Barraquer corneal f.
Troutman-Barraquer corneal fixation f.
Troutman-Barraquer iris f.

Troutman corneal f.
Troutman-Llobera fixation f.
Troutman-Llobera-Flieringa f.
Troutman microsurgery f.
Troutman superior rectus f.
Troutman tying f.
Truline f.
Trush grasping f.
Trylon hemostatic f.
T-shaped f.
tube-occluding f.
tubing f.
Tubinger gall stone f.
tubing introducer f.
tubular f.
Tucker bead f.
Tucker hallux f.
Tucker-McLane axis-traction f.
Tucker-McLane-Luikart f.
Tucker-McLane obstetrical f.
Tucker reach-and-pin f.
Tucker staple f.
Tucker tack and pin f.
Tudor-Edwards bone-cutting f.
Tuffier arterial f.
tumor f.
tumor-grasping f.
turbinate f.
Turnbull adhesion f.
Turner-Babcock tissue f.
Turner-Warwick-Adson f.
Turner-Warwick stone f.
Turrell rectal biopsy f.
Turrell specimen f.
Turrell-Wittner rectal biopsy f.
Tuttle dressing f.
Tuttle obstetrical f.
Tuttle-Singley thoracic f.
Tuttle thoracic f.
Tuttle thumb f.
Tuttle tissue f.
Twisk f.
two-stream irrigating f.
two-toothed f.
Tydings-Lakeside tonsillar f.
Tydings tonsillar f.
tying f.
tympanoplasty f.
Tyrrell foreign body f.
Ullrich-Aesculap f.
Ullrich bone-holding f.
Ullrich dressing f.
Ullrich-St. Gallen f.
Ultrata capsulorhexis f.
Universal f.
University of Kansas corneal f.
University of Michigan Mixter
  thoracic f.
upbiting biopsy f.
upbiting cup f.
up-cupped f.
upcurved basket f.
Uppsala gall duct f.
upturned f.
upward bent f.

Urbantschitsch nasal f.
ureteral catheter f.
ureteral isolation f.
ureteral stone f.
U-shaped f.
uterine artery f.
uterine biopsy punch f.
uterine-dressing f.
uterine-elevating f.
uterine-grasping f.
uterine-holding f.
uterine-manipulating f.
uterine-packing f.
uterine polyp f.
uterine specimen f.
uterine tenaculum f.
uterine vulsellum f.
utility f.
Utrata capsulorhexis f.
vaginal hysterectomy f.
Valin f.
Van Buren bone-holding f.
Van Buren sequestrum f.
Vanderbilt arterial f.
Vanderbilt deep-vessel f.
Vanderbilt University hemostatic f.
Vanderbilt University vessel f.
Vander Pool sterilizer f.
Van Doren uterine biopsy punch f.
Vannas fixation f.
Van Ruben f.
Van Struyken nasal f.
Vantage tube-occluding f.
Vantec grasping f.
Varco gallbladder f.
Varco thoracic f.
vascular tissue f.
vasectomy f.
vas isolation f.
Vaughn sterilizer f.
vectis cesarean f.
vena cava f.
Verbrugge bone-holding f.
Verhoeff capsular f.
Verhoeff capsule f.
Verhoeff cataract f.
vertical f.
vessel f.
Vick-Blanchard hemorrhoidal f.
Vickerall round ringed f.
Vickers ring-tip f.
Victor-Bonney f.
Vigger-5 eye f.
Virtus splinter f.
viscera-holding f.
visceral f.
vise f.
visual hemostatic f.
Vital-Adson tissue f.
Vital-Babcock tissue f.
Vital-Cushing tissue f.
Vital-Duval intestinal f.
Vital-Evans pelvic tissue f.
Vital general tissue f.
Vital intestinal f.

F

forceps (continued)
Vital lung-grasping f.
Vital needle holder f.
Vital-Potts-Smith f.
Vital-Wangensteen tissue f.
vitreous-grasping f.
V. Mueller biopsy f.
V. Mueller bone-cutting f.
V. Mueller laser Backhaus towel f.
V. Mueller laser Crile micro-
  arterial f.
V. Mueller laser micro-Allis f.
V. Mueller laser Rhoton
  microtying f.
V. Mueller laser Singley tissue f.
V. Mueller nonperforating towel f.
V. Mueller tying f.
V. Mueller-Vital laser Babcock f.
V. Mueller-Vital laser Potts-Smith f.
Vogler hysterectomy f.
Vogt toothed capsular f.
vomer septal f.
von Graefe fixation f.
von Graefe iris f.
von Graefe tissue f.
Von Mandach capsule fragment f.
Von Mandach clot f.
von Petz f.
Voris-Oldberg intervertebral disk f.
Vorse tube-occluding f.
Vorse-Webster f.
VPI-Ambrose resectoscope f.
vulsellum f.
Wachtenfeldt clip-applying f.
Wadsworth lid f.
Wainstock eye suturing f.
Waldeau fixation f.
Waldenstrom laryngeal f.
Waldeyer f.
Walker f.
Wallace cesarean f.
Walsham nasal f.
Walsham septal f.
Walsham septum-straightening f.
Walsh tissue f.
Walter splinter f.
Walther tissue f.
Walton-Allis tissue f.
Walton-Liston f.
Walton meniscal f.
Walton-Schubert uterine biopsy f.
Walzl hysterectomy f.
Wangensteen intestinal f.
Wangensteen tissue f.
Warthen f.
watchmaker f.
Watson duckbill f.
Watson tonsil-seizing f.
Watson-Williams ethmoid-biting f.
Watson-Williams nasal f.
Watson-Williams polyp f.
Watzke f.
Waugh-Brophy f.
Waugh dissection f.

Waugh dressing f.
Waugh tissue f.
wave-tooth f.
Weaver chalazion f.
Weck-Harms f.
Weck hysterectomy f.
Weck rectal biopsy f.
Weck towel f.
Weck uterine biopsy f.
Weeks eye f.
Weiger-Zollner f.
Weil-Blakesley ethmoidal f.
Weil ear f.
Weil ethmoidal f.
Weiner uterine biopsy f.
Weingartner ear f.
Weis chalazion f.
Weisman f.
Weiss f.
Welch Allyn anal biopsy f.
Weller cartilage f.
Weller meniscal f.
Wells f.
Welsh ophthalmic f.
Welsh pupil-spreader f.
Wertheim-Cullen compression f.
Wertheim-Cullen hysterectomy f.
Wertheim-Cullen kidney pedicle f.
Wertheim hysterectomy f.
Wertheim-Navratil f.
Wertheim uterine f.
Wertheim vaginal f.
Westermark-Stille f.
Westermark uterine dressing f.
Westmacott dressing f.
West nasal-dressing f.
Westphal gall duct f.
Westphal hemostatic f.
Wheeler plaque f.
Wheeler vessel f.
White-Lillie tonsillar f.
White-Oslay prostatic f.
White-Smith f.
White tonsillar f.
Whitney superior rectus f.
Wickman uterine f.
Wiener hysterectomy f.
Wies chalazion f.
Wiet otologic cup f.
Wikström arterial f.
Wilde-Blakesley ethmoidal f.
Wilde ear f.
Wilde ethmoidal exenteration f.
Wilde intervertebral disk f.
Wilde laminectomy f.
Wilde nasal-cutting f.
Wilde nasal-dressing f.
Wilder dilating f.
Wilde septal f.
Wilde-Troeltsch f.
Wilkerson intraocular lens-
  insertion f.
Willauer-Allis thoracic f.
Willauer-Allis tissue f.
Willauer intrathoracic f.

Willett placental f.
Willett placenta previa f.
Willett scalp flap f.
Williamsburg f.
Williams diskectomy f.
Williams gastrointestinal f.
Williams intestinal f.
Williams splinter f.
Williams tissue f.
Williams uterine f.
Williams vessel-holding f.
Wills Hospital ophthalmic f.
Wills utility f.
Wilmer iris f.
Wilson-Cook bronchoscope biopsy f.
Wilson-Cook colonoscope biopsy f.
Wilson-Cook gastroscope biopsy f.
Wilson-Cook grasping f.
Wilson-Cook hot biopsy f.
Wilson-Cook retrieval f.
Wilson-Cook tripod retrieval f.
Wilson vitreous foreign body f.
Winter-Nassauer placental f.
Winter ovum f.
Winter placental f.
wire-closure f.
wire-crimping f.
wire prosthesis-crimping f.
wire-pulling f.
wire-twisting f.
Wittner uterine biopsy f.
Wolf biopsy f.
Wolf biting-basket f.
Wolf cataract delivery f.
Wolf curved-basket f.
Wolf eye f.
Wolfson f.
Wolf uterine cuff f.
Woodward f.
Woodward-Potts intestinal f.
Woodward thoracic artery f.
Worth advancement f.
Worth muscle f.
Worth strabismus f.
wound f.
wound-clip f.
Wright-Rubin f.
Wrigley f.
W-shape f.
Wullstein ear f.
Wullstein-House f.
Wullstein-Paparella f.
Wullstein tympanoplasty f.
Wylie tenaculum f.
Wylie uterine f.
X-long cement f.
Yankauer ethmoidal f.
Yankauer-Little f.
Yasargil angled f.
Yasargil applying f.
Yasargil arterial f.
Yasargil bipolar f.
Yasargil clip-applying f.
Yasargil flat serrated ring f.
Yasargil microvessel clip-applying f.

Yasargil neurosurgical bipolar f.
Yasargil straight f.
Yeoman uterine f.
Yeoman uterine biopsy f.
Yeoman-Wittner rectal f.
Younge-Kevorkian f.
Younge uterine f.
Young intestinal f.
Young lobe f.
Young prostatectomy f.
Young prostatic f.
Young tongue f.
Young uterine f.
Z-clamp hysterectomy f.
Zeeifel angiotribe f.
Zenker f.
Zeppelin obstetrical f.
Ziegler ciliary f.
Zimmer-Hoen f.
Zimmer-Schlesinger f.
Zollinger multipurpose tissue f.

Ford
    F. clamp
    F. Hospital ventricular cannula
Ford-Deaver retractor
forearm
    f. flexion control strap
    f. tourniquet
Foregger
    F. bronchoscope
    F. laryngoscope
    F. rigid esophagoscope
Foregger-Racine adapter
foreign
    f. body bur
    f. body curette
    f. body cystoscopy forceps
    f. body eye forceps
    f. body locator
    f. body loop
    f. body magnet
    f. body needle
    f. body probe
    f. body remover
    f. body retrieval system
    f. body-retrieving forceps
    f. body screw
    f. body spud
ForeRunner
    F. automatic external defibrillator
        device
    F. coronary sinus guiding catheter
fork
    crus guide f.
    double-pronged f.
    Gardiner-Brown neurological
        tuning f.
    f. hammer
    Hardy implant f.
    Hardy 3-prong f.
    Hartmann tuning f.
    Jacobson f.
    Jannetta double-pronged f.
    Jarit tuning f.
    knife and f.

F

fork *(continued)*
  Leasure tuning f.
  magnesium tuning f.
  McCabe crus guide f.
  neurological tuning f.
  Okonek-Yasargil tumor f.
  Penn tuning f.
  Ralks tuning f.
  Rhoton 3-prong f.
  Rica tuning f.
  Riverbank Laboratories tuning f.
  Rydel-Seiffert tuning f.
  SMIC tuning f.
  Sugita f.
  three-prong f.
  tuning f.
Forker retractor
form
  Amoena breast f.
  breast f.
  Discrene breast f.
  Dow Corning external breast f.
  Jettmobile Tumble F.'s
  mastopexy f.
  Nearly Me breast f.
  Roth arch f.
  Spenco external breast f.
  Trulife silicone breast f.
  Vestibulator positioning tumble f.'s
  Yours Truly asymmetrical external breast f.
formaldehyde catgut suture
Formatray mandibular splint
Forma water-jacketed incubator
formboard
  Séguin f.
formed
  f. nonirrigating cystitome
Formex barium catheter
FormFlex
  F. formocresal lens
  F. intraocular lens
  F. lens loop
Foroblique
  F. bronchoscope
  F. bronchoscopic telescope
  F. endoscope
  F. fiberoptic esophagoscope
  F. lens
  F. microlens resectoscope
Forrester
  F. cervical collar brace
  F. clamp
  F. head halter
  F. head splint
Förster
  F. enucleation snare
  F. iris forceps
  F. photometer
  F. photoptometer
Forte ES instrument
Fortuna syringe
Fort urethral bougie
forward-cutting knife

forward-grasping forceps
forward-viewing endoscope
Foss
  F. anterior resection clamp
  F. bifid gallbladder retractor
  F. biliary retractor
  F. cardiovascular clamp
  F. cardiovascular forceps
  F. clamp forceps
  F. intestinal clamp
fossa curette
FossFill Health Pillow
Foster
  F. bed
  F. fracture frame
  F. scissors
  F. snare enucleator
  F. suture
Foster-Ballenger
  F.-B. forceps
  F.-B. nasal speculum
Fothergill suture
Fotofil
  F. activator light
  F. dental restorative material
Fotona
  F. Novalis ER:YAG laser
  F. Novalis R ruby laser
Fouli tourniquet
Foundation
  F. total hip system
  F. total knee system
fountain
  F. design prosthesis
  xenon cold light f.
four-bar
  f.-b. linkage prosthetic knee mechanism
  f.-b. polycentric knee prosthesis
four-beam laser Doppler probe
four-channel Aesculap ventriculoscope
four-degree-of freedom manipulator
four-eye catheter
four-flanged nail
four-footed lens
four-head camera
four-hole
  f.-h. anteromedial Alta straight plate
  f.-h. side plate
Fourier
  F. harmonic analysis
  F. transformation spectrum analyzer
  F. transform infrared spectroscopy
four-layer bandage
four-legged cage heart valve
four-loop
  f.-l. iris clip implant
  f.-l. iris fixated implant
four-lumen polyvinyl manometric catheter
four-mirror
  f.-m. goniolens
  f.-m. goniolens lens
Fournier tip
four-piece intraocular lens

four-point
　　f.-p. cervical brace
　　f.-p. fixation intraocular lens
　　f.-p. spreader bag
four-poster frame
four-prong
　　f.-p. finger speculum
　　f.-p. finger splint
　　f.-p. retractor
four-sided cutting needle
four-tailed
　　f.-t. bandage
　　f.-t. dressing
four-tap screw
four-wing
　　f.-w. Malecot drain
　　f.-w. Malecot retention catheter
Fowler
　　F. double-end curette
　　F. dressing
　　F. self-retaining retractor
　　F. urethral sound
Fowler-Zollner knife
Fox
　　F. aluminum eye shield
　　F. bipolar electrocautery forceps
　　F. clavicular splint
　　F. conformer
　　F. dermal curette
　　F. eyelid implant
　　F. eye speculum
　　F. hydrostatic irrigator
　　F. I&A unit
　　F. impactor-extractor
　　F. internal fixation device
　　F. postnasal balloon
　　F. prosthesis
　　F. spherical eye implant
　　F. tissue forceps
Fox-Blazina prosthesis
FPS
　　FPS system
Frackelton
　　F. fascial needle
　　F. wire threader
FracSure
　　F. apparatus
　　F. appliance
　　F. splint
　　F. unit
Fractomed splint
Fractura
　　F. Flex bandage
　　F. Flex cast
fracture
　　f. band
　　f. bar
　　f. bed
　　f. boot
　　f. chisel
　　f. computer-aided surgery
　　f. computer-aided surgery
　　　(FRACAS) system
　　f. fixation device
　　f. frame

　　f. reducing elevator
　　f. splint
　　f. table
fracture-banding apparatus
Fraenkel (*var. of* Fränkel)
Frag Commander ultrasonic pars plana
　　lensectomy system
Fragen
　　F. anterior commissure
　　　microlaryngoscope
　　F. carrier
　　F. laryngoscope
　　F. laryngoscope fiberoptic light
Fragmatome
　　CooperVision F.
　　F. flute syringe
　　Gill-Hess F.
　　Girard F.
　　F. tip
fragmentation/aspiration handpiece
fragmentation probe
fragment forceps
fragmentor
　　Lieberman f.
Frahm carver
Frahur
　　F. cartilage clamp
　　F. scissors
fraise
　　diamond f.
frame
　　Ace-Fischer f.
　　Alexian Brothers overhead
　　　fracture f.
　　Andrews spinal f.
　　anterior quadrilateral triplane f.
　　A-f. orthosis
　　Balkan fracture f.
　　Böhler-Braun fracture f.
　　Böhler reducing fracture f.
　　Boston Children's f.
　　Bradford fracture f.
　　Braun f.
　　Brown-Roberts-Wells head f.
　　Buck extension f.
　　Budde-Greenberg-Sugita stereotactic
　　　head f.
　　Charest head f.
　　Chick CLT operating f.
　　CHOP f.
　　Codman f.
　　Cole hyperextension fracture f.
　　Colles external fixation f.
　　Compass stereotactic f.
　　Cosman-Roberts-Wells (CRW)
　　　stereotactic f.
　　couch-mounted head f.
　　Crawford head f.
　　Delta external fixation f.
　　Denis Browne retractor oval
　　　sprocket f.
　　DePuy rainbow fracture f.
　　designs for vision f.
　　detachable stretcher f.
　　Dingman mouthgag f.

F

frame *(continued)*
Doctor Plymale lift fracture f.
double-ring f.
Elekta stereotactic head f.
Elgiloy f.
Erich facial fracture f.
Foster fracture f.
four-poster f.
fracture f.
fusion f.
Gardner-Wells fixation f.
Goldthwait fracture f.
Granberry hyperextension fracture f.
Greenberg retractor f.
Hall-Relton f.
halo fracture f.
halo head f.
Hastings f.
head f.
Heffington lumbar seat spinal
 surgery f.
Herzmark fracture f.
Hibbs fracture f.
Hitchcock stereotactic
 immobilization f.
Horsley-Clarke stereotactic f.
hyperextension fracture f.
Ilizarov f.
Irby head f.
Janes fracture f.
Jewett f.
Jones abduction f.
Joseph septal f.
Kessler traction f.
Komai stereotactic head f.
Laitinen stereotactic head f.
laminectomy f.
Leksell D-shaped stereotactic f.
Leksell-Elekta stereotactic f.
Leksell Model G stereotactic f.
Leksell stereotaxic f.
Lex-Ton lumbar laminectomy f.
Maddacrawler f.
Malcolm-Lynn C-RXF cervical
 retractor f.
Malcolm-Rand cranial x-ray f.
Mayfield fixation f.
Monticelli-Spinelli f.
mouthgag f.
MTL trial f.
Mussen f.
nitinol mesh-covered f.
nonferromagnetic MR-compatible f.
occluding fracture f.
Oculus trial f.
Olivier-Bertrand-Tipal f.
Ostby dam f.
overhead fracture f.
Pearson attachment to Thomas f.
Pelorus stereotactic f.
phantom f.
Pittsburgh triangular f.
Putti f.
quadraplegic standing f.

radiolucent spine f.
Radionics CRW stereotactic head f.
Rainbow fracture f.
Rand-Malcolm cranial x-ray f.
reducing fracture f.
Reichert-Mundinger-Fischer
 stereotactic f.
Reichert-Mundinger stereotactic
 head f.
Relton-Hall spinal f.
retractor oval sprocket f.
Richards Colles fracture f.
Risser f.
robotics-controlled stereotactic f.
Russell f.
self-retaining brain retractor f.
Slatis f.
sling f.
spinal turning f.
Stealth f.
stereotactic head f.
stereotactic localization f.
Stryker CircOlectric fracture f.
Stryker turning fracture f.
Sugita multipurpose head f.
Talairach stereotactic f.
Taylor spinal f.
Thomas fracture f.
Thomas hyperextension f.
Thompson hyperextension fracture f.
Todd-Wells stereotactic f.
trial fracture f.
triangular ankle fusion f.
vasocillator fracture f.
Vidal-Hoffman fixator f.
Watson-Jones f.
Whitman fracture f.
Wilson spinal f.
Wingfield fracture f.
Young rubber dam fracture f.
Zimcode traction f.
Zimmer fracture f.
frameless
f. air support therapy system
f. stereotaxy system
framer
F. finger extension bow
GTC repeated stereotactic
 localizer f.
F. splint
F. tendon passer
F. tendon-passing needle
Francer porcelain powder
Franceschetti corneal trephine
Franceschetti-type freeblade
Francis
F. knife spud
F. spud chalazion forceps
Francis-Gray wire crimper
Francke needle
Franco triflange ventilation tube
Frangenheim
F. biopsy punch forceps
F. hook forceps

F. hook punch
F. laparoscope

Frank
F. EKG lead placement system
F. XYZ orthogonal lead
F. XYZ orthogonal lead system

Fränkel, Fraenkel
F. appliance
F. cutting-tip forceps
F. esophagoscopy forceps
F. head band
F. laryngeal forceps
F. sinus probe
F. speculum
F. tampon forceps

Frankfeldt
F. diathermy snare
F. grasping forceps
F. hemorrhoidal needle
F. rectal snare
F. sigmoidoscope

Franklin
F. glasses
F. liver puncture needle
F. malleable retractor
F. spectacles

Franklin-Silverman
F.-S. biopsy cannula
F.-S. curette
F.-S. prostatic biopsy needle

Franseen liver biopsy needle
Franz
F. abdominal retractor
F. monophasic action potential catheter

Franzen needle guide
Fraser
F. depressor
F. forceps
F. Harlake respirometer

Frater
F. intracardiac retractor
F. suture

Frazier
F. aspirating tube
F. brain-exploring cannula
F. brain-exploring trocar
F. brain suction tube
F. Britetrac nasal suction tube
F. cerebral retractor
F. cordotomy hook
F. cordotomy knife
F. dural elevator
F. dural guide
F. dural hook
F. dural scissors
F. dural separator
F. fiberoptic suction tube
F. laminectomy retractor
F. lighted retractor
F. modified suction tube
F. monopolar cautery cord
F. nasal suction tube
F. nerve hook
F. osteotome

F. pituitary capsulectomy knife
F. skin hook
F. stylet
F. suction
F. suction cannula
F. suction elevator
F. suction tip
F. suction tip aspirator
F. suction tube
F. suction tube obturator
F. ventricular cannula
F. ventricular needle

Frazier-Adson osteoplastic clamp
Frazier-Fay retractor
Frazier-Ferguson
F.-F. aspirating tube
F.-F. ear suction tube

Frazier-Paparella mastoid suction tube
Frazier-Sachs clamp
Frederick
F. pneumothoracic needle
F. pneumothorax needle

Frederick-Miller tube
Fredricks mammary prosthesis
Free
F. & Active incontinence pant

freeblade
Franceschetti-type f.

Freedom
F. arthritis support
F. arthritis support for hand
F. Back Support
F. Cath
F. dental unit
F. Elastic Long Wrist Support
F. external catheter
F. knife
F. leg bag collection system
F. Micro Pro stimulator
F. Neutral Position Splint
F. Omni Progressive Splint
F. Pak Seven catheter
F. Palm guard
F. Progressive Resting Splint
F. Sportsfit Splint
F. stent
F. Thumbkeeper
F. Thumb spica cast
F. Thumb Stabilizer
F. T-tap leg bag
F. T-tap leg bag kit
F. Ultimate Grip Splint
F. USA Wristlet

FreeDop
F. Doppler monitor
F. portable Doppler unit

Free-Flow system prosthesis
Freegenol cement
Freehand neuroprosthetic system
free implant
FreeLock femoral fixation system
Freeman
F. Blue-Max cannula
F. capsular polisher
F. clamp

F

Freeman *(continued)*
- F. cookie cutter areola marker
- F. facelift retractor
- F. femoral component
- F. modular total hip prosthesis
- F. positioning cannula
- F. punctum plug
- F. rhytidectomy scissors
- F. transorbital leukotome

Freeman-Samuelson knee prosthesis
Freeman-Schepens scissors
Freeman-Swanson knee prosthesis
Freenseen rectal curette
Freer
- F. bone chisel
- F. double-end elevator
- F. dural dissector
- F. dural retractor
- F. lacrimal chisel
- F. nasal chisel
- F. nasal gouge
- F. nasal spatula
- F. nasal submucous knife
- F. periosteal elevator
- F. periosteotome
- F. septal elevator
- F. septal forceps
- F. septal knife
- F. skin hook
- F. skin retractor
- F. submucous chisel
- F. submucous retractor

Freer-Gruenwald punch forceps
Freer-Ingal nasal submucous knife
Freer-Sachs dissector
free-spinning probe
free-standing
- f.-s. implant
- f.-s. single crown
- f.-s. stent
- f.-s. tissue retraction bridge system

Freestyle
- F. aortic root bioprosthesis
- F. CAPD catheter adapter
- F. valve

Freeway Lite portable aerosol compressor
freezer
- CryoMed 1010A f.
- Gentle Jane Snap f.
- Kryo 10 model 10-20 f.

freezing point osmometer
Freezor cryocatheter
Freiberg
- F. cartilage knife
- F. hip retractor
- F. meniscectomy knife
- F. nerve root retractor
- F. traction
- F. tractor

Freiburg
- F. biopsy set
- F. mediastinoscope

Freidenwald-Guyton snare

Freidman splint
Freidrich-Ferguson retractor
Freimuth ear curette
Freitag stent
Frejka
- F. cast
- F. hip pillow
- F. jacket
- F. orthosis
- F. pillow splint
- F. traction

Frekatheter vena cava catheter
Frelex lens
French
- F. angiographic catheter
- F. catheter gauge
- F. chisel
- F. Cope loop nephrostomy catheter
- F. curve out-of-plane catheter
- F. cystoscope
- F. double-lumen catheter
- F. Foley catheter
- F. Gesco catheter
- F. hook spatula
- F. in-plane guiding catheter
- F. JR4 Schneider catheter
- F. lacrimal dilator
- F. lacrimal probe
- F. lacrimal spatula
- F. lock
- F. MBIH catheter
- F. mushroom-tip catheter
- F. needle holder
- F. Pharmacovigilance system
- F. pigtail nephrostomy catheter
- F. red-rubber Robinson catheter
- F. Robinson catheter
- F. rod bender
- F. SAL catheter
- F. scoop
- F. shaft catheter
- F. sheath
- F. Silastic Foley catheter
- F. sizing of catheter
- F. spring-eye needle
- F. S-shaped brain retractor
- F. steel sound
- F. stent
- F. Swan-Ganz balloon
- F. Teflon pyeloureteral catheter
- F. T-tube

French-eye
- F.-e. needle
- F.-e. Vital needle holder

French-Hanks uterine dilator
French-McCarthy endoscope
French-McRea dilator
French-pattern
- F.-p. forceps
- F.-p. osteotome
- F.-p. raspatory
- F.-p. spatula

French-Stern-McCarthy retractor
Frenckner curette

Frenckner-Stille
F.-S. curette
F.-S. punch
Frenta
F. enteral feeding bag
F. Mat feeding pump
F. System II feeding pump
frequency doubled neodymium:yttrium-aluminum-garnet laser
Fresenius
F. AG dialyzer
F. dialysis machine
F. Euro-Collins kit
F. F-40 filter
F. volumetric dialysate balancing system
Fresgen frontal sinus probe
FreshStart mammary support garment
Fresnel
F. goggles
F. lens
F. lens pusher
F. manipulating hook
F. nystagmus glasses
F. nystagmus spectacles
F. prism
F. zone plate
Freyer suprapubic drain
Frey-Freer bur
Frey-Sauerbruch rib shears
Frey tunneled eye implant
Frialit-2 system Frialloc transgingival threaded implant
FRIALITE-2 dental implant system
Friatec
F. implant
F. manual arthroscopy instrument
Fricke
F. arterial forceps
F. bandage
F. scrotal dressing
friction-fit adapter
friction lock pin
friction-reduced segmented table
Friedenwald
F. funduscope
F. ophthalmoscope
Friedländer incision marker
Friedman
F. bone rongeur
F. elevator
F. hand-held Hruby lens
F. knife guide
F. olive-tip vein stripper
F. perineal retractor
F. Phaco/IOL manipulator
F. rasp
F. rongeur forceps
F. splint
F. tantalum clip
F. vaginal retractor
Friedmann visual field analyzer
Friedman-Otis bougie à boule
Friedrich
F. clamp

F. raspatory
F. rib elevator
Friedrich-Petz
F.-P. clamp
F.-P. machine resector
Friend catheter
Friend-Hebert catheter
Friesner ear knife
Frigitronics
Cilco F.
F. colposcope
F. cryoprobe
F. cryosurgical unit
F. disposable cryosurgical stylet
F. freeze-thaw cryopexy probe
F. Mark II cryoextractor
F. nitrous oxide cryosurgery apparatus
F. vitrector
Frimberger-Karpiel
F.-K. 12 o'clock papillotome
F.-K. 12 O'Clock sphincterotome
Fritsch
F. abdominal retractor
F. catheter
Fritz
F. aspirator
F. vitreous transplant needle
frog
f. cortex remover
f. splint
frog-leg splint
Frohm mouthgag
Froimson splint
Frommer dilator
Fromm triangle orthopaedic device
front
f. build-up implant
f. support strap
f. wall needle
frontal
f. sinus cannula
f. sinus chisel
f. sinus curette
f. sinus dilator
f. sinus probe
f. sinus rasp
f. sinus wash tube
frontalis snare
front-entry guide
front-wheeled walker
Frost
F. scissors
F. stitch
F. suture
Frosted Flex earmold material
Fruehevald splint
Frumin valve
Frydman catheter
Frye aspirator
Frykholm
F. bone rongeur
F. goniometer
Fry nasal forceps

F

F-Scan foot force and gait analysis system
FSD colpostat
F-series
    F.-s. dialyzer
    F.-s. fluorescence spectrophotometer
FTO eye patch
Fuchs
    F. capsular forceps
    F. capsule forceps
    F. capsulotomy forceps
    F. extracapsular forceps
    F. iris forceps
    F. lancet-type keratome
    F. retinal detachment syringe
    F. surgical stool
    F. two-way eye syringe
Fuji
    F. AC2 storage phosphor computed radiology system
    F. dental cement
    F. FCR9000 computed radiology system
Fujica camera
Fujinon
    F. biopsy forceps
    F. CEG-FP-series videoelectroscope
    F. diagnostic laparoscope
    F. EB-410S bronchoscope
    F. EC-series video colonoscope
    F. ED-series duodenoscope
    F. ED7-XU2 videoduodenoscope
    F. EG-FP-series endoscope
    F. EG-series endoscope
    F. EG-series gastroscope
    F. EG7-series videoelectroscope
    F. ES-200ER sigmoidoscope
    F. EVE-series endoscope
    F. EVG-CT-series endoscope
    F. EVG-FP-series endoscope
    F. EVG-F-series endoscope
    F. EVG-series endoscope
    F. FD-series duodenoscope
    F. flexible bronchoscope
    F. flexible fiberoptic laparoscope
    F. flexible hysteroscope
    F. flexible sigmoidoscope
    F. FP-series endoscope
    F. FS-100ER sigmoidoscope
    F. GF-series gastroscope
    F. operating laparoscope
    F. 400-series super image video gastroscope
    F. SP-501 sonoprobe system
    F. UGI-FP-series video endoscope
    F. variceal injector
    F. 310XU videoduodenoscope
Fujita
    F. snake retractor
    F. suction cannula
Fukasaku pupil snapper hook
Fukuda humeral head retractor
Fukusaku spatula
Fukushima
    F. C-clamp clamp

    F. dissector
    F. malleable brain spatula
    F. monopolar malleable coagulator
    F. retractor
    F. ring-curette
    F. rongeur
Fulcast alloy
fulgurating electrode
full
    f. lower denture
    f. spine board
    f. upper denture
full-circle goniometer
full-curved clamp
full-dimpled Lucite eye implant
Fuller
    F. bivalve trach tube
    F. perianal shield
    F. rectal dressing
    F. silicone sponge
Fullerview
    F. flexible iris retractor
FullFlow catheter
full-hand splint
full-intensity needle
full-lumen esophagoscope
full-occlusal splint
full-radius resector
full-thickness implant
full-time occlusion eye patch
full-wave rectifier
fully-automatic atrioventricular Universal dual-channel pacemaker
fully constrained tricompartmental knee prosthesis
Fulpit tissue forceps
Fulton
    F. laminectomy rongeur
    F. mouthgag
    F. pediatric scissors
    F. retractor
Ful-Vue
    F.-V. ophthalmoscope
    F.-V. spot retinoscope
    F.-V. streak retinoscope
functional
    f. electronic peroneal brace
    f. fracture brace
    f. MRI
    f. orthotic
    f. resting position splint
fundal
    f. contact lens
    f. laser lens
fundal-focalizing lens
fundamental frequency indicator
fundus
    f. camera
    f. contact lens
    f. focalizing lens
funduscope
    Friedenwald f.
fundus-retinal camera

funnel
Esca Buess + fistula f.
stent f.
funnelform taper
Funsten supination splint
Furacin
F. gauze dressing
F. gauze holder
Furlong tendon stripper
Furlow cylinder passer
Furnas bayonet osteotome
Furness
F. anastomosis clamp
F. catheter
F. cornea-holding forceps
F. polyp forceps
Furness-Clute
F.-C. anastomosis clamp
F.-C. duodenal clamp
F.-C. pin
Furness-McClure-Hinton clamp
fused bifocal lens
fused-tip catheter
fusiform bougie

fusion
f. cage
f. frame
f. plate
Futch antral cannula
Futrex analyzer
Futura resectoscope sheath
Futuro
F. splint
F. wrist brace
F. wrist support
FyBron
F. calcium alginate dressing
Fyodorov
F. dipstick
F. eye implant
F. four-loop iris clip intraocular
lens
F. lens expressor
F. type I, II intraocular lens
F. type I, II lens implant
Fyodorov-Sputnik FFP contact
intraocular lens

F

G5

G5 Fleximatic massage/percussion unit
G5 Flimm Fighter percussor
G5 massage and percussion machine
G5 Mist-Ease nebulizer
G5 Neocussor percussor
G5 Porta-Plus muscle stimulator
G5 Vari-Tilt Adjustable Tilt-Board

G3PDH cDNA probe
Gaab endoscope
GaAs laser
Gabarro

G. board
G. retractor

Gabbay-Frater suture guide
Gabor probe
Gabriel

G. proctoscope
G. syringe
G. Tucker bougie
G. Tucker forceps
G. Tucker tube

gadolinium scan
Gaeltec catheter-tip pressure transducer
gaff
Gaffee speculum
Gaffney

G. ankle prosthesis
G. joint

gag (*See* mouthgag)

Brophy g.
Crowe-Davis mouth g.
Lane mouth g.
Millard mouth g.

Gaillard-Arlt suture
gait

g. belt
g. lock splint
g. lock splint brace
g. plate

gaiter brace
GAIT spacer
Galand

G. disk lens
G. in-the-bag lens

Galand-Knolle modified J-loop intraocular lens
Galante

G. hip guide
G. hip prosthesis

Galaxy

G. McManis hylo table
G. pacemaker

galeal forceps
Galen

G. bandage
G. dressing
G. Scan scanner
G. teleradiology system

Galetti articulator
Galezowski lacrimal dilator

Galilean

G. loupe
G. microscope

Galileo

G. evoked potential electroencephalograph
G. rigid hysteroscope

Galin

G. intraocular implant lens
G. intraocular lens implant
G. lens spatula
G. silicone bleb cup

gall

g. duct dilator
g. duct forceps
g. duct probe
g. duct scoop

Gall-Addison uterine manipulator
Gallagher

G. antral rasp
G. bipolar mapping probe
G. trocar

Gallannaugh bone plate
gallbladder

g. aspirator
g. cannula
g. forceps
g. retractor
g. ring clamp
g. scissors
g. scoop
g. spoon

Gallie

G. cryoenucleator
G. fusion-using cable
G. tendon passer

Gallini bone marrow aspiration needle
gallium-aluminum-arsenide laser
Galloway electrode
gallows

Killian suspension g.
G. splint

gallows-type retractor
gallstone

g. basket
g. dilator
g. forceps
g. probe
g. scoop

Galt

G. aspirating cannula
G. hand drill
G. skull trephine

Galtac device
Galton

G. ear whistle
G. galvanometer

galvanic

g. electrode stimulator
g. probe
g. skin response device
g. skin response meter

G

galvanometer
    d'Arsonval g.
    Einthoven string g.
    Galton g.
Galveston
    G. fixation with TSRH crosslink
    G. metacarpal brace
    G. plate
    G. splint
Gambale-Merrill bone-cutting forceps
Gambee suture
Gamboscope
    G. scope
Gambro
    G. AK10 machine
    G. catheter
    G. dialyzer
    G. dialyzer holder
    G. FH88H filter
    G. freezing bag
    G. hemodialyzer
    G. hemofiltration system
    G. Liendia plate
    G. oxygenator
Gambro-Lundia
    G.-L. coil dialyzer
    G.-L. Minor hemodialyzer
Gamgee dressing
gamma
    g. emitter
    g. knife
    g. probe
    g. scintillation camera
    G. trochanteric locking nail
    g. well counter
gamma-detecting probe
gamma-ray
    g.-r. counter
    g.-r. spectrometer
Gammatone II gamma camera
Gam-Mer
    G.-M. aneurysm clamp
    G.-M. bipolar coagulator
    G.-M. bone-cutting forceps
    G.-M. bur
    G.-M. chuck
    G.-M. clip applier
    G.-M. gouge
    G.-M. groover
    G.-M. medial esophageal retractor
    G.-M. minimallet
    G.-M. miniosteotome
    G.-M. nerve hook
    G.-M. oblique raspatory
    G.-M. occipital retractor
    G.-M. occlusion clamp
    G.-M. periosteal elevator
    G.-M. rasp
    G.-M. rongeur
    G.-M. spinal fusion curette
    G.-M. vise
Gammex
    G. RMI DAP meter
    G. RMI scanner
GAN-19 needle

Gandhi knife
Gandy clamp
ganglion
    g. injection needle
    g. scissors
Ganley splint
Gannetta dissector
Gans cyclodialysis cannula
Gant
    G. clamp
    G. gallbladder retractor
    G. rectal probe
gantry
    CT scan g.
Ganz-Edwards coronary infusion catheter
Ganzfeld
    G. electroretinograph
    G. stimulator
Garceau
    G. bougie
    G. ureteral catheter
Garcia
    G. aorta clamp
    G. aortic clamp
    G. endometrial biopsy set
Garcia-Ibanez M picture camera
Garcia-Novito eye implant
Garcia-Rock endometrial biopsy curette
Gard-all boot shoe
Gardiner-Brown neurological tuning fork
Gardlok neurosurgical sponge
Gardner
    G. bone chisel
    G. bone forceps
    G. chair
    G. headholder
    G. headrest
    G. hysterectomy forceps
    G. needle
    G. needle holder
    G. skull clamp
Gardner-Wells
    G.-W. fixation frame
    G.-W. headrest
    G.-W. traction tongs
Gardray dosimeter
Garfield-Holinger laryngoscope
Gariel pessary
Gariot articulator
Garland
    G. hysterectomy clamp
    G. hysterectomy forceps
Garlock spur crusher
garment
    Canfield facial plastics g.
    compression g.
    crotchless compression g.
    facial plastics g.
    FreshStart mammary support g.
    HK breast/torso g.
    Jobst pressure g.
    Marena by LySonix compression g.
    Medical Z post surgery g.
    pneumatic g.

PresSsion pneumatic g.
surgical compression g.
Garney rubber band applicator
Garren-Edwards gastric balloon
Garretson
G. bandage
G. dressing
Garrett
G. peripheral vascular retractor
G. vein passer
Garrigue
G. uterine-dressing forceps
G. vaginal retractor
G. weighted vaginal speculum
Garrison forceps
Garron spatula
garter
Goffman eye g.
G. shield
Gärtner tonometer
gas
G. Check blood analyzer
g. chromatograph
g. chromatography/mass spectroscopy
g. cylinder
g. discharge lamp
g. insufflator
g. isotope ratio mass spectrometer
g. laser
G. lyte ABG syringes
GaSampler Multilaminate Bag
Gaskell clamp
gasket
Seal-Tite adhesive g.
Gaskin fragment forceps
Gas-Pak jar
Gasparotti bevel tip
Gass
G. cataract-aspirating cannula
G. cervical punch
G. corneoscleral punch
G. dye applicator
G. I&A unit
G. muscle hook
G. neurosurgical light
G. retinal detachment cannula
G. retinal detachment hook
G. scleral marker
G. scleral punch
G. sclerotomy punch
G. vitreous-aspirating cannula
gastric
g. balloon
g. bubble
g. clamp
g. resection retractor
g. shield
g. tube
g. volvulus
gastrocamera
Bolex g.
cine g.
Exakta Varex g.
Olympus g.

gastroenterostomy
g. catheter
g. clamp
gastrofiberscope
Pentax FG-series ultrasound g.
GastrographH
G. ambulatory pH monitoring
system
G. Mark III pH analyzer
gastrointestinal
g. clamp
g. forceps
g. needle
g. surgical gut suture
g. surgical linen suture
g. surgical silk suture
gastrojejunostomy tube
gastroplasty stapler
Gastro-Port II feeding tube
Gastroreflex ambulatory pH monitor
Gastroscan motility system
gastroscope
ACMI g.
Benedict operating g.
Bernstein g.
Cameron omni-angle g.
Chevalier Jackson g.
disposable-sheath flexible g.
Eder g.
Eder-Bernstein g.
Eder-Chamberlin g.
Eder-Hufford g.
Eder-Palmer g.
Ellsner g.
end-viewing g.
Ewald g.
examining g.
fiberoptic g.
flexible g.
Fujinon EG-series g.
Fujinon GF-series g.
Fujinon 400-series super image
video g.
Herman-Taylor g.
Hirschowitz g.
Housset-Debray g.
Janeway g.
Jenning-Streifeneder g.
Kelling g.
Krentz g.
Mancke flex-rigid g.
Olympus GF-series g.
Olympus GIF-K-series g.
Olympus GIF-series g.
Olympus GIF-XQ-series flexible g.
Olympus GTF-series g.
Olympus OES-series g.
Olympus 2T-2000 twin-channel
therapeutic g.
pediatric g.
Pentax EUP-EC-series ultrasound g.
peroral g.
Schindler g.
Sielaff g.
Taylor g.

G

gastroscope *(continued)*
Tomenius g.
Universal g.
Wolf-Henning g.
Wolf-Knittlingen g.
Wolf-Schindler g.
gastrostomy
Beck g.
g. button
Depage-Janeway g.
feeding g.
g. feeding tube
Glassman g.
Kader g.
Microvasive One Step Button g.
Olympus g.
percutaneous endoscopic g. (PEG)
g. plug
Russell percutaneous endoscopic g.
Ssabanejeu-Frank g.
Surgitek One Step percutaneous
endoscopic g.
Witzel g.
Gatch bed
gate clip
Gates-Glidden
G.-G. bur
G.-G. drill
GateWay Y-adapter rotating hemostatic
valve
Gatlin gun drill guide
gator
G. drape
G. meniscal cutter
g. plastic orthosis
G. resector
G. shaver
Gatron nerve stimulator
Gaubatz rib retractor
Gauderer-Ponsky PEG
Gauder Silicon PEG catheter
Gau gastric balloon
gauge
American wire g.
Austin measuring g.
B&L pinch g.
Boley g.
bone screw depth g.
Bourdon tube pressure g.
Broggi-Kelman dipstick g.
calibrated depth g.
Charnley femoral condyle radius g.
Charnley socket g.
Cloward depth g.
Cloward L-W g.
Cloward spanner g.
CTS g.
Dacomed snap g.
depth g.
Dontrix g.
Durkan CTS g.
Edslab pressure g.
finger circumference g.
French catheter g.

Harris femoral head g.
isometric strain g.
Jamar hydraulic pinch g.
Knolle lens g.
Kundin wound measurement g.
leaf g.
LeVeen inflator with pressure g.
manual dermatome thickness g.
Marco radius g.
measuring g.
Mendez degree g.
mercury-in-Silastic strain g.
Neumann depth g.
orthopedic depth g.
oval piston g.
Padgett baseline pinch g.
pain threshold g.
Philips toe force g.
Pilling Excalibur g.
pinch g.
pinwheel sensation g.
pressure g.
Preston pinch g.
Reichert radius g.
Rocabado posture g.
Rosette strain g.
screw depth g.
Shepard incision depth g.
Silastic strain g.
Snap-Gauge g.
spanner g.
Stahl lens g.
standard wire g.
Steinert-Deacon incision g.
strain g.
Synthes mini-depth g.
Tinnant g.
Tycos g.
uniaxial strain g.
water g.
Gauje curved chisel
Gaulian knife guide
gauntlet bandage
Gauss hemostatic forceps
Gauthier
G. bicycle ergometer
G. retractor
Gautier ureteroscope
Gauvain brace
gauze
Adaptic g.
Aquaphor g.
Avant Gauze nonwoven g.
g. bandage
BIPP ribbon g.
Cover-Roll adhesive g.
Curafil hydrogel impregnated g.
g. dissector sponge
dry sterile g.
dry textile g.
finger g.
GraftCyte g.
Intersorb fine mesh g.
Intersorb six-ply absorbent roll
stretch g.

Intersorb wide mesh g.
KBM absorbent g.
Kling g.
KOMFORM coated g.
g. neck tie
Oxycel g.
g. pack
g. packer
g. pad carrier
PanoGauze hydrogel-impregnated g.
paraffin g.
petrolatum g.
plain g.
g. rosebud sponge
Safe-Wrap g.
g. scissors
sodium chloride-impregnated g.
Sof-Form conforming g.
Sta-tite 2ply elastic roll g.
g. stent
g. stent dressing
surgical steel g.
Surgicel g.
Surgitube tubular g.
tantalum g.
Teletrast g.
Telfa g.
g. tissue bag
Topper nonadherent g.
TransiGel hydrogel-impregnated g.
White Plume absorbent g.
g. wick
woven cotton g.
Xeroform g.

Gauztape bandage
Gauztex
    G. bandage
    G. dressing
Gavin-Miller
    G.-M. clamp
    G.-M. colon forceps
    G.-M. intestinal forceps
    G.-M. tissue forceps
Gavriliu gastric tube
Gaylor uterine biopsy forceps
Gaymar
    G. Thermacare warming unit
    G. water-circulating blanket
Gazayerli
    G. endoscopic retractor
    G. knot pusher
Gazayerli-Mediflex retractor
G-C
    G-C filling instrument
    G-C polishing strip
    G-C "SMOOTH CUT" diamond
      point
    G-C syringe
    G-C Vest investment material
    G-C wax carver
GDLH posterior spinal system
GD Regainer system
GDx nerve fiber analyzer
GE
    GE Advance PET scanner

GE CT Advantage scanner
GE CT Hi-Speed Advantage system
GE CT Max scanner
GE CT Pace scanner
GE 9800 CT system
GE Genesis CT scanner
GE GN 500-MHz scanner
GE GN300 7.5-T/89-mm bore
  multinuclear spectrometer
GE 9800 high-resolution CT
  scanner
GE HiSpeed Advantage helical CT
  scanner
GE Maxicamera gamma camera
GE MR Max scanner
GE MR Signa scanner
GE MR Vectra scanner
GE NMR spectrometer
GE Omega 500-MHz scanner
GE pacemaker
GE RT 3200 Advantage II
GE RT 3200 Advantage II
  ultrasound
GE Senographe 2000D
  mammography system
GE Signa 5.4 Genesis MR imager
GE Signa 5.5 Horizon EchoSpeed
  MR imager
GE Signa MR system
GE Signa 1.5-T magnet
GE single-axis SR-230 echoplanar
  scanner
GE single-axis SR-230 echoplanar
  system
GE single-detector SPECT-capable
  camera
GE Spiral CT scanner
GE Starcam single-crystal
  tomographic scintillation camera

gear shift pedicle probe
Geckeler screw
Geenan
    G. biliary cytology brush
    G. Endotorque
    G. Endotorque guide
    G. Endotorque guidewire
    G. Endotorque wire
    G. graduated dilation catheter
    G. pancreatic stent
Gehrung pessary
Geibel blade plate
Geiger
    G. cautery
    G. counter
    G. electrocautery
Geiger-Müller
    G.-M. counter
    G.-M. detector
    G.-M. tube
Geissendorfer
    G. rib retractor
    G. uterine forceps
gel
    g. cushion
    g. pack

G

gel *(continued)*
- g. pad
- g. sheeting
- g. stump sock
- g. suspension sleeve
- g. tubing
- g. warmer
- g. wound dressing

Gelastic bed

gelatin
- g. compression boot
- g. sponge
- g. sponge pad

gelatin-covered mesh stent

gelatin-resorcin-formalin
- g.-r.-f. glue
- g.-r.-f. tissue glue adhesive

gelatin-subbed slide

GelBand arm band

Geldmacher tendon-passing probe

gel-filled
- g.-f. bladder
- g.-f. implant
- g.-f. prosthesis

Gelfilm
- G. cap
- G. dressing
- G. forceps
- G. plate
- G. retinal implant

Gelfoam
- G. cookie
- G. cube
- fibrin glue-soaked G.
- G. pad
- G. pledget
- G. pressure forceps
- G. punch
- thrombin-soaked G.
- G. torpedo

Gel-Foam Ultra-Wedge cushion

Geliperm gel dressing

Gellhorn
- G. pessary
- G. uterine biopsy forceps
- G. uterine biopsy punch

Gellman instrumentation

Gellquist scissors

GellyComb bed

Gelocast
- G. dressing
- G. Unna boot

Gelpi
- G. abdominal retractor
- G. hysterectomy forceps
- G. perineal retractor
- G. self-retaining retractor
- G. vaginal retractor

Gelpi-Lowrie
- G.-L. hysterectomy forceps
- G.-L. retractor

gel-saline
- g.-s. mammary implant
- g.-s. Surgitek mammary prosthesis

Gel-Sole shoe insert

Gel-Syte wound dressing

GEL-U-SLEEP series III floatation mattress system

Gély suture

Gembase dental cement

Gemcem dental cement

Gemcore dental cement

Gem DR implantable defibrillator

Gemini
- G. clamp
- G. cup
- G. DDD pacemaker
- G. gall duct forceps
- G. hemostatic forceps
- G. hip
- G. hip system prosthesis
- G. Mixter forceps
- G. paired helical wire basket
- G. syringe
- G. thoracic forceps

GEM nonlatex medical bag

GEM-Premier point-of-care blood analyzer

Gene
- G. scissors
- G. Screen nylon membrane filter

Genell biopsy curette

GeneraBloc bite block

general
- g. closure needle
- g. closure suture
- G. Electric 400AC Maxicamera
- G. Electric Advantx system
- G. Electric Model RT-3200 ultrasound
- G. Electric pacemaker
- G. Electric Pass-C echocardiograph machine
- g. probe
- g. retractor
- g. tissue forceps
- g. utility scissors
- g. wire forceps

Generation
- G. II
- G. II all-in-one-hand control
- G. II KAFO
- G. II knee brace

generator
- Angeion 2000 ICD g.
- Aurora pulse g.
- ballistic energy g.
- banana plug dipolar g.
- Bird neonatal CPAP g.
- Birtcher electrosurgical g.
- Chardack-Greatbatch implantable cardiac pulse g.
- CO_2 g.
- computerized pattern g.
- Coratomic implantable pulse g.
- Cordis Theta Sequicor DDD pulse g.
- Cosmos II multiprogrammable dual-chamber cardiac pulse g.

CPI-PRx pulse g.
Cyberlith multiprogrammable
  pulse g.
deuterium-tritium g.
direct current g.
distal stimulation g.
Down flow g.
^{166}Dy g.
dysprosium-holmium (^{166}Dy-166Ho)
  in vivo g.
electric g.
electrostatic g.
electrosurgical g.
Endostat II bipolar/monopolar
  electrosurgical g.
Erbe ICC g.
extraction g.
Force 2 CEM g.
Force FX g.
Grass visual pattern g.
^{166}Ho in vivo g.
Instant Response technology g.
Intec AID cardioverter-
  defibrillator g.
Itrel I unipolar pulse g.
Itrel II quadripolar pulse g.
Lithoclast ballistic energy g.
Maxilith pacemaker pulse g.
Medstone STS shockwave g.
Medtronic Cardiorhythm Atakr g.
Medtronic pulse g.
Microlith pacemaker pulse g.
Microny SR+ single-chamber, rate-
  responsive pulse g.
Minilith pacemaker pulse g.
molybdenum-technetium g.
multiprogrammable pulse g.
NDM Power-Point electrosurgical g.
Neuro N-50 lesion g.
Optima pulse g.
Pacesetter Affinity SR g.
Pacesetter Synchrony III pulse g.
Pacesetter Trilogy DR+ pulse g.
Parama pulse wave g.
polyphase g.
Programalith III pulse g.
programmable pulse g.
radio frequency g.
Radionics radiofrequency lesion g.
Radionics stimulus g.
Regency SR+ pulse g.
resonance g.
Res-Q ICD g.
Scan Pattern g.
spark-gap shock wave g.
Spectrax SXT pulse g.
Stilith implantable cardiac pulse g.
supervoltage g.
Symmetry endobipolar g.
tantalum-178 g.
transurethral needle ablation of the
  prostate radio frequency g.
Trilogy DC, DR, SR pulse g.
Triphasix g.

Valleylab Force IC
  electrosurgical g.
Van de Graaf g.
ventricular demand pulse g.
Ventritex g.
Vivalith II pulse g.
x-ray g.
GenESA closed-loop delivery system
Genesis
  G. arthroplasty hardware
  G. 2000 carbon dioxide laser
  G. diamond blade
  G. II total knee system
  G. knee prosthesis
  G. lens
  G. unicompartmental knee
**Genesys Vertex variable angle gamma
  camera**
**Genetics Systems microplate reader
  spectrophotometer**
Genga bandage
genial advancement plate
Genie resin
genioplate
  Synthes g.
Genisis dual-chamber pacemaker
**Genitor mini-intrauterine insemination
  cannula**
GenJect
Genotropin
  G. MiniQuick
  G. pen
  G. system
  G. two-chamber cartridge
Gen-Probe
Gensini
  G. cardiac device
  G. coronary arteriography catheter
  G. Teflon catheter
gentamicin implant
Gentell
  G. foam wound dressing
  G. hydrogel dressing
  G. isotonic saline wet dressing
Gentex PDQ polycarbonate lens
gentian violet marking pen
GENTLE
  G. TOUCH Loop Ostomy System-4
  G. TOUCH System,
  Colostomy/Ileostomy Postoperative
  Kit
  G. TOUCH System, Urostomy
  Postoperative Kit
Gentle
  G. Jane Snap freezer
  G. Threads interference screw
  G. Touch colostomy appliance
  G. Touch colostomy/ileostomy
  postoperative system
Gentle-Flo suction catheter
GentleLASE
  G. laser
  G. laser system
Genucom
  G. ACL laxity analysis system

G

Genucom *(continued)*
G. arthrometer
G. knee flexion analysis system
Genuine
G. sheepskin crutches accessory kit
G. sheepskin elbow protector
G. sheepskin heel protector
Genupak tampon
Genutrain
G. knee brace
G. P3 active knee support
Geo-Matt
G.-M. contour cushion
G.-M. 30-degree body aligner
G.-M. gel cushion
G.-M. mattress
G.-M. PRT cushion
G.-M. wheelchair cushion
Geometric total knee prosthesis
George Washington strut
Georgiade
G. breast prosthesis
G. fixation device
G. rasp
G. visor
G. visor cervical traction
G. visor halo fixation apparatus
Georgia valve
Gerald
G. bayonet microbipolar
neurosurgical forceps
G. brain forceps
G. clamp
G. dressing forceps
G. monopolar forceps
G. straight microbipolar
neurosurgical forceps
G. tissue forceps
Gerber space maintainer
Gerbode
G. cardiovascular tissue forceps
G. mitral valvulotome
G. mitral valvulotomy dilator
G. modified Burford rib spreader
G. patent ductus clamp
G. rib spreader
G. sternal retractor
Gerdy intra-auricular loop
Gergoyie-Guggenheim olive
Gergoyie olive
Gerhardt table
geriatric
g. chair
g. chair trunk support
GeriMend skin tear therapy
Geristore dental implant
Germain needle holder
German lock
Gerow-Harrington heart-shaped distal
end retractor
Gerow Small-Carrion penile implant
Gerster
G. bone clamp
G. fracture appliance

G. traction bar
G. traction device
Gertie ball
Gerzog
G. bone hammer
G. bone mallet
G. ear knife
G. nasal speculum
Gerzog-Ralks knife
Gesco
G. aspirator
G. cannula
G. catheter
Gess cannula tip
Get-A-Grip grip
Getz
G. crown
G. root canal pin
G. rubber base
Geuder
G. corneal needle
G. implanter
G. keratoplasty needle
GFH alloy
GFS Mark II inflatable penile prosthesis
GF-UM3
G.-U. duodenoscope
G.-U. scanner
GF-UM30P linear-oriented radial
scanning echoendoscope
GFX2 coronary stent system
gfx coronary stent
Ghajar guide
Ghazi rib retractor
Gherini-Kauffman
G.-K. endo-otoprobe
G.-K. endo-otoprobe laser
GHM
GHM KLE II x-ray film holder
GHM polishing strip
Ghormley double cannula
GI
GI clamp
GI forceps
GI pop-off silk suture
GIA
GIA forceps
GIA II loading unit
Multifire GIA
GIA staple
GIA stapling device
Giannestras turnbuckle
Giannini needle holder
Gianturco
G. expandable metallic biliary stent
G. expanding metallic stent
G. metal urethral stent
G. occlusion coil
G. prosthesis
G. steel coil
G. wool-tufted wire coil
G. zigzag stent
Gianturco-Roehm bird's nest vena cava
filter

Gianturco-Rosch self-expandable biliary Z stent
Gianturco-Roubin
    G.-R. flexible coil stent
    G.-R. FlexStent coronary stent
Gianturco-Wallace-Anderson coil
Giardet corneal transplant scissors
Gibbon
    G. indwelling ureteral stent
    G. urethral catheter
Gibbs eye punch
Gibney
    G. boot
    G. dressing
    G. fixation bandage
Gibralter headrest
Gibson
    G. anterior chamber irrigator
    G. bandage
    G. dressing
    G. I&A unit
    G. inner ear shunt
    G. splint
    G. stone dislodger
Gibson-Balfour abdominal retractor
Gibson-Cooke sweat test apparatus
Gibson-Ross board
GiCi-400 Invader
Giertz
    G. rib guillotine
    G. rib shears
Giertz-Shoemaker rib shears
Giertz-Stille
    G.-S. rib shears
    G.-S. scissors
Giesy ureteral dilatation balloon
Gifford
    G. corneal applicator
    G. corneal curette
    G. fixation forceps
    G. iris forceps
    G. mastoid retractor
    G. needle holder
    G. scalp retractor
Gifford-Jansen mastoid retractor
GIF-HM endoscope
GIF-N-series fiberoptic pediatric endoscope
GIF-XP-series endoscope
GIF-XQ-series endoscope
Gigator hemorrhoidal ligator
Gigli
    G.-saw blade
    G. saw conductor
    G.-saw guide
    G.-saw handle
    G. solid-handle saw
    G. spiral saw wire
    G. wire saw
Gigli-Strully saw
G II Unloader ADJ knee brace
Gilbert
    G. cystic duct forceps
    G. pediatric balloon catheter

    G. plug-sealing catheter
    G. prosthesis
Gilbert-Graves speculum
Gilbert-type Bardex Foley catheter
Gildenberg biopsy forceps
Gilfillan humeral prosthesis
Giliberty
    G. acetabular prosthesis
    G. device
Gill
    G. biopsy brush
    G. blade
    G. corneal knife
    G. counterpressor
    G. curved iris forceps
    G. double I&A cannula
    G. double Luer-Lok cannula
    G. incision spreader
    G. incision-spreading forceps
    G. intraocular implant lens
    G. I respirator
    G. iris forceps
    G. iris knife
    G. needle
    G. pop-up arcuate diamond knife
    G. pressor counter
    G. renal tourniquet
    G. scissors
    G. sinus cannula
Gill-Arruga capsular forceps
Gill-Chandler iris forceps
Giller hearing aid
Gillespie obstetrical forceps
Gillette
    G. Blue Blade
    G. brace
    G. double-flexure ankle joint system
    G. joint
    G. joint orthosis
    G. joint prosthesis
    G. modification of ankle-foot orthosis
Gill-Fine corneal knife
Gill-Fuchs capsular forceps
Gill-Hess
    G.-H. blade
    G.-H. Fragmatome
    G.-H. iris forceps
    G.-H. knife
    G.-H. mules
    G.-H. scissors
Gillies
    G. bone hook
    G. dissecting forceps
    G. dural hook
    G. horizontal dermal suture
    G. implant
    G. nasal hook
    G. needle holder
    G. prosthesis
    G. single-hook skin retractor
    G. skin hook
    G. suture scissors
    G. tissue forceps
    G. zygoma elevator

G

Gillies *(continued)*
- G. zygoma hook
- G. zygomatic hook

Gillies-Converse skin hook
Gillies-Dingman hook
Gillmore needle
Gillquist
- G. suction curette
- G. suction tube

Gillquist-Oretorp-Stille
- G.-O.-S. dilator
- G.-O.-S. forceps
- G.-O.-S. knife
- G.-O.-S. needle holder
- G.-O.-S. probe

Gillquist-Stille arthroplasty suction tube
Gill-Safar forceps
Gill-Thomas locator
Gill-Welsh
- G.-W. aspirating cannula
- G.-W. capsular forceps
- G.-W. capsular polisher
- G.-W. cortex extractor
- G.-W. curette
- G.-W. double cannula
- G.-W. guillotine port
- G.-W. irrigating cannula
- G.-W. knife
- G.-W. lens loop
- G.-W. olive-tip cannula
- G.-W. scissors
- G.-W. spatula

Gill-Welsh-Morrison lens loop
Gill-Welsh-Vannas
- G.-W.-V. angled microscissors
- G.-W.-V. capsulotomy scissors

Gilmer
- G. dental splint
- G. tooth splint
- G. wire

Gilmore
- G. intraocular implant lens
- G. probe

Gil-Vernet
- G.-V. lumbotomy retractor
- G.-V. renal sinus retractor

Gimbel
- G. fountain cannula
- G. glove
- G. stabilizing ring

gingival clamp
gingivectomy knife
Gingrass-Messer pin
Ginsberg tissue forceps
Gio-occlusive dressing
GIP/Medi-Globe prototype needle
giraffe biopsy forceps
Girard
- G. anterior chamber needle
- G. cataract-aspirating needle
- G. corneoscleral forceps
- G. corneoscleral scissors
- G. Fragmatome
- G. Fragmatome probe
- G. irrigating cannula
- G. irrigating tip
- G. keratoprosthesis prosthesis
- G. phacofragmatome needle
- G. phakofragmatome
- G. scleral ring
- G. synechia spatula
- G. ultrasonic unit

Girard-Swan
- G.-S. knife
- G.-S. needle

girdle
- Ace halo pelvic g.
- compression g.
- Lipo-Medi g.
- male compression g.

Girdner probe
girth hitch
Gish
- G. autoinfuser
- G. micro YAG laser

Gissane
- G. spike
- G. spike nail

Givner lid retractor
Gizmo catheter
glabellar rasp
Glacier
- G. ceramic 4-in-1 knee cutting guide
- G. Pack

Gladiator shock suit
Gladstone-Putterman transmarginal rotation entropion clamp
Glaser laminectomy retractor
Glasgold Wafer chin implant
glass
- G. abdominal retractor
- g. bead
- g. bead sterilizer
- g. ionomer cement
- G. liver-holding clamp
- g. penile prosthesis
- g. pH electrode
- g. retracting rod
- g. sphere eye implant
- g. tract detector
- g. vaginal plug

Glasscock
- G. ear dressing
- G. scissors

Glasscock-House knife
Glasser fixation screw
glasses
- bifocal g.
- contact g.
- Crookes g.
- crutch g.
- Difei g.
- fiberoptic video g.
- Franklin g.
- Fresnel nystagmus g.
- Grafco magnifying g.
- Hallauer g.
- hyperbolic g.
- magnifying g.
- Masselon g.

nystagmus g.
presbyopia g.
protective g.
safety g.
trifocal g.
Wood g.
Worst corneal contact g.

Glassman
G. basket
G. bowel atraumatic clamp
G. brush
G. gastrostomy
G. intestinal clamp
G. liver-holding clamp
G. noncrushing gastroenterostomy
clamp
G. noncrushing gastrointestinal
clamp
G. noncrushing pickup forceps
G. pickup forceps
G. stone extractor
G. thin-point scissors

Glassman-Allis
G.-A. clamp
G.-A. intestinal forceps
G.-A. noncrushing common duct
forceps
G.-A. noncrushing intestinal forceps
G.-A. noncrushing tissue-holding
forceps

Glassman-Babcock forceps
glaucoma
g. drainage device
g. pencil
G. Wick

Gleason
G. headband
G. rasp
G. speculum

**Gleeson FloVAC Hi-Flo laparoscopic
suction-irrigation system**
Glegg nasal polyp snare
Glenn
G. diverticular forceps
G. shunt

Glenner
G. vaginal hysterectomy forceps
G. vaginal retractor

glenoid
g. alignment peg
g. drill
g. drill guide
g. fin broach
g. fixation screw

glenoid-reaming forceps
Gliadel wafer
GliaSite radiation therapy RTS system
Glick instrument
glide
Hessburg intraocular lens g.
intraocular lens g.
mushroom walker g.
Pearce intraocular g.
Sheets intraocular g.
Sheets lens g.

Glidecath hydrophilic coated catheter
Glidewire
angle-tip G.
G. catheter
G. Gold surgical guide wire
G. Gold surgical guidewire
long taper/stiff shaft G.
Microvasive G.
Radiofocus G.
Terumo G.

Glidex coated Percuflex catheter
gliding hinge joint

Glisson snare
global
g. force applicator
G. Fx shoulder fracture system
G. Therapeutics Freedom stent
G. Therapeutics V-Flex stent
G. total shoulder arthroplasty
G. total shoulder arthroplasty
system
G. total shoulder implant

globe prolapsus pessary
globular object forceps
Glomark fluorescent skin marker
Glori pressure earrings
Glo-Tip ERCP catheter
glottic prosthesis
glove, gloves
Biobrane g.
Biogel orthopaedic surgical g.
Biogel Sensor surgical g.
Biogel surgeons' g.
Dermapor g.
G. drain
Elastylon g.
electrode g.
Encore microptic powder-free latex
surgical g.
ESP radiation reduction
examination g.
finger flexion g.
F&L attenuating g.'s
flexion g.
Gimbel g.
Handeze fingerless g.
impact g.
Isotoner g.
Jobst g.
Kevlar g.'s
Kid G.
Life Liner stick- and cut-
resistant g.'s
Maxxus orthopaedic latex
surgical g.
Medak g.
Medarmor puncture-resistant g.'s
Micro-Touch Platex medical g.'s
Necelon surgical g.'s
neoprene g.
New ultra-thick powder-free latex
surgical g.
nitrile g.
Nouvisage Deep Hydration g.

G

glove *(continued)*
peripheral nerve g.
pressure g.
Push-Ease wheelchair g.
radial nerve g.
Repela surgical g.'s
Satin Plus g.
Skinsense g.
Surgtech g.'s
Tactyl 1 g.
Tactylon synthetic surgical g.
Thermal responsive non-latex nitrile
surgical g.
vinyl g.
Viro G.
weighted g.
Glove-n-Gel
G.-n.-G. amniotome
G.-n.-G. amniotomy kit
Glover
G. anastomosis forceps
G. auricular-appendage clamp
G. auricular clamp
G. bulldog clamp
G. coarctation clamp
G. coarctation forceps
G. curved clamp
G. curved forceps
G. infundibular rongeur forceps
G. modification of Brock aortic
dilator
G. patent ductus clamp
G. patent ductus forceps
G. rongeur
G. spoon-shaped anastomosis clamp
G. spoon-shaped forceps
G. suction tube
G. vascular clamp
Glover-DeBakey clamp
Glover-Stille clamp
gloves *(var. of* glove)
GLP7 film
GLS brace
Gluck rib shears
**Glucocheck Pocketlab II blood glucose
system**
Glucolet lancet device
glucometer
Accu-Chek II g.
Advantage g.
G. DEX blood glucose monitor
G. DEX system
Glucostar II g.
GlucoWatch g.
G. II
G. II home glucose monitoring
system
Mills Glucometer II g.
One Touch basic g.
gluconate
BIOPATCH antimicrobial dressing
with chlorhexidine g.
GlucoScan monitor
Glucostar II glucometer

GlucoWatch
G. bloodless glucose monitor
G. glucometer
G. glucose monitoring device
glue
BioGlue g.
Biolex wound g.
butyl cyanoacrylate g.
cyanoacrylate g.
ethyl cyanoacrylate g.
fibrin g.
gelatin-resorcin-formalin g.
Histoacryl g.
methyl cyanoacrylate g.
g. patch
Tisseel fibrin g.
Tisseel surgical g.
tissue g.
glued-on hard contact lens
glue-in suture
glutameter
EndoDynamics g.
glutaraldehyde-tanned
g.-t. bovine collagen tube
g.-t. bovine graft
g.-t. bovine heart valve
g.-t. porcine heart valve
Glutex glutaraldehyde neutralizer
glycerine syringe
glycerin-preserved graft
glycolide trimethylene carbonate material
GlyMed Camouflage system
GM alloy
gnathograph
Gnatholator
gnathologic instrument
gNomos stereotactic system
Gobble Plus removal instrument
Gobi dehumidifier
Gobin-Weiss loop
go-cart
Chailey g.-c.
Godart expirograph
Goddio disposable cannula
Godelo dilator
Godina vessel-fixation instrument
Godiva wax
Goebel-Stoeckel snare
Goelet double-ended retractor
Goeltec catheter
Goetz
G. bipolar electrode
G. cardiac device
Goffman
G. blue eye garter shield
G. eye garter
G. occluder
goggles
EndoShield mask and g.
Fresnel g.
stenopaic g.
swimmer's g.
Gohrbrand
G. cardiac dilator
G. valvulotome

Goidnich bone plate
goiter
- g. clamp
- g. dissector
- g. hook
- g. ligature carrier
- g. retractor
- g. scissors
- g. vulsellum forceps

goiter-seizing forceps
Golaski graft
Golaski-UMI vascular prosthesis
Golay gradient coil
gold
- g. bur
- g. burnisher
- G. deep-surgery forceps
- g. ear marker
- G. eyelid load implant
- G. hemostatic forceps
- g. needle
- G. pessary
- G. portable CO_2 laser
- G. probe
- G. Probe bipolar hemostasis catheter
- G. Probe electrohemostasis catheter
- G. Probe hemostasis therapy
- g. ring
- g. saw
- G. Series bone drilling system
- g. weight
- g. weight and wire spring implant material

Goldbacher
- G. anoscope
- G. anoscope speculum
- G. proctoscope
- G. rectal needle

Goldberg
- G. MPC mediastinoscope
- G. MPC operative enteroscope
- G. side port splitter

Goldblatt clamp
Golden
- G. Comfort orthotic
- G. Fitness orthotic
- G. Retriever

Goldenberg implant system
gold-handled chuck
Goldman
- G. bar
- G. cartilage punch
- G. curette
- G. guarded chisel
- G. guillotine nerve knife
- G. knife guide
- G. saw
- G. septal elevator
- G. septal scissors
- G. Universal nerve hook
- G. vaporizer

Goldman-Fox
- G.-F. gum scissors
- G.-F. knife
- G.-F. probe

Goldman-Kazanjian
- G.-K. nasal forceps
- G.-K. rongeur

Goldmann
- G. applanation tonometer
- G. capsulorrhexis forceps
- G. contact lens prism
- G. expressor
- G. goniolens
- G. knife needle
- G. macular contact lens
- G. multimirror lens
- G. multimirror lens implant
- G. perimeter
- G. three-mirror gonioscopy lens

Gold-Mules eye implant
gold-paneled chisel
Goldstein
- G. anterior chamber cannula
- G. anterior chamber irrigator
- G. anterior chamber syringe
- G. curette
- G. golf club spud
- G. Grasp atraumatic cervical stabilizer
- G. irrigating cannula
- G. lacrimal cannula
- G. lacrimal sac retractor
- G. lacrimal syringe
- G. Microspike approximator clamp
- G. refractor
- G. septal speculum

Goldthwait
- G. bar
- G. brace
- G. fracture appliance
- G. fracture frame

Goldvasser clamp
Goldwasser suture carrier
Golf
golf
- G. exercise system
- g. tee hollow titanium cannula
- g. tee-shaped polyvinyl prosthesis

golf-club spud
Golgi
- G. apparatus
- G. device

Goligher
- G. modification of the Berkeley-Bonney retractor
- G. speculum
- G. sternal-lifting retractor

Golub EKG lead
Gomco
- G. bell clamp
- G. bloodless circumcision clamp
- G. drain
- G. forceps
- G. suction tube
- G. thoracic drainage pump
- G. umbilical cord clamp
- G. uterine aspirator

Gomez gastric retractor
gonad shield

G

Gonin
    G. cautery
    G. marker
Gonin-Amsler scleral marker
goniofocalizing lens
goniogram
    Becker g.
goniolaser
    Thorpe four-mirror g.
goniolens
    Allen-Thorpe g.
    Barkan g.
    Cardona focalizing g.
    four-mirror g.
    Goldmann g.
    Koeppe g.
    g. lens
    PF Lee pediatric g.
    single-mirror g.
    Thorpe-Castroviejo g.
    Thorpe four-mirror g.
    Zeiss g.
goniometer
    Bailliart g.
    Carroll finger g.
    Conzett g.
    digital g.
    electronic g.
    EOC g.
    finger g.
    Frykholm g.
    full-circle g.
    Grafco g.
    International standard g.
    Jarit finger g.
    Mottgen g.
    orthopedic g.
    Osborne g.
    Polk finger g.
    Sammons biplane g.
    Sceratti g.
    Sedan g.
    Thole g.
    Tomac g.
    two-arm g.
    Universal g.
    Zimmer g.
goniophotography
Goniopora
    coralline hydroxyapatite G.
gonioprism
    Jacob-Swan g.
    Posner diagnostic g.
    Posner surgical g.
goniopuncture knife
gonioscope
    Barkan g.
    Heine g.
    Jacob-Swan g.
    Maine g.
    Nevada g.
    Sussman four-mirror g.
    Thorpe surgical g.
    Troncoso g.

    University of Michigan g.
    Zeiss g.
gonioscopic
    g. implant
    g. lens
    g. prism
goniotomy
    g. knife
    g. knife cannula
    g. needle holder
Gonzalez specialized dissecting cannula
Gooch
    G. mastoid retractor
    G. splint
Good
    G. antral rasp
    G. 'N Bed wedge
    G. obstetrical forceps
    G. retractor
    G. tonsillar scissors
Goodale-Lubin cardiac catheter
Goode
    G. Magne-Splint magnetic nasal
       splint
    G. Trim tube
    G. T-tube
    G. T-tube ventilating tube
Goodell uterine dilator
Goodfellow frontal sinus cannula
Goodhill
    G. cautery
    G. double-end curette
    G. hook
    G. knife
    G. prosthesis
    G. retractor
    G. strut introducer
    G. tonsillar forceps
Goodhill-Down knife
Goodhill-Pynchon tonsillar suction tube
GoodKnight 418 CPAP home-care system
Goodlite super headlight
Good-Reiner scissors
Goodwillie periosteal elevator
Goodwin bone clamp
Goodyear
    G. tonsillar knife
    G. tonsillar retractor
Goodyear-Gruenwald forceps
gooseneck
    g. chisel
    g. rongeur
    g. snare
Goosen vascular punch
Goot-Lite headband
Gordh needle
Gordon
    G. bead forceps
    G. ciliary forceps
    G. splint
    G. uterine forceps
    G. vulsellum forceps
Gore
    G. cast liner

G. cast liner material
G. Smoother Crucial Tool
G. subcutaneous augmentation
material
G. suture passer
G. thyroplasty device

Gore-Tex
G.-T. alloplastic material
G.-T. aortofemoral (AF) fistula
G.-T. baffle
G.-T. bifurcated vascular graft
G.-T. cardiovascular patch
G.-T. DualMesh Plus biomaterial
G.-T. FEP-Ringed vascular graft
G.-T. jump graft
G.-T. knee prosthesis
G.-T. limb
G.-T. MycroMesh Plus biomaterial
G.-T. nasal implant
G.-T. periodontal material
G.-T. peritoneal catheter
G.-T. regenerative material
G.-T. SAM facial implant
G.-T. shunt
G.-T. soft tissue patch
G.-T. stretch vascular graft
G.-T. strip
G.-T. surgical membrane
G.-T. suture
G.-T. tapered vascular graft
G.-T. vascular implant
G.-T. waterproof cast liner

gorget
Anthony g.
Teale g.

Gorlin pacing catheter
Gorney
G. dissector
G. facelift scissors
G. rhytidectomy scissors
G. septal suction elevator

Gorsch
G. needle
G. sigmoidoscope

GO scope
Gosnell scale
gossamer silk suture
Gosset
G. abdominal retractor
G. appendectomy retractor
G. self-retaininig retractor

Gosteyer punch
**Gotfried percutaneous compression
plating**
Gott
G. butterfly heart valve
G. cannula
G. implant
G. low-profile prosthesis
G. malleable retractor
G. shunt
G. tube

Gott-Balfour blade
Gott-Daggett heart valve prosthesis
Gottesman splash shield

Gott-Harrington blade
Gottschalk
G. middle ear aspirator
G. nasostat
G. transverse saw

Gott-Seeram blade
Goudet uterine scoop
Gouffon hip pin
gouge
Alexander mastoid bone g.
Andrews mastoid g.
annular g.
antral g.
AO g.
Army bone g.
Aufranc arthroplasty g.
Ballenger g.
Bishop mastoid g.
Boley dental g.
bone g.
Bowen g.
Bowls septal g.
Buch-Gramcko g.
Campbell arthroplasty g.
Capner g.
Cave scaphoid g.
Charnley g.
Chermel bone g.
Cobb spinal g.
Codman bone g.
concave g.
Cooper spinal fusion g.
Crane g.
curved g.
Dawson-Yuhl g.
Derlacki g.
Dix g.
Dontrix g.
Duray-Read g.
Flanagan spinal fusion g.
Freer nasal g.
Gam-Mer g.
Guy g.
Hibbs bone g.
Hibbs spinal fusion g.
hip arthroplasty g.
Hoen laminar g.
Holmes cartilage g.
Hough g.
hump g.
Jewett g.
Kezerian g.
Killian g.
Kuhnt g.
lacrimal sac g.
Lahey Clinic spinal fusion g.
Lexer g.
Lillie g.
long-handle offset g.
Lucas g.
Mannerfelt g.
Martin hip g.
mastoid g.
Metzenbaum g.
Meyerding curved g.

G

gouge *(continued)*
    Moe g.
    Moore spinal fusion g.
    Morgenstein g.
    Murphy g.
    nasal g.
    Neivert rocking g.
    Newport cartilage g.
    Nicola g.
    orthopedic g.
    Parkes hump g.
    Partsch bone g.
    Petanguy-McIndoe g.
    Pilling g.
    Putti arthroplasty g.
    Read g.
    Rica mastoid g.
    Richards-Cobb spinal g.
    Richards-Hibbs g.
    Rowen spinal fusion g.
    Rubin g.
    Schuknecht g.
    semicircular g.
    Sheehan g.
    SMIC mastoid g.
    Smith-Petersen bone g.
    Smith-Petersen curved g.
    spinal fusion g.
    spud g.
    g. spud
    Stacke g.
    Stagnara g.
    Stille bone g.
    Stille-Stiwer g.
    surgical g.
    swan-neck g.
    tendon g.
    Todd foreign body g.
    Trough g.
    Turner spinal g.
    Tworek Universal g.
    Ultra-Cut Cobb spinal g.
    Ultra-Cut Hibbs g.
    U. S. Army g.
    U X-Acto g.
    vomerine g.
    Walton foreign body g.
    Watson-Jones bone g.
    West bone g.
    West nasal g.
    Zielke scoliosis g.

Gould
    G. electromagnetic flowmeter
    G. ES 1000 recorder
    G. Godard pneumotachograph
    G. intraocular implant lens
    G. PentaCath thermodilution catheter
    G. polygraph
    G. polygraph gastric motility
      measuring device
    G. pressure monitor
    G. Statham pressure transducer
    G. suture
Gould-Brush 481 eight-channel recorder

Gouley
    G. dilator
    G. guide
    G. tunneled urethral sound
    G. whalebone filiform catheter
Goulian
    G. blade
    G. dermatome
    G. knife
Goulter device
Goutz catheter
Govons pituitary curette
Gowen decompression tube
gown
    Barrier g.
    Exami-Gown g.
GPX
    G. rotary instrument
grab bar
grabber
    Apple laparoscopic stone g.
    meniscal suture g.
    SunVideo frame g.
    Tab g.
Graber appliance
Grabow forceps
Grace plate 4-hole adapter
Gracey curette
gradient
    g. amplifier
    g. index lens
    g. sheet coil
grading of retinal nerve fiber layer
gradiometer
    axial g.
Gradle
    G. ciliary forceps
    G. corneal trephine
    G. eyelid retractor
    G. needle electrode
    G. refractor
    G. stitch scissors
graduated
    g. catheter
    g. compression stockings
    g. electronic decelerator
    g. Garrett dilator
Gradwohl sternal bone marrow aspirator
Graefe
    G. cataract knife
    G. cataract spoon
    G. curved iris forceps
    G. cystitome knife
    G. dressing forceps
    G. eye-fixation forceps
    G. eye speculum
    G. flexible cystitome
    G. instrument
    G. iris hook
    G. iris knife
    G. iris needle
    G. mules
    G. scarifier
    G. strabismus hook
    G. straight iris forceps

G. tissue forceps
G. tissue-grasping forceps
Graether
G. mushroom hook
G. pupil expander
G. refractor
G. retractor
Graf
G. cervical cordotomy knife
G. stabilization system
Grafco
G. breast pump
G. cannula
G. colostomy bag
G. cotton tip applicator
G. eye shield
G. goniometer
G. head mirror
G. ileostomy bag
G. incontinence clamp
G. laryngeal mirror
G. magnet
G. magnifying glasses
G. Martin laryngectomy tube
G. ophthalmoscope
G. otoscope
G. pelvic traction belt
G. percussion hammer
G. perineal lamp
G. pinwheel
G. seizure stick
G. tourniquet
G. tracheal tube brush
G. umbilical cord clamp
G. x-ray apron
Grafco-Halsted forceps
Graflex material
graft
accordion g.
G. ACE fixed-wire balloon catheter
acrylic g.
albumin-coated vascular g.
albuminized woven Dacron tube g.
AlloDerm dermal g.
AlloDerm processed tissue g.
aortic tube g.
Apligraf g.
Atrium hemodialysis g.
AV Gore-Tex g.
Banks bone g.
Bard PTFE g.
batten g.
Berens g.
bifurcated vascular g.
Biocoral g.
Biograft g.
BioGran resorbable synthetic bone g.
Bionit vascular g.
BioPolyMeric femoropopliteal bypass g.
BioPolyMeric vascular g.
Björk-Shiley g.
Blair-Brown g.
g. board

Bonfiglio bone g.
Boplant g.
bovine pericardium dural g.
Boyd bone g.
Braun g.
Braun-Wangensteen g.
brephoplastic g.
Brett bone g.
cable g.
Calcitite bone g.
Campbell g.
Carbo-Seal cardiovascular composite g.
g. carrier spoon
g. clamp
clip g.
Codivilla g.
collagen-impregnated knitted Dacron velour g.
compressed Ivalon patch g.
Cooley woven Dacron g.
coralline PBHA bone g.
coralline porous block hydroxyapatite bone g.
Corvita endoluminal g.
Corvita endovascular g.
Cotton cartilage g.
Cragg endoluminal g.
Creech aortoiliac g.
Crescent g.
Cryolife valvular g.
Dacron-covered stent g.
Dacron knitted g.
Dacron preclotted g.
Dacron Sauvage g.
Dacron tightly-woven g.
Dacron tube g.
Dacron tubular g.
Dacron velour g.
Dacron Weave Knit g.
Dardik umbilical g.
Davis g.
DeBakey g.
Dembone g.
Dermagraft g.
diamond inlay bone g.
Diastat vascular access g.
Distaflo bypass g.
double-velour knitted g.
Douglas g.
Dragstedt g.
g. driver
Edwards-Tapp arterial g.
Edwards woven Teflon aortic bifurcation g.
Esser g.
expanded polytetrafluoroethylene vascular g.
EXS femoropopliteal bypass g.
externally supported Dacron g.
Favaloro saphenous vein bypass g.
FEP-ringed Gore-Tex vascular g.
fiberglass g.
glutaraldehyde-tanned bovine g.
glycerin-preserved g.

G

graft *(continued)*
Golaski g.
Gore-Tex bifurcated vascular g.
Gore-Tex FEP-Ringed vascular g.
Gore-Tex jump g.
Gore-Tex stretch vascular g.
Gore-Tex tapered vascular g.
Grafton DBM bone g.
Graftpatch g.
Hancock pericardial valve g.
Hancock vascular g.
Hemashield collagen-enhanced g.
Hemashield vascular g.
Hybrid g.
IMA g.
Impra bypass g.
Impra Carboflo ePTFE vascular g.
Impra Flex vascular g.
Impra microporous PTFE
   vascular g.
Inclan g.
Intercede g.
Ionescu-Shiley pericardial valve g.
Ionescu-Shiley vascular g.
Ivalon compressed patch g.
Jeb g.
Kebab g.
Kiel g.
Kimura cartilage g.
knitted g.
Koenig g.
Krause-Wolfe g.
latex sponge g.
Lee g.
LifeCell AlloDerm acellular
   dermal g.
Lo-Por vascular g.
lyophilized g.
mandrel g.
Mangoldt epithelial g.
Marlex mesh g.
Marqez-Gomez conjunctival g.
McFarland tibial g.
McMaster bone g.
Meadox Microvel arterial g.
Meadox Microvel double-velour
   Dacron g.
Meadox vascular g.
g. measuring instrument
Mediform dural g.
Medtronic AneuRx stent g.
Mersilene g.
mesh g.
methyl methacrylate g.
Meyerding bone g.
Microknit patch g.
Microknit vascular g.
Microvel double velour g.
Millesi interfascicular g.
Milliknit g.
Mules g.
Nicoll bone g.
Ollier g.
Ollier-Thiersch g.

OsteoGen bone g.
Ostrup vascularized rib g.
Padgett mesh skin g.
Paladon g.
Papineau bone g.
paraffin g.
Paritene mesh g.
patch g.
Paufique g. knife
Peri-Guard vascular g.
PerioGlas synthetic bone g.
Perma-Flow coronary bypass g.
Perma-Seal dialysis access g.
Phemister onlay bone g.
pigskin g.
plasma TFE vascular g.
Plexiglas g.
Plystan g.
polyethylene g.
Poly-Plus Dacron vascular g.
polytetrafluoroethylene (PTFE)
   stent g.
polyurethane g.
polyvinyl g.
porcine g.
portacaval H g.
preclotted g.
Proplast g.
prosthetic g.
PTFE Gore-Tex g.
Rastelli g.
Rehne skin g. knife
Repliform g.
Reverdin g.
Ruese bone g.
Sauvage Bionit g.
Sauvage Dacron g.
Sauvage filamentous velour g.
seamless g.
Seddon nerve g.
Shea vein g. scissors
Sheen tip g.
Shiley Tetraflex vascular g.
sieve g.
Silastic g.
Silovi saphenous vein g.
Siloxane g.
in situ tricortical iliac crest block
   bone g.
Solvang g.
Speed osteotomy g.
sponge g.
spongiosa bone g.
spreader g.
St. Jude composite valve g.
strut g.
g. suction tube
Supramid g.
Talent stent g.
tarsoconjunctival composite g.
Teflon g.
Thiersch g.
Thomas extrapolated bar g.
tube g.
tunnel g.

Varivas loop g.
Varivas R vein g.
Vascutek gelseal vascular g.
Vascutek knitted vascular g.
Vascutek woven vascular g.
Velex woven Dacron vascular g.
velour collar g.
Venoflow PTFE g.
Vitagraft vascular g.
Wesolowski bypass g.
Wesolowski Teflon g.
Wheeler g.
Wolf g.
Wölfe-Krause g.
woven Dacron tube g.
XenoDerm g.

Graftac absorbable skin tack
Graftac-S skin stapler
GraftAssist vein and graft holder
GraftCyte
G. gauze
G. moist wound dressing
Graftmaster device
Grafton
G. bone grafting material
G. DBM bone graft
G. flexible sheet
G. moldable putty
Graftpatch graft
graft-seeking catheter
Graftskin
Apligraf G.
Graham
G. blunt hook
G. catheter
G. Clark silicone sponge
G. dural hook
G. muscle hook
G. nerve hook
G. pediatric scissors
G. rib contractor
G. scalene elevator
Grahamizer I exerciser
Graham-Kerrison punch
Gram cannula
Granberg cervical traction system
Granberry
G. finger traction bow
G. hyperextension fracture frame
G. splint
G. tongue depressor
Grand
G. Sahara dehumidifier
G. Stand support stand
Grandon cortex extractor set
GraNee needle
Granger articulator
Grant
G. aortic aneurysm clamp
G. dural separator
G. gallbladder retractor
G. needle holder
Grantham
G. lobotomy electrode
G. lobotomy needle

graphic level recorder
Graseby anesthesia pump
Grasp
Babcock Endo G.
Endo G.
grasper
atraumatic curved g.
Blakesley g.
bowel g.
Endo Babcock g.
endoscopic Babcock g.
Hansen g.
Hasson g.
laparoscopic g.
Lion's Claw g.
Lion's Paw g.
loose body g.
MetraGrasp ligament g.
Polaris reusable g.
three-pronged g.
tripod g.
grasper-cutter
Questus Leading Edge
arthroscopic g.-c.
grasping
g. biopsy forceps
g. clamp
g. forceps tip
G. Stitcher system
g. tripod forceps
Grass
G. electroencephalograph
G. force displacement fluid collector
G. Model S9 stimulator
G. neurodata system
G. neurostimulator
G. pressure-recording device
G. S88 muscle stimulator
G. visual pattern generator
Grasshopper positioner
grater
acetabular g.
grater-type reamer with Zimmer-Hudson shank
Gratloch wire bender
Graves
G. bivalve speculum
G. Britetrac vaginal speculum
G. Coldlite speculum
G. open-side vaginal speculum
gravity
g. infusion cannula
G. Lumbar Traction system
gravity-driven angle finder
Gravlee jet washer
Gray
G. arterial forceps
G. bone drill
G. clamp
G. cystic duct forceps
G. flexible intramedullary reamer
G. revision instrument system
G. surgical retractor
gray-scale ultrasonogram
Grayson corneal forceps

G

Grayton corneal forceps
Grazer blepharoplasty forceps
great
    G. Ormond Street pediatric tracheostomy tube
    g. toe implant
Greck ileostomy bag
Greco cutting block
Green
    G. automatic corneal trephine
    G. bulldog clamp
    G. capsular forceps
    G. cataract knife
    G. chalazion forceps
    G. corneal curette
    G. corneal dissector
    G. corneal knife
    G. corneal marker
    G. double spatula
    G. eye calipers
    G. eye needle holder
    G. eye shield
    G. fixation forceps
    G. goiter retractor
    G. iris replacer
    G. lens scoop
    G. lens spatula
    G. lid clamp
    G. mouthgag
    G. muscle hook
    G. muscle tucker
    G. optical crater marker
    G. pendulum scalpel
    G. refractor
    G. replacer spatula
    G. Sleeve compression device
    G. strabismus hook
    G. strabismus tucker
    G. suction tube forceps
    G. suction tube-holding clamp
    G. thyroid retractor
    G. tissue-grasping forceps
    G. tube-holding forceps
green
    g. braided suture
    g. laser
    g. Mersilene suture
    g. monofilament polyglyconate suture
Green-Armytage
    G.-A. hemostatic forceps
    G.-A. polythene rod
    G.-A. reamer
    G.-A. syringe
Greenberg
    G. bar
    G. clamp
    G. instrument holder
    G. Maxi-Vise adapter
    G. retracting system
    G. retractor frame
    G. retractor set
    G. Universal retractor
Greenberg-Sugita retractor

Greene
    G. endocervical curette
    G. needle
    G. placental curette
    G. uterine curette
Greenfield
    G. caval catheter
    G. needle
    G. titanium inferior vena cava (IVC) filter
    G. vena cava filter system
Green-Gould needle
Green-Kenyon corneal marker
Green-Sewall mouthgag
Greenwald
    G. Control Tip cystoscopic electrode
    G. cutting loop
    G. flexible endoscopic electrode
    G. needle
    G. retractor
    G. Roth Grip-Tip suture guide
    G. sound
Greenwood
    G. bipolar coagulation-suction forceps
    G. spinal trephine
Gregg cannula
Gregory
    G. baby profunda clamp
    G. carotid bulldog clamp
    G. external clamp
    G. forceps
    G. stay suture clamp
    G. vascular miniature clamp
Greiling gastroduodenal tube
Greissinger
    G. foot prosthesis
    G. Multi-Axis joint
    G. Multi-Axis joint implant
grenade
    bulb g.
Greven alligator forceps
Grey-Hess screen
Grey Turner forceps
Grice
    G. laparoscopic sump
    G. lift
    G. retractor
    G. suture needle
grid
    Amsler g.
    Bernell g.
    g. cabinet
    Hirji-Callandar g.
    g. maze board
    oscillating g.
    radiographic g.
    Shar-Tek foot positioning g.
Gridley intraocular lens
Grierson
    G. meniscal shaver
    G. tendon stripper
Grieshaber
    G. blade

G. calibrated corneal trephine
G. corneal needle
G. diamond-coated forceps
G. endo-illuminator
G. flexible iris retractor
G. internal limiting membrane
  forceps
G. iris forceps
G. iris needle
G. manipulator forceps
G. microbipolar coagulator
G. needle holder
G. ophthalmic needle
G. power injector system
G. ruby knife
G. self-retaining retractor
G. spring wire retractor
G. three-function manipulator
G. two-function manipulator
G. ultrasharp knife
G. vertical cutting scissors
G. vitreous scissors
Grieshaber-Balfour retractor
Griffin bandage lens dressing
Griffiths-Brown forceps
Grigor fiberoptic guiding catheter
grinder
  skin g.
Grinfeld cannula
GRIN lens
grip
  dowel g.
  Get-A-Grip g.
  Neo-Fit neonatal endotracheal
    tube g.
  polly power g.
  Posey g.
  screw g.
  Skil-Care cushion g.
Grip-Ease device
Gripp
  G. squeeze ball
  G. squeeze ball hand exerciser
Gripper
  G. acetabular cup prosthesis
  G. needle
  Steeper powered G.
Grip-Tip suture guide
GRIP torque device
Grizzard subretinal cannula
Groenholm
  G. lid retractor
  G. refractor
Groff electrosurgical knife
Grollman
  G. pigtail catheter
  G. pulmonary artery-seeking catheter
Gromley-Russell cannula
grommet
  g. bone liner
  g. drain tube
  Exmoor plastics aural g.
  g. myringotomy tube
  Shah g.
  Shepard g.

Silastic g.
Szulc g.
Twardon g.
g. ventilating tube
Groningen
  G. button
  G. voice prosthesis
grooved
  g. director
  g. silicone implant
  g. silicone sponge
  g. tying forceps
groover
  Alway g.
  Gam-Mer g.
groove suture
Groshong double-lumen catheter
Gross
  G. brain spatula
  G. coarctation clamp
  G. dressing forceps
  G. ductus spreader
  G. ear curette
  G. ear hook
  G. ear spoon
  G. ear spud
  G. hyoid-cutting forceps
  G. iris retractor
  G. patent ductus retractor
  G. probe
  G. sponge forceps
  G. spur crusher
**Grossan nasal irrigator tip with Water
  Pik**
Grosse-Kempf
  G.-K. bone drill
  G.-K. femoral nail
  G.-K. locking nail
  G.-K. tibial nail
Gross-Pomeranz-Watkins
  G.-P.-W. atrial retractor
  G.-P.-W. retractor
Grotena
  G. abdominal belt
  G. abdominal support
  G. lumbar belt
Grotting forceps
Grover
  G. Atra-grip clamp
  G. auricular appendage clamp
  G. meniscotome
  G. meniscus knife
Gruber
  G. bougie
  G. ear speculum
Gruca
  G. hip reamer
  G. spring
Gruca-Weiss spring
Gruening eye magnet
Gruenwald
  G. bayonet-dressing forceps
  G. dissecting forceps
  G. dressing forceps
  G. Durogrip forceps

G

Gruenwald *(continued)*
G. ear forceps
G. nasal-cutting forceps
G. nasal-dressing forceps
G. nasal punch
G. pituitary rongeur
G. retractor
G. tissue forceps
Gruenwald-Bryant
G.-B. nasal-cutting forceps
G.-B. nasal forceps
Gruenwald-Jansen forceps
Gruenwald-Love
G.-L. intervertebral disk rongeur
G.-L. neurosurgical forceps
Grundelach punch
Grüning magnet
Grüntzig
G. arterial balloon catheter
G. balloon
G. balloon angiography catheter
G. balloon dilator
G. femoral stiffening cannula
G. G, S dilating catheter
G. steerable catheter
Grüntzig-Dilaca catheter
Gruppe
G. wire crimper
G. wire-crimping forceps
G. wire prosthesis
GS-9
GS-9 blade
GS-9 needle
GSA-9 blade
GSB
GSB elbow prosthesis
GSB knee prosthesis
G&S electroejaculator
GSI 16 audiometer
G-suit device
GTC repeated stereotactic localizer framer
GTS
guided trephine system
GTS great toe system
TMS-1 videokeratoscope GTS
G-tube
button-type G.-t.
Guangzhou GD-1 prosthetic valve
guard
Albany eye g.
Attends pad and g.
BandageGuard half-leg g.
cannula g.
CastGuard g.
cataract knife g.
Cloward cervical drill g.
Codman skull perforator g.
Dignity Plus briefmates g.
drill g.
ether g.
eye knife g.
forceps g.
Freedom Palm g.

Hansen keratome g.
Horsley g.
intracardiac sucker g.
Joseph g.
keratome g.
Kneed-It knee g.
laser-assisted intrastromal keratomileusis cannula eye g.
LASIK eye g.
McDavid ankle g.
McDavid hinged knee g.
Midas Rex bur g.
Omed vented instrument g.
palm g.
Peri-Guard vascular graft g.
pin g.
plastic mouth g.
Progressive palm g.
Rubin-Wright forceps g.
scalpel g.
Somatics mouth g.
Storz Teflon forceps g.
tip g.
tooth g.
Twist-Lock drill g.
Ullrich drill g.
UltraPower bur g.
Wright-Rubin forceps g.
guarded
g. chisel
g. irrigating cystitome
g. osteotome
Guardian
G. AICD
G. DNA system
G. ICD
G. one-piece ostomy system: sterile drainage O.R. set
G. pacemaker
G. two-piece ostomy system
G. two-piece ostomy system: closed mini-pouch
G. two-piece ostomy system: closed pouch
G. two-piece ostomy system: drainable mini-pouch
G. two-piece ostomy system: drainable pouch
G. two-piece ostomy system: sterile drainage loop set
G. two-piece ostomy system stoma cap
G. two-piece ostomy system: stoma irrigator drain
G. two-piece ostomy system: urostomy pouch
G. walker
guard-ring tocodynamometer
Guardsman femoral interference screw
Guedel
G. airway
G. laryngoscope
G. laryngoscope blade
Guedel-Negus laryngoscope

Guell laser-assisted intrastromal keratomileusis (LASIK) cannula
Guepar
    G. II hinged knee prosthesis
Guest needle
Guggenheim
    G. adenoidal forceps
    G. scissors
Guggenheim-Gergoiye dilator
Guggenheim-Schuknecht scissors
Guglielmi detachable coil
Guibor
    G. canaliculus intubation set
    G. Expo eye bubble
    G. Expo flat eye bandage
    G. lacrimal drain
    G. shield
    G. Silastic tube
Guidant
    G. balloon
    G. CRM pacemaker
    G. guide wire
    G. guiding catheter
    G. Heart Rhythm Technologies Linear Ablation system
    G. stent
    G. TRIAD three-electrode energy defibrillation system
Guidant-CPI device
guide
    Accu-Line chamfer resection g.
    acetabular angle g.
    acetabular shell g.
    ACL drill g.
    Acufex alignment g.
    Acufex drill g.
    Adapteur multifunctional drill g.
    Adson drill g.
    Adson Gigli-saw g.
    AGC dual-pivot resection g.
    Amplatz tube g.
    anterior cruciate ligament drill g.
    antirotation g.
    AO stopped-drill g.
    Arrow true torque wire g.
    Arthrex drill g.
    Arthrex tibial tunnel g.
    Bailey Gigli-saw g.
    Barraquer wire g.
    barrel g.
    Blair Gigli-saw g.
    bone g.
    Borchard Gigli-saw g.
    bougie g.
    Bow & Arrow cannulated drill g.
    Bullseye femoral g.
    Caldwell g.
    cartilage g.
    catheter g.
    CCK femoral stem provisional g.
    chamfer g.
    Clayman intraocular g.
    Cloward drill g.
    Codman g.
    Concept tibial g.

    Cone g.
    contoured anterior spinal plate drill g.
    Cook stereotaxic g.
    Cooper basal ganglia g.
    Cor-Flex wire g.
    Cosman-Nashold spinal stereotaxic g.
    Cottle bone g.
    Cottle cartilage g.
    Cottle knife g.
    Crockard sublaminar wire g.
    cruciate ligament g.
    Cushing Gigli-saw g.
    Cushing saw g.
    Davis saw g.
    Delta Recon proximal drill g.
    disposable measuring g.
    distal femoral cutting g.
    drill g.
    eccentric drill g.
    Eccentric Isotac tibial g.
    Eriksson g.
    Eschenbach low vision rehabilitation g.
    extramedullary alignment g.
    E-Z g.
    femoral intermedullary g.
    femoral notch g.
    Ferciot wire g.
    filiform g.
    fixed-offset g.
    Flexguide intubation g.
    g. forceps
    Franzen needle g.
    Frazier dural g.
    Friedman knife g.
    front-entry g.
    Gabbay-Frater suture g.
    Galante hip g.
    Gatlin gun drill g.
    Gaulian knife g.
    Geenan Endotorque g.
    Ghajar g.
    Gigli-saw g.
    Glacier ceramic 4-in-1 knee cutting g.
    glenoid drill g.
    Goldman knife g.
    Gouley g.
    Greenwald Roth Grip-Tip suture g.
    Grip-Tip suture g.
    guidepin g.
    gutter g.
    Guyon curved catheter g.
    hand-held drill g.
    Harrison forked-type strut g.
    Harris precoat neck osteotomy g.
    Hewson ligament drill g.
    hollow needle g.
    House strut g.
    House wire g.
    humeral cutting g.
    IM/EM tibial resection g.

G

guide *(continued)*
    Interson biopsy needle g.
    intramedullary g.
    Iowa pudendal needle g.
    Iowa trumpet needle g.
    Jonesco bone wire g.
    Joseph saw g.
    Kazanjian g.
    Lebsche saw g.
    LeFort filiform g.
    Levin drill g.
    ligature g.
    Lipscomb-Anderson drill g.
    long nail-mounted drill g.
    L-resection g.
    Lunderquist-Ring torque g.
    Maggi disposable biopsy needle g.
    measuring g.
    microdrilling g.
    MOD femoral drill g.
    Modny g.
    Morrissey Gigli-saw g.
    Mumford Gigli-saw g.
    needle point suture passer/incision
      closure g.
    Neivert knife g.
    nut alignment g.
    Oshukova collapsible bougie g.
    Palmer cruciate ligament g.
    patellar drill g.
    patellar reamer g.
    patellar resection g.
    picket fence g.
    Pilotip catheter g.
    Pilot suturing g.
    g. pin
    pin g.
    Poppen Gigli-saw g.
    ProTrac ACL tibial g.
    Puddu drill g.
    pudendal needle g.
    punch g.
    Rand-Wells pallidothalmomectomy g.
    Raney Gigli-saw g.
    rear-entry ACL drill g.
    Reece osteotomy g.
    Rhinelander g.
    Richards drill g.
    Roth Grip-Tip suture g.
    Savary-Gilliard wire g.
    Scanlan ligature g.
    scaphoid screw g.
    Schlesinger Gigli-saw g.
    Scott-RCE osteotomy g.
    Slick stylette endotracheal tube g.
    Slidewire extension g.
    Stader pin g.
    stationary angle g.
    Stewart cruciate ligament g.
    Stille Gigli-saw g.
    stoma-centering g.
    straight catheter g.
    surgical instrument g.
    suture g.

    targeting drill g.
    TEGwire g.
    telescopic view g.
    telescoping g.
    TFE-coated wire g.
    The Asta-Cath female catheter g.
    tibial cutter g.
    tissue anchor g. (TAG)
    Todd stereotaxic g.
    Todd-Wells g.
    Todt-Heyer cannula g.
    TraceHybrid wire g.
    Tracer hybrid wire g.
    Trailblazer screw g.
    TrueTorque wire g.
    trumpet needle g.
    Tucker vertebrated g.
    tunnel drill g.
    Tworek screw g.
    Unis Universal g.
    Urbanski strut g.
    Uslenghi drill g.
    Van Buren catheter g.
    Wilson-Cook standard wire g.
    wire g.
    g. wire
guided trephine system (GTS)
Guidefather catheter
guideline
    Böhler g.
    Hartel g.
    Letournel g.
guidepin, guide pin
    AO g.
    g. guide
guider
    NL3 g.
guidewire, guide wire *(See also* wire)
    ACS Amplatz g.
    ACS Hi-Torque Balance g.
    ACS LIMA g.
    Amplatz Super Stiff g.
    Amplatz Super Stiff g.
    angled g.
    angle-tip g.
    argon g.
    beaded g.
    Beath g.
    Becton Dickinson g.
    Bentson Glidewire g.
    Cannu-Flex g.
    cannula with pre-loaded 0.35-inch g.
    Cardiometrics Flow-wire g.
    catheter g.
    Choice PT g.
    Commander angioplasty g.
    ControlWire g.
    Cook straight g.
    Coons Super Stiff long-tip g.
    Cope mandrel g.
    Cor-Flex g.
    Critikon g.
    Crosswire nitinol hydrophilic g.
    Crosswire PTCA g.
    Dasher g.

delivery g.
Doppler g.
Doppler-tipped angioplasty g.
drill-tipped g.
Eder-Puestow g.
Elastorc catheter g.
EnTre g.
ERCP g.
exchange g.
extra-stiff g.
extra-support g.
FasTrac hydrophilic-coated g.
flexible g.
flexible-tip Bentsen g.
Flex Tip g.
FloMap g.
floppy tip g.
floppy-tipped g.
FloWire Doppler g.
fluid-filled pressure monitoring g.
Geenan Endotorque g.
Glidewire Gold surgical g.
heparin-coated g.
Hi-Per Flex exchange g.
Hi-Torque Flex-T g.
Hi-Torque Floppy exchange g.
Hi-Torque Floppy II g.
Hi-Torque Floppy intermediate g.
Hi-Torque Standard g.
hydrophilic-coated g.
hydrophilic polymer-coated
  steerable g.
Hydro Plus coated g.
Hyperflex flexible g.
inclination g.
J exchange g.
J Rosen g.
J-tip g.
J-tipped g.
Kadir Hi-Torque g.
Lubriglide-coated g.
Lumenator injectable g.
Lumina g.
Lunderquist g.
Magic Torque g.
Magnum g.
Medi-Tech g.
micropuncture g.
Microvasive Geenen Endotorque g.
Microvasive Glidewire g.
nail-driving g.
Newton LLT g.
New Yorker g.
nitinol g.
nonconductive g.
Pathfinder exchange g.
PDT g.
Phantom cardiac g.
Placer g.
Platinum Plus g.
Preceder interventional g.
Premo g.
Pressure Guard g.
Radiofocus catheter g.
Reflex SuperSoft steerable g.

Roadrunner PC g.
Rosen J-guide g.
Rotacs g.
Saf-T J g.
Schwarten LP g.
Seeker g.
silk g.
slipper-tipped g.
SOF-T g.
Sones g.
stainless steel g.
steerable angioplastic g.
straight g.
Superselector Y-K g.
Surpass g.
Taper g.
tapered torque g.
Teflon-coated g.
Terumo hydrophilic g.
Terumo/Meditech g.
Terumo-Radiofocus hydrophilic
  polymer-coated g.
tip-deflecting g.
Ultra-Select nitinol PTCA g.
USCI Hyperflex g.
Veriflex g.
Wholey Hi-torque modified-J g.
Wilson-Cook Protector g.
Wilson-Cook Tracer g.
Zebra exchange g.
guiding
  g. cannula
  g. catheter
Guild-Pratt rectal speculum
Guilford
  G. brace
  G. scissors
Guilford-Schuknecht wire-cutting scissors
Guilford-Wright
  G.-W. bivalve speculum
  G.-W. bur
  G.-W. bur saw
  G.-W. clip
  G.-W. crurotomy knife
  G.-W. curette
  G.-W. cutting block
  G.-W. double-edged knife
  G.-W. drum elevator
  G.-W. duckbill elevator
  G.-W. elevator knife
  G.-W. fenestrometer
  G.-W. flap knife
  G.-W. footplate pick
  G.-W. forceps
  G.-W. incudostapedial knife
  G.-W. meatal retractor
  G.-W. middle ear instrument
  G.-W. prosthesis
  G.-W. roller knife
  G.-W. scissors
  G.-W. stapes pick
  G.-W. suction tube
  G.-W. Teflon wire piston
  G.-W. wire cutter
Guilford-Wullstein bur saw

guillotine
  g. adenotome
  Ballenger-Sluder g.
  Charnley femoral inlay g.
  g. cutting tip
  Giertz rib g.
  Lilienthal rib g.
  Myles g.
  Poppers tonsillar g.
  Sauerbruch rib g.
  g. scissors
  Sluder-Sauer tonsillar g.
  Sluder tonsillar g.
  SMIC tonsillar g.
  tonsil g.
  tonsillar g.
  Van Osdel g.
  g. vitrectomy instrument
  Zipster rib g.
guillotine-type cutter
guillotome forceps
guilt screen
Guimaraes
  G. implantable contact lens
    manipulator
  G. ophthalmic flap spatula
Guiot-Talairach construct
Guisez tube
Guist
  G. enucleation hemostat
  G. enucleation scissors
  G. fixation forceps
  G. speculum
  G. sphere eye implant
Guist-Black eye speculum
Guist-Bloch speculum
Gulani
  G. triple function laser-assisted
    intrastromal keratomileusis cannula
  G. triple function LASIK cannula
Guldmann Overhead Trac system
Guleke bone rongeur
Gullstrand
  G. lens
  G. lens loupe
  G. ophthalmoscope
  G. six-surface eye model
  G. slit-lamp
  G. slit lamp
Gullstrand-Zeiss lens loupe
gum
  g. elastic bougie introducer
  G. Machine oral irrigator
gun
  Arthrex meniscal dart g.
  Bard Biopty g.
  BD g.
  Biofix arrow g.
  biopsy g.
  Biopty g.
  Bone Injection g.
  caulking g.
  Cobe staple g.
  Cook biopsy g.
  coring biopsy g.

  electron g.
  EnhanCement g.
  enhancement g.
  Harris cement g.
  Heaf g.
  heat g.
  introducer g.
  Lidge cement g.
  Mentor injector g.
  Messing root canal g.
  Miltex g.
  modified caulking g.
  Moss T-anchor needle introducer g.
  Promag 2.2 biopsy g.
  Reflex g.
  rivet g.
  seam-sealer g.
  skin g.
  spring-loaded biopsy g.
  surgical stapling g.
Gunderson
  G. bone forceps
  G. muscle recession forceps
Gundry cannula
Gunnar-Hey roller forceps
Gunning jaw splint
GunSlinger shoulder orthosis
Gunston-Hult knee prosthesis
Gunston polycentric knee prosthesis
Guppe forceps
Gusberg
  G. cervical biopsy curette
  G. cervical cone curette
  G. endocervical biopsy curette
  G. endocervical biopsy punch
  G. hysterectomy clamp
  G. uterine forceps
Gussenbauer
  G. clamp
  G. suture
Gustilo knee prosthesis
Gustilo-Kyle
  G.-K. cementless total hip
    arthroplasty
  G.-K. total hip
  G.-K. total knee
gut
  g. clamp
  g. suture
Gutgemann
  G. auricular appendage clamp
  G. auricular appendage forceps
Gutglass
  G. hemostat
  G. hemostatic cervical forceps
Guthrie
  G. card
  G. eye-fixation hook
  G. iris hook
  G. retractor
  G. skin hook
Guthrie-Smith
  G.-S. apparatus
  G.-S. bed
Gutierrez-Najar grasping forceps

gutta-percha point
gutter
    g. guide
    G. speculum
Guttmann
    G. obstetrical retractor
    G. vaginal retractor
    G. vaginal speculum
guy
    G. gouge
    g. suture
    G. tenotomy knife
Guyon
    G. curettage
    G. curved catheter guide
    G. dilating bougie
    G. dilating sound
    G. dilator
    G. exploratory bougie
    G. kidney clamp
    G. ureteral catheter
    G. urethral sound
    G. vessel clamp
Guyon-Benique urethral sound
Guyon-Péan vessel clamp
guy-steading suture
Guyton
    G. corneal transplant trephine
    G. electrode
    G. scissors
    G. suturing forceps
Guyton-Clark
    G.-C. forceps
    G.-C. fragment forceps
Guyton-Friedenwald suture
Guyton-Lundsgaard
    G.-L. cataract knife
    G.-L. keratome
    G.-L. scalpel
    G.-L. sclerotome
Guyton-Maumenee speculum
Guyton-Minkowski potential acuity meter
Guyton-Noyes fixation forceps
Guyton-Park eye speculum
Guzman-Blanco epiglottic retractor
Gwathmey
    G. hook
    G. suction tube

G/W Heel Lift, Inc. orthosis
Gx-99 vibratory endermatherapie system
GX cephalometer
gym
    g. ball
    hand g.
    limb g.
    total g.
    Zuni g.
gymball
    Exertools g.
Gymnastik ball
Gymnic ball
Gyn-A-Lite vaginal speculum
Gynaspir vacuum curettage
Gynecare
    G. Thermachoice uterine balloon therapy system
    G. Verascope hysteroscopy system
Gynefold
    G. prolapse pessary
    G. retrodisplacement pessary
Gynex
    G. extended-reach needle
    G. iris hook
Gynkotek pump
GynoSampler endometrial aspirator
Gyno Sampler endometrial sampling device
Gynoscann
Gynos perineometer
Gypsona
    G. cast
    G. plaster dressing
    G. rapid-setting cast material
Gyratome
Gyroscan
    ACS G.
    G. HP Philips 15S whole-body system
    Philips G.
    G. S15 scanner
    G. superconducting MRI
    T Philips ACS-II G.
Gysi articulator

G

H-1
    H-1 catheter
    H-1 MR spectroscopy
HA
    hydroxyapatite
    HA adhesive
    HA membrane
    Proplast HA
Haab
    H. after-cataract knife
    H. eye knife
    H. eye magnet
    H. knife needle
    H. scleral resection knife
Haag-Streit
    H.-S. 900 cobalt blue filter
    H.-S. distometer
    H.-S. Endo-Set
    H.-S. keratometer
    H.-S. ophthalmometer
    H.-S. pacemeter
    H.-S. slit lamp
Haberer
    H. gastrointestinal forceps
    H. intestinal clamp
    H. spatula
Haberer-Gili forceps
Haberman
    H. feeder
    H. suction elevator
HA-biointegrated dental implant system
Hackett
    H. sacral belt
    H. sacroiliac cinch belt
HA-coated
    H.-c. hip implant
    H.-c. Micro-Vent implant
    H.-c. root-form dental implant
Hadeco
    H. ES100VX mini Doppler
    H. intraoperative Doppler
    H. MiniDop Doppler
Hader
    H. aneroid sphygmomanometer
    H. bar clip
    H. dental attachment
    H. implant bar
Hadfield hand board
Hadlock table
Hadow balloon
Haefliger cleaver
Haeggstrom antral trocar
Haemogram blood loss monitor
Haemolite
    H. autologous blood recovery
      system
    Cell Saver H.
Haemonetics
    H. Cell Saver
    H. Cell Saver system
Haemoson ultrasound Doppler
Haenig irrigating scissors

Haering
    H. esophageal prosthesis
    H. tube
Haftelast self-adhering bandage
Hagan surface suction tube
Hagar probe
Hagedorn
    H. needle holder
    H. operation suture needle
Hagenbarth clip-applying forceps
Hagfer needle holder
Hagie
    H. pin
    H. pin nail
    H. wrench
Haglund
    H. plaster scissors
    H. spreader
    H. vaginal speculum
Haglund-Stille
    H.-S. plaster spreader
    H.-S. vaginal speculum
Hagner
    H. bag catheter
    H. hemostatic bag
    H. urethral bag
Hague cataract lamp
Hahn
    H. bone nail
    H. cannula
    H. screw
Hahnenkratt
    H. aspirator
    H. backing
    H. dental clasp
    H. lingual bar
    H. matrix band
    H. orthodontic wire
    H. retainer
    H. root canal pin
    H. root canal post
    H. temporary crown
Haid
    H. cervical plate
    H. Universal bone plate
    H. Universal bone plate system
Haidinger brush
Haifa camera
Haig-Ferguson obstetrical forceps
Haight
    H. pediatric rib spreader
    H. pulmonary retractor
    H. rib retractor
Haight-Finochietto
    H.-F. rib retractor
    H.-F. rib spreader
Haig obstetrical forceps
Haik eye implant
Haiman tonsillar electrode
Haimovici arteriotomy scissors
Haines arachnoid dissector
hair transplant punch

H

Haitz canaliculus punch
Hajek
- H. antral punch forceps
- H. antral retractor
- H. antral rongeur
- H. cannula
- H. downbiting rongeur
- H. elevator
- H. lip retractor
- H. mallet
- H. septal chisel
- H. upbiting rongeur

Hajek-Ballenger
- H.-B. septal dissector
- H.-B. septal elevator

Hajek-Claus rongeur
Hajek-Koffler
- H.-K. bone punch forceps
- H.-K. laminectomy rongeur
- H.-K. reversible punch
- H.-K. sphenoidal forceps
- H.-K. sphenoidal punch
- H.-K. sphenoidal rongeur

Hajek-Skillern sphenoidal punch
Hakansson bone rongeur
Hakansson-Olivecrona rongeur
Hakim
- H. catheter
- H. high-pressure valve
- H. precision valve
- H. reservoir
- H. shunt
- H. tube
- H. valve system

Hakim-Cordis pump
Hakko Dwellcath catheter
Hakler forceps
Halberg
- H. clip
- H. contact lens forceps
- H. indirect ophthalmoscope
- H. trial clip occluder

Haldane
- H. apparatus
- H. tube

Haldane-Priestly tube
Hale obstetrical forceps
Hales piesimeter
half
- h. Jimmie
- h. ring

half-and-half nail
half-circle plate
half-curved clamp
half-intensity needle
half-moon retractor
Halifax
- H. fine adjustment instrument
- H. interlaminar clamp
- H. interlaminar clamp system
- H. placement forceps
- H. wrench

Hall
- H. air drill
- H. arthrotome

- H. bone bur
- H. dermatome
- H. double-hole spinal stapler
- H. driver
- H. intrauterine device
- H. large bone instrument
- H. mandibular implant system
- H. mastoid bur
- H. Micro-Aire drill
- H. modified Moe hook
- H. modular acetabular reamer system
- H. Neurairtome drill
- H. Orthairtome drill
- H. Osteon drill system kit
- H. Osteon irrigation kit
- H. power drill
- H. prosthetic heart valve
- H. sacral anchor
- H. sagittal saw
- H. screwdriver
- H. self-holding introducer
- H. series 4 large bone instrument
- H. spinal screw
- H. step-down drill
- H. Surgairtome II drill
- H. surgical drill
- H. valvulotome
- H. Versipower drill
- H. Versipower oscillating saw
- H. Versipower reamer
- H. Versipower reciprocating saw

Hallach comedo extractor
Hallauer
- H. glasses
- H. spectacles

Hallberg forceps
Hall-Chevalier stripper
Hall-Dundar drill
Halle
- H. bone curette
- H. chisel
- H. dural knife
- H. ethmoidal curette
- H. infant nasal speculum
- H. septal elevator
- H. septal needle
- H. sinus curette
- H. trigeminus knife
- H. vascular spatula

Hall-effect strain transducer
Halle-Tieck nasal speculum
Hall-Fish Hyfrecator
Hallin carotid endarterectomy shunt
Hall-Kaster
- H.-K. heart valve
- H.-K. tilting-disk valve prosthesis

Hallman tunneler
Hall-Morris biphase screw
Hallpike-Blackmore ear microscope
Hall-Relton frame
hallux
- h. forceps
- h. valgus orthosis

halo
Ace low-profile MR h.
Ace Mark III h.
h. apparatus
h. brace
Bremer h.
Brown-Roberts-Wells head ring h.
H. catheter
h. cervical orthosis
h. cervical traction system
H. CO$_2$ laser system
h. femoral traction device
h. fracture frame
h. gravity traction device
h. head frame
h. hoop device
Houston h.
Lerman non-invasive h.
h. retractor
h. retractor system
h. traction device
h. tractor
h. vest
Halocath catheter
halogen
h. coaxial ophthalmoscope
h. dual lightsource
h. lamp
h. light source
H. otoscope
halo-Ilizarov distraction instrumentation
halo-ring adapter
Haloscale respirometer
haloscope
phase-difference h.
halothane analyzer
halo-vest orthosis
Halsey
H. mosquito forceps
H. nail scissors
H. needle
H. Vital needle holder
Halsey-Webster needle holder
Halsted
H. arterial forceps
H. curved mosquito clamp
H. curved mosquito forceps
H. hemostatic mosquito forceps
H. mattress suture
H. Micro-Line arterial forceps
H. mosquito hemostat
H. mules
H. strabismus scissors
H. straight mosquito clamp
Halsted-Swanson tendon-passing forceps
halter
Cerva crane h.
deluxe head h.
DePuy head h.
Diskard head h.
disposable head h.
Forrester head h.
head h.
neck-wrap h.
Repro head h.

standard head h.
TMJ h.
Upper 7 model head h.
Zimfoam head h.
Zimmer head h.
Zyler head h.
Hamas upper limb prosthesis
hamate finder
Hamblin minimagnet
Hamburger-Brennan-Mahorner thyroid retractor
Hamby
H. brain retractor
H. clip-applying forceps
H. right-angle clip applier
H. rod
H. twist drill
H. wire threader
Hamby-Hibbs retractor
Hamer scalpel
Hamilton
H. bandage
H. deep-surgery forceps
H. pelvic traction screw tractor
H. tongue depressor
H. ventilator
Hamilton-Forewater amniotomy hook
Hamilton-Steward catheter
Hamilton-Thorn motility analyzer
Hamm
H. fulgurating electrode
H. resectoscope electrode
hammer
Babinski percussion h.
Berliner neurological h.
Berliner percussion h.
Buck neurological h.
Buck percussion h.
cervical/lumbar h.
Cloward h.
Dejerine-Davis percussion h.
Dejerine percussion h.
Epstein neurological h.
h. forceps
fork h.
Gerzog bone h.
Grafco percussion h.
Hibbs h.
House tapping h.
intranasal h.
Kirk bone h.
Kirk orthopaedic h.
Küntscher h.
Lucae bone h.
Millet test h.
Monreal reflex h.
neurological percussion h.
orthopedic h.
percussion h.
Quisling intranasal h.
Rabiner neurological h.
reflex h.
Rica bone h.
slide h.
sliding h.

H

hammer *(continued)*
SMIC bone h.
Smith-Petersen h.
surgical h.
tapping h.
Taylor percussion h.
Taylor reflex h.
Traube neurological h.
Tromner percussion h.
Wartenberg neurological h.
Williger h.
Hammersmith
H. heart valve
H. mitral valve prosthesis
hammer-type acupuncture needle
Hamming-Hahn filter
hammock
h. bandage
h. dressing
Mersilene gauze h.
Hammond
H. alloy
H. orthodontic splint
H. winged retractor blade
Hamou
H. colpomicrohysteroscope
H. contact microhysteroscope
H. endoscope
H. hysteroscope
H. microcolpohysteroflator
Hampton
H. electrosurgical unit
H. needle holder
Hamrick
H. suction dissector
H. suction elevator
Hanafee catheter
Hanastome microkeratome
Hanau
H. 130-21 articulator
H. face bow
Hancke/Vilmann biopsy handle instrument
Hancock
H. aortic valve prosthesis
H. bioprosthetic heart valve
H. coronary perfusion catheter
H. embolectomy catheter
H. fiberoptic catheter
H. heterograft heart valve
H. hydrogen detection catheter
H. luminal electrophysiologic recording catheter
H. mitral valve prosthesis
H. modified orifice valve
H. M.O. II porcine bioprosthesis
H. pericardial valve graft
H. porcine heterograft
H. porcine valve
H. temporary cardiac pacing wire
H. thermodilution catheter
H. vascular graft
H. wedge-pressure catheter

hand
h. block
h. brace
Brueckmann lead h.
h. cock-up snare
h. cock-up splint
h. cone
h. cuff
h. drill
h. exercise ball
h. exerciser
Freedom arthritis support for h.
h. gym
H. Helper device
H. Helper hand exerciser
lead h.
Myobock artificial h.
Naeser laser home treatment program for the h.
pediatric retractor malleable wire h.
h. retractor
h. surgery rasp
h. trephine
Vaduz h.
h. volumeter
Winter Helping H.
Handages
Hand-Aid
H.-A. arterial wrist support
H.-A. strapping material
hand-assisted laparoscopic surgery
hand-control cautery
hand-crimped stent
Hand-E-Vent
Handeze fingerless glove
hand-held
h.-h. drill guide
h.-h. exploring electrode probe
h.-h. eye magnet
h.-h. fundus camera
h.-h. Hruby lens
h.-h. mapping probe
h.-h. nebulizer
h.-h. retractor
h.-h. rotary prism
h.-h. trephine
handheld dynamometer
hand-holder
Tupper h.-h.
HandiCare adult disposable pant and pad system
Handi-Cath catheter kit
Handisol phototherapy device
handle
Acufex h.
autopsy h.
Bard-Parker h.
Barton traction h.
bayonet h.
Beaver h.
blade h.
B-P surgical h.
Bruening esophagoscopy forceps h.
Charnley brace h.
Cloward cross-bar h.

Cloward double-hinge cervical
retractor h.
Cloward dowel h.
Corwin knife h.
Cottle protected knife h.
DORC h.
DuraLite h.
Dynagrip blade h.
ear knife h.
Elliot trephine h.
endoscopic electrode h.
FloGUN suction/irrigation control h.
Gigli-saw h.
Hardy lateral knife h.
hexagonal h.
House myringotomy knife h.
insulated knife h.
Klein-Delrin Luer-Lok h.
knife h.
knurled h.
laryngeal knife h.
laryngeal mirror h.
Luikart-Bill traction h.
Lynch laryngeal knife h.
Marino rotatable transsphenoidal
knife h.
Marlow Primus h.
Morse instrument h.
myringotomy knife h.
Ortho-Grip silicone rubber h.
Parker-Bard h.
protected knife h.
rotatable transsphenoidal knife h.
Rusch laryngoscope h.
safety h.
saw h.
scalpel h.
Stiwer scalpel h.
stone basket screw mounted h.
Storz ear knife h.
Strully Gigli-saw h.
surgical h.
Thera-Band h.
Therap-Loop door h.
Tip-Trol h.
T-pin h.
traction h.
tympanum perforator h.
Universal chuck h.
V. Mueller Tip-Trol h.
V. Mueller Universal h.

handleless clamp
hand-mounted stent
handpiece
A-Dec h.
AMO Series 4 phaco h.
AVIT h.
B-mode h.
Cavitron I&A h.
Chayes h.
ClearCut 2 electrosurgical h.
collimated beam h.
CooperVision irrigation/aspiration h.
CUSA system 200 straight
autoclavable h.

Densco dental h.
Dermacerator h.
Dermastat dermatology h.
Doriot h.
DynaSurg electric h.
Dynatrak h.
Emesco h.
Endo-Gripper endodontic h.
Excaliber h.
fragmentation/aspiration h.
Hexascan computerized
dermatology h.
Imperator h.
infusion h.
Kaessman h.
KaVo dental h.
Kelman irrigating h.
Kerr M4 safety h.
Kurtin h.
Lares dental h.
Lightning high-speed vitrectomy h.
Litton dental h.
McIntyre infusion h.
Micro oral surgery h.
micropigmentation h.
MicroSeal ophthalmic h.
Microstat h.
M4 safety h.
Neuroguide optical h.
oral surgery h.
Packer Wick extrusion h.
phacoemulsification h.
PhotoDerm PL h.
ProFinesse II ultrasonic h.
reciprocating power h.
Revelation h.
rotosteotome rotary h.
Sabra OMS 45 dental h.
SITE Phaco II h.
soft-tipped extrusion h.
Sonop h.
Storz h.
SureScan scanning h.
Surgitek h.
Titan slow-speed h.
Wullstein contra-angle h.

hand-roller
Lundy tubing h.-r.
hands
H. Free knee retractor system
Otto Bock system electric h.
handset
Force GSU laparoscopic h.
hand-sutured closure
CEM handswitching nosecone
Handy
H. II articulator
H. non-mydriatic video fundus
camera
Handy-Buck extension tractor
Haney
H. needle driver

H

365

hanger
    Adjusta-Rak h.
    Conveen bag h.
Hanger prosthesis
hanging cast sling
Hank-Dennen obstetrical forceps
Hankins lucite ovoid
Hanks-Bradley uterine dilator
Hanks uterine dilator
Hanley-McDermott pelvimeter
Hannahan
    H. bur
    H. forceps
Hanna trephine
Hann filter
Hannon endometrial curette
Hannover needle holder
Hansatome
    Chiron H.
Hansen
    H. grasper
    H. keratome
    H. keratome guard
Hansen-Street
    H.-S. anchor plate
    H.-S. pin
    H.-S. self-broaching nail
    H.-S. solid intramedullary nail
Hanslik patellar prosthesis
Hanson speed bracket
Hans Rudolph three-way valve
Hapad
    H. felt insert
    H. longitudinal metatarsal arch pad
    H. metatarsal insole
    H. shoe insert
Hapex bioactive material
Hapset
    H. bone graft plaster material
    H. hydroxyapatite bone graft plaster
haptic
    h. area implant
    h. area lens
    Coburn h.
    modified C-loop h.
    modified J-loop h.
    h. plate lens
    PMMA h.
    Slant h.
haptic-fixated intraocular lens
haptic-sec lens
hard
    h. contact lens
    h. mallet
    h. palate retractor
    h. socket
    h. tissue replacement-malleable facial
      implant
    h. x-ray imaging spectrometer
Hardesty
    H. tendon hook
    H. tenotomy hook
Hardt-Delima osteotome

hardware
    Genesis arthroplasty h.
    TiMesh h.
Hardy
    H. aluminum crutch
    H. bayonet curette
    H. bayonet dressing forceps
    H. bayonet enucleator
    H. bayonet neurosurgical bipolar
      forceps
    H. bivalve speculum
    H. hypophysial curette
    H. implant fork
    H. lateral knife handle
    H. lensometer
    H. lip retractor
    H. microbipolar forceps
    H. microdissector
    H. microsurgical bayonet bipolar
      forceps
    H. microsurgical enucleator
    H. modification of Bronson-Ray
      curette
    H. nasal bivalve speculum
    H. pituitary dissector
    H. pituitary spoon
    H. 3-prong fork
    H. rongeur
    H. sellar punch
    H. suction tube
    H. transsphenoidal mirror
Hardy-Duddy
    H.-D. speculum
    H.-D. vaginal retractor
Hardy-Rand-Rittler plate
Hare
    H. compact traction splint
    H. splint device
    H. traction device
harelip
    h. forceps
    h. needle
    h. traction bow
Har-el pharyngeal tube
Hargin antral trocar
Hargis periosteal elevator
Hariri-Heifetz microsurgical system
Harken
    H. auricular clamp
    H. ball heart valve
    H. cardiovascular forceps
    H. erysiphake
    H. heart needle
    H. prosthesis
    H. prosthetic valve
    H. rib retractor
    H. rib spreader
    H. valvulotome
Harken-Cooley forceps
Harken-Starr valve
Harloff cart
Harlow plate
Harm
    H. cage
    H. posterior cervical plate

Harman
    H. eye dressing
    H. fixation forceps
Harmon chisel
harmonic
    h. attenuation table
    H. scalpel
    h. scissors
Harmonie
    H. Classic Plus brief
    H. underpad
Harms
    H. corneal forceps
    H. microtying forceps
    H. suture-tying forceps
    H. trabeculotome
    H. trabeculotomy probe
    H. tying forceps
    H. utility forceps
    H. vessel forceps
Harms-Moss anterior thoracic instrumentation
Harms-Tubingen tying forceps
harness
    Heart Hugger sternum support h.
    Kicker Pavlik h.
    Pavlik h.
    Rhino Cruiser Pavlik h.
    Rhino Kicker Pavlik h.
    SecureEasy endotracheal h.
    Wheaton Pavlik h.
    Zuni h.
Harold
    H. Crowe drill
    H. Hayes eustachian bougie
Harpenden
    H. handgrip dynamometer
    H. skinfold calipers
    H. stadiometer
Harper
    H. cervical laminectomy punch
    H. periosteal elevator
Harpoon suture anchor
Harrah lung clamp
Harrington
    H. bladder retractor
    H. Britetrac retractor
    H. clamp forceps
    H.-Deaver retractor
    H. deep surgical scissors
    H. distraction instrumentation
    H. dual square-ended rod
    H. erysiphake
    H. flat wrench
    H. hook clamp
    H. hook driver
    H. lung-grasping forceps
    H. pedicle hook
    H. protractor
    H. rod and hook system
    H. rod instrumentation
    H. rod instrumentation distraction outrigger device
    H. spinal elevator
    H. spinal instrumentation
    H. splanchnic retractor
    H. spreader
    H. strut
    H. sympathectomy retractor
    H. thoracic forceps
    H. tonometer
    H. vulsellum forceps
Harrington-Carmalt clamp
Harrington-Flocks multiple pattern
Harrington-Kostuik
    H.-K. distraction device
    H.-K. instrumentation
Harrington-Mayo
    H.-M. scissors
    H.-M. tissue forceps
Harrington-Mixter
    H.-M. thoracic clamp
    H.-M. thoracic forceps
Harrington-Pemberton sympathectomy retractor
Harris
    H. band
    H. brace-type reamer
    H. broach
    H. catheter
    H. cemented hip prosthesis
    H. cement gun
    H. center-cutting acetabular reamer
    H. condylocephalic nail
    H. condylocephalic rod
    H. dissector
    H. femoral head gauge
    H. footprint mat
    H. Hemi Arm sling
    H. hip nail
    H. implant
    H. medullary nail
    H. Micromini prosthesis
    H. modified J-loop intraocular lens
    H. plate
    H. precoat neck osteotomy guide
    H. precoat prosthesis
    H. protrusio shell
    H. rigid quadriped intraocular lens
    H. separator
    H. snare
    H. splint sling
    H. suture-carrying forceps
    H. tonsillar knife
    H. trephine
    H. uterine injector (HUI)
    H. wire tier
    H. wire tightener
Harris-Galante
    H.-G. cup
    H.-G. hip replacement acetabular component
    H.-G. I porous-coated acetabular component
    H.-G. porous acetabular component
    H.-G. porous-coated femoral component
    H.-G. porous hip prosthesis
Harris-Kronner uterine manipulator/injector (HUMI)

H

Harrison
- H. bone-holding forceps
- H. capsular knife
- H. chalazion retractor
- H. forked-type strut guide
- H. implant
- H. interlocked mesh dressing
- H. interlocked mesh prosthesis
- H. myringoplasty knife
- H. suture-removing scissors
- H. tucker

Harrison-Nicolle polypropylene peg
Harrison-Shea
- H.-S. curette
- H.-S. knife

Harris-Sinskey microlens hook
Harris-Smith anterior interbody drill
Harshill rectangle
Hart
- H. extension finger splint
- H. pediatric three-mirror lens

Hartel guideline
Hartinger Coincidence refractionometer
Hartley
- H. implant
- H. mammary prosthesis

Hartmann
- H. adenoidal curette
- H. alligator forceps
- H. biopsy punch
- H. bone rongeur
- H. clamp
- H. dewaxer speculum
- H. ear-dressing forceps
- H. ear polyp forceps
- H. ear punch
- H. ear rongeur
- H. ear speculum
- H. eustachian catheter
- H. hemostat
- H. hemostatic mosquito forceps
- H. knife
- H. mastoid rongeur
- H. mosquito hemostatic forceps
- H. nasal conchotome
- H. nasal-cutting forceps
- H. nasal-dressing forceps
- H. nasal polyp forceps
- H. nasal punch
- H. nasal speculum
- H. tonsillar dissector
- H. tonsillar punch
- H. tonsillar punch forceps
- H. tuning fork
- H. uterine biopsy forceps

Hartmann-Citelli
- H.-C. alligator forceps
- H.-C. ear punch
- H.-C. ear punch forceps

Hartmann-Corgill ear forceps
Hartmann-Gruenwald nasal-cutting forceps
Hartmann-Herzfeld
- H.-H. ear forceps
- H.-H. ear rongeur

Hartmann-Noyes nasal-dressing forceps
Hartmann-Proctor ear forceps
Hartmann-Weingärtner ear forceps
Hartmann-Wullstein ear forceps
Hartstein
- H. iris cryoretractor
- H. irrigating iris retractor
- H. irrigator
- H. refractor

Hartzler
- H. ACS coronary dilation catheter
- H. ACX II catheter
- H. balloon catheter
- H. dilatation catheter
- H. Excel catheter
- H. LPS dilatation catheter
- H. Micro-600 catheter
- H. Micro II angioplasty balloon
- H. Micro II catheter
- H. Micro XT catheter
- H. rib retractor
- H. RX-14 balloon catheter
- H. Ultra-Lo-Profile catheter

Harvard
- H. cannula
- H. 2 dual-syringe pump
- H. microbore intravenous extension set
- H. needle

harvester
- Brandel cell h.
- multiple automated sample h.
- OsteoHarvester bone h.
- TomTec cell h.

Harvey
- H. Elite stethoscope
- H. Stone clamp
- H. vapor sterilizer
- H. wire-cutting scissors

Hashizume endoscopic ligator kit
Hashmat shunt
Hashmat-Waterhouse shunt
Haslinger
- H. bronchoscope
- H. endoscope
- H. esophagoscope
- H. headholder
- H. headrest
- H. laryngoscope
- H. palate retractor
- H. tip forceps
- H. tracheobronchoesophagoscope
- H. tracheoscope
- H. uvular retractor

Hasner
- H. lid forceps
- H. valve

Hassan-type port
Hasson
- H. balloon uterine elevator cannula
- H. blunt port
- H. bullet-tip forceps
- H. grasper
- H. grasping forceps
- H. laparoscope

H. laparoscopic trocar
H. needle-nose forceps
H. open-laparoscopy cannula
H. retractor
H. ring forceps
H. spike-tooth forceps
H. stable access cannula
H. uterine manipulator
Hasson-Eder laparoscopy cannula
Hastings frame
Hasund appliance
hat
measuring h.
Hatch
H. catheter
H. chisel
H. clamp
Hatcher pin
hatchet
black h.
California h.
Nordent h.
Hatfield bone curette
HA-threaded hexlock implant
Hatt
H. golf-stick elevator
H. spoon
Haugh ear forceps
Hausmann
H. vascular clamp
H. weight rack
H. Work-Well work hardening
system
Hautmann ileoneobladder
Haven skin graft hook
Haverfield
H. brain cannula
H. hemilaminectomy retractor
Haverfield-Scoville hemilaminectomy
retractor
Haverhill
H. clamp
H. dermal abrader
H. needle
Haverhill-Mack clamp
Havlicek
H. spiral cannula
H. trocar
Hawkeye suture needle
Hawkins
H. breast localization needle
H. cervical biopsy forceps
Hawkins-Akins needle
Hawks-Dennen obstetrical forceps
Hawksley random zero mercury
sphygmomanometer
Hawley
H. appliance
H. bite plate
H. chart
H. retainer
H. table
Hayden
H. footplate pick
H. palate elevator

H. probe
H. tonsillar curette
Hayek oscillator
Hayes
H. anterior resection clamp
H. anterior resection forceps
H. colon clamp
H. intestinal clamp
H. Martin forceps
H. vaginal speculum
Hayes-Olivecrona forceps
Hayman dilator
Haynes
H. brain cannula
H. 25 material
H. pin
H. retractor
H. scissors
Haynes-Griffin mandibular splint
Haynes-Stellite implant metal prosthesis
Hays
H. finger retractor
H. hand retractor
H. pharyngoscope
Hayton-Williams
H.-W. forceps
H.-W. mouthgag
HBT Sleuth
HCH disk
HCMI chiropractic system
HD
HD II total hip prosthesis
HD Secura dialyzer
HDI
HDI ultrasound
HDI 1000, 3000, 5000 ultrasound
system
head
Austin Moore h.
h. of bed
Biolox ball h.
h. brace
Bruening-Storz diagnostic h.
Bruening-Work diagnostic h.
cobalt-chromium h.
h. coil
contra-angle h.
coupling h.
h. extractor
h. fixation device
h. frame
h. halter
h. halter cervical traction
h. holder
h. lamp
Matroc femoral h.
h. mirror
Morse h.
MRI probe h.
Omniflex h.
Rhoton-Merz rotatable coupling h.
h. ring
rotatable coupling h.
Series-II humeral h.
h. sling

H

head *(continued)*
    h. spoon separator
    Storz-Bruening diagnostic h.
    Vitox femoral h.
    Work-Bruening diagnostic h.
    Ziramic femoral h.
    Zirconia orthopaedic prosthetic h.
    Zyranox femoral h.
headband
    Bosworth h.
    Gleason h.
    Goot-Lite h.
    plagiocephaly h.
    Pynchol h.
    Sluder h.
    Storz face shield h.
    Worrall h.
headgear
    horizontal pull h.
    Kloehn h.
    Kurz pulsation orthodontic h.
headholder
    AMSCO h.
    Bayless neurosurgical h.
    Derlacki-Juers h.
    Gardner h.
    Haslinger h.
    integrated h.
    Malcolm-Rand carbon-composite h.
    Mayfield-Kees h.
    Mayfield radiolucent h.
    Mayfield skull-pin h.
    Mayfield tic h.
    Methodist Hospital h.
    Parkinson h.
    pin h.
    pinion h.
    radiolucent cranial pin h.
    Shampaine h.
    Sugita h.
headhunter visceral angiography catheter
headlamp
    Keeler Magnalite fiberoptic h.
    Keeler video h.
    MTA h.
headlight
    Clip-Lite clip-on h.
    Cogent LightWear h.
    Goodlite super h.
    Heine UBL 100 h.
    high beam fiberoptic h.
    Keeler fiberoptic h.
    Klaar h.
    LightWear h.
    Orascoptic fiberoptic h.
    Quadrilite 6000 fiberoptic h.
    Welch Allyn single fiber
      illumination h.
Headmaster collar
head/moisture exchanger
headrest, head rest
    adjustable h.
    Adson h.
    Brown-Roberts-Wells h.

    Craig h.
    doughnut h.
    Gardner h.
    Gardner-Wells h.
    Gibralter h.
    Haslinger h.
    horseshoe h.
    Lempert rongeur h.
    Light h.
    Light-Veley h.
    Mayfield-Kees h.
    Mayfield pediatric horseshoe h.
    Mayfield radiolucent h.
    Mayfield swivel horseshoe h.
    McConnell orthopaedic h.
    Multipoise h.
    neurosurgical h.
    pin h.
    pinion h.
    Richards h.
    Roberts h.
    Shea h.
    Storz adjustable h.
    Veley h.
heads-up imaging system
Heaf gun
Healey revision acetabular component
healing
    h. screw
    h. shoe
Healon injection cannula
Healos
    H. synthetic bone grafting material
Healthdyne
    H. apnea monitor
    H. pulse oximeter
    H. ventilator
Healthflex orthotic
Healthier gel seating cushion
Health O Meter Scale
HealthShield antimicrobial mediastinal
  wound drainage catheter
Healy
    H. gastrointestinal forceps
    H. intestinal forceps
    H. suture-removing forceps
    H. uterine biopsy forceps
Healy-Jako pediatric subglottiscope
Heaney
    H. clamp
    H. endometrial biopsy curette
    H. hysterectomy forceps
    H. hysterectomy retractor
    H. suture
    H. tissue forceps
    H. uterine curette
    H. vaginal retractor
    H. Vital needle holder
Heaney-Kantor hysterectomy forceps
Heaney-Rezek forceps
Heaney-Simon
    H.-S. hysterectomy forceps
    H.-S. hysterectomy retractor
    H.-S. vaginal retractor
Heaney-Stumf forceps

hearing
- h. aid
- h. aid amplifier
- h. aid microphone
- h. protection device
- h. protector

Hearn needle
Hearst dilator
Heart
- H. Aid 80 defibrillator
- H. Aide Plus monitor
- H. Hugger sternum support harness
- H. pillow
- H. pillow infuser
- H. Rate 1-2-3 monitor
- H. Technology Rotablator

heart
- air-driven artificial h.
- Akutsu III total artificial h.
- ALVAD artificial h.
- artificial h.
- Baylor total artificial h.
- electromechanical artificial h.
- Hershey total artificial h.
- implantable artificial h.
- Jarvik-7, -8, 2000 artificialh.
- Jarvik 2000 artificial h.
- Liotta total artificial h.
- h. needle
- orthotopic biventricular artificial h.
- orthotopic univentricular artificial h.
- h. pacemaker
- Penn State total artificial h.
- Phoenix total artificial h.
- h. pump
- RTV total artificial h.
- Symbion/CardioWest 100 mL total artificial h.
- Symbion Jarvik-7 artificial h.
- Symbion total artificial h.
- University of Akron artificial h.
- Utah total artificial h.
- h. valve

HeartCard
- H. cardiac event recorder
- H. monitor

heart-lung resuscitator
HeartMate
- H. implantable pneumatic left ventricular assist system
- H. implantable ventricular assist device
- H. left ventricular assist system
- H. portable pump

Heartport
- H. catheter system
- H. endoaortic clamp
- H. Endocoronary Sinus catheter
- H. Endovenous drainage cannula
- H. Port-Access system

HeartPort-Endoclamp balloon cannula
HeartPort PrecisionOP system
HEARTrac I Cardiac Monitoring system
HeartSaver VAD
Heartwire

heat
- h. gun
- h. and moisture exchanger
- h. pad

heated tracheostomy collar
heater
- h. probe
- resistance wire h.
- Snowden-Pencer internal h.

heat-expandable stent
Heath
- H. chalazion curette
- H. chalazion forceps
- H. clip
- H. clip-removing forceps
- H. clip-removing scissors
- H. follicle expressor
- H. mallet
- H. mules
- H. nasal forceps
- H. punctum dilator
- H. suture-cutting scissors
- H. suture scissors
- H. trephine flap dissector
- H. wire cutter
- H. wire-cutting scissors

HeatProbe device
heavy
- h. cross-slot screwdriver
- h. monofilament suture
- h. retention suture
- h. septal scissors
- h. silk retention suture
- h. wire suture

heavy-duty pliers with side-cutter
heavy-gauge suture
HeavyMed ball
Hebra
- H. blade
- H. chalazion curette
- H. corneal curette
- H. hook

Hecht fascia lata forceps
Heck screw
Hedblom
- H. costal elevator
- H. rib retractor

Hedgehog
- Sonic H.

Hedges Corneal Wetting Pak
Hedstrom file
Hedwig
- H. introducer
- H. lumen finder

heel
- h. cup
- h. cushion
- H. Free splint
- H. Hugger therapeutic heel stabilizer
- h. lift
- h. pillow
- rubber walking h.
- h. sleeve
- soft ankle, cushioned h.

heel (*continued*)
    H. Spur Special orthosis
    Thomas h.
    walking h.
    wedge adjustable cushioned h. (WACH)
Heelbo decubitus protector
HeelCare cushion
Heeler inflatable heel protector
Heelift suspension boot
Heermann
    H. alligator forceps
    H. chisel
    H. ear forceps
Heffernan nasal speculum
Heffington
    H. lumbar seat
    H. lumbar seat spinal surgery frame
Hefty Bite pin cutter
Hegar
    H. bougie
    H. needle
    H. needle holder
    H. rectal dilator
    H. uterine dilator
Hegar-Baumgartner
    H.-B. needle
    H.-B. needle holder
Hegar-Goodell dilator
Hegar-Mayo-Seeley needle holder
Hegar-Olsen needle holder
Hegemann scissors
Hegenbarth
    H. clip
    H. clip-applying forceps
Hegenbarth-Adams clip
Hegenbarth-Michel clip-applying forceps
Hegge pin
He Hook chopper
Heidbrink expiratory spill valve
Heidelberg
    H. arm
    H. fixation forceps
    H. laser tomographic scanner
    H. retinal flowmeter
Heidelberg-R table
Heifitz
    H. aneurysm clip
    H. carotid occluder
    H. cerebral aneurysm clamp
    H. clip applier
    H. cup serrated ring forceps
    H. microclip
    H. retractor
    H. skull perforator
    H. spatula
Heifitz-Weck clip
Heightronic stadiometer
Heiming kidney stone forceps
Heimlich
    H. chest drainage valve
    H. heart valve
    H. tube
    H. Vygon pneumothorax valve

Heimlich-Gavrilu gastric tube
Hein
    H. raspatory
    H. rongeur
Heine
    H. gonioscope
    H. Lambda 100 retinometer
    H. penlight
    H. UBL 100 headlight
Heinkel sigmoidoscope
Heiss
    H. arterial forceps
    H. hemostatic forceps
    H. mastoid retractor
    H. soft tissue retractor
    H. vulsellum forceps
Heister mouthgag
Heitz-Boyer clamp
Hejnosz radium colpostat
Helanca seamless tube prosthesis
Helfrick anal retractor
helical
    h. coil
    h. coil stent
    h. computed tomographic angiogram
    h. CT
    h. CT scanner
    h. PTCA dilatation catheter
    h. suture
    h. tube saw
helical-ridged ureteral stent
helical-tip Halo catheter
helicoid endosteal implant
Heliodent dental x-ray unit
Heliodorus bandage
Helios diagnostic imaging system
Helioseal
Helistat absorbable collagen hemostatic sponge
Helitene absorbable collagen hemostatic agent
helium-cadmium diagnostic laser
helium-filled balloon catheter
helium-neon aiming laser
Helix
    H. camera
    H. endocervical curette
    H. multihead nuclear imaging system
    H. PTCA dilatation catheter
    H. uterine biopsy curette
helix
    h. balloon
heliX
    h. knot pusher
Heller
    H. biopsy forceps
    H. probe
Hellige electrocardiographic recorder
helmet
    collimator h.
    cooling h.
    plagiocephaly h.
Helmholtz
    H. double-surface coil

H. keratometer
H. ophthalmoscope
H. speculum
Helmont speculum
Helmstein balloon
HELP system
Helsper
H. laryngectomy button
H. tracheostomy vent tube
Helveston
H. "Great Big Barbie" retractor
H. scleral marking ruler
Helvestoon hook
hemacytometer
Hemaduct wound drain
hemadynamometer
Hemaflex
H. PTCA sheath with obturator
H. pure collage hemostat
H. sheath
Hemagard collection tube
Hemaquet
H. introducer
H. PTCA sheath with obturator
Hemashield
H. collagen-enhanced graft
H. vascular graft
HemAssist blood substitute
hematology rocker
Hematome system
Hemex prosthetic valve
hemiambulator walker
hemi-interpositional implant
hemiknee
hemilaminectomy
h. blade
h. retractor
hemiprosthesis
single-stemmed silicone h.
Hemi sling
hemisphere eye implant
hemispherical pusher
Hemocal hemoperfusion cartridge
Hemoccult
H. II
H. Sensa slide
Hemoclear dialyzer
Hemoclip-applying forceps
Hemoclip clamp
hemoconcentrator
Biofilter cardiovascular h.
HemoCue
H. blood glucose analyzer
H. blood glucose system
H. blood hemoglobin analyzer
H. glucose meter
H. hemoglobin photometer
H. microcurette
hemocytometer
Coulter MD 16 h.
Neubauer h.
hemodialysis concentrate
hemodialysis catheter
hemodialyzer
Altra Flux h.

1550 Baxter h.
Biospal h.
2008E h.
Gambro h.
Gambro-Lundia Minor h.
Polyflux h.
Redy h.
Hemofreeze blood bag
hemoheater
Vickers Treonic h.
Hemoject
H. injection catheter
H. needle
Hemokart hemoperfusion cartridge
Hem-o-lok polymer ligating clip
**Hemopad sterile absorbable collagen
hemostat**
Hemophan membrane
Hemopump
Johnson & Johnson H.
Medtronic H.
Nimbus H.
**Hemopure oxygen-based therapeutic
system**
hemorrhoidal
h. clamp
h. forceps
h. ligator
h. needle
hemostasis
h. scalp clip
h. silver clip
hemostat
Actifoam h.
Actifoam active h.
Adson h.
Allis h.
Avitene microfibrillar collagen h.
Avtifoam active h.
blackened h.
Blohmka tonsillar h.
blunt-nose h.
Boettcher h.
broadbill h. with push fork
Carmalt h.
Collastat OBP microfibrillar
collagen h.
Collier-DeBakey h.
Corboy h.
Corwin tonsillar h.
Crafoord h.
Crile gall h.
curved Kelly h.
curved mosquito h.
Dandy scalp h.
Davis h.
Dean tonsil h.
Deaver h.
Endo-Avitene microfibrillar
collagen h.
fine-tipped mosquito h.
Guist enucleation h.
Gutglass h.
Halsted mosquito h.
Hartmann h.
Hemaflex pure collage h.

H

373

hemostat *(continued)*
    Hemopad sterile absorbable collagen h.
    Hemotene absorbable collagen h.
    Instat collagen absorbable h.
    Instat MCH microfibrillar collagen h.
    Jackson tracheal h.
    Kelly h.
    Kocher h.
    Lahey h.
    Lewis h.
    Lothrop h.
    Lowsley h.
    Mathrop h.
    Mayo h.
    McWhorter h.
    Meigs h.
    microfibrillar collagen h.
    Mixter h.
    mosquito h.
    Nu-Knit absorbable h.
    Ochsner h.
    Ormco orthodontic h.
    orthopedic h.
    Perdue h.
    Providence Hospital h.
    Raimondi h.
    Rankin h.
    Rochester-Ochsner h.
    Rochester-Péan h.
    Sawtell h.
    Sawtell-Davis h.
    Schnidt h.
    Shallcross h.
    straight mosquito h.
    Surgicel fibrillator absorbable h.
    Surgicel Nu-Knit absorbable h.
    Thrombogen absorbable h.
hemostatic
    h. bag
    h. catheter
    h. cervical forceps
    h. clamp
    h. clip
    h. clip applier
    h. clip-applying forceps
    h. eraser
    h. neurosurgical forceps
    h. occlusive leverage device
    h. puncture closure device
    h. suture
    h. tissue forceps
    h. tonsillar forceps
    h. tonsillectome
    h. tracheal forceps
HemoTec
    H. activated clotting time monitor
    H. ACT machine
Hemotene absorbable collagen hemostat
Hemovac
    H. Hydrocoat drain
    H. suction device
    H. suction tube

Henahan elevator
Hendel guided osteotome
Henderson
    H. bone chisel
    H. clamp approximator
    H. self-retaining retractor
Henderson-Haggard inhaler
Hendon venoclysis cannula
Hendren
    H. cardiovascular clamp
    H. cardiovascular forceps
    H. ductus clamp
    H. megaureter clamp
    H. pediatric forceps
    H. pediatric retractor blade
    H. ureteral clamp
Hendrickson
    H. bag
    H. lithotrite
    H. suprapubic drain
Henke
    H. punch forceps
    H. punch forceps tip
    H. tonsillar dissector
Henke-Stille conchotome
Henley
    H. carotid retractor
    H. dilator
    H. retractor blade
    H. subclavian artery clamp
    H. vascular clamp
Henner
    H. endaural elevator
    H. endaural retractor
    H. T-model endaural retractor
Henning
    H. cardiac dilator
    H. cast spreader
    H. instrument set
    H. mallet
    H. meniscal retractor
    H. plaster spreader
    H. system
Henning-Keinkel stomach probe
Henny laminectomy rongeur
Henrotin
    H. retractor
    H. vulsellum
    H. vulsellum forceps
    H. weighted vaginal speculum
Henry
    H. ciliary forceps
    H. instrument tray
    H. Schein excavator
    H. Schein filling instrument
Henschke
    H. afterloader
    H. colpostat
    H. seed applicator
Henschke-Mauch SNS lower limb prosthesis
Henson CFS 2000 perimeter
Henton
    H. suture needle

H. tonsillar needle
H. tonsillar suture hook
Hepacon
H. cannula
H. catheter
HEPA filter
Hepamed-coated Wiktor stent
heparin
h. arterial filter
h. lock
Heparinase test cartridge
heparin-bonded
h.-b. Bott-type tube
heparin-coated
h.-c. catheter
h.-c. guidewire
h.-c. Palmaz-Schatz stent
heparin-flushing needle
heparin-induced extracorporeal lipoprotein precipitation system
HepatAssist
H. bioartificial liver
H. bioartificial liver system
hepatic artery infusion pump
hepatofugal porto-systemic venous shunt
Heraeus
H. LaserSonics InfraGuide
H. LaserSonics laser
Herbert
H. Adams coarctation clamp
H. bone screw
H. knee prosthesis
H. scaphoid screw
H. sclerotomy knife
H. screw fixator
Herbert-Whipple bone screw
Herchenson esophageal cytology collector
Hercules
H. drop-adjusting table
H. plaster shears
H. power injector
H. table
Herculite XRV lab system
Herculon suture
Herczel
H. dissector
H. periosteal elevator
H. raspatory elevator
H. rib elevator
H. rib rasp
H. rib raspatory
Herff
H. clamp
H. clip
H. membrane-puncturing forceps
Herget biopsy forceps
Heritage hip system
Hermann bone-holding forceps
Herman-Taylor gastroscope
Hermes
H. Evolution tricompartmental knee system
H. total knee system

Hermetic
H. external ventricular drainage system
H. external ventricular and lumbar drainage systems
H. II drainage management system
hermetically-sealed pacemaker
Hermitex bandage
Hernandez-Ros bone staple
hernia
h. retractor
h. stapler
Herniamesh
H. surgical mesh
H. surgical plug
herniotome
Cooper h.
Heros chiropody sponge
Herrick
H. kidney clamp
H. kidney forceps
H. lacrimal plug
H. pedicle clamp
H. silicone lacrimal implant
Herring tube
Hersbury anterior chamber intraocular lens
Hersh
H. LASIK retreatment forceps
H. LASIK retreatment spatula
Hershey
H. left ventricular assist device
H. total artificial heart
Hertel
H. bougie urethrotome
H. exophthalmometer
H. kidney stone forceps
H. nephrostomy speculum
H. ophthalmometer
H. rigid dilator stone forceps
H. rigid kidney stone forceps
Hertzler
H. baby rib retractor
H. rib spreader
Hertzog
H. lens spatula
H. pliable probe
Herzenberg bolt
Herzfeld ear forceps
Herzmark fracture frame
Herz meniscal tendon forceps
Hess
H. capsular forceps
H. diplopia screen
H. iris forceps
H. lens scoop
H. lens spoon
H. nerve root retractor
H. serrefine
H. tonsil expressor
Hess-Barraquer iris forceps
Hessburg
H. corneal shield
H. eye shield
H. intraocular lens glide

H

Hessburg *(continued)*
 H. lacrimal needle
 H. lens-inserting forceps
 H. subpalpebral lavage system
 H. vacuum trephine
Hessburg-Barron vacuum trephine
HESSCO 300, 500 series
Hessel-Nystrom pin
Hesseltine
 H. umbilical cord clamp
 H. Umbili Clip
Hess-Gill iris forceps
Hess-Horwitz iris forceps
Hessing brace
Hess-Lee screen
heterograft
 bovine h.
 Hancock porcine h.
 h. implant
 h. prosthesis
heteroscope
Hetherington circular saw
Hetter pyramid tip
Hevesy polyp forceps
Hewitt mouthgag
Hewlett-Packard
 H.-P. 78720 A SDN monitor
 H.-P. biplane 5-MHz probe
 H.-P. Codemaster defribrillator
 H.-P. color flow imager
 H.-P. defibrillator
 H.-P. ear oximeter
 H.-P. Echo-Doppler machine
 H.-P. 5 MHz phased-array TEE
 system
 H.-P. omniplane 5-MHz probe
 H.-P. phased-array imaging system
 H.-P. scanner
 H.-P. 2500 Sonos ultrasound
 H.-P. Sonos 1000, 1500 ultrasound
 system
 H.-P. ultrasound unit
Hewson
 H. breakaway pin
 H. drill
 H. ligament drill guide
 H. ligature passer
 H. suture passer
Hewson-Richards reamer
hex
 h. bar
 h. implant
 h. socket wrench
hexagonal
 h. handle
 h. handle osteotome
 h. wrench
hexagon snare
hexapolar catheter
**Hexascan computerized dermatology
 handpiece**
Hexastat
Hexcel
 H. cast dressing

 H. total condylar knee system
 H. total condylar prosthesis
Hexcelite
 H. cast
 H. mesh
 H. sheet splint
Hex-Fix
 H.-F. Add-A-Clamp
 H.-F. monolateral external fixator
 H.-F. system
 H.-F. Universal swivel clamp
hexhead
 h. bolt
 h. pin
 h. screwdriver
HEX heat applicator
Hex-Lock abutment
Hexon illumination system
Hextend plasma volume expander
Heyer-Pudenz valve
Heyer-Robertson suprapubic drain
Heyer-Schulte
 H.-S. antisiphon device
 H.-S. brain retractor
 H.-S. breast implant
 H.-S. breast prosthesis
 H.-S. catheter
 H.-S. disposal bag
 H.-S. hydrocephalus shunt
 H.-S. Jackson-Pratt wound-drainage
 reservoir
 H.-S. lens implant
 H.-S. microscope
 H.-S. Pour-Safe exudate bag
 H.-S. PVC kit
 H.-S. Rayport muscle biopsy clamp
 H.-S. rhinoplasty implant
 H.-S. silicone kit
 H.-S. Small-Carrion sizing set
 H.-S. valve
 H.-S. wedge-suction reservoir
 H.-S. wound drain
Heyer-Schulte-Fischer ventricular cannula
Heyer-Schulte-Ommaya CSF reservoir
Heyer-Schulte-Pudenz cardiac catheter
**Heyer-Schulte-Spetzler lumbar peritoneal
 shunt**
Hey-Groves needle
Heyman
 H. nasal-cutting forceps
 H. nasal forceps
 H. nasal scissors
Heyman-Knight nasal dressing forceps
Heyman-Paparella angular scissors
Heyman-Simon
 H.-S. capsule
 H.-S. source
Heyner
 H. curette
 H. dilator
 H. double cannula
 H. double needle
 H. expressor
 H. forceps

Heyns abdominal decompression apparatus
Hey skull saw
Heywood-Smith
    H.-S. dressing forceps
    H.-S. gallbladder forceps
    H.-S. sponge-holding forceps
HF
    HF dialyzer
    HF infrared laser
H-file
    engine H.-f.
    Mity engine H.-f.
HGM
    HGM argon green laser
    HGM Endo-Otoprobe
    HGM intravitreal laser
    HGM ophthalmic laser
    HGM Spectrum K1 krypton yellow
      & green laser
HG Multilock hip prosthesis
HGP
    HGP II acetabular component
    HGP II acetabular cup
H-H
    H.-H. neonatal shunt
    H.-H. open-end alimentation catheter
    H.-H. Rickham cerebrospinal fluid
      reservoir
    H.-H. shunt introducer
Hi
    All-Purpose Boot H.
    H. Speed Pulse lavage
    H. Vac tubing
Hi5 Torq Flow catheter
Hibbs
    H. biting forceps
    H. bone chisel
    H. bone curette
    H. bone-cutting forceps
    H. bone gouge
    H. bone-holding forceps
    H. chisel elevator
    H. clamp
    H. costal elevator
    H. fracture appliance
    H. fracture frame
    H. hammer
    H. mallet
    H. mouthgag
    H. osteotome
    H. periosteal elevator
    H. scoop
    H. self-retaining laminectomy
      retractor
    H. spinal curette
    H. spinal fusion gouge
    H. spinal retractor blade
    H. sponge
Hibbs-Spratt spinal fusion curette
Hickman
    H. indwelling right atrial catheter
    H. line
    H. percutaneous introducer
    H. tunneled catheter

Hickman-Broviac catheter
Hicks lugged plate
HICOR system
Hidalgo catheter
hi-density foam
Hiebert
    H. esophageal suture spoon
    H. vascular dilator
Hieshima coaxial catheter
Higbee vaginal speculum
Higgins
    H. bag
    H. catheter
Higginson irrigation syringe
high
    h. beam fiberoptic headlight
    h. density polyethylene
    H. Flex D 700 S bubble
      oxygenator
    h. flux dialyzer
    H. Frequency Oscillatory ventilator
    H. Oxygen PRM resuscitator
high-air-loss bed
high-capacity
    h.-c. fluid warmer
    h.-c. silicone drain
high-compliance latex balloon
high-diameter dilator
high-energy
    h.-e. bent-beam linear accelerator
    h.-e. laser
high-fidelity micromanometric catheter
high-field
    h.-f. open MRI scanner
    h.-f. system
high-flow
    h.-f. catheter
    h.-f. coaxial cannula
    h.-f. regulator
high-force Sundt clip system
high-frequency
    h.-f. jet ventilator
    h.-f. miniature probe
    h.-f. miniprobe
    h.-f. oscillation ventilator
    h.-f. tweezer-type epilator
    h.-f. ultrasound biomicroscope
high-humidity
    h.-h. face mask
    h.-h. tracheostomy collar
    h.-h. tracheostomy mask
    h.-h. tracheostomy shield
high-impedance, low-threshold lead
high-Knight brace
Highlighter
    Esenbach H.
Highlight spectral indirect ophthalmoscope
high-muscular-resistance bed
high-pass filter
high-performance liquid chromatograph
high-pressure liquid chromatograph
high-purity germanium detector
high-resolution
    h.-r. brain SPECT system

H

high-resolution *(continued)*
    h.-r. linear array transducer
    h.-r. multileaf collimator
    h.-r. probe
    h.-r. real-time scanner
high-risk needle
high-sensitivity collimator
high-speed
    h.-s. dermabrader
    h.-s. diamond three-tiered depth cutting bur
    h.-s. diamond wheel bur
    h.-s. drill
    h.-s. electrical tissue morcellator
    h.-s. microdrill
    h.-s. rotation dynamic angioplasty catheter
    h.-s. tungsten carbide bur
    h.-s. two-grit bur
high-torque
    h.-t. bur
    h.-t. wire
High-Vision surgical telescope
high-voltage
    h.-v. electron microscope
    h.-v. transformer
high-volume evacuator
HIHA tendon implant
Hilal
    H. coil
    H. embolization apparatus
    H. microcoil
    H. modified headhunter catheter
hilar clamp
Hildebrandt uterine hemostatic forceps
Hildreth
    H. coagulator
    H. electrocautery
    H. electrode
    H. ocular cautery
    H. transilluminator
Hildyard nasal forceps
Hilgenreiner brace
Hilger facial nerve stimulator
Hilight Advantage System CT scanner
Hill
    H. Air-Drop HA90C table
    H. Air-Flex table
    H. nasal raspatory
    H. rectal retractor
Hill-Bosworth saw
Hill-Ferguson rectal retractor
Hillis
    H. eyelid retractor
    H. fetal stethoscope
    H. perforator
    H. refractor
Hi-Lo
    H.-L. Jet tracheal tube
HiLo
    H. BodyTable
    H. MultiPro table
    H. PowerTilt
HI-LOO Power lift

Hilsinger tonsillar knife
Hilton
    H. self-retaining infusion cannula
    H. sutureless infusion cannula
HIMAC system
Himalaya dressing forceps
Himmelstein
    H. pulmonary valvulotome
    H. sternal retractor
Hinderer
    H. cartilage forceps
    H. malar prosthesis
hindfoot orthosis
hinge
    h. articulator
    Camber axis h.
    Compass h.
    Dee elbow h.
    elbow h.
    implant h.
    h. joint
    Kinematic rotating h.
    Lacey rotating h.
    offset h.
    Rancho swivel h.
    Weser dental h.
hinged
    h. articulated fixator
    h. articulator
    h. cast
    h. constrained knee prosthesis
    h. great toe replacement prosthesis
    h. implant
    h. implant prosthesis
    h. Thomas splint
    h. total knee prosthesis
hinged-leaflet vascular prosthesis
hinge-knee prosthesis
hingeless heart valve prosthesis
Hingson-Edwards needle
Hingson-Ferguson needle
Hinkle-James rectal speculum
Hinz tongs
hip
    anthropometric total h.
    h. arthroplasty gouge
    Bio-Groove h.
    Biomet h.
    Corin total h.
    h. disarticulation prosthesis
    Gemini h.
    h. guidance orthosis
    Gustilo-Kyle total h.
    Howmedica PCA textured h.
    Leinbach head and neck total h.
    Link anatomical h.
    PCA total h.
    Precision Osteolock total h.
    h. skid
    h. spica cast
    h. spica dressing
HIPciser abduction splint
Hi-Per
    H.-P. cardiac device

H.-P. Flex exchange guidewire
H.-P. Flex exchange wire
hipGRIP pelvic positioning system
hip-knee-ankle orthosis
hip-knee orthosis
Hipokrat bimodular shoulder system
Hippel trephine
Hippocrates bandage
Hipp & Sohn dental scissors
hipRAP pelvic positioning system
Hircoe denture base material
HiRider motorized lift wheelchair
Hirji-Callandar grid
Hirsch
    H. hypophyseal punch
    H. hypophysis punch forceps
    H. mucosal clamp
Hirschberg electromagnet magnet
Hirschman
    H. anoscope
    H. anoscope rectal speculum
    H. hemorrhoidal forceps
    H. hooked cannula
    H. iris hook
    H. iris spatula
    H. jeweler's forceps
    H. lens forceps
    H. lens manipulator
    H. lens spatula
    H. nasoendoscope
    H. pile clamp
    H. proctoscope
    H. retractor
Hirschman-Martin proctoscope
Hirschowitz
    H. gastroduodenal fiberscope
    H. gastroscope
Hirschtick utility shoulder splint
Hirst
    H. obstetrical forceps
    H. placental forceps
    H. spore trap
Hirst-Emmet
    H.-E. obstetrical forceps
    H.-E. placental forceps
His
    H. bundle catheter
Hishida pine-needle sound
Hispeed CT scanner
Hi-Star midfield MRI system
Histoacryl glue
Histofreezer cryosurgical system
Hitachi
    H. 704, 717 analyzer
    H. 737, 747 autoanalyzer
    H. convex-convex biplane probe
    H. convex ultrasound probe
    H. CT, MR scanner
    H. EUB-515C ultrasound console
    H. EUB-405 imaging system
    H. fingertip ultrasound probe
    H. F-series fluorescence
      spectrophotometer
    H. H-series electron microscope
    H. linear ultrasound probe

H. Open MRI system
H. Open MRI System scanner
H. transrectal ultrasound probe
H. transvaginal ultrasound probe
H. UB 420 digital ultrasound
  system
H. ultrasound
H. U-series spectrophotometer
Hita-Rite stadiometer
hitch
    ankle h.
    girth h.
Hitchcock stereotactic immobilization
  frame
HiTec insufflator
Hi-Top
    H.-T. foot/ankle brace
    H.-T. shoe
Hi-Torque
    H.-T. Flex-T guidewire
    H.-T. Floppy exchange guidewire
    H.-T. Floppy guide catheter
    H.-T. Floppy II guidewire
    H.-T. Floppy intermediate guidewire
    H.-T. Floppy with Pro/Pel
    H.-T. Standard guidewire
Hitselberger-McElveen neural dissector
Hittenberger prosthesis
Hix-Fix fracture fixation system
Hixon-Oldfather prediction table
HK
    HK binder
    HK breast/torso garment
    HK pad
    HK sheet
HKAFO prosthesis
Hobbs
    H. dilatation balloon catheter
    H. needle
    H. polypectomy snare
    H. sheath brush
    H. stent set
    H. stone basket
hockey-stick
    h.-s. catheter
    h.-s. electrosurgical probe
Hockin lucite ovoid
Hodge
    H. obstetrical forceps
    H. pessary
Hodgen
    H. apparatus
    H. hip splint
    H. leg splint
Hodlick needle holder
Hodrocollator gel pack
hoe
    Hough h.
    Hough-Saunders stapes h.
    Joe's h.
    Nordent h.
    stapes h.
Hoefer GS 300 laser densitometer
Hoefflin suture passer
Hoek-Bowen cement removal system

H

Hoen
 H. alligator forceps
 H. bayonet forceps
 H. dressing forceps
 H. dural separator
 H. grasping forceps
 H. hemilaminectomy retractor
 H. hemostatic forceps
 H. intervertebral disk rongeur
 H. laminar gouge
 H. laminectomy rongeur
 H. laminectomy scissors
 H. nerve hook
 H. periosteal elevator
 H. periosteal raspatory
 H. pituitary rongeur
 H. scalp forceps
 H. scalp retractor
 H. skull plate
 H. tissue forceps
 H. ventricular cannula
 H. ventricular needle

Hoffer
 H. corneal marker
 H. forward-cutting knife cannula
 H. ridged intraocular lens
 H. ridged lens implant

Hoffmann
 H. apex fixation pin
 H. ear punch forceps
 H. ear rongeur
 H. external fixation device
 H. external fixation system
 H. external fixator
 H. eye implant
 H. II compact external fixation
  component
 H. ligament clamp
 H. mini-lengthening fixation device
 H. scleral fixation pick
 H. traction device
 H. transfixion pin

Hoffmann-Osher-Hopkins plaster knife
Hoffmann-Pollock forceps
Hoffmann-Vidal external fixation device
Hoffrel transesophageal probe
Hoff towel clamp
Hofmeister
 H. drainage bag
 H. endometrial biopsy curette

Hogness box
Hohmann
 H. bone lever
 H. clamp
 H. osteotome
 H. retractor

Hohmann-Aldinger bone lever
Hohn
 H. catheter
 H. vessel dilator

hoist
 Temco h.

Hoke
 H. lumbar brace/corset

 H. osteotome
 H. spoon

Hoke-Martin tractor
Hoke-Roberts spoon
Holcombe gastric tourniquet
Hold-and-Hold positioner
Holden uterine curette
holder
 A1-Askari needle h.
 Abbey needle h.
 Adson dural needle h.
 Aesculap needle h.
 Alabama-Green eye needle h.
 Alabama needle h.
 Allen well leg h.
 Alvarado surgical knee h.
 Anchor needle h.
 Andrews rigid chest support h.
 Anis-Barraquer needle h.
 Anis needle h.
 Anspach leg h.
 Arruga eye h.
 Arruga needle h.
 arthroscopic ankle h.
 arthroscopic leg h.
 Aslan needle h.
 Axhausen needle h.
 Azar needle h.
 baby Barraquer needle h.
 baby Crile needle h.
 baby Crile-Wood needle h.
 Bard leg bag h.
 Barraquer baby needle h.
 Barraquer curved h.
 Barraquer eye needle h.
 Barraquer-Troutman needle h.
 Baumgartner needle h.
 Baum-Metzenbaum sternal needle h.
 Baum tonsillar needle h.
 bayonet needle h.
 Bechert-Sinskey needle h.
 Belin needle h.
 Berry sternal needle h.
 Bethea sheet h.
 Bihrle dorsal clamp-T-C needle h.
 Birks Mark II micro cross-action h.
 Birks Mark II needle h.
 Björk-Shiley heart valve h.
 bladebreaker h.
 Blair-Brown needle h.
 Bodkin thread h.
 bone-graft h.
 Bookler swivel-ball laparoscopic
  instrument h.
 boomerang needle h.
 Bovie h.
 Boyce needle h.
 Boynton needle h.
 Bozeman-Finochietto needle h.
 Bozeman needle h.
 Bozeman-Wertheim needle h.
 Bumgardner dental h.
 Bunt forceps h.
 Capillary System slide h.
 Carb-Bite needle h.

cardiovascular needle h.
Castroviejo-Barraquer needle h.
Castroviejo blade h.
Castroviejo-Kalt eye needle h.
Castroviejo needle h.
Castroviejo razor h.
Catalano needle h.
catheter guide h.
catheter leg tube h.
catheter waist tube h.
Cath-Secure catheter h.
Cath-Secure Dual Tab h.
CBI stereotactic head h.
Charnley trochanter h.
Cherf leg h.
Circon leg h.
clamp h.
Clerf needle h.
Cohan needle h.
Colles needle h.
Collier needle h.
Collins leg h.
Comfit endotracheal tube h.
Converse needle h.
Cooley Vital microvascular
  needle h.
Corboy needle h.
Cottle needle h.
Craig headrest h.
Crile-Murray needle h.
Crile needle h.
Crile-Wood needle h.
Crile-Wood-Vital needle h.
Crockard suction tube h.
curved micro-needle h.
Dainer-Kaupp needle h.
Dale drainage bulb and g-tube h.
Dale Foley catheter legband h.
Dale gastrostomy tube h.
Dale nasal dressing h.
Dale secondary wound dressing
  and h.
Dale tapeless wound dressing h.
Dale tracheostomy tube h.
Dean knife h.
DeBakey Vital needle h.
Dees h.
delicate needle h.
DeMartel-Wolfson clamp h.
Derf eye needle h.
Derf Vital needle h.
Derlacki ossicle h.
DeRoyal catheter tube h.
diamond grip needle h.
Diamond-Jaw needle h.
Donaghy angled suture needle h.
Doyen needle h.
Drummond hook h.
Eber h.
Eiselsberg-Mathieu needle h.
Elliot femoral condyle h.
Ellis needle h.
Endo-Assist disposable needle h.
Endo-Assist endoscopic needle h.
Eriksson-Paparella h.

Ermold needle h.
E-series needle h.
eye needle h.
E-Z hold adhesive/stretchable strap
  catheter tube h.
Ferguson bone h.
Ferris Smith needle h.
Finochietto needle h.
foot h.
French-eye Vital needle h.
French needle h.
Furacin gauze h.
Gambro dialyzer h.
Gardner needle h.
Germain needle h.
GHM KLE II x-ray film h.
Giannini needle h.
Gifford needle h.
Gillies needle h.
Gillquist-Oretorp-Stille needle h.
goniotomy needle h.
GraftAssist vein and graft h.
Grant needle h.
Greenberg instrument h.
Green eye needle h.
Grieshaber needle h.
Hagedorn needle h.
Hagfer needle h.
Halsey Vital needle h.
Halsey-Webster needle h.
Hampton needle h.
Hannover needle h.
head h.
Heaney Vital needle h.
Hegar-Baumgartner needle h.
Hegar-Mayo-Seeley needle h.
Hegar needle h.
Hegar-Olsen needle h.
Hodlick needle h.
hook h.
Hosel needle h.
House-Urban temporal bone h.
Huang vein h.
Hufnagel-Ryder needle h.
Hyde needle h.
Ilg microneedle h.
Ilg needle h.
instrument h.
intracardiac needle h.
I-tech cannula h.
I-tech needle h.
Ivy needle h.
Jacobson spring-handled needle h.
Jacobson-Vital needle h.
Jaffe needle h.
Jako laryngeal needle h.
Jameson needle h.
Jannetta bayonet needle h.
Jannetta bayonet-shaped needle h.
Jannetta needle h.
Jarcho tenaculum h.
Jarit forceps h.
Jarit microsurgical needle h.
Jarit sternal needle h.
Jarit wire h.

H

holder *(continued)*
Johnson prostatic needle h.
Jones IMA needle h.
Jordan-Caparosa h.
Juers-Derlacki Universal head h.
Julian needle h.
Kalman needle h.
Kalt-Arruga needle h.
Kalt eye needle h.
Kalt-Vital needle h.
Keeler-Catford micro jaws needle h.
Kilner needle h.
Knolle needle h.
Langenbeck needle h.
Lapides h.
laryngoscope chest support h.
laser Heaney needle h.
laser Julian needle h.
leg h.
Lenny Johnson surgical-assist
  knee h.
Leonard Arms instrument h.
Lewy chest h.
Lewy laryngoscope h.
Lichtenberg needle h.
limb h.
Lindley needle h.
lion jaw bone h.
Lundia dialyzer h.
Malis needle h.
Margraf beam aligning film h.
Marquette 3-channel laser h.
Masing needle h.
Mason leg h.
Masson-Luethy needle h.
Masson-Mayo-Hegar needle h.
Masson needle h.
Masson-Vital needle h.
mat h.
Mathieu needle h.
Mathieu-Olsen needle h.
Mathieu-Stille needle h.
Mayo-Hegar curved-jaw needle h.
Mayo needle h.
McAllister needle h.
McIntyre fish-hook needle h.
McPherson microsurgery eye
  needle h.
Metzenbaum needle h.
MGH needle h.
Micra needle h.
microneedle h.
microstaple h.
microsurgical needle h.
microvascular needle h.
Millin boomerang needle h.
Mills microvascular needle h.
mirror h.
Murray h.
needle h.
Neivert needle h.
Neo-Fit neonatal endotracheal
  tube h.
nerve h.

Neumann razor blade fragment h.
neurosurgical head h.
neurosurgical needle h.
New Orleans needle h.
Octopus h.
O'Gawa needle h.
Okmian microneedle h.
Olsen-Hegar needle h.
Olympic needle h.
Osher needle h.
OSI arthroscopic well-leg leg h.
Paparella monkey-head h.
Paton eye needle h.
Pilling needle h.
pin h.
Pittman needle h.
Portmann speculum h.
Posilok instrument h.
Potts-Smith needle h.
press plate needle h.
prostatic needle h.
prosthetic valve h.
Punctur-Guard Revolution safety
  needle h.
Quinn h.
Ravich needle h.
razor blade h.
Reill needle h.
Reverdin h.
Rhoton bayonet needle h.
Rhoton microneedle h.
Rica forceps h.
Rinn XCP film h.
Rochester needle h.
rod h.
Rogers needle h.
Rubio needle h.
Ryder needle h.
Sarot needle h.
Sarot-Vital needle h.
Scanlan microneedle h.
Schaefer sponge h.
Schlein shoulder h.
Shea speculum h.
Sheehan-Gillies needle h.
sheet h.
Silber microneedle h.
Sims sponge h.
Sinskey needle h.
speculum h.
Spetzler needle h.
S-P needle h.
spring-handled needle h.
spring needle h.
Stangel modified Barraquer
  microsurgical needle h.
Stanzel needle h.
Steinmann h.
Stenstrom nerve h.
Stephenson needle h.
sterile forceps h.
sternal needle h.
Stevens needle h.
Stevenson needle h.

Stille-French cardiovascular
  needle h.
Storz head h.
Storz needle h.
Stratte needle h.
Sugita head h.
Surcan knee h.
Surcan leg h.
SurgAssist surgical leg h.
suture h.
Swan eye needle h.
Swiss blade h.
swivel joint suture h.
tapered-spring needle h.
Taylor catheter h.
T-C needle h.
temporal bone h.
tenaculum h.
Tennant eye needle h.
Tennant thumb-ring needle h.
Texas Scottish Rite Hospital
  hook h.
The Dale tracheostomy tube h.
Thomas Long-Term endotracheal
  tube h.
three-point head h.
Tilderquist needle h.
Toennis needle h.
Tomac vest-style h.
Torres needle h.
Trake-Fit tracheal tube h.
trochanter h.
Troutman-Barraquer needle h.
Troutman needle h.
Tru-Cut biopsy needle h.
Turchik instrument h.
Turner-Warwick needle h.
Twisk needle h.
Universal head h.
Universal speculum h.
Vacutainer h.
valve h.
vascular needle h.
VBH head h.
Vickers needle h.
Vital-Baumgartner needle h.
Vital-Castroviejo eye needle h.
Vital-Cooley French-eye needle h.
Vital-Cooley general tissue h.
Vital-Cooley intracardiac needle h.
Vital-Cooley microvascular needle h.
Vital-Cooley neurosurgical needle h.
Vital-Crile-Wood needle h.
Vital-DeBakey cardiovascular
  needle h.
Vital-Derf eye needle h.
Vital-Finochietto needle h.
Vital French-eye needle h.
Vital-Halsey eye-needle h.
Vital-Heaney needle h.
Vital-Jacobson spring-handled
  needle h.
Vital-Julian needle h.
Vital-Kalt eye needle h.
Vital-Masson needle h.

Vital-Mayo-Hegar needle h.
Vital microsurgery needle h.
Vital microvascular needle h.
Vital-Mills vascular needle h.
Vital-Neivert needle h.
Vital neurosurgical needle h.
Vital-New Orleans needle h.
Vital-Olsen-Hegar needle h.
Vital-Rochester needle h.
Vital-Ryder needle h.
Vital-Sarot needle h.
Vital-Stratte needle h.
Vital-Wangensteen needle h.
Vital-Webster needle h.
V. Mueller laser Rhoton
  microneedle h.
V. Mueller-Vital laser Heaney
  needle h.
V. Mueller-Vital laser Julian
  needle h.
Vogel-Bale-Hohner head h.
Wangensteen needle h.
Wangensteen-Vital needle h.
washer h.
Watanabe pin h.
Watson heart value h.
Web needle h.
Webster-Halsey needle h.
Webster-Kleinert needle h.
Webster needle h.
Webster-Vital needle h.
Wehbe arm h.
Weisenbach sterile forceps h.
well-leg h.
Wertheim needle h.
Williams Uni-Quad leg h.
Wister forceps h.
Wolf-Castroviejo needle h.
Worcester instrument h.
Yasargil bayonet needle h.
Yasargil microneedle h.
Young boomerang needle h.
Young-Hryntschak boomerang
  needle h.
Young-Millin boomerang needle h.
Young needle h.
Zollinger leg h.
Zweifel needle h.

holding
  h. clip
  h. forceps
  h. mitt

Holinger
  H. anterior commissure laryngoscope
  H. applicator
  H. bronchoscopic magnet
  H. bronchoscopic telescope
  H. cannula
  H. curved scissors
  H. endoscopic magnet
  H. hook-on folding laryngoscope
  H. hourglass anterior commissure
    laryngoscope
  H. infant bougie
  H. infant bronchoscope

Holinger *(continued)*
    H. infant esophageal speculum
    H. infant esophagoscope
    H. infant laryngoscope
    H. laryngeal dissector
    H. modified Jackson laryngoscope
    H. needle
    H. open-end aspirating tube
    H. slotted laryngoscope
    H. specimen forceps
    H. ventilating fiberoptic
      bronchoscope
Holinger-Benjamin laser diverticuloscope
Holinger-Garfield laryngoscope
Holinger-Hurst bougie
Holinger-Jackson bronchoscope
Holladay posterior capsular polisher
Hollander clog
Hollenback carver
HolliGard seal closed stoma pouch
Hollister
    H. bridge suture bolster
    H. circumcision device
    H. clamp
    H. collecting device
    H. colostomy bag
    H. colostomy irrigator
    H. disposable Convex insert
    H. drainage bag
    H. external catheter
    H. First Choice pouch
    H. Hot/Ice knee blanket
    H. irrigator drain
    H. laryngoscope
    H. medial adhesive bandage
    H. replacement filters pouch cover
    H. self-adhesive catheter
    H. urostomy bag
    H. wound exudate absorber
Holllister Incorporated
hollow
    h. cannula
    h. chisel
    h. cutter
    h. fiber capillary dialyzer
    h. filter dialyzer (HF dialyzer)
    h. lucite pessary
    h. mill
    h. needle
    h. needle guide
    h. Silastic disk heart valve
    h. sphere prosthesis
    h. visceral tonometer
hollow-object forceps
hollow-sphere orbital implant
Holman
    H. flushing apparatus
    H. lung retractor
Holman-Mathieu salpingography cannula
Holmes
    H. cartilage gouge
    H. chisel
    H. fixation forceps

    H. nasopharyngoscope
    H. scissors
holmium
    h. laser
    h. laser lithotriptor
    h. yttrium aluminum garnet laser
      (Ho:YAG laser, holmium yttrium
      aluminum garnet laser)
holmium:YAG laser
holmium:yttrium-argon-garnet laser
Holofax
    H. Oxford retroillumination cataract
      camera
Hologic
    H. 1000 (2000) QDR densitometer
    H. 1000 QDR dual-energy
      absorptiometer
    H. QDR 1000W dual-energy x-ray
      absorptiometry scanner
    H. 2000 scanner
Holscher nerve retractor
Holter
    H. connector
    H. diary
    H. distal atrial catheter
    H. distal catheter passer
    H. distal peritoneal catheter
    H. elliptical valve
    H. external drainage system
    H. high-pressure valve
    H. hydrocephalus shunt system
    H. in-line shunt filter
    H. introducer
    H. lumboperitoneal catheter
    H. medium-pressure valve
    H. mini-elliptical valve
    H. monitor
    H. pump
    H. pump clamp
    H. shunt
    H. straight valve
    H. traction
    H. tube
    H. ventricular catheter
    H. ventriculostomy reservoir
Holter-Hausner
    H.-H. catheter
    H.-H. valve
Holter-Rickham ventriculostomy reservoir
Holter-Salmon-Rickham ventriculostomy
reservoir
Holter-Selker ventriculostomy reservoir
Holth
    H. corneoscleral punch
    H. cystitome
    H. punch forceps
    H. scleral punch
    H. sclerectomy punch
Holth-Rubin punch
Holt self-retaining catheter
Holtz endometrial curette
Holzbach
    H. abdominal retractor
    H. hysterectomy forceps

Holzheimer
    H. mastoid retractor
    H. skin retractor
Homan retractor
HomeKair
    H. bed
    H. D.M.S.
Homepump infusion system
Homer localizaton needle
Homerlok needle
Homestretch lumbar traction
HomeTrac
home uterine activity monitor
Homiak radium colpostat
HomMed
    H. monitoring system
Homochron monitor
homogeneous screen
homogenizer
    Polytron PT 3000 h.
    Potter-Elvehjem h.
    Wheaton tissue h.
homograft
    Cryolife h.
    denatured h.
    h. implant
    h. implant material
    h. prosthesis
homonuclear spin system
Honan
    H. balloon
    H. cuff
    H. manometer
    H. sphygmometer
Honeywell recorder
Hood
    H. dissector
    H. electrodermatome
    H. Laboratories Eccovision acoustic
      rhinometer
    H. manual dermatome
    H. stoma stent
    H. truss
hood
    laminar flow h.
    Oxyhood oxygen h.
    Oxypod oxygen h.
    surgical h.
hooded transilluminator
Hood-Graves vaginal speculum
Hood-Westaby T-Y stent
Hook
    H. hemi-harness shoulder
      immobilizer
hook (*See also* buttonhook)
    Abramson h.
    Adson angular h.
    Adson blunt dissecting h.
    Adson brain h.
    Adson dissecting h.
    Adson dural h.
    Allport h.
    Amenabar discission h.
    anchor h.

Anderson suture pusher and
  double h.
Andre h.
angled discission h.
h. approximator
Arruga extraction h.
Ashbell h.
attic h.
Aufranc h.
Azar lens h.
ball nerve h.
ball-tip nerve h.
Bane h.
Barr crypt h.
Barr rectal fistular h.
Barton double h.
Bellucci h.
Berens scleral h.
Bethune nerve h.
biangled h.
bifid h.
Billeau ear h.
Birks Mark II h.
Blair palate h.
h. blocker
blunt dissecting h.
blunt iris h.
blunt nerve h.
boat h.
Bobechko sliding barrel h.
Boettcher tonsillar h.
bone h.
Bonn iris h.
Bonn microiris h.
Bose tracheostomy h.
Boyes-Goodfellow h.
Bozeman h.
Braun decapitation h.
Braun obstetrical h.
Brimfield cannulated grasping h.
Brown h.
Bryant mitral h.
Buck h.
Burch h.
button h.
buttressed h.
canted finger h.
Carroll bone h.
Carroll skin h.
Caspar h.
Catalano muscle h.
caudal h.
cautery h.
C-D h.
Chavasse squint h.
Chavasse strabismus h.
Chernov tracheostomy h.
Clayman iris h.
cleft palate sharp h.
closed Cotrel-Dubousset h.
Cloward cautery h.
Cloward dural h.
coarctation h.
cold knife h.
Collier-Martin h.

hook (*continued*)
  Colver examining h.
  Colver retractor h.
  compression h.
  Converse hinged skin h.
  corkscrew dural h.
  corneal h.
  Cotrel-Dubousset closed h.
  Cottle double h.
  Cottle-Joseph h.
  Cottle nasal h.
  Cottle skin h.
  cranial Jacobs h.
  Crawford h.
  Crile nerve h.
  crural h.
  crypt h.
  Culler rectus muscle h.
  Cushing dural h.
  Cushing gasserian ganglion h.
  Cushing nerve h.
  cystic h.
  Daily fixation h.
  Dandy nerve h.
  Davis h.
  Day ear h.
  destructive obstetrical h.
  Dingman zygomatic h.
  discission h.
  dissecting h.
  distraction h.
  h. distractor
  Dohlman incus h.
  double h.
  double-pronged Cottle h.
  double-pronged Fomon h.
  double-tenaculum h.
  down-angle h.
  downsized circular laminar h.
  Doyen rib h.
  Drews-Sato suture-pickup h.
  drop-entry (closed body) h.
  Drummond h.
  Dudley rectal h.
  Dudley tenaculum h.
  dural h.
  ear h.
  Edwards-Levine h.
  Edwards rectal h.
  Effler-Groves h.
  Emmet tenaculum h.
  h. expressor
  expressor h.
  extraction h.
  Feaster lens h.
  fenestration h.
  Ferszt dissecting h.
  fibroid h.
  finger h.
  Fink oblique muscle h.
  Fink-Scobie h.
  Finsen tracheal h.
  Finsen wound h.
  Fisch dural h.

  fistula h.
  fixation twist h.
  flat tenotomy h.
  Fomon nasal h.
  footplate h.
  h. forceps
  Frazier cordotomy h.
  Frazier dural h.
  Frazier nerve h.
  Frazier skin h.
  Freer skin h.
  Fresnel manipulating h.
  Fukasaku pupil snapper h.
  Gam-Mer nerve h.
  Gass muscle h.
  Gass retinal detachment h.
  Gillies bone h.
  Gillies-Converse skin h.
  Gillies-Dingman h.
  Gillies dural h.
  Gillies nasal h.
  Gillies skin h.
  Gillies zygoma h.
  Gillies zygomatic h.
  goiter h.
  Goldman Universal nerve h.
  Goodhill h.
  Graefe iris h.
  Graefe strabismus h.
  Graether mushroom h.
  Graham blunt h.
  Graham dural h.
  Graham muscle h.
  Graham nerve h.
  Green muscle h.
  Green strabismus h.
  Gross ear h.
  Guthrie eye-fixation h.
  Guthrie iris h.
  Guthrie skin h.
  Gwathmey h.
  Gynex iris h.
  Hall modified Moe h.
  Hamilton-Forewater amniotomy h.
  Hardesty tendon h.
  Hardesty tenotomy h.
  Harrington pedicle h.
  Harris-Sinskey microlens h.
  Haven skin graft h.
  Hebra h.
  Helvestoon h.
  Henton tonsillar suture h.
  Hirschman iris h.
  Hoen nerve h.
  h. holder
  Hosmer Dorrance h.
  House crural h.
  House incus h.
  House oval-window h.
  House plate h.
  House strut h.
  House tragus h.
  Hunkeler ball-point h.
  h. impactor
  instant skin h.

intermediate C-D h.
intracapsular lens expressor h.
intraocular h.
iris h.
irrigating iris h.
Isola spinal implant system h.
IUD remover h.
Jackson tracheal h.
Jacobs cranial h.
Jacobson blunt h.
Jaeger strabismus h.
Jaffe iris h.
Jaffe lens-manipulating h.
Jaffe-Maltzman h.
Jaffe microlens h.
Jako fine ball-tip h.
Jako-Kleinsasser ball-tip h.
Jameson muscle h.
Jameson strabismus h.
Jannetta h.
Jardine h.
Jarit bone h.
Jarit palate h.
jaw h.
Johnson skin h.
Jordan h.
Joseph nasal h.
Joseph single-prong h.
Joseph skin h.
Joseph tenaculum h.
Juers h.
Katena boat h.
Keene compression h.
Kelly uterine tenaculum h.
Kelman irrigation h.
Kelman manipulator h.
Kennerdell-Maroon h.
Kennerdell-Maroon-Jameson h.
Kennerdell muscle h.
Kennerdell nerve h.
Kilner goiter h.
Kilner skin h.
Kimball nephrostomy h.
Kincaid right-angle h.
Kirby double-fixation muscle h.
Klapp tendon h.
Kleinert-Kutz skin h.
Kleinsasser h.
Klemme dural h.
Klintskog amniotomy h.
Knapp iris h.
h. knife
Kratz iris push-pull h.
Krayenbuehl dural h.
Krayenbuehl nerve h.
Krayenbuehl vessel h.
Kuglen manipulating iris h.
Küntscher nail-extracting h.
Lahey Clinic dural h.
Lambotte bone h.
laminar C-D h.
Lange fistular h.
Lange plastic surgery h.
Laqua black line retinal h.
large ball nerve h.

Leader iris h.
Leader vas h.
Leatherman alar h.
Leatherman compression h.
Leinbach olecranon h.
lens h.
Levy-Kuglen iris h.
Lewicky microlens h.
Lillie attic h.
Lillie ear h.
Linton vein h.
Loughnane prostatic h.
Lucae h.
lyre-shaped finger h.
Madden sympathectomy h.
Magielski h.
Maidera-Stern suture h.
Malgaigne patellar h.
Malis nerve h.
h. manipulator
Manson double-ended strabismus h.
Marino rotatable transsphenoidal
  right-angle h.
Martin rectal h.
Maumenee iris h.
Mayo fibroid h.
McIntyre irrigating iris h.
McMahon nephrostomy h.
McReynolds lid-retracting h.
Meyerding skin h.
microball h.
microiris h.
Microlens h.
micronerve h.
microscopic h.
microsurgical ear h.
microvessel h.
Millard thimble h.
mitral h.
Miya h.
Moe alar h.
Morgenstein h.
Morrison skin h.
Moss h.
Muelly h.
multispan fracture h.
Murphy ball-end h.
muscle h.
nasal polyp h.
Neivert nasal polyp h.
nerve pull h.
neutral h.
Newell nucleus h.
Newhart h.
New tracheostomy h.
New tracheotomy h.
Nova jaw h.
Nugent iris h.
oblique muscle h.
O'Brien rib h.
obstetrical decapitating h.
Ochsner h.
O'Connor flat tenotomy h.
O'Connor muscle h.
Oesch h.

H

hook *(continued)*
 open C-D h.
 ophthalmic h.
 Osher irrigating implant h.
 oval-window h.
 Pajot decapitating h.
 palate h.
 Paul tendon h.
 PCL-oriented placement marking h.
 pear-shaped nerve h.
 pediatric C-D h.
 pediatric TSRH h.
 pedicle h.
 pedicle C-D h.
 Penn swivel h.
 Pickrell h.
 plain ear h.
 Praeger iris h.
 Pratt crypt h.
 Pratt cystic h.
 Pratt rectal h.
 Pucci-Seed h.
 h. pusher
 Rainin iris h.
 Rainin lens h.
 Ramsbotham decapitating h.
 Rappazzo iris h.
 rectal h.
 retinal detachment h.
 h. retractor
 retractor h.
 Rhoton nerve h.
 ribbed h.
 Rica cerumen h.
 Richards bone h.
 right-angle h.
 Rogozinski h.
 Rolf muscle h.
 Rollet strabismus h.
 Rosser crypt h.
 h. rotary scissors
 rotatable transsphenoidal right-
   angle h.
 Russian four-pronged fixation h.
 Sachs dural h.
 Sadler bone h.
 Saunders-Paparella stapes h.
 Scanlan micronerve h.
 Scanlan microvessel h.
 Scheer h.
 Schnitman skin h.
 Schuknecht stapes h.
 Schwartz cervical tenaculum h.
 scleral h.
 scleral twist fixation h.
 Scobee oblique muscle h.
 Scoville blunt h.
 Scoville curved nerve h.
 Scoville dural h.
 Scoville retractor h.
 Searcy fixation h.
 Selby II h.
 Selverstone cordotomy h.
 Shambaugh endaural h.

 Shambaugh fistula h.
 Shambaugh microscopic h.
 sharp h.
 Sharpley h.
 Shea fenestration h.
 Shea fistular h.
 Shea oblique h.
 Shea stapes h.
 Sheets iris h.
 Shepard reversed iris h.
 side-opening laminar h.
 Simon fistula h.
 single h.
 Sinskey iris h.
 Sinskey lens-manipulating h.
 Sinskey microlens h.
 Sisson spring h.
 skin h.
 sliding barrel h.
 Sluder sphenoidal h.
 Smellie obstetrical h.
 SMIC cerumen h.
 Smith expressor h.
 Smith lid-retracting h.
 Smithwick ganglion h.
 Smithwick nerve h.
 Smithwick sympathectomy h.
 spatula h.
 h. spatula
 Speare dural h.
 Speer suture h.
 split-finger h.
 spring h.
 square-ended h.
 squint h.
 Stallard scleral h.
 Stamler side-port fixation h.
 stapes h.
 Stevens muscle h.
 Stevens tenotomy h.
 Stewart crypt h.
 Stewart rectal h.
 Stille coarctation h.
 St. Martin-Franceschetti cataract h.
 Storz iris h.
 Storz twist h.
 strabismus h.
 straight nerve h.
 Strandell-Stille tendon h.
 Strully dural twist h.
 strut bar h.
 Suraci elevator h.
 suture pickup h.
 sympathectomy h.
 Tauber ligature h.
 tenaculum h.
 tendon h.
 Tennant anchor lens-insertion h.
 Tennant iris h.
 tenotomy h.
 Texas Scottish Rite Hospital trial h.
 Toennis dural h.
 Tomas iris h.
 Tomas suture h.
 tonsillar h.

top-entry (open body) h.
Torchia-Kuglen h.
Torchia lens h.
tracheal h.
tracheostomy h.
tracheotomy h.
tragus House h.
triple h.
TSRH buttressed laminar h.
TSRH circular laminar h.
TSRH pedicle h.
tubal h.
twist fixation h.
two-pronged dural h.
Tyrrell iris h.
Tyrrell skin h.
Tyrrell tympanic membrane h.
UCLA CAPP TD h.
University of Kansas h.
up-angle h.
vas h.
Visitec angled lens h.
Visitec corneal suture
  manipulating h.
Visitec double iris h.
Visitec straight lens h.
V. Mueller blunt h.
Volkmann bone h.
Volkmann vas h.
von Graefe muscle h.
von Graefe strabismus h.
von Szulec h.
Wagener h.
Walsh h.
Weary nerve h.
Welch Allyn h.
Wiener corneal h.
Wiener scleral h.
Wiener suture h.
Wilder foreign body h.
Wilder lens h.
Y-h.
Yankauer h.
Yasargil spring h.
Zaufel-Jansen ear h.
Zielke bifid h.
Zoellner h.
zygoma h.
Zylik-Joseph h.

hooked
  h. catheter
  h. intramedullary nail
  h. knife
  h. medullary nail
  h. needle
hook-end intramedullary pin
hook-on
  h.-o. bronchoscope
  h.-o. folding laryngoscope
hook-rod
  Cotrel-Dubousset h.-r.
  Isola h.-r.
  TSRH h.-r.
**hook-to-screw L4-S1 compression
  construct**

hook-type
  h.-t. dermal curette
  h.-t. eye implant
hookwire needle
Hooper pediatric scissors
Hoopes corneal marker
Hope
  H. processor
  H. resuscitation bag
  H. resuscitator
Hopener clamp
Hopkins
  H. angle-view 30-degree optical
    system
  H. aortic forceps
  H. aortic occlusion clamp
  H. arthroscope
  H. dilator
  H. direct-vision telescope
  H. forward-oblique telescope
  H. Hospital periosteal raspatory
  H. hysterectomy clamp
  H. II optical system
  H. II rod lens
  H. lateral telescope
  H. nasal endoscopy telescope
  H. pediatric telescope
  H. Percuflex drainage catheter
  H. plaster knife
  H. retrospective telescope
  H. rigid telescope
  H. rod
  H. rod lens system
  H. rod lens telescope
  H. sigmoidoscope
  H. straight-view optical system
  H. tympanoscope
Hopkins-Cushing periosteal elevator
Hopp
  H. anterior commissure laryngoscope
    blade
  H. laryngoscope
Hopp-Morrison laryngoscope
Horgan
  H. center blade
  H. retractor
Horgan-Coryllos-Moure rib shears
Horgan-Wells rib shears
Horico
  H. diamond instrument
  H. disk
Horizon
  H. AutoAdjust CPAP system
  H. nasal CPAP system
  H. surgical ligating and marking
    clip
horizontal
  h. drain attachment device
  h. flexible bar retractor
  h. pull headgear
  h. ring curette
  h. tube attachment device
Horn endo-otoprobe laser
horopter
  Vieth-Mueller h.

H

horseshoe
   h. headrest
   h. heel pad
   h. magnet
   h. tourniquet
horseshoe-shaped pad
Horsley
   H. bone cutter
   H. bone-cutting forceps
   H. bone wax
   H. cranial bone rongeur
   H. dural knife
   H. dural separator
   H. elevator
   H. guard
   H. spine cutter
   H. suture
   H. trephine
Horsley-Clarke
   H.-C. stereotactic apparatus
   H.-C. stereotactic frame
Horsley-Stille
   H.-S. bone-cutting forceps
   H.-S. rib shears forceps
hose
   Juzo h.
   TED h.
   thromboembolic disease (TED) h.
Hosel
   H. needle holder
   H. retractor
Hosemann
   H. choledochus forceps
   H. choledochus knife
Hosford
   H. double-ended lacrimal dilator
   H. foreign body spud
   H. meibomian gland expressor
Hosford-Hicks
   H.-H. needle
   H.-H. transfer forceps
hosiery
   Spa Champion PowerSox for Men gradient pressure therapy h.
   Spa Ready-To-Wear gradient pressure therapy h.
   Spa SoftBasics gradient pressure therapy h.
   Spa UltraSilk Sheers gradient pressure therapy h.
Hoskins
   H. beaked Colibri forceps
   H. fine straight forceps
   H. fixation forceps
   H. microstraight forceps
   H. miniaturized micro straight forceps
   H. nylon suture laser lens
   H. razor fragment blade
   H. straight microiris forceps
   H. suture forceps
Hoskins-Barkan goniotomy infant lens
Hoskins-Castroviejo corneal scissors
Hoskins-Dallas intraocular lens-inserting forceps

Hoskins-Drake implant
Hoskins-Luntz forceps
Hoskins-Skeleton
   H.-S. fine forceps
   H.-S. grooved broad-tipped forceps
Hoskins-Westcott tenotomy scissors
Hosmer
   H. above-knee rotator
   H. Dorrance hook
   H. single-axis locking knee
   H. voluntary control (VC4) four-bar knee orthosis
   H. WALK prosthesis
   H. weight-activated locking knee
   H. weight-activated locking knee prosthesis
Hosmer-Dorrance voluntary control four-bar knee mechanism
Hospal Biospal filter
Hospidex microtiter plate
hospital
   h. bed
   Texas Scottish Rite H.
Hossli suction tube
host tissue forceps
hot
   h. biopsy forceps
   h. cathode x-ray tube
   h. flexible forceps
   h. knife
   h. moist pack
   h. pad
   h. salt sterilizer
   H. Sampler disposable hot biopsy forceps
   h. water bottle
   h. wet pack
Hotchkiss ear suction tube
Hot/Ice
   H. cold therapy cooler
   H. System III
   H. System III knee blanket
HOTLINE
   H. blood and fluid warmer
   H. fluid-warming device
Hotsy
   H. high-temperature cautery
Hottentot apron
hot-tip laser
hot-tipped catheter
hot-water circulating suit
hot-wire
   h.-w. anemometer
   h.-w. pneumotachometer
   h.-w. respirometer
Hotz ear probe
Hough
   H. anterior crurotomy nipper
   H. bed
   H. chisel
   H. crurotomy saw
   H. curette
   H. drape
   H. drum scraper
   H. fascial knife

H. gouge
H. hoe
H. incision knife
H. middle ear instrument
H. oval-window excavator
H. scissors
H. spatula
H. spatula elevator
H. stapedectomy footplate pick
H. stapedial footplate auger
H. Teflon cutter
H. whirlybird
H. whirlybird excavator
H. whirlybird knife
Hough-Boucheron ear speculum
Hough-Cadogan
    H.-C. footpedal suction control
    H.-C. suction tube
Hough-Derlacki mobilizer
Hough-Powell digitizer
Hough-Rosen knife
Hough-Saunders
    H.-S. excavator
    H.-S. stapes hoe
Houghton rongeur
Hough-Wullstein
    H.-W. bur saw
    H.-W. crurotomy saw bur
Hounsfield unit
24-hour
    24-h. ambulatory gastric pH monitor
    24-h. esophageal pH probe
hourglass anterior commissure
  laryngoscope
hour-glass dressing
Hourin tonsillar needle
House
    H. adapter
    H. alligator crimper forceps
    H. alligator grasping forceps
    H. alligator scissors
    H. alligator strut forceps
    H. bur
    H. calipers strut
    H. chisel
    H. crural hook
    H. cup forceps
    H. detachable blade
    H. dissector
    H. ear curette
    H. ear elevator
    H. ear forceps
    H. ear knife
    H. ear separator
    H. endaural elevator
    H. endolymphatic shunt
    H. endolymphatic shunt tube
    H. endolymphatic shunt tube
      introducer
    H. excavator
    H. Gelfoam press
    H. Gelfoam pressure forceps
    H. grading system
    H. grasping forceps
    H. hand-held double-end retractor

H. implant
H. incudostapedial joint knife
H. incus hook
H. knife blade
H. lacrimal dilator
H. lancet knife
H. malleus nipper
H. measuring rod
H. middle ear instrument
H. middle ear mirror
H. miniature forceps
H. myringoplasty knife
H. myringotomy knife
H. myringotomy knife handle
H. neurovascular clip
H. obtuse pick
H. ophthalmic blade
H. oval-cup forceps
H. oval-window hook
H. oval-window pick
H. piston
H. piston prosthesis
H. piston wire
H. plate hook
H. pressure forceps
H. and Pulec otic-periotic shunt
H. round knife
H. sickle knife
H. stapes curette
H. stapes elevator
H. stapes needle
H. stapes speculum
H. strut calipers
H. strut forceps
H. strut guide
H. strut hook
H. strut pick
H. sucker irrigator
H. suction tube
H. tantalum prosthesis
H. tapping hammer
H. Teflon-coated elevator
H. Teflon cutting block
H. tragus hook
H. T-tube irrigator
H. tympanoplasty curette
H. tympanoplasty knife
H. wire guide
H. wire loop
H. wire stapes prosthesis
House-Barbara
    H.-B. pick
    H.-B. shattering needle
House-Baron suction tube
House-Bellucci alligator scissors
House-Bellucci-Shambaugh alligator
  scissors
House-Billeau ear loop
House-Buck curette
House-Crabtree
    H.-C. dissector
    H.-C. dissector pick
House-Delrin cutting block
House-Derlacki chisel

H

House-Dieter
 H.-D. eye forceps
 H.-D. malleus nipper
House-Hough excavator
House-Paparella stapes curette
Housepian
 H. aneurysm clip
 H. clip-applying forceps
 H. sellar punch
Houser
 H. cul-de-sac irrigator tube
 H. silicone T-tube
House-Radpour
 H.-R. suction irrigator
 H.-R. suction tube
House-Rosen
 H.-R. knife
 H.-R. needle
House-Saunders middle ear curette
House-Sheehy knife curette
House-Stevenson
 H.-S. suction irrigator
 H.-S. suction tube
House-Urban
 H.-U. marker
 H.-U. microsurgery cine camera
 H.-U. middle fossa retractor
 H.-U. temporal bone holder
 H.-U. tube
 H.-U. UEM-100 cine camera
 H.-U. vacuum rotary dissector
House-Urban-Pentax camera
House-Urban-Stille camera
House-Wullstein
 H.-W. cup ear forceps
 H.-W. perforating bur
Houspian clip-applying forceps
Housset-Debray gastroscope
Houston
 H. halo
 H. halo cervical traction
 H. halo traction collar
 H. nasal osteotome
Houtz endometrial curette
Hoverbed bed
Hoveround HVR 100 power control programmable wheelchair
[166]**Ho in vivo generator**
Howard
 H. closing forceps
 H. corneal abrader
 H. Jones needle
 H. spinal curette
 H. spiral stone dislodger
 H. stone basket
 H. tonsillar forceps
 H. tonsil-ligating forceps
Howard-DeBakey aortic aneurysm clamp
Howard-Flaherty spiral stone dislodger
Howard-Schatz laser
Howarth nasal raspatory
Howell
 H. biliary aspiration needle
 H. biopsy aspiration needle

 H. rotatable BII papillotome
 H. rotatable BII sphincterotome
Howland lock
Howmedica
 H. Centrax head replacement
 H. cerclage
 H. Duracon implant
 H. hip fracture stem
 H. HNR system
 H. Kinematic II knee prosthesis
 H. Microfixation System drill bit
 H. Microfixation System forceps
 H. Microfixation Sytem plate cutter
 H. monotube
 H. monotube external rotator
 H. PCA textured hip
 H. pediatric osteotomy system
 H. Simplex P cement
 H. total ankle system
 H. Unitrax hip fracture system
 H. Universal compression screw
Howorth
 H. elevator
 H. osteotome
 H. prosthesis
 H. toothed retractor
Howse-Coventry hip prosthesis
Howtek Scanmaster DX scanner
Hoxworth
 H. clip
 H. forceps
Hoya
 H. AR-570 autorefractor
 H. HDR objective refractometer
 H. MRM objective refractometer
Ho:YAG laser
Hoyer
 H. lift
 H. snare
Hoyt
 H. deep-surgery forceps
 H. hemostatic forceps
Hoytenberger tissue forceps
HP
 HP M1350A fetal monitor
 HP OmniPlane TEE imaging transducer
 HP SONOS 5500 ultrasound imaging system
HP1035 gel heel protector
HPC guide wire
HPS II total hip prosthesis
Hruby
 H. contact implant
 H. contact lens
 H. laser
Hryntschak catheter
H-series healing shoe
H-shaped plate
HSS total condylar knee prosthesis
HTO fixator
HTR-MFI
 H.-M. chin implant
 H.-M. curved implant
 H.-M. malar implant

H.-M. onlay facial augmentation
  implant
H.-M. paranasal implant
H.-M. premaxillary implant
H.-M. ramus implant
H.-M. straight implant
H-TRON plus V100 insulin infusion
  pump
HTR-PMI implant
HTR polymer
Huang
  H. Universal arm retractor
  H. Universal flexible arm
  H. vein holder
Hubbard
  H. airplane vent tube
  H. bolt
  H. corneoscleral forceps
  H. electrode
  H. hydrotherapy tank
  H. plate
  H. retractor
Hubbard-Nylok bolt
Hubell meatoscope
Huber
  H. forceps handle
  H. point needle
  H. probe
HubGuard IV cushion pad
Hub saw
Huco diamond knife
Hudgins salpingography cannula
Hudson
  H. adapter
  H. All-Clear nasal cannula
  H. bone drill
  H. bone retractor
  H. brace bur
  H. brain forceps
  H. cerebellar attachment
  H. cerebellar extension
  H. clamp
  H. conical bur
  H. cranial bur
  H. cranial drill
  H. cranial forceps
  H. dressing forceps
  H. Hydrofloat cushion
  H. Lifesaver resuscitator
  H. Multi-Vent
  H. rongeur forceps
  H. shank
  H. tissue forceps
  H. TLSO brace
  H. T Up-Draft II disposable
    nebulizer
  H. type oxygen mask
Hudson-Jones knee cage brace
Huegli
  H. meatoscope
  H. meatotome
Hueter
  H. bandage
  H. perineal dressing
Huey scissors

Huffman
  H. infant vaginal speculum
  H. infant vaginoscope
Huffman-Graves
  H.-G. adolescent vaginal speculum
  H.-G. vaginal speculum
Huffman-Huber
  H.-H. infant urethrotome
  H.-H. infant vaginoscope
Hufford esophagoscope
Hufnagel
  H. aortic clamp
  H. commissurotomy knife
  H. implant
  H. low-profile heart prosthesis
  H. mitral valve forceps
  H. prosthetic valve
Hufnagel-Kay heart valve
Hufnagel-Ryder needle holder
Hu-Friedy
  H.-F. dental bur
  H.-F. elevator
  H.-F. PermaSharp suture
  H.-F. suction tip aspirator
Huger diamond-back nasal scissors
Hugger
  Bair H.
Hugg-L-O pillow
Hughes
  H. eye implant
  H. fulguration electrode
Hugly aspirating tube
HUI
  Harris uterine injector
  HUI catheter
  HUI Mini-Flex
  HUI Mini-Flex uterine injector
Huibregtse
  H. biliary stent
  H. biliary stent set
Huibregtse-Katon
  H.-K. ERCP catheter
  H.-K. needle knife
  H.-K. papillotome
  H.-K. sphincterotome
Hulbert
  H. electrosurgical knife
  H. endo-electrode set
Hulka
  H. clip
  H. clip applier
  H. clip forceps
  H. tenaculum forceps
  H. uterine cannula
  H. uterine manipulator
  H. uterine tenaculum
Hulka-Clemens clip
Hulka-Kenwick
  H.-K. uterine-elevating forceps
  H.-K. uterine elevator
  H.-K. uterine-manipulating forceps
Hulten-Stille cannula
HumatroPen
Humby knife
Hume aortic clamp

H

humeral
  h. cutting guide
  h. impactor
  h. reamer
  h. retractor
  h. saw

HUMI
  Harris-Kronner uterine manipulator/injector
  HUMI cannula
  HUMI uterine manipulator/injector

HumidAire heated humidifier
HumidFilter heat and moisture exchanger
humidifier
  Bard-Parker U-Mid/Lo h.
  Bennett Cascade II Servo controlled heated h.
  bubble h.
  cold-mist h.
  Fischer & Paykel HC100 heated h.
  Fisher-Paykel heated h.
  HumidAire heated h.
  Hygroscopic Condenser h.
  jet h.
  Mistogen passover h.
  MRT tidal h.
  OEM 503 h.
  Ohio Bubble h.
  passover h.
  room h.

Humid-Vent Port 1 elbow connector
Hummer
  H. microdebrider
  H. V Sputter coater

Hummingbird wand
hump
  h. forceps
  h. gouge

Humphrey
  H. ATLAS Eclipse corneal topography system
  H. automatic keratometer
  H. automatic refractor
  H. B-scan
  H. coronary sinus-sucker suction tube
  H. lens analyzer
  H. Mastervue corneal topography system
  H. perimeter
  H. retinal imager
  H. visual field analyzer

Humphries
  H. aortic aneurysm clamp
  H. reverse-curve aortic clamp

Humphriss binocular balance
Hundley knee knife
Hunkeler
  H. ball-point hook
  H. frown incision marker
  H. intraocular lens
  H. lightweight intraocular lens implant

Hunsaker
  H. jet ventilation tube
  H. Mon-Jet tube anesthesia system

Hunstad
  H. Handle flow control
  H. infusion needle
  H. Quik-Clik device
  H. tumescent anesthesia system

Hunt
  H. angiographic trocar
  H. angled serrated ring forceps
  H. angled-tip forceps
  H. arachnoid dissector
  H. bipolar forceps
  H. bladder retractor
  H. chalazion forceps
  H. chalazion scissors
  H. colostomy clamp
  H. grasping forceps
  H. metal sound
  H. needle
  H. organizer
  H. tumor forceps
  H. vessel forceps

Hunter
  H. balloon
  H. one-piece all-PMMA intraocular lens
  H. open cord tendon implant
  H. separator
  H. splinter forceps
  H. tendon prosthesis
  H. tendon rod
  H. uterine curette

Hunter-Satinsky clamp
Hunter-Sessions
  H.-S. balloon
  H.-S. vena cava-occluding balloon catheter

Hunt-Lawrence pouch
Huntleigh bubble pad mattress
Hunt-Reich secondary cannula
Hunt-Yasargil pituitary forceps
Hupp tracheal retractor
Hurd
  H. bipolar diathermy electrode
  H. bone-cutting forceps
  H. bone forceps
  H. septal bone-cutting forceps
  H. septal elevator
  H. septum-cutting forceps
  H. suture needle
  H. tonsillar dissector
  H. tonsillar pillar retractor
  H. turbinate electrode

Hurd-Morrison dissector
Hurdner tissue forceps
Hurd-Weder tonsillar dissector
Hurson
  H. flexible pressure clamp
  H. flexible retractor
  H. flexible sliding clamp

Hurst
  H. bullet-tip esophageal dilator

H. mercury-filled dilator
H. mercury-filled esophageal bougie
Hurst-Maloney dilator
Hurst-Tucker pneumatic dilator
Hurteau forceps
Hurtig dilator
Hurwitt catheter
Hurwitz
H. esophageal clamp
H. intestinal clamp
H. thoracic trocar
Huse cannula
Husen button
Husk mastoid rongeur
Hustead epidural needle
Hutch evacuator
Hutchins biopsy needle
Hutchinson iris retractor
Huxley respirator
huygenian eyepiece
Huzly
H. applicator
H. aspirator
HV
H. NightSplint splint
H. SoftSplint splint
HVF ventilator
Hyams scleral knife
Hybond N+ nylon membrane
hybrid
H. capture system
h. fixation of hip replacement
component
H. graft
h. prosthesis
HybridFit
H. total hip system
H. total knee system
hyCare G hydrogel dressing
hyCure
h. collagen hemostatic wound
dressing
hyCURE wound care powder
Hyde
H. astigmatism ruler
H. double-curved corneal forceps
H. "frog" irrigating cannula
H. irrigator & aspirator unit
H. needle holder
Hyde-Osher keratometric ruler
HydraClense sitz bath
hydraclip
Hydracon contact lens
HydraCross TLC PTCA catheter
Hydradjust
H. IV table
H. urology system
Hydragran absorption dressing
Hydrajaw insert
Hydrasoft contact lens
Hydrasorb foam wound dressing
hydraulic
h. capillary infusion system
h. hand dynamometer

h. knee unit prosthesis
h. vein stripper
Hydra Vision
H. V. ES urologic system
H. V. IV urology system
H. V. Plus
H. V. Plus urologic system
Hydro
H. Bonnet
H. Plus
H. Plus coated guidewire
H. Soothe recliner
H. TherAblator ablator
hydroactive dressing
Hydro-Bell
Hydro-Tone H.-B.
HydroBlade keratome
HydroBrush keratome
Hydro-Cast
H.-C. dental mold
H.-C. reliner
HydroCath central venous catheter
Hydrocol
H. sacral wound dressing
Hydrocollator
H. heating unit
H. pad
H. steam pack
hydrocollator
h. pack
hydrocolloid occlusive dressing
Hydrocurve lens
HydroDerm transparent dressing
hydrodiascope
Hydro-Dissection tip
hydrodissector
cortical cleaving h.
Mectra h.
Nezhat-Dorsey Trumpet Valve h.
Pearce nucleus h.
Trumpet Valve h.
HYDRO-EASE
H.-E. II gel flotation mattress
overlay
H.-E. I water flotation mattress
overlay
hydrofiber dressing
HydroFlex
H. irrigation system
Hydroflex
H. penile prosthesis
H. penile semirigid implant
H. sphincter
hydrofloat cushion
Hydrofloss electronic oral irrigator
hydrogel
H. expansile intraocular lens
h. sheet
SkinTegrity h.
Stericare glycerin h.
THINSite topical wound dressing
with BioFilm h.
H. wound dressing
Hydrogel-coated PTCA balloon catheter
Hydrojette aspirator

H

hydrokeratome
  Visijet h.
Hydrokinetic Vichy shower
Hydrolene polymer
Hydrolyser
  H. microcatheter
hydromassage table
Hydromer
  H. coated polyurethane stent
  H. grafted catheter
Hydron
  H. burn Bandage
  H. lens
hydrophilic
  h. contact lens
  h. dilator
  h. polymer-coated steerable
   guidewire
  h. polyurethane foam dressing
  h. tent
hydrophilic-coated
  h.-c. guide wire
  h.-c. guidewire
hydrophobic barrier pen
hydrophone
  Imotec needle h.
  needle h.
HydroPlus stent
hydropolymer pad
hydrosector
  Reddick-Saye h.
Hydrosight lens
Hydro-Splint II
hydrostatic
  h. bag
  h. balloon
  h. balloon catheter
  h. bed
  h. dilator
  h. dissector
HydroSurg laparoscopic irrigator
hydrotherapy tub
HydroThermAblator system
Hydro-Tone Hydro-Bell
Hydrotrack underwater treadmill
Hydroview
  H. foldable IOL
  H. lens
Hydroxial hip prosthesis
hydroxyapatite (HA)
  h. adhesive
  h. bead
  h. coated implant
  h. implant material
  Interpore h.
  Interpore 200 porous h.
  LPPS h.
  h. ocular implant
  h. orbital implant
  h. ossicular prosthesis
hydroxyapatite-coated stem
HyFil hydrogel dressing
Hyflex X-File instruments
Hyfrecator
  Birtcher H.

  H. coagulator
  Hall-Fish H.
Hyfrecutter
Hygroscopic
  H. Condenser humidifier
hygroscopic heat and moisture exchanger
Hylamer
  H. acetabular liner
  H. orthopaedic bearing polymer
Hylashield
Hylinks clip
Hylin rasp
Hymes
  H. double-lumen catheter
  H. meatal clamp
Hymes-Timberlake electrode
Hymlek portable chest tube
hyoid-cutting forceps
Hypafix retention tape
Hypan tent
hyperalimentation catheter
hyperbaric
  h. bed
  h. boot
  h. chamber
hyperbolic glasses
hyperextension
  h. brace
  h. fracture frame
Hyperex thoracic orthosis
Hyperflex
  H. flexible guidewire
  H. tracheostomy tube
Hypergel
  H. hydrogel wound dressing
Hyper-Oxy portable hyperbaric chamber
HyperPACS system
Hypertie bandage
Hypobaric
  H. transfemoral system
  H. transtibial system
hypodermic needle
hypogastric artery forceps
hypophyseal forceps
hypophysectomy forceps
hypophysial curette
Hypospray jet injection needle
Hypotherm Gel Kap
hypothermia
  h. blanket
  h. mattress
  h. oxygen warmer
Hyrax appliance
Hysorb wound dressing
hysterectomy
  h. clamp
  h. forceps
  h. kit
  h. retractor
hysterofiberscope
  Olympus flexible h.
hysterosalpingography catheter
hysteroscope
  ACMI Micro-H h.
  AMSCO h.

Baggish h.
Baloser h.
Circon ACMI h.
contact h.
diagnostic h.
Elmed h.
examining h.
fiberoptic h.
Fujinon flexible h.
Galileo rigid h.
Hamou h.
Karl Storz 15 French flexible h.
Liesegang LM-FLEX 7 flexible h.
MicroSpan h.
Olympus h.

OPERA Star SL h.
Scopemaster contact h.
h. sheath
Storz h.
Valle h.
Van Der Pas h.
hysteroscopic insufflator
Hysteroser
    H. contact hysteroscopy system
Hysto-vac drain
Hy-Tape
    H.-T. adhesive
    H.-T. latex-free surgical tape
HY-TEC automated allergy diagnostic system

H

3-I
-I. dental implant
-I. tapper

I&A
irrigating and aspirating
irrigation and aspiration
I&A coaxial cannula
I&A instrument
I&A kit
I&A machine
McIntyre I&A system
Simcoe I&A system
I&A system

IAB
940 I. Catheter
I. catheter

IABP
intraaortic balloon pump

Ialo photocoagulator

Iamin hydrating gel wound dressing

I-beam
I.-b. cement punch
I.-b. hemiarthroplasty hip prosthesis
Jergesen I.-b.
I.-b. Press-Fit punch

IBF
IBF knee instrument
IBF total knee instrumentation

IBM
IBM field-cycling research relaxometer
IBM NMR spectrometer
IBM Speech Server clinical reporting system

I-bolt
Texas Scottish Rite Hospital I.-b.

Icarex 25 Med mirror reflex lens camera

I-Cath
Firlit-Sugar intermittent catheter I.-C.

IC bed

ICD
implantable cardioverter-defibrillator
intracervical device
Cadence biphasic ICD
dual-chamber ICD
Guardian ICD
Telectronics Guardian ATP II ICD
transthoracically implanted ICD
Ventritex Cadence ICD
Vitatron Diamond ICD

ice
i. bag
i. clot evacuator
N'ice Stretch night splint suspension system with Sealed I.
I. Wedge hot/cold therapy wrap

I.C.E. Down cold pack

Iceflex Endurance suction suspension sleeve

ICE-Magic pain reduction kit

Iceman
I. cold therapy pad
I. continuous cold therapy unit

Iceross
I. Comfort Plus silicone gel liner
I. silicone socket

ICEROSS sleeve
ice-tong calipers

ICEX
I. 4-hole lock
I. socket

ICLH apparatus
Icofly infusion needle
Iconoclast

ICP
I. Camino bolt
I. catheter

ICP-T fiberoptic ICP monitoring catheter

ICTP RIA kit
ICV-10 ventilator
ICV reservoir

Ideal
I. cardiac device
I. tourniquet

Idecap dialyzer
Identifit hip prosthesis
IDI corneoscope
IDIS angiography system
ID-Micro typing system
I-Flow nerve block infusion kit

Iglesias
I. continuous-flow resectoscope
I. dilator
I. electrode
I. evacuator
I. fiberoptic resectoscope
I. microlens resectoscope

Igloo Heatshield system
iiRAD DR1000C digital radiographic system

IKI catgut suture

I-knife
Alcon I.-k.

Ikuta
I. clamp approximator
I. fixation device

IL
IL 1640 blood gas/electrolyte system
IL MED laser

IL-282 co-oximeter
ILA-series stapling device
ILA stapler

ileoneobladder
Hautmann i.
W-shaped i.

ileostomy
i. appliance
i. bag

Ilex
Biofreeze with I.

iLEX stomal seal
Ilfeld
    I. brace
    I. splint
Ilg
    I. capsular forceps
    I. curved micro tying forceps
    I. insertion forceps
    I. lens loop
    I. lens loupe
    I. microneedle holder
    I. needle
    I. needle holder
    I. probe
    I. push/pull
iliac
    i. artery stent
    i. clamp
    i. forceps
    i. graft separator
    i. screw
iliac-femoral cannula
Iliff
    I. blepharochalasis forceps
    I. clamp
    I. lacrimal probe
    I. lacrimal trephine
Iliff-Park speculum
Iliff-Wright fascia needle
iliosacral
    i. and iliac fixation construct
    i. screw
Ilizarov
    I. circular external fixator
    I. device
    I. distractor
    I. external ring fixator
    I. frame
    I. hybrid fixator
    I. limb-lengthening system
    I. ring
    I. screw
Illinois needle
Illiterate E chart
Illouz
    I. modified tip
    I. standard tip
    I. suction cannula
Illumen-8, -9 guiding catheter
Illumina
    I. Pro Series CO_2 surgical laser system
    I. Pro series laparoscopic laser
illuminated
    i. probe
    i. speculum
    i. suction needle
illuminating stylet
illuminator
    Barkan i.
    Britetrac i.
    Cogent XL i.
    DyoBrite i.
    fiberoptic surgical field i.
    intramedullary i.

    Light Commander xenon i.
    Luxo surgical i.
    Mammo Mask i.
    Novar oral i.
    Pelosi i.
    Pilling fiberoptic i.
    slit i.
    suspended operating i.
    XL i.
I.L.MED instrument
Ilopan disposable syringe
ILUS catheter
IM
    IM Jaws alligator forceps
    IM nail
    IM tendon stripper
IMA
    IMA graft
    IMA retractor
    IMA scissors
image
    i. analysis system
    I. custom external breast prosthesis
    i. Orthicon tube
Imagecath rapid exchange angioscope
ImageNet image digitizing system
image-processing unit
imager
    Acuson 128EP i.
    Digirad 2020 TC i.
    Digital fundus i.
    Digital slit-lamp i.
    Drystar dry i.
    flat-panel megavoltage i.
    GE Signa 5.4 Genesis MR i.
    GE Signa 5.5 Horizon EchoSpeed MR i.
    Hewlett-Packard color flow i.
    Humphrey retinal i.
    Integris V3000 i.
    Kodak 1200 Digital Science medical i.
    Magnes 2500 WH i.
    Magnetom SP MRI i.
    NeuroScan 3D i.
    Signa i.
    Sonos ultrasound i.
    Tesla Signa magnetic resonance i.
    I. Torque selective catheter
Image-View system
imaging
    blood flow i.
    Bucky high-contrast i.
    cine-magnetic resonance i.
    cine magnetic resonance i. (cine MRI)
    color-flow Doppler real-time 2-D blood flow i.
    Color Power Angio i.
    i. densitometer
    diffusion-weighted MR i.
    Doppler transesophageal color flow i.
    dynamic contrast-enhanced magnetic resonance i.

echoplanar magnetic resonance i.
endorectal surface-coil MR i.
Exceltech i.
fast-imaging steady precession
  sequence three-dimensional
  magnetic resonance i.
Integris cardiovascular i.
LaparoScan laparoscopic ultrasonic i.
Magnes magnetic source i.
magnetic resonance i. (MRI)
magnetic source i.
MedMorph III patient video i.
Niamtu video i.
phased-array body-coil MR i.
radionucleotide i.
Restore hair replacement i.
Resurface laser resurfacing i.
technetium (Tc)-99m sestamibi
  tomographic i.
three-dimensional fast spin-echo
  magnetic resonance i.
Tissue Specific i.
ultrafast magnetic resonance i.

imaging-angioplasty balloon catheter
Imagyn
  I. microlaparoscope
  I. surgical stapler
Imatron
  I. CT bone mineral phantom
  I. C-100 Ultrafast CT scanner
  I. Fastrac C-100 cine x-ray CT
    scanner
  I. system
imbedded microtransducer
IMCOR
  I. implant
  I. No-Touch implant placement
    system
IMED
  IMED Gemini PC-2 volumetric
    controller
  IMED Gemini PC-2 volumetric
    pump
  IMED infusion device
  IMED infusion pump
IM/EM
  IM/EM tibial resection guide
  IM/EM tibial resection stylus
Imex
  I. antepartum monitor
  I. Pocket-Dop OB Doppler
  I. scleral implant
  I. StethoDop
Imexdop CT Doppler
Imexlab vascular diagnostic system
Imhoff tank
IMMA lens
ImmEdge Pen
immediate
  I. Implant Impression system
  I. Impression implant
  I. Load implant
  i. postoperative prosthesis
  I. Response Mobile Analysis blood
    analysis system

Immergut
  I. suction-coagulation tube
  I. suction tube
immersible video camera
immersion bath
immobilization jacket
immobilizer
  arm and shoulder i.
  Comfort wrist i.
  Ezy Wrap shoulder i.
  Hook hemi-harness shoulder i.
  Kapp Surgical Instrument surgical
    knee i.
  knee i.
  long leg i.
  Olympic Neostraint i.
  QuickCast wrist i.
  shoulder abduction i.
  sternooccipitomanubrial i.
  Tab-Strap knee i.
  Trimline knee i.
  Velpeau shoulder i.
  Watco 2001 knee i.
  Westfield-style acromioclavicular i.
  Zinco Gunslinger II shoulder i.
immobilizing bandage
Immulite Dynamic Duo analyzer
immunoadsorption column
immunoanalyzer
  Labotech micro-plated i.
immunocytometer
immunomagnetic bead
Immunomedics system
Immunomount
immunonephelometer
  BNA-100-Behring Diagnostics i.
immunostainer
  Shandon Candenza i.
  Ventana 320 automated i.
immunoturbidimetry analyzer
Imotec needle hydrophone
Imount
  I. instrumentation
  I. instruments
IMP
  IMP bone screw targeter
  IMP Femur Finder
  IMP surgical leg pedestal
  IMP turnstile casting stand
  IMP Universal lateral positioner
IMPAC PDQ abutment
impact
  i. glove
  I. lithotriptor system
  i. mitt
  I. modular porous prosthesis
  I. modular total hip system
impactor
  Bio-Moore II stem i.
  Cloward bone graft i.
  Cloward dowel i.
  Cohort spinal i.
  Dawson-Yuhl i.
  electromechanical i.
  femoral i.

impactor *(continued)*
  hook i.
  humeral i.
  Judet i. for acetabular cup
  Küntscher i.
  lateral gutter i.
  Moe i.
  mushroom i.
  orthopedic i.
  i. plate
  Pollock wimp wire i.
  Raylor bone i.
  i. rod
  rotating air i.
  rotating arm i.
  shell i.
  Smith-Petersen i.
  spondylophyte i.
  vertebral body i.
impactor-extractor
  Fox i.-e.
ImPad inflation pad
Impax PACS system
IMP-Capello
  I.-C. arm support
  I.-C. slimline abduction pillow
impedance
  i. electrode
  i. phlebograph
Imperator handpiece
Imperatori laryngeal forceps
Imperial alloy
impermeable dressing
Imperson catheter
impervious
  i. sheet
  i. stockinette
  i. U-sheet
Impex
  I. aspiration & injection needle
  I. diamond radial keratotomy knife
Impex/Lerner foldable lens removing set
Impingement-Free tibial guide system
impingement rod
ImplaMed
  I. gold screw
  I. implant system
implant
  accessory eye i.
  accordion i.
  acorn-shaped eye i.
  acrylic ball eye i.
  acrylic conformer eye i.
  Acufex-Suretac i.
  Acuflex intraocular lens i.
  adjustable breast i.
  Advent i.
  Aequalis humeral head i.
  afterloading i.
  alar-columellar i.
  Allen-Braley lens i.
  Allen ePTFE ocular i.
  Allen eye i.
  Allen orbital i.

Allen Supramid i.
Alpar intraocular lens i.
Amelogen dental i.
AMO scleral i.
anchor endosteal i.
anterior chamber acrylic i.
AO/ASIF orthopaedic i.
Appolionio eye lens i.
Arenberg-Denver inner-ear valve i.
Arion i.
Arnett Lefort i.
Arroyo i.
Arruga eye i.
Arruga-Moura-Brazil orbital i.
articulated chin i.
artificial joint i.
Ashworth-Blatt i.
A-type dental i.
Avanta soft skeletal i.
Azar Tripod eye i.
Baerveldt glaucoma i.
Baerveldt seton i.
BAK/C cervical interbody fusion i.
BAK/Proximity interbody fusion i.
Balnetar i.
Bannon-Klein i.
Bard i.
Barkan infant lens i.
Barraquer i.
Bechert intraocular lens i.
Beekhuis-Supramid mentoplasty augmentation i.
Berens conical eye i.
Berens orbital i.
Berens pyramidal eye i.
Berens-Rosa scleral i.
Berens sphere eye i.
Bicon dental i.
Bicoral i.
Bietti eye i.
bifocal eye i.
bilumen mammary i.
Binder submalar i.
Binkhorst collar stud lens i.
Binkhorst eye i.
Binkhorst four-loop iris-fixated i.
Binkhorst lens i.
Binkhorst two-loop intraocular lens i.
BioCare i.
Biocell anatomical reconstructive mammary i.
Biocell RTV breast i.
Biocell textured i.
Bioceram two-stage series II endosteal dental i.
Biodel i.
BioDIMENSIONAL saline-filled i.
Bio-eye hydroxyapatite ocular i.
Biofix biodegradable i.
BioHorizon i.
Biomatrix ocular i.
Biomet custom i.
bioresorbable i.
BioSphere suture anchor i.

Bio-Vent i.
Biovert ceramic i.
bivalve nasal splint i.
blade endosteal i.
blade-form i.
Blair-Brown i.
i. blank
Boberg-Ans lens i.
Bonaccolto eye i.
Bonaccolto orbital i.
BoneSource i.
Bosker transmandibular i.
bovine collagen i.
Boyd orbital i.
Branemark endosteal i.
Branemark osseointegration i.
Braun i.
Brawner orbital i.
breast i.
Brink PeriPyriform i.
Brown-Dohlman Silastic corneal i.
build-up eye i.
Bunker i.
Calcitek i.
calcium phosphate ceramic i.
candle vaginal cesium i.
carbon i.
Cardona focalizing fundus lens i.
Cardona goniofocalizing i.
carpal lunate i.
Carrion-Small penile i.
cartilage i.
Castroviejo acrylic eye i.
Celestin i.
celluloid i.
ceramic endosteal i.
CeraOne abutment i.
Charnley i.
Chatzidakis i.
chessboard i.
chin i.
Choyce Mark VIII eye i.
chromium-cobalt alloy i.
Clarion multi-strategy cochlear i.
Clayman lens i.
cobalt-chromium i.
cobalt-chromium-molybdenum alloy
  metal i.
cobalt-chromium-tungsten-nickel alloy
  metal i.
Coburn anterior chamber intraocular
  lens i.
Coburn Mark IX eye i.
cochlear i.
Cogan-Boberg-Ans lens i.
collagen i.
i. collar
columellar i.
Combi-40 cochlear i.
Complete i.
condylar i.
conical eye i.
contact shell i.
Contigen Bard collagen i.
Continuum knee system i.

Contour Profile Natural saline
  breast i.
Contour Profile silicone breast i.
conventional reform eye i.
conventional shell-type eye i.
Cooper i.
Copeland intraocular lens i.
Corail HA-coated stem hip i.
corneal i.
Corning i.
corrected cosmetic contact shell
  eye i.
cosmetic contact shell i.
Cox-Uphoff i.
Cronin mammary i.
Cryo-Barrages vitreous i.
CUI columellar i.
CUI dorsal i.
CUI malar i.
CUI rhinoplasty i.
curl-back shell eye i.
curvilinear chin i.
Custodis i.
custom-contoured i.
Cutler eye i.
Cutter i.
cylinder-type i.
3D Accuscan facial i.
Dacron i.
Dacron-backed i.
Dannheim eye i.
DeBakey i.
defibrillator i.
Deflux system i.
dental i.
De Paco i.
DePuy orthopaedic i.
Dermostat orbital i.
DeWecker eye i.
Doherty spherical eye i.
Donnheim i.
dorsal columellar i.
dorsal column stimulator i.
double-lumen breast i.
double-plate Molteno i.
double-stem i.
Dow Corning i.
Dragstedt i.
D-shaped i.
dual-compartment gel-inflatable
  mammary i.
Duehr-Allen eye i.
Duracon knee i.
Dura-II concealable penile i.
dural i.
Durallium i.
Durapatite i.
Duros leuprolide i.
DynaFlex penile i.
Edwards Teflon intracardiac i.
Ehmke platinum Teflon i.
i. elastomer shell
electrical i.
endodontic endosteal i.
endo-osseous dental i.

implant *(continued)*
 Endopore i.
 endosseous HA i.
 endosseous hydroxyapatite i.
 epilepsy i.
 Epstein collar stud acrylic i.
 EPTFE i.
 Esser i.
 esthetic Taylor mandibular angle i.
 Ethrone i.
 E-type dental i.
 Ewald-Walker knee i.
 Ewing eye i.
 expandable breast i.
 expanded polytetrafluoroethylene
  (EPTFE) i.
 expansible infrastructure endosteal i.
 extended anatomical high-profile
  malar i.
 Extrafil breast i.
 extraoral bone-anchored i.
 eye spherical i.
 facial i.
 fascia lata i.
 feathered extended malar i.
 fenestra i.
 Ferguson i.
 Fibrel gelatin matrix i.
 Fine magnetic i.
 finger joint i.
 Finney penile i.
 fixed bearing knee i.
 fixed mandibular i.
 Flatt i.
 flexible digital i.
 flexible Dualens i.
 flexible rod penile i.
 Flexi-Flate penile i.
 Flexi-Rod II penile i.
 Flowers Mandibular Glove i.
 Flowers Tear Trough i.
 i. forceps
 four-loop iris clip i.
 four-loop iris fixated i.
 Fox eyelid i.
 Fox spherical eye i.
 free i.
 free-standing i.
 Frey tunneled eye i.
 Frialit-2 system Frialloc
  transgingival threaded i.
 Friatec i.
 front build-up i.
 full-dimpled Lucite eye i.
 full-thickness i.
 Fyodorov eye i.
 Fyodorov type I, II lens i.
 Galin intraocular lens i.
 Garcia-Novito eye i.
 gel-filled i.
 Gelfilm retinal i.
 gel-saline mammary i.
 gentamicin i.
 Geristore dental i.

 Gerow Small-Carrion penile i.
 Gillies i.
 Glasgold Wafer chin i.
 glass sphere eye i.
 Global total shoulder i.
 Gold eyelid load i.
 Goldmann multimirror lens i.
 Gold-Mules eye i.
 gonioscopic i.
 Gore-Tex nasal i.
 Gore-Tex SAM facial i.
 Gore-Tex vascular i.
 Gott i.
 great toe i.
 Greissinger Multi-Axis joint i.
 grooved silicone i.
 Guist sphere eye i.
 HA-coated hip i.
 HA-coated Micro-Vent i.
 HA-coated root-form dental i.
 Haik eye i.
 haptic area i.
 hard tissue replacement-malleable
  facial i.
 Harris i.
 Harrison i.
 Hartley i.
 HA-threaded hexlock i.
 helicoid endosteal i.
 hemi-interpositional i.
 hemisphere eye i.
 Herrick silicone lacrimal i.
 heterograft i.
 hex i.
 Heyer-Schulte breast i.
 Heyer-Schulte lens i.
 Heyer-Schulte rhinoplasty i.
 HIHA tendon i.
 i. hinge
 hinged i.
 Hoffer ridged lens i.
 Hoffmann eye i.
 hollow-sphere orbital i.
 homograft i.
 hook-type eye i.
 Hoskins-Drake i.
 House i.
 Howmedica Duracon i.
 Hruby contact i.
 HTR-MFI chin i.
 HTR-MFI curved i.
 HTR-MFI malar i.
 HTR-MFI onlay facial
  augmentation i.
 HTR-MFI paranasal i.
 HTR-MFI premaxillary i.
 HTR-MFI ramus i.
 HTR-MFI straight i.
 HTR-PMI i.
 Hufnagel i.
 Hughes eye i.
 Hunkeler lightweight intraocular
  lens i.
 Hunter open cord tendon i.
 Hydroflex penile semirigid i.

hydroxyapatite coated i.
hydroxyapatite ocular i.
hydroxyapatite orbital i.
3-I dental i.
IMCOR i.
Imex scleral i.
Immediate Impression i.
Immediate Load i.
Implantech Binder i.
Implantech facial i.
Implantech Flowers i.
Implantech Mittelman i.
Implantech Terino i.
Imtec premounted threaded i.
IMZ endosteal i.
inlay i.
I. Innovations titanium screw
Insall-Burstein intracondylar total
  knee i.
Intacs corneal ring i.
Integral Omniloc i.
Intermedics intraocular lens i.
Interpore osteointegrated i.
interstitial i.
intracochlear i.
intraocular lens i.
intraorbital i.
Iovision i.
Iowa orbital i.
ITI-Bonefit endosseous i.
ITI dental i.
Ivalon lucite orbital eye i.
Ivalon sponge eye i.
Jardon-Straith chin i.
Jardon-Straith nasal i.
joint i.
Jonas i.
Jordan eye i.
K i.
Keragen i.
Kerato-Lens i.
Kinetik great toe i.
King orbital i.
Klockner i.
Koenig total great toe i.
Koeppe intraocular lens i.
Kratz i.
Kratz-Sinskey intraocular lens i.
Krause-Wolfe i.
Kryptok bifocal lens i.
Lacey total knee i.
LaminOss i.
Landegger orbital i.
LaPorta great toe i.
large-pore polyethylene i.
Lash-Loeffler i.
Lawrence first metatarsophalangeal
  joint i.
Lemoine orbital i.
lens i.
Levitt eye i.
Lifecath peritoneal i.
Lincoff scleral sponge i.
Linkow blade i.
Little intraocular lens i.

Liverpool elbow i.
Loptex laser intraocular lens i.
Lovac fundal contact lens i.
Lovac six-mirror gonioscopic lens i.
low-profile breast i.
Lucite sphere i.
lucite sphere i.
Luhr i.
lumbar anterior root stimulator i.
lunate i.
Lyda-Ivalon-Lucite i.
MacIntosh i.
Maestro i.
i. magnet
magnetic eye i.
malar i.
malleable facial i.
mammary i.
Marlex mesh i.
i. material
McCannel i.
McCutchen hip i.
McGhan breast i.
McGhan eye i.
McGhan facial i.
Medallion intraocular lens i.
MedDev gold eyelid i.
Medical Optics eye i.
Medical Optics intraocular lens i.
Medical Workshop intraocular
  lens i.
Medicornea Kratz intraocular lens i.
Medpor biomaterial i.'s
Medpor facial i.
Medpor malar i.
Medpor reconstructive i.
Medpor surgical i.'s
Melauskas acrylic orbital i.
Meme mammary i.
Meniscus Arrow i.
Mentor malleable semirigid penile i.
Mentor Siltex i.
meridional i.
Mersilene i.
meshed ball i.
mesostructure i.
metacarpophalangeal i.
metal-backed acetabular component
  hip i.
metal hemi-toe i.
metal orthopaedic i.
methyl methacrylate beads i.
methyl methacrylate eye i.
Mettelman prejowl chin i.
Micro-Lok i.
Micro-Vent i.
Micro-Vent^2 i.
middle ear i.
Mini-Matic i.
Miragel i.
Mittelman i.
3M mammary i.
mobile bearing knee i.
modular i.
Molteno double-plate i.

implant (*continued*)
    Molteno drainage eye i.
    motility eye i.
    Mueller shield eye i.
    Muhlberger orbital i.
    Mules eye i.
    multichannel cochlear i.
    Naden-Rieth i.
    nasal dorsal i.
    needle endosteal i.
    Neer II total shoulder system i.
    NeuFlex metacarpophalangeal joint i.
    NeuroControl Freehand i.
    NexGen knee i.
    Nexus i.
    Niebauer i.
    Niebauer-Cutter i.
    Nobel Biocare i.
    Nobelpharma i.
    Nocito i.
    Novagold mammary i.
    Nucleus 22 cochlear i.
    Nucleus multichannel cochlear i.
    Octa-Hex i.
    Oculo-Plastik ePTFE ocular i.
    Ollier-Thiersch i.
    O'Malley self-adhering lens i.
    Omniloc dental i.
    onlay i.
    Ophtec occlusion i.
    optic i.
    oral i.
    orbital floor i.
    Organon percutaneous E2 i.
    orthotic attachment i.
    Osseodent dental i.
    osseointegrated oral i.
    Osseotite two-stage procedure i.
    osseous i.
    OsteoGen HA dental i.
    Osteogen resorbable osteogenic
      bone-filling i.
    Osteonics-HA coated femoral i.
    Osteoplate i.
    Padgett i.
    Panje i.
    paraffin i.
    Paragon Complete i.
    Partnership i.
    Pasqualini i.
    patch i.
    patella-resurfacing i.
    patient-matched i.
    peanut eye i.
    Pearce vaulted-Y lens i.
    pectoralis muscle i.
    pedicle i.
    penile i.
    percutaneous dorsal column
      stimulator i.
    Periotest i.
    PhacoFlex II foldable intraocular
      lens i.
    Phystan i.

    piggyback i.
    pin i.
    Pisces i.
    planar I mesh i.
    planoconvex eye i.
    plastic sphere eye i.
    Platina intraocular lens i.
    platinum eyelid i.
    Plexiglas eye i.
    PMI i.
    PMMA i.
    Polaris adjustable spinal cage i.
    polyethylene sphere i.
    polyglycolide i.
    polylactide i.
    polymer tooth replica i.
    polymethyl methacrylate i.
    Polystan i.
    polytetrafluoroethylene (PTFE) i.
    polyurethane-coated silicone breast i.
    polyvinyl sponge i.
    Porex Medpor i.
    Porex paranasal i.
    Porex PHA i.
    porous polyethylene i.
    posterior chamber lens i.
    Precision-Cosmet intraocular lens i.
    Press-Fit i.
    processed carbon i.
    ProOsteon synthetic bone i.
    Proplast preformed facial i.
    Proplast-Teflon disk i.
    Protek joint i.
    PTFE-containing i.
    pyramidal eye i.
    Radin-Rosenthal i.
    radiocarpal i.
    Radovan breast i.
    ramus blade i.
    ramus endosteal i.
    Rastelli i.
    Rayner-Choyce eye i.
    reform eye i.
    Replace system tapered i.
    Restore bone i.
    Restore dental i.
    Restore orthobiologic soft-tissue i.
    Restore threaded i.
    retinal Gelfilm i.
    Reuter bobbin i.
    Reverdin i.
    reverse-shape i.
    rhinoplasty i.
    Ridley anterior chamber lens i.
    Ridley Mark II lens i.
    Rizzo dorsal i.
    Roberts dental i.
    Rodin orbital i.
    root-form dental i.
    Rosa-Berens orbital i.
    Ruedemann eye i.
    Ruiz plano fundal lens i.
    saline-filled anatomical breast i.
    saline-filled round breast i.
    SAM facial i.

Sargon i.
Sauerbruch i.
Schepens hollow hemisphere i.
Schocket tube i.
scleral buckle eye i.
scleral buckler i.
screw-type i.
Screw-Vent i.
S-D-Sorb E-Z TAC i.
Seeburger i.
seed i.
self-tapping screw-type i.
semishell eye i.
Septopal i.
serrefine i.
Severin i.
Sgarlato hammertoe i.
Shearing posterior chamber
  intraocular lens i.
shelf-type i.
shell eye i.
Shepard intraocular lens i.
SHIP hammertoe i.
SHIP-Shaw rod hammertoe i.
Shirakable nasal i.
Sichel movable orbital i.
Sichi i.
Silastic chin i.
Silastic corneal eye i.
Silastic Cronin i.
Silastic eye i.
Silastic finger i.
Silastic midfacial malar i.
Silastic penile i.
Silastic rhinoplasty i.
Silastic scleral buckle i.
Silastic scleral buckler eye i.
Silastic silicone rubber i.
Silastic subdermal i.
Silastic testicular i.
Silastic toe i.
silicone buckling i.
silicone button eye i.
silicone elastomer rubber ball i.
silicone-filled anatomical breast i.
silicone-filled mammary i.
silicone-filled round breast i.
silicone-gel breast i.
silicone meshed motility i.
silicone MP i.
silicone nasal strut i.
silicone pad eye i.
silicone rod i.
silicone sleeve eye i.
silicone sponge i.
silicone strip eye i.
silicone textured mammary i.
silicone tire eye i.
Siloxane i.
Siltex mammary i.
Simcoe-AMO eye i.
Simcoe intraocular lens i.
single-channel cochlear i.
single-stage screw i.
single-tooth subperiosteal i.

Sinskey lens i.
Sinterlock i.
i. site dilator
Sled i.
i. sleeve
sleeve i.
Small-Carrion Silastic rod for
  penile i.
SmartScrew bioabsorbable i.
Smith orbital floor i.
smooth staple i.
Snellen conventional reform eye i.
SoftForm facial i.
soft silicone sphere i.
solid silicone buttock i.
solid silicone with Supramid
  mesh i.
Spectra-System i.
Spectrum Designs facial i.
spherical eye i.
Sphero Flex i.
spiral endosteal i.
Spline Twist microtextured
  titanium i.
split-thickness i.
i. sponge
sponge i.
stainless steel i.
STAR-LOCK Press-Fit cylinder i.
Startanius blade i.
Star/Vent one-stage dental screw i.
Steri-Oss endosteal dental i.
Stone eye i.
Straith chin i.
Straith nasal i.
Strampelli i.
S-type dental i.
subdermal i.
submucosal i.
subperiosteal i.
SuperCat self-tapping i.
superficial i.
I. Support Systems titanium screw
Supramid i.
Supramid-Allen i.
surface eye i.
Surgibone i.
Surgicel i.
Surgitek Flexi-Flate II penile i.
Surgitek mammary i.
Sustain HA-coated screw i.
Sustain hydroxyapatite biointegrated
  dental i.
Sutter hinged great toe i.
Swanson carpal lunate i.
Swanson carpal scaphoid i.
Swanson finger joint i.
Swanson great toe i.
Swanson metacarpophalangeal i.
Swanson radial head i.
Swanson radiocarpal i.
Swanson Silastic i.
Swanson small joint i.
Swanson trapezium i.
Swanson ulnar head i.

implant (*continued*)
    Swanson wrist joint i.
    Swede-Vent TL self-tapping external
      hex i.
    Swiss MP joint i.
    Syed-Neblett i.
    Syed template i.
    tantalum mesh eye i.
    tapered Micro-Vent i.
    Taper-Lock external hex i.
    Techmedica i.
    Teflon mesh i.
    Teflon orbital floor i.
    tendon i.
    Tennant Anchorflex lens i.
    Tensilon i.
    Terino anatomical chin i.
    testicular i.
    Tevdek i.
    TG Osseotite single-stage
      procedure i.
    TheraSeed i.
    thick-walled Dacron-backed i.
    Thiersch i.
    ThreadLoc i.
    TiMesh patient configured titanium
      craniomaxillofacial i.
    TiOblast dental i.
    i. tire
    tire eye i.
    titanium alloy i.
    titanium plasma sprayed dental i.
    Tobin anatomical malar prosthetic i.
    tobramycin-impregnated PMMA i.
    total top i.
    Townley i.
    transmandibular i.
    transosseous i.
    transosteal pin i.
    trapezium i.
    trial i.
    Trilucent breast i.
    triple-lumen i.
    Troncoso gonioscopic lens i.
    Troutman eye i.
    T-type dental i.
    tunneled eye i.
    Twist MTX i.
    Ultex lens i.
    unicompartmental knee i.
    Unilab Surgibone surgical i.
    ureteral i.
    Uribe orbital i.
    Usher Marlex mesh i.
    U-type dental i.
    VA magnetic orbital i.
    Varigray i.
    Varilux lens i.
    Vitallium eye i.
    Vitrasert intraocular i.
    Vivosil i.
    VoCoM thyroplasty i.
    Volk conoid i.
    Walter Reed i.

    WasherLoc i.
    Weber hip i.
    Weck-cel i.
    Weil i.
    Weil-modified Swanson i.
    Wheeler spherical eye i.
    wire mesh eye i.
    Wolf i.
    Wölfe-Krause i.
    Zang metatarsal cap i.
    Zeichner i.
    Zest subperiosteal i.
    Zoladex i.
    Zyderm collagen i.
    Zyplast i.
implantable
    i. artificial heart
    i. atrial defibrillator
    i. automatic cardioverter-defibrillator
    i. cardioverter-defibrillator (ICD)
    i. cardioverter/defibrillator catheter
    i. infusion port
    i. neural stimulator
    i. osmotic pump
    i. pacemaker
    i. silicone microballoon
    i. vascular access device (IVAD)
**Implantaid Di-Lock cardiac lead
  introducer**
implantation forceps
implant-borne prosthesis
Implantech
    I. Binder implant
    I. facial implant
    I. Flowers implant
    I. Mittelman implant
    I. SE-100 smoke aspiration tip
    I. Terino implant
implanted
    i. infusion pump
    i. pacemaker
implanter
    Geuder i.
    Wallner interstitial prostate i.
implant material (*See also* material)
    acrylic i. m.
    allogeneic lyophilized bone graft i.
      m.
    bioceramic i. m.
    Bonaccolto monoplex orbital i. m.
    bone i. m.
    celluloid i. m.
    corundum ceramic i. m.
    cyanoacrylate fixed orbital silicone
      sleds i. m.
    Dermostat eye i. m.
    Edwards Teflon intracardiac patch i.
      m.
    Expander mammary i. m.
    Fletching femoral hernia i. m.
    homograft i. m.
    hydroxyapatite i. m.
    Keolar i. m.
    Lash-Loeffler penile i. m.
    Lincoff sponge i. m.

Linkow dental i. m.
L-rod i. m.
methyl methacrylate i. m.
Ommaya reservoir i. m.
Paladon i. m.
paraffin i. m.
Pearman penile i. m.
polyether i. m.
polyethylene i. m.
polyurethane i. m.
polyvinyl i. m.
Scialom dental i. m.
Shearing posterior chamber i. m.
shell i. m.
Small-Carrion penile i. m.
solid buckling i. m.
solid silicone exoplant i. m.
Spitz-Holter valve i. m.
sponge silicone i. m.
Stimoceiver i. m.
Szulc orbital i. m.
tissue mandrel i. m.
titanium i. m.
transcatheter umbrella i. m.
tunnel-type i. m.
Usher Marlex mesh i. m.
Vitallium i. m.
implant-retained denture
implant-supported
i.-s. fixed prosthesis
i.-s. overdenture
Implast
I. bone cement
I. bone cement adhesive
Implatome dental tomography system
Implens intraocular lens
Import vascular access port with Bio-Glide
Impra
I. bypass graft
I. Carboflo ePTFE vascular graft
I. collagen-impregnated Dacron prosthesis
I. Flex vascular graft
I. microporous PTFE vascular graft
I. peritoneal catheter
impregnated
i. dressing
i. electrode
Impregum impression material
impression
i. material syringe
I. mattress
i. tonometer
Impress Softpatch urinary pad
IMProv cement
impulse
i. inertial exercise trainer
I. oxygen conserving device
IMSC five-hole nail
IMSI-Metripond operating room table
Imtec
I. BioBarrier membrane
I. premounted threaded implant
IMVbird

IMx PSA system
IMZ
IMZ endosteal implant
IMZ implant system
in
In Charge diabetes control system
in situ tricortical iliac crest block bone graft
in situ valve-cutter kit
in situ valve scissors
in vitro fertilization micropipette
in vivo H' magnetic resonance spectroscopy
Inaba and Ezaki dissector
inactive electrode
Inamura small incision capsulorrhexis forceps
INC
inside-the-needle catheter
Inc.
Cardiac Pacemaker, I.
Medical support Systems, I.
Orthopedic Systems I. (OSI)
SERTEC International, I.
Yellow Springs Instrument Co., I. (YSI)
incandescent
i. endoscope lamp
i. sheath
Incardia valve system
InCare
I. brace
I. pelvic floor therapy office system
INCA system
Incavo wire passer
Incenti-neb nebulizer
incentive spirometer
In-Ceram
I.-C. Alumina bonding
I.-C. Cerestore bonding
I.-C. Dicor bonding
I.-C. Empress bonding
I.-C. Fortress bonding
I.-C. Optec bonding
I.-C. Spinell bonding
Incert
I. bioabsorbable implantable sponge
I. sponge
Incise drape
incision
i. dilator
i. knife
i. retractor
i. spreader
Incisor arthroscopic blade
Inclan graft
inclination guidewire
inclinometer
Incono bag
incontinence clamp
Incorporated
Holllister I.
incubator
double-walled i.

incubator *(continued)*
    Forma water-jacketed i.
    Ohmeda Care-Plus i.
incudostapedial joint knife
incus replacement prosthesis
Indeflator
    ACS I.
indentation tonometer
indenter
    diamond pyramid i.
independent jaw
in-depth shoe
Indermil tissue adhesive
index
    bispectral i.
    Sokolow electrocardiographic i.
indexed splint
Index Knobber II massage tool
Indiana
    I. reamer
Indian club needle
India rubber suture
indicator
    AccuAngle i.
    Berens-Tolman ocular
      hypertension i.
    finger i.
    fundamental frequency i.
    Neesone root canal depth i.
    ocular hypertension i.
    Pio root canal depth i.
indifferent electrode
indirect
    i. laser ophthalmoscope
    i. retainer
indocyanine green angiogram
Indomitable scanner
Indong Oh prosthesis
industrial
    i. spectacles
    I. Work brace
indwelling
    16Ch, 18Ch i. silicone catheter
    i. Foley catheter
    i. nonvascular shunt
    i. subclavian catheter
    i. transcutaneous vascular access
      device
    i. ureteral stent
    i. venous catheter
Inerpan flexible burn dressing
inertial suction sampler
In-Exsufflator respiratory device
infant
    i. abdominal retractor
    i. abduction splint
    i. Ambu resuscitator
    i. biopsy forceps
    i. bronchoscope
    i. dilator
    i. esophagoscope
    i. eyelid retractor
    i. female catheter
    I. Flow nasal CPAP system

    i. Karickhoff laser lens
    i. male catheter
    i. nasal cannula assembly
    i. passive mitt
    i. rib retractor
    i. rib shears
    I. Star high-frequency 500/950
      ventilator
    i. telescope
    i. three-mirror laser lens
    i. urethrotome
    i. urethrotome blade
    i. ventilation monitor
infantometer
    Infantrac i.
    Measure Mat i.
Infantrac infantometer
In-Fast
    I.-F. bone screw system
    I.-F. cystourethropexy
inferior
    i. vena cava catheter
    i. vena cava clip
    i. vena cava umbrella filter
InFerno moist heat therapy
infiltration cannula
infiltrator
    Klein i.
    I. local drug delivery device
Infiniti
    I. catheter
    I. catheter introducer system
Infinity
    I. hip system
    I. modular hip prosthesis
    I. sensor
    I. stirrups
InFix interbody fusion system
inflatable
    i. elbow splint
    i. Foley bag catheter
    i. mammary prosthesis
    i. Mentor penile prosthesis
    i. penile prosthesis
    i. thoracic lumbosacral orthosis
    i. tourniquet cuff
    i. tracheal tube cuff
inflated balloon
inflator
    Bonney retrograde i.
    LeVeen i.
    Ogden-Senturia eustachian i.
    rapid cuff i.
inflow cannula
InfraGuide
    I. delivery system
    Heraeus LaserSonics I.
infraguide tip
infrared
    i. applicator
    i. coagulator
    i. laser-Doppler flowmeter
    i. light-emitting diode
    i. liver scanner

i. optometer
i. ray photocoagulator
infrared-beam diode laser
Infrasonics ventilator
Infumed pump
infundibular
i. forceps
i. punch
InfuO.R. drug delivery pump
Infusaid
I. catheter
I. Infuse-a-Port
I. infusion pump
I. needle
InfusaSleeve
I. II catheter
Kaplan-Simpson I.
LocalMed I.
Infuse-A-Cath catheter
Infuse-a-Port
I.-a.-P. catheter
Infusaid I.-a.-P.
I.-a.-P. port
I.-a.-P. pump
I.-a.-P. vascular access system
infuser, infusor
Alton Deal pressure i.
ANNE anesthesia i.
BP Cuff pressure i.
Critikon pressure i.
Dento-Infuser i.
Ethox Surgi-Press pressure i.
Heart pillow i.
MicroFuse I.
Ohio pressure i.
Paragon i.
Parker micropump insulin i.
PCA i.
pen pump insulin i.
Single-Day Baxter i.
Travenol i.
Infuset
I. GP syringe
I. T fluid delivery system
infusible pressure infusion bag
infusion
i. cannula
i. catheter
i. device
i. handpiece
i. port
i. pump
i. suction vitreous cutter
i. tube
infusion/infiltration cannula
infusor (var. of infuser)
Infu-Surg pressure infuser bag
Ingals
I. antral cannula
I. flexible silver cannula
I. nasal speculum
I. rectal injection cannula

Inge
I. laminar spreader
I. laminectomy retractor
Ingersoll
I. adenoid curette
I. tonsillar needle
Ingold M-series glass electrode pH monitor
Ingraham-Fowler
I.-F. clip-applying forceps
I.-F. cranium clip
I.-F. tantalum clip
Ingraham skull punch
Ingram
I. bicycle seat
I. catheter
I. trocar
ingress/egress cannula
inguinal truss
inhalation
i. breath unit
i. cannula
inhalator
OIC emergency oxygen i.
Oxy-Quik Mark IV oxygen i.
inhaler
AeroChamber bronchial i.
AeroChamber metered-dose i.
AERx electronic i.
breath-operated i.
Chiesi powder i.
Diskhaler i.
Diskus i.
dry-powder i.
Easi-Breathe i.
FOII powder i.
Henderson-Haggard i.
Inhalet i.
InspirEase i.
Junker i.
metered-dose i. (MDI)
Nebuhaler i.
Orion i.
Oxford miniature vaporizer i.
Rondo i.
Schimelbusch i.
Spinhaler i.
Spiral Mark V portable ultrasonic drug i.
Turbuhaler i.
ultrasound i.
Inhalet inhaler
inherent filter
inhibitor
PREMIX-SLIP premixed instrument milk lubricant and rust i.
vaporizing rust i.
initial incision retractor
initiator drill
InjecAid system
Injectate probe
injection
i. cannula
i. electrode catheter

Innovation plate

injection *(continued)*
 i. gold probe
 i. needle
Injectoflex respirator jet
injector
 Amplatz i.
 auto i.
 automatic twin syringe i.
 Bioject jet i.
 Cordis i.
 Dermo-Jet high-pressure i.
 Dyonics syringe i.
 EpiE-Z Pen epinephrine i.
 extractor i.
 E-Z Ject i.
 E-Z 'Jector i.
 Fujinon variceal i.
 Harris uterine i. (HUI)
 Hercules power i.
 HUI Mini-Flex uterine i.
 Lakatos Teflon i.
 Marcon-Haber varices i.
 Medi-Jector i.
 Medrad automated power i.
 Medrad contrast medium i.
 Medrad Mark IV angiographic i.
 Medrad power angiographic i.
 Miller ratchet i.
 Mill-Rose esophageal i.
 Mini-Flex flexible Harris uterine i.
 modified Mark IV R-wave-triggered
   power i.
 Olympus 13 L i.
 Peninject 2.25 i.
 power i.
 pressure i.
 PulseSpray i.
 Renovist II i.
 Robinject needle i.
 Rowden uterine manipulator i.
   (RUMI)
 Syrijet Mark II Needleless I.
 Taveras i.
 Teflon i.
 Tubex i.
 uterine i.
 Virag i.
ink
 Bonney blue i.
inlay implant
inlet
 Berry rotating i.
 Fish i.
 i. forceps
in-line
 i.-l. blood gas monitor
 i.-l. trap
 i.-l. venous pressure monitor
Inmed whistle tip urethral catheter
inner
 i. heel wedge
 i. lip plate
InnerDyne trocar

innerspring
 Nylex II Convoluted i.
Innervision MR scanner
Innoboot night splint
Innomed
 I. arthroplasty measuring system
 I. Assistant Free surgical instrument
 I. bone curette
Innova
 I. feminine incontinence treatment
   system
 I. home incontinence therapy system
 I. pelvic floor stimulator
Innovasive Devices ROC XS suture
 anchor
Innovative Medical Products Steri-Clamp
InnovaTome microkeratome device
Innovator Holter system
Innsbruck electrode
Inokucki vascular stapler
inorganic dental cement
Inoue
 I. balloon catheter
 I. self-guiding balloon
Inpersol peritoneal dialysis set
InPouch TV subculture kit
input
 i. device
 I. PS introducer
Inrad HiLiter ultrasound-enhanced stylet
Inro
 I. surgical nail
Inronail
 I. fingernail prosthesis
 I. toenail prosthesis
INRO surgical nail
Insall-Burstein
 I.-B. II modular knee system
 I.-B. intracondylar total knee
   implant
 I.-B. knee prosthesis
 I.-B. posterior stabilizer
Insall-Burstein-Freeman total knee
 instrumentation
insemination
 i. dish
 intrauterine i. (IUI)
insert
 articular i.
 Bidet toilet i.
 clamp i.
 Dischler rectoscopic suction i.
 Durasul polyethylene, high wear
   resistant acetabular i.
 Endostat calibration pod i.
 Energy Plus shoe i.
 FemSoft urethral i.
 Fogarty i.
 Fogarty-Hydragrip i.
 Fogarty-Softjaw i.
 Gel-Sole shoe i.
 Hapad felt i.
 Hapad shoe i.
 Hollister disposable Convex i.
 Hydrajaw i.

Johnson & Johnson PFC cruciate-substituting i.
New York University i.
Orthex Relievers shoe i.
Osteonics Scorpio i.
Poly-Dial i.
POWERPoint orthotic shoe i.
P.R. heat moldable i.
Profix confirming tibial i.
Reliance urinary control i.
retainer i.
Roho solid seat i.
Softjaw i.
S-ROM Poly-Dial i.
Sur-Fit disposable Convex i.
urinary control urethral i.
Warm'N'Form i.
inserter, insertor
AMO-PhacoFlex lens and i.
Buck femoral cement restrictor i.
cement restrictor i.
cement spacer i.
DDT lock screw i.
deluxe FIN pin i.
diaphragm i.
Kirschner wire i.
Lehner II i.
Lens-Eze i.
Moon-Robinson prosthesis i.
Mport lens i.
Prodigy lens i.
Robinson-Moon prosthesis i.
Shaffner orthopaedic i.
spacer i.
Storz i.
subperiosteal glass bead i.
Texas Scottish Rite Hospital hook i.
twist-in drain tube i.
Tytan tube i.
ventilation tube i.
insertion forceps
inside-the-needle
i.-t.-n. catheter (INC)
i.-t.-n. infusion catheter
Insight
I. knee positioning and alignment system
InSIGHT manometry system
insole
Comf-Orthotic 3/4 length i.
Comf-Orthotic sports replacement i.
Darco moldable i.
Diab-A-Foot rocker i.
Diab-A-Pad i.
Diab-A-Sole i.
Diabetic Diagnostic I.
D-Soles i.
EMED i.
Ever-Flex i.
Flexi-Therm diabetic diagnostic i.
Hapad metatarsal i.
Kinetic Wedge molded i.
molded postpartum i.
Orthex reliever i.

PAL Diasole i.
Plexidure i.
Poron 400 i.
PPT MXL soft molded i.
PPT Plastazote i.
PPT RX firm molded i.
ProThotics i.
PumpPals shoe i.'s
silicone i.
Spenco i.
S-Soles i.
TechnoGel i.
Viscoped i.
inspirator
Inspire
Medtronic I.
InspirEase
I. device
I. inhaler
inspirometer
Inspiron
I. Instromedix computer
I. small inspiratory training device
Inspirx incentive spirometer
Insta-Mold
I.-M. ear protection device
I.-M. silicone ear impression material
Insta-Nerve device
instant
i. cold pack
I. Fever Tester thermometer
I. Response technology generator
i. skin hook
Insta-Pulse heart rate monitor
Insta-Putty silicone ear plug
InstaScan scanner
Instat
I. collagen absorbable hemostat
I. collagen absorbable hemostatic agent
I. MCH microfibrillar collagen hemostat
Insta-Temp
Diatek 9000 I.-T.
InstaTrak
I. system
I. System image-guided surgery
Instead feminine protection cup
InStent
I. CarotidCoil stent
INSTRA-mate instrument-holding spring
Instron machine
instrument
Abradabloc dermabrasion i.
Accu-Line distal femoral resection i.
Accu-Line patellar i.
Accurate Surgical and Scientific I.'s (ASSI)
AccuSharp i.
activating adjusting i. (AAI)
Acufex MosaicPlasty i.
Alcon Surgical i.'s
American Hydron i.'s
arterial oscillator endarterectomy i.

instrument *(continued)*

Arthrotek Ellipticut hand i.'s
Ascon i.'s
A13 Sequel programmable behind-the-ear hearing i.
ASSI S&T microsurgical i.
Atlas orthogonal percussion i.
Austin middle ear i.
Auto Ref-keratometer i.
AxyaWeld i.
Ayerst i.'s
BabyBeat ultrasound i.
BackBiter i.
Backlund stereotactic i.
Bard BladderScan bladder volume i.
i. basket
bibeveled cutting i.
Biomer microsuturing i.
Biophysic Ophthascan S i.
bone abduction i.
Bone Grafter i.
Britetrac fiberoptic i.
Carl Zeiss i.'s
Carter Tubal Assistant surgical i.
Ceprate SC I. II
cervical range-of-motion i.
Chang Quick Chop combo ophthalmic i.
Cheshire-Poole-Yankauer suction i.
chiropractic adjusting i.
Clarke stereotactic i.
ClearCut 2 i.
Cloward i.
Cobb spinal i.
i. coding tape
Collis TDR i.
conization i.
contour-facilitating i.
Cooley neonatal i.
Corex i.
CRIT-LINE i.
cryosurgical i.
currycomb i.
Daisy I&A i.
Daniel EndoForehead i.
Delcom filling i.
diamond i.
Diamond-Lite cardiovascular i.
Diamond-Lite titanium i.
digitized i.
Disk-Criminator i.
Dix double-ended i.
Dolphin i.
DORC backflush i.
DORC surgical i.'s
DSP Micro Diamond-Point microsurgery i.
Dualine digital hearing i.
Duette double lumen ERCP i.
Dwyer i.
Dyonics arthroscopic i.
EarCheck Pro i.
Eckardt Heme-Stopper i.
ECTRA carpal tunnel i.

Endoflex endoscopy i.
Endoloop chromic ligature suture i.
EndoMax advanced laparoscopic i.
endosonography i.
Endo Stitch i.
Endotrac endoscopy i.
EndoWrist i.
ESI Lite-Pipe fiberoptic i.
ESI Lite-Pipe plastic surgery i.
eXcel-DR disposable/reusable i.
Exprin DQ1 biopsy i.
falloposcope endoscopic i.
FirstStep tibial osteotomy i.'s
Fleming conization i.
Forte ES i.
Friatec manual arthroscopy i.
G-C filling i.
Glick i.
gnathologic i.
Gobble Plus removal i.
Godina vessel-fixation i.
GPX rotary i.
Graefe i.
graft measuring i.
Guilford-Wright middle ear i.
guillotine vitrectomy i.
Halifax fine adjustment i.
Hall large bone i.
Hall series 4 large bone i.
Hancke/Vilmann biopsy handle i.
Henry Schein filling i.
i. holder
Horico diamond i.
Hough middle ear i.
House middle ear i.
Hyflex X-File i.
I&A i.
IBF knee i.
I.L.MED i.
Imount i.
Innomed Assistant Free surgical i.
IOLAB titanium i.
ionization i.
IOS immunodiagnostic testing i.
ISI laparoscopic i.
Isse Endo Brow i.
ITD-FG dental diamond i.
Johnson Endobag i.
Jordan middle ear i.
Jordan strut-measuring i.
Kapp surgical i.
Karl Ilg i.'s
Keeler cryosurgical i.
Kerato-Kontours i.'s
Kimberley diamond i.
KinetiX i.
Kirkland i.
Kirschner surgical i.
Kitner blunt dissecting i.
knot-tying i.
Koh ultramicro i.
Kos middle ear i.
Krwawicz cataract cryosurgical i.
Küntscher nail i.
K x-ray fluorescence i.

Ladmore plastic filling i.
LapTie i.
LapTie endoscopic knot-tying i.
ligature-passing i.
Lusk i.
MacKinnon-Dellon Diskriminator i.
I. Makar biodegradable interference
  screw
Malis bipolar i.
Marlow Primus i.
Matsuda titanium surgical i.'s
McCabe measuring i.
McCall i.
McGee middle ear i.
mechanical radial-scanning i.
Medicon i.
3M filling i.
Micro-Aire pneumatic power i.
Micro Diamond-Point
  microsurgery i.
micro-Doppler i.
Micromedics surgical i.
Micro-Three microsurgery i.
Midas Rex pneumatic i.
Millet neurological test i.
Miracompo filling i.
Mitek SuperAnchor i.
Mity Roto rotary i.
M4 Kerr Safety Hedstrom i.
Model TC2-64B pulsed-range gated
  Doppler i.
Monarch II bleaching i.
Monogram total knee i.
myoma fixation i.
NeoKnife electrosurgical i.
Neuro-Trace i.
Newport medical i.
Nicolet Compass
  electromyography i.
Nordent filling i.
Nucleotome Endoflex i.
oblique-forward-viewing i.
Obwegeser orthognathic surgery i.'s
OPG-Gee i.
Ortho-Athrex i.
orthopedic cutting i.
OrthoVise orthopaedic i.
Paparella middle ear i.
Partnership i.
pencil-grip i.
Pen-Probe i.
pistol-grip i.
Plastibell compression i.
plugging i.
point-search i.
Polaris reusable laparoscopic i.
polytome i.
Precision tack i.
ProFile variable taper rotary i.
ProLine endoscopic i.
PROloop i.
pulsed-range gated Doppler i.
Purstring disposable i.
Quantec endodontic i.
Quinton suction biopsy i.

Radionics bipolar i.
Rancho external fixation i.
reciprocal planing i.
reduction i.
Reichert Ultramatic Rx Master
  Phoroptor refracting i.
Retinomax refractometry i.
i. retrieval container
RingLoc i.
Rizzuti-Bonaccolto i.'s
Rizzuti-Fleischer i.'s
Rizzuti-Kayser-Fleischer i.'s
Rizzuti-Lowe i.'s
Rizzuti-Maxwell i.'s
Rizzuti-Soemmering i.
Roboprep G i.
Rosenberg gynecomastia dissection i.
Rosen middle ear i.
rotary cutting i.
Ruggles surgical i.
Rumex titanium i.'s
Safco diamond i.
Salinger reduction i.
Scheer middle ear i.
Schlesinger i.
Schneider PTCA i.
Schuknecht middle ear i.
ScoliTron i.
screwdriver i.
Semmes-Weinstein monofilament i.
Sensonic plaque removal i.
Sharpoint cutting i.
Shea middle ear i.
single-beveled cutting i.
single-plane i.
single-reference-point i.
SITE I&A i.
slotted i.
small-diameter endosonographic i.
Smith-Miller-Patch cryosurgical i.
Snowden-Pencer laparoscopic
  cholecystectomy i.
Sofamor spinal i.
solid-state i.
spark-gap i.
SpeedReducer i.
Splintrex i.
spring loaded biopsy i.
i. stabilizer pad
Steele filling i.
stereotaxic i.
Stratus i.
strut measuring i.
Surgi-Tron thoracoscopic i.
Sutcliffe laser shield and
  retracting i.
Sutherland rotatable microsurgery i.
Suture Assistant i.
suturing i.
Take-apart i.
Tessier craniofacial i.
test handle i.
The Treaser surgical i.
Thomas Kapsule i.'s
Todd-Wells stereotaxic i.

instrument *(continued)*
    topographic scanning/indocyanine green angiography combination i.
    Ultra-Cut Cobb spinal i.
    ultrasonic bone-cutting i.
    UniPuls electrostimulation i.
    Unitech i.'s
    Universal nasal i. handle
    ureteral visualization i.
    Uroloop i.
    UTAS 2000 electroretinography i.
    Valleylab laparoscopic i.
    VAPORbar i.
    VAPORloop i.
    Vibrasonic hearing i.
    Wallach minifreezer cryosurgical i.
    Wiet graft-measuring i.
    Wigand endoscopic i.
    Wright-Guilford middle ear i.
    XP peritympanic hearing i.
    XQ video i.
    Yasargil-Aesculap i.

instrumentation
    Accu-Line knee i.
    advanced breast biopsy i. (ABBI)
    anterior distraction i.
    AO fixateur interne i.
    AO notched i.
    ArthroPlastics ankle i.
    Baxter V. Mueller laparoscopic i.
    biofeedback i.
    Bio-Moore II i.
    Caspar anterior i.
    C-D i.
    compression U-rod i.
    Cotrel-Dubousset i. (CDI)
    Cotrel-Dubousset pedicle screw i.
    Cotrel-Dubousset pedicular i.
    Cotrel-Dubousset spinal i.
    craniofacial i.
    distraction i.
    double Zielke i.
    Dwyer i.
    dynamic compression plate i.
    Edwards i.
    EEG and PSG i.
    EndoMax endoscopic i.
    Gellman i.
    halo-Ilizarov distraction i.
    Harms-Moss anterior thoracic i.
    Harrington distraction i.
    Harrington-Kostuik i.
    Harrington rod i.
    Harrington spinal i.
    IBF total knee i.
    Imount i.
    Insall-Burstein-Freeman total knee i.
    InSurg laparoscopic i.
    interspinous segmental spinal i.
    Jacobs locking hook spinal rod i.
    Kambin i.
    Kambin-Gellman i.
    Kaneda anterior spinal i.
    Karl Storz i.

    Kostuik-Harrington spinal i.
    I. Laboratory system
    Louis i.
    L-rod i.
    lumbosacral spine transpedicular i.
    Luque II segmental spinal i.
    Luque semirigid segmental spinal i.
    Microvasive i.
    MIDA CoroNet i.
    Midas Rex i.
    modular i.
    Moss i.
    Moss-Miami spinal i.
    Mueller laparoscopic i.
    multiple hook assembly C-D i.
    Passport i.
    posterior distraction i.
    posterior hook-rod spinal i.
    Putti-Platt i.
    Russell-Taylor interlocking nail i.
    sacral spine modular i.
    sacral spine Universal i.
    segmental spinal i.
    Smith-Richards i.
    Steffee spinal i.
    stereotactic i.
    Stryker power i.
    TAG i.
    Texas Scottish Rite Hospital (TSRH) i.
    Zielke pedicular i.

instrument-grasping forceps
instruments
InstruWipes surgical sponge
insufflation device
insufflator
    Bonney i.
    Buckstein colonic i.
    colonic i.
    Dench i.
    DyoPneumatic i.
    Eder i.
    gas i.
    HiTec i.
    hysteroscopic i.
    Kelly i.
    Kidde tubal i.
    laparoscopic i.
    Medicam 900 i.
    Milex vaginal i.
    Neal i.
    Op-Pneu i.
    Pneumomat laparoscopic i.
    Semm Pelvi-Pneu i.
    Sieger i.
    Snowden-Pencer i.
    Stille i.
    Storz Laparoflator i.
    variable flow i.
    Venturi i.
    Weber colonic i.
    Wisap i.
Insuflon insulin delivery device
insulated
    i. bayonet forceps

i. curved scissors
i. electrode needle
i. gate field-effect transistor
i. knife handle
i. monopolar forceps
i. straight scissors
i. tissue forceps

InsulScan
Insul-Sheath vaginal speculum sheath
InSurg
I. common bile duct (CBD) basket
I. laparoscopic instrumentation
I. LapTie needle driver suturing device

InSync
I. cardiac stimulator
inSync miniform
Intac
In-Tac bone anchoring system
Intacs
I. corneal ring implant
I. intrastromal corneal ring

Intact
I. catheter
I. xenograft valve

Intec
I. AID cardioverter-defibrillator generator
I. implantable defibrillator

Integra
I. artificial skin
I. catheter
I. II balloon
I. skin replacement system
I. tissue expander

integral
I. distal centralizer
I. hip system
I. Interlok femoral prosthesis
I. Omniloc implant
i. uniformity scintillation camera

integrated
I. Ankle orthotic ankle joint
i. automatic stone-tissue detection system
i. electromyography
i. headholder
i. lead system
i. life support system
i. sideport access portal

Integriderm mattress
Integris
I. cardiac imaging system
I. cardiovascular imaging
I. 3000 scanner
I. V3000 imager

Integrity
I. acetabular cup
I. acetabular cup prosthesis
I. acetabular cup screw
I. neutral liner
I. shell

InteguDerm dressing

Intelect
I. Legend stimulator
I. 600MP microcurrent stimulator
Intellicath pulmonary artery catheter
Intelliject pump
IntelliJet fluid management system
intensified
I. Radiographic Imaging System
i. radiographic imaging system scanner

intensifier
C-arm image i.
OEC-Diasonics mobile C-arm image i.

intensifying screen
Inteq
I. small joint suturing system
I. TFC repair kit
Interad whole body CT scanner
Interax total knee system
interbody
i. fusion rasp
i. graft tamp
intercalary allograft
intercardiac sucker
Intercede graft
Interceed
I. absorbable adhesion barrier
I. barrier material
Interceptor M3 triple-channel, solid-state monitor
interchangeable
i. vein stripper
i. vein stripper olive
intercostal
i. catheter
i. drain
i. trocar
interdental splint
interdigitating coil stent
interface
I. arterial blood filter
Monarch Mini Mask nasal i.
Quicknet monitor i.
ShearGuard low-friction i.
interference
i. barrier filter
i. screw
interferential
i. stimulator
i. therapy
interferometer
Fizeau-Tolansky i.
Interfit-Pharmacea Intermedic intraocular lens
InterFix
I. RP threaded spinal fusion "cage" device
I. titanium threaded spinal fusion cage
Interflux intraocular lens
interfragmentary
i. lag screw
i. plate
InterGard knitted collagen

interimplant papillary template
interlaminar clamp
Interlink
    I. injection cap
    I. threaded lock cannula
interlocking
    i. detachable coil
    i. sound
Interlok primary femoral component
INtermate
    Baxter I.
intermaxillary wire
intermediate
    i. C-D hook
    i. splint
Intermedics
    I. atrial antitachycardia pacemaker
    I. Cyberlith X multiprogrammable pacemaker
    I. intraocular lens implant
    I. intraocular tonometer
    I. lens
    I. lithium-powered pacemaker
    I. Marathon dual-chamber rate-responsive pacemaker
    I. natural hip system
    I. Natural-Knee knee prosthesis
    I. phaco I & A unit
    Pharmacia I.
    I. Quantum unipolar pacemaker
    I. RES-Q implantable cardioverter-defibrillator
    I. Stride pacemaker
    I. Thinlith II pacemaker

intermittent
    i. extremity pump
    i. flow machine
internal
    i. cervical device
    i. ear prosthesis
    i. fiberoptic cable
    i. fixation device
    i. fixation spring
    i. hex-thread connection
    i. monitor
    i. nucleus hydrodelineation needle
    i. tibial torsion brace
International
    I. Biomedical Mode 745-100 microcapillary infusion system
    I. compression system
    I. standard goniometer
    I. 10-20 system
Inter-Op acetabular prosthesis
interosseous wire
Interpore
    I. bone replacement material
    I. ceramic material
    I. hydroxyapatite
    I. IMZ implant system
    I. osteointegrated implant
    I. 200 porous hydroxyapatite
Interpret ultrasound catheter
interprobe system

interrupted pledgeted suture
Interseal acetabular cup
intersegmental table
Intersept cardiotomy reservoir
Interson biopsy needle guide
Intersorb
    I. absorptive burn pad
    I. fine mesh gauze
    I. six-ply absorbent roll stretch gauze
    I. wide mesh gauze
interspace
    i. shaper
    i. width marker
    I. YAG laser lens
Interspec XL ultrasound
interspinous
    i. cable
    i. segmental spinal instrumentation
Interstate spatula
interstitial implant
Intertach
    I. II pacer
    I. pacemaker
Intertech
    I. anesthesia breathing circuit
    I. Mapleson D nonrebreathing circuit
    I. nonrebreathing modified Jackson-Rees circuit
    I. Perkin-Elmer gas sampling line
Intertherapy intravascular ultrasound
Intertron therapy microprocessor
intervener
    Love-Gruenwald i.
interventional catheter
intervertebral
    i. curette
    i. disk forceps
    i. disk rongeur
    i. spreader
Interzeag bowl perimeter
intestinal
    i. anastomosis clamp
    i. anastomosis forceps
    i. bag
    i. closing forceps
    i. decompression trocar
    i. holding forceps
    i. occlusion clamp
    i. occlusion retractor
    i. plication needle
    i. resection clamp
    i. ring clamp
    i. tissue forceps
in-the-bag lens
in-the-ear (ITE)
    i.-t.-e. hearing aid
    i.-t.-e. listening device
Intimax
    I. biliary catheter
    I. cholangiography catheter
    I. occlusion catheter
    I. vascular catheter

intraaortic
- i. balloon assist device
- i. balloon catheter
- i. balloon pump (IABP)
- i. counterpulsation balloon

IntraArc 9963 arthroscopic power system

intraarterial
- i. cannula
- i. chemotherapy catheter

intracapsular
- i. lens expressor
- i. lens expressor hook
- i. lens forceps
- i. lens loop

intracardiac
- i. accelerometer
- i. cannula
- i. catheter
- i. needle holder
- i. retractor
- i. sucker
- i. sucker guard
- i. suction tube
- i. sump tube

intracardial shunt
Intracath catheter
intracavitary afterloading applicator
Intracell
- I. mechanical muscle device
- I. myofascial trigger-point device
- I. Sprinter stick

intracerebral depth electrode
intracervical
- i. bag
- i. device (ICD)

intracochlear implant
Intracone intramedullary reamer
intracorneal lens
intracoronal retainer
intracoronary
- i. Doppler flow wire
- i. guiding catheter
- i. perfusion catheter
- i. stent

intracranial
- i. pressure catheter
- i. pressure Express digital monitor
- i. pressure monitoring device
- i. pressure monitor screw

IntraDop
- Doppler I.
- I. intraoperative Doppler
- I. probe

Intraducer
- I. peritoneal cannula
- I. peritoneal catheter

intraductal
- i. imaging catheter
- i. ultrasound
- i. ultrasound probe

intradural retractor
IntraEAR Round Window u Cath RWuCath
Intrafix tibial fastener

Intraflex
- I. intramedullary pin
- I. intramedullary pin extractor

intragastric
- i. balloon
- i. cannula
- i. continuous pH-meter meter

intraligamentary syringe
IntraLuminal
- I. Safe-Steer guidewire system

intraluminal
- i. probe
- i. reference electrode
- i. stapler
- i. suture
- i. ultrasound

intrameatal
- i. earphone
- i. electrode

Intramed angioscopic valvulotome
Intramedic PE-50 polyethylene tubing
intramedullary
- i. alignment rod
- i. ANK nail
- i. bar
- i. broach
- i. brush
- i. canal plug
- i. catheter
- i. drill
- i. fixation device
- i. guide
- i. illuminator
- i. (IM) nail
- i. pin
- i. reamer
- i. Rush rod
- i. supracondylar multihole nail

Intran
- I. disposable intrauterine pressure measurement
- I. intrauterine pressure measurement catheter

intranasal
- i. bivalve splint
- i. hammer

intraocular
- i. balloon
- i. hook
- i. irrigating forceps
- i. lens (IOL)
- i. lens cannula
- i. lens dialer
- i. lens folder
- i. lens forceps
- i. lens glide
- i. lens implant
- i. tension recorder

Intra-Op autotransfusion system
intraoperative ultrasonic probe
IntraOptics
- I. intraocular lens
- I. lensometer

intraoral
- i. fracture appliance

intraoral *(continued)*
    i. stent
    i. titanium mandibular distraction
      device
intraorbital implant
intraosseous needle
intrapartum monitor
intraperitoneal onlay mesh
intrapleural
    i. catheter
    i. sealed drainage unit
intraportal endovascular ultrasonography
Intra-Prostatic stent
Intrascan ultrasound
intrascapular roll
Intrasil catheter
IntraSite
    I. gel applipak
    I. gel wound dressing
IntraSonix TULIP laser device
Intrasound
    Medtronic Pulsor I.
intraspinal drug infusion system
IntraStent
    I. DoubleStent biliary endoprosthesis
    I. DoubleStrut biliary endoprosthesis
intrathoracic forceps
intraurethral
    i. coil
    i. prostatic bridge catheter
intrauterine
    i. balloon cannula
    i. balloon-type cannula
    i. catheter (IUC)
    i. device (IUD)
    i. insemination (IUI)
    i. insemination cannula
    i. insemination cannula with
      mandrel
    i. insemination catheter
    i. pessary
    i. pressure catheter
    i. pressure monitor
intravaginal ring
intravascular
    i. catheter electrode
    i. Doppler-tipped guide wire
    i. stent
    i. ultrasound catheter
intravenous
    i. accurate control device
    i. needle
    i. pacing catheter
    i. Soluset
    i. ultrasound catheter
intravenous-enhanced MRI
intraventricular
    i. pressure monitoring catheter
intravitreal
    i. cryoprobe
    i. laser

Intrepid
    I. balloon catheter

    I. percutaneous transluminal
      coronary angioplasty catheter
    I. PTCA catheter
intrinsic transverse connector
Intro Deuce double-lumen introducer
introducer
    ACS percutaneous i.
    Allen spherical eye i.
    Angestat hemostasis i.
    Angetear tear-away i.
    Atkinson i.
    Avanti i.
    Cardak percutaneous catheter i.
    Carter spherical eye i.
    catheter i.
    i. catheter
    Check-Flo i.
    Ciaglia percutaneous tracheostomy i.
    Cook micropuncture i.
    Cook Peel-Away i.
    Cope-Saddekni i.
    Davol pacemaker i.
    Desilets i.
    Desilets-Hoffman pacemaker i.
    Dumon-Gilliard prosthesis i.
    Encapsulon sheath i.
    endolymphatic shunt tube i.
    entrapment sack i.
    Eric Lloyd i.
    Eschmann endotracheal tube i.
    Excalibur i.
    FasTrac i.
    Goodhill strut i.
    gum elastic bougie i.
    i. gun
    Hall self-holding i.
    Hedwig i.
    Hemaquet i.
    H-H shunt i.
    Hickman percutaneous i.
    Holter i.
    House endolymphatic shunt tube i.
    I. II sheath
    Implantaid Di-Lock cardiac lead i.
    Input PS i.
    Intro Deuce double-lumen i.
    Littleford Spector i.
    Maryfield i.
    Micropuncture Peel-Away i.
    Morgan vent tube i.
    Moss T-anchor needle i.
    Neuroguide peel-away catheter i.
    Nottingham i.
    P.D. Access with Peel-Away
      needle i.
    peel-away i.
    Pennine-O'Neil urinary catheter i.
    pull-apart i.
    Ramses diaphragm i.
    Razi cannula i.
    Richardson polyethylene tube i.
    i. sheath
    silicone i.
    Speck i.
    sphere i.

split-sheath i.
stent i.
Storz vent tube i.
SupraFoley suprapubic i.
Taut percutaneous i.
Tuohy-Borst side-arm i.
UMI transseptal Cath-Seal
  catheter i.
Uni-Shunt with reservoir i.
USCI i.
ventricular catheter i.
Weaver trocar i.
Wellwood-Ferguson i.
introducing forceps
Introl bladder neck support prosthesis
Intron A multidose pen
intubation laryngoscope
Invacare
I. APM
I. APM mattress
I. padded shower chair
I. vinyl transfer bench
I. wheelchair
Invader
GiCi-400 I.
invaginator
Lempert i.
invalid
i. chair
i. cushion
i. ring
inverted
i. buttoned device
i. cone bur
i. U-pouch ileal reservoir
inverter
Barrett appendix i.
Damian i.
Mayo-Boldt i.
I. vitrectomy system
Wangensteen tissue i.
Invertrac equipment
Investa suture
INVOS
INVOS 3100 cerebral oximeter
INVOS 3100 cerebral oximeter
  monitoring system
INVOS transcranial cerebral
  oximeter
INX stent
Inyo nail
Ioban
I. antimicrobial incise drape
I. 2 iodophor cesarean sheet
I. Steri-drape
Iocare titanium needle
iodine
i. catgut suture
i. cup
iodized surgical gut suture
iodochromic catgut suture
Iodoflex
I. absorptive dressing
I. solid gel pad
iodoform-impregnated plastic sheet

iodophor-impregnated adhesive wrap
iodophor Steri-drape
Iodosorb absorptive dressing
Iogel intraocular lens
IOL
intraocular lens
AC IOL
  anterior chamber intraocular lens
accommodative IOL
IOL dialer
Hydroview foldable IOL
Kearney side-notch IOL
MemoryLens IOL
Staar low-diopter IOL
Staar Toric IOL
IOLAB
I. Azar intraocular lens
I. I&A photocoagulator
I. irrigating needle
I. Slimfit lens
I. taper-cut needle
I. taper-point needle
I. titanium instrument
I. titanium needle
Iomed Phoresor electrode
ion
i. chromatograph
i. laser
i. pump
Ionalyzer analyzer
Ionescu-Shiley
I.-S. aortic valve prosthesis
I.-S. artificial cardiac valve
I.-S. pericardial patch
I.-S. pericardial valve
I.-S. pericardial valve graft
I.-S. pericardial xenograft
I.-S. vascular graft
Ionescu tri-leaflet valve
Ionguard titanium modular head
  component
ionization
i. counter
i. instrument
ion-selective electrode
ion-sensitive field-effect transistor
ion-specific field effect transducer
Iontophor drug delivery system
iontophoresis
Dynaphor i.
i. electrode
iontophoretic applicator
Ioptex
I. intraocular lens
I. TabOptic lens
IOS immunodiagnostic testing instrument
Iovision implant
Iowa
I. membrane forceps
I. orbital implant
I. pudendal needle guide
I. State fixation forceps
I. stem
I. total hip prosthesis
I. trumpet

Iowa *(continued)*
>   I. trumpet needle guide
>   I. University periosteal elevator

Iowa-Mengert membrane forceps
IPAS
>   IPAS flexible cannula
>   IPAS syringe

IPC boots
IPCO-Partridge defibrillator
I-plate
>   Syracuse anterior I.-p.

I-Plus humeral brace
IPOP cast dressing
ipos
>   i. arch support system
>   i. heel relief orthosis
>   i. heel relief shoe

Irby head frame
Irene lens
Irex
>   I. Exemplar ultrasound
>   I. Exemplar ultrasound scanner

iridectomy scissors
iridium
>   i. needle
>   i. prosthesis

iridium-192 stent
iridocapsular intraocular lens
iridocapsulotomy scissors
iridodialysis spatula
iridotomy scissors
IRIS
>   I. OcuLight SLx indirect
>   ophthalmoscope delivery system
>   I. 10,000 overlay
>   I. pressure-reduction mattress
>   I. scanner

iris
>   i. bipolar forceps
>   i. claw lens
>   i. expressor
>   i. hook
>   i. hook cannula
>   i. knife
>   i. lens manipulator
>   i. microforceps
>   i. needle
>   I. Oculight SLx MicroPulse laser
>   i. repositor
>   i. retractor
>   i. scissors
>   i. spatula
>   i. suture microforceps
>   i. tissue forceps

iris-clip intraocular lens
Iriscorder recorder
iris-supported intraocular lens
IRMA blood gas analysis system
iron
>   Böhler i.
>   I. Intern retractor
>   Jewett bending i.
>   i. lung

>   Lusskin subungual hematoma i.
>   Pineda LASIK Flap I.

Irox endocardial pacing leads
irradiator
>   portable blood i.

Irri-Cath suction system
irrigating
>   i. cannula
>   i. catheter
>   i. cystitome
>   i. dialer
>   i. iris hook
>   i. lens loop
>   i. lens manipulator
>   i. mushroom retractor
>   i. notched spatula
>   i. probe
>   i. sheath
>   i. tip
>   i. uterine curette
>   i. vectis loop

irrigating and aspirating *(var. of*
irrigation and aspiration) **(I&A)**
irrigating-aspirating *(var. of* irrigation and
aspiration)
irrigating/aspirating
>   i. cannula
>   i. vectis

irrigating-positioning needle
irrigation
>   i. bipolar system
>   i. catheter

**irrigation and aspiration, irrigating-
aspirating, irrigating and aspirating,
irrigation-aspiration (I&A)**
irrigator
>   anterior chamber i.
>   antral i.
>   Barraquer i.
>   Baumrucker clamp i.
>   Bishop-Harman anterior chamber i.
>   Carabelli i.
>   Dento-Spray oral i.
>   DeVilbiss eye i.
>   Doss automatic percolator i.
>   Endo-Flo i.
>   endoscopic i.
>   Fink cul-de-sac i.
>   Fisch bone drill i.
>   Fluvog i.
>   Fox hydrostatic i.
>   Gibson anterior chamber i.
>   Goldstein anterior chamber i.
>   Gum Machine oral i.
>   Hartstein i.
>   Hollister colostomy i.
>   House-Radpour suction i.
>   House-Stevenson suction i.
>   House sucker i.
>   House T-tube i.
>   Hydrofloss electronic oral i.
>   HydroSurg laparoscopic i.
>   Irrijet i.
>   Kelman i.
>   Kemp i.

laser-assisted intrastromal
  keratomileusis flap i.
LASIK flap i.
Lukens double-channel i.
LySonix Delta Tip i.
McKenna Tide-Ur-Ator i.
Moncrieff anterior chamber i.
nasal i.
Nezhat i.
olive-tipped i.
Ortholav pulsed i.
Perio Pik i.
Perry ostomy i.
Pro Pulse i.
Radpour i.
Radpour-House suction i.
Randolph i.
Rollet anterior chamber i.
Shambaugh i.
Shea i.
Shooter Saeed multiband i.
sinus i.
Sterling-Sylva i.
Stopko i.
Stryker suction i.
suction i.
Sylva anterior chamber i.
Thornwald antral i.
Valentine i.
Vidaurri i.
Water Pik i.
Wells i.
Younge i.
Zimmer suction i.
Irrigo syringe
Irrijet
  I. DS irrigation system
  I. DS wound irrigation device
  I. irrigator
Irrivac syringe
Irvine
  I. corneal scissors
  I. I&A unit
  I. probe-pointed scissors
  I. viable organ-tissue transport
    system
IS1000 gel documentation imaging
system
Isaacs endometrial cell sampler
ISAH
  ISAH stereotactic immobilizing mask
I-S artificial cardiac valve
Isberg scleral plug
ISCH-DISH
  ISCH-DISH CFT pressure relieving
    seat surface
  ISCH-DISH Plus cushion
ischial
  i. containment socket
  i. weightbearing brace
  i. weightbearing prosthesis
ischial-gluteal weightbearing socket
iseikonic lens

Iselin forceps
Ishihara
  I. I-Temp cautery
  I. IV slit lamp
  I. pseudoisochromatic plate
  I. test chart book
ISI laparoscopic instrument
ISOBAR barostat distension device
Isobex dynamometer
Isocam
  I. scintillation imaging system
  I. SPECT imaging system
isochromatic plate
Isocon camera
isodiametric bipolar screw-in lead
isoelastic
  i. pelvic prosthesis
  i. rip clamp
Isoflex
  I. bed
  I. mattress
Isoflow pump
isokinetic Unex III exerciser
Isola
  I. fixation system
  I. hook-rod
  I. spinal implant system
  I. spinal implant system accessory
  I. spinal implant system anchor
  I. spinal implant system component
  I. spinal implant system eye rod
  I. spinal implant system hook
  I. spinal implant system iliac screw
  I. spinal instrumentation system
  I. vertebral screw
  I. wire
isolation
  i. bag
  i. face mask
  i. forceps
isolator
  I. blood culture system
  I. lysis-centrifugation tube
  Vickers i.
isolette
  Airshields i.
  double-bubble i.
Isolex 300i stem cell selection system
Isomet
  I. low speed saw
  I. Plus precision saw
isometer
  CA-5000 drill-guide i.
  tension i.
Isometer bone graft placement site
detector
isometric strain gauge
Isoprene plastic splint
Iso-Quadron exerciser
Isosal syringe
Isostent
  Bx I.
Isotac pilot wire

Isotechnologies
    I. B-200 back testing and rehabilitation system
    I. B-200 low back machine
Iso-Thermex 16-channel electronic thermometer
Isotoner glove
isotonic machine
isotopic pulse generator pacemaker
Isovis wound protector
Israel
    I. Benzedrine vaporizer
    I. blunt rake retractor
    I. camera
    I. nasal rasp
    I. suction tube
    I. tongue depressor
    I. tonsillar dissector
Isse Endo Brow instrument
i-STAT
    i.-S. hand-held analyzer
    i.-S. system
Itard eustachian catheter
ITC
    ITC radiopaque balloon catheter
ITD-FG dental diamond instrument
ITE
    in-the-ear
    ITE listening device
I-tech
    I.-t. cannula
    I.-t. cannula holder
    I.-t. cannula tray
    I.-t. intraocular foreign body forceps
    I.-t. needle holder
    I.-t. splinter forceps
    I.-t. tying forceps
I-tech-Castroviejo bladebreaker
ITI
    ITI dental implant
    ITI dental implant system
ITI-Benefit endosseous implant
ITO laser pen
Ito needle
Itrel
    I. II, III spinal cord stimulation system
    I. II quadripolar pulse generator
    I. I unipolar pulse generator
    I. programmed transmitter-receiver
ITVAD
IUC
    intrauterine catheter
IUD
    intrauterine device

    ParaGard T380 copper IUD
    IUD remover hook
IUI
    intrauterine insemination
    IUI disposable cannula
    IUI catheter
IV
    IV Align
    IV catheter
    IV needle
IVAC
    IVAC device
    IVAC 831 drip controller
    IVAC needleless IV system
    IVAC Temp Plus II thermometer
    IVAC ventilator
    IVAC volumetric infusion pump
IVAD
    implantable vascular access device
Ivalon
    I. compressed patch graft
    I. dressing
    I. embolic sponge
    I. foam
    I. lucite orbital eye implant
    I. prosthesis
    I. sponge
    I. sponge eye implant
    I. suture
    I. wire coil
Ivan
    I. laryngeal applicator
    I. nasopharyngeal applicator
IVEC-10 neurotransmitter analyzer
IV-enhanced MRI
Iverson dermabrader
Ives
    I. anoscope
    I. rectal speculum
Ives-Fansler anoscope
I.V. House wound cover
Ivinsco cervical dilator
Ivocryl resin
ivory
    I. rubber dam clamp
IVT percutaneous catheter introducer sheath
Ivy
    I. loop
    I. mastoid rongeur
    I. needle holder
    I. wire
Iwabuchi clip
Iwashi clamp approximator
Iwata-Ricky gonioscopic lens

J

J board
J exchange guidewire
J exchange wire
J needle
J orthogonal electrode
J pad
J Rosen guidewire
J-24 cervical orthosis
J-35 hyperextension orthosis
J-45 contraflexion orthosis
J-55
J-55 postfusion brace
J-55 postfusion orthosis
J-59 Florida brace
Jabaley scissors
Jabaley-Stille scissors
Jaboulay button
JACE
JACE continuous passive motion ankle system
JACE hand continuous passive motion unit
JACE knee brace
JACE shoulder exerciser
JACE W550 continuous passive motion (CPM) wrist device
JACE-STIM
JACE-STIM electrical stimulator
JACE-STIM electrotherapy unit
Jack
J. Frost hot/cold pack
jacket
body j.
Bonchek-Shiley cardiac j.
Boston soft body j.
Calot j.
cervicothoracic j.
cuirass j.
Daily cooling j.
Frejka j.
immobilization j.
Kydex body j.
Lexan j.
Low Profile plastic body j.
LS⁴ custom spinal j.
Medtronic cardiac cooling j.
Minerva back j.
Minerva plastic j.
Orfizip body j.
Orthoplast j.
plaster-of-Paris j.
Prenyl j.
Radix-Raney j.
Raney j.
Risser wedging j.
Royalite body j.
Sayre j.
Vitrathene j.
Von Lackum transection shift j.
Willock respiratory j.
Wilmington plastic j.

jacket-type chest dressing
Jackman
J. coronary sinus electrode catheter
J. orthogonal catheter
Jackson
J. alligator grasping forceps
J. anterior commissure laryngoscope
J. approximation forceps
J. aspirating tube
J. biopsy forceps
J. bite block
J. bone clamp
J. bone-extension clamp
J. bone-holding clamp
J. broad staple forceps
J. bronchial dilator
J. button forceps
J. cane-shaped tracheal tube
J. cone-shaped tracheal tube
J. conventional foreign body forceps
J. costophrenic bronchoscope
J. cross-action forceps
J. cylindrical-object forceps
J. double-concave rat-tooth forceps
J. double-prong forceps
J. down-jaw forceps
J. dressing forceps
J. dull-pointed forceps
J. dull rotation forceps
J. endoscopic forceps
J. esophageal dilator
J. esophageal scissors
J. esophageal shears
J. esophagoscope
J. fenestrated peanut-grasping forceps
J. fiberoptic slide laryngoscope
J. flexible upper lobe bronchus forceps
J. forward-grasping forceps
J. full-lumen bronchoscope
J. globular object forceps
J. head-holding forceps
J. hemostatic forceps
J. hollow-object forceps
J. imaging table
J. infant biopsy forceps
J. intervertebral disk rongeur
J. lacrimal intubation set
J. laryngeal applicator
J. laryngeal applicator forceps
J. laryngeal atomizer
J. laryngeal basket forceps
J. laryngeal-dressing forceps
J. laryngeal-grasping forceps
J. laryngeal punch forceps
J. laryngeal ring-rotation forceps
J. laryngeal scissors
J. laryngectomy tube
J. laryngofissure forceps
J. laryngostat
J. magnification ruler set

J

Jackson *(continued)*
J. open-end aspirating tube
J. papilloma forceps
J. perichondrial elevator
J. pin-bending costophrenic forceps
J. punch
J. punch forceps
J. radiopaque bougie
J. ring-jaw forceps
J. ring-rotation forceps
J. rod
J. self-retaining goiter retractor
J. sharp-pointed rotation forceps
J. side-curved forceps
J. silver tracheostomy tube
J. sister-hook forceps
J. sliding laryngoscope
J. spinal surgery table
J. sponge carrier
J. square punch tip
J. staging system
J. standard bronchoscope
J. standard laryngoscope
J. staple bronchoscope
J. steel-stem woven filiform bougie
J. tendon-seizing forceps
J. tracheal bistoury
J. tracheal bistoury knife
J. tracheal bougie
J. tracheal dilator
J. tracheal hemostat
J. tracheal hemostatic forceps
J. tracheal hook
J. tracheal retractor
J. tracheal scalpel
J. tracheal tenaculum
J. tracheal tube
J. tracheoscope
J. tracheotomic bistoury
J. triangular brass dilator
J. triangular-punch forceps
J. tunneler
J. turbinate scissors
J. vaginal retractor
J. vaginal speculum
J. velvet-eye aspirating tube
J. warning stop tube
Jackson-Moore shears
Jackson-Mosher cardiospasm dilator
Jackson-Plummer dilator
Jackson-Pratt
J.-P. bifurcated drain extension
J.-P. catheter
J.-P. dissector
J.-P. flat drain kit
J.-P. Gold wound drain
J.-P. Hemaduct drain
J.-P. hysterectomy kit
J.-P. large-volume round silicone drain kit
J.-P. large-volume suction reservoir
J.-P. PVC kit
J.-P. round PVC drain
J.-P. silicone flat drain

J.-P. silicone round drain
J.-P. suction drain
J.-P. suction tube
J.-P. T-tube drain
Jackson-Rees
J.-R. apparatus
J.-R. circuit
J.-R. endotracheal tube
Jackson-Trousseau dilator
Jacobaeus thoracoscope
Jacobaeus-Unverricht thoracoscope
Jacob capsule fragment forceps
Jacobs
J. biopsy forceps
J. capsular fragment forceps
J. chuck adapter
J. chuck drill
J. clamp
J. cranial hook
J. distraction rod
J. locking hook spinal rod
J. locking hook spinal rod instrumentation
J. snap-lock chuck
J. T-handled chuck
J. uterine tenaculum
J. vulsellum
J. vulsellum forceps
Jacobsen template
Jacobson
J. bayonet-shaped scissors
J. bipolar forceps
J. bladder retractor
J. blood vessel probe
J. blunt hook
J. bulldog clamp
J. counter-pressure elevator
J. curette
J. dressing forceps
J. endarterectomy spatula
J. fork
J. goiter retractor
J. hemostatic forceps
J. microbulldog clamp
J. microscissors
J. mosquito forceps
J. spring-handled needle holder
J. spring-handled scissors
J. suture pusher
J. vas deferens probe
J. vessel clamp
J. vessel knife
J. vessel punch
Jacobson-Potts vessel clamp
Jacobson-Vital needle holder
Jacobs-Palmer laparoscope
Jacob-Swan
J.-S. gonioprism
J.-S. gonioscope
J.-S. gonioscopic prism
J.-S. goniotomy pliers
Jacobus mammotome
Jacoby heel splint

Jacques
- J. catheter
- J. gastric tube

Jade Audio-Starr hearing aid

Jaeger
- J. acuity card
- J. eye chart
- J. keratome
- J. keratome knife
- J. LE3000 treadmill
- J. lid retractor
- J. metal lid plate
- J. reading chart
- J. strabismus hook

Jaeger-Whiteley catheter

Jaffe
- J. capsulorhexis forceps
- J. Cilco lens
- J. eyelid speculum
- J. intraocular spatula
- J. iris hook
- J. laser blepharoplasty and facial resurfacing set
- J. lens-manipulating hook
- J. lens spatula
- J. microlens hook
- J. needle holder
- J. one-piece all-PMMA intraocular lens
- J. suturing forceps
- J. wire lid retractor

Jaffe-Bechert nucleus rotator

Jaffe-Givner lid retractor

Jaffe-Maltzman
- J.-M. hook
- J.-M. lens manipulator

Jager meniscal forceps

Jagwire wire

Jahnke anastomosis clamp

Jahnke-Barron heart support net

Jahnke-Cook-Seeley clamp

jail
- stent j.

Jako
- J. clamp
- J. facial nerve monitor
- J. fine ball-tip hook
- J. knot pusher
- J. laryngeal forceps
- J. laryngeal knife
- J. laryngeal mirror
- J. laryngeal needle holder
- J. laryngeal probe
- J. laryngeal suction tube
- J. laryngoscope
- J. laser aspirating tube
- J. laser retractor
- J. laser trocar
- J. microlaryngeal cup forceps
- J. microlaryngeal grasping forceps
- J. microlaryngeal scissors
- J. microlaryngoscope
- J. suction-irrigator
- J. suction tube
- J. transilluminator

Jako-Cherry laryngoscope

Jako-Kleinsasser
- J.-K. ball-tip hook
- J.-K. knife
- J.-K. microforceps
- J.-K. microscissors

Jako-Pilling laryngoscope

Jalaguier-Reverdin needle

Jamar
- J. hydraulic hand dynamometer
- J. hydraulic pinch gauge

James
- J. lumbar peritoneal catheter
- J. wound-approximation forceps

Jameson
- J. eye calipers
- J. facelift scissors
- J. muscle clamp
- J. muscle hook
- J. muscle recession forceps
- J. needle holder
- J. strabismus forceps
- J. strabismus hook
- J. strabismus needle
- J. tracheal muscle forceps

Jameson-Metzenbaum scissors

Jameson-Werber scissors

Jamshidi
- J. adult needle
- J. liver biopsy needle

Jamshidi-Kormed bone marrow biopsy needle

Janacek reimplantation set

Janelli clip

Janes
- J. fracture appliance
- J. fracture frame

Janet bladder swab

Janeway
- J. gastroscope
- J. sphygmomanometer

Jannetta
- J. alligator grasping forceps
- J. aneurysm neck dissector
- J. angular elevator
- J. angular knife
- J. bayonet forceps
- J. bayonet needle holder
- J. bayonet scissors
- J. bayonet-shaped needle holder
- J. bayonet-shaped scissors
- J. double-pronged fork
- J. duckbill elevator
- J. hook
- J. microbayonet forceps
- J. needle holder
- J. posterior fossa retractor
- J. probe
- J. sterilizing rack

Jannetta-Kurze dissecting scissors

Jansen
- J. bayonet dressing forceps
- J. bayonet ear forceps
- J. bayonet nasal forceps
- J. bayonet rongeur

J

Jansen *(continued)*
J. bone curette
J. bone rongeur
J. clamp
J. dissecting forceps
J. dressing forceps
J. ear rongeur
J. mastoid raspatory
J. mastoid retractor
J. monopolar forceps
J. mouthgag
J. nasal-dressing forceps
J. periosteotome
J. scalp retractor
J. thumb forceps
Jansen-Cottle rongeur
Jansen-Gifford mastoid retractor
Jansen-Gruenwald forceps
Jansen-Middleton
J.-M. nasal-cutting forceps
J.-M. punch forceps
J.-M. rongeur
J.-M. scissors
J.-M. septal forceps
J.-M. septal punch
J.-M. septotomy forceps
J.-M. septum-cutting forceps
Jansen-Mueller forceps
Jansen-Newhart mastoid probe
Jansen-Sluder mouthgag
Jansen-Struyken septal forceps
Jansen-Wagner mastoid retractor
Jansen-Zaufel rongeur
Japanese
J. Bruening anastigmatic aural magnifier
J. erection ring
J. fingertrap
J. suction tip
Japonicum laminaria
Jaquet apparatus
jar
bubble j.
Gas-Pak j.
Jarabak arch wire
Jarabak-type archwire
Jarcho
J. pressometer
J. self-retaining uterine cannula
J. tenaculum forceps
J. tenaculum holder
J. uterine tenaculum
Jardine hook
Jardon eye shield
Jardon-Straith
J.-S. chin implant
J.-S. nasal implant
Jarell forceps
Jarit
J. air injection cannula
J. anterior resection clamp
J. bipolar coagulator
J. bladebreaker
J. bone hook

J. brain forceps
J. cartilage clamp
J. comedo extractor
J. cross-action retractor
J. disposable cannula
J. disposable trocar
J. dissecting scissors
J. endarterectomy scissors
J. finger goniometer
J. flat-tip scissors
J. forceps holder
J. hand surgery osteotome
J. intestinal clamp
J. lacrimal cannula
J. lower lateral scissors
J. mallet
J. meniscal clamp
J. microstitch scissors
J. microsurgery scissors
J. microsurgical needle holder
J. microsuture tying forceps
J. mosquito forceps
J. palate hook
J. P.E.E.R. retractor
J. periosteal elevator
J. peripheral vascular scissors
J. pin cutter
J. plaster knife
J. plaster shears
J. renal sinus retractor
J. reverse adenoid curette
J. rotator
J. Rotator endoscope
J. spring-wire retractor
J. sterilizer forceps
J. sternal needle holder
J. stitch scissors
J. tendon-pulling forceps
J. three-prong cast spreader
J. tube-occluding forceps
J. tuning fork
J. utility shears
J. wire holder
J. wire-pulling forceps
Jarit-Allis tissue forceps
Jarit-Crafoord forceps
Jarit-Dandy forceps
Jarit-Deaver retractor
Jarit-Graves vaginal speculum
Jarit-Kerrison rongeur
Jarit-Liston bone-cutting forceps
Jarit-Mason cast breaker
Jarit-Pederson vaginal speculum
Jarit-Poole abdominal suction tube
Jarit-Ruskin rongeur
Jarit-Yankauer suction tube
Jarvik-7, -8, 2000 artificial heart
Jarvik 2000 artificial heart
Jarvis
J. hemorrhoidal forceps
J. pile clamp
J. snare
Jasbee esophagoscope
JAS elbow motion device
Jasin Frontal Ostent stent

J

Jatene arterial switch valve
Jatene-Macchi prosthetic valve
Javal
    J. keratometer
    J. ophthalmometer
Javerts
    J. placental forceps
    J. polyp forceps
Javid
    J. bypass clamp
    J. bypass tube
    J. carotid clamp
    J. carotid shunt
    J. catheter
jaw
    j. exerciser
    j. hook
    independent j.
    j. rongeur
    j. spreader
    j. spring clip
Jay
    J. Care wheelchair seating system
    J. J2 wheelchair
    J. Rave cushion
    J. seating system
    J. Triad cushion
    J. Xtreme cushion
Jayco H2 lactose breath analyzer
Jayles forceps
Jazbi tonsillar dissector
Jeanie Rub Massager
Jeb graft
Jedmed
JedMed TRI-GEM microscope
Jefferson self-retaining retractor
Jeffrey introducer set
Jehle coronary perfusion catheter
jejunal feeding tube
jejunostomy
    needle catheter j.
    percutaneous endoscopic j.
Jelco
    J. intravenous catheter
    J. intravenous stylet
    J. needle
Jelenko
    J. arch bar
    J. facial fracture appliance
    J. pliers
    J. splint
jelly dressing
Jelm two-way catheter
Jelonet dressing
JEM-100B and 100S electron microscope
Jena colposcope
Jena-Schiotz tonometer
Jenkins chisel
Jennings
    J. Loktite mouthgag
Jennings-Skillern mouthgag
Jenning-Streifeneder gastroscope
Jenny mammary prosthesis
Jensen
    J. capsular polisher

    J. capsular scratcher
    J. intraocular lens forceps
    J. lens-inserting forceps
Jensen-Thomas I&A cannula
Jentzer trephine
Jerald forceps
Jergensen reamer
Jergensen-Trinkle reamer
Jergesen I-beam
jerkin plethysmograph
Jervey
    J. capsular fragment forceps
    J. iris forceps
Jesberg
    J. aspirating tube
    J. grasping forceps
    J. infant bronchoscope
    J. laryngectomy clamp
    J. oval esophagoscope
    J. upper esophagoscope
Jesco scissors
jet
    Doppler color j.
    j. humidifier
    Injectoflex respirator j.
    j. nebulizer
    Riwomat respirator j.
    J. shield
    j. stylet
    J. Vac cement dispenser
Jet-Air splint
Jetco spray cannula
Jeter
    J. lag screw
    J. position screw
Jettmobile Tumble Forms
Jewel
    J. AF implantable defibrillator
    J. Atrial fibrillation dual chamber
      device
    J. pacer-cardioverter-defibrillator
    J. PCD
jeweler's
    j. bipolar forceps
    j. pickup forceps
    j. tweezers
Jewett
    J. bar
    J. bending iron
    J. bone chip packer
    J. bone extractor
    J. contraflexion brace
    J. contraflexion orthosis
    J. double-angled osteotomy plate
    J. driver
    J. electrode
    J. fracture appliance
    J. frame
    J. gouge
    J. hip nail
    J. hyperextension brace
    J. nail plate
    J. pickup screw
    J. post-fusion brace

Jewett (*continued*)
    J. post-fusion orthosis
    J. prosthesis
    J. slotted plate
    J. socket reamer
    J. thoracolumbosacral orthosis
    J. urethral sound
    J. uterine dilator
    J. uterine sound
Jewett-Benjamin
    J.-B. cervical brace
    J.-B. cervical orthosis
JF-1T Olympus adult duodenoscope
JF-200 duodenoscope
JFB III endoscope
JF-IT20 duodenoscope
JF-V10 duodenoscope
J-hook electrosurgical probe
Jiffy tube
jig
    Ace-Hershey halo j.
    chamfer j.
    Charnley tibial onlay j.
    cutting j.
    external-alignment compression j.
    extramedullary tibial alignment j.
    fixation j.
    Osteonics j.
    Plexiglas j.
    precompression j.
jigsaw blade
Jimmie
    half J.
Jimmy
    J. dislodger
    J. dissector
    J. John colonic irrigation system
Jinotti
    J. closed suctioning system
    J. dual-purpose catheter
J & J
    Johnson & Johnson
JJIS stent
JL
    JL catheter
JL4
    Judkins left 4
JL4, JL5 catheter
J-loop
    J.-l. electrode
    J.-l. posterior chamber intraocular
    lens
J-Maxx stent
JMS injection needle
J-needle
    Unimar J.-n.
Joal lens
Job Attitude Scale
Jobert de Lamballe suture
Jobson-Horne
    J.-H. cotton applicator
    J.-H. probe
Jobson-Pynchon tongue depressor

Jobst
    J. air band
    J. appliance
    J. athrombic pump system
    J. athrombotic pump
    J. boot
    J. extremity pump
    J. glove
    J. mammary support dressing
    J. postoperative air-boot
    J. pressure garment
    J. prosthesis
    J. sleeve
    J. UlcerCare dressing
    J. VPGS stockings
Jobstens neurostimulator
Jobst-Stride support stockings
Jobst-Stridette support stockings
Joel scanning electron microscope
Joe's
    J. hoe
    J. hoe retractor
Johannson
    J. hip nail
    J. lag screw
Johannson-Stille
    J.-S. cystotomy trocar
    J.-S. lag screw
John
    J. A. Tucker mediastinoscope
    J. Bunn Mini-Mist nebulizer
    J. Green calipers
    J. Green pendulum scalpel
    J. Weiss forceps
Johns
    J. Hopkins bulldog clamp
    J. Hopkins coarctation clamp
    J. Hopkins gallbladder forceps
    J. Hopkins gallbladder retractor
    J. Hopkins gall duct forceps
    J. Hopkins hemostatic forceps
    J. Hopkins modified Potts clamp
    J. Hopkins occluding forceps
    J. Hopkins serrefine forceps
    J. Hopkins stone basket
Johnson
    J. brain tumor forceps
    J. canaliculus wire
    J. cervical thoracic orthosis
    J. cheek retractor
    J. coagulation suction tube
    J. dental band
    J. double cannula
    J. Endobag instrument
    J. erysiphake
    J. evisceration knife
    J. gauze sponge
    J. hook retractor
    J. intestinal tube
    J. & Johnson (J & J)
    J. & Johnson Band-Aid sterile
    drape
    J. & Johnson biliary stent
    J. & Johnson coronary stent
    J. & Johnson dressing

J. & Johnson gauze sponge
J. & Johnson Hemopump
J. & Johnson non-stick pads
J. & Johnson PFC cruciate-
  substituting insert
J. & Johnson PFC Sigma system
J. & Johnson saliva ejector
J. & Johnson tourniquet
J. & Johnson waterproof tape
J. Kydex chairback orthosis
J. prostatic needle holder
J. ptosis forceps
J. ptosis knife
J. screwdriver
J. skin hook
J. spatula
J. stone dislodger
J. swab sampler
J. thoracic forceps
J. total hip stabilization orthosis
J. twin-wire appliance
J. ureteral stone basket
J. ventriculogram retractor
Johnson-Bell erysiphake
Johnson-Kerrison punch
Johnson-Tooke corneal knife
Johnston
J. clamp
J. gastrostomy plug
J. infant dilator
J. LASIK flap applanator
joint
A rotating j.
artificial hip j.
Cam Lock knee j.
j. cinch
CUI j.
Delrin j.
j. distraction cuff
Fillauer dorsiflexion assist ankle j.
Fillauer PDC ankle j.
Gaffney j.
Gillette j.
gliding hinge j.
Greissinger Multi-Axis j.
hinge j.
j. implant
Integrated Ankle orthotic ankle j.
Klenzak double-channeled ankle j.
Klenzak knee j.
Metasul j.
Oklahoma ankle j.
Ottoback 3R65 children's hydraulic
  knee j.
Ottoback 3R45 modular knee j.
Perlstein j.
Scotty stainless ankle j.
Tamarack flexure j.
temporomandibular j. (TMJ)
T rotating j.
Joint-Jack finger splint
Jo-Kath catheter
joker
j. dissector
j. elevator

Jolly uterine dilator
Jomed stent
Jonas
J. implant
J. penile prosthesis
Jonas-Graves vaginal speculum
Jonathan Livingston Seagull patella
  prosthesis
Jonell
J. countertraction finger splint
J. thumb splint
Jones
J. abduction frame
J. adenoid curette
J. arm splint
J. brace
J. cervical knife
J. dissecting scissors
J. dressing
J. forearm splint
J. hemostatic forceps
J. IMA diamond knife
J. IMA epicardial retractor
J. IMA forceps
J. IMA kit
J. IMA needle holder
J. IMA scissors
J. keratome
J. lacrimal canaliculus dilator
J. metacarpal splint
J. nasal splint
J. needle holder
J. pin
J. punctum dilator
J. Pyrex tube
J. suspension traction
J. tear duct tube
J. thoracic clamp
J. towel clamp
J. towel forceps
J. traction splint
Jonesco
J. bone wire guide
J. wire suture needle
Joplin
J. bone-holding forceps
J. tendon passer
J. tendon stripper
J. toe prosthesis
Jordan
J. canal elevator
J. canal incision knife
J. capsular knife
J. eye implant
J. hook
J. middle ear instrument
J. needle
J. perforating bur
J. stapedectomy knife
J. strut forceps
J. strut-measuring instrument
J. wire loop dilator
Jordan-Caparosa holder
Jordan-Day
J.-D. cutting bur

J

Jordan-Day *(continued)*
 J.-D. dermatome
 J.-D. drill
 J.-D. fenestration bur
 J.-D. polishing bur
Jordan-Hermann chisel
Jordan-Rosen
 J.-R. curette
 J.-R. elevator
Jorgenson
 J. dissecting scissors
 J. gallbladder scissors
 J. retractor
 J. thoracic scissors
Joseph
 J. angular knife
 J. antral perforator
 J. bayonet saw
 J. bistoury knife
 J. button-end knife
 J. cervical knife
 J. chisel
 J. double-edged knife
 J. guard
 J. measuring ruler
 J. nasal brace
 J. nasal elevator
 J. nasal hook
 J. nasal knife
 J. nasal rasp
 J. nasal raspatory
 J. nasal saw
 J. nasal scissors
 J. nasal splint
 J. periosteal elevator
 J. periosteal raspatory
 J. periosteotome
 J. punch
 J. saw guide
 J. saw protector
 J. septal bar
 J. septal clamp
 J. septal fracture appliance
 J. septal frame
 J. septal splint
 J. serrated scissors
 J. single-prong hook
 J. skin hook
 J. skin hook retractor
 J. tenaculum hook
 J. wound retractor
Josephberg probe
Joseph-Farrior saw
Joseph-Killian septal elevator
Joseph-Maltz
 J.-M. angular nasal saw
 J.-M. knife
 J.-M. scissors
Josephson
 J. quadpolar mapping electrode
 J. quadripolar catheter
Joseph-Stille saw

Joseph-Verner
 J.-V. raspatory
 J.-V. saw
JoStent coronary stent
Jostra
 J. arterial blood filter
 J. cardiotomy reservoir
 J. catheter
joule counter
Jousto dropfoot splint, skid orthosis
Joyce-Loebl Magiscan image analysis system
Joystick retractor
J-periosteal elevator
JR
 JR catheter
JR4, JR5 catheter
J-scope esophagoscope
J-shaped
 J.-s. endoscope
 J.-s. I&A cannula
 J.-s. tube
JS Quick-fill system
J-tip guidewire
J-tipped guidewire
Judd
 J. cannula
 J. clamp
 J. cystoscope
 J. strabismus forceps
 J. suture forceps
 J. trocar
 J. urethroscope
Judd-Allis
 J.-A. clamp
 J.-A. intestinal forceps
 J.-A. intestinal retractor
 J.-A. tissue forceps
Judd-DeMartel gallbladder forceps
Judd-Mason
 J.-M. bladder retractor
 J.-M. prostatic retractor
Judet
 J. dissector
 J. hip prosthesis
 J. impactor for acetabular component
 J. impactor for acetabular cup
 J. strut
Judkins
 J. coronary catheter
 J. curve LAD catheter
 J. curve LCX catheter
 J. curve STD catheter
 J. guiding catheter
 J. left coronary catheter
 J. left 4 (JL4) catheter
 J. left (JL) catheter
 J. right coronary catheter
 J. right (JR) catheter
 J. torque-control catheter
 J. USCI catheter
Judkins left 4 (JL4)
Judson-Smith manipulator

Juers
   J. crimper forceps
   J. ear curette
   J. hook
   J. lingual forceps
   J. wire crimper
Juers-Derlacki Universal head holder
Juers-Lempert
   J.-L. endaural rongeur
   J.-L. rongeur forceps
Juevenelle clamp
jugular venous catheter
jugum forceps
Julian
   J. cystoresectoscope
   J. needle holder
   J. splenorenal forceps
   J. thoracic artery forceps
Julian-Damian
   J.-D. clamp
   J.-D. thoracic forceps
Julian-Fildes clamp
jumbo forceps
junctional pacemaker
junction field-effect transistor
Jung
   J. Autostainer XL

   J. CV 5000 Robotic Coverslipper
   J. microtome knife
Junior Tompkins portable aspirator
Junker inhaler
Junod boot
Jurasz laryngeal forceps
Jurgan
   J. pin
   J. pin ball
   J. Pin Ball pin protector
   J. pin-ball system
Jutte tube
Jux-A-Cisor exerciser
juxtaglomerular apparatus
Juzo
   J. hose
   J. shrinker
   J. stockings
Juzo-Hostess two-way stretch
   compression stockings
J-Vac
   J-V. bulb suction reservoir
   J-V. catheter
   J-V. closed wound drainage system
   J-V. drain
J-wire
   safety J-w.

J

K

K blade
K dissector sponge
K implant
K pack
K pad
K reamer
K root canal file
K stylet
K wire
K wire driver
K x-ray fluorescence instrument

Kþer Knit patch
Kffttnerblunt dissector
K-37 pediatric arterial blood filter
KAAT II Plus intra-aortic balloon pump
Kader

K. fishhook needle
K. gastrostomy
K. intestinal spatula

Kadesky forceps
Kadir Hi-Torque guidewire
Kaessman handpiece
Kaessmann nail
KAFO

Generation II KAFO
KAFO prosthesis

Kahler

K. bronchial biopsy forceps
K. bronchoscopic forceps
K. bronchus-grasping forceps
K. double-action tip
K. laryngeal biopsy forceps
K. polyp forceps

Kahn

K. scissors
K. tenaculum forceps
K. traction tenaculum
K. trigger cannula
K. uterine cannula
K. uterine dilator

Kahn-Graves vaginal speculum
Kahre-Williger periosteal elevator
Kaiser speculum
Kalamarides dural retractor
Kal-Dermic suture
Kaleidoscope chair
Kalginate calcium alginate wound dressing
Kalinowski

K. ear speculum
K. perforator
K. rasp

Kalinowski-Verner

K.-V. ear speculum
K.-V. rasp

Kalish

K. Duredge wire cutter
K. Duredge wire extender
K. Duredge wire extractor

Kalk

K. electrode
K. esophagoscope
K. palpitation probe

Kallassy

K. ankle support
K. brace
K. orthosis

kallikrein-inhibiting unit
Kall modification of Silverman needle
Kallmorgen vaginal spatula
Kalman

K. filter
K. needle holder
K. occluding forceps
K. tube-occluding forceps

Kalos pacemaker
Kalt

K. capsular forceps
K. corneal needle
K. eye needle
K. eye needle holder
K. eye spoon
K. needle holder clamp
K. vein needle

Kalt-Arruga needle holder
Kaltenborn-Evjenth Concept Wedge mobilization wedge
Kaltostat

K. Fortex dressing
K. hydrofiber wound packing
K. rope
K. wound packing dressing
K. wound packing material

Kalt-Vital needle holder
Kambin-Gellman instrumentation
Kambin instrumentation
Kamdar microscissors
Kamerling

K. Capsular 90 lens
K. one-piece all-PMMA intraocular lens

Kaminsky

K. catheter
K. stent

Kamppeter anomaloscope
KAM Super Sucker
Kanavel

K. apparatus
K. brain-exploring cannula
K. cock-up splint
K. conductor
K. table

Kanavel-Senn retractor
Kandel stereotactic apparatus
Kane

K. obstetrical clamp
K. umbilical cord clamp

Kaneda

K. anterior scoliosis system
K. anterior spinal instrumentation
K. anterior spinal system

Kaneda *(continued)*
  K. anterior spine stabilizing device
  K. distraction device
  K. distractor
  K. rod
Kangaroo
  K. feeding pump
  K. silicone gastrostomy feeding tube
kangaroo tendon suture
Kangnian acupuncture needle
Kangoo Thera-P bar
Kansas
  K. City band truss
  K. University corneal forceps
Kantor
  K. circumcision clamp
  K. forceps
Kantor-Berci video laryngoscope
Kantrowitz
  K. dressing forceps
  K. hemostatic clamp
  K. pacemaker
  K. thoracic clamp
  K. thoracic forceps
  K. tissue forceps
Kap
  Hypotherm Gel K.
  Kold K.
Kaplan
  K. PenduLaser laser
  K. resectoscope
  K. tracheostomy needle
Kaplan-Simpson InfusaSleeve
Kapp
  K. clip
  K. forceps
  K. microarterial clamp
  K. microclamp
  K. surgical instrument
  K. Surgical Instrument prosthetic
    knee
  K. Surgical Instrument surgical knee
    immobilizer
  K. Surgical Instrument total hip
    calipers
  K. Surgical Instrument total knee
    retractor
Kapp-Beck
  K.-B. bronchial clamp
  K.-B. coarctation clamp
  K.-B. colon clamp
  K.-B. forceps
Kapp-Beck-Thomson clamp
Kaprelian easy-access tweezers
Kaps operating microscope
Kara
  K. cataract-aspirating cannula
  K. cataract needle
  K. erysiphake
Karakashian-Barraquer scissors
Karamar-Mailatt tarsorhaphy clamp
Karaya
  K. adhesive ileostomy appliance
  K. dressing

  K. electrode
  K. seal ileostomy stomal bag
  K. self-adhesive conductive material
Karickhoff
  K. diagnostic lens
  K. double cannula
  K. keratoscope
  K. laser lens
Karl
  K. Ilg instruments
  K. Storz Calcutript
  K. Storz Calcutript endoscope
  K. Storz coagulator
  K. Storz flexible endoscope
  K. Storz flexible ureteropyeloscope
  K. Storz 15 French flexible
    hysteroscope
  K. Storz instrumentation
  K. Storz light source connector
  K. Storz lithotriptor
  K. Storz-Lutzeyer lithotriptor
  K. Storz pediatric bronchoscopy
    system
  K. Storz reusable multi-function
    valve trocar take-apart scissors
    forceps
Karlin microknife
Karmen
  K. cannula
  K. catheter
Karmody
  K. vascular spring retractor
  K. venous scissors
Karolinska-Stille punch
Karp
  K. aortic punch
  K. aortic punch forceps
Karras angiography needle
Kartchner carotid artery clamp
Kartch pigtail probe
Kartush
  K. insulated retractor
  K. stimulus dissection elevator
  K. tympanic membrane patcher
Karwetsky U-bow activator
Kasai peritoneal venous shunt
Kasdan retractor
Kashiwabara laryngeal mirror
Kaslow gastrointestinal tube
Kaster mitral valve prosthesis
kastRAP wrap
Kataya seal closed stoma pouch
Katena
  K. boat hook
  K. cannula
  K. double-edged sapphire blade
  K. forceps
  K. iris spatula
  K. Quick Switch I/A system
  K. ring
  K. speculum
  K. trephine
Katena-Barron trephine
Katon catheter
Katsch chisel

Katzeff cartilage scissors
Katzen
    K. flap unzipper
    K. infusion wire
    K. long balloon dilatation catheter
Katzenstein rectal cannula
Katzin
    K. corneal transplant scissors
    K. trephine
Katzin-Barraquer
    K.-B. Colibri forceps
    K.-B. corneal forceps
Katzin-Long balloon
Katzin-Troutman scissors
Kaufer type II retractor
Kaufman
    K. adapter
    K. catheter
    K. clip applier
    K. ENT forceps
    K. III anti-incontinence prosthesis
    K. II vitrector
    K. incontinence device
    K. kidney clamp
    K. male urinary incontinence prosthesis
    K. type II retractor
    K. vitrector
    K. vitreophage
KaVo
    K. dental handpiece
    K. oral surgery system
Kawasumi infusion set
Kay
    K. aortic anastomosis clamp
    K. rhinolaryngeal stroboscope
Kaycel towel
Kay-Cross suction tip suction tube
Kaye
    K. blepharoplasty scissors
    K. facelift scissors
    K. fine-dissecting scissors
    K. tamponade balloon
Kay-Lambert clamp
Kayser-Fleischer ring
Kay-Shiley
    K.-S. disk valve prosthesis
    K.-S. heart valve
Kay-Suzuki
    K.-S. heart valve
    K.-S. prosthesis
Kazanjian
    K. action-type osteotome
    K. bone-cutting forceps
    K. cutting forceps
    K. guide
    K. nasal forceps
    K. nasal hump forceps
    K. nasal splint
    K. scissors
    K. T-bar
    K. tooth button
Kazanjian-Cottle forceps
Kazanjian-Goldman rongeur

K-Blade
    K.-B. microsurgical blade
KBM
    KBM absorbent gauze
    KBM cotton ball
    KBM gauze swab
K/B prosthesis
K-Caps
K-Centrum anterior spinous fixation system
KDC-Healthdyne nonfluorescent spotlight
KD chin prosthesis
KDF-2.3
    KDF-2.3 intrauterine insemination cannula
    KDF-2.3 intrauterine insemination catheter
Keane Mobility bed
Kean-M-4 occluder
Kearney
    K. side-notch intraocular lens
    K. side-notch IOL
Kearns
    K. bag catheter
    K. bladder dilator
Kebab graft
K-edge filter
keel
    Deltafit K.
    McNaught k.
    Montgomery laryngeal k.
    k. stent
Keeler
    K. camera
    K. cryoextractor
    K. cryophake
    K. cryophake unit
    K. cryosurgical instrument
    K. cryosurgical unit
    K. extended round tip forceps
    K. fiberoptic headlight
    K. intraocular foreign body grasping forceps
    K. intravitreal scissors
    K. lamp
    K. lancet tip
    K. lightsource stand
    K. Magnalite fiberoptic headlamp
    K. microscissors
    K. micro spear tip
    K. ophthalmoscope
    K. panoramic lens
    K. panoramic loupe
    K. panoramic surgical telescope
    K. pantoscope
    K. prism
    K. prosthesis
    K. Pulsair noncontact tonometer
    K. puncture tip
    K. razor tip
    K. retinoscope
    K. retractable blade
    K. round tip
    K. ruby knife
    K. spotlight lens loupe

K

Keeler *(continued)*
    K. Tearscope
    K. triple-facet tip
    K. ultrasonic cataract removal lancet
    K. video headlamp
    K. wide-angle lens loupe
Keeler-Amoils
    K.-A. curved cataract probe
    K.-A. glaucoma probe
    K.-A. long-shank retinal probe
    K.-A. microcurved cataract probe
    K.-A. ophthalmic cryosystem
    K.-A. ophthalmic long-shank probe
    K.-A. ophthalmic Machemer retinal probe
    K.-A. ophthalmic straight cataract probe
    K.-A. ophthalmic vitreous probe
Keeler-Amoils-Machemer retinal probe
Keeler-Catford
    K.-C. micro jaws needle holder
Keeler-Fison tissue retractor
Keeler-Galilean surgical loupe
Keeler-Keislar lacrimal cannula
Keeler-Konan Specular microscope
Keeler-Meyer diamond knife
Keeler-Pierse eye speculum
Keeler-Rodger iris retractor
Keeley vein stripper
Keene
    K. compression hook
    K. obturator
Keen Edge disposable biopsy forceps
keeper
    line k.
    Nelson line k.
Keer aneurysm clip
Kees clip applier
Kegel perineometer
Kehr
    K. gallbladder tube
    K. T-tube
Keisler lacrimal cannula
Keith
    K. abdominal needle
    K. drain
Keithley clamp kit
Keitzer infant urethrotome
Keizer-Lancaster
    K.-L. eye speculum
    K.-L. lid retractor
Keizer lid retractor
Kelikian foot dressing
Kellan
    K. capsular sparing system
    K. hydrodissection cannula
    K. sutureless incision blade
Keller-Blake leg splint
Keller cephalometric device
Kelley-Goerss Compass stereotactic system
Kelling gastroscope
Kellman-Elschnig spatula
Kellogg tongue depressor

Kelly
    K. abdominal retractor
    K. arterial forceps
    K. clamp
    K. curette
    K. cystoscope
    K. direct-vision adenotome
    K. dressing forceps
    K. endoscope
    K. fistular scissors
    K. hemostat
    K. hemostatic forceps
    K. inflatable T-tube
    K. insufflator
    K. intestinal needle
    K. orifice dilator
    K. ovum forceps
    K. placental forceps
    K. polypus forceps
    K. proctoscope
    K. punch
    K. rectal speculum
    K. sigmoidoscope
    K. sphincter dilator
    K. sphincteroscope
    K. stereotactic system
    K. tissue forceps
    K. tube
    K. urethral forceps
    K. uterine dilator
    K. uterine scissors
    K. uterine tenaculum
    K. uterine tenaculum hook
    K. vulsellum
Kelly-Descemet membrane punch
Kelly-Gray
    K.-G. uterine curette
    K.-G. uterine forceps
Kelly-Murphy forceps
Kelly-Rankin forceps
Kelly-Sims vaginal retractor
Kelly-Wick vascular tunneler
Kelman
    K. air cystotome
    K. aspirator
    K. Cry-O-Cadet
    K. cryoextractor
    K. cryophake
    K. cryosurgical unit
    K. cyclodialysis cannula
    K. cystitome
    K. cystitome knife
    K. dipstick
    K. double-bladed cystotome
    K. flexible tripod lens
    K. I&A unit
    K. II three-point fixation rigid tripod intraocular lens
    K. implantation forceps
    K. intraocular forceps
    K. iris retractor
    K. irrigating handpiece
    K. irrigation hook
    K. irrigator
    K. irrigator forceps

K. knife-cannula cystotome
K. knife cystotome
K. manipulator hook
K. Multiflex II intraocular lens
K. needle
K. Omnifit intraocular lens
K. PC 27LB CapSul lens
K. phacoemulsification unit
K. Phaco-Emulsifier
K. Quadraflex intraocular lens
K. S-flex intraocular lens
K. tip
Kelman-Cavitron I&A unit
Kelman-McPherson
K.-M. corneal forceps
K.-M. microtying forceps
K.-M. suture forceps
K.-M. tissue forceps
K.-M. tying forceps
Kelocote sheeting
Kel retractor
Kelsey
K. pile clamp
K. unloading exercise therapy
Kelsey-Fry bone awl
Kelvin Sensor pacemaker
Kempf internal screw fixation
Kemp irrigator
Ken
K. driver
K. Drive sleeve
K. screwdriver
K. sliding nail
Kendall
K. A-V impulse system
K. compression stockings
K. endotracheal tube cuff
K. McGaw Intelligent pump
K. sequential compression device
K. Ventex wound dressing system
Kenna knee scale
Kennedy
K. bar
K. LAD
K. ligament augmentation device
K. sinus pack
K. spillproof cup
K. vulsellum forceps
Kennedy-Cornwell bladder evacuator
Kennerdell
K. bayonet forceps
K. medial orbital retractor
K. muscle hook
K. nerve hook
K. spatula
Kennerdell-Maroon
K.-M. dissector
K.-M. duckbill elevator
K.-M. hook
K.-M. orbital retractor
K.-M. probe
Kennerdell-Maroon-Jameson hook
Kennett tenaculum
Kenny crutch
Kenny-Howard splint

Kensey atherectomy catheter
Kent forceps
Kenwood
K. finger cot
K. laparotomy sponge
Keofeed feeding tube
Keolar implant material
Keracor laser
KeraCorneoScope scope
Keragen implant
Kerascan
keratectomy scissors
keratographer
Keravue k.
keratoiridoscope scope
Kerato-Kontours instruments
Kerato-Lens implant
Keratolux fixation device
keratome
Agnew k.
Atkinson k.
Bard-Parker k.
Beaver blade k.
Berens partial k.
k. blade
Castro-Martinez k.
Castroviejo angled k.
Czermak k.
Daily k.
Draeger modified k.
filamentary k.
Fink-Rowland k.
Fuchs lancet-type k.
k. guard
Guyton-Lundsgaard k.
Hansen k.
HydroBlade k.
HydroBrush k.
Jaeger k.
Jones k.
Kirby k.
Kirby-Duredge k.
Lancaster k.
Landolt k.
Lichtenberg k.
Martinez k.
Martinez-Castro k.
McCaslin wave-edge k.
McReynolds k.
McReynolds-Castroviejo k.
McReynolds pterygium k.
Rowland k.
SatinSlit k.
Storz k.
Storz-Duredge k.
Thomas k.
Tri-Beeled trapezoidal k.
UltraShaper k.
UniShaper single-use k.
Wiener k.
keratometer
Autoref k.
Bausch & Lomb manual k.
Canon automatic k.
Canon auto refraction k.

K

keratometer *(continued)*
Haag-Streit k.
Helmholtz k.
Humphrey automatic k.
Javal k.
k. lens
manual k.
Marco manual k.
Osher surgical k.
OV-1 surgical k.
Storz k.
surgical k.
Terry k.
Topcon k.
Keratom excimer laser system
keratoplasty scissors
keratoprosthesis
Eckardt temporary k.
Lander wide-field temporary k.
PHEMA core-and-skirt k.
keratoscope
Karickhoff k.
Klein self-luminous k.
Placido k.
Polack k.
van Loonen operating k.
wire-loop k.
keratotomy forceps
KeraVision
K. Intacs intracorneal ring
Keravue keratographer
Kerlix
K. bandage roll
K. cast pad
K. cast padding
K. dressing
K. gauze bandage
K. laparotomy sponge
K. packing sponge
K. super sponge
K. wrap
Kern
K. bone-holding clamp
K. bone-holding forceps
K. miniforceps
Kernan-Jackson coagulating bronchoscope
Kerner dental mirror
Kern-Lane bone-holding forceps
Kerpel bone curette
Kerr
K. abduction splint
K. clip applier
K. electro-torque drill
K. Endopost
K. hand drill
K. K-Flex file
K. M4 safety handpiece
Kerrison
K. bone punch
K. cervical rongeur
K. forceps
K. laminectomy punch
K. lumbar rongeur
K. mastoid rongeur

K. microrongeur
K. retractor
Kerrison-Costen rongeur
Kerrison-Ferris Smith rongeur
Kerrison-Jacoby punch
Kerrison-Morgenstein rongeur
Kerrison-Rhoton sellar punch
Kerrison-Schwartz rongeur
Kerrison-Spurling rongeur
Kershner one-step micro capsulorhexis forceps
Kersting colostomy clamp
Kesilar cannula
Kesling
K. appliance
K. tooth-spacing spring
Kessel osteotomy plate
Kessler
K. external fixator
K. metacarpal distractor
K. podiatry rasp
K. prosthesis
K. stitch
K. traction frame
Kessler-Kleinert suture
Kestler ambulatory head tractor
Kestrel disinfector
Ketac
K. Fil cement
K. liner
K. Silver cement
Keuch pupil dilator
Kevlar gloves
Kevorkian
K. endocervical curette
K. endometrial curette
K. uterine biopsy forceps
Kevorkian-Younge
K.-Y. cervical biopsy forceps
K.-Y. endocervical biopsy curette
K.-Y. uterine applicator
K.-Y. uterine biopsy forceps
K.-Y. uterine curette
key
Allen-type hex k.
K. periosteal elevator
K. rasp
ResCue K.
keyboard
ErgoLogic k.
Kinesis k.
keyed
k. filling device
k. supracondylar plate
Keyes
K. bone-splitting chisel
K. cutaneous biopsy punch
K. cutaneous trephine
K. dermatologic punch
K. lithotrite
K. skin punch
K. vulvar punch
Keyes-Ultzmann-Luer cannula
keyhole punch

KeyMed
- K. advanced oesophageal dilator set
- K. automatic reprocessor
- K. dilator
- K. disposable variceal injection needle
- K. esophageal tube
- K. fiberoptic scope
- K. unit

Keys-Briston type spline
Keys-Kirschner traction bow
keystone
- k. last
- K. Plus oxygenator concentrator
- K. splint

keyway
- OEC lag screw component with k.

Kezerian
- K. chisel
- K. curette
- K. gouge

K-file
- Mity K.-f.
- nitinol K.-f.

K-Fix fixator system
K-Flexofile
- K.-F. Batt tip
- K.-F. file

KF ring
K-Gar umbilical clamp
Khan-Jaeger clamp
Khodadad
- K. clamp
- K. clip
- K. microclamp
- K. microclip
- K. microclip forceps

Khosia cautery
Khouri hydrodissection cannula
kibisitome
- k. cystitome

kick bucket
Kicker
- K. Pavlik harness

Kidd
- K. cystoscope
- K. trocar
- K. U-tube

Kidde
- K. nebulizer
- K. tourniquet
- K. tourniquet cuff
- K. tubal insufflator
- K. uterine cannula

Kid-Dee-Lite orthosis
Kidde-Robbins tourniquet
Kid Gloves
Kid-Kart wheelchair
kidney
- Ask-Upmark k.
- Duo-Klex artificial k.
- Elmar artificial k.
- k. internal splint
- k. internal splint/stent
- k. internal stent

- k. internal stent catheter
- k. pedicle clamp
- k. pedicle forceps
- k. retractor
- k. stone forceps
- k. suturing needle

kidney-elevating forceps
Kido suprapubic trocar
Kiefer clamp
Kiel graft
Kielland forceps
Kiene bone tamp
Kiethly-DAS series 500 data-acquisition system
Kifa
- K. clip
- K. green, grey, red, yellow catheter

Killearn rongeur
Killey molar retractor
Killian
- K. antral cannula
- K. antrum cannula
- K. cutting forceps tip
- K. dissector
- K. double-articulated forceps tip
- K. frontal sinus chisel
- K. gouge
- K. laryngeal spatula
- K. nasal cannula
- K. nasal speculum
- K. probe
- K. rectal speculum
- K. septal compression forceps
- K. septal elevator
- K. septal speculum
- K. suspension gallows
- K. suspension gallows apparatus
- K. tonsillar knife
- K. tube

Killian-Claus chisel
Killian-Eichen cannula
Killian-Halle nasal speculum
Killian-Jameson forceps
Killian-King goiter retractor
Killian-Lynch suspension laryngoscope
Killian-Reinhard chisel
Killip wire
Kilner
- K. chisel
- K. elevator
- K. goiter hook
- K. malar lever
- K. mouthgag
- K. nasal retractor
- K. needle holder
- K. skin hook
- K. skin hook retractor
- K. suture carrier

Kilner-Dott mouthgag
Kilpatrick retractor
Kilp lens
Kimball
- K. catheter
- K. nephrostomy hook

Kimberley diamond instrument

K

Kimpton vein spreader
Kim-Ray
    K.-R. Greenfield antiembolus filter
    K.-R. Greenfield vena cava filter
Kimura
    K. cartilage graft
    K. platinum spatula
Kimwipes wipe
KinAir
    K. III, TC low-air-loss bed
    K. IV mattress
Kinamed Exact-Fit ATH system
Kincaid right-angle hook
Kin-Con
    K.-C. device
    K.-C. isokinetic exercise system
Kinder Design pedo forceps
Kindt
    K. arterial clamp
    K. carotid clamp
Kinematic
    K. facebow
    K. II condylar and stabilizer total
    knee system
    K. II rotating-hinge knee system
    K. II rotating-hinge total knee
    prosthesis
    K. rotating hinge
    K. rotating-hinge total knee
Kinemax
    K. modular condylar and stabilizer
    total knee system
    K. Plus knee prosthesis
    K. Plus total knee system
    K. removable fixation peg
    K. spacer
Kinemetric guide system
Kinesis
    K. keyboard
    K. reagent kit
kinestatic charge detector
kinesthesiometer
KineTec
    K. clubfoot CPM exerciser
    K. hip CPM machine
kinetic
    k. continuous passive motion device
    k. rehabilitation device
    K. Wedge molded insole
    K. Wedge orthotic
Kinetik
    K. great toe implant
    K. great toe implant system
Kinetix
KinetiX
    K. instrument
    K. ventilation monitor
Kinetron muscle strengthening apparatus
KINEX anatomic specimen stand
King
    K. adenoidal punch
    K. cardiac bioptome
    K. cardiac device
    K. cervical brace
    K. clamp

    K. connector adapter
    K. corneal trephine
    K. double-umbrella closure system
    K. fluff rolls & sponge
    K. guiding catheter
    K. of Hearts event recorder
    K. of Hearts Holter monitor
    K. interlocking device
    K. multipurpose coronary graft
    catheter
    K. orbital implant
    K. self-retaining goiter retractor
    K. suture needle
    K. tissue forceps
    K. wound forceps
King-Armstrong unit
King-Hurd
    K.-H. retractor
    K.-H. tonsillar dissector
King-Prince
    K.-P. knife
    K.-P. muscle forceps
    K.-P. recession forceps
Kingsley
    K. grasping forceps
    K. orthodontic plate
    K. splint
    K. Steplite foot
kink-resistant peritoneal catheter
KINS
    KINS all-in-one cotton brief
    KINS draw sheet
    KINS fitted mattress protector
    KINS liner
    KINS prefolded flat 100% cotton
    flannelette diaper
    KINS pull-on waterproof bloomer
    KINS pull-on waterproof pant
    KINS soaker pad
Kinsella-Buie lung clamp
Kinsella periosteal elevator
Kinsey atherectomy catheter
KIP laser
Kirby
    K. angulated iris spatula
    K. capsular forceps
    K. cataract knife
    K. corneoscleral forceps
    K. curved zonular separator
    K. cylindrical zonular separator
    K. double-ball separator
    K. double-fixation muscle hook
    K. eye tissue forceps
    K. fixation forceps
    K. flat zonular separator
    K. hook expressor
    K. intracapsular lens expressor
    K. intracapsular lens forceps
    K. intracapsular lens loop
    K. intracapsular lens spoon
    K. intraocular lens loop
    K. intraocular lens loupe
    K. iris forceps
    K. keratome
    K. lens dislocator

K. lens forceps
K. lid retractor
K. refractor
K. scissors
Kirby-Arthus fixation forceps
Kirby-Bracken iris forceps
Kirby-Duredge
K.-D. keratome
K.-D. knife
Kirchner
K. retractor
Kirk
K. bone hammer
K. mallet
K. orthopaedic hammer
Kirkheim-Storz urethrotome
Kirkland
K. cement
K. cement dressing
K. curette
K. instrument
K. knife
K. periodontal pack
K. retractor
Kirklin
K. atrial retractor
K. fence
K. sternal awl
Kirkpatrick tonsillar forceps
Kirmisson
K. periosteal elevator
K. periosteal raspatory
Kirschenbaum
K. foot positioner
K. retractor
Kirschner
K. abdominal retractor
K. bone drill
K. boring wire
K. device
K. extension bow
K. femoral canal plug
K. guiding probe
K. hip replacement system
K. II-C shoulder system
K. II-C shoulder system stem
K. integrated shoulder system
K. interlocking intramedullary nail
K. Medical Dimension hip replacement
K. Medical Dimension hip replacement system
K. pin fixation
K. skeletal traction
K. surgical instrument
K. suture
K. total shoulder prosthesis
K. traction apparatus
K. traction bow nut
K. Universal self-centering captive-head bipolar component
K. wire (K wire, K-wire)
K. wire cutter
K. wire drill
K. wire fixation

K. wire inserter
K. wire pin
K. wire splint
K. wire spreader
K. wire tightener
K. wire traction
K. wire traction bow
K. wire tractor
Kirschner-Balfour abdominal retractor
Kirschner-Ullrich forceps
Kirwan
K. bipolar coagulator
K. bipolar electrosurgical forceps
K. coaptation ophthalmic bipolar forceps
K. cranioblade
K. iris curved ophthalmic bipolar forceps
K. iris straight ophthalmic bipolar forceps
K. jeweler's curved ophthalmic bipolar forceps
K. jeweler's insulated straight ophthalmic bipolar forceps
Kirwan-Adson ophthalmic bipolar forceps
Kirwan-Nadler-style coaptation ophthalmic bipolar forceps
Kirwan-Tenzel ophthalmic bipolar forceps
Kish
K. urethral catheter
K. urethral illuminated catheter set
Kishi lens
kissing
k. balloon
k. stent
Kistner
K. plastic tracheostomy tube
K. probe
K. tracheal button
kit
ABI PRISM Dye Terminator Cycle Sequencing Ready Reaction K.
Adjust-A-Flow colostomy irrigation k.
Amplicor typing k.
Apdyne phenol applicator k.
Arrow pneumothorax k.
Assess esophageal testing k.
Bard Sequence II Plus incontinent skin care k.
Bard-Steigmann-Goff variceal ligation k.
Bergland-Warshawski phaco/cortex k.
BFO K.
BIO101MERmaid k.
Biosearch jejunostomy k.
BiPort hemostasis introducer sheath k.
Boehringer k.
Brimms Quik-Fix denture repair k.
brush biopsy k.
Burnett Pap smear k.
"cake mix" k.

K

kit *(continued)*

Camino OLM intracranial pressure monitoring k.
Camino postcraniotomy subdural pressure monitoring k.
Carey-Coons biliary endoprosthesis k.
carpal tunnel surgery relief k.
Cartmill feeding tube k.
Ceramco porcelain k.
cervical block k.
Circulon System Step 1, 2 venous ulcer k.
clear PVC tube & connector k.
CloseSure procedure k.
Cloward anterior fusion k.
Cloward PLIF II k.
Cloward posterior lumbar interbody fusion k.
Codman IMA k.
Coloplast deluxe irrigation k.
combination cone/tube irrigator k.
Concept CTS Relief k.
Confide HIV test k.
ConQuest male continence system leg bag k.
contour defect molding k.
Cordis lead conversion k.
Crystar porcelain k.
CTS Relief k.
Cyfra 21-1 IRMA k.
Davol sterile female cath k.
Debut ear piercing k.
Dentifix denture repair k.
Denver percutaneous access k.
diabetic orthosis k.
Diethrich coronary artery bypass k.
Digital Care k.
Dover midstream urine collection k.
Dynacor enema cleansing k.
DynaPak electrode k.
Elastafit tubing k.
Enemette enema cleansing k.
ERx Avulsed Tooth k.
Etch-Master k.
Euro-Collins multiorgan perfusion k.
Exerball k.
Extended Wear self-adhering urinary external catheter starter k.
FACE k.
Fergus percutaneous introducer k.
Fillauer Scottish Rite orthosis k.
Flexiflo Inverta-PEG gastrostomy k.
Flexiflo Lap G laparoscopic gastrostomy k.
Flexiflo Lap J laparoscopic jejunostomy k.
Flexiflo over-the-guidewire gastrostomy k.
Fome-Cuf laser k.
Freedom T-tap leg bag k.
Fresenius Euro-Collins k.

GENTLE TOUCH System, Colostomy/Ileostomy Postoperative K.
GENTLE TOUCH System, Urostomy Postoperative K.
Genuine sheepskin crutches accessory k.
Glove-n-Gel amniotomy k.
Hall Osteon drill system k.
Hall Osteon irrigation k.
Handi-Cath catheter k.
Hashizume endoscopic ligator k.
Heyer-Schulte PVC k.
Heyer-Schulte silicone k.
hysterectomy k.
I&A k.
ICE-Magic pain reduction k.
ICTP RIA k.
I-Flow nerve block infusion k.
InPouch TV subculture k.
Inteq TFC repair k.
Jackson-Pratt flat drain k.
Jackson-Pratt hysterectomy k.
Jackson-Pratt large-volume round silicone drain k.
Jackson-Pratt PVC k.
Jones IMA k.
Keithley clamp k.
Kinesis reagent k.
KLS-Martin modular neuro k.
Ko-Lec-Pac urinary collection k.
Lacrimedics occlusion starter k.
Laitinen high-precision stereotactic-assisted radiation therapy k.
Laitinen percutaneous tumor biopsy k.
Lang jet adjustor k.
Laserscope discography k.
latex tube & connector k.
Lingeman k.
Lymwrap lymphedema bandaging k.
Malis brain retractor k.
Mallinckrodt ultra tag labeling k.
Marlen biliary drainage k.
Massachusetts Vision K.
Master K.
McGhan fill k.
MediCordz tubing k.
Medscand Pap smear k.
Merit Final Flexion K.
MERmaid k.
Metra PS procedure k.
Micro E irrigation k.
Micro 100 irrigation k.
microvascular STA-MCA k.
modular temPPTthotic k.
Moss G-tube PEG k.
neonatal internal jugular puncture k.
Nerve Block Infusion K.
No Pour Pak suction catheter k.
Oncor ApopTaq K.
One Time dressing k.
Ortho diaphragm k.
Osteo-Lock endodontic stabilization k.

ototome irrigation k.
Otovent autoinflation k.
Ott-Mayo channel sampling k.
palmar swab k.
Panda NCJ k.
parallel pin k.
PB-FOxS pediatric femoral
  sensor k.
pelvic reconstruction k.
Percufix catheter cuff k.
percutaneous access k.
percutaneous catheter introducer k.
Per-fit percutaneous tracheostomy k.
Perry Noz-Stop k.
Persona monitoring k.
Portex Per-fit tracheostomy k.
Posey bar k.
Preci-Vertix k.
Prep-IM hip bone preparation k.
Pro-Vent ABG k.
Pro-Vent arterial blood sampling k.
Pulsator dry heparin arterial blood
  gas k.
Pulse-Pak infusion k.
QIAmp tissue k.
Quick-Sil starter k.
Radiofocus introducer B k.
radioimmunoassay k.
resistive chair exercise k.
Rosenberg meniscal repair k.
Russell gastrostomy k.
Sacks-Vine gastrostomy k.
sensory stimulation k.
Set-Op myringotomy k.
Shearing suction k.
Shiley distention k.
Shofu porcelain stain k.
shunt k.
Sigma TMB assay k.
Sims Per-fit percutaneous
  tracheostomy k.
in situ valve-cutter k.
Starlite endodontic implant starter k.
stereotactic-assisted radiation
  therapy k.
Stomate low-profile gastrostomy k.
StoneRisk diagnostic monitoring k.
Straith nasal splint k.
Sub-4 Platinum Plus wire k.
Tacticon peripheral neuropathy k.
thermodilution catheter introducer k.
Tisseel VH k.
Toomey syringe k.
Tri-Port hemostasis introducer
  sheath k.
tuboplasty surgical k.
Tum-E-Vac gastric lavage k.
UMI amniocentesis k.
UniPort hemostasis introducer
  sheath k.
Unna-Flex Plus venous ulcer k.
ureteral brush biopsy k.
Varioligator k.
Versa-PEG gastrostomy k.

Vesica percutaneous bladder neck
  suspension k.
Vesica Sling K.
Wilson-Cook feeding tube k.
Wood colonic k.
Wound-Evac k.
Xomed sinus irrigation k.
Kitchen postpartum gauze packer
Kit-Green
  FastRNA K.-G.
Kitner
  K. blunt dissecting instrument
  K. blunt dissector
  K. clamp
  K. dissecting scissors
  K. goiter forceps
  K. retractor
  K. thyroid-packing forceps
Kiwisch bandage
Kjelland
  K. blade
  K. obstetrical forceps
Kjelland-Barton forceps
Kjelland-Luikart obstetrical forceps
Klaar headlight
Klaff septal speculum
Klammt elastic open activator
Klapp tendon hook
Klatskin liver biopsy needle
Klauber band setter
Klause antral punch
Klause-Carmody antral punch
Klearway
Klebanoff
  K. bougie
  K. common duct sound
  K. gallstone scoop
Kleegman
  K. cannula
  K. dilator
Kleen-Needle system
KleenSpec
  K. disposable anoscope
  K. disposable laryngoscope
  K. disposable vaginal speculum
  K. fiberoptic disposable
    sigmoidoscope
  K. forceps
  K. otoscope adapter
Kleer base plate
Kleesattel
  K. elevator
  K. raspatory
Klein
  K. cannula tip
  K. curved cannula
  K. 1-hole infiltrator tip
  K. infiltration needle
  K. infiltrator
  K. multihole infiltrator tip
  K. pump
  K. punch
  K. self-luminous keratoscope
  K. transseptal introducer sheath
  K. ventilation tube

K

Klein-Delrin Luer-Lok handle
Kleinert-Kutz
    K.-K. bone cutter
    K.-K. bone-cutting forceps
    K.-K. bone file
    K.-K. bone rongeur
    K.-K. clamp
    K.-K. clamp approximator
    K.-K. dissector
    K.-K. elevator
    K.-K. hook retractor
    K.-K. microclip
    K.-K. rasp
    K.-K. rongeur forceps
    K.-K. skin hook
    K.-K. synovectomy rongeur
    K.-K. tendon forceps
    K.-K. tendon-passing forceps
    K.-K. tendon retriever
    K.-K. tendon-retrieving forceps
Kleinert-Ragnell retractor
Kleinert splint
Kleinsasser
    K. anterior commissure laryngoscope
    K. hook
    K. knife
    K. lens loop
    K. microlaryngeal scissors
    K. operating laryngoscope
    K. probe
    K. retractor
Kleinsasser-Riecker laryngoscope
Kleinschmidt appendectomy clamp
Klemme
    K. appendectomy retractor
    K. dural hook
    K. gasserian ganglion retractor
    K. laminectomy retractor
Klenzak
    K. brace
    K. double-channeled ankle joint
    K. double-upright splint
    K. knee joint
Kleppinger bipolar forceps
Klevas clamp
KLI
    KLI bipolar forceps
    KLI laprocator laparoscope
    KLI monopolar forceps
Klima-Rosegger sternal needle
Kliners alar retractor
Kling
    K. adhesive dressing
    K. fluff roll
    K. gauze
    K. gauze bandage
    K. gauze dressing
    K. sponge
Klinikum-Berlin tubing clamp
Klinkenbergh-Loth scissors
Klintmalm clamp
Klintskog amniotomy hook
Klip
    Taut Safety K.
Klippel retractor set

Klockner implant
Kloehn
    K. facebow
    K. headgear
Klondike bed
Kloti vitreous cutter
KLS
    KLS Centre-Drive screw
    KLS Centre-Drive screwdriver
KLS-Martin
    KLS-M. Centre-Drive screw
    KLS-M. modular neuro kit
    KLS-M. modular osteosynthesis system
Klutch denture adhesive
Klute clamp
KM-1 breast pump
KMC femoral stem prosthesis
KMP
    KMP femoral stem prosthesis
    KMP fenestrated femoral stem
KM-series
    KM-s. liner
    KM-s. shell
KMW/PC femoral prosthesis
Knapp
    K. blade
    K. cataract knife
    K. cataract spoon
    K. cyclodialysis spatula
    K. cystitome
    K. eye speculum
    K. iris hook
    K. iris knife
    K. iris knife needle
    K. iris probe
    K. iris repositor
    K. iris scissors
    K. iris spatula
    K. lacrimal sac retractor
    K. lens loop
    K. lens scoop
    K. lens spoon
    K. refractor
    K. strabismus scissors
    K. trachoma forceps
Knapp-Culler speculum
Knapp-Luer trachoma forceps
Knead-A-Ball exerciser
knee
    k. bolster
    k. brace splint
    cadaveric k.
    k. cage brace
    49er k. brace
    k. extension orthosis
    Genesis unicompartmental k.
    Gustilo-Kyle total k.
    Hosmer single-axis locking k.
    Hosmer weight-activated locking k.
    k. immobilizer
    k. immobilizer splint
    Kapp Surgical Instrument prosthetic k.
    Kinematic rotating-hinge total k.

Korn Cage k.
Link Endo-Model rotational k.
Mauch Swing and Stance
  hydraulic k.
k. MD brace
Miller-Galante unicompartmental k.
Noiles posterior stabilized k.
Noiles rotating hinge k.
Otto Bock modular rotary
  hydraulic k.
Otto Bock Safety constant-
  friction k.
PCA modular total k.
PCA revision total k.
PCA unicompartmental k.
PC Performer k.
K. Pillo pillow
pneumatic 4-bar linkage k.
PolymerFriction total k.
k. positioner
Press-Fit condylar total k.
k. retractor
self-aligning k.
K. Signature System
single-axis friction k.
single-axis locking k.
Stanmore total k.
Total Knee 2100 prosthetic k.
Ultimate k.
variable axis k.
k. wedge
weight-activated locking k.
knee-ankle-foot orthosis
knee-ankle orthosis
knee-bearing prosthesis
kneecap stabilizer
KneeCrank
Kneed-It
  K.-I. knee guard
  K.-I. kneeguard
knee-foot-ankle orthosis
kneeguard
  Kneed-It k.
kneeRAP wrap
knife, pl. **knives**
Abraham tonsillar k.
ACL graft k.
Adson dural k.
Agnew canaliculus k.
A-K diamond k.
Alcon A-OK crescent k.
Alcon A-OK phacoemulsification
  slit k.
Alcon A-OK ShortCut k.
Aleman meniscotomy k.
Alexander otoplasty k.
Allen-Barkan k.
Allen-Hanbury k.
amputation k.
Anderson double-end k.
angular k.
arachnoid k.
Arenberg endolymphatic sac k.
Arthro-Lok k.
arthroscopy k.

ASICO multi-angled diamond k.
Atkins tonsillar k.
Austin dental k.
Austin dissection k.
Austin sickle k.
Auth k.
Ayre cone k.
Ayre-Scott cervical cone k.
Backhaus cervical k.
backward-cutting k.
Bailey-Glover-O'Neill
  commissurotomy k.
Bailey-Morse mitral k.
Bailey round k.
Ballenger cartilage k.
Ballenger mucosal k.
Ballenger nasal k.
Ballenger septal k.
Ballenger swivel k.
Bard-Parker k.
Barkan goniotomy k.
Barker Vacu-tome suction k.
Baron ear k.
Barraquer corneal k.
Barraquer keratoplasty k.
Barrett uterine k.
bayonet k.
Beard lid k.
Beaver blade cataract k.
Beaver blade discission k.
Beaver cataract k.
Beaver ear k.
Beaver goniotomy needle k.
Beaver tonsillar k.
Beaver Xstar k.
Beck tonsillar k.
Beer canaliculus k.
Beer cataract k.
Bellucci lancet k.
Berens cataract k.
Berens glaucoma k.
Berens iris k.
Berens keratoplasty k.
Berens ptosis k.
Berens sclerotomy k.
Bickle microsurgical k.
Bircher meniscus k.
Bishop-Harman k.
bistoury k.
blade k.
k. blade
bladebreaker k.
Blair-Brown skin graft k.
Blair cleft palate k.
Blake gingivectomy k.
Blount k.
Bock k.
Bodenham-Blair skin graft k.
Bodenham-Humby skin graft k.
Bodian discission k.
Bonta mastectomy k.
Bosher commissurotomy k.
Bowman eye k.
Braithwaite skin graft k.
Brock mitral valve k.

K

knife *(continued)*

Brock pulmonary valve k.
Brophy bistoury k.
Brophy cleft palate k.
Brown-Blair skin graft k.
Brown cleft palate k.
Buck myringotomy k.
Bucy cordotomy k.
Burford-Lebsche sternal k.
button-end k.
Caltagirone skin graft k.
Canad meniscal k.
canal k.
canaliculus k.
Canfield tonsillar k.
k. cannula cystitome
capsular k.
Carter septal k.
cartilage k.
cast k.
Castroviejo discission k.
Castroviejo ophthalmic k.
Castroviejo twin k.
Castroviejo-Wheeler discission k.
cataract k.
Catlin amputation k.
Cave cartilage k.
Celita Elite k.
Celita Sapphire k.
cervical cone k.
chalazion k.
circle k.
clasp k.
Cobbett skin graft k.
cold coning k.
Collin amputation k.
Collings electrosurgery k.
Colver tonsillar k.
Concept arthroscopic k.
Converse nasal k.
cordotomy k.
corneal k.
cornea-splitting k.
Cornman dissecting k.
Cottle double-edged nasal k.
Crescent plaster k.
Crile cleft palate k.
Crile gasserian ganglion k.
Cronin palate k.
Crosby k.
Culbertson canal k.
Curdy sclerotome k.
Cushing dural hook k.
Cusick goniotomy k.
k. cystotome
Davidoff cordotomy k.
Daviel chalazion k.
Day tonsillar k.
Dean capsulotomy k.
Dean iris k.
Dean tonsillar k.
DeLee laparotrachelotomy k.
Dench ear k.
DePalma k.

Derlacki capsular k.
Dermot-Pierce ball-tipped k.
Derra commissurotomy k.
Derra guillotine k.
D'Errico laminar k.
Desmarres iris k.
Desmarres paracentesis k.
Deutschman cataract k.
Devonshire k.
Diamatrix trapezoidal diamond k.
diamond blade k.
diamond-dusted k.
diamond phaco k.
Diamontek k.
diathermy k.
Dintenfass-Chapman ear k.
discission k.
dissection k.
k. dissector
dissector k.
double-edged sickle k.
double-ended flap k.
Douglas tonsillar k.
Down epiphyseal k.
Downing cartilage k.
drum elevator k.
Dupuytren k.
Duredge k.
Duredge-Paufique k.
ear furuncle k.
EdgeAhead crescent k.
EdgeAhead phaco slit k.
k. electrode
electronic k.
Elschnig cataract k.
Elschnig corneal k.
Elschnig pterygium k.
epiretinal delamination diamond k.
Equen-Neuffer laryngeal k.
Esmarch plaster k.
eye k.
facial nerve k.
Farrior-McHugh ear k.
Farrior otoplasty k.
Farrior septal cartilage stripper k.
Farrior sickle k.
Farrior triangular k.
Feaster radial keratotomy k.
feather k.
Ferris Robb tonsillar k.
Fine-Gill corneal k.
Fisher tonsillar k.
flap k.
Fletcher tonsillar k.
Foerster capsulotomy k.
Fomon double-edge k.
k. and fork
forward-cutting k.
Fowler-Zollner k.
Frazier cordotomy k.
Frazier pituitary capsulectomy k.
Freedom k.
Freer-Ingal nasal submucous k.
Freer nasal submucous k.
Freer septal k.

Freiberg cartilage k.
Freiberg meniscectomy k.
Friesner ear k.
gamma k.
Gandhi k.
Gerzog ear k.
Gerzog-Ralks k.
Gill corneal k.
Gill-Fine corneal k.
Gill-Hess k.
Gill iris k.
Gill pop-up arcuate diamond k.
Gillquist-Oretorp-Stille k.
Gill-Welsh k.
gingivectomy k.
Girard-Swan k.
Glasscock-House k.
Goldman-Fox k.
Goldman guillotine nerve k.
goniopuncture k.
goniotomy k.
Goodhill k.
Goodhill-Down k.
Goodyear tonsillar k.
Goulian k.
Graefe cataract k.
Graefe cystitome k.
Graefe iris k.
Graf cervical cordotomy k.
Green cataract k.
Green corneal k.
Grieshaber ruby k.
Grieshaber ultrasharp k.
Groff electrosurgical k.
Grover meniscus k.
Guilford-Wright crurotomy k.
Guilford-Wright double-edged k.
Guilford-Wright elevator k.
Guilford-Wright flap k.
Guilford-Wright incudostapedial k.
Guilford-Wright roller k.
Guy tenotomy k.
Guyton-Lundsgaard cataract k.
Haab after-cataract k.
Haab eye k.
Haab scleral resection k.
Halle dural k.
Halle trigeminus k.
k. handle
Harrison capsular k.
Harrison myringoplasty k.
Harrison-Shea k.
Harris tonsillar k.
Hartmann k.
Herbert sclerotomy k.
Hilsinger tonsillar k.
Hoffmann-Osher-Hopkins plaster k.
hook k.
hooked k.
Hopkins plaster k.
Horsley dural k.
Hosemann choledochus k.
hot k.
Hough fascial k.
Hough incision k.

Hough-Rosen k.
Hough whirlybird k.
House ear k.
House incudostapedial joint k.
House lancet k.
House myringoplasty k.
House myringotomy k.
House-Rosen k.
House round k.
House sickle k.
House tympanoplasty k.
Huco diamond k.
Hufnagel commissurotomy k.
Huibregtse-Katon needle k.
Hulbert electrosurgical k.
Humby k.
Hundley knee k.
Hyams scleral k.
Impex diamond radial keratotomy k.
incision k.
incudostapedial joint k.
iris k.
Jackson tracheal bistoury k.
Jacobson vessel k.
Jaeger keratome k.
Jako-Kleinsasser k.
Jako laryngeal k.
Jannetta angular k.
Jarit plaster k.
Johnson evisceration k.
Johnson ptosis k.
Johnson-Tooke corneal k.
Jones cervical k.
Jones IMA diamond k.
Jordan canal incision k.
Jordan capsular k.
Jordan stapedectomy k.
Joseph angular k.
Joseph bistoury k.
Joseph button-end k.
Joseph cervical k.
Joseph double-edged k.
Joseph-Maltz k.
Joseph nasal k.
Jung microtome k.
Keeler-Meyer diamond k.
Keeler ruby k.
Kelman cystitome k.
Killian tonsillar k.
King-Prince k.
Kirby cataract k.
Kirby-Duredge k.
Kirkland k.
Kleinsasser k.
Knapp cataract k.
Knapp iris k.
KOI diamond k.
Korte plaster k.
Kreissl meatotomy k.
Krull acetabular k.
Kyle crypt k.
Ladd k.
Lancaster k.
Lance k.
lancet k.

K

knife *(continued)*
Landolt eye k.
Lange blade k.
Lange cartilage k.
Langenbeck flap k.
Langenbeck resection k.
Lang eye k.
Lanigan cartilage k.
laryngeal k.
Laseredge microsurgical k.
Lebsche sternal k.
Lee cartilage k.
Lee-Cohen k.
Leksell gamma k.
Leland-Jones tonsillar k.
Leland tonsillar k.
Lempert k.
ligamentum teres k.
Lillie tonsillar k.
Lindvall meniscectomy k.
Lindvall-Stille meniscal k.
Lipschiff k.
Lister k.
Liston amputation k.
Liston phalangeal k.
Lorez PC/TC ultra-sharp k.
Lothrop tonsillar k.
Lowe-Breck cartilage k.
Lowell glaucoma k.
Lowe microtome k.
Lucae ear perforation k.
Lundsgaard k.
Lundsgaard-Burch k.
Lynch obtuse-angle laryngeal k.
Lynch right-angle k.
Lynch straight k.
Lynch tonsillar k.
MacCallum k.
Machemer scleral k.
MacKenty cleft palate k.
Magielski bayonet canal k.
Maltz button-end k.
Maltz cartilage k.
Mandelbaum ear k.
Marcks k.
margin-finishing k.
Martinez corneal dissector k.
Maumenee goniotomy k.
Mayo k.
McCabe canal k.
McCaslin k.
McGee tympanoplasty k.
McHugh facial nerve k.
McHugh-Farrior canal k.
McHugh flap k.
McKeever cartilage k.
McMurray tenotomy k.
McPherson-Wheeler eye k.
McPherson-Ziegler microiris k.
McReynolds-Castroviejo pterygium k.
McReynolds pterygium k.
Mead lancet k.
meniscal k.
meniscectomy k.

Mercer cartilage k.
Merrifield k.
Metzenbaum septal k.
Meyer Swiss diamond lancet k.
Meyer Swiss diamond wedge k.
Meyhöffer eye k.
Micra k.
microiris k.
micrometer k.
microsurgical k.
Midas Rex k.
Millette tonsillar k.
Millette-Tyding k.
Miltex ligature k.
Mitchell cartilage k.
Monahan-Lewis k.
Moncorps k.
Moorehead ear k.
Morgenstein periosteal k.
Moritz-Schmidt k.
Murphy plaster k.
Myocure k.
myringoplasty k.
myringotomy k.
nasal k.
Neff meniscal k.
Neivert tonsillar k.
Neoflex bendable k.
Newman uterine k.
Niche k.
Niedner commissurotomy k.
Nordent periodontic k.
Nunez-Nunez mitral stenosis k.
OIU cold k.
Olivecrona trigeminal k.
Olk membrane peeler k.
Optima diamond k.
Orandi k.
Oretorp retractable k.
orthopedic k.
Osher diamond k.
Osher micrometer cataract k.
Pace hysterectomy k.
Page tonsillar k.
Paparella canal k.
Paparella-House k.
Paparella incudostapedial joint k.
Paparella sickle k.
paracentesis k.
Parasmillie k.
Parker serrated discission k.
Parker tenotomy k.
Paufique corneal k.
Paufique-Duredge k.
Paufique graft k.
Paufique keratoplasty k.
Phaco-4 diamond step k.
pick k.
plaster k.
platelet-shaped k.
Politzer angular ear k.
Politzer-Ralks k.
Pope rectal k.
Potter modified k.
Potter sickle k.

Potts expansile k.
pterygium k.
ptosis k.
pull k.
Quantum enhancement k.
Questus Leading Edge sheathed
  arthroscopy k.
radial keratotomy k.
Ralks reversible k.
Rayport dural k.
razor blade k.
Reese ptosis k.
Rehne skin graft k.
Reiner plaster k.
retrograde k.
retrograde-cutting hook-shaped k.
Rhein Advantage diamond k.
Rhein clear corneal diamond k.
Rica trigeminal k.
Ridlon plaster k.
right-angle k.
Rish cartilage k.
Rizzuti-Spizziri cannula k.
Robb tonsillar k.
Robertson tonsillar k.
Robinson flap k.
Rochester mitral stenosis k.
rocker k.
Roentgen k.
Roger septal k.
roller k.
Rosen cartilage k.
Rosen ear incision k.
round ruby k.
Royce bayonet ear k.
ruby diamond k.
Ryerson tenotome k.
Salenius meniscal k.
sapphire k.
Sarot k.
SatinCrescent implant k.
SatinShortCut implant k.
SatinSlit implant k.
Sato corneal k.
scarifier k.
Schanz k.
Scheer elevator k.
Scheie goniopuncture k.
Scheie goniotomy k.
Scholl meniscal k.
Schuknecht roller k.
Schuknecht sickle k.
Schultze embryotomy k.
Schwartz cordotomy k.
scleral resection k.
sculp k.
Seiler tonsillar k.
Sellor mitral valve k.
semilunar cartilage k.
septal k.
serrated fine-cutting k.
Sexton ear k.
Shaffer modification of Barkan k.
Shambaugh k.
Shambaugh-Lempert k.

sharp k.
Sharpoint k.
Shea incision k.
Sheehy canal k.
Sheehy-House k.
Sheehy myringotomy k.
Sheehy round k.
Sherman k.
ShortCut A-OK small-incision k.
Sichel iris k.
sickle k.
Silver k.
Silverstein round k.
Silverstein sickle k.
Simon fistula k.
Simons cleft palate k.
Sims k.
skiving k.
slit blade k.
Sluder k.
SMIC sternal k.
Smillie meniscal cartilage k.
Smith cartilage k.
Smith cataract k.
Smith cordotomy k.
Smith-Fisher cataract k.
Smith-Green cataract k.
Speed-Sprague k.
Spizziri cannula k.
k. spud
stapedectomy k.
Stealth DBO free-hand diamond k.
Stecher arachnoid k.
Step-Knife diamond blade k.
sternal k.
Stewart cartilage k.
stiletto k.
stitch-removing k.
Stiwer furuncle k.
Storz cataract k.
Storz-Duredge steel cataract k.
Storz folding-handle ear k.
Storz sheath-handle ear k.
straight tympanoplasty k.
Strayer meniscal k.
Stryker cartilage k.
Stryker-School meniscal k.
Suker spatula k.
Swan discission k.
Swan spade-type needle k.
Swets goniotomy k.
swift-cut phaco incision k.
swivel k.
sword k.
Tabb double-ended flap k.
Tabb ear k.
Tabb myringoplasty k.
Tabb pick k.
Taylor k.
tendon k.
teres k.
testing drum k.
thermal k.
Thiersch skin graft k.
Thornton T-incision diamond k.

K

knife *(continued)*
    Tiemann-Meals tenolysis k.
    Tobold laryngeal k.
    Toennis dural k.
    tonsillar k.
    Tooke angled corneal k.
    Tooke iris k.
    Tooke-Johnson corneal k.
    Torchia corneal k.
    trifacet k.
    trigeminal k.
    triple-edge diamond-blade k.
    Troilius capsulotomy k.
    Troutman corneal k.
    Troutman-Tooke corneal k.
    Tubby tenotomy k.
    Tweedy canaliculus k.
    twin k.
    Tydings tonsillar k.
    tympanoplasty k.
    Ullrich fistula k.
    Ullrich uterine k.
    UltraCision ultrasonic k.
    Unicat k.
    Unigraft k.
    Unitome k.
    upward-cutting triangular k.
    Vacu-tome k.
    Vannas abscess k.
    Vaughan abscess k.
    vessel k.
    Vic hair transplant k.
    Vic Vallis running hair k.
    Virchow brain k.
    Virchow cartilage k.
    Virchow skin graft k.
    Visitec circular k.
    Visitec crescent k.
    Visitec EdgeAhead phaco slit k.
    Visitec stiletto k.
    V-lance eye k.
    Wagner k.
    Walb k.
    Wallace-Maloney k.
    Walton ear k.
    Watson skin graft k.
    wave-edge k.
    Weber canaliculus k.
    Weber iris k.
    Webster skin graft k.
    Weck k.
    Wheeler discission k.
    Wheeler iris k.
    Wheeler malleable-shape k.
    Wilder cystitome k.
    Williams cartilage k.
    Woodruff spatula k.
    Wright-Guilford double-edged k.
    Wright-Guilford elevator k.
    Wright-Guilford flap k.
    Wright-Guilford incudostapedial k.
    Wright-Guilford roller k.
    Wullstein double-edged k.
    X-Acto utility k.
    XKnife k.
    Yamanda k.
    Yasargil arachnoid k.
    Yund ligamentum teres k.
    Ziegler iris k.
knife-pick
Knight
    K. biopsy needle
    K. brace
    K. nasal-cutting forceps
    K. nasal scissors
    K. nasal septum-cutting forceps
    K. polyp forceps
    K. septal forceps
    K. septum-cutting forceps
    K. turbinate forceps
Knighton-Crawford forceps
Knighton hemilaminectomy self-retaining retractor
Knighton-Kerrison punch
Knight-Sluder nasal forceps
Knight-Taylor
    K.-T. brace
    K.-T. and Williams spinal orthosis
Knit-Rite suspension sleeve
knitted
    k. Dacron
    k. graft
    k. prosthesis
    k. sewing ring
    k. Teflon prosthesis
    k. vascular prosthesis
knives *(pl. of* knife*)*
Knobble massager
Knoche tube
Knodt distraction rod
Knolle
    K. anterior chamber irrigating cannula
    K. capsular polisher
    K. capsular scraper
    K. capsular scratcher
    K. capsule polisher
    K. dipstick
    K. lens cortex spatula
    K. lens gauge
    K. lens implantation forceps
    K. lens nucleus spatula
    K. lens speculum
    K. needle holder
Knolle-Kelman
    K.-K. cannulated cystitome
    K.-K. sharp cystitome
Knolle-Pearce
    K.-P. cannula
    K.-P. irrigating lens loop
    K.-P. vectis
Knolle-Shepard lens forceps
Knolle-Volker lens-holding forceps
knot
    k. pusher
    k. tier
knot-holding forceps
knotting forceps
knot-tying instrument

Knowles
    K. bandage scissors
    K. hip pin
    K. pin nail
Knuckle Benders
knuckle-bender splint
knurled handle
Knutsson
    K. penile clamp
    K. urethrography clamp
Knuttsen bending film
Koagamin dressing
Koala intrauterine pressure catheter
Kobak needle
Kobayashi
    K. retractor
    K. vacuum extractor
Koby cataract forceps
Koch
    K. chopper
    K. nucleus hydrolysis needle
    K. phaco manipulator
    K. phaco manipulator/splitter
Kocher
    K. arterial forceps
    K. artery forceps
    K. bladder retractor
    K. bladder spatula
    K. blade retractor
    K. bone retractor
    K. brain spoon
    K. bronchocele sound
    K. depressor
    K. gallbladder retractor
    K. goiter director
    K. goiter dissector
    K. grooved director
    K. hemostat
    K. hemostatic forceps
    K. intestinal clamp
    K. kidney-elevating forceps
    K. Micro-Line intestinal forceps
    K. periosteal dissector
    K. periosteal elevator
    K. probe
    K. raspatory
    K. self-retaining goiter retractor
Kocher-Crotti self-retaining goiter
    retractor
Kocher-Langenbeck retractor
Kocher-Ochsner hemostatic forceps
Kocher-Wagner retractor
Koch-Julian sphincterotome
Koch-Mason dressing
Koch-Salz nucleus splitter
Kock
    K. ileal reservoir
    K. nipple
Kodak
    K. 1200 Digital Science medical
      imager
    K. Ektachem autoanalyzer
    K. Ektachem 700 machine
    K. XAR-5 x-ray film

    K. X-Omatic C-1 cassette
    K. XRP-1 x-ray film
Kodel
    K. polyester elbow protector
    K. sling
Kodex drill
Koeberlé forceps
Koeller illumination system
Koenig
    K. elevator
    K. graft
    K. grooved director
    K. metatarsal broach
    K. MPJ implant and arthroplasty
      system
    K. MPJ prosthesis
    K. nail-splitting scissors
    K. probe
    K. rasp
    K. raspatory
    K. tonsillar swab
    K. total great toe implant
    K. vascular forceps
    K. vein retractor
Koenig-Stille scissors
Koeppe
    K. diagnostic lens
    K. goniolens
    K. gonioscopic lens
    K. intraocular lens implant
    K. lamp
Koerte
    K. gallstone forceps
    K. retractor
Koffler-Hajek
    K.-H. laminectomy rongeur
    K.-H. sphenoidal punch
Koffler-Lillie septal forceps
Koffler septal forceps
Kogan
    K. endocervical speculum
    K. endospeculum
    K. endospeculum forceps
    K. urethra speculum
KOH
    KOH colpotomizer system
Kohlman urethral dilator
Kohn needle
Koh ultramicro instrument
KOI diamond knife
KoKo
    K. Rhythm PC-Based ECG
    K. spirometer
Kokowicz raspatory
Kolb
    K. bronchial forceps
    K. trocar
Kold
    K. Kap
    K. Kompress cold pack
    K. Wrap
    K. Wrap cold compression bandage
    K. Wrap freezable compress

K

Kold (*continued*)
    K. Wrap general use sterile burn dressing & emergency wound cover
Ko-Lec-Pac urinary collection kit
Kollagen dressing
Koln clip
Kolobow membrane lung
Kolodny
    K. clamp
    K. forceps
Komai stereotactic head frame
Koman-Nair iris repositor
KOMFORM coated gauze
Konan
    K. SP8000 image analysis system
    K. SP8000 noncontact specular microscope
Koneg retractor
Konica scanner
Konig bar chart
Konigsberg
    K. catheter
    K. 5-channel solid-state catheter assembly
    K. microtransducer
Kontack temporary crown
Kontron
    K. balloon catheter
    K. electrode
    K. intra-aortic balloon
    K. intra-aortic balloon pump
    K. TFT 45.6 rotor
Kooijman eye model
Kool Kit cold therapy pack
koolPAK pack
Koontz hernia needle
Kopan breast lesion localization needle
Kopetzky sinus bur
Korex cork sheet
Kormed disposable liver biopsy needle
Korn
    K. Cage knee
    K. Cage knee brace
koroscope
Koros EndoMax scissors
Korotkoff sound
Korte
    K. abdominal spatula
    K. gallstone forceps
    K. plaster knife
    K. retractor
Korte-Wagner retractor
Korth ureterotome
Kos
    K. attic cannula
    K. chisel
    K. crimper forceps
    K. curette
    K. ear suction tube
    K. elevator
    K. middle ear instrument
    K. pick

Koslowski
    K. hip nail
    K. microforceps
Kostuik
    K. internal spine fixation system
    K. rod
    K. screw
Kostuik-Harrington
    K.-H. anterior distraction system
    K.-H. device
    K.-H. distraction system
    K.-H. spinal instrumentation
Kowa
    K. angiographic camera
    K. fluorescein system
    K. FM-500 laser flare meter
    K. fundus camera
    K. hand camera
    K. hand-held slit lamp
    K. laser flare-cell photometer
    K. Optimed slit lamp
    K. PRO II retinal camera
    K. RC-XV fundus camera
Kowa-Optimed camera
Koylon foam rubber dressing
Kozlinski retractor
Kozlowski tube
K-Pratt dilator
KR-7000P auto-kerato-refractometer
Krackow
    K. HTO blade staple
    K. suture
Kraff
    K. capsular polisher
    K. capsule polisher curette
    K. cortex cannula
    K. intraocular utility forceps
    K. lens-inserting forceps
    K. nucleus lens loop
    K. nucleus splitter
    K. suturing forceps
    K. tying forceps
Kraff-Osher lens forceps
Kraff-Utrata
    K.-U. capsulorrhexis forceps
    K.-U. intraocular utility forceps
    K.-U. tear capsulotomy forceps
Krahn exophthalmometer
Krakau tonometer
Kramer
    K. direct-vision telescope
    K. ear speculum
    K. forceps
    K. operating laryngoscope
Kramer-Collins Spore trap
Kramp scissors
Krasky retractor
Krasnov lens
Kratz
    K. aspirating speculum
    K. capsular scraper
    K. capsular scratcher
    K. cystitome
    K. diamond-dusted needle
    K. elliptical-style lens

K. implant
K. iris push-pull hook
K. lens-inserting forceps
K. modified J-loop intraocular lens
K. polisher
K. posterior chamber intraocular lens

Kratz-Barraquer wire lid speculum
Kratz-Jensen
  K.-J. capsular scratcher
  K.-J. polisher
Kratz-Johnson modified J-loop intraocular lens
Kratz-Sinskey intraocular lens implant
Krause
  K. angular oval punch
  K. antral trocar
  K. arm rest
  K. biopsy forceps
  K. ear polyp snare
  K. esophagoscopy forceps
  K. laryngeal snare
  K. nasal polyp snare
  K. nasal snare cannula
  K. oval punch tip
  K. punch forceps
  K. punch forceps tip
  K. square-basket tip
  K. Universal forceps
Krause-Davis spatula
Krause-Wolfe
  K.-W. graft
  K.-W. implant
  K.-W. prosthesis
Krayenbuehl
  K. dural hook
  K. nerve hook
  K. vessel hook
Krego elevator
Kreiger-Spitznas vibrating scissors
Kreischer bone chisel
Kreiselman
  K. infant warmer
  K. resuscitation unit
Kreissl meatotomy knife
Kremer
  K. excimer laser
  K. fixation forceps
  K. triple-optical zone corneal marker
  K. two-point fixation forceps
Krentz
  K. gastroscope
  K. photogastroscope
Kretschmer retractor
Kretz
  K. Combison 330 ultrasound scanner
  K. ultrasound system
Kreuscher semilunar cartilage scissors
Kreutzmann
  K. cannula
  K. trocar
Krieger
  K. wide-field fundus lens

Krinkle gauze roll
Krinsky-Prince accommodation ruler
Kristeller
  K. vaginal retractor
  K. vaginal speculum
Kristiansen eyelet lag screw
Krogh
  K. apparatus spirometer
Krol esophageal dilator
Krol-Koski tracheal dilator
Kromayer lamp
Kron
  K. bile duct dilator
  K. bile duct probe
Kronecker aneurysm needle
Kronendonk pin
Kroner apparatus
Kronfeld
  K. eyelid retractor
  K. micropin forceps
  K. pin
  K. refractor
  K. surface electrode
  K. suturing forceps
Krönlein-Berke retractor
Krönlein hemostatic forceps
Kronner
  K. external fixation device
  K. Manipujector
  K. Manipujector uterine manipulator/injector
Krosnick vesicourethral suspension clamp
Krueger instrument stop
Krukenberg
  K. pigment spindle forceps
  K. sponge
Krull acetabular knife
Krumeich-Barraquer
  K.-B. lasitome
  K.-B. microkeratome
Krumeich stereoscope
Krupin
  K. eye disk
  K. valve with disk
Krupin-Denver
  K.-D. eye valve
Krwawicz
  K. cataract cryosurgical instrument
  K. cataract extractor
Kry-Med
  K.-M. cryopexy unit
  K.-M. 300 probe
Kryo 10 model 10-20 freezer
Kryptok bifocal lens implant
krypton red laser
KS 5 ACL brace
K/S-Allis forceps
KSK articulator
KSO brace
K-Sponge
  K.-S. hydrocellulose sponge
  K.-S. II
KT1000 foot stabilizer
KT1000, 2000 knee ligament arthrometer
KT1000/s surgical arthrometer

KTK laminaria tent
KTP
  KTP laser
  KTP laser probe
KTP/532
  KTP/532 laser
  KTP/532 surgical laser
  KTP/532 surgical laser system
KTP/Nd:YAG
  KTP/Nd:YAG laser
  KTP/Nd:YAG XP surgical laser
    system
KTP/YAG
  KTP/YAG laser
  KTP/YAG surgical laser system
K-Tube tube
Kuda
  K. endoscope
  K. laparoscope
  K. retractor
  K. shaver
Kudo elbow component
Kugel
  K. hernia patch
  K. mesh
Kuglen
  K. angled lens manipulator
  K. irrigating lens manipulator
  K. lens retractor
  K. manipulating iris hook
  K. push/pull
  K. refractor
  K. straight lens manipulator
Kuhlman
  K. cervical brace
  K. cervical traction device
Kuhn
  K. endotracheal tube
  K. mask
Kuhn-Bolger
  K.-B. angled curette
  K.-B. seeker
Kuhne coverglass forceps
Kuhnt
  K. capsular forceps
  K. capsule forceps
  K. corneal scarifier
  K. fixation forceps
  K. gouge
Kulvin-Kalt
  K.-K. iris forceps
  K.-K. mules
Kulzer inlay system
Kummel intestinal spatula
Kumpe catheter
Kundin wound measurement gauge
Küntscher
  K. cloverleaf nail
  K. drill
  K. extractor
  K. femur guide pin
  K. finisher
  K. hammer
  K. impactor
  K. intramedullary nail

  K. nail driver
  K. nail extender
  K. nail-extracting hook
  K. nail instrument
  K. nail set
  K. rod
  K. shaft reamer
  K. traction apparatus
  K. traction device
Küntscher-Hudson brace
Kunzli orthopaedic sports shoe
Kurer anchor
Kurlander orthopaedic wrench
Kurosaka interference-fit screw
Kurtin
  K. handpiece
  K. planing dermabrasion brush
  K. vein stripper
  K. wire brush
Kurze
  K. dissecting scissors
  K. dissector
  K. microbiopsy forceps
  K. micrograsping forceps
  K. microscissors
  K. pickup forceps
  K. suction-irrigator
  K. suction tube
Kurz pulsation orthodontic headgear
Kurzweil reading machine
Kusch'kin Ace wheelchair
**Kushner-Tandatnick endometrial biopsy
  curette**
Küstner
  K. suture
  K. tenaculum
  K. uterine tenaculum forceps
Kuttner
  K. dissector
  K. wound stretcher
Kutzmann clamp
Kuyper-Murphy sternal retractor
Kwapis
  K. interdental forceps
  K. ligature carrier
  K. subcondylar retractor
Kwik
  K. Board IV and arterial line
    stabilizer
  K. wax
Kwik-Skan monitor
K wire
  Kirschner wire
K-wire
  Kirschner wire
  percutaneous K-wire
Kwitko
  K. conjunctival spreader
  K. lens spatula
Kydex
  K. body jacket
  K. brace
Kyle
  K. applicator

K. crypt knife
K. nasal speculum

kyphosis brace
K-Y pliers

K

laboratory automation system
Laborde
    L. forceps
    L. tracheal dilator
Labotech micro-plated immunoanalyzer
Labtron stethoscope
labyrinth curette
LaCarrere
    L. electrode
    L. electrodiaphake
lace
    no-tie stretch l.
    spyrolace shoe l.
lace-on brace
L.A. cervical orthosis
Lacey
    L. prosthesis
    L. rotating hinge
    L. total knee implant
lacidem suture
Lack tongue retractor
Lacor tube
Lacricath lacrimal duct catheter
lacrimal
    l. apparatus
    l. awl
    l. balloon catheter
    l. canaliculus dilator
    l. duct probe
    l. duct T-tube
    l. intubation probe
    l. irrigating cannula
    l. needle
    l. osteotome
    l. sac bur
    l. sac chisel
    l. sac gouge
    l. sac retractor
    l. sac rongeur
    l. sound
    l. stent
    l. trephine
Lacrimedics occlusion starter kit
Lactina Select breast pump
Lactomer
    L. absorbable subcuticular skin staple
    L. copolymer absorbable stapler
    L. skin staple material
LactoSorb
    L. plating system
    L. resorbable craniomaxillofacial fixation
    L. resorbable fixation device
    L. resorbable fixation system
LAD
    ligament augmentation device
    Kennedy LAD
LADARVision
    L. excimer laser system
Ladarvision Platform

Ladd
    L. calipers
    L. elevator
    L. fiberoptic system
    L. intracranial pressure monitor
    L. intracranial pressure sensor
    L. knife
    L. lid clamp
    L. raspatory
ladder
    finger l.
    shoulder l.
Ladmore plastic filling instrument
Lady & Sir dignity plus pant
LAE cast
Laerdal
    L. infant resuscitator
    L. Resusci Folding Bag II
Lafayette skinfold calipers
LaForce
    L. adenotome
    L. adenotome blade
    L. golf-club knife spud
    L. hemostatic tonsillectome
LaForce-Grieshaber adenotome
LaForce-Stevenson adenotome
LaForce-Storz adenotome
LAGB system - Lap-Band adjustable gastric banding system
Lagleyze needle
Lagrange
    L. eye scissors
    L. sclerectomy scissors
Lagrange-Letoumel hip prosthesis
lag screw
Lahey
    L. arterial forceps
    L. bag
    L. bronchial clamp
    L. Carb-Edge scissors
    L. catheter
    L. Clinic dural hook
    L. Clinic nerve root retractor
    L. Clinic skull trephine
    L. Clinic spinal fusion gouge
    L. Clinic thin osteotome
    L. delicate scissors
    L. dissecting forceps
    L. dissecting scissors
    L. drain
    L. gall duct forceps
    L. goiter retractor
    L. goiter-seizing forceps
    L. goiter tenaculum
    L. goiter vulsellum forceps
    L. hemostat
    L. hemostatic forceps
    L. ligature carrier
    L. ligature passer
    L. lock arterial forceps
    L. needle
    L. operating scissors

L

Lahey *(continued)*
    L. thoracic clamp
    L. thoracic forceps
    L. thyroid retractor
    L. thyroid scissors
    L. thyroid tenaculum forceps
    L. thyroid tissue traction forceps
    L. thyroid traction vulsellum forceps
    L. Y-tube
    L. Y-tube tube
Lahey-Babcock forceps
Lahey-Péan forceps
Lahey-Sweet dissecting forceps
Laidley double-catheterizing cystoscope
Laing
    L. concentric hip cup
    L. osteotomy plate
Laird spatula
LAIS laser
Laitinen
    L. CT guidance system
    L. high-precision stereotactic-assisted radiation therapy kit
    L. percutaneous tumor biopsy kit
    L. stereotactic head frame
    L. stereotactic system
Lajeune hemostatic forceps
Lakatos Teflon injector
Lakeside
    L. cotton roll
    L. nasal scissors
Lalonde
    L. bone clamp
    L. delicate hook forceps
    L. extra fine skin hook forceps
    L. tendon approximator
LA4072 low-air-loss overlay
Lamb cannula
Lambda
    L. Omni Stanicor pacemaker
    L. Physik EMG 103 laser
    L. Plus PDL 1, 2 laser system
lambdoidal suture
Lambert
    L. aortic clamp
    L. chalazion forceps
Lambert-Berry rib raspatory
Lambert-Heiman scissors
Lambert-Kay
    L.-K. anastomosis forceps
    L.-K. aortic clamp
    L.-K. vascular clamp
Lambert-Lowman
    L.-L. bone clamp
    L.-L. chisel
Lambone
    L. demineralized laminar bone
    L. freeze dried bone
Lambotte
    L. bone chisel
    L. bone-holding clamp
    L. bone-holding forceps
    L. bone hook
    L. elevator

    L. exhaust system
    L. fibular forceps
    L. osteotome
    L. rib raspatory
Lambotte-Henderson osteotome
Lambrinudi splint
lamellar blade
laminar
    l. air flow unit
    l. C-D hook
    l. dissector
    l. elevator
    l. flow hood
    l. flow system
laminaria
    l. cervical tent
    Dilapan l.
    Japonicum l.
    l. seaweed obstetrical cervical dilator
lamina spreader
laminectomy
    l. blade
    l. chisel
    l. frame
    l. raspatory
    l. rongeur
    l. self-retaining retractor
    l. wedge sponge
Laminex needle
LaminOss
    L. implant
    L. implant system
Lamis
    L. Autofuse infusion pump
    L. infusion system
    L. patellar clamp
Lamitrode lead
Lamont
    L. elevator
    L. nasal rasp
    L. nasal saw
lamp
    Aero-Kromayer l.
    Alzheimer l.
    Bausch-Lomb-Thorpe slit l.
    Bausch & Lomb-Thorpe slit l.
    Binner head l.
    Birch l.
    Birch-Hirschfeld l.
    black light l.
    900 BQ slit l.
    Campbell slit l.
    carbon arc l.
    clamp l.
    Coburn-Rodenstock slit l.
    Coherent LaserLink slit l.
    Davis l.
    Duke-Elder l.
    Eldridge-Green l.
    examining l.
    Faro coolbeam l.
    Finsen l.
    fluorescent l.
    gas discharge l.

Grafco perineal l.
Gullstrand slit l.
Haag-Streit slit l.
Hague cataract l.
halogen l.
head l.
incandescent endoscope l.
Ishihara IV slit l.
Keeler l.
Koeppe l.
Kowa hand-held slit l.
Kowa Optimed slit l.
Kromayer l.
Marco slit l.
mouth l.
Nightingale examining l.
Nikon zoom photo slit l.
Nitra l.
Posner slit l.
quartz l.
Quick-Lite l.
Reichert slit l.
Rodenstock slit l.
Rusch laryngoscope l.
Rycroft l.
sigmoidoscope replacement l.
slit l.
Specular reflex slit l.
Thorpe slit l.
Topcon SL-E series slit l.
tungsten-halogen l.
Universal Mack l.
Universal slit l.
Uviolite l.
VG slit l.
V-slit l.
Wood l.
xenon l.
Zeiss carbon arc slit l.

Lancaster
L. eye magnet
L. eye speculum
L. keratome
L. knife
L. lid speculum
L. ocular transilluminator
L. red-green screen
L. sclerotome

Lancaster-O'Connor
L.-O. forceps
L.-O. speculum

lance
Rolf l.

Lanceford prosthesis
Lance knife
lancet
l. blade
Cleanlet l.
Keeler ultrasonic cataract removal l.
l. knife
Laser L.
Lipectron ultrasonic l.
Meyer Swiss diamond knife l.
Microlance blood l.
Pharmacia l.

Phazet l.
Surelite blood l.
suture l.
l. suture
Swan l.
ultrasonic cataract removal l.

lancet-shaped
l.-s. biopsy forceps
l.-s. electrode

Landau
L. dilator
L. speculum
L. trocar
L. vaginal retractor

Landegger orbital implant
Landers
L. biconcave lens
L. contact lens
L. irrigating vitrectomy ring
L. vitrectomy lens forceps

Landers-Foulks
L.-F. prosthesis
L.-F. temporary keratoprosthesis lens

Lander wide-field temporary keratoprosthesis
Landmark midline catheter
Landolt
L. C acuity chart
L. cannula
L. C ring
L. enucleation scissors
L. eye knife
L. keratome
L. spreader
L. spreading forceps

Landon
L. colpostat
L. forceps
L. narrow-bladed retractor

Landry
L. vein light
L. vein light venoscope

Lane
L. bone-holding clamp
L. bone-holding forceps
L. bone lever
L. bone screw
L. cleft palate needle
L. dissector
L. fasciatome
L. fracture plate
L. gastroenterostomy clamp
L. gastrointestinal forceps
L. intestinal clamp
L. intestinal forceps
L. mouth gag
L. mouthgag
L. periosteal elevator
L. periosteal raspatory
L. rectal catheter
L. retractor
L. screwdriver
L. screw-holding forceps
L. suturing needle
L. tissue forceps

L

Lane *(continued)*
    L. towel clamp
    L. ureteral meatotomy electrode
Lanex medium screen
Lang
    L. dissector
    L. eye knife
    L. eye scoop
    L. eye speculum
    L. iris forceps
    L. jet adjustor kit
    L. suture
Lange
    L. antral punch
    L. approximation forceps
    L. blade
    L. blade knife
    L. bone elevator
    L. bone retractor
    L. cartilage knife
    L. fistular hook
    L. mouthgag
    L. plastic surgery hook
    L. skinfold calipers
Lange-Converse nasal root rongeur
Lange-Hohmann
    L.-H. bone lever
    L.-H. bone retractor
Langenbeck
    L. bone-holding forceps
    L. flap knife
    L. metacarpal amputation saw
    L. needle holder
    L. periosteal elevator
    L. periosteal raspatory
    L. periosteal retractor
    L. resection knife
Langenbeck-Cushing vein retractor
Langenbeck-Green retractor
Langenbeck-Mannerfelt retractor
Langenbeck-O'Brien raspatory
Langerman diamond knife system
Langinate impression material
language acquisition device
Lanier clinical reporting system
Lanigan cartilage knife
Lantiseptic skin protectant
Lanz
    L. low-pressure cuff endotracheal
    tube
    L. pressure regulating valve
    L. tracheostomy tube
lap
    l. pad
    L. Sac
    l. tape
LAP-13 Ranfac cholangiographic catheter
laparator
    Weck high-flow l.
Laparocam
    Storz L.
Laparofan
    L. pneumoperitoneum device
    L. smoke evacuator

Laparolift system
Laparomed
    L. cholangiogram device
    L. cholangiogram vacuum system
    L. suture-applier device
LaparoSAC
    L. obturator
    L. single-use obturator and cannula
    L. trocar
LaparoScan laparoscopic ultrasonic
  imaging
laparoscope
    ACMI Transvaginal Hydro l.
    American Medical Source l.
    AMS autoclavable l.
    Cabot Medical Corporation
    diagnostic l.
    Cabot Medical Corporation
    operating l.
    Circon ACMI diagnostic l.
    Daniel double-punch laser l.
    3Dscope l.
    Dyonics rod lens l.
    Eder l.
    EL2-LS2 flexible video l.
    Elmed diagnostic l.
    Elmed operating l.
    flexible video l.
    Frangenheim l.
    Fujinon diagnostic l.
    Fujinon flexible fiberoptic l.
    Fujinon operating l.
    Hasson l.
    Jacobs-Palmer l.
    KLI laprocator l.
    Kuda l.
    Marlow Surgical Technologies, Inc.
    diagnostic l.
    Marlow Surgical Technologies, Inc.
    operating l.
    Menghini-Wildhirt l.
    MiniSite l.
    offset operating l.
    Olympus diagnostic l.
    Olympus operating l.
    Polaris l.
    Richard Wolf Medical Instruments
    diagnostic l.
    Richard Wolf Medical Instruments
    operating l.
    Ruddock l.
    Sharplav l.
    Solos endoscopy diagnostic l.
    Stoltz l.
    Storz diagnostic l.
    Storz operating l.
    Surgiview multi-use disposable l.
    USA Series Distortion Free
    Hydro l.
    Weerda l.
    Wildhirt l.
    Wisap diagnostic l.
    Wisap operating l.
    Wolf insufflation l.

zero-degree l.
Ziskie operating l.

laparoscopic
l. Allis clamp
l. cannula
l. cholangiography catheter
l. Doppler probe
l. forceps
l. grasper
l. insufflator
l. needle driver
l. pneumodissector
l. retraction system
l. scissors
l. sleeve
l. tie clip

LaparoSonic coagulating shears

Laparostat
Olsen self-retaining L.

laparotomy
l. sponge
l. sponge ring

Laparo Vac I&A system

Lap-Band gastric banding system

Lapides
L. catheter
L. collecting bag
L. holder
L. ileostomy bag
L. needle

Lapidus
L. alternating air-pressure mattress
L. bed

Laplace
L. forceps
L. liver retractor

LaPorta great toe implant

lapping tool

Lapras catheter

Lapra-Ty suture

Lapro-Clip
L.-C. ligating clip
L.-C. ligating clip system

Lapro-Loop device

LapSac collection sack

LAPSE monitor

LapTie
L. endoscopic knot-tying instrument
L. instrument

LapTop cushion

Lapwall
L. laparotomy sponge
L. wound protector

Laqua black line retinal hook

Lar-A-Jext laryngectomy tube

Lardennois button

Laredo-Bard needle

Lares dental handpiece

large
l. antral cannula
l. ball nerve hook
l. bowel curette
l. nail spicule bur
l. uterine curette

large-angled forceps

large-base quad cane

large-bore
l.-b. bile duct endoprosthesis
l.-b. cannula
l.-b. catheter
l.-b. heat probe
l.-b. imaging system scanner
l.-b. magnet
l.-b. slotted aspirating needle

large-caliber nonabsorbable suture

large-channel
l.-c. endoscope
l.-c. therapeutic duodenoscope

large-diameter optics intraocular lens

large-loop electrode

large-lumen catheter

large-pore polyethylene implant

large-tip electrode

Large vena cava clamp (Alfred M. Large)

large-volume
l.-v. round silicone drain
l.-v. suction reservoir

LaRivetti-Levinson intraluminal shunt

LaRocca nasolacrimal tube

LaRoe undermining forceps

Larrey
L. bandage
L. dressing

Larry
L. rectal director
L. rectal probe

Larsen
L. tendon forceps
L. tendon-holding forceps

laryngeal
l. applicator
l. applicator forceps
l. atomizer
l. basket forceps
l. biopsy forceps
l. bronchial grasping forceps
l. cannula
l. curette forceps
l. dilator
l. dissector
l. grasping forceps
l. knife
l. knife handle
l. mask
l. mask airway
l. mirror
l. mirror handle
l. probe
l. punch forceps
l. retractor
l. rotation forceps
l. saw
l. scissors
l. snare
l. sponge carrier
l. sponging forceps
l. stent
l. syringe
l. trocar

L

463

laryngeal-bronchial telescope
laryngectomy clamp
laryngofissure
    l. forceps
    l. retractor
Laryngoflex reinforced endotracheal tube
laryngonasopharyngoscope
    Berci-Ward l.
laryngopharyngoscope
    Berci-Ward l.
    Proctor l.
    Stuckrad magnifying l.
laryngoscope
    adult l.
    adult reverse-bevel l.
    Albert-Andrews l.
    Andrews infant l.
    anterior commissure l.
    Atkins-Tucker shadow-free l.
    baby Miller l.
    Belscope l.
    Benjamin binocular slimline l.
    Benjamin-Lindholm
      microsuspension l.
    Benjamin pediatric operating l.
    Bizzarri-Guiffrida l.
    l. blade
    Briggs l.
    Broyles anterior commissure l.
    Broyles optical l.
    Broyles wasp-waist l.
    Bullard intubating l.
    Burton l.
    l. chest support holder
    Chevalier Jackson l.
    Clerf l.
    commissure l.
    Dedo-Jako l.
    Dedo laser l.
    Dedo-Pilling l.
    direct l.
    disposable l.
    dual distal-lighted l.
    ESI l.
    fiberoptic slide l.
    Fink l.
    Finnoff l.
    Flagg l.
    folding l.
    Foregger l.
    Fragen l.
    Garfield-Holinger l.
    Guedel l.
    Guedel-Negus l.
    Haslinger l.
    Holinger anterior commissure l.
    Holinger-Garfield l.
    Holinger hook-on folding l.
    Holinger hourglass anterior
      commissure l.
    Holinger infant l.
    Holinger modified Jackson l.
    Holinger slotted l.
    Hollister l.
    hook-on folding l.

Hopp l.
Hopp-Morrison l.
hourglass anterior commissure l.
intubation l.
Jackson anterior commissure l.
Jackson fiberoptic slide l.
Jackson sliding l.
Jackson standard l.
Jako l.
Jako-Cherry l.
Jako-Pilling l.
Kantor-Berci video l.
Killian-Lynch suspension l.
KleenSpec disposable l.
Kleinsasser anterior commissure l.
Kleinsasser operating l.
Kleinsasser-Riecker l.
Kramer operating l.
laser l.
Lewy anterior commissure l.
Lewy suspension l.
Lindholm operating l.
Lundy l.
Lynch suspension l.
Machida fiberoptic l.
MacIntosh l.
Magill l.
Mantel l.
Miller l.
mirror l.
multipurpose l.
Negus l.
Olympus ENF-P-series l.
optical l.
Ossoff-Karlan-Dedo l.
Ossoff-Karlan-Jako l.
Ossoff-Karlan laser l.
Ossoff-Karlen l.
pencil-handled l.
polio l.
l. profilometer
reverse-bevel l.
Rica anesthetic l.
Rica anterior commissure l.
Rica infant l.
Riecker-Kleinsasser l.
Roberts self-retaining l.
rotating l.
Rusch l.
Sanders intubation l.
self-retaining l.
shadow-free l.
Shapshay-Healy operating l.
Shapshay-Healy phonatory l.
Siker mirror l.
sliding l.
slotted l.
SMIC anterior commisure l.
standard Jackson l.
Stange l.
Storz anterior commissure l.
Storz-Hopkins l.
Storz infection ventilation l.
Storz-Riecker l.
straight-blade l.

suspension l.
Tucker anterior commissure l.
Tucker-Holinger l.
Tucker-Jako l.
Tucker mid-lighted optic slide l.
Tucker slotted l.
wasp-waist l.
Weerda distending operating l.
Welch Allyn l.
Wisconsin l.
Wis-Foregger l.
Wis-Hipple l.
Yankauer l.

laryngostat
Jackson l.
Lewy l.
Priest wasp-waist l.
Proctor l.
Proctor-Hellens l.
Roman l.

laryngostroboscope
Nagashima LS-3 l.

larynx
American artificial l.
artificial l.
Cooper-Rand intraoral artificial l.
electronic artificial l.
external auditory l.
Nu-Vois artificial l.
Xomed intraoral artificial l.

Lasag
L. contact lens

LASAG microruptor

Laschal suture scissors

LaseAway
L. laser
L. ruby laser system
L. ruby Nd:YAG laser
L. Smooth Touch laser

LASER
LASER I bubble system

laser
acupuncture l.
ADD'Stat l.
Aesculap argon ophthalmic l.
Aesculap excimer l.
Aesculap-Meditec excimer l.
Albarran l.
alexandrite l.
AMO YAG 100 l.
ArF excimer l.
argon blue l.
argon-fluoride l.
argon green l.
argon ion l.
argon-krypton l.
argon pump dye l.
argon-pumped tunable dye l.
ArthroGuide carbon dioxide l.
ArthroProbe l.
Articu-Lase l.
atheroblation l.
Aura desktop l.
l. balloon
balloon-centered argon l.

Biophysic Medical YAG l.
Britt argon pulsed l.
Britt BL-12 l.
Britt krypton l.
Britt pulsed argon l.
Candela pulsed dye l.
Candela ScleroLaser l.
carbon dioxide (CO_2) l.
Cardona l.
Carl Zeiss YAG l.
Cavitron l.
CB Diode/532 l.
CB Erbium/2.94 l.
char-free carbon dioxide l.
Chromaser dermatology l.
l. CHRP rigid fiberscope system
Chrys surgical CO_2 l.
Cilco argon l.
Cilco Frigitronics l.
Cilco Hoffer Laseridge l.
Cilco krypton l.
Cilco Lasertek argon l.
Cilco YAG l.
ClearView CO_2 l.
Coherent 7910 l.
Coherent 920 argon l.
Coherent carbon dioxide l.
Coherent EPIC l.
Coherent Medical YAG l.
Coherent Novus Omni
multiwavelength l.
Coherent Selecta 7000 l.
Coherent UltraPulse 5000C l.
cold beam l.
continuous-wave argon l.
continuous-wave diode l.
cool-tip l.
CoolTouch Nd:YAG l.
Cooper argon l.
Cooper LaserSonics l.
CooperVision argon l.
CooperVision YAG l.
copper bromide l.
copper vapor pulsed l.
CO_2 Sharplan l.
coumarin-flashlamp-pumped pulsed-
dye l.
coumarin pulsed dye l.
CrTmEr:YAG l.
Crystalase alexandrite DP l.
Crystalase erbium 2 l.
CTE:YAG l.
Culpolase l.
Cynosure l.
l. delivery catheter
Derma 20 Er:YAG l.
Derma K combination Er:YAG &
CO_2 l.
l. diode
diode pumped Nd:YAG l.
Diomed surgical diode l.
l. Doppler flowmeter
l. Doppler flowmetry
l. Doppler perfusion monitor
l. Doppler velocimeter

L

laser *(continued)*

Dornier Medilas H holmium:YAG endourology l.
dye yellow l.
Dynatronics Model 1620 l.
EC-5000 excimer l.
Eclipse holmium l.
Eclipse TMR l.
Endo-Lase C0₂ l.
Epic l.
EpiLaser hair removal l.
EpiTouch l.
erbium CrystaLase l.
erbium Renaissance l.
erbium:YAG l.
erbium:YAG infrared l.
ErCr:YAG l.
Er:YAG l.
esthetic CO₂ l.
Evergreen Lasertek l.
ExciMed UV200 excimer l.
excimer cool l.
excimer gas l.
excimer ultraviolet l.
L. Extensometer
FeatherTouch CO₂ l.
l. fiber
L. Fiber Director
FiberLase l.
l. flare meter
flashlamp pulsed Nd:YAG l.
flashlamp pumped pulsed dye l.
fluorescence-guided "smart" l.
Fotona Novalis ER:YAG l.
Fotona Novalis R ruby l.
frequency doubled neodymium:yttrium-aluminum-garnet l.
l. fume absorber
GaAs l.
gallium-aluminum-arsenide l.
gas l.
Genesis 2000 carbon dioxide l.
GentleLASE l.
Gherini-Kauffman endo-otoprobe l.
Gish micro YAG l.
Gold portable CO₂ l.
green l.
l. Heaney needle holder
helium-cadmium diagnostic l.
helium-neon aiming l.
Heraeus LaserSonics l.
HF infrared l.
HGM argon green l.
HGM intravitreal l.
HGM ophthalmic l.
HGM Spectrum K1 krypton yellow & green l.
high-energy l.
holmium l.
holmium:YAG l.
holmium:yttrium-argon-garnet l.
Horn endo-otoprobe l.
hot-tip l.

Howard-Schatz l.
Ho:YAG l., holmium yttrium aluminum garnet l.
  holmium yttrium aluminum garnet laser
Hruby l.
Illumina Pro series laparoscopic l.
IL MED l.
infrared-beam diode l.
intravitreal l.
ion l.
Iris Oculight SLx MicroPulse l.
l. Julian needle holder
Kaplan PenduLaser l.
Keracor l.
KIP l.
Kremer excimer l.
krypton red l.
KTP l.
KTP/532 l.
KTP/Nd:YAG l.
KTP/532 surgical l.
KTP/YAG l.
LAIS l.
Lambda Physik EMG 103 l.
L. Lancet
l. laryngoscope
LaseAway l.
LaseAway ruby Nd:YAG l.
LaseAway Smooth Touch l.
laser l.
Laserex Era 4106 YAG l.
LaserHarmonic l.
Laserscope KTP/532 l.
LaserSonics Paragon l.
Lasertek YAG l.
Lassag Micropter II l.
Lastec System angioplasty l.
Lateralase l.
lateral-firing l.
l. lens
Lightblade l.
Lightstic 180 (or 360) fiberoptic l.
liquid organic dye l.
Lithognost flash-lamp pulsed dye l.
l. lithotriptor
l. lithotriptor basket
low-energy l.
LPK-80 II argon l.
Lumonics YAG l.
Luxar NovaPulse CO₂ l.
MC-7000 multi-wavelength ophthalmic l.
Medilas fiberTome l.
Medilas Nd:YAG surgical l.
Meditech l.
MedLite Q-Switched neodymium-doped yttrium-aluminum-garnet l.
MedLite Q-Switched YAG l.
MEL 60 excimer l.
MEL 70 flying spot l.
MEL 60 scanning l.
Merimack 1040 CO₂ l.
l. microlaryngeal cup forceps
l. microlaryngeal grasping forceps

Microlase transpupillary diode l.
l. microprobe mass analyzer
MicroProbe ophthalmic l.
l. microscope
microsecond pulsed flashlamp
  pumped dye l.
mid-infrared pulsed l.
Mira AGL-400 l.
l. mirror
Mochida CO_2 Medi-Laser l.
mode-locked l.
Moeller l.
molectron l.
MultiLase D copper vapor l.
MultiLase Nd:YAG surgical l.
Myriadlase Side-Fire l.
Nanolas Nd:YAG l.
NaturaLase erbium l.
NaturaLase Er:YAG l.
Nd:YAG l.
  neodymium-doped yttrium-
    aluminum-garnet laser
  neodymium:yttrium-aluminum-
    garnet laser
Nd:YLF l.
neodymium l.
neodymium-doped yttrium-aluminum-
  garnet l. (Nd:YAG laser)
neodymium:YAG l. (Nd:YAG)
neodymium:yttrium-aluminum-
  garnet l. (Nd:YAG laser)
neodymium:yttrium-lithium-fluoride
  photodisruptive l.
Neurolase microsurgical CO_2 l.
Nidek EC-1000, -5000 excimer l.
Nidek Laser System l.
NovaLine Litho-S DUV excimer l.
NovaPulse CO_2 l.
Novascan scanning headpiece l.
Novatec LightBlade l.
OcuLight SLx ophthalmic l.
oculocutaneous l.
OmniMed argon-fluoride excimer l.
OmniPulse holmium l.
OmniPulse-MAX holmium l.
Ophthalas argon/krypton l.
Ophthalas krypton l.
Opmilas CO_2 multipurpose l.
Opmilas 144 surgical l.
l. optometer
orange dye l.
orthogonal l.
OtoLam l.
l. ovary forceps
Palomar E2000 l.
Paragon l.
PBI Medical copper vapor l.
PBI MultiLase D copper vapor l.
PC EDO ophthalmic office l.
Pegasus Nd:YAG surgical l.
PhotoDerm PL,VL l.
photodisrupting l.
PhotoGenica LPIR with TKS l.
PhotoGenica T^{10} l.
PhotoGenica V l.

PhotoGenica VLS pulsed dye l.
Photon l.
PhotoPoint l.
photovaporizing l.
Polaris 1.32 Nd:YAG l.
Polytec LaseAway Q-switched
  ruby l.
potassium titanyl phosphate l.
Prima KTP/532 l.
l. probe
Prolase II lateral firing Nd:YAG l.
Prostalase l.
pulsed metal vapor l.
pulsed tunable dye l.
pulsed yellow dye l.
PulseMaster l.
Pulsolith coumarin pulsed-dye l.
pumped dye l.
QS alexandrite l.
Q-switched alexandrite l.
Q-switched Er:YAG l.
Q-switched Nd:YAG l.
Q-switched neodymium:YAG l.
Q-switched neodymium:yttrium
  aluminum-garnet l.
Q-switched ruby l.
red l.
red-beam l.
RevitaLase erbium cosmetic l.
rhodamine l.
l. rod
rotational ablation l.
ruby l.
l. scalpel
scanning excimer l.
ScleroPLUS LongPulse dye l.
Sharplan argon l.
Sharplan CO_2 l.
Sharplan Medilas Nd:YAG
  surgical l.
Sharplan SilkTouch flashscan
  surgical l.
SharpLase Nd:YAG l.
SideFire l.
Silhouette endoscopic l.
SilkTouch l.
SITE argon l.
Skinlight erbium yttrium-aluminum-
  garnet l.
Skinlight Er:YAG l.
SLT CL MD/Dual Contact l.
SLT Contact MTRL l.
smart l.
SoftLight l.
Spectranetics l.
Spectra-Physics argon l.
Spectra-Physics microsurgical l.
spectroscopy-directed l.
Spectrum K1 l.
Spectrum ruby l.
SPTL vascular lesion l.
Star X carbon dioxide l.
stereotaxic l.
Storz l.
Summit excimer l.

L

laser *(continued)*
Summit Omnimed excimer l.
Summit SVS Apex l.
Summit UV 200 Excimed l.
Surgica K6 l.
surgical l.
Surgicenter 40 CO_2 l.
Surgilase 150 high-powered CO_2 l.
Surgilase 55W l.
Surgipulse XJ 150 CO_2 l.
Tactilaze angioplasty l.
Takata l.
l. taper
TEC 2100 positioning l.
TE MOO mode beam l.
thulium-holmium-chromium:yttrium-
aluminum-garnet (THC:YAG) l.
thulium-holmium:YAG l.
Topaz CO_2 l.
tracker-assisted PRK l.
transpupillary l.
Trimedyne holmium l.
l. tubal scissors
tunable dye l.
L. Tweezers
UltraFine erbium l.
UltraLine l.
UltraPulse CO_2 l.
UltraPulse surgical l.
UroGold l.
Urolase CO_2 l.
VEINLASE captured-pulse l.
VersaLight l.
VersaPulse holmium l.
VersaPulse Select l.
visual endoscopically controlled l.
Visulas argon C l.
Visulas Nd:YAG l.
Visulas YAG C l.
VISX 2020 excimer l.
Wild l.
Xanar 20 Ambulase CO_2 l.
XeCl excimer l.
xenon-chloride excimer l.
YAG l.
yttrium-aluminum-garnet laser
yttrium-aluminum-garnet l. (YAG
laser)
Zeiss H l.
Zeiss MD l.
Zeiss Opmilas surgical l.
Zeiss Visulas 690s l.
Zyoptix l.
laser-adjustable lens
laser-assisted
l.-a. intrastromal keratomileusis
aspiration spoon
l.-a. intrastromal keratomileusis
cannula
l.-a. intrastromal keratomileusis
cannula eye guard
l.-a. intrastromal keratomileusis flap
irrigator

Laserdish
L. electrode
L. pacing lead
laser-Doppler
l.-D. flowmetry probe
l.-D. Periflux PF-3 probe
l.-D. spectroscopy
Laseredge microsurgical knife
Laserex Era 4106 YAG laser
Laserflo
L. BPM
L. BPM laser Doppler monitor
Laserflow
L. blood perfusion monitor
L. BPM^2 real time cerebral
perfusion monitor
L. Doppler probe
LaserHarmonic laser
Laseridge
Cilco Hoffer L.
L. Optics lens
LaserMed laser pointer
LaserPen
Laserprobe-PLR Plus
LaserScan LSX excimer laser system
Laserscope
L. discography kit
L. disposable Endostat fiber
L. KTP 532
L. KTP/532 laser
L. YAG 1064
**Laser-Shield XII wrapped endotracheal
tube**
Lasersonic ACMI Ultraline
LaserSonics
L. EndoBlade
L. Nd:YAG LaserBlade scalpel
L. Paragon laser
L. SurgiBlade
Lasertek YAG laser
Laser-Trach endotracheal tube
Lasertripter
Candela MDA-200 L.
Lasertubus tracheal tube
LaserTweezers
Lasette laser finger perforator
Lash-Loeffler
L.-L. implant
L.-L. penile implant material
L.-L. penile prosthesis
LASIK
L. aspiration spoon
L. eye guard
L. flap irrigator
L. spear
lasitome
Krumeich-Barraquer l.
Lassag Micropter II laser
lasso
lens l.
l. snare
last
bunion l.
keystone l.
Lastec System angioplasty laser

lata
　　Fascian human fascia l.
　　Suspend Tutoplast processed
　　　fascia l.
　　Tutoplast fascia l.
latent pacemaker
lateral
　　l. guide pin
　　l. gutter impactor
　　l. microlens telescope
　　l. osteotome
　　l. positioner
　　l. screw
　　l. trap suture
　　l. wall retractor
Lateralase laser
lateral-firing laser
LaTeX
　　L. device
latex
　　l. bag
　　l. balloon
　　l. catheter
　　l. drain
　　l. O band
　　l. rubber tourniquet strap
　　l. sponge graft
　　l. tube & connector kit
　　l. wheelchair cushion
Latham
　　L. appliance
　　L. bowl
Lathbury cotton applicator
lathe-cut polymethyl methacrylate
　　intraocular lens
Latis catheter
Latrobe soft palate retractor
Latson multipurpose catheter
Lattimer Silastic testicular prosthesis
Laufe
　　L. aspirating curette
　　L. cervical dilator
　　L. divergent outlet forceps
　　L. obstetrical forceps
　　L. portable uterine evacuator
　　L. uterine polyp forceps
Laufe-Barton-Kjelland obstetrical forceps
Laufe-Barton-Kjelland-Piper obstetrical
　　forceps
Laufe-Barton obstetrical forceps
Laufe-Novak
　　L.-N. diagnostic curette
　　L.-N. gynecologic curette
Laufe-Piper
　　L.-P. obstetrical forceps
　　L.-P. uterine polyp forceps
Laufe-Randall gynecologic curette
Laufman forceps
Laurens-Alcatel nuclear powered
　　pacemaker
Laurer forceps
Laurus needle driver
Lavacuator gastric evacuator
lavage
　　bone l.

　　Easi-Lav gastric l.
　　Hi Speed Pulse l.
　　pulsatile jet l.
　　Pulsavac l.
　　pulse l.
　　Simpulse pulsing l.
　　Tum-E-Vac gastric l.
lavaging catheter
Laval advancement forceps
LaVeen helical stripper
Lawford speculum
Lawrence
　　L. deep forceps
　　L. first metatarsophalangeal joint
　　　implant
　　L. hemostatic forceps
Lawrie modified circumflex scissors
Lawson-Thornton plate
Lawton
　　L. corneal scissors
　　L. forceps
Lawton-Balfour self-retaining retractor
Lawton-Schubert biopsy forceps
Lawton-Wittner cervical biopsy forceps
Layden infant lens
layer
　　Dermanet wound contact l.
　　grading of retinal nerve fiber l.
　　Profore wound contact l.
　　SPTL-1b vascular lesion l.
Layman tongue depressor
Lazar microsuction forceps
LBE cast
LB 9501 luminometer
L-buttress plate
L-Cath
　　L-C. peripherally inserted neonatal
　　　catheter
LCC lung compression clamp
LCS
　　LCS mobile bearing knee system
　　LCS total knee system
LC strip
LDD delivery system
LDS
　　LDS clip
　　LDS clip applier
LDU brace
Le
　　Le Bag
　　Le Bag urinary pouch
　　Le Blond R diamond dental bur
　　Le Fort follower
　　Le Grand-Gullstrand eye model
Lea
　　L. shield
　　L. Symbol chart
lead
　　Accufix pacemaker l.
　　AngeFlex l.
　　l. apron
　　barbed epicardial pacing l.
　　barb-tip l.
　　bifurcated J-shaped tined atrial
　　　pacing and defibrillation l.

L

lead *(continued)*
Biotronik l.
l. block
l. bra
Cadence TVL nonthoracotomy l.
capped l.
CapSure cardiac pacing l.
Cardifix EZ cardiac pacing l.
CCS endocardial pacing l.
Cordis Ancar pacing l.'s
CPI endocardial defibrillation rate-
sensing pacing l.
CPI Endotak SQ electrode l.
CPI porous tined-tip bipolar
pacing l.
CPI Sentra endocardial l.
CPI Sweet Tip l.
deep brain l.
dual coil transvenous l.
dual octapolar l.
dual quadrapolar l.
EASYTRAK coronary venous l.
Ela ventricular pacing l.
endocardial balloon l.
endocardial cardiac l.
Endotak C transvenous l.
Endotak C tripolar
pacing/sensing/defibrillation l.
Endotak DSP l.
epicardial l.
l. eye shield
Fast-Pass endocardial l.
finned pacemaker l.
fishhook l.
floating l.
Frank XYZ orthogonal l.
Golub EKG l.
l. hand
high-impedance, low-threshold l.
Irox endocardial pacing l.'s
isodiametric bipolar screw-in l.
Lamitrode l.
Laserdish pacing l.
left ventricular transvenous l.
Lewis l.
limb l.
Medtronic Spring l.
Medtronic Transvene endocardial l.
modified chest l.
monitor l.'s
myocardial l.
Nehb D l.
nonintegrated transvenous
defibrillation l.
nonintegrated tripolar l.
octapolar l.
Oscor atrial l.
Oscor pacing l.'s
Osypka atrial l.
over-the-wire pacing l.
Pacesetter Tendril DX pacing l.
l. pellet marker
permanent cardiac pacing l.
Permathane l.

l. plate
Polyrox Fractal active fixation l.
Retrox Fractal active fixation l.
reversed arm l.'s
scalar l.'s
screw-in l.
screw-on l.
segmented ring tripolar l.
single-pass l.
Stela electrode l.
l. suture
Sweet-Tip bipolar l.
temporary pervenous l.
Tendril DX implantable pacing l.
ThinLine EZ bipolar cardiac
pacing l.
three-turn epicardial l.
Transvene-RV l.
transvenous defibrillator l.
tripolar l.
two-turn epicardial l.
Unipass endocardial pacing l.
unipolar J-tined passive-fixation l.
**Leadbetter-Politano ureteral implant
prosthesis**
Leadcare handheld blood lead analyzer
Leader
L. iris hook
L. vas hook
L. vas isolation forceps
Leader-Kohlman dilator
lead-filled mallet
lead-shot tie suture
leaf
l. gauge
l. splint
leaflet retractor
leaf-spring brace
Leahey
L. chalazion forceps
L. clamp
L. marginal chalazion forceps
L. suture forceps
Leake Dacron mandible prosthesis
Leander
L. chiropractic table
L. motorized flexion table
L. 79-Series distraction table
LEAP balloon material
Leasure
L. aspirator
L. nasal forceps
L. round punch tip
L. tracheal retractor
L. tuning fork
leather
L. antegrade valvulotome
l. orthosis
L. retrograde valvulotome
Leather-Karmody in-situ valve scissors
Leatherman
L. alar hook
L. compression hook
L. trochanteric retractor
Leaver sclerotomy forceps

LeBag reservoir
Lebensohn chart
Lebsche
    L. forceps
    L. raspatory
    L. rongeur
    L. saw guide
    L. sternal chisel
    L. sternal knife
    L. sternal punch
    L. sternal shears
    L. wire saw
LeCocq brace
Lectromed urinary investigation system
LED
    light-emitting diode
Ledor pigtail catheter
Ledraplastic exercise ball
Lee
    L. bracket
    L. bronchus clamp
    L. cartilage knife
    L. cryoprobe
    L. diamond bur
    L. double-ended retractor
    L. graft
    L. lingual button
    L. microvascular clamp
    L. needle
    L. orthodontic resin
    L. & Westcott needle
leeches
    Biopharm l.
Lee-Cohen
    L.-C. knife
    L.-C. septal elevator
Leeds-Keio ligament prosthesis
Leeds-Northrup Speedomax recorder
Lee-Fischer plastic bracket
LEEP Redi-kit
Lees
    L. arterial forceps
    L. nontraumatic forceps
    L. vascular clamp
    L. wedge resection clamp
Leff
    L. alloy
    L. stethoscope
Lefferts
    L. bone-cutting forceps
    L. rib shears
    L. rib spreader
LeFort
    L. dilator
    L. filiform
    L. filiform bougie
    L. filiform guide
    L. male catheter
    L. speculum
    L. suture
    L. urethral catheter
    L. urethral sound
    L. urethral ultrasound
    L. uterine sound

left
    l. coronary catheter
    l. heart catheter
    l. Judkins catheter
    l. long leg brace
    l. ventricular assist device (LVAD)
    l. ventricular bypass pump
    l. ventricular sump catheter
    l. ventricular transvenous lead
left-handed cornea scissors
left-to-right shunt
leg
    l. brace
    l. holder
    l. positioner
    l. sling
Legacy Series 2000 Cavitron/Kelman
    phaco-emulsifier aspirator
Legasus Sport CPM device
Legend pacemaker
Legen self-retaining retractor
legging
    traction l.
Legg osteotome
legholder
    lithotomy l.
    Low Profile l.
    Prep-Assist l.
    Surbaugh l.
leg-holding device
Legueu
    L. bladder retractor
    L. kidney retractor
    L. spatula
Lehman
    L. aortographic catheter
    L. cardiac device
    L. pancreatic manometry catheter
    L. ventriculography catheter
Lehner
    L. II inserter
    L. II loader
Lehnhardt Universal cap
Leibinger
    L. 3-D bone plate
    L. E-Z flap
    L. Locking system
    L. Micro Dynamic mesh
    L. Micro Plus plate
    L. Micro Plus screw
    L. Micro System drill bit
    L. Micro System plate cutter
    L. Micro System plate-holding
       forceps
    L. miniplate system
    L. mini Würzburg plate
    L. Mini Würzburg screw
    L. plating
    L. plating system
    L. Profyle hand system
    L. titanium mini Würzburg implant
       system
    L. titanium Würzburg mandibular
       reconstruction system

L

Lenny Johnson (handwritten)

Leibinger *(continued)*
- L. Würzburg plate
- L. Würzburg screw

Leica
- L. microscope
- L. vibrating knife microtome

Leicaflex camera
Leigh capsular forceps
Leighton needle
Leinbach
- L. device
- L. head and neck endoprosthesis
- L. head and neck total hip
- L. hip prosthesis
- L. olecranon hook
- L. olecranon screw
- L. osteotome

Leios pacemaker
Leisegang colposcope
Leiske intraocular lens
Leiter tube
Leitz
- L. image analysis system
- L. microscope
- L. 1600 Saw microtome

Leivers
- L. blade
- L. mouthgag

Lejeune
- L. cotton applicator
- L. thoracic forceps

Leksell
- L. arc
- L. bone rongeur
- L. cardiovascular rongeur
- L. D-shaped stereotactic frame
- L. gamma knife
- L. gamma knife target series
- L. grooved director
- L. laminectomy rongeur
- L. Micro-Stereotactic system
- L. Model G stereotactic frame
- L. punch
- L. rongeur forceps
- L. selector
- L. stereotactic device
- L. stereotactic gamma unit
- L. stereotactic system
- L. stereotaxic frame
- L. sternal approximator
- L. sternal spreader
- L. trephine

Leksell-Elekta stereotactic frame
Leksell-Stille thoracic rongeur
Leland
- L. refractor
- L. tonsillar knife

Leland-Jones
- L.-J. forceps
- L.-J. tonsillar knife
- L.-J. vascular clamp

Lell
- L. bite block
- L. biteblock

- L. esophagoscope
- L. laryngofissure saw
- L. tracheal tube

LeMaitre-Bookwalter dilator
LeMaitre Glow 'N Tell tape
Lema strap
Lembert suture
Lem-Blay circumcision clamp
Lemmon
- L. blade
- L. intimal dissector
- L. needle
- L. rib contractor
- L. self-retaining sternal retractor
- L. sternal approximator
- L. sternal elevator
- L. sternal spreader

Lemmon-Russian forceps
Lemoine
- L. forceps
- L. orbital implant
- L. serrefine

Lemoine-Searcy
- L.-S. anchor
- L.-S. fixation anchor loop
- L.-S. fixation anchor loupe

Lemole
- L. atrial valve self-retaining retractor
- L. mitral valve retractor

lemon squeezer
lemon-squeezer obstetrical elevator
Lempert
- L. bone curette
- L. bone rongeur
- L. diamond-dust polishing bur
- L. endaural curette
- L. endaural rongeur
- L. excavator
- L. fenestration bur
- L. fine curette
- L. heavy elevator
- L. invaginator
- L. knife
- L. malleus cutter
- L. malleus nipper
- L. malleus punch
- L. narrow elevator
- L. perforator
- L. periosteal elevator
- L. retractor
- L. rongeur forceps
- L. rongeur headrest

Lempert-Beckman-Colver endaural speculum
Lempert-Colver
- L.-C. endaural speculum
- L.-C. retractor

Lempert-Juers rongeur
Lempert-Storz
- L.-S. lens
- L.-S. lens loop
- L.-S. loupe

Lempka vein stripper
Lems lens

Lenard ray tube
Lennarson tube
Lenny Johnson surgical-assist knee
  holder
Lenox
    L. bucket
    L. Hill Spectralite knee brace
lens
    Abraham contact l.
    Abraham iridectomy laser l.
    Abraham peripheral button
      iridotomy l.
    Abraham YAG laser l.
    AC l.
    AccuGel l.
    acrylic l.
    AcrySof foldable intraocular l.
    Acuvue bifocal l.
    Acuvue disposable contact l.
    Acuvue Etafilcon A l.
    Adaptar "no-line" contact l.
    Advent Flurofocon contact l.
    Albarran l.
    Alcon intraocular l.
    Alien WildEyes l.
    Allen-Braley intraocular l.
    Allergan-Simcoe C-loop
      intraocular l.
    all-in-the-bag intraocular l.
    all-PMMA one-piece C-loop
      intraocular l.
    Amenabar l.
    Amercal intraocular l.
    Amercal-Shepard intraocular l.
    American Medical Optics (AMO)
      Baron l.
    amnifocal l.
    AMO Advent contact l.
    AMO Array foldable intraocular l.
    AMO intraocular l.
    AMO Phacoflex II foldable
      intraocular l.
    AMO Sensar intraocular l.
    Amsoft l.
    Anis staple l.
    anterior chamber intraocular l. (AC
      IOL, AC-IOL)
    Aquaflex contact l.
    Aquasight l.
    Arnott one-piece all-PMMA
      intraocular l.
    Array foldable intraocular l.
    Arruga l.
    aspherical ophthalmoscopic l.
    aspheric cataract l.
    aspheric viewing l.
    auxiliary l.
    Azar Mark II intraocular l.
    bag-fixated intraocular l.
    Bagolini l.
    Baikoff l.
    bandage soft contact l.
    Barkan gonioscopic l.
    Barkan infant l.
    Barkan operating l.

    Baron intraocular l.
    Barraquer J-loop intraocular l.
    Barrett hydrogel intraocular l.
    Bausch & Lomb Optima l.
    Bausch & Lomb Surgical L161U l.
    Bechert one-piece all-PMMA
      intraocular l.
    Beebe l.
    biconcave contact l.
    biconvex intraocular l.
    bicylindrical l.
    Bietti l.
    bifocal intracorneal l.
    Binkhorst collar stud intraocular l.
    Binkhorst-Fyodorov l.
    Binkhorst mustache lens
      intraocular l.
    Binkhorst two-loop l.
    Binkhorst two modified J-loops
      intraocular l.
    biomicroscopic indirect l.
    Bi-Soft l.
    bispherical l.
    Bloodshot WildEyes l.
    Blumenthal intraocular l.
    Boberg l.
    Boberg-Ans intraocular l.
    Boston Envision l.
    Bowling l.
    Boys-Smith laser l.
    Burian-Allen contact l.
    Byrne expulsive hemorrhage l.
    l. cannula
    capsular-style l.
    Capsulform l.
    Cardona fiberoptic diagnostic l.
    Carl Zeiss l.
    cast-molded PMMA intraocular l.
    catadioptric l.
    CeeOn heparinized intraocular l.
    Centra-Flex l.
    central retinal l.
    CGI-1 contact l.
    Charles contact l.
    Charles intraocular l.
    Charles irrigating l.
    Chiroflex C11UB l.
    Choyce Mark intraocular l.
    Choyce Mark VIII l.
    Choyce-Tennant l.
    Ciba Soft l.
    Ciba Thin l.
    Cibathin l.
    Cilco intraocular l.
    Cilco MonoFlex PMMA l.
    Cilco Optiflex intraocular l.
    Cilco posterior chamber
      intraocular l.
    Cilco-Simcoe II l.
    Cilco Slant l.
    Cilco-Sonometrics l.
    CIMA*flex* 411 foldable silicone l.
    Clayman intraocular l.
    l. clip
    C-loop posterior chamber l.

L

lens (*continued*)

closed-loop intraocular l.
Coburn equiconvex l.
Coburn intraocular l.
Coburn Optical Industries-Feaster intraocular l.
Coburn-Storz intraocular l.
Cogan-Boberg-Ans l.
Collamer intraocular l.
L. Comfort ultrasound cleaning and disinfecting system
compressible acrylic intraocular l.
compression-molded PMMA intraocular l.
condensing l.
contact bandage l.
contact low-vacuum l.
CooperVision-Cilco-Kelman multiflex all-PMMA intraocular l.
CooperVision-Cilco Novaflex anterior chamber intraocular l.
CooperVision PMMA-ACL Flex l.
Copeland anterior chamber intraocular l.
Copeland radial loop intraocular l.
Copeland radial panchamber UV l.
coquille plano l.
Crookes l.
crystalline l.
CSI l.
cylindrical l.
Darin l.
diagnostic fiberoptic l.
diopter l.
direct gonioscopic l.
disk lens intraocular l.
dispersing l.
Donnheim l.
Doubra l.
Drews l.
Dubroff radial loop intraocular l.
Dulaney intraocular implant l.
Duragel l.
Durasoft 2 contact l.
Durasoft toric l.
Dura-T l.
E Clips prescription computer l.
Edge III hydrogel contact l.
Emcee l.
Emery l.
endocapsular artificial lens intraocular l.
l. enucleation scoop
Epstein collar stud acrylic l.
Epstein-Copeland l.
Epstein intraocular l.
Epstein posterior chamber l.
ERG-Jet disposable contact l.
Ernest-McDonald soft intraocular l.
Eschenback Optik l.
etafilcon A disposable contact l.
European in-the-bag l.
l. expressor
extended-wear soft contact l.

EZ.1 multifocal contact l.
EZVue violet haptic intraocular l.
Falcon l.
Feaster Dualens intraocular l.
Feaster dual-placement intraocular l.
Fechtner intraocular l.
Flexcon l.
flexible fluoropolymer contact l.
flexible-loop anterior chamber intraocular l.
flexible-loop posterior chamber intraocular l.
Flexlens l.
Flexner-Worst iris claw l.
F/M base curve contact l.
foldable intraocular l.
folding l.
FormFlex formocresal l.
FormFlex intraocular l.
Foroblique l.
four-footed l.
four-mirror goniolens l.
four-piece intraocular l.
four-point fixation intraocular l.
Frelex l.
Fresnel l.
Friedman hand-held Hruby l.
fundal contact l.
fundal-focalizing l.
fundal laser l.
fundus contact l.
fundus focalizing l.
fused bifocal l.
Fyodorov four-loop iris clip intraocular l.
Fyodorov-Sputnik FFP contact intraocular l.
Fyodorov type I, II intraocular l.
Galand disk l.
Galand in-the-bag l.
Galand-Knolle modified J-loop intraocular l.
Galin intraocular implant l.
Genesis l.
Gentex PDQ polycarbonate l.
Gill intraocular implant l.
Gilmore intraocular implant l.
l. glide cutter
glued-on hard contact l.
Goldmann macular contact l.
Goldmann multimirror l.
Goldmann three-mirror gonioscopy l.
goniofocalizing l.
goniolens l.
gonioscopic l.
Gould intraocular implant l.
gradient index l.
Gridley intraocular l.
GRIN l.
Gullstrand l.
hand-held Hruby l.
haptic area l.
haptic-fixated intraocular l.
haptic plate l.
haptic-sec l.

hard contact l.
Harris modified J-loop intraocular l.
Harris rigid quadriped intraocular l.
Hart pediatric three-mirror l.
Hersbury anterior chamber
    intraocular l.
Hoffer ridged intraocular l.
l. hook
Hopkins II rod l.
Hoskins-Barkan goniotomy infant l.
Hoskins nylon suture laser l.
Hruby contact l.
Hunkeler intraocular l.
Hunter one-piece all-PMMA
    intraocular l.
Hydracon contact l.
Hydrasoft contact l.
Hydrocurve l.
Hydrogel expansile intraocular l.
Hydron l.
hydrophilic contact l.
Hydrosight l.
Hydroview l.
IMMA l.
l. implant
l. implantation forceps
Implens intraocular l.
infant Karickhoff laser l.
infant three-mirror laser l.
Interfit-Pharmacea Intermedic
    intraocular l.
Interflux intraocular l.
Intermedics l.
Interspace YAG laser l.
in-the-bag l.
intracorneal l.
intraocular l. (IOL)
IntraOptics intraocular l.
Iogel intraocular l.
IOLAB Azar intraocular l.
IOLAB Slimfit l.
Ioptex intraocular l.
Ioptex TabOptic l.
Irene l.
iridocapsular intraocular l.
iris claw l.
iris-clip intraocular l.
iris-supported intraocular l.
iseikonic l.
Iwata-Ricky gonioscopic l.
Jaffe Cilco l.
Jaffe one-piece all-PMMA
    intraocular l.
J-loop posterior chamber
    intraocular l.
Joal l.
Kamerling Capsular 90 l.
Kamerling one-piece all-PMMA
    intraocular l.
Karickhoff diagnostic l.
Karickhoff laser l.
Kearney side-notch intraocular l.
Keeler panoramic l.
Kelman flexible tripod l.

Kelman II three-point fixation rigid
    tripod intraocular l.
Kelman Multiflex II intraocular l.
Kelman Omnifit intraocular l.
Kelman PC 27LB CapSul l.
Kelman Quadraflex intraocular l.
Kelman S-flex intraocular l.
keratometer l.
Kilp l.
Kishi l.
Koeppe diagnostic l.
Koeppe gonioscopic l.
Krasnov l.
Kratz elliptical-style l.
Kratz-Johnson modified J-loop
    intraocular l.
Kratz modified J-loop intraocular l.
Kratz posterior chamber
    intraocular l.
Krieger wide-field fundus l.
Landers biconcave l.
Landers contact l.
Landers-Foulks temporary
    keratoprosthesis l.
large-diameter optics intraocular l.
Lasag contact l.
laser l.
laser-adjustable l.
Laseridge Optics l.
l. lasso
lathe-cut polymethyl methacrylate
    intraocular l.
Layden infant l.
Leiske intraocular l.
Lempert-Storz l.
Lems l.
Lester notch intraocular l.
Levick one-piece all-PMMA
    intraocular l.
Lewicky intraocular l.
Lieb-Guerry cataract implant l.
Lindstrom Centrex l.
Lindstrom modified J-loop, three-
    piece reverse PMMA optic
    intraocular l.
Liteflex l.
Little-Arnott tripod intraocular l.
long-wearing contact l.
l. loop
loop-fixated intraocular l.
l. loop forceps
Lovac fundal contact l.
Lovac gonioscopic l.
Lovac six-mirror gonioscopic l.
low-power optics for myopic
    correction l.
Lynell intraocular l.
Machemer flat l.
Machemer infusion contact l.
Machemer magnifying vitrectomy l.
macular contact l.
Mainster-HM retinal laser l.
Mainster retinal laser l.
Mainster-S retinal laser l.
Mainster Ultra Field PRP laser l.

L

lens *(continued)*

Mainster-WF retinal laser l.
Mainster wide-field l.
Maltese cross l.
Mandelkorn suture lysis l.
l. manipulator
March laser l.
Mark IX l.
Mazzocco silicone intraocular l.
McGhan l.
McLean prismatic fundus laser l.
Meditech bandage contact l.
Mehta intraocular l.
MemoryLens foldable intraocular l.
meniscal posterior concave
 intraocular l.
Mentor ORC MemoryLens l.
meter l.
MiniQuad XL l.
3M intraocular l.
l. mitral heart valve
modified C-loop intraocular l.
modified J-loop, posterior chamber
 intraocular l.
Momosi spider lens intraocular l.
Monoflex l.
Morgan therapeutic l.
Multi-Optics l.
multiple-piece intraocular l.
narrow l.
Neolens l.
New Orleans l.
NewVues l.
Nikon aspheric l.
Nikon SMZ 2T magnifying l.
Nokrome bifocal l.
Nova Aid l.
Nova Curve l.
Novaflex intraocular l.
Nova Soft II l.
Nuvita l.
NuVue l.
objective l.
Oculaid l.
ocular Gamboscope l.
O'Malley-Pearce-Luma l.
Omnifit intraocular l.
one-piece plate haptic silicone
 intraocular l.
L. Opacities Classification System
 II
open l.
open-loop intraocular l.
Ophtec Co. l.
Optical Radiation intraocular l.
2-Optifit toric l.
Optiflex intraocular l.
Optima contact l.
Opti-Vu l.
Opt-Visor l.
ORC posterior chamber
 intraocular l.
orthoscopic l.
O'Shea l.

Osher-Fresnel intraocular l.
Osher pan-fundus l.
Osher surgical posterior pole l.
Packard intraocular l.
Palmer l.
Palmer-Buono contact l.
panchamber UV l.
Pannu II intraocular l.
PanoView Optics l.
parfocal defraction l.
PBII blue loop l.
PC-IOL l.
Pearce-Keates bifocal intraocular l.
Pearce posterior chamber
 intraocular l.
Pearce Tripod cataract l.
Pearce Tripod intraocular l.
pediatric Karickhoff laser l.
pediatric three-mirror laser l.
Permalens l.
Perspex CQ intraocular l.
Perspex CQ-Shearing-Simcoe-
 Sinskey l.
Peyman-Green vitrectomy l.
Peyman special optics for low
 vision l.
Peyman-Tennant-Green l.
Peyman wide-field l.
PhacoFlex II intraocular l.
Phakic 6 l.
Pharmacia Intermedics ophthalmics
 intraocular l.
Pharmacia Visco J-loop l.
piggyback contact l.
plano l.
planoconcave l.
planoconvex l.
planoconvex nonridge l.
Platina clip l.
plus power l.
PMMA hard contact l.
PMMA intraocular l.
Pointer one-piece all-PMMA
 intraocular l.
polypropylene intraocular l.
Posner diagnostic l.
posterior chamber intraocular l.
posterior convex intraocular l.
Precision Cosmet l.
prismatic contact l.
prismatic gonioscopic l.
prismatic goniotomy l.
Prokop intraocular l.
prosthetic l.
punctal l.
l. pusher
QuadPediatric fundus l.
Rappazzo intraocular l.
Rayner l.
Rayner-Choyce intraocular l.
Red Reflex Lens Systems l.
retroscopic l.
reverse intraocular l.
Revolution l.
right-angled telescopic l.

rigid gas-permeable contact l.
rigid intraocular l.
Ritch contact l.
Ritch nylon suture laser l.
Ritch trabeculoplasty laser l.
Rodenstock panfundus l.
Rohm and Haas PMMA
  intraocular l.
Roussel-Fankhauser contact l.
Ruiz fundal contact l.
Ruiz fundal laser l.
Ruiz plano fundal l.
Sableflex anterior chamber
  intraocular l.
sapphire l.
SaturEyes contact l.
Sauflon PW hydrophilic contact l.
Schachar l.
Scharff l.
SeeQuence disposable contact l.
self-stabilizing vitrectomy l.
semiflexible intraocular l.
semirigid intraocular l.
Severin multiple closed-loop
  intraocular l.
Shah-Shah intraocular l.
Shearing J-Loop intraocular l.
Shearing posterior chamber
  intraocular l.
Shearing S-style anterior chamber
  intraocular l.
Sheets closed-loop posterior chamber
  intraocular l.
Shepard flexible anterior chamber
  intraocular l.
Shepard Universal intraocular l.
short C-loop intraocular l.
Siepser intraocular l.
Signet Optical l.
silica contact l.
silicone elastomer l.
Silsoft extended wear contact l.
silvered contact l.
Simcoe C-loop intraocular l.
SingleStitch PhacoFlex l.
Sinskey J-loop intraocular l.
Slant haptic intraocular l.
Slimfit l.
Smith intraocular implant l.
Snellen soft contact l.
Soflens contact l.
SoFlex l.
soft contact l.
soft intraocular l.
SoftSITE high add aspheric
  multifocal contact l.
Sola Optical USA Spectralite high-
  index l.
Sola VIP l.
Sovereign bifocal l.
l. spatula
Spectralite Transitions l.
spherocylindrical l.
l. spoon
Staar foldable intraocular l.

Staar implantable contact l.
Staar Toric l.
Stableflex l.
Stankiewicz iris clip intraocular l.
Starr Surgical polyimide loop
  intraocular l.
Stokes l.
Storz Capsulor blue intraocular l.
Strampelli l.
Super Field NC slit lamp l.
Supramid l.
Surefit intraocular l.
Surevue contact l.
Surgidev Leiske anterior chamber
  intraocular l.
Sutherland l.
Tano double-mirror peripheral
  vitrectomy l.
Tennant Anchorflex anterior chamber
  intraocular l.
The Sensar foldable acrylic
  posterior chamber intraocular l.
Thorpe four-mirror goniolaser l.
Thorpe four-mirror vitreous fundus
  laser l.
Thorpe gonioprism l.
Thorpe plastic l.
three-footed lens intraocular l.
three-mirror contact l.
three-mirror intraocular l.
three-piece acrylic intraocular l.
three-piece modified J-loop
  intraocular l.
three-piece silicone intraocular l.
three-point fixation intraocular l.
Tillyer bifocal l.
T-lens therapeutic contact l.
Tolentino prism l.
Tolentino vitrectomy l.
Topcon aspheric l.
toric intraocular l.
Touchlite zoom l.
tripod intraocular l.
Trokel l.
Trokel-Peyman laser l.
Troncoso tubular l.
Trupower aspherical l.
Truvision Omni l.
Ultex l.
UltraCon rigid gas permeable
  contact l.
Ultra mag l.
Ultra view SP slit lamp l.
ultraviolet-blocking intraocular l.
uniplanar intraocular l.
Univision low-vision microscopic l.
Urrets-Zavalia retinal surgical l.
uvea-fixated intraocular l.
uvea-supported intraocular l.
Uvex l.
UVR-absorbing intraocular l.
Varigray l.
Varilux Infinity l.
Varilux Plus l.
Viscolens l.

L

lens *(continued)*
    Vision Tech l.
    Visitec Company l.
    Volk conoid l.
    Volk high-resolution aspherical l.
    Volk panretinal l.
    Volk QuadrAspheric fundal l.
    Volk SuperField aspherical l.
    Volk SuperPupil NC l.
    Volk Super Quad 160 pan retinal l.
    Wang l.
    Weber-Elschnig l.
    Wesley-Jessen l.
    Wild l.
    Wise iridotomy laser l.
    Wise sphincterotomy laser l.
    Worst gonioprism contact l.
    Worst lobster-claw l.
    Worst Medallion l.
    Yalon intraocular l.
    Yannuzzi fundus laser l.
    Youens l.
    Zeiss aspheric l.
    Zeiss-Gullstrand l.
    Ziski iris clip intraocular l.
    Zoeffle soft intraocular l.
LensCheck Advanced Logic lensometer
lensed fiber-tip laser delivery catheter
Lens-Eze inserter
Lensmeter
    L. 701
    L. lensometer
lensometer
    Allergan-Humphrey l.
    AMO l.
    Carl Zeiss l.
    Coburn l.
    Hardy l.
    IntraOptics l.
    LensCheck Advanced Logic l.
    Lensmeter l.
    Marco l.
    Reichert l.
    Reichert-Lenschek advanced logic l.
    Topcon LM P5 digital l.
    Zeiss LA 110 projection l.
lens-threading forceps
Lente silver nitrate probe
Lent photolaparoscope
Lentulo spiral drill
Leo
    L. Bathlifter
    L. Schwartz sponge-holding forceps
Leon
    L. cobra cannula
    L. cobra tip
Leonard
    L. arm
    L. arm device
    L. Arms instrument holder
    L. forceps
Leone expansion screw
LePad breast exam training pad

Lepley-Ernst tracheal tube
Leptos pacemaker
Lere bone mill
Leriche
    L. hemostatic forceps
    L. spatula
    L. tissue forceps
Lerman
    L. hinge brace
    L. non-invasive halo
Lermoyez nasal punch
LeRoy
    L. clip-applying forceps
    L. infant scalp clip
    L. ventricular catheter
LeRoy-Raney scalp clip
L'Esperance
    L. erysiphake
    L. needle
Lester
    L. A. Dine camera
    L. fixation forceps
    L. Jones tube
    L. lens manipulator
    L. muscle forceps
    L. notch intraocular lens
Lester-Burch eye speculum
Letournel
    L. acetabular fracture bone plate
    L. guideline
leucocyte detection strip
leukocyte automatic recognition computer
LeukoNet filter
Leukopore tape
leukoscope
Leukos pacemaker
Leukotape P sports tape
leukotome
    Bailey l.
    Dorsey transorbital l.
    Freeman transorbital l.
    Lewis l.
    Lours l.
    Love l.
    McKenzie l.
    Nosik transorbital l.
    Tworek transorbital l.
Leukotrap
    L. RC storage system
    L. red cell collector
    L. red cell storage system
Leung endoscopic nasal biliary drainage set
Leur-par collimator
Leurs nasal rasp
Leusch atraumatic obturator
Levant stone dislodger
LeVasseur-Merrill retractor
levator snare
LeVeen
    L. ascites shunt
    L. catheter
    L. dialysis shunt
    L. inflation syringe
    L. inflator

L. inflator with pressure gauge
L. peritoneal shunt
L. peritoneovenous shunt
L. plaque cracker
L. plaque-cracker
L. valve

Level
L. Anchorage appliance
L. Anchorage system
L. I normothermic irrigating system
L. One normothermic IV fluid set

Levenson tissue forceps

lever
Alexander bone l.
Bennett bone l.
bone l.
Bristow l.
Buck-Gramcko bone l.
Charnley femoral l.
Cottle bone l.
Hohmann-Aldinger bone l.
Hohmann bone l.
Kilner malar l.
Lane bone l.
Lange-Hohmann bone l.
Murphy bone l.
Murphy-Lane l.
Norrbacka-Stille l.
l. pessary
Sellheim obstetrical l.
Tager l.
Torpin obstetrical l.
Verbrugge-Mueller bone l.
Wagner bone l.
Watson-Jones bone l.

Levick one-piece all-PMMA intraocular lens

Levin
L. drill guide
L. duodenal tube
L. thermocouple cordotomy electrode
L. tube catheter

Levin-Davol tube

Levine
L. curetting spud
L. foreign body spud

Levinthal surgery retractor
Levis arm splint
Levitt eye implant
Levora fixation forceps
Levret forceps

Levy
L. articulating retractor
L. perineal retractor
L. & Rappel foot orthosis

Levy-Kuglen
L.-K. iris hook
L.-K. lens manipulator

Levy-Okun stripper

Lewicky
L. capsular scraper
L. cortex extractor
L. formed cystitome
L. intraocular lens
L. IOL spatula

L. microlens hook
L. needle
L. self-retaining chamber maintainer
L. threaded infusion cannula

Lewin
L. baseball finger splint
L. bone-holding clamp
L. bone-holding forceps
L. bunion dissector
L. elevator
L. sesamoidectomy dissector
L. spinal-perforating forceps

Lewin-Stern
L.-S. finger splint
L.-S. thumb splint

Lewis
L. dental mirror
L. expandable adjustable prosthesis
L. hemostat
L. intramedullary device
L. laryngectomy tube
L. lead
L. lens loop
L. lens scoop
L. leukotome
L. mouthgag
L. nail
L. nasal rasp
L. Pair-Pak needle
L. periosteal elevator
L. periosteal raspatory
L. recording cystometer
L. retractor
L. septal forceps
L. suspension device
L. tongue depressor
L. tonsillar hemostatic forceps
L. tonsillar screw
L. tonsillar snare
L. ureteral stone isolation forceps
L. vertical slot bracket

Lewis-Leigh
L.-L. positive-pressure nonrebreathing valve

Lewis-Resnik punch
Lewkowitz
L. lithotomy forceps
L. ovum forceps
L. placental forceps

Lewy
L. anterior commissure laryngoscope
L. chest holder
L. laryngoscope holder
L. laryngostat
L. suspension apparatus
L. suspension device
L. suspension laryngoscope
L. Teflon glycerine-mixture injection needle
L. Teflon glycerine-mixture syringe

Lewy-Holinger Teflon injection needle
Lewy-Rubin Teflon glycerine-mixture injection needle
Lexan jacket

Lexer
  L. chisel
  L. dissecting scissors
  L. gouge
  L. osteotome
  L. tissue forceps
Lexer-Durotip dissecting scissors
Lex-Ton lumbar laminectomy frame
Leycom volume conductance catheter
Leydig drain
Leyla
  L. flexible arm
  L. self-retaining brain retractor
  L. self-retaining tractor bar
Leyla-Yasargil self-retaining retractor
Leyro-Diaz thoracic forceps
Lezinski Flex-HA PORP ossicular chain prosthesis
Lezius suction tube
L-F Uniflex diathermy electrosurgical unit
LGM filter
L-hook electrosurgical probe
Libbe lower bowel evacuation device
Liberty
  L. CMC thumb brace
  L. One splint
  L. spinal system
Lichtenberg
  L. corneal trephine
  L. keratome
  L. needle holder
Lichtwicz
  L. abdominal trocar
  L. antral cannula
  L. antral needle
  L. antral trocar
Lichtwicz-Bier antral needle
LICO
  L. disposable penlight
  L. Hertel exophthalmometer
lid
  l. clamp
  l. everter
  l. expressor
  l. forceps
  l. plate
  l. retractor
  l. scalpel
  l. speculum
Liddicoat aortic valve retractor
Liddle aortic clamp
LidFix speculum
Lidge cement gun
Lido
  L. Active Multijoint system
  L. Lift
  L. Multi Joint II isokinetic dynamometer
  L. Passive Multijoint system
  L. WorkSET work simulator
Lidoback isokinetic dynamometry system
Lido-Pen Auto-Injector
Liebel-Flarsheim CT 9000 contrast delivery system

Lieberman
  L. abrader
  L. aspirating speculum
  L. fragmentor
  L. K-Wire speculum
  L. MicroFinger manipulator
  L. phaco crusher
  L. proctoscope
  L. sigmoidoscope
  L. suturing forceps
  L. tying forceps
  L. Wire Aspirating Speculum with V-shape blades
Lieberman-Pollock double corneal forceps
Lieb-Guerry
  L.-G. cataract implant lens
  L.-G. forceps
Liebreich probe
Lieppman
  L. microcystitome
  L. sharp cystitome
  L. spatula
Liesegang LM-FLEX 7 flexible hysteroscope
LIFE
  LIFE Imaging System and White Light bronchoscope
Life
  L. Care pump
  L. Liner stick- and cut-resistant gloves
  L. Suit
Life-Air 1000 hypothermic therapy system
Lifecare ventilator
Lifecath
  L. catheter
  L. peritoneal implant
LifeCell AlloDerm acellular dermal graft
Lifecore Restore wide diameter implant system
Lifeline electrode
Life-Lok clamp
LIFE-Lung fluorescence endoscopy system
Lifemask infant resuscitator
Lifemed
  L. blood tubing
  L. cannula
  L. catheter
  L. heterologous heart valve
Life-O-Matt
Life-Pack 5 cardiac monitor
Lifepath AAA endovascular graft system
LifePort infusion set
Lifesaver disposable resuscitator bag
life-saving tube
LifeScan blood glucose monitoring system
Lifescope 12 bedside monitor
Lifestream
  L. centrifugal pump
  L. coronary dilation catheter
Lifestride treadmill
Life-Tech flowmeter

lift
> BTE dynamic l.
> Easy Pivot patient l.
> Grice l.
> heel l.
> HI-LOO Power l.
> Hoyer l.
> Lido L.
> M/L l.
> pneumatic chair l.
> Sabina l.
> shoe l.

LiftALERT electronic device
lifter
> tissue l.
> Totallift-II l.
> waltzing areolar l.
> Yasargil tissue l.

LiF thermoluminescence dosimeter
LiftMate patient transfer device
Ligaclip
> Ethicon L.
> L. MCA multiple-clip applier
> L. surgical clip

ligament
> l. augmentation device (LAD)
> l. button
> l. clamp
> Dacron synthetic l.
> Zenotech synthetic l.

ligament-grasping forceps
ligamentum
> l. flavum forceps
> l. teres knife

Ligamentus
> L. Ankle ankle orthotic
> L. Ankle orthosis

Ligand plus 1, 2, 3, noninvasive monitor
Ligapak suture
Lig-A-Ring separator
LigaSure vessel sealing system
ligating and dividing stapler
ligation device
ligator
> Arrequi laparoscopic knot pusher l.
> Barron hemorrhoidal l.
> Centrix PDQ l.
> Clarke-Reich l.
> DDV l.
> endoscopic band l.
> Gigator hemorrhoidal l.
> hemorrhoidal l.
> Lurz-Goltner l.
> McGivney hemorrhoidal l.
> Microvasive Speedband Superview l.
> NAMI DDV l.
> Preston-Hopkins l.
> RapidFire multiple band l.
> rubber band l.
> Rudd l.
> Saeed Six-Shooter multi-band l.
> Salvatore umbilical cord l.
> Sanford l.
> Scanlan l.

> Speedband multiple band l.
> Stiegmann-Goff Clearvue endoscopic l.
> Tucker hemorrhoidal l.
> Twist-Mate l.

ligature
> l. cannula
> l. carrier
> Desault l.
> l. director
> l. forceps
> l. guide
> l. needle
> l. passer
> Potts l.
> l. scissors
> Speedband l.
> Surgiwip suture l.
> Tahoe Surgical Instruments l.
> l. tie wire
> l. tucker

ligature-carrying forceps
ligatureless bracket
ligature-locking pliers
ligature-passing instrument
Light
light
> AMSCO l.
> Barkan l.
> bili l.
> Brite Lite III l.
> l. carrier
> Castle surgical l.
> Chick surgical l.
> Clar head l.
> Co-Axa l.
> cobalt blue l.
> Cogent l.
> L. Commander xenon illuminator
> l. cross-slot screwdriver
> dermatologic ultraviolet l.
> l. electron microscope
> l. emitter
> floor-standing surgical l.
> Floxite mirror l.
> Fotofil activator l.
> Fragen laryngoscope fiberoptic l.
> Gass neurosurgical l.
> L. headrest
> Landry vein l.
> Lumiwand l.
> Maglite l.
> l. monitoring probe
> MultArray l.
> Murphy l.
> overhead l.
> l. pen
> l. pipe
> l. pipe pick
> l. pipette
> pulsed l.
> Right Light examination l.
> Serdarevic Circle of L.
> Solar Beam medical examination l.
> L. Talker device

L

light *(continued)*
    ultraviolet l.
    l. wire appliance
    Witt dental l.
    Wood l.
Lightblade laser
light-curing resin
lighted
    l. retractor
    l. speculum
    l. stent
    l. stylet
light-emitting diode (LED)
Lighthouse ET-DRS acuity chart
Lightning high-speed vitrectomy handpiece
LighTouch Neonate thermometer
lightsource
    halogen dual l.
Lightspeed file
Lightstic 180 (or 360) fiberoptic laser
Light-Veley
    L.-V. apparatus
    L.-V. bur
    L.-V. cranial drill
    L.-V. headrest
LightWare micro retractor
LightWear headlight
Lightweight and portable Sullivan nasal CPAP
Ligmajet
    L. syringe
Liguory endoscopic nasal biliary drainage set
LIH hook pin
Liks Russian disk rotation heart valve
Lilienthal
    L. probe
    L. rib guillotine
    L. rib spreader
Lilienthal-Sauerbruch
    L.-S. retractor
    L.-S. rib spreader
Lillehei
    L. pacemaker
    L. retractor
    L. valve-grasping forceps
Lillehei-Cruz-Kaster valve prosthesis
Lillehei-Kaster
    L.-K. cardiac valve prosthesis
    L.-K. mitral valve prosthesis
    L.-K. pivoting disk
    L.-K. pivoting-disk prosthetic valve
Lillehei-Warden catheter
Lillie
    L. antral trocar
    L. attic cannula
    L. attic hook
    L. ear hook
    L. frontal sinus probe
    L. gouge
    L. intestinal forceps
    L. nasal speculum
    L. rectus tendon clamp

    L. retractor
    L. rongeur
    L. tissue-holding forceps
    L. tonsillar knife
    L. tonsillar scissors
Lillie-Killian septal forceps
Lillie-Koffler tool
Lilliput neonatal oxygenator
LIMA-Lift
LIMA-Loop
Limb
limb
    L. and elbow protector
    Gore-Tex l.
    l. gym
    l. holder
    l. lead
    Trowbridge TerraRound sports l.
limited-contact dynamic compression plate
limiter
    Becker 655 motion control l.
LINAC
    linear accelerator
    Varian LINAC
LINAC-based radiosurgical system
Linatrix suture
Lin clamp
Lincoff
    L. design of Storz scleral buckling balloon catheter
    L. lens sponge
    L. scleral sponge implant
    L. sponge implant material
    L. sponge rod
Lincoln-Metzenbaum scissors
Lincoln pediatric scissors
Lindbergh pump
Linde
    L. cryogenic probe
    L. cryoprobe
    L. Xi-scan
Lindeman
    L. bone cutter
    L. self-retaining uterine vacuum cannula
    L. transfusion needle
Lindeman-Silverstein
    L.-S. Arrow tube
    L.-S. ventilation tube
Lindermann bur
Lindholm
    L. microlaryngoscope
    L. operating laryngoscope
    L. tracheal tube
Lindholm-Stille elevator
Lindley
    L. needle holder
    L. scissors
Lindner
    L. anastomosis clamp
    L. corneoscleral suture
    L. cyclodialysis spatula
    L. cyclodialysis spoon

Lindorf
>L. lag screw
>L. position screw

Lindsay-Rea forceps

Lindstrom
>L. arcuate incision marker
>L. astigmatic marker
>L. Centrex lens
>L. lens-insertion forceps
>L. modified J-loop, three-piece reverse PMMA optic intraocular lens
>L. Star nucleus manipulator

Lindstrom-Chu aspirating speculum
Lindvall meniscectomy knife
Lindvall-Stille
>L.-S. meniscal knife

line
>Codman ICP monitoring l.
>Hickman l.
>Intertech Perkin-Elmer gas sampling l.
>l. keeper
>Nafion dryer l.
>oxygen supply l.
>Pall leukogard-6 arterial l.
>peripherally inserted central catheter l.
>PICC l.
>Seraflo blood l.
>Tycos pressure infusion l.
>Wackenheim clivus canal l.

linear
>l. accelerator (LINAC)
>l. accelerator system (LINAC system)
>l. accelerator unit
>l. array-hydrophone assembly
>l. array transducer
>l. convex array scanner
>l. hearing aid
>L. hip stem
>l. in-line ligature carrier
>L. KGT tonometer
>l. 35-MHz transducer
>l. potentiometer
>l. scissor punch
>l. stapler
>l. stapling device
>L. total hip system
>l. variable-differential transducer
>l. variable differential transformer

linear-type echoendoscope
Lineback adenoidal punch
linen suture
liner
>Ac'cents permanent lash l.
>Ardee denture l.
>Calcipulpe cavity l.
>cast l.
>Cavitec cavity l.
>Cavoline cavity l.
>Conveen Security+male external catheter & l.

DePuy acetabular l.
Dignity Plus l.
elevated rim acetabular l.
Enduron acetabular l.
Fillauer prosthesis l.
Fillauer silicone suspension l.
Gore cast l.
Gore-Tex waterproof cast l.
grommet bone l.
Hylamer acetabular l.
Iceross Comfort Plus silicone gel l.
Integrity neutral l.
Ketac l.
KINS l.
KM-series l.
OrthoGel l.
Ortho-Wick foam l.
polyethylene l.
Polysorb l.
provisional l.
Pulpdent cavity l.
Reflection l.
rubber bite l.
Silosheath gel l.
SlimLine fitted l.
splint l.
TEC l.
Teflon l.
Tempo denture l.
Tubulitec cavity l.

Lingeman
>L. kit
>L. 3-in-1 procedure drape
>L. TUR drape

lingoscope
lingual
>l. arch
>l. bar
>l. cortical plate
>l. forceps
>l. spatula
>l. wire

Link
link
>L. anatomical hip
>L. approximator
>L. cementless reconstruction hip prosthesis
>L. custom partial pelvis replacement system
>L. Endo-Model rotational knee
>L. Endo-Model rotational knee system
>L. Lubinus AP hip system
>L. Lubinus SP II total hip replacement system
>L. microporous hip stem
>L. MP hip noncemented reconstruction prosthesis
>L. Saddle Prosthesis Endo-Model hip replacement system
>L. stack split splint
>L. toe splint
>Waldmar l.

L

Linkow
- L. blade implant
- L. dental implant material

Link-Plus retention pin

Linnartz
- L. forceps
- L. intestinal clamp
- L. stomach clamp

Linn-Graefe iris forceps

Linson electronic cell counter

lint-free sponge

Linton
- L. elastic stockings
- L. esophageal tube
- L. splanchnic retractor
- L. tourniquet
- L. tourniquet clamp
- L. vein hook
- L. vein stripper

Linton-Blakemore needle

Linton-Nachlas tube

Lintro-Scan scanner

Linvatec
- L. absorbable screw
- L. arthroscopic infusion pump
- L. bioabsorbable interference screw
- L. cannula
- L. driver
- L. meniscal BioStinger anchor suture
- L. wrist arthroscopy traction tower

Linvotec microdebrider

Linx
- L. extension wire
- L. guidewire extension
- L. guidewire extension cardiac device

Linx-EZ cardiac device

lion
- l. forceps
- l. hearing aid
- l. jaw bone holder
- l. jaw tenaculum

lion-head clamp

Lionheart catheter

lion-jaw
- l.-j. bone-holding forceps
- l.-j. clamp

Lion's
- L. Claw grasper
- L. Paw grasper

Liotta-BioImplant LPB prosthetic valve

Liotta total artificial heart

lip
- l. clamp
- l. retractor
- l. traction bow

Lipectron
- L. ultrasonic lancet
- L. ultrasonic scalpel

Lipisorb dressing

lipodissector

Lipo-Medi girdle

liposhaver

Liposorber
- L. cholesterol filter
- L. LA-15 system

Lipovacutainer cannister

Lipowitz metal

Lippes loop intrauterine device

Lippman hip prosthesis

Lippy modified prosthesis

Lipschiff knife

Lipschwitz needle

Lipscomb-Anderson drill guide

Lipshultz epididymovasostomy microdissection scissors

liquid
- L. Embolic system
- l. organic dye laser
- l. scintillation spectrometer
- l. scintillation spectrophotometer
- l. vitreous-aspirating cannula

LISCO sponge

Liss CES device

Listening Glass hearing aid

Lister
- L. bandage
- L. bandage scissors
- L. conjunctival forceps
- L. dressing
- L. knife
- L. lens manipulator
- L. mules

Lister-Burch eye speculum

List needle

Liston
- L. amputation knife
- L. bone-cutting forceps
- L. phalangeal knife
- L. plaster-of-Paris scissors
- L. shears
- L. splint

Liston-Key bone-cutting forceps

Liston-Key-Horsley
- L.-K.-H. forceps
- L.-K.-H. rib shears

Liston-Littauer
- L.-L. bone-cutting forceps
- L.-L. rongeur

Liston-Luer-Whiting rongeur

Liston-Ruskin shears

Liston-Stille bone-cutting forceps

Lite
- L. blade

Liteflex lens

Lite-Gait partial weight-bearing gait therapy device

Liteguard mini-defibrillator

LiteNest portable seating system

Lite-Pipe
- Millard L.-P.

lithium
- l. iodine battery
- l. pacemaker

lithium-powered pacemaker

Lithoclast
- L. ballistic energy generator

L. lithotriptor
Swiss L.
Lithognost flash-lamp pulsed dye laser
Lithospec lithotriptor
Lithostar
L. lithotripsy unit
L. lithotriptor
L. Plus
Lithostat
lithotomy
l. forceps
l. legholder
lithotripsy table
lithotriptor, lithotripter
Breakstone l.
Calcusplit pneumatic l.
Calcutript electrohydraulic l.
Candela laser l.
Circon-ACMI l.
Diasonics Therasonic l.
Direx Tripter X-1 l.
Dormia gallstone l.
Dormia waterbath l.
Dornier compact l.
Dornier extracorporeal shock-wave l.
Dornier HM-series l.
Dornier MPL 9000 gallstone l.
EDAP LT.1 l.
electrohydraulic l.
electromagnetic l.
extracorporeal piezoelectric l.
extracorporeal shock wave l.
holmium laser l.
Karl Storz l.
Karl Storz-Lutzeyer l.
laser l.
Lithoclast l.
Lithospec l.
Lithostar l.
manual l.
Medispec Econolith spark plug l.
Medstone extracorporeal shock-wave l.
Modulith SL 20 l.
MonoLith single-piece mechanical l.
Northgate SD-3 dual-purpose l.
Pentax l.
percutaneous ultrasonic l.
piezoelectric shock wave l.
pneumoballistic l.
l. probe
Pulsolith laser l.
second generation l.
shock wave l.
Siemens Lithostar Plus System C l.
Sonolith 3000 l.
Sonotrode l.
Storz Monolith l.
Therasonics l.
third generation l.
tubeless l.
ultrasonic l.
water cushion l.

lithotriptoscope
Ravich l.
lithotrite
Alcock l.
Bigelow l.
Hendrickson l.
Keyes l.
Löwenstein l.
Lowsley l.
Marmite l.
Ravich l.
Reliquet l.
Teale gorget l.
Wolf l.
Lithovac master suction system
Littauer
L. bone-cutting forceps
L. ciliary forceps
L. dissecting scissors
L. ear-dressing forceps
L. ear polyp forceps
L. nasal-dressing forceps
L. rongeur
L. stitch scissors
L. suture scissors
Littauer-Liston bone-cutting forceps
Littauer-West
L.-W. cutting forceps
L.-W. rongeur
Littell cannula
Litt forceps
Littig strut AFO
Little
L. cargo vest
L. intraocular lens implant
L. Ones Pediatric Urine Collector
L. Ones SUR-FIT flexible wafer, white collar
L. Ones SUR-FIT pediatric belt
L. retractor
Little-Arnott tripod intraocular lens
Littleford Spector introducer
Littler
L. dissecting scissors
L. suture-carrying scissors
Littlewood tissue forceps
Littmann
L. defibrillation pad
L. ECG electrode
L. galilean magnification changer
L. Master Classic II stethoscope
Litton dental handpiece
Litvak-Pereyra ligature needle
Litwak
L. cannula
L. clamp
L. mitral valve scissors
Litwin scissors
liver
l. biopsy needle
l. coil
HepatAssist bioartificial l.
l. retractor
liver-holding clamp
Livermore trocar

L

Livernois
    L. lens-holding forceps
    L. pickup and folding forceps
Liverpool
    L. elbow implant
    L. knee prosthesis
live splint
Living Air XL-15 unit
Livingston
    L. forceps
    L. intramedullary bar
    L. peribulbar wedge
Lixiscope scope
LIZ-88 ablation unit
Ljunggren-Stille tenotome
LKB/Wallach
    LKB/W. 1277 automatic gamma
      counter
    LKB/W. scintillation counter
LKB/Wallac 1217 Rackbeta equipment
LLETZ/LEEP loop electrode
LLL brace
Llobera fixation forceps
Llorente dissecting forceps
Lloyd
    L. adapter
    L. adapter counterbore
    L. bronchial catheter
    L. chiropractic table
    L. double catheter
    L. esophagoscopic catheter
    L. flexion distraction table
    L. nail driver
    L. nail extractor
Lloyd-Davies
    L.-D. clamp
    L.-D. occlusion forceps
    L.-D. rectal scissors
    L.-D. sigmoidoscope
    L.-D. stirrups
LMA-Unique disposable laryngeal mask
  airway
L'Nard
    L. boot
    L. long opponens hand and wrist
      orthosis
    L. Multi-Podus orthosis
    L. thoracolumbosacral orthosis
Lo
    Lo Bak spinal support
    Lo Bak spinal support prosthesis
loader
    Lehner II l.
lobectomy
    l. forceps
    l. scissors
lobe-grasping forceps
lobe-holding forceps
Lobell splinter forceps
Lobenstein-Tarnier forceps
lobotomy
    l. electrode
    l. needle
lobster bone-reduction forceps
lobster-tail catheter

lobster-type clamp
local gradient coil
localizer
    Berman l.
    FlashPoint optical l.
    Risser l.
    Roper-Hall l.
    Suetens-Gybels-Vandermeulen
      angiographic l.
    Urrets-Zavalia l.
localizing
    l. electrode
    l. probe
LocalMed
    L. catheter infusion sleeve
    L. InfusaSleeve
locator
    ASIS femoral head l.
    Berman foreign body l.
    Bronson-Turner foreign body l.
    foreign body l.
    Gill-Thomas l.
    Neosono MC apex l.
    Odontometer electronic apex l.
    Porex nerve l.
    Root ZX apex l.
    Roper-Hall l.
    saddle l.
    Staodyn Insight point l.
    Sweet l.
    ToDyeFor root canal l.
locator-stimulator
    Neuro-Pulse nerve l.-s.
LOC guidewire extension
lock
    L. Clamshell device
    Codman disposable ICP l.
    English l.
    French l.
    German l.
    heparin l.
    Howland l.
    ICEX 4-hole l.
    Luer cannula l.
    l. needle
    pivot l.
    sliding l.
Locke bone clamp
Lockhart-Mummery
    L.-M. probe
    L.-M. retractor
lock-in amplifier
locking
    l. clamp
    l. device
    l. nut
    l. peg
    l. prosthesis
    l. reconstruction plate
    l. screw
    l. stylet
Lockjaw arch bar
Lockwood
    L. clamp

L. intestinal forceps
L. tissue forceps
Lockwood-Allis
    L.-A. intestinal forceps
    L.-A. tissue forceps
Loc-Light lumbar support belt
Loctoplate
Loewi suspension device
Lofberg
    L. thyroid retractor
    L. vaginal speculum
Lofric disposable urethral catheter
Lofstrand
    L. brace
    L. crutch
Logan
    L. dissector
    L. lacrimal sac self-retaining
    retractor
    L. lip traction bow
    L. periosteal elevator
LogiCal pressure transducer system
logMAR chart
Lok-it screwdriver
Lok-Mesh bonding base
Lok-screw double-slot screwdriver
lollipop stick
Lombard-Beyer
    L.-B. forceps
    L.-B. rongeur
Lombard-Boies mastoid rongeur
Lombard rongeur
Lombart
    L. radioscope
    L. tonometer
Londermann corneal trephine
London
    L. College foil carrier
    L. narrow-bladed retractor
    L. tissue forceps
Lone
    L. Star retractor
    L. Star retractor system
long
    l. above-elbow cast
    l. ACE fixed-wire balloon catheter
    l. arm navicular cast
    l. arm splint
    l. atraumatic retractor
    L. Beach stereotactic robot
    l. below-elbow cast
    L. Brite Tip guiding catheter
    l. coarse bur
    l. double upright brace
    L. Island College Hospital placental
    forceps
    l. leg brace
    l. leg cylinder cast
    l. leg immobilizer
    l. leg plaster
    l. leg plaster cast
    l. leg posterior molded splint
    l. leg splint
    l. leg walking cast
    l. nail-mounted drill guide

l. needle
l. occluder
l. scalpel
L. Skinny over-the-wire balloon
catheter
l. taper/stiff shaft Glidewire
l. tissue forceps
long-bore collimator
Longdwel
    L. catheter needle
    L. Teflon catheter
Longevity V-Lign hip prosthesis
long-handle
    l.-h. curette
    l.-h. offset gouge
longitudinal spinal bar
long-jaw basket forceps
Longmire-Mueller curved valvulotome
Longmire-Storm clamp
Longmire valvulotome
long-nosed sphincterotome
long-span rigid plate
long-stretch bandage
long-term
    l.-t. ambulatory physiologic
    surveillance monitor
    l.-t. internal jugular catheter
long-wearing contact lens
Lonnecken tube
Look
    L. capsular polisher
    L. cortex extractor
    L. cystitome
    L. I&A coaxial cannula
    L. irrigating lens loop
    L. irrigating vectis
    L. micropuncture device
    L. retrobulbar needle
    L. suture
loop (*See also* loupe)
    Adler tripronged lens error l.
    Amenabar lens l.
    angled lens l.
    angled nucleus removal l.
    Atwood l.
    Aus-Jena-Gullstrand lens l.
    Axenfeld nerve l.
    l. ball electrode
    Beck twisted wire snare l.
    Beebe lens l.
    Berens lens l.
    Berger l.
    Berget lens l.
    Billeau ear l.
    Billeau-House ear l.
    bipolar urological l.
    Blair-Ivy l.
    blind l.
    Bunnell finger l.
    Callahan lens l.
    Cannon endarterectomy l.
    Castroviejo lens l.
    Clayman-Knolle irrigating lens l.
    l. curette
    cutting l.

L

loop (continued)
    Diaflex retrieval l.
    Duncan l.
    ear l.
    Electrodes l.
    Elschnig-Weber l.
    finger l.
    Flynn lens l.
    foreign body l.
    FormFlex lens l.
    Gerdy intra-auricular l.
    Gill-Welsh lens l.
    Gill-Welsh-Morrison lens l.
    Gobin-Weiss l.
    Greenwald cutting l.
    l. & hook strapping
    House-Billeau ear l.
    House wire l.
    Ilg lens l.
    intracapsular lens l.
    irrigating lens l.
    irrigating vectis l.
    Ivy l.
    Kirby intracapsular lens l.
    Kirby intraocular lens l.
    Kleinsasser lens l.
    Knapp lens l.
    Knolle-Pearce irrigating lens l.
    Kraff nucleus lens l.
    Lemoine-Searcy fixation anchor l.
    Lempert-Storz lens l.
    lens l.
    Lewis lens l.
    Look irrigating lens l.
    lyodura l.
    McKenzie leukotomy l.
    Medevice surgical l.
    Meyer temporal l.
    nucleus delivery l.
    nucleus removal l.
    nylon l.
    Oculus lens l.
    Olympus resectoscope l.
    Pearce-Knolle irrigating lens l.
    physiologic endometrial
      ablation/resection l. (PEARL)
    pressure length l.
    Ransford l.
    l. retractor
    retrieval l.
    l. scaler
    Schroeder tenaculum l.
    l. scissors
    l. shunt
    Simcoe double-end lens l.
    Simcoe II posterior chamber nucleus
      delivery l.
    Simcoe nucleus lens l.
    Snellen lens l.
    soft wire l.
    spring wire l.
    Stierlen lens l.
    Storz Universal lens l.
    Sur-Fit l.

    Surgitite ligating l.
    Teflon Silastic l.
    tenaculum hook l.
    toe l.
    tonsillar l.
    tonsillectome l.
    Torchia vectis l.
    tri-pronged l.
    twisted wire snare l.
    two-angled polypropylene l.
    unipolar cutting l.
    Uresil radiopaque silicone-band
      vessel l.'s
    vaginal speculum l.
    vascular l.
    vectis l.
    Vedder l.
    vessel l.
    Visitec nucleus removal l.
    V. Mueller vascular l.
    Ward-Lempert lens l.
    Weber-Elschnig lens l.
    Wilder lens l.
    wire l.
    Zein l.
loop-fixated intraocular lens
loop-over wrap
loop-tipped electrode
loop-type
    l.-t. snare forceps
    l.-t. stone-crushing forceps
Loopuyt needle
loose
    l. body grasper
    l. body suction forceps
Lopez enteral valve
Lopez-Reinke tonsillar dissector
Lo-Por
    L.-P. tracheal tube
    L.-P. vascular graft
    L.-P. vascular graft prosthesis
LoPresti
    L. fiberoptic esophagoscope
    L. panendoscope
Lo-Profile
    L.-P. balloon
    L.-P. II balloon catheter
    L.-P. steerable dilatation catheter
    L.-P. urostomy pouch
Loptex laser intraocular lens implant
LORAD
    LORAD StereoGuide
Lorad
    L. Stereo Guide prone breast
      biopsy system
    L. Stereo Guide stereotactic breast
      biopsy system
    L. SteroGuide
Lord
    L. cup
    L. total hip prosthesis
Lordan chalazion forceps
Lord-Blakemore tube
Lordoticiser
    Posture Pump L.

Lore
    L. subglottic forceps
    L. suction tube
    L. suction tube-holding forceps
    L. suction tube and tip-holding
    forceps
Lore-Lawrence tracheotomy tube
Lorenz
    L. brace
    L. chisel
    L. gauze packer
    L. Micro-Power dense bone drilling
    and cutting system
    L. osteosynthesis system
    L. PC/TC scissors
    L. plating system
    L. reamer
    L. screw
    L. SMO prosthesis
    L. titanium screws and plate
Lorez PC/TC ultra-sharp knife
lorgnette occluder
Lorie
    L. antral trephine
    L. cheek retractor
Loring ophthalmoscope
Lorna nonperforating towel clamp
Loth-Kirschner drill
Lothrop
    L. dissector
    L. hemostat
    L. ligature forceps
    L. tonsillar knife
    L. tonsillar retractor
    L. uvular retractor
Lotman Visometer
Lo-Trau side-cutting needle
Lottes
    L. pin
    L. reamer
    L. triflange intramedullary nail
Loughnane prostatic hook
Louis instrumentation
Louisville elevator
Lounsbury placental curette
loupe (*See also* loop)
    Arlt lens l.
    Bausch & Lomb Duoloupe lens l.
    Beebe l.
    Berens lens l.
    binocular l.
    Callahan lens l.
    Castroviejo lens l.
    Codman magnifying l.
    corneal monocular l.
    Daviel lens l.
    Denlan magnifying l.
    Duoloupe lens l.
    Elschnig-Weber l.
    fiberoptic l.
    Galilean l.
    Gullstrand lens l.
    Gullstrand-Zeiss lens l.
    Ilg lens l.
    Keeler-Galilean surgical l.

    Keeler panoramic l.
    Keeler spotlight lens l.
    Keeler wide-angle lens l.
    Kirby intraocular lens l.
    Lemoine-Searcy fixation anchor l.
    Lempert-Storz l.
    Magill magnifying l.
    l. magnification
    Magni-Focuser lens l.
    magnifying l.
    Mark II Magni-Focuser l.
    May hook-on lens l.
    New Orleans lens l.
    nucleus delivery l.
    nucleus removal l.
    ocular Gamboscope l.
    operating l.
    Opticaid lens l.
    Opt-Visor l.
    panoramic l.
    prism l.
    Simcoe II PC nucleus delivery l.
    surgical l.
    Troutman lens l.
    Wilder l.
    Zeiss-Gullstrand l.
    Zeiss lens l.
    Zeiss operating field l.
Lours leukotome
Loute wire tightener
Lovac
    L. fundal contact lens
    L. fundal contact lens implant
    L. gonioscopic lens
    L. six-mirror gonioscopic lens
    L. six-mirror gonioscopic lens
    implant
Love
    L. leukotome
    L. nasal splint
    L. nasopharyngeal retractor
    L. nerve root retractor
    L. pituitary rongeur
    L. uvula retractor
Love-Adson periosteal elevator
Love-Gruenwald
    L.-G. alligator forceps
    L.-G. cranial rongeur
    L.-G. intervener
    L.-G. intervertebral disk rongeur
    L.-G. laminectomy rongeur
    L.-G. pituitary forceps
    L.-G. pituitary rongeur
Lovejoy retractor
Love-Kerrison
    L.-K. rongeur
    L.-K. rongeur forceps
Lovelace
    L. bladder forceps
    L. gallbladder traction forceps
    L. hemostatic forceps
    L. lung-grasping forceps
    L. thyroid-traction vulsellum forceps
    L. tissue forceps

L

Lovelace *(continued)*
    L. traction lung forceps
    L. traction tissue forceps
Loversan infusion set
Lovitt-Uhler modification of Jewett post-fusion brace
low
    l. impedance thermocouple
    l. margin standard abutment
    l. outlet forceps
    L. Profile legholder
    L. Profile plastic body jacket
    l. profile plate
    L. Profile walker
    l. quarter Blucher shoe
low-air-loss bed
Löw-Beer forceps
low-compliance balloon
low-contact
    l.-c. dynamic compression plate
    l.-c. stress plate
LowDye
    L. strapping
    L. taping
Lowe-Breck cartilage knife
Lowell
    L. glaucoma knife
    L. pleural needle
Lowe microtome knife
Löwenberg forceps
low-energy
    l.-e. collimator
    l.-e. laser
Löwenstein lithotrite
lower
    l. gall duct forceps
    l. lateral forceps
    l. limb prosthesis
Lowette needle
Lowette-Verner needle
low-flow
    l.-f. circuit
    l.-f. regulator
low-flux cuprammonium dialyzer
low-grade suction unit
Lowis
    L. intervertebral disk forceps
    L. periosteal elevator
Lowman
    L. bone-holding clamp
    L. bone-holding forceps
    L. chisel
    L. hand retractor
    L. rongeur
Lowman-Gerster bone clamp
Lowman-Hoglund
    L.-H. chisel
    L.-H. clamp
Lown cardioverter
low-pass filter
low-power optics for myopic correction lens
low-pressure voice prosthesis

low-profile
    l.-p. angioplasty balloon
    l.-p. balloon-positioning catheter
    l.-p. breast implant
    l.-p. mitral heart valve
    l.-p. prosthesis
    l.-p. R-K marker
low-profile, port implantable port
low-resistance rolling seal spirometer
Lowsley
    L. grasping forceps
    L. hemostat
    L. lithotrite
    L. prostate retractor
    L. prostatic forceps
    L. prostatic tractor
    L. retractor with hand-sutured closure
    L. ribbon-gut needle
    L. stone crusher
    L. suprapubic tractor
    L. urethroscope
Lowsley-Luc forceps
Lowsley-Peterson
    L.-P. cystoscope
    L.-P. endoscope
low-speed
    l.-s. Christmas tree diamond bur
    l.-s. rotation angioplasty catheter
    l.-s. tapered carbide bur
low-surface reactive Boglass
low-viscosity
    l.-v. bone cement
low-vision
    l.-v. aid
    l.-v. enhancement system
LPK-80 II argon laser
L-plate
    L.-p. plate
    Synthes mini L.-p.
LPPS
    LPPS hydroxyapatite
    LPPS hydroxyapatite adhesive
LPS
    LPS balloon
L-resection guide
LR needle
L-rod
    L.-r. implant material
    L.-r. instrumentation
    Luque L.-r.
LSC 7000 curved array transducer
LS⁴ custom spinal jacket
L-shaped
    L.-s. aneurysm clip
    L.-s. cautery
    L.-s. elevator
    L.-s. miniplate
    L.-s. plate
LSI silver self-adhesive disposable electrode
LSK One Disposable microkeratome
LSR patent-pending bedside monitor
L stylet

LSU
>LSU reciprocation-gait orthosis
>LSU reciprocation-gait orthosis brace

L.T. Jones tear duct tube
LTK system
LT V-105 implantable cardioverter-defibrillator
LTX PTCA catheter
Lubafax dressing
Lubinus
>L. acetabular component
>L. AP hip system
>L. knee prosthesis
>L. SP II
>L. SP II anatomically adapted hip system

Lübke-Berci VersaLite
Lübke uterine vacuum cannula
Lubri-Flex
>L.-F. ureteral stent
>L.-F. urologic stent

Lubriglide-coated guidewire
Luc
>L. ethmoidal forceps
>L. forceps
>L. nasal-cutting forceps
>L. septal forceps
>L. septum-cutting forceps

Lucae
>L. bayonet
>L. bayonet dressing forceps
>L. bayonet ear forceps
>L. bayonet tissue forceps
>L. bone hammer
>L. bone mallet
>L. dissecting forceps
>L. ear forceps
>L. ear perforation knife
>L. ear probe
>L. ear speculum
>L. eustachian catheter
>L. hook
>L. mastoid mallet

Lucas
>L. alveolar curette
>L. chisel
>L. gouge

Lucchese mitral valve dilator
lucite
>l. sphere implant
>L. sphere implant

Luck
>L. bone drill
>L. bone saw
>L. fasciatome

Luck-Bishop saw
Lu corneal marker
Ludwig
>L. middle ear applicator
>L. sinus applicator

Luedde exophthalmometer
Luer
>L. bone curette
>L. bone rongeur
>L. cannula lock
>L. connection
>L. connector
>L. curette forceps
>L. double-ended tracheal retractor
>L. eye speculum
>L. hemorrhoidal forceps
>L. lock fitting
>L. mallet
>L. needle
>L. reconstruction plate
>L. rongeur forceps
>L. scoop
>L. speaking tube
>L. S-shaped retractor
>L. suction cannula adapter
>L. syringe
>L. thoracic rongeur
>L. tracheal cannula
>L. tracheal tube

luer
>positioner l.

Luer-Friedman bone rongeur
Luer-Hartmann rongeur
Luer-Koerte gallstone scoop
Luer-Liston-Wheeling rongeur
Luer-Lok
>L.-L. adapter
>L.-L. B-D syringe
>L.-L. jet ventilator connector
>L.-L. male adapter plug
>L.-L. needle
>L.-L. port
>L.-L. stopcock

Luer-Stille rongeur
Luer-Whiting
>L.-W. forceps
>L.-W. rongeur
>L.-W. rongeur forceps

Luhr
>L. fixation plate
>L. implant
>L. implant screw
>L. mandibular plate
>L. maxillofacial fixation system
>L. MCS bone plate
>L. microbone plate
>L. microfixation cranial plate
>L. microfixation system
>L. Microfixation System drill bit
>L. Microfixation System plate cutter
>L. Microfixation System plate-holding forceps
>L. Microfixation System pliers
>L. microplate
>L. minifixation bone plate
>L. miniplate
>L. MRS system
>L. pan fixation system
>L. pan plate
>L. Vitallium micromesh plate
>L. Vitallium screw

Luikart-Bill
>L.-B. forceps
>L.-B. traction handle

Luikart forceps

L

Luikart-Kjelland
    L.-K. obstetrical forceps
Luikart-McLane obstetrical forceps
Luikart-Simpson obstetrical forceps
Lukens
    L. aspirator
    L. bone wax dressing
    L. cannula
    L. catgut suture
    L. collecting tube
    L. collector
    L. double-channel irrigator
    L. double-ended tracheal retractor
    L. epiglottic retractor
    L. needle
    L. orthodontic band
    L. thymus retractor
    L. trap
Lulu clamp
Lumaguide infusion catheter
lumbar
    l. anterior root stimulator implant
    l. aortography needle
    l. corset
    l. intersomatic fusion expandable cage
    l. orthosis
    l. pedicle screw
    l. peritoneal catheter
    l. port
    l. puncture needle
    l. retractor
    l. roll
    l. subarachnoid catheter
Lumbard airway
lumbosacral
    l. corset
    l. fusion elevator
    l. orthosis
    l. spine transpedicular instrumentation
    l. support pelvic traction
lumbotomy retractor
lumbrical bar
Lumelec pacing catheter
lumen
    l. cannula
    l. finder
Lumenator injectable guidewire
Lumex
    L. lightweight wheelchair
    L. Preferred Care recliner
    L. shower bed
    L. shower stretcher
    L. Tilt-in-Space reclining wheelchair
    L. walker
Lumi alloy
Lumina
    L. guidewire
    L. operating telescope
    L. rod lens arthroscope
luminal stent
Lumina-SL telescope
luminometer
    LB 9501 l.

Lumiscan scanner
Lumiwand light
Lumix dental x-ray unit
Lumonics YAG laser
Lunar
    L. DPX densitometer
    L. DPX dual-energy absorptiometer
    L. DPX total-body scanner
    L. Expert densitometer
lunate
    l. implant
    l. prosthesis
Lunax Boot
Lund-Dodick punch
Lunderquist
    L. catheter
    L. coat hanger wire
    L. guidewire
Lunderquist-Ring torque guide
Lundholm
    L. plate
    L. screw
Lundia dialyzer holder
Lundsgaard
    L. blade
    L. knife
    L. rasp
    L. sclerotome
Lundsgaard-Burch
    L.-B. corneal rasp
    L.-B. knife
    L.-B. sclerotome
Lundy
    L. fascial needle
    L. laryngoscope
    L. tubing hand-roller
Lundy-Irving caudal needle
Luneau retinoscopy rack
lung
    artificial l.
    l. dissecting scissors
    l. exclusion clamp
    l. imaging fluorescence endoscope
    iron l.
    Kolobow membrane l.
    membrane artificial l.
    l. retractor
    Sci-Med Life Systems, Inc. membrane artificial l.
    l. tissue forceps
lung-grasping forceps
lungmotor
Luntz-Dodick punch
Luomanen oral airway
Luongo
    L. curette
    L. hand retractor
    L. needle
    L. septal elevator
    L. sphenoid irrigating cannula
Luque
    L. cerclage wire
    L. fixation device
    L. II fixation system
    L. II plate

L. II screw
L. II segmental spinal instrumentation
L. L-rod
L. rectangle
L. rod
L. semirigid segmental spinal instrumentation
L. sublaminar wire
Lurz-Goltner ligator
Lusk instrument
Lusskin
L. bone drill
L. subungual hematoma iron
Luster investment material
Luther-Peter
L.-P. lid everter
L.-P. retractor
Lutz
L. automatic reprocessor
L. septal forceps
Luxar
L. NovaPulse CO$_2$ laser
L. Silhouette noninvasive body appearance equipment
Luxation patellar saw
Luxator extractor
Lux culture dish
Luxo
L. illuminated magnifier
L. surgical illuminator
Luxtec
L. fiberoptic system
L. illuminated surgical telescope
L. surgical telescope
Luys separator
LVAD
left ventricular assist device
vented-electric HeartMate LVAD
LV apex cannula
LVAS implantable pump
LX
BiPAP Duet LX
LX needle
Lyda-Ivalon-Lucite implant
Lyman-Smith
L.-S. toe drop brace
L.-S. tractor
Lymphapress compression therapy
LymphoScan
L. nuclear imaging system
L. nuclear imaging system scanner
Lymwrap lymphedema bandaging kit

Lynch
L. blunt dissector
L. cup-shaped curette forceps
L. curette
L. electrode
L. laryngeal dissector
L. laryngeal forceps
L. laryngeal knife handle
L. mucosa separator plate
L. obtuse-angle laryngeal knife
L. right-angle knife
L. scissors
L. septal splint
L. spatula
L. straight knife
L. suspension apparatus
L. suspension laryngoscope
L. tonsillar dissector
L. tonsillar knife
Lynco
L. biomechanical orthotic system
L. foot orthosis
Lynell intraocular lens
Lynx OTW catheter
lyodura loop
LYOfoam
L. A water resistant dressing
L. C dressing
L. T dressing
Lyo-Ject
Cardizem L.-J.
Lyon
L. forceps
L. ring
L. tube
lyophilized graft
Lyra laser system
Lyrelle patch
lyre-shaped finger hook
LySonix
L. 250 aspirator
L. 2000 complete ultrasonic surgical system
L. Delta Tip irrigator
L. Post-Operative patient system
L. TTD Cannula System
L. 2000 ultrasonic surgical system
L. 2000 ultrasound device
Lyster water bag
Lyte Fit orthotic
Lytle metacarpal splint
LZT crystal

L

3M

3M Clean Seals waterproof bandage
3M Coban LF self-adherent wrap
3M drape
3M filling instrument
3M intraocular lens
3M limb isolation bag
3M mammary implant
3M matrix tape
3M Microdon dressing
3M Micropore surgical tape
3M microvascular anastomotic coupling device
3M No Sting barrier film
3M Reston self-adhering foam pad & roll
3M scanner
3M small aperture Steri-Drape drape
3M SoftCloth adhesive wound dressing
3M Tegaderm HP high MVTR transparent dressing
3M Tegaderm transparent dressing with absorbent pad
3M Tegapore wound contact material
3M Tegasorb hydrocolloid dressing
3M Vi-drape

M4

M4 Kerr Safety Hedstrom instrument
M4 safety handpiece

M4-400 Freedom blade

MA

MA 53 two-channel audiometer

MA-1 respirator

MAC

MAC cervical collar

Macaluso stent remover

MacAusland

M. bone mallet
M. chisel
M. dissector
M. finishing-ball reamer
M. finishing-cup reamer
M. hip skid
M. muscle retractor

MacAusland-Kelly retractor

Macbeth ColorChecker

MacCallum knife

MacCarty forceps

MacDonald

M. dissector
M. gastric clamp
M. periosteal elevator

Macewen

M. drill
M. saw

Macey tendon carrier

MacGregor

M. conjunctival forceps

M. mules
M. osteotome

Machat

M. adjustable aspirating wire speculum
M. double-ended marker
M. superior flap LASIK marker

Machemer

M. calipers
M. diamond-dust-coated foreign body forceps
M. diamond-dusted forceps
M. flat lens
M. infusion contact lens
M. magnifying vitrectomy lens
M. scleral knife
M. VISC vitrector
M. vitreous cutter

Machida

M. fiber-duodenoscope
M. fiberoptic laryngoscope
M. flexible endoscope
M. light source connector
M. nasolaryngoscope

machine

A2008 ABGII hemodialysis m.
Accuray Neurotron 1000 m.
AK-10 dialysis m.
Aloka echocardiograph m.
Berkeley suction m.
Biodex isokinetic testing m.
Bird m.
borazone blade cutting m.
Brown-Bovari m.
Bruel & Kjaer 1860 ultrasound m.
Burdick Eclipse ECG m.
bypass m.
CamStar exercise m.
Catalyst m.
Cavitron m.
Cavitron-Kelman phacoemulsification m.
cobalt megavoltage m.
Cobe-Stockert heart-lung m.
constant passive-motion m. (CPMM)
cooling m.
CooperVision I&A m.
Corometrics-Aloka echocardiograph m.
Corometrics Model 900SC in-office mammography m.
CPM m.
Craoford-Senning heart-lung m.
Cybex m.
Danniflex CPM m.
demand flow m.
Drake-Willard hemodialysis m.
Drake-Willock dialysis m.
endoscopic sewing m.
Endotek m.
Epilatron hair-removal m.

M

machine *(continued)*
Euro Precision Technology submicron lathe m.
Exerstrider m.
Faxitron x-ray m.
Finapres Dinamap blood pressure m.
focused, segmented, ultrasound m.
Fresenius dialysis m.
Gambro AK10 m.
General Electric Pass-C echocardiograph m.
G5 massage and percussion m.
HemoTec ACT m.
Hewlett-Packard Echo-Doppler m.
I&A m.
Instron m.
intermittent flow m.
Isotechnologies B-200 low back m.
isotonic m.
KineTec hip CPM m.
Kodak Ektachem 700 m.
Kurzweil reading m.
Mayo-Gibbon heart-lung m.
MB-900 AC m.
MDA ultrasound-assisted lipoplasty m.
Medicamat ultrasound-assisted lipoplasty m.
MedX functional testing m.
MedX knee m.
MedX Mark II lumbar extension m.
MedX stretch m.
megavoltage m.
Mentor ultrasound-assisted lipoplasty m.
Morwel ultrasound-assisted lipoplasty m.
Narco esophageal motility m.
Narkomed anesthesia m.
NervePace nerve conduction testing m.
neutron therapy m.
Nova II m.
Orthion traction m.
Orthopantomograph-series panoramic x-ray m.
OsseoCare m.
OsteoPower drilling and cutting m.
Panelipse panoramic x-ray m.
Panex-E (Panoral) panoramic x-ray m.
Panorex panoramic x-ray m.
PC-1000 panoramic x-ray m.
Philips ultrasound m.
Portadial kidney m.
Primus prostate m.
Puritan-Bennett BiLevel Knight Star 335 m.
remote control afterloading m.
ResMed CPAP Sullivan III m.
Respironics BiPAP m.
Respironics CPAP m.
Respitrace m.

Rife m.
SDU-400 EchoView ultrasound m.
Sebbin ultrasound-assisted lipoplasty m.
SMEI ultrasound-assisted lipoplasty m.
Sono-stat Plus EMG m.
Stat Scrub handwasher m.
Status-X m.
Surgilav m.
Surgitron ultrasound-assisted lipoplasty m.
TECA-TD20 EMG m.
TENS m.
Toshiba echocardiograph m.
Toshiba electrocardiography m.
Ventana Immuno-automated m.
VersaClimber exercise m.
Visual-Tech m.
Wikco ankle m.

Machlett collimator
Macima reusable underpad
MacIntosh
M. blocker
M. fiberoptic laryngoscope blade
M. implant
M. laryngoscope
M. tibial plateau prosthesis
Maciol suture needle set
Mack
M. ear plug
M. lingual tonsillar tonsillectome
M. serrefine
M. tonometer
MacKay
M. contour self-retaining retractor
M. nasal splint
MacKay-Marg tonometer
MacKenty
M. cleft palate knife
M. laryngectomy tube
M. periosteal elevator
M. scissors
M. septal elevator
M. sphenoidal punch
M. tissue forceps
MacKenty-Converse periosteal elevator
Mackenzie polygraph
MacKinnon-Dellon
M.-D. Diskriminator
M.-D. Diskriminator instrument
Mackler intraluminal tube
MacKool
M. capsule retractor
M. system
Mackray short-cuffed endobronchial tube
Maclaren mobile buggy
Maclay tonsillar scissors
Mac-Lee enema bag
Macmed pediatric intramedullary nail
MacNab-English shoulder prosthesis
MacNamara cataract spoon
Macon Hospital speculum
MacQuigg-Mixter forceps
MacRae flap flipper/retreatment spatula

Macro-5 camera
Macrofit hip prosthesis
macromanipulators
    Microbeam I, II, III, IV m.
macro-mesh mesh
Macroplastique implantable device
MacroVac vacuum
macular contact lens
Macula retinoscope
MaculoScope scope
MacVicar double-end strabismus
  retractor
MAC-VU electrocardiograph
Madajet
    M. XL jet-injection anesthesia
      system
    M. XL local anesthesia system
Madayag biopsy needle
Maddacare child bath seat
Maddacrawler frame
Maddapult Asissto-Seat
Madden
    M. dissector
    M. forceps
    M. intestinal clamp
    M. ligature carrier
    M. sympathectomy hook
Madden-Potts
    M.-P. intestinal forceps
    M.-P. tissue forceps
Maddox
    M. caudal needle
    M. LASIK spatula
    M. prism
    M. rod
    M. rod occluder
Madoff suction tube
madreporic
    m. coral
    m. hip prosthesis
Madsen OB822 clinical audiometer
Maestro
    M. implant
    M. implantable cardiac pacemaker
    M. system
MAFO
    MAFO cane
magazine clip
Magellan monitor
Magerl
    M. hook-plate system
    M. plate-screw system
Maggi
    M. disposable biopsy needle guide
Magic
    M. microcatheter
    M. Torque guidewire
    M. Wand vibrator
Magicap
    Coltene M.
Magic-Wall stent
Magielski
    M. bayonet canal knife
    M. coagulating forceps
    M. coagulation cautery

    M. coagulator
    M. elevator
    M. hook
    M. needle
    M. stapes chisel
    M. tonsillar forceps
    M. tonsil-seizing forceps
Magielski-Heermann strut forceps
Magill
    M. catheter forceps
    M. circuit
    M. endotracheal catheter
    M. endotracheal forceps
    M. laryngoscope
    M. magnifying loupe
    M. orthodontic band
    M. Safety Clear endotracheal tube
Maglinte catheter
Maglite light
MagMag breast pump
Magna-Finder locating device
MagnaPod pain relief magnet
Magna-Site locating system
Magna-SL scanner
Magnassager massage tool
Magnatherm
    M. pulsed therapy high-frequency
      unit
    M. SSP electromagnetic therapy
      unit
Magnathotics orthotic
Magnatone hearing aid
MagneCore magnetic therapy
MAGneedle
    M. controller
    M. driver
    M. puller
Magnes
    M. biomagnetometer
    M. biomagnetometer system
    M. magnetic source imaging
    M. 2500 WH imager
    M. 2500 whole-blood scanner
magnesium tuning fork
magnet
    air-core m.
    Alnico Magneprobe m.
    Atlas-Storz eye m.
    Berman m.
    Bonaccolto m.
    bronchoscopic m.
    Bronson m.
    Bronson-Magnion eye m.
    Coronet m.
    C-shaped resistive m.
    doughnut m.
    ear m.
    Eindhoven m.
    elbow m.
    Equen stomach m.
    eye m.
    Fe-Ex orogastric tube m.
    Firlene eye m.
    foot m.
    foreign body m.

M

magnet *(continued)*
    GE Signa 1.5-T m.
    Grafco m.
    Gruening eye m.
    Grüning m.
    Haab eye m.
    hand-held eye m.
    Hirschberg electromagnet m.
    Holinger bronchoscopic m.
    Holinger endoscopic m.
    horseshoe m.
    implant m.
    Lancaster eye m.
    large-bore m.
    MagnaPod pain relief m.
    Magnex m.
    Mellinger m.
    Mueller giant eye m.
    nonenclosed m.
    Norris tip m.
    open m.
    original Sweet eye m.
    Oxford m.
    pancake MRI m.
    passively shimmed
     superconducting m.
    Patel intraocular m.
    Ralks eye m.
    rare earth intraocular m.
    Schumann giant eye m.
    Scientronics m.
    shim m.
    shimmed m.
    short-bore m.
    m. splint
    Storz m.
    Storz-Atlas eye m.
    suction m.
    superconducting m.
    surgical power m.
    Sweet eye m.
    Sweet original m.
    Szulc eye m.
    Tectonic m.
    Tesla m.
    m. therapy
    Thomas m.
    Trowbridge-Campau eye m.
    tubular m.
    Walker m.
    Wildgen-Reck metal locator m.
    m. wire

magnetic
    m. bead
    m. cup
    m. extractor
    m. eye implant
    m. eye probe
    m. induction device
    m. internal ureteral stent
    m. jaw tracking device
    m. mat pad
    m. microsphere
    m. motion transducer

    m. resonance cholangiopancreatogram
    m. resonance endoscope
    m. resonance imaging (MRI)
    m. resonance imaging-guided
     focused ultrasound sector
     transducer
    m. resonance imaging scan
    m. resonance spectroscopy
    m. retriever
    m. shielded cabin
    m. source imaging
    m. stimulator
    m. support belt
    M. Surgery system
    m. wrap

magnetically activated cell sorter
Magnetom
    M. Open system
    M. scanner
    M. SP MRI imager
    M. Vision MR system
magnetometer probe
Magnetrode cervical unit
Magnetron MRI system
magnet-tipped flexible catheter
Magnex
    M. Alpha MR system
    M. magnet
    M. MR scanner
magnifier
    anastigmatic aural m.
    aural m.
    Bruening Japanese anastigmatic
     aural m.
    Bruening-Storz anastigmatic aural m.
    Circline m.
    Japanese Bruening anastigmatic
     aural m.
    Luxo illuminated m.
    Optelec Passport m.
    Storz-Bruening anastigmatic aural m.
Magni-Focuser lens loupe
magnifying
    m. colonoscope
    m. glasses
    m. loupe
Magnum
    M. bariatric patient system bed
    M. 800 bed
    M. chisel
    M. curette
    M. guidewire
    M. 101 Plus table
Magnum-Meier system
Magnuson
    M. abduction humeral splint
    M. circular twin saw
    M. double counter-rotating saw
    M. single circular saw
    M. strut
    M. twist drill
    M. valve prosthesis
Magnuson-Cromie prosthesis

Magovern-Cromie
    M.-C. ball-cage prosthetic valve
    M.-C. prosthesis
Magovern heart valve
Magrina-Bookwalter
    M.-B. vaginal Deaver blade
    M.-B. vaginal retractor
    M.-B. vaginal retractor ring
Magstim 200 stimulator
Maguire-Harvey vitreous cutter
Mahoney
    M. dilator
    M. intranasal antral speculum
Mahorner
    M. dilator
    M. thyroid retractor
Mahurkar
    M. curved extension catheter
    M. dual-lumen femoral dialysis catheter
    M. fistular needle
Maico Gamma hearing aid
Maico-MA 20 audiometer
Maidera-Stern suture hook
Maier
    M. dressing forceps
    M. polyp forceps
    M. sponge forceps
    M. uterine forceps
Mailler
    M. colon forceps
    M. cut-off forceps
    M. intestinal forceps
    M. rectal forceps
Maine gonioscope
Maingot
    M. clamp
    M. gallbladder tube
    M. hysterectomy forceps
main pancreatic duct stent
Mainstay urologic soft tissue anchor
Mainster
    M. retinal laser lens
    M. Ultra Field PRP laser lens
    M. wide-field lens
Mainster-HM retinal laser lens
Mainster-S retinal laser lens
Mainster-WF retinal laser lens
maintainer
    anterior chamber m.
    Blumenthal anterior chamber m.
    Fary anterior chamber m.
    filter m.
    Gerber space m.
    Lewicky self-retaining chamber m.
    self-retaining chamber m.
Mainz
    M. pouch
    M. pouch urinary reservoir
Maisonneuve
    M. bandage
    M. urethrotome
Maison retractor
Majewski nasal curette
Major amblyoscope

Makar coagulator
Maki scissors
Maklakoff tonometer
Makler
    M. cannula
    M. counting chamber
    M. insemination device
    M. reusable semen analysis chamber
    M. sperm counting device
Mala-paedic shoe
malar
    m. implant
    m. periosteum-SMAS flap fixation suture
Malcolm-Lynn
    M.-L. C-RXF cervical retractor frame
    M.-L. radiolucent spinal retraction system
Malcolm-Rand
    M.-R. carbon-composite headholder
    M.-R. cranial x-ray frame
    M.-R. radiolucent headrest and retraction system
male
    m. catheter
    m. compression girdle
    m. condom
    m. washer
Malecot
    M. four-wing catheter
    M. four-wing drain
    M. nephrostomy catheter
    M. nephrostomy tube
    M. reentry catheter
    M. self-retaining urethral catheter
    M. Silastic catheter
    M. suprapubic cystostomy catheter
    M. two-wing catheter
    M. two-wing drain
Malette-Spencer coronary cannula
Malgaigne
    M. apparatus
    M. clamp
    M. patellar hook
Malibu cervical orthosis
Maliniac
    M. nasal brace
    M. nasal rasp
    M. nasal retractor
Malis
    M. angled bayonet forceps
    M. bipolar coagulating/cutting system
    M. bipolar coagulation forceps
    M. bipolar cutting forceps
    M. bipolar instrument
    M. bipolar irrigating forceps
    M. bipolar microcoagulator
    M. brain retractor kit
    M. cerebellar retractor
    M. cerebral retractor
    M. clip applier
    M. CMC-III electrosurgical system
    M. CMC-II PC bipolar coagulator

Malis *(continued)*
    M. cup forceps
    M. curette
    M. dissector
    M. electrocoagulation unit
    M. elevator
    M. hinge clamp
    M. irrigating bipolar CMC III
    M. irrigating forceps stylet
    M. irrigation tubing set
    M. jeweler bipolar forceps
    M. ligature passer
    M. needle holder
    M. nerve hook
    M. neurosurgical scissors
    M. solid state coagulator
    M. titanium microsurgical forceps
Malis-Frazier suction tube
Malis-Jensen
    M.-J. bipolar forceps
    M.-J. microbipolar forceps
Malith pacemaker
malleable
    m. blade
    m. blade retractor
    m. copper retractor
    m. facial implant
    m. metal finger splint
    m. microsurgical suction device
    m. multipore suction tube
    m. passing needle
    m. probe
    m. prosthesis
    m. ribbon retractor
    m. spatula
    m. stainless steel retractor
    m. stylet
    m. sucker
malleolar gel sleeve
Malleoloc anatomic ankle orthosis
Malleotrain ankle support
mallet
    Bakelite m.
    Bergman m.
    Blount nylon m.
    bone m.
    Boxwood m.
    brass m.
    Brown m.
    Carroll aluminum m.
    cervical m.
    Chandler m.
    Children's Hospital m.
    copper m.
    Cottle m.
    Crane m.
    Doyen bone m.
    fiber m.
    Gerzog bone m.
    Hajek m.
    hard m.
    Heath m.
    Henning m.
    Hibbs m.

    Jarit m.
    Kirk m.
    lead-filled m.
    Lucae bone m.
    Lucae mastoid m.
    Luer m.
    MacAusland bone m.
    Mead m.
    Meyerding m.
    nasal m.
    No Bounce m.
    nylon face m.
    nylon head m.
    Ombrédanne m.
    polyethylene-faced m.
    Ralks m.
    Rica bone m.
    Richards combination m.
    Rissler m.
    Rush m.
    slotted m.
    SMIC surgical m.
    Smith-Petersen m.
    solid copper head m.
    standard pattern m.
    Steinbach m.
    Stille m.
    surgical m.
    Surgical No Bounce m.
    Swanson m.
    White m.
malleus
    m. cutter
    m. forceps
    m. nipper
malleus-footplate assembly
malleus-incus prosthesis
malleus-stapes assembly
Mallinckrodt
    M. angiographic catheter
    M. endotracheal tube
    M. Laser-Flex tube
    M. scanner
    M. sensor system
    M. ultra tag labeling kit
    M. vertebral catheter
Mallory-Head
    M.-H. Interlok calcar trimmer
    M.-H. Interlok primary femoral
      component
    M.-H. Interlok rasp
    M.-H. Interlok reamer
    M.-H. modular acetabular template
    M.-H. modular calcar system
    M.-H. porous primary femoral
      prosthesis
Mallory RM-1 cell pacemaker
Malm-Himmelstein pulmonary
  valvulotome
Malmö hip splint
Maloney
    M. catheter
    M. endo-otoprobe
    M. mercury-filled esophageal dilator
    M. no-hole lens manipulator

M. tapered mercury-filled esophageal bougie
M. tapered-tip dilator
Maloney-Hurst dilator
Maloney-type bougie
malsensing pacemaker
Malström
M. cup
M. vacuum extractor
Malström-Westman cannula
Malteno glaucoma artificial valve
Maltese cross lens
Maltz
M. bayonet saw
M. button-end knife
M. cartilage knife
M. nasal rasp
M. needle
M. retractor
Maltz-Anderson nasal rasp
Maltz-Lipsett nasal rasp
Maltzman needle
Malvern analyzer
Mammalok localization needle
mammary
m. implant
m. prosthesis
m. support dressing
mammary-coronary tissue forceps
Mammatech breast prosthesis
mammographic view box
Mammo-Lume view box
Mammo Mask illuminator
Mammomat C3 mammography system
mammometer
Mammopatch gel self adhesive
Mammoscan digital imaging system
Mammospot
Mammotest
M. Plus breast biopsy system
Mammotome
M. biopsy system
M. core biopsy device
mammotome
Biopsys m.
Jacobus m.
Rogers m.
Mammotrax
MAMTAT probe
Manan cutting needle
Manashil sialography catheter
Manche
M. LASIK forceps
M. LASIK speculum
Manchester
M. knee replacement
M. LDR implant system
M. nasal osteotome
M. ovoid
Manchu cotton dressing
Mancke
M. flex-rigid gastroscope
Mancusi-Ungaro scissors
Mandelbaum
M. cannula

M. catheter
M. ear knife
Mandelkorn suture lysis lens
mandibular
m. advancement appliance
m. angle fracture intraoral open reduction microplate
m. angle fracture intraoral open reduction screw
m. arch bar
m. body retractor
m. bridging plate
m. mesh
m. miniplate
m. orthopaedic repositioning appliance
m. overdenture
m. positioning device
m. sheet
m. staple bone plate
mandrel, mandril
m. graft
intrauterine insemination cannula with m.
steam-shaping m.
mandrin
m. dilator
wire m.
Mangat curvilinear chin prosthesis
Mangoldt epithelial graft
Mangum knot pusher
Manhattan Eye & Ear
M. E. & E. corneal dissector
M. E. & E. probe
M. E. & E. spatula
M. E. & E. suturing forceps
ManHood absorbent pouch
Mani cerebral catheter
manifold
M. II slot-blot apparatus
Morse m.
three-stopcock m.
Manipujector
Kronner M.
manipulation board
manipulator
Barrett flange lens m.
Barrett irrigating lens m.
button lip lens m.
button-tip m.
ClearView uterine m.
Drysdale nucleus m.
Feaster lens m.
four-degree-of freedom m.
Friedman Phaco/IOL m.
Gall-Addison uterine m.
Grieshaber three-function m.
Grieshaber two-function m.
Guimaraes implantable contact lens m.
Hasson uterine m.
Hirschman lens m.
hook m.
Hulka uterine m.
iris lens m.

M

manipulator *(continued)*
    irrigating lens m.
    Jaffe-Maltzman lens m.
    Judson-Smith m.
    Koch phaco m.
    Kuglen angled lens m.
    Kuglen irrigating lens m.
    Kuglen straight lens m.
    lens m.
    Lester lens m.
    Levy-Kuglen lens m.
    Lieberman MicroFinger m.
    Lindstrom Star nucleus m.
    Lister lens m.
    Maloney no-hole lens m.
    McIntyre irrigating iris m.
    Microbeam m.
    multi-coordinate m.
    Osher nucleus lens m.
    Pelosi uterine m.
    Ramirez m.
    Rappazzo intraocular m.
    RUMI uterine m.
    Sinskey lens m.
    Smith-Leiske lens m.
    uterine m.
    Vico angled m.
    Visitec vico m.
    ZUMI uterine m.
manipulator/injector
    Harris-Kronner uterine m./i. (HUMI)
    HUMI uterine m./i.
    Kronner Manipujector uterine m./i.
    Zinnanti uterine m./i.
manipulator/splitter
    Koch phaco m.
Mannerfelt
    M. chisel
    M. gouge
    M. raspatory
    M. retractor
Mann forceps
Manning
    M. forceps
    M. retractor
Mannis
    M. suture
    M. suture probe
manometer
    Capsuel CPAP m.
    catheter-tipped m.
    DeVilbiss CPAP m.
    Dinamap ultrasound blood
      pressure m.
    Ethitek's automated protection m.
    Honan m.
    M. stopcock
    Tycos m.
    Validyne m.
    ventilator pressure m.
manometer-tipped catheter
manometric
    m. catheter
    m. sensor

manoptoscope
Mansfield
    M. Atri-Pace 1 catheter
    M. balloon
    M. balloon dilatation catheter
    M. bioptome
    M. forceps
    M. orthogonal electrode catheter
    M. Polaris electrode
    M. Scientific dilatation balloon
      catheter
Mansfield-Webster
    M.-W. catheter
    M.-W. deflectable curve catheter
Manson-Aebli corneal section scissors
Manson double-ended strabismus hook
Mansson urinary pouch
Mantel laryngoscope
Mantisol drain
Mantis retrograde forceps
Mantoux needle
Mantz rectal dilator
manual
    m. dermatome
    m. dermatome brush
    m. dermatome thickness gauge
    m. esthesiometer
    m. keratometer
    m. lithotriptor
    m. osteotome
    m. resuscitation bag
    m. retractor
    m. wheelchair
many-tailed
    m.-t. bandage
    m.-t. dressing
MAPF
    MAPF femoral stem prosthesis
    MAPF (textured surface) femoral
      stem
Maple Leaf orthosis
Mapper hemostasis EP mapping sheath
mapping/ablation catheter
mapping catheter
Maquet operating table
Maramed
    M. Miami fracture brace system
    M. ThermoFlex
Marathon guiding catheter
Marax dilator
Marbach episiotomy scissors
Marble bone pin
March
    M. laser lens
    M. laser sclerostomy needle
Marchac forehead template
March-Barton forceps
Marcks knife
Marco
    M. ARK-2000 refractor
    M. chart projector
    M. lensometer
    M. manual keratometer
    M. prism exophthalmometer
    M. radius gauge

M. slit lamp
M. SurgiScope
Marcon colon decompression set
Marcon-Haber varices injector
Marcuse
M. forceps
M. tube clamp
Mardis-Dangler ureteral stent set
Mardis soft stent
Marena by LySonix compression garment
Marex MRI system
marginal
m. chalazion forceps
m. clamp
margin-finishing knife
Margolis appliance
Margraf beam aligning film holder
Margulies
M. coil
M. intrauterine device
Marici bronchoscope
Marino
M. rotatable transsphenoidal enucleator
M. rotatable transsphenoidal horizontal-ring curette
M. rotatable transsphenoidal knife handle
M. rotatable transsphenoidal right-angle hook
M. rotatable transsphenoidal round dissector
M. rotatable transsphenoidal spatula dissector
M. rotatable transsphenoidal vertical-ring curette
M. transsphenoidal curette
Marin reamer
Marion
M. drain
M. oxygen resuscitation system
M. screw
Marion-Reverdin needle
Mark
M. II Chandler total knee retractor
M. II concave total knee retractor
M. II distal femur distractor
M. II femoral component extractor
M. III halo system
M. II Kodros radiolucent awl
M. II lateral collateral ligament retractor
M. II Magni-Focuser loupe
M. II modular weighted retractor
M. II PCL retractor
M. II Sorrells hip arthroplasty retractor system
M. II "S" total knee retractor
M. II Stubbs short-prong collateral ligament retractor
M. II Stulberg hip positioner
M. II tibial component extractor
M. II wide PCL knee retractor
M. II Wixson hip positioner

M. II "Z" knee retractor
M. IV Moss decompression-feeding catheter
M. IX lens
M. VII cooling vest
Mark-7 intrauterine sound
Markell
M. brace boot
M. Mobility Health clogs
M. Mobility Shoes
M. open-toe shoe
M. tarso medius straight shoe
M. tarso pronator outflare shoe
marker
Accu-Line surgical m.
Amsler scleral m.
Anastomark flexible coronary graft m.
Arrowsmith corneal m.
astigmatic m.
biprong muscle m.
Bores radial m.
Brems Astigmatism M.
Castroviejo corneal transplant m.
Castroviejo scleral m.
m. catheter
Chayet corneal m.
Codman m.
corneal transplant m.
Dell astigmatism m.
Desmarres m.
Donahoo m.
Dulaney LASIK m.
facelift flap m.
fecal m.
Feldman radial keratotomy m.
fiducial m.
fine-line tissue m.
Fink biprong m.
Fink muscle m.
Freeman cookie cutter areola m.
Friedländer incision m.
Gass scleral m.
Glomark fluorescent skin m.
gold ear m.
Gonin m.
Gonin-Amsler scleral m.
Green corneal m.
Green-Kenyon corneal m.
Green optical crater m.
Hoffer corneal m.
Hoopes corneal m.
House-Urban m.
Hunkeler frown incision m.
interspace width m.
Kremer triple-optical zone corneal m.
lead pellet m.
Lindstrom arcuate incision m.
Lindstrom astigmatic m.
low-profile R-K m.
Lu corneal m.
Machat double-ended m.
Machat superior flap LASIK m.
McDonald optic zone m.

M

marker *(continued)*
  Mendez corneal m.
  metallic skin m.
  Mickey and Minnie surgical m.
  MicroMark tissue m.
  Neumann double corneal m.
  Neumann-Shepard corneal m.
  Nordin-Ruiz trapezoidal m.
  O'Brien m.
  O'Connor m.
  ocular m.
  Oshar-Neumann 8-line corneal m.
  oval optical zone m.
  Perone laser-assisted intrastromal
    keratomileusis (LASIK) m.
  Price radial m.
  radial keratotomy m.
  radiopaque end m.
  retroreflective m.
  RK m.
  roentgenographic opaque m.
  round optical zone m.
  Ruiz adjustable m.
  Ruiz-Shepard m.
  Saunders-Paparella m.
  scleral m.
  Shepard optical center m.
  Simcoe corneal m.
  Sitzmarks radiopaque m.
  skin m.
  Skin Skribe m.
  SklarScribe skin m.
  Soll suture and incision m.
  Squeeze-Mark surgical m.
  Storz radial incision m.
  tantalum-ball m.
  tape m.
  Thornton corneal m.
  Thornton K3-7991 360 degree
    arcuate m.
  Thornton low-profile m.
  T-incision m.
  TLS surgical m.
  trephine m.
  vein graft ring m.
  Visitec RK zone m.
  Vismark surgical skin m.
  window rasp m.
Markham biopsy needle
Markham-Meyerding hemilaminectomy
  retractor
marking
  m. pen
  m. scissors
Markley
  M. orthodontic wire
  M. retention pin
  M. retractor
Markwalder
  M. bone rongeur
  M. rib forceps
  M. rib rongeur
Marlen
  M. biliary drainage kit

  M. colostomy appliance
  M. ileostomy bag
  M. leg bag
  M. SkinShield adhesive skin barrier
  M. UltraLite system
Marlen's Ultra one-piece pouch
Marlex
  M. band
  M. bandage
  M. mesh
  M. mesh graft
  M. mesh implant
  M. mesh prosthesis
  M. mesh snare
  M. methyl methacrylate prosthesis
  M. methyl methacrylate sandwich
  M. suture
Marlin
  M. cervical collar
  M. cervical orthosis
  M. thoracic catheter
Marlow
  M. disposable cannula
  M. disposable trocar
  M. Primus handle
  M. Primus instrument
  M. Primus shaft
  M. Primus tip
  M. Surgical Technologies, Inc.
    diagnostic laparoscope
  M. Surgical Technologies, Inc.
    operating laparoscope
Marmite lithotrite
Marmor modular knee prosthesis
maroon
  M. lip curette
  m. spoon
Maroon-Jannetta dissector
Marqez-Gomez conjunctival graft
Marquardt bone rongeur
Marquest Respirgard II nebulizer
Marquette
  M. Case-12 electrocardiographic
    system
  M. 3-channel laser holder
  M. electrocardiograph
  M. 8000 Holter monitor
  M. Holter recorder
  M. Responder 1500 multifunctional
    defibrillator
  M. Series 8000 Holter analyzer
  M. treadmill
Marritt dilator
Marrs intrauterine catheter
MARS
  Modular Acetabular Revision System
    MARS revision acetabular
    component
Marshall V-suture
Marshik
  M. tonsillar forceps
  M. tonsil-seizing forceps
Marstock apparatus

Marsupial
- M. belt
- M. pouch

Martel
- M. conductor
- M. intestinal clamp

Marten hair eye brush

Martin
- M. abdominal retractor
- M. ballpoint scissors
- M. bandage
- M. bipolar coagulation forceps
- M. blade
- M. bur
- M. cartilage chisel
- M. cartilage clamp
- M. cartilage forceps
- M. cartilage scissors
- M. cheek retractor
- M. dermal curette
- M. diamond wire cutter
- M. endarterectomy stripper
- M. hip gouge
- M. laryngectomy tube
- M. lip retractor
- M. meniscal forceps
- M. muscle clamp
- M. nasopharyngeal biopsy forceps
- M. nasopharyngeal forceps
- M. nerve root retractor
- M. palate retractor
- M. pelvimeter
- M. rectal hook
- M. rectal hook retractor
- M. rectal speculum
- M. rubber dressing
- M. snare
- M. Surefit lens pusher
- M. tenaculum
- M. throat scissors
- M. thumb forceps
- M. tissue forceps
- M. tracheostomy tube
- M. uterine fistula probe
- M. uterine needle
- M. uterine sound
- M. uterine tenaculum forceps
- M. vaginal retractor
- M. vaginal speculum
- M. Vigorimeter

Martinez
- M. corneal dissector knife
- M. corneal transplant centering ring
- M. corneal trephine blade
- M. disposable corneal trephine
- M. double-ended corneal dissector
- M. keratome
- M. scleral centering ring
- M. universal interstitial template

Martinez-Castro keratome

Martini bone curette

Marx
- M. bridging plate system
- M. needle

Maryan biopsy punch forceps

Maryfield
- M. introducer
- M. introducer catheter

Mary Jane breast pump

Maryland
- M. bridge
- M. monopolar electrosurgical dissector

Masciuli silicone sponge

Mascot indirect ophthalmoscope

Masimo SET pulse oximeter

Masing needle holder

mask
- AccuroX m.
- AeroChamber face m.
- Aquaplast m.
- Armstrong CPR m.
- bag and m.
- bridgeless m.
- Cold Compress m.
- convolution m.
- CP2 Inflat-A-Mask inflatable sinus m.
- EndoShield m.
- face m.
- Finney m.
- high-humidity face m.
- high-humidity tracheostomy m.
- Hudson type oxygen m.
- ISAH stereotactic immobilizing m.
- isolation face m.
- Kuhn m.
- laryngeal m.
- meter m.
- mouth m.
- nonrebreathing m.
- OEM Venturi MixOMask m.
- open face m.
- Orfit m.
- oxygen m.
- partial rebreathing m.
- Patil-Syracuse m.
- PEP m.
- Petit facial m.
- Phantom nasal m.
- RB face m.
- RBS face m.
- rebreathing m.
- Rendell-Baker Soucek m.
- reservoir face m.
- Rudolph m.
- SCRAM face m.
- SealEasy resuscitation m.
- surgical m.
- Swiss Therapy eye m.
- Venti m.
- ventilated m.
- Venturi m.

Masket
- M. forceps
- M. phaco spatula

Mason
- M. leg holder
- M. splint
- M. suction tube

M

Mason (*continued*)
M. tonsil suction dissector
M. vascular clamp
Mason-Allen
M.-A. hand splint
M.-A. snare
Mason-Auvard weighted vaginal speculum
Mason-Judd
M.-J. bladder retractor
M.-J. self-retaining retractor
Mason-Likar 12-lead EKG system
Mason-School aspirating needle
mass
m. flow controller
m. spectrometer
m. spectrophotometer
m. spectrophotometric detector
Massachusetts Vision Kit
massager
Cryocup ice m.
Jeanie Rub M.
Knobble m.
Morfam M.
Saso Variable Speed M.
The Original Backknobber muscle m.
Thera Cane m.
Massage Time Pro hydromassage table
Masselon
M. glasses
M. spectacles
Masseran trepan bur
Massie
M. driver
M. extractor
M. II nail
M. II plate
M. nail assembly
M. screwdriver
M. sliding nail
M. sliding nail tube
Massiot polytome
Masson
M. fascial needle
M. fascial stripper
M. fasciatome
M. needle holder
Masson-Luethy needle holder
Masson-Mayo-Hegar needle holder
Masson-Vital needle holder
MAST
military antishock trousers
MAST pants
MAST suit
MAST trousers
mastectomy skin flap retractor
Mastel
M. compass-guided arcuate keratotomy system
M. diamond compass
M. trifaceted diamond blade
master
Balance M.

m. cement
M. Flow Pumpette
M. Flow Pumpette pump
M. Kit
NeuroCom balance m.
Pro Balance M.
M. screwdriver
SMART Balance M.
SpaceLabs Event M.
M. step foot prosthesis
Masterbrace 3 functional ACL knee brace
MasterCraft hearing aid
MasterFlex pump
Masters intestinal clamp
Masterson
M. hysterectomy forceps
M. pelvic clamp
Masters-Schwartz
M.-S. intestinal clamp
M.-S. liver clamp
Master-Stim interferential stimulator
masticatory apparatus
Mastin
M. goiter forceps
M. muscle clamp
M. muscle forceps
mastoid
m. bur
m. catheter
m. chisel
m. curette
m. dressing
m. gouge
m. probe
m. rongeur
m. searcher
m. self-retaining retractor
m. suction tube
mastopexy form
Masy angioscope
mat
Dermafit massage m.
Harris footprint m.
m. holder
Scoot-Gard m.
Secur-Its silicon cushion m.
silicone-spiked m.
sting m.
Matas vessel band
Matchett-Brown
M.-B. hip endoprosthesis
M.-B. prosthesis
M.-B. stem rasp
material (*See also* implant material, implant material, implant material)
ACCO impression m.
AccuGel impression m.
Accu-Mix impression m.
Acuflex impression m.
Adaptic II dental restorative m.
Agarloid impression m.
Algee impression m.
alginate impression m.
Algitec impression m.

allogeneic m.
alloplastic graft m.
Aneuroplast acrylic m.
Apligraf skin graft m.
Apligraf venous ulcer graft m.
Astron investment m.
Audisil silicone ear mold m.
Augmen bone-grafting m.
Aurovest investment m.
Avitene hemostatic m.
Biobrane/HF graft m.
biocompatible spacing m.
Bioglass bone substitute m.
Biograft bovine heterograft m.
BioMend periodontal m.
Bioplastique augmentation m.
Biovert implant m.
bone substitute m.
Carboplast II sheet orthotic m.
Carbo-Seal graft m.
Carbo-Zinc skin barrier m.
Castorit investment m.
Celestin graft m.
Cellolite m.
Codman cranioplastic m.
Coe impression m.
Coe investment m.
collagen hemostatic m.
Collagraft bone graft matrix m.
Coltene impression m.
Coltex impression m.
Compafill MH dental restorative m.
Compalay dental restorative m.
Compamolar dental restorative m.
cranioplastic acrylic cranioplasty m.
Cristobalite investment m.
Crossfire polyethylene m.
Cutinova Cavity wound filling m.
cyanographic contrast m.
cyanographin contrast m.
Dentemp filling m.
Dentloid impression m.
Dermalogen m.
Derma-Sil impression m.
DermAssist wound filling m.
Dermatell hydrocolloid dressing m.
Dextran-70 barrier m.
Diviplast impression m.
DualMesh m.
Duplicone silicone dental
  impression m.
Durafill dental restorative m.
Durapatite bone replacement m.
Dur-A-Sil ear impression m.
Duraval Hook & Loop strap m.
DYNAfabric m.
DynaLEAP balloon m.
Elgiloy clip m.
Embarc bone repair m.
Endo-Avitene collagen hemostatic m.
Endur bonding m.
Epicel skin graft m.
Estilux dental restorative m.
Evazote cushioning m.
Fastcure denture repair m.

Fermit-N occlusal hole blockage m.
Flexistone impression m.
FlowGel barrier m.
Fotofil dental restorative m.
Frosted Flex earmold m.
G-C Vest investment m.
glycolide trimethylene carbonate m.
gold weight and wire spring
  implant m.
Gore cast liner m.
Gore subcutaneous augmentation m.
Gore-Tex alloplastic m.
Gore-Tex periodontal m.
Gore-Tex regenerative m.
Graflex m.
Grafton bone grafting m.
Gypsona rapid-setting cast m.
Hand-Aid strapping m.
Hapex bioactive m.
Hapset bone graft plaster m.
Haynes 25 m.
Healos synthetic bone grafting m.
Hircoe denture base m.
implant m.
Impregum impression m.
Insta-Mold silicone ear
  impression m.
Interceed barrier m.
Interpore bone replacement m.
Interpore ceramic m.
Kaltostat wound packing m.
Karaya self-adhesive conductive m.
Lactomer skin staple m.
Langinate impression m.
LEAP balloon m.
Luster investment m.
MediFlex earmold m.
Medpor allograft m.
Medpor alloplastic m.
Medpor block facial structure
  building m.
MP-35 clip m.
3M Tegapore wound contact m.
Multidex wound-filling m.
MycroMesh graft m.
Omega splinting m.
Ommaya reservoir implant m.
Omniflex impression m.
Opotow filling m.
Optisson contrast m.
OrthoDyn bone substitute m.
Orthoglass splint m.
Ortho-Jel impression m.
OsteoGen bone grafting m.
Osteogenics BoneSource synthetic
  bone replacement m.
OsteoGraf bone grafting m.
OsteoGraf/D bone grafting m.
OsteoGraf/LD bone grafting m.
OsteoGraf/N-Block grafting m.
Palfique Estelite tooth shade
  resin m.
Paradentine dental restorative m.
Pearlon impression m.
PE LITE m.

M

material *(continued)*
>PerioGlas m.
>Perma-Cryl denture base m.
>PermaMesh m.
>PermaSoft reline m.
>Permatone denture m.
>Phynox cobalt alloy clip m.
>plastic wax m.
>Platorit investment m.
>Poloxamer 407 barrier m.
>Polyviolene polyester suture m.
>PolyWic wound filling m.
>Porites coral m.
>Porocoat m.
>precollagenous filamentous m.
>ProOsteon implant graft m.
>Proplast I, II porous implant m.
>Protegen m.
>Protouch m.
>Provit filling m.
>Ramitec bite m.
>reline m.
>Rema-Exakt investment m.
>Reprodent acrylic tooth m.
>SAM facial implant m.
>Scutan temporary splint m.
>SeamGuard staple line m.
>Septosil impression m.
>ShowerSafe protector m.
>Sili-Gel impression m.
>Silon silicone thermoplastic splinting m.
>SR-Isosit dental restorative m.
>SR-Ivocap denture m.
>SR-Ivolen impression m.
>SR-Ivoseal impression m.
>Stellite ring m.
>subcutaneous augmentation m.
>Surgamid polyamide suture m.
>Surgical Nu-Knit absorbable hemostatic m.
>Tru-Chrome band m.
>TrueBlue background m.
>twisted cotton nonabsorbable surgical suture m.
>Wirosol investment m.
>Wirovest investment m.
>Zenotech graft m.

Mathews
>M. drill point
>M. hand drill
>M. load drill
>M. osteotome
>M. rectal speculum

Mathieu
>M. double-ended retractor
>M. foreign body forceps
>M. needle
>M. needle holder
>M. pliers
>M. raspatory
>M. tongue forceps
>M. urethral forceps

Mathieu-Horton-Devine flip-flap

Mathieu-Olsen needle holder
Mathieu-Stille needle holder
Mathrop hemostat
Mathys prosthesis
matrix
>ACCOR dental m.
>m. band
>Collagraft bone graft m.
>demineralized bone m.
>DuraGen absorbable dural graft m.
>Dynafill graft biomedium mineralized bone m.
>m. Grafton putty
>NeoDura m.
>Osteovit bone m.
>PermaMesh hydroxyapatite woven sheet m.
>m. retainer
>Walser m.

Matroc femoral head
Matrol femoral head prosthesis
Matson
>M. raspatory
>M. rib elevator
>M. rib stripper

Matson-Alexander
>M.-A. raspatory
>M.-A. rib elevator
>M.-A. rib stripper

Matson-Mead
>M.-M. apicolysis retractor
>M.-M. periosteum stripper

Matson-Plenk raspatory
Matsuda
>M. titanium surgical instruments

matte black forceps
Matthew
>M. cross-leg clamp
>M. forceps

matting
>Dycem roll m.

Mattis corneal scissors
Mattison-Upshaw retractor
Mattox aortic clamp
Mattox-Potts scissors
mattress
>AccuMax self-adjusting pressure management m.
>AIR-O-EASE static air flotation m.
>Airsoft dry replacement m.
>Akros extended-care m.
>AkroTech m.
>apnea alarm m.
>Babytherm IC gel m.
>Bedge antireflux m.
>Bio Core therapeutic m.
>Clinisert m.
>Comfort nylon m.
>convoluted foam m.
>Critical care m.
>D.A.D. m.
>DeCube therapeutic m.
>Dermasoft m.
>Dräger thermal gel m.

DynaGuard APM alternating pressure m.
Econo-Float Water flotation m.
eggcrate m.
FirstStep m.
foam cube m.
Geo-Matt m.
Huntleigh bubble pad m.
hypothermia m.
Impression m.
Integriderm m.
Invacare APM m.
IRIS pressure-reduction m.
Isoflex m.
KinAir IV m.
Lapidus alternating air-pressure m.
MaxiFloat DFP, EF, LFP m.
MaxiFloat pressure-reduction m.
Medisupra m.
Medline Aero-Flow II air m.
Medline deluxe air m.
Medline Saf-T-Side m.
Neuropedic multidensity m.
Neuropedic neurolon m.
NewLife therapeutic m.
Nirvana pressure-reducing m.
OptiMax Supreme pressure-reduction m.
Orthoderm convertible m.
overlay m.
PressureGuard IV alternating pressure m.
ProForm maxim pressure reduction m.
ProForm maxim-VE pressure reduction m.
Q-Star IV pressure-relief m.
Q-Star Voyager pressure-reduction m.
Recovercare System 3 low-air, loss-alternating pressure m.
RIK Defender prevention m.
RIK fluid m.
Roho m.
SeCure therapeutic m.
Silhouette therapeutic m.
Sof.Care m.
Sofflex m.
Sof-Matt pressure reducing m.
SPR.Plus II m.
static air m.
Stop-Leak gel flotation m.
m. suture
m. system
Tempur-Med hospital replacement m.
Tempur-Pedic pressure relieving Swedish m.
Tempur-Plus m.
T-Foam m.
TheraRest m.
Tri-Float pressure reduction m.
UltraForm therapeutic m.
Unitek I decubitus m.

Mattrix spinal cord stimulation system
Maturna bra system
Matzenauer vaginal speculum
Mauch
    M. double-sheathed plastic wash pipe
    M. GaitMaster system
    M. Swing and Stance hydraulic knee
Mauermayer
    M. resectoscope
    M. stone punch
Maumenee
    M. capsular forceps
    M. corneal forceps
    M. cross-action capsular forceps
    M. erysiphake
    M. goniotomy cannula
    M. goniotomy knife
    M. iris hook
    M. straight-action capsular forceps
    M. Suregrip forceps
    M. tissue forceps
    M. vitreous-aspirating needle
    M. vitreous sweep spatula
Maumenee-Barraquer vitreous sweep spatula
Maumenee-Colibri corneal forceps
Maumenee-Park
    M.-P. erysiphake
    M.-P. eye speculum
Maunder oral screw mouthgag
Maunoir iris scissors
Max
    M. FiberScan laser system
    M. Fine scissors
    M. Fine tying forceps
    M. Force balloon dilatation catheter
    M. Force TTS biliary balloon dilatation catheter
    M. Plus MR scanner
    M. ventilator
Maxair Autohaler
Maxam suture
MaxBloc bite block
MaxCast
    M. cast
    M. fiberglass casting tape
Maxenon 300 watt xenon light source
MaxiCare
    M. adult disposable contoured brief
    M. adult disposable undergarment
    M. disposable underpad
Maxi-Driver driver
MaxiFloat
    M. DFP, EF, LFP mattress
    M. pressure-reduction mattress
    M. pressure reduction mattress model DFP+/DXP+
    M. pressure reduction mattress model EF/EX
    M. wheelchair cushion
MaxiFlo breathable disposable underpad
Maxilift Combi patient lifting system

M

Maxilith
 M. pacemaker
 M. pacemaker pulse generator
maxillary
 m. arch bar
 m. disimpaction forceps
 m. fracture forceps
 m. prosthesis
 m. removable implant-retained
 denture
 m. sinus cannula
maxillofacial
 m. bone screw
 m. osteotome
 m. plating system
maxillomandibular elastic
Maxillume 250 watt quartz halogen
 light source
Maxima
 M. II TENS unit
 M. II transcutaneous electrical nerve
 stimulator
 M. Plus plasma resistant fiber
 oxygenator
Maxim modular knee system
Maxi-Myst
 M.-M. nebulizer system
 M.-M. vaporizer
Max-I-Probe
 M.-I.-P. endodontic irrigation syringe
 M.-I.-P. irrigation probe
Maxisorb test plate
Maxon absorbable suture
Maxorb alginate wound dressing
Max-Relax pillow
Maxum
 M. Carr-Locke angled forceps
 M. reusable endoscopic forceps
Maxwell 3D field simulator
Maxxum balloon catheter
Maxxus orthopaedic latex surgical glove
May
 M. anatomical bone plate
 M. hook-on lens loupe
 M. kidney clamp
 M. ophthalmoscope
Maydl pessary
Mayer
 M. forceps
 M. nasal splint
 M. orthotic
 M. pessary
 M. speculum
Mayfield
 M. aneurysm clamp
 M. aneurysm forceps
 M. bayonet osteotome
 M. CIS-RE aneurysm clip
 M. clip applicator
 M. disposable skull pin
 M. fixation frame
 M. head clamp
 M. head rest
 M. malleable brain spatula

 M. miniature clip applier
 M. pediatric horseshoe headrest
 M. pediatric horseshoe pad
 M. radiolucent base unit
 M. radiolucent headholder
 M. radiolucent headrest
 M. retractor
 M. skull clamp adapter
 M. skull clamp pin
 M. skull-pin headholder
 M. spinal curette
 M. surgical headrest system
 M. swivel horseshoe headrest
 M. temporary aneurysm clip applier
 M. three-pin skull clamp
 M. tic headholder
Mayfield/ACCISS stereotactic device
Mayfield-Kees
 M.-K. clip
 M.-K. headholder
 M.-K. headrest
 M.-K. skull fixation apparatus
 M.-K. table attachment
Mayo
 M. abdominal retractor
 M. bone-cutting forceps
 M. catgut needle
 M. common duct probe
 M. common duct scoop
 M. coronary perfusion cannula
 M. coronary perfusion tip
 M. curved scissors
 M. cystic duct scoop
 M. external vein stripper
 M. fibroid hook
 M. gallbladder scoop
 M. gall duct scoop
 M. gallstone scoop
 M. goiter ligature carrier
 M. hemostat
 M. instrument table
 M. instrument tray
 M. intestinal needle
 M. kidney clamp
 M. kidney pedicle forceps
 M. kidney stone probe
 M. knife
 M. linen suture
 M. long dissecting scissors
 M. needle holder
 M. operating scissors
 M. perfusing "O" ring
 M. round blade scissors
 M. semiconstrained elbow prosthesis
 M. stand
 M. straight scissors
 M. tissue forceps
 M. total ankle prosthesis
 M. trocar needle
 M. trocar-point needle
 M. ureter isolation forceps
 M. uterine probe
 M. uterine scissors
 M. vessel clamp

Mayo-Adams
    M.-A. appendectomy retractor
    M.-A. self-retaining retractor
Mayo-Boldt inverter
Mayo-Collins
    M.-C. appendectomy retractor
    M.-C. double-ended retractor
    M.-C. mastoid retractor
Mayo-Gibbon heart-lung machine
Mayo-Guyon
    M.-G. kidney clamp
    M.-G. vessel clamp
Mayo-Harrington
    M.-H. dissecting scissors
    M.-H. forceps
    M.-H. scissors
Mayo-Hegar curved-jaw needle holder
Mayo-Lexer scissors
Mayo-Lovelace
    M.-L. abdominal retractor
    M.-L. spur crusher
    M.-L. spur crushing clamp
Mayo-Myers external vein stripper
Mayo-New scissors
Mayo-Noble dissecting scissors
Mayo-Ochsner
    M.-O. cannula
    M.-O. forceps
    M.-O. trocar
Mayo-Potts dissecting scissors
Mayo-Robson
    M.-R. gallstone scoop
    M.-R. gastrointestinal forceps
    M.-R. intestinal clamp
Mayo-Russian gastrointestinal forceps
Mayo-Simpson retractor
Mayo-Sims dissecting scissors
Mayo-Stille operating scissors
Mazlin intrauterine device
Mazzariello-Caprini
    M.-C. stone forceps
    M.-C. stone forceps sterilizing case
Mazzocco
    M. flexible lens forceps
    M. silicone intraocular lens
MB-900 AC machine
MBE cast
MBF3 infrared laser-Doppler flowmeter
MB&J
    MB&J hip drape
    MB&J knee positioner
M-brace corneal trephine
MBS snap-on orthotic
MC-7000 multi-wavelength ophthalmic laser
McAllister
    M. needle holder
    M. scissors
MCAS modular clip application system
McAtee
    M. apparatus
    M. olecranon compression screw device
McBratney aspirating speculum

McBride
    M. cup
    M. femoral prosthesis
    M. pin
    M. plate
    M. tripod pin traction
McBride-Moore prosthesis
McBurney
    M. fenestrated retractor
    M. thyroid retractor
McCabe
    M. antral retractor
    M. canal knife
    M. crurotomy saw
    M. crus guide fork
    M. facial nerve dissector
    M. flap knife dissector
    M. measuring instrument
    M. parotidectomy retractor
    M. perforation rasp
    M. posterior fossa retractor
McCabe-Farrior rasp
McCaffrey positioner
McCain
    M. TMJ arthroscopic system
    M. TMJ cannula
    M. TMJ curette
    M. TMJ forceps
McCall instrument
McCannel
    M. implant
    M. ocular pressure reducer
    M. suture
McCarthy
    M. bladder evacuator
    M. catheter
    M. coagulation electrode
    M. continuous-flow resectoscope
    M. diathermic knife electrode
    M. endoscope
    M. Foroblique operating telescope
    M. Foroblique panendoscope cystoscope
    M. fulgurating electrode
    M. infant electrotome
    M. loop operating electrode
    M. microlens resectoscope
    M. miniature electrotome
    M. miniature loop electrode
    M. miniature resectoscope
    M. miniature telescope
    M. multiple resectoscope
    M. panendoscope
    M. punctate electrotome
    M. visual hemostatic forceps
McCarthy-Alcock forceps
McCarthy-Campbell miniature cystoscope
McCaskey
    M. antral catheter
    M. antral curette
    M. sphenoid cannula
McCaslin
    M. knife
    M. needle
    M. wave-edge keratome

M

McClamary elevator
McCleery-Miller
    M.-M. intestinal anastomosis clamp
    M.-M. locking device
McClintoch brace
McClintock
    M. placental forceps
    M. uterine forceps
McClure iris scissors
McCollough
    M. elevator
    M. internal tibial torsion brace
    M. osteotome
    M. rasp
    M. tying forceps
McConnell
    M. orthopaedic headrest
    M. shoulder positioner
McCool capsule retractor
McCoy
    M. septal forceps
    M. septum-cutting forceps
McC panendoscope
McCrea
    M. cystoscope
    M. dilator
    M. infant sound
McCullough
    M. externofrontal retractor
    M. hysterectomy clamp
    M. strabismus forceps
    M. suture-tying forceps
    M. suturing forceps
McCurdy staphylorrhaphy needle
McCutchen
    M. hip implant
    M. SLT hip prosthesis
McDavid
    M. ankle guard
    M. hinged knee guard
    M. knee brace
McDermott
    M. clip
    M. extractor
    M. Surgiclip
McDonald
    M. bone plate
    M. cerclage
    M. dissector
    M. expressor
    M. gastric clamp
    M. lens-folding forceps
    M. optic zone marker
McDougal prostatectomy clamps
McDowell
    M. mouthgag
    M. needle
McElroy curette
McElveen-Hitselberger neural dissector
McFadden
    M. cross-legged clip
    M. Surgiclip
    M. Vari-Angle aneurysm clip
    M. Vari-Angle clip applier
McFadden-Kees clip

McFarland tibial graft
MCF shoulder orthosis
McGannon
    M. iris retractor
    M. lens forceps
    M. refractor
McGaw
    M. plastic bottle
    M. skinfold calipers
    M. tape measure
    M. volumetric pump
McGee
    M. canal elevator
    M. ear piston prosthesis
    M. footplate pick
    M. middle ear instrument
    M. oval-window rasp
    M. platinum/stainless steel piston
    M. prosthesis needle
    M. raspatory
    M. splint
    M. tympanoplasty knife
    M. wire-closure forceps
    M. wire crimper
    M. wire-crimping forceps
McGee-Caparosa wire crimper
McGee-Paparella wire-crimping forceps
McGee-Priest
    M.-P. wire-closure forceps
    M.-P. wire crimper
    M.-P. wire forceps
McGee-Priest-Paparella forceps
McGehee elbow prosthesis
McGhan
    M. breast implant
    M. breast prosthesis
    M. eye implant
    M. facial implant
    M. fill kit
    M. lens
    M. plastic surgical needle
    M. tissue expander
McGill
    M. forceps
    M. neurological percussor
    M. retractor
McGinnis balloon system
McGivney
    M. hemorrhoidal forceps
    M. hemorrhoidal ligator
McGlamry elevator
McGoey-Evans acetabular cup
McGoey Vitallium punch
McGoon
    M. cannula
    M. coronary perfusion catheter
McGovern nipple
McGowan-Keeley tube
McGowan needle
McGravey tissue forceps
McGregor
    M. conjunctival forceps
    M. needle
McGuire
    M. clamp

M. conformer
M. corneal scissors
M. I&A system
M. marginal chalazion forceps
M. pelvic positioner
M. rib spreader
M. tendon tucker
McHenry tonsillar forceps
McHugh
M. facial nerve knife
M. flap knife
M. oval speculum
McHugh-Farrior canal knife
McIndoe
M. bone-cutting forceps
M. dissecting forceps
M. dressing forceps
M. elevator
M. nasal chisel
M. rasp
M. raspatory
M. retractor
M. rongeur forceps
M. scissors
McIntire splint
McIntosh
M. double-lumen hemodialysis catheter
M. suture-holding forceps
McIntyre
M. anterior chamber cannula
M. coaxial cannula
M. coaxial I&A system
M. fish-hook needle holder
M. guarded cystitome
M. guarded irrigating cystitome set
M. I&A needle
M. I&A system
M. infusion handpiece
M. infusion set
M. irrigating iris hook
M. irrigating iris manipulator
M. irrigating spatula
M. irrigation/aspiration needle
M. lacrimal cannula
M. microhook
M. nylon cannula connector
M. reverse cystotome
M. suture tamper
M. truncated cone
McIntyre-Binkhorst irrigating cannula
McIver nephrostomy catheter
McIvor mouthgag
McKay ear forceps
McKee
M. brace
M. femoral prosthesis
M. speculum
M. table
M. totally constrained elbow prosthesis
M. tri-fin nail
McKee-Farrar
M.-F. acetabular cup
M.-F. hip prosthesis

McKeever
M. cartilage knife
M. patellar cap prosthesis
McKenna
M. Tide-Ur-Ator evacuator
M. Tide-Ur-Ator irrigator
McKenzie
M. AirBack support
M. bone drill
M. cervical roll
M. clamp
M. clip-applying forceps
M. cranial drill
M. enlarging bur
M. hemostasis clip
M. leukotome
M. leukotomy loop
M. lumbar roll
M. night roll
M. perforating twist drill
M. silver brain clip
M. V-clip
McKerman-Adson forceps
McKerman-Potts forceps
McKernan-Adson forceps
McKernan forceps
McKernan-Potts forceps
McKesson
M. mouthgag
M. mouth probe
M. pneumothorax apparatus
M. suction bottle unit
McKinley EpM pump
McKinney
M. eye speculum
M. fixation ring
McKissock keyhole areolar template
McLane
M. obstetrical forceps
M. pile forceps
McLane-Luikart obstetrical forceps
McLane-Tucker-Kjelland forceps
McLane-Tucker-Luikart forceps
McLane-Tucker obstetrical forceps
McLaughlin
M. carpal scaphoid screw
M. hip plate
M. laser mirror
M. laser vaginal measuring rod
M. nail
M. osteosynthesis device
M. quartz rod
M. speculum
McLean
M. capsular forceps
M. capsulotomy scissors
M. clamp
M. muscle-recession forceps
M. ophthalmic forceps
M. prismatic fundus laser lens
M. suture
M. tonometer
McLearie bone forceps
McLeod padded clavicular splint
McLight PCL brace

McMahon nephrostomy hook
McMaster bone graft
McMurray tenotomy knife
McMurtry-Schlesinger shunt tube
McNaught
    M. keel
    M. prosthesis
McNealey-Glassman
    M.-G. clamp
    M.-G. visceral retainer
McNealey-Glassman-Mixter
    M.-G.-M. clamp
    M.-G.-M. forceps
McNealey visceral retractor
McNealy-Glassman-Babcock forceps
McNeill-Goldmann
    M.-G. blepharostat
    M.-G. blepharostat ring
    M.-G. scleral ring
McNutt
    M. driver
    M. extractor
MCP finger joint prosthesis
McPherson
    M. angled forceps
    M. bent forceps
    M. corneal forceps
    M. corneal section scissors
    M. eye speculum
    M. iris spatula
    M. irrigating forceps
    M. lens forceps
    M. microbipolar forceps
    M. microconjunctival scissors
    M. microcorneal forceps
    M. microiris forceps
    M. microsurgery eye needle holder
    M. microsuture forceps
    M. microtenotomy scissors
    M. straight bipolar forceps
    M. suture-tying forceps
    M. trabeculotome
    M. tying iris forceps
McPherson-Castroviejo
    M.-C. corneal section scissors
    M.-C. forceps
    M.-C. microcorneal scissors
McPherson-Pierse
    M.-P. microcorneal forceps
    M.-P. microsuturing forceps
McPherson-Vannas
    M.-V. iris scissors
    M.-V. microiris scissors
McPherson-Westcott
    M.-W. conjunctival scissors
    M.-W. stitch scissors
McPherson-Wheeler
    M.-W. blade
    M.-W. eye knife
McPherson-Ziegler microiris knife
M-C prosthesis
McQueen vitreous forceps
McQuigg
    M. clamp
    M. forceps

McQuigg-Mixter bronchial forceps
McReynolds
    M. driver
    M. extractor
    M. eye spatula
    M. keratome
    M. lid-retracting hook
    M. pterygium keratome
    M. pterygium knife
    M. pterygium scissors
McReynolds-Castroviejo
    M.-C. keratome
    M.-C. pterygium knife
McShirley amalgamator
McSpadden compactor
M-cup vacuum extraction device
MCW cement adhesive
McWhinnie
    M. electrode
    M. tonsillar dissector
McWhorter
    M. hemostat
    M. tonsillar forceps
McXIM file
MD2 Doppler
MDA ultrasound-assisted lipoplasty
  machine
MD brace
MDI
    metered-dose inhaler
MDILO device
MDS
    MDS adhesive
    MDS microdebrider
    MDS Truspot articulating film
Meacham-Scoville forceps
Mead
    M. bone rongeur
    M. bridge remover
    M. crown remover
    M. dental rongeur
    M. Johnson tube
    M. lancet knife
    M. mallet
    M. periosteal elevator
Meadox
    M. Dacron mesh
    M. Dardik Biograft
    M. graft sizer
    M. ICP monitor
    M. Microvel arterial graft
    M. Microvel double-velour Dacron
      graft
    M. Surgimed catheter
    M. Surgimed Doppler probe
    M. Teflon felt pledget
    M. vascular graft
    M. woven velour prosthesis
Meadox-Cooley woven low-porosity
  prosthesis
measure
    McGaw tape m.
Measure Mat infantometer

measurement
    Intran disposable intrauterine pressure m.

measurer
    Bunnell digital exertion m.
    Pach-Pen corneal thickness m.

measuring
    m. gauge
    m. guide
    m. hat
    m. rod

measuring-mounting catheter
Measuroll suture
meat
    m. forceps
    m. hook retractor

meatal
    m. clamp
    m. dilator
    m. sound

meat-grasping forceps
meatoscope
    Hubell m.
    Huegli m.

meatotome
    Bunge ureteral m.
    Ellik m.
    Huegli m.
    Riba electrical ureteral m.

meatotomy
    m. electrode
    m. scissors

mechanical
    m. articulated arm
    m. device
    m. finger
    m. finger forceps
    m. joint apparatus
    m. longitudinal/sector scanning echoendoscope
    m. percussor
    m. radial-scanning instrument
    m. respirator
    m. rotating probe
    m. separator
    m. ventilator
    m. vitrector

mechanically assisted respirator
mechanic's
    m. pin
    m. waste dressing

mechanism
    adjustable leg and ankle repositioning m.
    disengagement m.
    four-bar linkage prosthetic knee m.
    Hosmer-Dorrance voluntary control four-bar knee m.
    MicroStable liner locking m.
    Noiles rotating-hinge knee m.
    patient-operated selector m.
    rotating m.
    spring m.
    sunburst m.
    terminal extensor m.

mechanized scissors
Meckel rod
Mecon-I hearing aid
meconium aspirator
Mecring acetabluar prosthesis
Mectra
    M. hydrodissector
    M. I&A system
    M. Tissue Sample Retainer

Medak glove
Medallion
    M. intraocular lens implant
    M. lens expressor

Medarmor puncture-resistant gloves
Medasonics
    M. transcranial Doppler

MedaSonics ultrasound BF4A, BF5A stethoscope
Meda 2500 TENS unit
MED^{next} bone dissecting system
MedCam Pro Plus video camera
Med-Co flexible catheter
Medcor pacemaker
MEDDARS cardiac catheterization analysis system
MedDev gold eyelid implant
Medela
    M. Apgar timer
    M. breast pump
    M. Dominant vacuum delivery pump
    M. manual breast pump
    M. membrane regulator

Medelec
    M. DMG 50 Teflon-coated monopolar electrode
    M. five-channel neurophysiological device

Medelec-Van Gogh electroencephalographic recording system
Medena continent ileostomy catheter
Medevice
    M. surgical loop
    M. surgical paws

Medex
    M. Protege 3010 syringe infusion pump
    M. Secure system
    M. transducer

Med-Fit cranial-sacral table
Medfusion (1001, 2001) syringe infusion pump
MedGraphics
    M. CPE 2000 electronically braked bicycle
    M. CPX/D metabolic cart

Medgraphics body plethysmograph
Medi-aire
    Bard M.-a.

medial
    m. bicortical screw
    m. heel-and-sole wedge
    m. heel wedge

M

medial (*continued*)
    m. sole wedge
    m. unicortical screw
mediaometer
mediastinal
    m. cannula
    m. catheter
    m. drain
    m. sump filter
    m. tube
mediastinoscope
    Carlens m.
    Freiburg m.
    Goldberg MPC m.
    John A. Tucker m.
mediastinoscopy aspirating needle
Medi-Band bandage
Medi-Breather IPPB device
medical
    m. adhesive remover
    m. ankle orthosis
    m. cyclotron
    M. Design brace
    M. Dynamics 5990 needle
      arthroscope
    m. gas analyzer
    M. genuine sheepskin pad
    M. Optics eye implant
    M. Optics intraocular lens implant
    M. Resources hydrophilic wound
      dressing
    M. support Systems, Inc.
    M. Workshop intraocular lens
      implant
    M. Z post surgery garment
Medicam
    M. camera
    M. 900 insufflator
    M. light source
Medicamat
    M. ultrasound-assisted lipoplasty
      machine
    M. ultrasound device
Medici aerosol adhesive tape remover
   dressing
medicinal nebulizer
Medicon
    M. contractor
    M. instruments
    M. rib retractor
    M. rib spreader
    M. ultrasonic liposuction device
    M. wire-twister forceps
Medicon-Jackson rectal forceps
Medicon-Packer mosquito forceps
MediCordz tubing kit
Medicornea Kratz intraocular lens
   implant
Medicus bed
Medicut
    M. cannula
    M. catheter
    M. intravenous needle

Medi-Duct ocular fluid management
   system
Medifil collagen hemostatic wound
   dressing
Mediflex
    M. Gazayerli retractor
    M. MD-7 endoscopic video system
Mediflex-Bookler device
MediFlex earmold material
Mediflow
    M. waterbase pillow
    M. Waterpillow
Mediform dural graft
Medi-graft vascular prosthesis
Medigraphics 2000 analyzer
Medi-Ject needle free insulin injection
   system
Medi-Jector
    M.-J. adapter
    M.-J. Choice
    M.-J. injector
Medilas
    M. fiberTome laser
    M. Nd:YAG surgical laser
MEDILOG
    M. ambulatory ECG recorder
    M. 4000 ambulatory ECG recorder
MedImage scanner
Medi-Mist nebulizer
Medina
    M. ileostomy catheter
    M. tube
Meding
    M. tonsil enucleator tonometer
    M. tonsil enucleator tonsillectome
Medinol NIRside slotted stent
Med-I-Pad underpad
Medi Plus compression stockings
Medipore
    M. dressing cover
    M. Dress-it dressing
    M. H soft cloth surgical tape
MediPort
    M. implanted vascular device
    M. infusion vascular access device
MediPort-DL (double-lumen) catheter
Medi-Quet tourniquet
Medi-Rip dressing
MediRule measuring device
Medisense
    M. Pen 2 blood glucose meter
    M. Pen 2 self blood glucose
      monitor
Mediskin
    M. hemostatic sponge
    M. porcine biological wound
      dressing
MEDIS off-line quantitative coronary
   angiogram
Medison scanner
Medisorb drug delivery system
MediSpacer
    Airlife M.
Medispec Econolith spark plug
   lithotriptor

Medi-Stim stimulator
Medi-Strumpf stockings
Medisupra mattress
Medisystems fistular needle
Meditape tape
meditation bench
Medi-Tech
    M.-T. arterial dilatation catheter
    M.-T. bipolar probe
    M.-T. catheter system
    M.-T. fascial dilator
    M.-T. flexible stiffening cannula
    M.-T. guidewire
    M.-T. IVC filter
    M.-T. multipurpose basket
    M.-T. occlusion balloon catheter
    M.-T. sheath
    M.-T. steerable catheter
    M.-T. stone basket
    M.-T. wire
Meditech
    M. bandage contact lens
    M. laser
Medi-Tech-Mansfield dilating catheter
Medi-Trace electrode
Meditrode iontophoresis Transvene
    electrode
Meditron EL-100 Endolav
medium
    m. below-elbow cast
    m. forceps
medium-energy collimator
Medi vascular stockings
MediVators DSD-91P endoscope
    reprocessor
Medivent
    M. self-expanding coronary stent
    M. vascular stent
MedJet microkeratome
Medline
    M. Aero-Flow II air mattress
    M. Alpha subacute care bed
    M. deluxe air mattress
    M. Derma-Gel dressing
    M. gauze sponge
    M. gel/foam wheelchair cushion
    M. Lap-pal safety cushion
    M. lateral stabilizer
    M. Packing strips
    M. positioner
    M. roll
    M. Saf-T-Side mattress
    M. wedge
MedLite
    M. Q-Switched neodymium-doped
      yttrium-aluminum-garnet laser
    M. Q-Switched YAG laser
Med-Logics ML Microkeratome
Medmetric KT-1000 knee laxity
    arthrometer
Medmont M600 perimeter
MedMorph
    M. III patient video imaging
Med-Neb respirator
Mednext bone dissecting system

Medoc-Celestin
    M.-C. endoprosthesis prosthesis
    M.-C. tube
Medoff
    M. sliding femoral plate
    M. sliding fracture plate
Medos
    M. mechanical circulatory support
      system
    M. valve
Medos-Hakim valve
Medpacific LD 5000 Laser-Doppler
    perfusion monitor
Medpor
    M. allograft material
    M. alloplastic material
    M. biomaterial implants
    M. biomaterial wedge
    M. block facial structure building
      material
    M. facial implant
    M. malar implant
    M. reconstructive implant
    M. surgical implants
Medrad
    M. angiographic catheter
    M. automated power injector
    M. contrast medium injector
    M. Mark IV angiographic injector
    M. Mrinnervu endorectal colon
      probe
    M. Mrinnervu endorectal colon
      probe coil
    M. power angiographic injector
Medrafil wire suture
Medscand
    M. cervical spatula
    M. Cytobrush Plus cell collector
    M. cytology brush
    M. endometrial brush
    M. Pap smear kit
Meds eye protector
Medspec
    M. MR imaging system
    M. MR imaging system scanner
Medstone
    M. extracorporeal shock-wave
      lithotriptor
    M. IRIS system
    M. STS lithotripsy system
    M. STS shockwave generator
Medtel pacemaker
Medtronic
    M. Activa tremor-control therapy
    M. Activitrax rate-responsive
      unipolar ventricular pacemaker
    M. AneuRx stent graft
    M. automated coagulation timer
    M. AVE S660 coronary stent
    M. balloon catheter
    M. Bestent stent
    M. bipolar pacemaker
    M. cardiac cooling jacket
    M. Cardiorhythm Atakr generator
    M. Chardack pacemaker

M

Medtronic *(continued)*
  M. corkscrew electrode pacemaker
  M. defibrillator implant support device
  M. demand pacemaker
  M. Elite II pacemaker
  M. external cardioverter-defibrillator
  M. external/internal pacemaker
  M. external tachyarrhythmia control device
  M. Hancock II tissue valve
  M. Hemopump
  M. Hemopump system
  M. Inspire
  M. Interactive Tachycardia Terminating system
  M. Interstim sacral nerve stimulation system
  M. interventional vascular stent
  M. Jewel AF arrhythmia management device
  M. Jewel 7219C, D device
  M. Jewel Plus Active Can defibrillator
  M. Micro Jewel cardioverter-defibrillator system
  M. Micro Jewel defibrillator
  M. Micro Jewel II
  M. Minix pacemaker
  M. Pacette pacemaker
  M. prosthetic valve
  M. pulse generator
  M. Pulsor Intrasound
  M. Pulsor Intrasound system
  M. radiofrequency receiver
  M. RF 5998 pacemaker
  M. spinal cord stimulation system
  M. SPO pacemaker
  M. SP 502 pacemaker
  M. Spring lead
  M. Symbios pacemaker
  M. SynchroMed implantable pump
  M. temporary pacemaker
  M. Thera "i-series" cardiac pacemaker
  M. tip
  M. Transvene 6937 electrode catheter
  M. Transvene endocardial lead
  M. Transvene endocardial lead system
  M. tremor control therapy device
Medtronic-Alcatel pacemaker
Medtronic-Byrel-SX pacemaker
Medtronic-Hall
  M.-H. device
  M.-H. heart valve prosthesis
  M.-H. monocuspid tilting-disk valve
  M.-H. prosthetic heart valve
  M.-H. tilting-disk valve prosthesis
Medtronic-Hancock device
Medtronic.Kappa 400 pacemaker
Medtronic-Laurens-Alcatel pacemaker

Medtronics Sequestra 1000 autotransfusion system
Medtronic-Zyrel pacemaker
medullary
  m. canal reamer
  m. nail
  m. pin
  m. rod
Medwatch telemetry system
Med-Wick
  M.-W. medication delivery system
  M.-W. nasal pack
MedX
  M. camera
  M. functional testing machine
  M. knee machine
  M. Mark II lumbar extension machine
  M. physical therapy device
  M. scanner
  M. stretch machine
Meek
  M. pelvic traction belt
  M. snare
Meeker
  M. deep-surgery forceps
  M. gallbladder forceps
  M. gallstone clamp
  M. hemostatic forceps
  M. intestinal forceps
  M. monopolar electrosurgical dissector
  M. right-angle clamp
Meek-style clavicular strap
Meek-Wall
  M.-W. dermatome
  M.-W. microdermatome
Meerschaum probe
Mefix adhesive tape
MEG
  MEG head-based coordinate system
  MEG sensor
Mega-Air bed
MegaDyne
  M. all-in-one hand control
  M. arthroscopic hook electrode
  M. cautery
  M. electrocautery pencil
  M. E-Z clean cautery tip
MegaDyne/Fann E-Z clean laparoscopic electrode
MegaFlo infusion set
MegaLink biliary stent
Megarcart electrocardiograph
Megasource penile prosthesis
Mega Tilt and Turn bed
megaureter clamp
megavoltage machine
Mehta intraocular lens
meibomian
  m. expressor forceps
  m. gland expressor
Meier magnum system
Meigs
  M. endometrial curette

M. hemostat
M. retractor
M. suture
M. uterine curette

MEL

MEL 60 excimer laser
MEL 70 flying spot laser
MEL 60 scanning laser

Melauskas acrylic orbital implant
Melaware flatware
Meller

M. cyclodialysis spatula
M. lacrimal sac retractor

Mellinger

M. eye speculum
M. fenestrated blades speculum
M. magnet

Mellinger-Axenfeld eye speculum
Melmed blood freezing bag
Melotte metal
Melt elevator
Meltzer

M. adenoid punch
M. nasopharyngoscope
M. tonsillar punch

membrane

m. artificial lung
barrier m.
biobarrier m.
BioGen nonporous barrier m.
Bio-Gide resorbable barrier m.
BioMend collagen m.
Biopore m.
collagen m.
m. delamination wedge
Duralon-UV nylon m.
elastic silicone m.
EPTFE augmentation m.
m. forceps
Gore-Tex surgical m.
HA m.
Hemophan m.
Hybond N+ nylon m.
Imtec BioBarrier m.
MSI nylon m.
m. oxygenator
m. peeler
m. perforator
polysulfone m.
Preclude pericardial m.
Preclude peritoneal m.
Preclude spinal m.
REGENTEX GBR-200 m.
Seprafilm bioresorbable m.
Sodium hyaluronate-based
  bioresorbable m.
m. tack
TefGen-FD guided tissue
  regeneration m.
ultrafiltration m.
Viresolve ultrafiltration m.

membrane-puncturing forceps
Meme

M. breast prosthesis
M. mammary implant

Memokath catheter
memory

M. basket
m. board
m. catheter
m. exercise card
M. II cushion
m. splint

MemoryLens

M. foldable intraocular lens
M. IOL

MemoryTrace

M. AT
M. AT ambulatory cardiac monitor

Memotherm

M. colorectal stent
M. Flexx biliary stent

Mendel ligature forceps
Mendez

M. astigmatism dial
M. corneal marker
M. cystitome
M. degree calipers
M. degree gauge
M. multi-purpose LASIK forceps
M. ultrasonic cystotome

Mendez-Schubert aortic punch
Menge pessary
Mengert membrane-puncturing forceps
Menghini

M. cannula
M. liver biopsy needle

Menghini-type coring bevel
Menghini-Wildhirt

M.-W. laparoscope
M.-W. peritoneoscope

meniscal

m. basket forceps
m. clamp
m. curette
m. cutter
m. hook scissors
m. knife
m. mirror
m. posterior concave intraocular
  lens
m. repair needle
m. retractor
m. spoon
m. staple
m. suture grabber

meniscectomy

m. blade
m. knife
m. probe
m. scissors

meniscotome

Bowen-Grover m.
Drompp m.
Dyonics m.
Grover m.
Ruuska m.
Smillie m.

M

Meniscus
    M. Arrow implant
    M. Mender II system
Menlo Care catheter
Mentanium vitreoretinal instrument set
Mentor
    M. absorbent pouch
    M. Alpha 1 inflatable penile prosthesis
    M. biliary stent
    M. bladder pacemaker
    M. breast prosthesis
    M. B-VAT II monitor
    M. B-VAT visual acuity chart
    M. Contour Genesis ultrasonic assisted lipoplasty system
    M. coudé catheter
    M. Curved eraser
    M. Exeter ophthalmoscope
    M. female self-catheter
    M. fine-focus microscope
    M. Foley catheter
    M. Foley catheter with comfort sleeve
    M. GFS penile prosthesis
    M. injector gun
    M. IPP penile prosthesis
    M. malleable penile prosthesis
    M. malleable semirigid penile implant
    M. Mark II penile prosthesis
    M. ORC MemoryLens lens
    M. prostate biopsy needle
    M. Self-Cath penile prosthesis
    M. Self-Cath soft catheter
    M. Siltex implant
    M. Spectrum contour expander
    M. straight catheter
    M. Tele-Cath ileal conduit sampling catheter
    M. tissue expander
    M. ultrasound-assisted lipoplasty machine
    M. ultrasound device
    M. Wet-Field cautery
    M. Wet-Field cordless coagulator
    M. Wet-Field electrocautery
    M. Wet-Field eraser
Mentor-Maumenee Suregrip forceps
Mentor-Urosan external catheter
Menuet
    M. Compact primary urodynamic nerve fiber analyzer
    M. Compact urodynamic testing device
Mepiform self-adherent silicone dressing
Mepilex foam dressing
Mepitel
    M. contact-layer wound dressing
    M. nonadherent silicone dressing
Mepore absorptive dressing
Mercedes
    M. tip
    M. tip cannula

Mercer cartilage knife
Mercier
    M. catheter
    M. sound
Merck respirator
mercury
    m. bougie
    m. cell-powered pacemaker
mercury-filled
    m.-f. dilator
    m.-f. esophageal bougie
mercury-in-rubber strain gauge plethysmograph
mercury-in-Silastic strain gauge
mercury-weighted
    m.-w. dilator
    m.-w. rubber bougie
Meridian
    M. intersegmental table
    M. pacemaker
    M. ST femoral implant component
meridional
    m. implant
    m. refractometer
Merimack 1040 CO$_2$ laser
Merit-B periodontal probe
Merit Final Flexion Kit
Merlin
    M. arthroscopy blade
    M. bendable blade
    M. stone forceps
Merlis obstetrical excavator
MERmaid kit
Merocel
    M. epistaxis packing
    M. sponge
    M. surgical spear
    M. tampon
Merogel
    M. dressing
    M. nasal packing
    M. stent
Merriam forceps
Merrifield knife
Merrill-Levassier retractor
Merrimack laser adapter
Merry
    M. Walker
    M. Walker ambulation device
Mershon
    M. band pusher
    M. spring
Mersilene
    M. band
    M. braided nonabsorbable suture
    M. gauze hammock
    M. graft
    M. implant
    M. Kessler stitch
    M. mesh
    M. mesh dressing
    M. mesh sling
    M. tape
Mersilk suture

Merthiolate
    M. dressing
    M. swab
Mertz keratoscopy ring
Merz
    M. aortic punch
    M. hysterectomy forceps
Merz-Vienna nasal speculum
Mesalt sodium chloride-impregnated
   dressing
mesh
    Auto Suture surgical m.
    Bard-Marlex m.
    Bard Sperma-Tex preshaped m.
    Brennen biosynthetic surgical m.
    craniomaxillofacial m.
    Dacron m.
    Dexon polyglycolic acid m.
    Dexon surgically knitted m.
    DualMesh hernia m.
    Dumbach mini m.
    Dumbach regular m.
    Dumbach titanium m.
    Epicon m.
    Ethicon m.
    Flared patch m.
    m. graft
    Herniamesh surgical m.
    Hexcelite m.
    intraperitoneal onlay m.
    Kugel m.
    Leibinger Micro Dynamic m.
    macro-mesh m.
    mandibular m.
    Marlex m.
    Meadox Dacron m.
    Mersilene m.
    micro m.
    mixed m.
    m. myringotomy tube
    Parietex composite m.
    Permacol m.
    polyamide m.
    polyglactin m.
    polyglycolic m.
    polypropylene m.
    polytetrafluoroethylene (PTFE) m.
    Prolene m.
    sintered titanium m.
    skin graft expander m.
    Sperma-Tex preshaped m.
    stainless steel m.
    m. stent
    m. stent prosthesis
    Supramid polyamide m.
    surgical metallic m.
    Surgipro hernia m.
    m. suture
    SynMesh m.
    synthetic m.
    tantalum m.
    Teflon m.
    TiMesh cranial m.
    TiMesh orbital m.
    TiMesh titanium m.

    titanium m.
    Trelex natural m.
    Visilex polypropylene m.
meshed ball implant
mesher
    Collin m.
    skin graft m.
    Tanner m.
    Zimmer skin graft m.
Meshgraft skin expander
mesocaval
    m. H-graft shunt
mesonephric drain
mesostructure implant
Messerklinger
    M. endoscope
    M. sinus endoscopy set
Messing root canal gun
Meta
    M. DDDR pacemaker
    M. II pacemaker
    M. MV cardiac pacemaker
    M. rate-responsive pacemaker
metabolator
    Sanborn m.
metabolic
    m. cart
    m. heat load stimulator
metacarpal
    m. broach
    m. double-ended retractor
    m. saw
metacarpophalangeal
    m. implant
    m. prosthesis
MetaFluor system
metal
    m. adapter
    m. ball-tip catheter
    m. band
    m. band suture
    m. bar retractor
    m. bucket-handle prosthesis
    m. cannula
    m. clip
    Co-Cr-W-Ni alloy implant m.
    d'Arcet m.
    m. electrode
    m. femoral head prosthesis
    m. Fox shield
    m. frame reinforced plastic bracket
    m. hemi-toe implant
    m. hybrid orthosis
    Lipowitz m.
    Melotte m.
    m. needle
    m. orthopaedic implant
    m. oxide semiconductor field-effect
      transistor
    m. pin
    m. reconstruction plate
    m. ruler
    m. scleral shield
    m. sewing ring
    m. splint

M

metal *(continued)*
> m. tongue depressor
> M. Z stent

metal-augmented polymer stent

metal-backed
> m.-b. acetabular component hip implant
> m.-b. socket

metal-ball tip cannula

metal-coated stent

Metalift crown and bridge removal system

Metaline dressing

metallic
> m. clip
> m. frontal needle
> m. pointer
> m. screw
> m. skin marker
> m. staple
> m. stent
> m. suture
> m. tip cannula

metallic-tip catheter

metallograft

metal-olive dilator

metal-on-metal articulating intervertebral disk prosthesis

metal-tipped stent pusher

Metaport catheter

Metasul
> M. hip joint component
> M. hip prosthesis
> M. joint
> M. metal-on-metal hip prosthesis system

metatarsal
> m. cookie
> m. stem broach

metatarsophalangeal endoprosthesis

Metavox hearing aid

Metcalf spring drop brace

Metcher eye speculum

Metcoff pediatric biopsy needle

meter
> Accu-Chek III blood glucose m.
> Aleo m.
> Assess peak flow m.
> Astech peak flow m.
> AvocetPT rapid prothrombin time m.
> BioTrainer exercise m.
> Chemstrip MatchMaker blood glucose m.
> clip force m.
> Cybex finger-clip pulse m.
> electromagnetic flow m.
> ExacTech blood glucose m.
> exposure m.
> Fisher Accumet pH m.
> galvanic skin response m.
> Gammex RMI DAP m.
> Guyton-Minkowski potential acuity m.
> HemoCue glucose m.
> intragastric continuous pH-meter m.
> Kowa FM-500 laser flare m.
> laser flare m.
> m. lens
> m. mask
> Medisense Pen 2 blood glucose m.
> Miles Encore QA glucose m.
> Narkotest m.
> One-Touch blood glucose m.
> OxiFlow m.
> oxygen saturation m.
> peak flow m.
> Peakometer urinary flow-rate m.
> Periflux PF 1 D blood-flow m.
> photovolt pH m.
> potential acuity m.
> reciprocal ohm m.
> Roentgen m.
> sound level m.
> Statham electromagnetic flow m.
> Supreme II blood glucose m.
> SureStep glucose m.
> Synectics 6000 digital pH m.
> TruZone peak flow m.
> urinary drainage bag and urine m.
> US 1005 uroflow m.
> Venturi m.
> Wright peak flow m.
> Youlten nasal inspiratory peak flow m.

metered-dose inhaler (MDI)

Metermatic nasal nebulizer

methacrylate
> polymethyl m. (PMMA)

Methodist
> M. Hospital headholder
> M. vascular suction tube

methyl
> m. cyanoacrylate glue
> m. methacrylate bead
> m. methacrylate beads implant
> m. methacrylate block
> m. methacrylate cement adhesive
> m. methacrylate cranioplastic plug
> m. methacrylate ear stent
> m. methacrylate eye implant
> m. methacrylate graft
> m. methacrylate implant material
> m. methacrylate spacer

Metico forceps

MetraGrasp ligament grasper

MetraPass suture passer

Metra PS procedure kit

Metras bronchial catheter

MetraTie knot pusher

Metrecom
> M. device
> M. digitizer

metric ophthalmoscope

MetriTray system soaking tray

Metrix
> M. atrial defibrillation system
> M. implantable atrioverter

metrizamide-filled balloon

MetroFlex endoscopic cart
metronoscope
Metron Plus dispenser
Mettelman prejowl chin implant
Mettler
    M. Dia-Sonic electrosurgical unit
    M. electrotherapy
Mett tube
Metzelder modification activator
Metzel-Wittmoser forceps
Metzenbaum
    M. chisel
    M. delicate scissors
    M. dissecting scissors
    M. gouge
    M. long scissors
    M. needle holder
    M. operating scissors
    M. septal knife
    M. tonsillar forceps
Metzenbaum-Lipsett scissors
Metzenbaum-Tydings forceps
Meurig Williams spinal fusion plate
MEVA probe
Mevatron 74 linear accelerator
Mewissen infusion catheter
Mexican bat
Meyer
    M. biliary retractor
    M. cervical orthosis
    M. cyclodiathermy needle
    M. olive-tipped vein stripper
    M. spiral vein stripper
    M. Swiss diamond knife lancet
    M. Swiss diamond lancet knife
    M. Swiss diamond wedge knife
    M. temporal loop
Meyerding
    M. bone graft
    M. bone skid
    M. chisel
    M. curved gouge
    M. finger retractor
    M. hip skid
    M. laminectomy blade
    M. mallet
    M. osteotome
    M. prosthesis
    M. retractor blade
    M. saw-toothed curette
    M. self-retaining laminectomy
       retractor
    M. shoulder skid
    M. skin hook
Meyerding-Deaver retractor
Meyer-Schwickerath coagulator
Meyhöffer, Meyhoeffer
    M. bone curette
    M. chalazion curette
    M. eye knife
M-F heel protector
MG
    MG II knee prosthesis
    MG II total hip system
    MG II total knee system

MGH
    MGH knee prosthesis
    MGH needle holder
    MGH osteotome
    MGH periosteal elevator
    MGH uterine vulsellum forceps
    MGH vulsellum
MGM glenoidal punch
Miami
    M. Acute Care cervical collar
    M. Acute Care cervical traction
    M. cervical fracture brace
    M. J cervical collar
    M. "J" collar cervical traction
    M. TLSO scoliosis brace
MIBB breast biopsy system
MIC
    MIC bolus gastrostomy tube
    MIC gastroenteric tube
    MIC jejunal tube
    MIC jejunostomy tube
mica spectacles
MICA 3x sleeve
Michel
    M. aortic clamp
    M. clip-applying forceps
    M. clip-removing forceps
    M. pick
    M. rhinoscopic mirror
    M. scalp clip
    M. skin clip
    M. suture clip
    M. tissue forceps
Michele trephine
Michelson infant bronchoscope
Michelson-Sequoia air drill
Michel-Wachtenfeldt clip
Michigan University intestinal forceps
Mick
    M. afterloading needle
    M. prostate template
    M. seed applicator
    M. TP-200 applicator
MIC-Key gastrostomy tube
Mickey and Minnie surgical marker
Micor catheter
Micra
    M. knife
    M. needle holder
Micrins
    M. forceps
    M. microsurgical suture
Micro
    M. Delta system
    M. Diamond-Point microsurgery
       instrument
    M. E irrigation kit
    M. FET isometric force
       dynamometer
    M. 100 irrigation kit
    M. Link endoscope fiber
    M. Minix pacemaker
    M. One pneumatonometer
    M. oral surgery handpiece
    M. Plus plating system

M

Micro *(continued)*
- M. Plus screw
- M. Plus spirometer
- M. punctum plug
- M. Series wire driver
- M. Stent II

micro
- m. mesh
- m. round-tip needle
- m. scissors
- m. Westcott scissors

Micro-6 ureteroscope
micro-adaption plate
Micro-Aire
- M.-A. bur
- M.-A. drill
- M.-A. facial plating system
- M.-A. oscillating bone saw
- M.-A. osteotome
- M.-A. pneumatic power instrument
- M.-A. pulse lavage system
- M.-A. surgical instrument system

microAir turn-Q-plus
micro-Allis forceps
microamperage electrical nerve stimulator
microamps TENS unit
microanalyzer
- electronic m.
- electron probe x-ray m.

microanastomosis
- m. approximator
- m. clip

microarterial
- m. clamp
- m. forceps

microaspirator
- Ergo m.

microball hook
microballoon
- implantable silicone m.
- m. probe
- Rand m.

microbayonet
- m. forceps
- m. rasp
- m. scoop

Microbeam
- M. I, II, III, IV macromanipulators
- M. manipulator

microbiopsy forceps
microbipolar forceps
microblade
- Beaver m.
- Sharptome m.

microbone curette
microbore Tygon tube
microbronchoscopic
- m. grasping forceps
- m. tissue forceps

microbulldog
- m. clamp
- m. clip

microcalipers
- Storz m.

Microcap scalpel
Micro-Cast collimator
microcatheter
- Cardima Pathfinder m.
- Hydrolyser m.
- Magic m.
- Prowler m.
- Renegade m.
- Terumo SP hydrophilic-polymer-coated m.
- Tracker m.
- UltraLite flow-directed m.

microcautery unit
Microcell
- M. alternating pressure pad
- M. chamber

microcentrifuge
- Compac m.

MicroChoice electric powered surgical system
microclamp
- disposable m.
- m. forceps
- Kapp m.
- Khodadad m.

Microclens wipe
microclip
- m. forceps
- Heifitz m.
- Khodadad m.
- Kleinert-Kutz m.
- Williams m.
- Yasargil m.
- Zylik m.

microcoagulator
- Malis bipolar m.
- Polar-Mate bipolar m.

microcoil
- ACT M.
- endothelin-1 platinum-Dacron m.
- Hilal m.
- platinum m.
- platinum-Dacron m.

micro-Colibri forceps
microcolpohysteroflator
- Hamou m.

microcomputer upper limb exerciser
microconjunctival scissors
microconnector
- titanium m.

microcorneal
- m. forceps
- m. scissors

microcrimped prosthesis
microcup
- m. pituitary forceps

microcurette
- Accurette m.
- HemoCue m.
- Rhoton m.
- Ruggles m.

microcurrent electrode
microcut bandsaw

microcystitome
Lieppman m.
microdebrider
Hummer m.
Linvotec m.
MDS m.
Radnoid m.
Stryker m.
Wizard m.
microdensitometer
Vickers M85a m.
microdermabrader
Pelle Peel m.
microdermatome
Meek-Wall m.
MicroDigitrapper apnea recorder
MicroDigitrapper-HR fingertrap
MicroDigitrapper-S
M.-S. apnea screening device
M.-S. fingertrap
MicroDigitrapper-V fingertrap
microdilution system
microdissecting forceps
microdissector
Crockard m.
Hardy m.
Rhoton m.
Yasargil m.
Microdon dressing
micro-Doppler instrument
microdressing forceps
microdrill
high-speed m.
Shea m.
microdrilling guide
microelectrode
tungsten m.
microendoprope
Toshiba m.
microendoscope
Omegascope OM2/070 flexible m.
ophthalmic laser m.
Toshiba m.
microendoscopic
m. optical catheter
m. test card
microextractor forceps
MicroFet2 muscle testing device
microfibrillar
m. collagen
m. collagen hemostat
Microfil silicone-rubber injection compound
microfilter
Minnpure m.
Microflo test strip
Micro-Flow compactor
MicroFlow phacoemulsification needle
Microfoam
M. dressing
M. surgical tape
microforceps
Adson m.
Anis m.
Birks-Mathelone m.

Collis m.
iris m.
iris suture m.
Jako-Kleinsasser m.
Koslowski m.
Nicola m.
Rhoton m.
Scanlan m.
Sparta m.
V. Mueller laser Rhoton m.
Yasargil m.
Microfuge tube
MicroFuse Infuser
Microgel surface-enhanced ventilation tube
Microglass pH electrode
Micro-Glide corneal suture
microgonioscope
micrograft dilator
Micro-Guide catheter
microguidewire
Transcend m.
Microgyn II urinary incontinence device
Micro-Halogen otoscope
micro-Halstead arterial forceps
microhandpiece
MicroHartzler ACS balloon catheter system
microhemostat
O'Brien-Storz m.
microhook
Bonn m.
McIntyre m.
Shambaugh-Derlacki m.
Simcoe m.
microhysteroscope
Hamou contact microhysteroscope
Micro-Imager high-resolution digital camera
microimpactor
Codman m.
microimplant
Artecoll injectable m.
Bioplastique injectable m.
silicone m.
microinjection
microiris
m. hook
m. knife
m. scissors
microirrigator
Stryker m.
Microjet-based cutting and debriding device
Microjet Quark portable pump
micro-jewelers monopolar forceps
microkeratome
Barraquer m.
Barraquer-Carriazo m.
Carriazo-Barraquer m.
Chiron ACS m.
Corneal Shaper m.
FlapMaker disposable m.
Hanastome m.
Krumeich-Barraquer m.

M

microkeratome *(continued)*
LSK One Disposable m.
MedJet m.
Med-Logics ML M.
ML M.
ONE Disposable m.
Ruiz m.
Summit Krumeich-Barraquer M.

microknife
Karlin m.

Microknit
M. patch graft
M. vascular graft
M. vascular graft prosthesis

Microlance blood lancet

MicroLap
M. endoscope
M. Gold microlaparoscopy system

microlaparoscope
Imagyn m.

microlaryngeal
m. endotracheal tube
m. grasping forceps
m. laser probe
m. scissors

microlaryngoscope
Abramson-Dedo m.
anterior commissure m.
Dedo-Jako m.
Fragen anterior commissure m.
Jako m.
Lindholm m.

Microlase
M. transpupillary diode
M. transpupillary diode laser

Microlens
M. cystourethroscope
M. direct-vision telescope
M. Foroblique telescope
M. hook
M. urethroscope

Microlet
M. electrode needle
M. Vaculance

Micro-Line arterial forceps

Microlith
M. pacemaker pulse generator
M. P pacemaker

Microloc
M. knee prosthesis
M. knee system

Micro-Lok implant

Microloop spirometer

microloupe

microlumbar diskectomy retractor

MicroLux video camera system

Microlyzer Gas analyzer

micromanipulator
microscope-mounted m.
MicroSpot m.
self-centering m.
UniMax 2000 laser m.

micromanometer
m. catheter
m. catheter system

MicroMark tissue marker

MicroMax
M. centrifuge
M. drill system
M. speed drill

Micromedics surgical instrument

micromesh sheeting

micrometer
diamond m.
m. knife
Tolman m.
ultrasonic m.

MicroMewi multiple sidehole infusion catheter

Micro-Mill knee instrument system

micromirror
Apfelbaum m.
Silverstein m.

MicroMirror gold sensor

Micro-Mist disposable nebulizer

MicroMite anchor suture

micromosquito
m. curved scissors
m. straight scissors

micromultiplane transesophageal echocardiographic probe

Micron
M. bobbin ventilation tube
M. Res-Q implantable cardioverter-defibrillator

micronebulizer
Bird m.

microneedle
m. holder
m. holder forceps

micronerve hook

microneurosurgical forceps

micron needle

Microny SR+ single-chamber, rate-responsive pulse generator

Micro-One dissecting forceps

microphone
hearing aid m.
Sennheiser electric condenser ME 40-3 m.

MicroPhor iontophoretic drug delivery system

microphthalmoscope

micropigmentation handpiece

micropin
m. forceps
Pischel m.

micropipette
in vitro fertilization m.

micropituitary
m. rongeur
m. scissors

microplate
C-shaped m.
Luhr m.
mandibular angle fracture intraoral open reduction m.

Microplate fixation
micropoint
    m. needle
    m. suture
Micropore
    M. surgical tape dressing
    M. tape
MicroProbe
    Endo Optics M.
    M. integrated laser and endoscope
    system
    M. ophthalmic laser
Micro-Probe tip
microprocessor
    Intertron therapy m.
Micro-Pulsar TENS unit
micropuncture
    m. guidewire
    m. introducer needle
Micropuncture Peel-Away introducer
Microputor II
microrasp
    Scanlan m.
microraspatory
    Yasargil m.
microreciprocating saw
microretractor
    flexible arm m.
microrongeur
    Davol m.
    Kerrison m.
microruler
    Stecher m.
microruptor
    LASAG m.
microsagittal saw
Microsampler device
microscalpel
    Oasis feather m.
microscanner
    pQCT m.
microscissors
    Collis m.
    curved conventional m.
    DORC microforceps and m.
    Gill-Welsh-Vannas angled m.
    Jacobson m.
    Jako-Kleinsasser m.
    Kamdar m.
    Keeler m.
    Kurze m.
    Rhoton m.
    round-tip m.
    Scanlan m.
    Shutt m.
    straight m.
    Twisk m.
    V. Mueller laser Rhoton m.
    Yasargil m.
  microscope
    Accu-Scope m.
    acoustic m.
    analytical electron m. (AEM)
    Beckerscope binocular m.
    BHTU m.

Bio-Optics specular m.
Bitumi monobjective m.
cine m.
Cohan-Barraquer m.
confocal m.
conventional transmission
  electron m.
CooperVision m.
corneal m.
Czapski m.
EIE 150F operating m.
electron m.
ELMISKOP 101 electron m.
endothelial specular m.
Fiberlite m.
fiberoptic m.
Galilean m.
Hallpike-Blackmore ear m.
Heyer-Schulte m.
high-voltage electron m.
Hitachi H-series electron m.
JedMed TRI-GEM m.
JEM-100B and 100S electron m.
Joel scanning electron m.
Kaps operating m.
Keeler-Konan Specular m.
Konan SP8000 noncontact
  specular m.
laser m.
Leica m.
Leitz m.
light electron m.
Mentor fine-focus m.
Moller m.
nailfold capillary m.
Olympus BHT-2 m.
Olympus CBK fluorescence m.
Omni 2 m.
OM 2000 operating m.
operating m.
OpMI PRO magis surgical m.
OpMi VISU 200 m.
Optiphot-2UD m.
Optique m.
Philips CM 12 electron m.
pneumatic m.
Project Research Ophthalmic
  specular m.
Pro-Koester wide-field SCM m.
Protégé Plus m.
real-time confocal scanning laser m.
Rheinberg m.
scanning laser acoustic m.
scanning slit confocal m.
scanning transmission electron m.
scanning tunneling m.
Seiler MC-M900 surgical m.
slit-lamp m.
SMZ zoom stereo m.
stereoscopic m.
Storz m.
surgical m.
tandem scanning confocal m.
Topcon SP-series non-contact
  specular m.

M

microscope *(continued)*
transmission electron m.
Universal electron m.
Urban m.
Varimic 900 m.
video specular m.
Weck m.
Wild M 690 m.
Wild operating m.
x-ray tomographic m.
Zeiss Axioskop m.
Zeiss-Barraquer cine m.
Zeiss-Barraquer surgical m.
Zeiss-Contraves operating m.
Zeiss IDO3 phase-contrast m.
Zeiss-Jena surgical m.
Zeiss operating m.
Zeiss OpMi CSI surgical m.
Zeiss OpMi MDO ophthalmic
surgical m.
Zeiss S9 electron m.
microscope-mounted micromanipulator
microscopic
m. hook
m. scissors
microscopy
double-immunofluorescence m.
electron m.
microscrew
Barouk m.
MicroSeal
M. nebulizer
M. ophthalmic handpiece
Storz M.
**microsecond pulsed flashlamp pumped
dye laser**
Microsect
M. curette
M. shaver
microserrefine
Storz m.
MicroShape keratome system
Micro-Sharp blade
microshaver
Stryker m.
MICROS infusion system
MicroSmooth probe
Microsnap hemostatic forceps
Microsoftrac catheter
**Micro-Soft Stream sidehole infusion
catheter**
Microson hearing aid
MicroSpan
M. capnometer
M. hysteroscope
M. minihysteroscopy system
M. sheath
microspatula
Osher malleable m.
microspectroscope
microsphere
Embosphere m.
magnetic m.

paramagnetic m.
Super-Bright m.
Microspike
M. approximator
M. approximator clamp
microsponge
Alcon m.
M. delivery system
Teardrop m.
M. Teardrop sponge
Weck-cel m.
MicroSpot micromanipulator
Micross
M. dilatation catheter
M. SL balloon
MicroStable liner locking mechanism
microstaple
Barouk m.
m. holder
Microstar dialysis system
Microstat
M. handpiece
M. ultrasonic nebulizer
Microstent II
MicroStim 100 TENS device
microstomia prevention appliance
microsurgery
transanal endoscopic m.
microsurgical
m. biopsy forceps
m. dissector
m. ear hook
m. ear pick
m. grasping forceps
m. knife
m. needle holder
m. retractor
m. scissors
m. tying forceps
microsuture
Sharpoint m.
microsyringe
MicroTach pneumotachometer
Microtek
M. cupped forceps
M. Heine otoscope
M. scissors
microtenotomy scissors
MicroTeq portable belt
micro-thin plastic fiber
Microthin P2 pacemaker
Micro-Three microsurgery instrument
MicroTip
M. catheter
M. phaco tip
microtip
m. bipolar jeweler's forceps
m. pressure transducer
microtissue forceps
microtitration plate reader
microtome
Cryo-Cut m.
Leica vibrating knife m.
Leitz 1600 Saw m.
Stadie-Riggs m.

microtonometer
    Computon m.
Micro-Touch Platex medical gloves
Micro-Tracer
    M.-T. portable ECG
    M.-T. portable EKG
microtransducer
    imbedded m.
    Konigsberg m.
Micro-Transducer catheter
Microtron
    M. accelerator
    racetrack M.
Micro-Two forceps
microtying forceps
MicroTymp2 hand-held tympanometer
MicroTymp tympanometric device
MicroVac catheter
microvascular
    m. clamp
    m. clamp-applying forceps
    m. clip
    m. modified Alm retractor
    m. needle holder
    m. scissors
    m. STA-MCA kit
    m. tying forceps
Microvasive
    M. Altertome
    M. biliary device
    M. biliary stent system
    M. controlled radial expansion
        esophageal dilator
    M. disposable alligator-shaped
        forceps
    M. 5F minisnare
    M. Geenen Endotorque guidewire
    M. Glidewire
    M. Glidewire guidewire
    M. instrumentation
    M. One Step Button
    M. One Step Button gastrostomy
    M. papillotome
    M. radial jaw biopsy forceps
    M. retrieval balloon
    M. Rigiflex balloon catheter
    M. Rigiflex balloon dilator
    M. Rigiflex through-the-scope
        balloon
    M. Rigiflex TTS balloon
    M. sclerotherapy needle
    M. Speedband Superview ligator
    M. stent
    M. Ultraflex esophageal stent
        system
    M. ultratome
Microvel
    M. double velour graft
    M. prosthesis
Microvena
    M. Amplatz Goose Neck snare
    M. Das Angel Wings occluder
Micro-Vent
    M.-V. implant
    M.-V. implant system

Micro-Vent^2 implant
MicroVent ventilator
microvessel hook
MicroView sheath-based IVUS catheter
Microvit
    M. cutter
    M. probe
    M. probe system
    M. scissors
    M. vitrector
microvitrector
microvitreoretinal
    m. blade
    m. spatula
Microwec scissors
microweld
Microwell
MicroWrist
Micro-Z neuromuscular stimulator
micturition bag
MIDA
    MIDA CoroNet instrumentation
    MIDA 1000 monitoring system
Midas
    M. Rex bur guard
    M. Rex craniotome
    M. Rex drill
    M. Rex instrumentation
    M. Rex instrumentation system
    M. Rex knife
    M. Rex pneumatic instrument
    M. Rex Quick-Connect system
midcavity forceps
middle
    m. ear aspirator
    m. ear calipers
    m. ear chisel
    m. ear excavator
    m. ear implant
    m. ear ring curette
    m. ear strut forceps
    m. ear suction cannula
    m. fossa retractor
    m. palatine suture
Middledorf retractor
Middledorpf splint
Middlesex-Pointe retractor
Middleton
    M. adenoid curette
    M. rongeur
midgastric electrode
midget MRI scanner
mid-infrared pulsed laser
Midland tilt table
Midline Hi-Lo Mat Platform
Midmark 413 power female procedure
    chair
midoccipital electrode
midstream aortogram catheter
Mighty Bite Zimmon lateral biopsy cup
    forceps
Mignon cataract extractor
Mijnhard electrical cycloergometer
Mikaelsson catheter
Mikros pacemaker

M

Mikro-Tip
  M.-T. angiocatheter
  M.-T. micromanometer-tipped
   catheter
  M.-T. transducer
Mikulicz
  M. abdominal retractor
  M. crusher
  M. drain
  M. liver retractor
  M. pack
  M. pad
  M. peritoneal clamp
  M. peritoneal forceps
  M. spatula
  M. sponge
  M. tonsillar forceps
Mikulicz-Radecki
  M.-R. clamp
  M.-R. drain
Milan uterine curette
Milch resection plate
Miles
  M. antral curette
  M. bone chisel
  M. Encore QA glucose meter
  M. punch biopsy forceps
  M. rectal clamp
  M. retractor
  M. skin clip
  M. Teflon clip
  M. vena cava clip
  M. V.I.P. 300 vacuum infiltration
   processor
Milette-Tyding dissector
Milewski driver
Milex
  M. forceps
  M. Jel-Jector vaginal applicator
  M. pessary
  M. retractor
  M. spatula
  M. vaginal insufflator
military antishock trousers (MAST)
mill
  hollow m.
  Lere bone m.
  OrthoBlend powered bone m.
Millar
  M. Doppler catheter
  M. micromonometer catheter
  M. Mikro-Tip catheter pressure
   transducer
  M. MPC-500 catheter
  M. pigtail angiographic catheter
  M. urodynamic catheter
Millard
  M. clamp
  M. Lite-Pipe
  M. mouth gag
  M. mouthgag
  M. thimble hook
Millenia
  M. balloon catheter

  M. percutaneous transluminal
   coronary angioplasty (PTCA)
   catheter
Millennium
  M. CX microsurgical system
  M. LX microsurgical system
  M. oxygen concentrator
Mille Pattes screw
Miller
  M. articulating forceps
  M. bayonet forceps
  M. bone file
  M. bougie
  M. bracket positioner
  M. curette
  M. cystoscope
  M. dental elevator
  M. dilator
  M. dissecting scissors
  M. endotracheal tube
  M. fiberoptic laryngoscope blade
  M. laryngoscope
  M. operating scissors
  M. rasp
  M. ratchet injector
  M. rectal forceps
  M. rectal scissors
  M. retractor
  M. scale
  M. septostomy catheter
  M. tonsillar dissector
  M. vaginal speculum
Miller-Abbott
  M.-A. catheter
  M.-A. double-lumen intestinal tube
Miller-Apexo elevator
Miller-Galante
  M.-G. hip prosthesis
  M.-G. revision knee system
  M.-G. total knee system
  M.-G. unicompartmental knee
Miller-Senn
  M.-S. double-ended retractor
Miller-vac drain
Millesi
  M. interfascicular graft
  M. scissors
Millet
  M. needle
  M. neurological test instrument
  M. test hammer
Millette tonsillar knife
Millette-Tyding knife
Millex
  M. GS-series filter
  M. GV-series filter
Millie female urinal
Milligan
  M. double-ended dissector
  M. self-retaining retractor
  M. speculum
Milliknit
  M. arterial prosthesis
  M. Dacron prosthesis

M. graft
M. vascular graft prosthesis
millimeter ruler
Millin
M. bladder neck spreader
M. bladder spatula
M. boomerang needle holder
M. capsular forceps
M. clamp
M. ligature-guiding forceps
M. prostatectomy forceps
M. retropublic bladder retractor
M. self-retaining retractor
M. suction tube
M. T-shaped forceps
Millin-Bacon
M.-B. bladder neck spreader
M.-B. bladder self-retaining retractor
M.-B. retropubic prostatectomy
retractor
milliner's needle
millinery bag
milling cutter
Millipore
M. suture
M. ultrafree-CL centrifugal filter
Milli-Q water purification system
Mill-Rose
M.-R. cytology brush
M.-R. esophageal injector
M.-R. flexible endoscopic overtube
M.-R. RiteBite biopsy forceps
M.-R. spiral stone basket
M.-R. Surebrite biopsy forceps
M.-R. tube
Mills
M. circumflex scissors
M. coronary endarterectomy set
M. coronary endarterectomy spatula
M. dressing
M. Glucometer II glucometer
M. microvascular needle holder
M. operative peripheral angioplasty
catheter
M. tissue forceps
M. valvulotome
Milroy-Piper suction tube
Milteck scissors
Miltex
M. bone saw
M. disposable biopsy punch
M. gun
M. ligature knife
M. nail nipper
M. pump
M. retractor
M. rib spreader
M. wire twister
Milwaukee
M. scoliosis brace
M. scoliosis orthosis
M. snare

Mi-Mark
M.-M. disposable endocervical
curette
M.-M. endocervical curette set
MindSet toe splint
Miner osteotome
Minerva
M. back jacket
M. cast
M. collar
M. orthosis
M. plastic jacket
M. robot
M. system
Mingograf
M. 62 6-channel electrocardiograph
M. electroencephalograph
M. 82 recorder
Mingograph
MINI
M. 6000 C-arm
mini
m. applier
m. Bio-Phase suture anchor
M. Cliplamp
m. Hoffmann external fixation
system
M. II, II+ automatic implantable
cardioverter defibrillator
m. lag screw
M. Orbita plate
M. speech processor
m. trephine
m. Vidas automated immunoassay
system
m. Würzburg Flexplates
craniomaxillofacial plating system
m. Würzburg screw
m. Würzburg standard
craniomaxillofacial plating system
Mini-Acutrak small-bone fixation system
miniapplier
miniature
m. blade
m. bulldog clamp
m. centrifugal fast analyzer
m. intestinal forceps
m. loop electrode
m. probe
m. sound
m. ultrasound suction device
miniaturized ultrasound catheter probe
Mini-Bag Plus container
miniballoon
MiniBard catheter
minibasket
Shutt m.
Wilson-Cook m.
miniBIRD position tracker
miniblade
Beaver miniblade
minibladebreaker
Troutman-Barraquer m.
miniclip
Stangel fallopian tube m.

M

minicoil
minicurette
minicut bandsaw
mini-defibrillator
    Liteguard m.-d.
Minidop ES-100VX Pocket Doppler
mini-echo sounder
mini-endoscope
mini-excimer
    Compak-200 m.-e.
Mini-Fibralux pocket otoscope
minifixator
    Pennig m.
Mini-Flex
    M.-F. flexible Harris uterine injector
    HUI M.-F.
miniforceps
    Kern m.
miniform
    inSync m.
minigraft dilator
Miniguard
    M. adhesive patch
    M. stress incontinence device
MiniHEART nebulizer
mini-Hoffmann external fixator
mini-Hohmann retractor
26 MiniII device
mini-keratoplasty stitch scissors
mini-Lambotte osteotome
minilaparoscope
    Aslan 2-mm m.
    Pixie m.
minilaparotomy Falope-ring applicator
mini-Lexer osteotome
Minilith
    M. pacemaker
    M. pacemaker pulse generator
miniloop
    Olympus HX-21L detachable m.
Minilux pocket otoscope
minimagnet
    Hamblin m.
minimallet
    Gam-Mer m.
Mini-Matic implant
Minimax 200 watt light source
MiniMed
    M. continuous glucose monitoring
      system
    M. III infusion pump
MiniMedBall hand exerciser
mini-meniscus blade
Mini-Motionlogger Actigraph
Mini-Neb nebulizer
mini-ophthalmic drape
mini-Orthofix fixator
miniosteotome
    Gam-Mer m.
mini-ovoid
MiniOX
    M. 1A, 1000 oxygen analyzer
    M. I, II, III, 100-IV oxygen
      monitor
    M. V pulse oximeter

miniplate
    L-shaped m.
    Luhr m.
    mandibular m.
    Storz m.
    m. strut
    titanium m.
    two-hole m.
    Vitallium m.
mini-pouch
    CenterPointLock two-piece ostomy
      system: closed m.-p.
    CenterPointLock two-piece ostomy
      system: drainable m.-p.
    closed m.-p.
    Filter Security closed m.-p.
    Guardian two-piece ostomy system:
      closed m.-p.
    Guardian two-piece ostomy system:
      drainable m.-p.
    Premier drainable m.-p.
    Sur-Fit M.-p.
miniprobe
    high-frequency m.
Mini-Profile dilatation catheter
minipump
    Alzer Model 2001 osmotic m.
    osmotic m.
MiniQuad XL lens
MiniQuick
    Genotropin M.
minirazor bladebreaker
mini-retractor
    R-Med m.-r.
miniscope
    Candela m.
MiniSite laparoscope
minisnare
    Microvasive 5F m.
Minispace IUI catheter
MiniSpacer
    Airlife Dual Spray M.
ministaple
    Bio-R-Sorb resorbable poly-L-lactic
      acid m.
    Richards m.
MiniStim TENS unit
mini-Stryker power drill
mini-Sugita clip
Mini-tip culturette
minivise
mini-Wright peak flowmeter
Minix pacemaker
Minneapolis hip prosthesis
Minnesota
    M. impedance cardiograph
    M. retractor
    M. thermal disk temperature testing
      device
    M. tube
Minnpure microfilter
Minos air drill
Minuet DDD pacemaker

MIP
> MIP anatomic overlay
> MIP reusable cover

Mipron digital computer-assisted calipers
Mira
> M. AGL-400 laser
> M. cautery
> M. coagulator
> M. diathermy
> M. drill
> M. electrocautery
> M. encircling element
> M. endovitreal cryopencil
> M. female trochanteric reamer
> M. femoral head reamer
> M. photocoagulator
> M. silicone rod
> M. unit

Mira-Charnley reamer
Miracompo filling instrument
Miracon
Mirage
> M. nasal ventilation mask system
> M. over-the-wire balloon catheter
> M. spinal system

Miragel
> M. implant
> M. sponge

Miralene suture
MIRALVA applicator
Mirasorb sponge
Miratract
mirror
> Articu-Lase laser m.
> bayonet transsphenoidal m.
> Buckingham m.
> m. cannula
> contact lens training m.
> curved laryngeal m.
> curved magnifying m.
> DenLite illuminated hand-held m.
> M. DPS
> Everclear laryngeal m.
> fiberoptic lighted m.
> Grafco head m.
> Grafco laryngeal m.
> Hardy transsphenoidal m.
> head m.
> m. holder
> House middle ear m.
> Jako laryngeal m.
> Kashiwabara laryngeal m.
> Kerner dental m.
> laryngeal m.
> m. laryngoscope
> laser m.
> Lewis dental m.
> McLaughlin laser m.
> meniscal m.
> Michel rhinoscopic m.
> Neovision micro m.
> Oliair mouth m.
> Olyco mouth m.
> Olympia mouth m.

> m. optical system
> Poh mouth m.
> polygon m.
> rhinoscopic m.
> SMIC mouth m.
> Stiwer laryngeal m.
> straight laryngeal m.
> straight magnifying m.

mirror-based reflective optics
Mischler-Pudenz shunt
Mischler shunt
Misdome-Frank curette
Mishima-Hedbys attachment pacemeter
Mishler
> M. dual-chamber valve
> M. flushing valve

Miskimon cerebellar self-retaining retractor
Missouri catheter
Misstique female external urinary collector
mist
> M. 14-gauge Eubanks instrument series
> m. tent

Mistette nasal spray pump
Mistogen
> M. nebulizer
> M. passover humidifier

Misty-Neb nebulizer
Mitamura fine ceramic heart valve
Mitchel-Adam clamp
Mitchel aortotomy clamp
Mitchell
> M. cartilage knife
> M. osteotome
> M. stone basket
> M. ureteral stone dislodger

Mitchell-Diamond biopsy forceps
Mitek
> M. anchor appliance
> M. asorbable bone anchor
> M. Fastin threaded anchor
> M. GII Easy Anchor
> M. GII Snap-pak
> M. GII suture anchor
> M. GII suture anchor system
> M. GL anchor
> M. Knotless anchor
> M. Ligament anchor
> M. Micro anchor
> M. Micro QuickAnchor
> M. Mini GII anchor
> M. Mini GLS anchor
> M. Mini QuickAnchor
> M. Panalok anchor
> M. Panalok RC anchor/Snap-Pak
> M. QuickAnchor device
> M. Rotator cuff anchor
> M. SuperAnchor instrument
> M. Tacit threaded anchor
> M. Vapr tissue removal system

Mithoefer-Jansen mouthgag
mitochondrial ethanol oxidase system

M

Mitraflex
    M. sterile spyrosorbent multilayer wound dressing
mitral
    m. hook
    m. valve dilator
    m. valve-holding forceps
    m. valve retractor
    m. valve scissors
Mitrathane wound dressing
Mitroflow
    M. pericardial prosthetic valve
    M. PeriPatch cylinders
Mitsubishi
    M. angioscope
    M. angioscopic catheter
mitt
    holding m.
    impact m.
    infant passive m.
    motion control m.
    paraffin m.
Mittelman implant
Mittlemeir ceramic hip prosthesis
Mitutoyo Digimatic calipers
Mity
    M. engine H-file
    M. Gates Glidden file
    M. Hedström file
    M. K-file
    M. plugger
    M. Roto rotary instrument
    M. spreader
    M. Turbo File file
Mityvac
    M. extractor
    M. obstetric vacuum extractor cup
    M. Super M cup
    M. vacuum delivery system
mixed mesh
Mixter
    M. arterial forceps
    M. baby hemostatic forceps
    M. brain biopsy punch
    M. common duct irrigating Dilaprobe
    M. common duct irrigating Dilaprobe dilator
    M. common duct probe
    M. Dilaprobe probe
    M. dilating probe
    M. dissector
    M. gallbladder forceps
    M. gall duct probe
    M. gallstone forceps
    M. hemostat
    M. irrigating probe
    M. ligature-carrier clamp
    M. mosquito forceps
    M. operating scissors
    M. pediatric hemostatic forceps
    M. thoracic clamp
    M. thoracic forceps
    M. tube
    M. ventricular needle

Mixter-McQuigg forceps
Mixter-O'Shaughnessy
    M.-O. dissecting forceps
    M.-O. hemostatic forceps
    M.-O. ligature forceps
Mixter-Paul
    M.-P. arterial forceps
    M.-P. hemostatic forceps
Mixtner catheter
Miya
    M. hook
    M. hook ligament carrier
    M. hook ligature carrier
Mizuho surgical Doppler
Mizutani laminaria tent
Mizzy needle
MKG knee support
MKII automated scanner
MKIII
    Digitrapper MKIII
MK IV ophthalmoscope
MKM
    MKM AutoPilot
    MKM AutoPilot stereotactic system
MKS II knee brace
Mladick
    M. concave cannula
    M. convex cannula
M/L lift
ML Microkeratome
MLR+ camera
MM-6000 colposcope
MMG
    MMG Easycath
    MMG Ready Cath
MMG/O'Neil
    MMG/O'Neil intermittent catheter system
    MMG/O'Neil sterile field urinary catheter system
M-mode sector transducer
MMS low-profile acetabular cup
Moberg
    M. bone plate
    M. chisel
    M. forceps
    M. osteotome
    M. retractor
Moberg-Stille
    M.-S. forceps
    M.-S. retractor
Mobetron
    M. electron beam system
    M. intraoperative radiation therapy treatment system
    M. mobile, self-shielded electron accelerator
mobile
    m. air chair
    m. bearing knee implant
    M. dilator storage tray
    m. electroconvulsive therapy apparatus
Mobilimb CPM device

mobilizer
Derlacki ear m.
Derlacki-Hough m.
Hough-Derlacki m.
Therabite m.
Mobin-Uddin
M.-U. sieve
M.-U. umbrella vena cava filter
Mobitz type I, II
Moblvac suction unit
Mochida CO₂ Medi-Laser laser
MOD
M. femoral drill guide
M. unicompartmental knee system
model
M. 500F electromagnetic flowmeter
foot m.
Gullstrand six-surface eye m.
M. IL 750, AA spectrophotometer
Kooijman eye m.
Le Grand-Gullstrand eye m.
M. 3-60 mass spectroscopy
Rem-air 750 XL, XXL m.
M. TC2-64B pulsed-range gated
Doppler instrument
M. 5500 vapor pressure osmometer
modeling carver
mode-locked laser
modified
m. birdcage coil
m. caulking gun
m. chest lead
m. CIF needle
m. C-loop haptic
m. C-loop intraocular lens
m. electron-beam CT scanner
m. Grace plate
m. Harrington rod
m. J-loop haptic
m. J-loop, posterior chamber
intraocular lens
m. Mark IV R-wave-triggered
power injector
m. Moore hip locking prosthesis
m. Oppenheimer splint
m. Rashkind PDA occluder
m. Robert Jones dressing
m. sclerectomy punch
m. spatula needle
m. suction tube
m. Younge forceps
m. zinc oxide-eugenol cement
m. Z-stent
Modny
M. drill
M. guide
M. pin
Modulap
M. probe
modular
M. Acetabular Revision System
(MARS)
M. acetabular revision system
m. Austin Moore hip prosthesis
m. calcar replacement stem

m. head remover
m. implant
m. instrumentation
m. Iowa Precoat total hip prosthesis
m. Lenbach hip system
M. One pneumatonometer
m. S-ROM total hip system
m. temPPTthotic kit
m. total hip prosthesis
module
AIM 7 thermocouple input m.
A-Lastic m.
Capnostat Mainstream carbon
dioxide m.
CUSA electrosurgical m.
dialysate preparation m.
Nd:YAG m.
Peak gait m.
SAM m.
Modulith
M. SL20 device for ESWL
M. SL 20 lithotriptor
Modulock
M. posterior spinal fixation
M. posterior spinal fixation device
Modulus CD anesthesia system
Moe
M. alar hook
M. bone curette
M. gouge
M. impactor
M. intertrochanteric plate
M. modified Harrington rod
M. nail
M. osteotome
M. subcutaneous rod
Moehle
M. cannula
M. corneal forceps
Moeller laser
Moeltgen flexometer
Moersch
M. bronchoscope
M. bronchoscopic forceps
M. cardiospasm dilator
M. electrode
M. esophagoscope
Moffat-Robinson bone pate collector
Mogen circumcision clamp
Mohr
M. finger splint
M. pinchcock clamp
moist
m. interactive dressing
moistened fine mesh gauze dressing
moisture
m. chamber
m. exchanger
moisture-retentive dressing
Mojave-Mini dehumidifier
molar bracket
mold
acrylic m.
Altchek vaginal m.
Aquaplast m.

M

mold *(continued)*
    Biothotic orthotic m.
    Counsellor vaginal m.
    CRYO rubber m.
    filter m.
    flavine wool m.
    Hydro-Cast dental m.
    Silastic m.
    silicone m.
    sodium alginate wool m.
    Swyrls swim m.
    Teflon m.

molded
    m. ankle-foot orthosis
    M. Bulb closed wound drainage reservoir
    m. postpartum insole

molding sock
Mold-In-Place back support
molectron laser
molecular sieve
moleskin
    m. bandage
    m. padding
    m. traction hitch dressing

Molestick padding
Molina
    M. mandibular distractor
    M. mandibular distractor set
    M. needle catheter

Moller microscope
Mollison
    M. mastoid rongeur
    M. self-retaining retractor

Molnar disk
Molt
    M. curette
    M. dissector
    M. mouthgag
    M. No. 4 elevator
    M. pedicle forceps
    M. periosteal elevator

Molteno
    M. double-plate implant
    M. drainage eye implant
    M. implant drainage device
    M. seton
    M. shunt tube

Moltz-Storz tonsillectome
molybdenum
    m. anode
    m. rotating-anode x-ray tube
    m. target tube

molybdenum-technetium generator
Mo-Mark curette
Momberg
    M. tourniquet
    M. tube

Momma-Too Maternity Support
Momosi spider lens intraocular lens
Monaco broach
Monaghan
    M. respirator
    M. 300 ventilator

Monahan-Lewis knife
Monaldi
    M. drain
    M. drainage system

Monarch
    M. II bleaching instrument
    M. IOL delivery system
    M. knee brace
    M. Mini Mask nasal interface

Monark
    M. bicycle
    M. bicycle ergometer
    M. Rehab Trainer

Mon-a-Therm
    M.-a.-T. thermocouple
    M.-a.-T. 6510 two-channel thermometer

Moncorps knife
Moncrieff
    M. anterior chamber irrigating cannula
    M. anterior chamber irrigator

MO needle
monitor
    Accucap CO_2/O_2 m.
    Accu-Chek Easy glucose m.
    Accu-Chek II Freedom blood glucose m.
    Accucom cardiac output m.
    Accutorr A1 blood pressure m.
    Accutorr bedside m.
    Accutracker blood pressure m.
    actocardiotocograph fetal m.
    Acuson V5M transesophageal echocardiographic m.
    Aequitron apnea m.
    AlphaCare m.
    ambulatory electrogram m. (AEM)
    antepartum m.
    apnea m.
    AR+ portable heart m.
    Arrhythmia Net m.
    Arvee model 2400 infant apnea m.
    automatic single-needle m. (ASN)
    Baby Dopplex 3000 antepartum fetal m.
    Bear NUM-1 tidal volume m.
    Bedfont carbon monoxide m.
    Behavior Assessment System for Children m.
    Biocon impedance plethysmography cardiac output m.
    Biotrack coagulation m.
    BladderScan m.
    blood perfusion m.
    Brackmann facial nerve m.
    Camino fiberoptic ICP m.
    Capintec nuclear VEST m.
    Capnogard capnograph m.
    Capnomac Ultima m.
    cardiac m.
    cardiac-apnea m.
    CardioBeeper CB-12L m.
    Cardiocap 5-patient m.
    CardioDiary heart m.

Cardioguard 4000
electrocardiographic m.
Cardiotach fetal m.
cardiovascular m.
Cardiovit AT-10 m.
CDI 2000 blood gas m.
cerebral function m.
Codman ICP m.
Codman intracranial pressure m.
Colin ambulatory BP m.
Colin STBP-780 stress test blood
pressure m.
Commucor A+V Patient m.
Companion 2 blood glucose m.
Contimed II pelvic floor muscle m.
Coremetrics fetal apnea m.
Corometrics maternal/fetal m.
Cortexplorer cerebral blood flow m.
CO2SMO m.
Cricket pulse oximetry m.
Criticare comprehensive vital
sign m.
Criticare ETCO$_2$/SpO$_2$ m.
Criticare 507-series noninvasive
blood pressure m.
Datex infrared CO$_2$ m.
DeltaTrac II metabolic m.
DeVilbiss Mini-Dop fetal m.
DeVilbiss OB-Dop fetal m.
Digitrapper Mark III sleep m.
Dinamap Plus vital signs m.
Doppler blood flow m.
Doppler Cavin m.
Doppler ultrasonic fetal heart m.
Doppler ultrasound m.
Doptone fetal m.
dosimetrist radiation beam m.
Duet glucose control m.
DynaPulse 5000A ambulatory blood
pressure m.
EarCheck m.
EcoCheck oxygen m.
EdenTec 2000W in-home
cardiorespiratory m.
electrocardiographic
transtelephonic m.
Endotek OM-3 Urodata m.
Endotek UDS-1000 m.
endotracheal cardiac output m.
Engstrom multigas m.
Escort 300A defibrillator/pacer m.
Eucotone m.
external m.
Fetal Dopplex m.
Fetalert fetal heart rate m.
fetal heart rate m.
FetalPulse Plus m.
Fetasonde fetal m.
Finapres blood pressure m.
Flo-Stat fluid m.
FreeDop Doppler m.
Gastroreflex ambulatory pH m.
Glucometer DEX blood glucose m.
GlucoScan m.
GlucoWatch bloodless glucose m.

Gould pressure m.
Haemogram blood loss m.
Healthdyne apnea m.
Heart Aide Plus m.
HeartCard m.
Heart Rate 1-2-3 m.
HemoTec activated clotting time m.
Hewlett-Packard 78720 A SDN m.
Holter m.
home uterine activity m.
Homochron m.
24-hour ambulatory gastric pH m.
HP M1350A fetal m.
Imex antepartum m.
infant ventilation m.
Ingold M-series glass electrode
pH m.
in-line blood gas m.
in-line venous pressure m.
Insta-Pulse heart rate m.
Interceptor M3 triple-channel, solid-
state m.
internal m.
intracranial pressure Express
digital m.
intrapartum m.
intrauterine pressure m.
Jako facial nerve m.
KinetiX ventilation m.
King of Hearts Holter m.
Kwik-Skan m.
Ladd intracranial pressure m.
LAPSE m.
laser Doppler perfusion m.
Laserflo BPM laser Doppler m.
Laserflow blood perfusion m.
Laserflow BPM^2 real time cerebral
perfusion m.
m. leads
Life-Pack 5 cardiac m.
Lifescope 12 bedside m.
Ligand plus 1, 2, 3,
noninvasive m.
long-term ambulatory physiologic
surveillance m.
LSR patent-pending bedside m.
Magellan m.
Marquette 8000 Holter m.
M. Master M. support
Meadox ICP m.
Medisense Pen 2 self blood
glucose m.
Medpacific LD 5000 Laser-Doppler
perfusion m.
MemoryTrace AT ambulatory
cardiac m.
Mentor B-VAT II m.
MiniOX I, II, III, 100-IV
oxygen m.
Moor MBF3D m.
Mortara ELI 100 12-lead m.
MRL blood pressure m.
MRM-2 oxygen consumption m.
Multinex ID gas m.
Myotone EMG m.

M

monitor *(continued)*
    MyoTRac2 EMG m.
    Myotrace neuromuscular block m.
    Nazorcap capnographic
      respiratory m.
    Nellcor N-499 fetal oxygen
      saturation m.
    Nellcor Nl0 ETCO$_2$/SpO$_2$ m.
    Nellcor Symphony N-3100
      noninvasive blood pressure m.
    neonatal m.
    Neo-trak 515A neonatal m.
    nerve-integrity m.
    NervePace nerve conduction m.
    Neuroguide m.
    Neurosign 100 nerve m.
    Nicolet Nerve Integrity M. (NIM-2)
    nocturnal penile tumescence m.
    noise level m.
    noninvasive continuous cardiac
      output m.
    NOxBOX II m.
    Ohio Vortex respiration m.
    Ohmeda 5250 respiratory gas m.
    Omega 5600 noninvasive blood
      pressure m.
    Omron Hem-601 automatic digital
      wrist blood pressure m.
    Omron/Marshall 97 automatic
      oscillometric digital blood
      pressure M.
    One Touch blood glucose m.
    Oxisensor fetal oxygen
      saturation m.
    Paratrend 7 continuous blood
      gas m.
    Passport bedside m.
    patient dose m.
    perfusion m.
    Pick and Go m.
    picture-in-picture m.
    Pocket-Dop fetal heart rate m.
    Polar Vantage XL heart rate m.
    Polar wrist m.
    Porta-Resp m.
    Press-Mate model 8800T blood
      pressure m.
    Pressore wrapping pressure m.
    PressureSense m.
    Pressurometer blood pressure m.
    ProDynamic m.
    Propaq Encore vital signs m.
    Puritan-Bennett 7250 metabolic m.
    Quik Connect fetal m.
    radiation beam m.
    Rascal II anesthetic gas m.
    respiratory function m.
    RigiScan penile tumescence and
      rigidity m.
    Rossmax automatic wristwatch blood
      pressure m.
    Scholar II vital sign m.
    Seer cardiac m.
    SentiLite neurological m.
    Sentinel-4 neurological m.
    Silverstein facial nerve m.
    sleep apnea m.
    Sonicaid Axis m.
    Sonicaid system 8000 fetal m.
    SpaceLabs Holter m.
    Spir-O-Flow peak flow m.
    Stat-Temp II liquid crystal
      temperature m.
    Steritek ICP mini m.
    SureStep glucose m.
    Surveyor m.
    TC CO$_2$ m.
    TempTrac temperature m.
    Terumo Doppler fetal heart rate m.
    Thermograph temperature m.
    TINA m.
    Toitu cardiovascular m.
    Tracer Blood Glucose m.
    transcutaneous carbon dioxide m.
    transcutaneous oxygen m.
    Transonic laser Doppler
      perfusion m.
    Trans-Scan 2100 noninvasive
      physiological m.
    transtelephonic exercise m.
    Tri-Met apnea m.
    ultrasound m.
    Vantage Performance m.
    VentCheck m.
    ventricular arrhythmia m.
    Verner-Smith m.
    VEST ambulatory ventricular
      function m.
    VIA arterial blood gas and
      chemistry m.
    video m.
    ViewSite video m.
    virtual labor m.
    Wakeling fetal heart m.
    WinABP ambulatory blood
      pressure m.
    Xomed-Treace nerve integrity m.
monitoring probe
MonitorMate monitor arm
MoniTorr
    M. CIP lumbar catheter
    M. ICP CSF drainage and
      monitoring system
Moniz carotid siphon
Monk hip prosthesis
Monks malar elevator
monoangle chisel
monoballoon
monoblock femoral component
monocortical screw
Monocryl
    M. poliglecaprone suture
monocular
    m. bandage
    m. eye dressing
    m. indirect ophthalmoscope
    m. patch
Monod punch forceps

monofilament
- m. absorbable suture
- m. clear suture
- m. green suture
- m. nylon suture
- m. polypropylene suture
- Semmes-Weinstein nylon m.
- m. skin suture
- m. snare wire
- SofTip m.
- m. steel suture
- m. wire suture

Monofixateur external fixator
Monoflex lens
monofoil catheter
Monogram total knee instrument
Monoject
- M. bone marrow aspirator
- M. laceration irrigation tray

Monojector fingerstick device
MonoLith single-piece mechanical lithotriptor
Monolyth oxygenator
monomer filter
monopolar
- m. cautery
- m. coagulating forceps
- m. electrocautery
- m. insulated forceps
- m. temporary electrode
- m. tissue forceps

Monopty needle
Monorail
- M. angioplasty catheter
- M. guide wire
- M. imaging catheter
- M. Piccolino catheter
- M. Speedy balloon

Monoscopy
- M. locking trocar
- M. locking trocar with Woodford spike

Monosof suture
monostrut
- M. Bjödork-Shiley valve
- m. cardiac valve prosthesis
- M. heart valve

monotube
- Howmedica m.

Monotube external fixator system
Monreal reflex hammer
Montague
- M. abrader
- M. proctoscope
- M. sigmoidoscope

Montando tube
Montefiore tracheal tube
Montenovesi
- M. cranial forceps
- M. cranial rongeur

Montgomery
- M. esophageal tube
- M. laryngeal keel
- M. laryngeal stent
- M. Safe-T-Tube

- M. salivary bypass tube
- M. speaking valve
- M. Stomeasure device
- M. strap
- M. strap dressing
- M. thyroplasty implant system
- M. tracheal cannula
- M. tracheal fenestrator
- M. tracheal T-tube
- M. tracheal tube
- M. tracheostomy
- M. T-tube
- M. vaginal speculum

Montgomery-Bernstine speculum
Montgomery-Lofgren tapered Safe-T-Tube
Monticelli-Spinelli
- M.-S. circular external fixation system
- M.-S. distractor
- M.-S. frame

Montreal positioner
Montrose dressing applicator
Moody fixation forceps
Moolgaoker forceps
Moon
- M. Boot
- M. Boot brace
- M. rectal retractor
- M. Walker

Moon-Robinson
- M.-R. prosthesis inserter
- M.-R. stapes prosthesis

Moonwalker weightbearing system
Moore
- M. adjustable nail
- M. blade plate
- M. bone drill
- M. bone elevator
- M. bone reamer
- M. bone retractor
- M. direction finder
- M. disk
- M. driver
- M. femoral neck prosthesis
- M. fixation pin
- M. gallbladder spoon
- M. gall duct scoop
- M. gallstone scoop
- M. hip endoprosthesis system
- M. hip endoprosthesis system stem
- M. hip prosthesis
- M. hollow chisel
- M. hooked extractor
- M. lens-inserting forceps
- M. measuring rod
- M. nail extractor
- M. nail set
- M. osteotome
- M. prosthesis extractor
- M. prosthesis-mortising chisel
- M. raspatory
- M. sliding nail plate
- M. spinal fusion gouge
- M. stem rasp
- M. template

M

Moore *(continued)*
    M. thoracoscope
    M. tracheostomy button
    M. tube
Moore-Blount
    M.-B. driver
    M.-B. extractor
    M.-B. plate
    M.-B. screwdriver
Moorehead
    M. cheek retractor
    M. dental retractor
    M. dissector
    M. ear knife
    M. elevator
    M. lid clamp
    M. periosteotome
Moore-Troutman corneal scissors
Moore-Wilson hyperopic conformer
Moorfields
    M. curette
    M. cystitome
Moor MBF3D monitor
MOP-Videoplan morphometric system
Moran-Karaya
    M.-K. disk
    M.-K. ring
    M.-K. sheet
morcellator
    Cook tissue m.
    Diva laparoscopic m.
    electric tissue m.
    electromechanical m.
    Elmore tissue m.
    high-speed electrical tissue m.
    motorized m.
    OPERA Star m.
    rotating m.
    Semm m.
    Steiner electromechanical m.
    tissue m.
morcellizer
    Rubin septal m.
    Yarmo m.
Morch
    M. respirator
    M. swivel adapter
    M. swivel tracheostomy tube
    M. ventilator
Moren-Moretz vena cava clip
Moreno gastroenterostomy clamp
Moretsky LASIK hinge protector
   fixation ring
Moretz
    M. clip
    M. prosthesis
    M. Tiny Tytan ventilation tube
    M. Tytan ventilation tube
Morfam Massager
Morgan
    M. proctoscope
    M. therapeutic lens
    M. vent tube introducer
Morgan-Boehm proctoscope

Morganstern
    M. aspiration/injection system
    M. continuous-flow operating
      cystoscope
Morgenstein
    M. blunt forceps
    M. gouge
    M. hook
    M. periosteal knife
    M. spatula
Morgenstein-Kerrison rongeur
Moria
    M. obturator
    M. one-piece speculum
    M. trephine
Moria-France dacryocystorhinostomy
   clamp
Moritz-Schmidt
    M.-S. knife
    M.-S. laryngeal forceps
Morpho exerciser
Morrell crown remover
Morris
    M. aortic clamp
    M. biphase screw
    M. cannula
    M. forceps
    M. mitral valve spreader
    M. retractor
    M. Silastic thoracic drain
    M. splint
    M. thoracic catheter
Morrison-Hurd
    M.-H. pillar retractor
    M.-H. tonsillar dissector
Morrison skin hook
Morrissey Gigli-saw guide
Morrow-Brown needle
Morscher
    M. anterior cervical plate
    M. titanium cervical plate
Morsch-Retec respirator
Morse
    M. backward-cutting aortic scissors
    M. blade
    M. head
    M. instrument handle
    M. manifold
    M. modified Finochietto retractor
    M. sternal retractor
    M. sternal spreader
    M. stopcock
    M. suction tube
    M. taper
    M. taper lock of modular hip
      implant component
    M. taper stem
    M. towel clip
    M. valve retractor
Morse-Andrews suction tube
Morse-Ferguson suction tube
Morson
    M. forceps
    M. trocar
Mortara ELI 100 12-lead monitor

mortising chisel
Morton
    M. bandage
    M. ophthalmoscope
    M. stone dislodger
    M. toe support
Mortson V-shaped clip
Morwel
    M. cannula
    M. silhouette suction apparatus
    M. ultrasound-assisted lipoplasty
     machine
    M. ultrasound device
Mosaic
    M. cardiac bioprosthesis
    M. valve
MOS capacitor
Mose concentric ring
Moseley
    M. fasciatome
    M. glenoid rim prosthesis
Mosher
    M. bag
    M. dilator
    M. drain
    M. esophagoscope
    M. ethmoid curette
    M. ethmoid punch forceps
    M. intubation tube
    M. Life Saver antichoke suction
     device
    M. lifesaver retractor
    M. life-saving tracheal suction tube
    M. nasal speculum
    M. strip
    M. urethral speculum
mosquito
    m. hemostat
    m. hemostatic clamp
    m. hemostatic forceps
    m. lid clamp
Moss
    M. balloon triple-lumen gastrostomy
     tube
    M. cage
    M. decompression feeding catheter
    M. feeding tube
    M. fixation system
    M. gastric decompression tube
    M. gastrostomy tube
    M. G-tube PEG kit
    M. hook
    M. instrumentation
    M. Mark IV tube
    M. Miami load-sharing spinal
     implant system
    M. nasal tube
    M. rod
    M. Suction Buster
    M. Suction Buster catheter
    M. Suction Buster tube
    M. suction buster tube
    M. T-anchor needle
    M. T-anchor needle introducer
    M. T-anchor needle introducer gun

Mossbauer spectrometer
Moss-Harms basket
Moss-Miami spinal instrumentation
Mosso sphygmomanometer
Motech cage
mother-baby
    m.-b. endoscope
    m.-b. endoscope system
mother-daughter endoscope
Mother Jones dressing
Mother-To-Be
    M.-T.-B. abdominal support
    M.-T.-B. Support Maternity Support
motility eye implant
motion
    controlled ankle m. (CAM)
    m. control mitt
motion-compensating format converter
Motivator FTR2000 exerciser
motorized
    m. meniscal shaver
    m. morcellator
Moto-tool
    Dremel M.-t.
Mot-R-Pak vitrectomy system
Mott
    M. double-ended retractor
    M. raspatory
Mottgen goniometer
Moule screw pin
Moult
    M. curette
    M. mouth prop
Moulton lacrimal duct tube
Mount intervertebral disk forceps
Mount-Mayfield aneurysm forceps
Mount-Olivecrona
    M.-O. clip applier
    M.-O. forceps
Mouradian
    M. humeral fixation system
    M. humeral rod
Moure-Coryllos rib shears
Moure esophagoscope
MouseMitt Keyboarders wrist support
Mouse Nest mouse rest
mouse-tooth
    m.-t. clamp
    m.-t. forceps
Mousseau-Barbin esophageal tube
moustache dressing
mouth
    m. gag
    m. lamp
    m. mask
mouthgag, mouth gag
    Boettcher-Jennings m.
    Boyle-Davis m.
    Brophy m.
    Brown-Davis m.
    Brown-Fillebrown-Whitehead m.
    Brown-Whitehead m.
    Collis m.
    Crowe-Davis m.
    Dann-Jennings m.

M

mouthgag *(continued)*
- Davis-Crowe m.
- Davis ring m.
- Denhardt m.
- Denhardt-Dingman m.
- Dilner-Doughty m.
- Dingman m.
- Dingman-Millard m.
- Dott m.
- Dott-Kilner m.
- Doxen m.
- Doyen-Jansen m.
- Ferguson m.
- Ferguson-Ackland m.
- Ferguson-Brophy m.
- Ferguson-Gwathmey m.
- m. frame
- Frohm m.
- Fulton m.
- Green m.
- Green-Sewall m.
- Hayton-Williams m.
- Heister m.
- Hewitt m.
- Hibbs m.
- Jansen m.
- Jansen-Sluder m.
- Jennings Loktite m.
- Jennings-Skillern m.
- Kilner m.
- Kilner-Dott m.
- Lane m.
- Lange m.
- Leivers m.
- Lewis m.
- Maunder oral screw m.
- McDowell m.
- McIvor m.
- McKesson m.
- Millard m.
- Mithoefer-Jansen m.
- Molt m.
- Negus m.
- Newkirk m.
- oral screw m.
- oral speculum m.
- palate-type m.
- Proetz m.
- Proetz-Jansen m.
- Pynchon m.
- Rabbit m.
- Ralks-Davis m.
- Rew-Wyly m.
- Roser m.
- Roser-Koenig m.
- Seeman-Seiffert m.
- side m.
- Sluder-Ferguson m.
- Sluder-Jansen m.
- Sydenham m.
- Thackray m.
- m. tongue depressor blade
- m. tooth plate
- Trousseau m.

- Wesson m.
- Whitehead m.
- Whitehead-Jennings m.
- Wolf Loktite m.

mouthguard
- Oxyguard oxygenating m.

MouthGuard oral protector

mouthpiece
- E-Z-Guard m.

Moxa heat therapy

Moynihan
- M. bile duct probe
- M. clip
- M. gallstone probe
- M. gallstone scoop
- M. intestinal forceps
- M. kidney pedicle forceps
- M. respirator
- M. speculum
- M. towel clamp
- M. towel forceps

Moynihan-Navratil forceps

MP-35 clip material

MP-A-1 catheter

MP-A-2 catheter

M-Pact
- M.-P. cast cutter
- M.-P. cast spreader
- M.-P. flexible orthotic

MPC
- MPC automated intravitreal scissors
- MPC coagulation forceps

MPD stent

MPL
- MPL aspirating syringe
- MPL dental needle
- MPL Hypo intraosseous needle

MPM
- MPM bandage
- MPM conductive hydrogel dressing
- MPM GelPad dressing
- MPM hydrogel dressing
- MPM I multi-parameter monitoring system
- MPM multilayer dressing

MPO Active walking Multi Podus boot

Mport
- M. foldable lens placement system
- M. lens inserter

MPR drain catheter

MP video endoscopic lens attachment

MR
- MR 290 humidification chamber
- MR proton spectroscopy
- MR simulator

MRI
- magnetic resonance imaging
  - dynamic contrast-enhanced MRI
  - Excelart short-bore MRI
  - functional MRI
  - Gyroscan superconducting MRI
  - intravenous-enhanced MRI
  - IV-enhanced MRI
  - multiplanar MRI
  - MRI probe head

proton-density-weighted MRI
rectal coil MRI
MRI scan
Siemens Vision MRI
surface-coil MRI
ThromboScan MRI
ultrafast MRI

MRL
    MRL blood pressure monitor
    MRL oximeter
MRM-2 oxygen consumption monitor
Mr. PainAway Health-Up TENS unit
MRT tidal humidifier
MSC-2001 ECG
MS Classique balloon dilatation catheter
M-series bur (M-1, M-2, etc.)
MSI nylon membrane
M.S. splint
MST cryoprobe
Mt.
    Mt. Clemens Hospital clip applier
    Mt. Sinai skull clamp pin
MTA
    M. brace
    M. headlamp
MTC Ventcontrol ventricular catheter
M-TEC 2000 surgical system
MTL trial frame
MTM 2 bur
MTS electrohydraulic piston
M-type extractor
Mucat
    M. cervical sampler
    M. cervical sampling device
Muck tonsillar forceps
mucosal
    m. elevator
    m. separator plate
mucotome
    Castroviejo-Steinhauser m.
    Norelco m.
mucous forceps
Mueller
    M. alkaline battery cautery
    M. aortic clamp
    M. bronchial clamp
    M. bur
    M. catheter
    M. coronary perfusion cannula
    M. curette
    M. Currentrol cautery
    M. electric corneal trephine
    M. electrocautery
    M. electronic tonometer
    M. eye shield
    M. eye speculum
    M. fixation device
    M. forceps
    M. giant eye magnet
    M. lacrimal sac retractor
    M. laparoscopic instrumentation
    M. needle
    M. pediatric clamp
    M. refractor
    M. saw

    M. shield eye implant
    M. suction tube
    M. telescope
    M. tongue blade
    M. total hip prosthesis
    M. Ultralite brace
    M. vena cava clamp
Mueller-Balfour self-retaining retractor
Mueller-Charnley hip prosthesis
Mueller-Frazier suction tube
Mueller-Hinton-supplemented agar plate
Mueller-LaForce adenotome
Mueller-Markham patent ductus forceps
Mueller-Poole suction tube
Mueller-Pynchon suction tube
Mueller-type
    M.-t. acetabular cup
    M.-t. femoral head replacement
Mueller-Yankauer suction tube
Muelly hook
Muenster cast
Muer anoscope
Mufson-Cushing retractor
Muhlberger
    M. orbital implant
    M. orbital prosthesis
Mühlemann periodontometer
Mui
    M. Scientific 6-channel esophageal
      pressure probe
    M. Scientific pressurized capillary
      infusion system
Muir
    M. hemorrhoidal forceps
    M. rectal cautery clamp
    M. rectal speculum
Muirhead-Little pelvic rest tractor
Muirhead pelvic rest
Muldoon
    M. lacrimal dilator
    M. lacrimal probe
    M. lid retractor
    M. meibomian forceps
    M. tube
mules
    Bishop-Harman m.
    Colibri m.
    M. eye implant
    Gill-Hess m.
    Graefe m.
    M. graft
    Halsted m.
    Heath m.
    Kulvin-Kalt m.
    Lister m.
    MacGregor m.
    Paton-Berens m.
    M. prosthesis
    M. scoop
    M. vitreous sphere
MULE upper limb exerciser
Mulholland growth guidance system
Mullan
    M. percutaneous trigeminal ganglion
      microcompression set

M

Mullan *(continued)*
    M. trigeminal ganglion
      microcompression set
    M. wire
Müller tray
Mulligan
    M. anastomosis clamp
    M. cervical biopsy punch
    M. dissector
    M. Silastic prosthesis
Mullins
    M. blade
    M. cardiac device
    M. sheath system
    M. tongue depressor
    M. transseptal catheter
    M. transseptal catheterization sheath
MultArray light
Multi
    M. Dopplex II
    M. Dopplex II Doppler
    M. Dopplex MDI vascular test unit
    M. Podus foot system
multi-access catheter
multiaxial screw
multiaxis foot
Multibite
    M. multiple sample biopsy forceps
MultiBoot orthosis
multicellular stent
multichannel
    m. analyzer
    m. cochlear implant
    m. signal averager
Multiclip disposable ligating clip device
multi-coordinate manipulator
Multicor
    M. Gamma pacemaker
    M. II cardiac pacemaker
multicoupled loop-gap resonator
multicrystal gamma camera
Multidex
    M. maltodextrin wound dressing
    M. wound-filling material
multidimensional
    m. analysis
    M. Scalogram Analysis
Multi-Dimensional Voice Program 4305
multidirectional distractor
MultiDop XS system
multielectrode
    m. basket catheter
    m. impedance catheter
    m. probe
multifilament
    m. steel suture
Multifire
    M. Endo GIA stapling device
    M. Endo hernia clip applier
    M. GIA
    M. GIA-series stapler
    M. TA-series stapler
multifire clip applicator

Multi-Fit Luer-Lok control tonsillar
    syringe
multiflanged Portnoy catheter
Multiflex catheter
Multi-Flex stent
MultiGuide mandibular distractor
MultiLase
    M. D copper vapor laser
    M. Nd:YAG surgical laser
multilayer design catheter
multilead electrode
multileaf
    m. collimating system
    m. collimator
    M. collimator device
MultiLight system
Multilink stent
Multilith pacemaker
multiload
    M. Cu-375 intrauterine device
    m. occlusive clip applicator
multiloaded
multiloaded clip applier
Multi-Lock
    M.-L. hand operating table
    M.-L. knee brace
multilumen
    m. manometric catheter
    m. probe
Multi-Med triple-lumen infusion catheter
Multinex ID gas monitor
Multi-Optics lens
MultiPad absorptive dressing
multiparameter sensor
multiparticle cyclotron
multiplanar
    m. mandibular distractor
    m. MRI
multiplane intracavitary probe
multiple
    m. automated sample harvester
    m. hook assembly C-D
      instrumentation
    m. jointed digitizer scanner
    M. Parameter telemetry device
multiple-piece intraocular lens
multiple-pin hole occluder
multiple-point electrode
multiplex catheter
Multi-Ply reusable electrode
multipoint contact plate
Multipoise headrest
multipolar
    m. bipolar cup
    m. electrode catheter
    m. impedance catheter
Multi-Pro 2000 biopsy needle
multiprogrammable
    m. pacemaker
    m. pulse generator
multiprong rake retractor
MultiPro table
Multipulse 1000 compression pump
multipurpose
    m. ball electrode

m. breathing circuit
m. catheter
m. clamp
m. forceps
m. laryngoscope
m. retractor
m. valve
multirod collimator
multisensor catheter
multisensory
m. ballpit
m. structured light range digitizer scanner
multispan fracture hook
Multispatula cervical sampling device
MultiSPIRO system
Multistim electrode catheter
multistrand suture
multitoothed cartilage forceps
multivane intensity modulation compensator
Multi-Vent
Hudson M.-V.
multiwire
m. gamma camera
m. proportional chamber
Mumford Gigli-saw guide
Munchen endometrial biopsy curette
Mundie placental forceps
Munich-Crosstreet anoscope
Munro
M. brain scissors
M. self-retaining retractor
Muraco vaporizer
Murdock eye speculum
Murdock-Wiener eye speculum
Murdoon eye speculum
Murless
M. fetal head extractor
M. head extractor forceps
M. head retractor
Murphy
M. ball-end hook
M. ball reamer
M. bone lever
M. bone skid
M. brace
M. button
M. chisel
M. common duct dilator
M. gallbladder retractor
M. gouge
M. intestinal needle
M. light
M. osteotome
M. plaster knife
M. punch
M. rake retractor
M. scissors
M. sling
M. splint
M. tonsillar forceps
Murphy-Balfour
M.-B. center blade
M.-B. retractor

Murphy-Johnson anastomosis button
Murphy-Lane
M.-L. bone elevator
M.-L. bone skid
M.-L. lever
Murphy-Péan hemostatic forceps
MurphyScope neurologic device
Murray
M. forceps
M. holder
M. knee prosthesis
Murray-Jones arm splint
Murray-Thomas arm splint
Murtagh self-retaining infant scalp retractor
muscle
m. biopsy clamp
m. forceps
m. hook
m. and neurological stimulation electrotherapy device
muscular tube
Museholdt nasal-dressing forceps
Museux
M. tenaculum
M. tenaculum forceps
M. uterine forceps
M. vulsellum forceps
Museux-Collins uterine vulsellum forceps
mush clamp
mushroom
m. catheter
m. impactor
m. walker glide
Musial tissue forceps
Musken tonometer
muslin dressing
Mussen frame
mustache dressing
Mustang steerable guide wire
Mustarde
M. awl
M. forceps
MVB blade
MVR blade
MVS
MVS cannula
MVS Phaco-Emulsifier
MVV ventilator
MX2-300 xenon quality light source
MycroMesh
M. + biomaterial
M. graft material
M. Plus biomaterial
myelography needle
Myelo-Nate
M.-N. needle
M.-N. set
Myerson
M. antral trocar
M. biting punch
M. biting tip
M. bronchial forceps
M. electrode
M. laryngeal forceps

M

Myerson *(continued)*
    M. laryngectomy saw
    M. resin
    M. wash tube
Myerson-Moncrieff cannula
Mylar catheter
Myles
    M. antral curette
    M. guillotine
    M. guillotine adenotome
    M. guillotine tonsillectome
    M. hemorrhoidal clamp
    M. hemorrhoidal forceps
    M. nasal forceps
    M. nasal punch
    M. nasal speculum
    M. sinus cannula
    M. tonsillectome snare
Myles-Ray speculum
Mynol endodontic cement
Myobock artificial hand
myocardial
    m. clamp
    m. dilator
    m. electrode
    m. lead
    M. Protection system
myochronoscope
Myocure
    M. blade
    M. blade scalpel
    M. knife
    M. phacoblade
myodynamometer
myoelectric prosthesis
Myoexorciser II, III portable EMG device
Myoexorciser 1000 recorder
myograph
    acoustic m.
    M. 2000 neuromuscular function analyzer

Myogyn II stimulator
Myojector
myokinesimeter
myoma
    m. fixation instrument
    m. screw
myomatome
    Segond m.
myometer
Myopulse muscle stimulator
MyoScan sensor
myoscope
myosthenometer
Myosynchron muscle stimulator
MYOterm XP cardioplegia delivery system
Myotest train-of-four nerve stimulator
Myotone EMG monitor
MyoTRac
    M. biofeedback incontinence training device
    M. EMG
MyoTRac2 EMG monitor
Myotrace neuromuscular block monitor
Myowire
    M. II cardiac electrode
Myriadlase Side-Fire laser
myringoplasty knife
myringotome
    barbed m.
    Buck m.
    Rica m.
    SMIC m.
myringotomy
    m. drain tube
    m. knife
    m. knife blade
    m. knife handle
Myrtle leaf probe
Mystic balloon catheter
M-Zole 7 Dual Pack

Nabatoff vein stripper
Nabors probe
Nachlas gastrointestinal tube
Nachlas-Linton
    N.-L. esophagogastric balloon
    tamponade device
    N.-L. tube
Naclerio diaphragm retractor
Nada-Chair Back-Up portable back sling
Naden-Rieth
    N.-R. implant
    N.-R. prosthesis
Nadler
    N. bipolar coaptation forceps
    N. superior radial scissors
Naegele obstetrical forceps
Naeser laser home treatment program
  for the hand
Nafion dryer line
Nagahara
    N. karate chopper
    N. phaco chopper
Nagaraja endoscopic nasal biliary
  drainage set
Nagashima
    N. antroscope trocar
    N. electrogustometer
    N. electronystagmograph
    N. LS-3 laryngostroboscope
    N. right-angle antroscope
Nagel anomaloscope
Nager
    N. palatal needle
    N. tonsillar needle
Nagielski needle
nail
    antegrade/retrograde compression n.
    Augustine boat n.
    Bickel intramedullary n.
    Biomet ankle arthrodesis n.
    blind medullary n.
    boat n.
    Böhler hip n.
    Brooker double-locking unreamed
      tibial n.
    Brooker-Wills n.
    cannulated n.
    Capener n.
    Chandler unreamed interlocking
      tibial n.
    closed Küntscher n.
    cloverleaf n.
    crutch and belt femoral closed n.
    Curry hip n.
    Delitala T-nail n.
    Delta Recon n.
    Derby n.
    diamond n.
    Dooley n.
    double-ended n.
    n. drill
    elastic stable intramedullary n.

Ender n.
Engel-May n.
flexible intramedullary n.
fluted Sampson n.
fluted titanium n.
four-flanged n.
Gamma trochanteric locking n.
Gissane spike n.
Grosse-Kempf femoral n.
Grosse-Kempf locking n.
Grosse-Kempf tibial n.
Hagie pin n.
Hahn bone n.
half-and-half n.
Hansen-Street self-broaching n.
Hansen-Street solid intramedullary n.
Harris condylocephalic n.
Harris hip n.
Harris medullary n.
hooked intramedullary n.
hooked medullary n.
IM n.
IMSC five-hole n.
INRO surgical n.
Inro surgical n.
intramedullary ANK n.
intramedullary (IM) n.
intramedullary supracondylar
  multihole n.
Inyo n.
Jewett hip n.
Johannson hip n.
Kaessmann n.
Ken sliding n.
Kirschner interlocking
  intramedullary n.
Knowles pin n.
Koslowski hip n.
Küntscher cloverleaf n.
Küntscher intramedullary n.
Lewis n.
Lottes triflange intramedullary n.
Macmed pediatric intramedullary n.
Massie II n.
Massie sliding n.
McKee tri-fin n.
McLaughlin n.
medullary n.
Moe n.
Moore adjustable n.
Neufeld n.
n. nipper
noncannulated n.
Nylok self-locking n.
Nystroem hip n.
Nystroem-Stille hip n.
OEC-Kuntscher Interlocking
  Pathfinder n.
Orthofix intramedullary n.
OrthoSorb pin n.
Palmer bone n.
Peterson n.

N

nail *(continued)*
    Pidcock n.
    n. plate
    Pugh self-adjusting n.
    Recon n.
    ReVision n.
    R-T n.
    Rush intramedullary n.
    Russell-Taylor delta tibial n.
    Russell-Taylor interlocking
      medullary n.
    Rydell n.
    Sampson fluted n.
    Schneider intramedullary n.
    n. scissors
    Seidel humeral locking n.
    Slocum-Smith-Petersen n.
    slotted n.
    Smillie n.
    Smith-Petersen cannulated n.
    Smith-Petersen femoral neck n.
    Smith-Petersen transarticular n.
    spring-loaded n.
    Staples osteotomy n.
    Steinmann extension n.
    supracondylar n.
    Sven Johansson femoral neck n.
    Synthes titanium elastic n.
    Temple University n.
    Terry n.
    Thatcher n.
    Thornton n.
    Tiemann n.
    titanium elastic n.
    True/Flex intramedullary n.
    Uniflex intramedullary n.
    Venable-Stuck n.
    Vesely n.
    Vesely-Street n.
    Vitallium n.
    V-medullary n.
    Watson-Jones n.
    Webb bolt n.
    Williams interlocking Y n.
    Z-fixation n.
    Zickel n.
    Zimmer telescoping n.
nail-bending device
nail-cutting forceps
nail-driving guidewire
nail-extracting forceps
nailfold capillary microscope
nail nipper
    Turnbull n. n.
nail-nipper scissors
nail-pulling forceps
Nakamura brace
Nakao
    N. Ejector biopsy forceps
    N. snare I and II
Nakayama
    N. anastomosis apparatus
    N. clamp
    N. microvascular stapler

    N. ring
    N. staple
Na-K exchange pump
Nalebuff-Goldman strut
Nalzene filter
Namic
    N. angiographic syringe
    N. catheter
    N. localization needle
NAMI DDV ligator
Nanolas Nd:YAG laser
Nanos 1 pacemaker
napkin ring calcar allograft
Naraghi-DeCoster reduction clamp
Narco
    N. Biosystems rectilinear recorder
    N. esophageal motility machine
    N. Physiograph-6B recorder
Narcomatic flowmeter
Narkomed anesthesia machine
Narkotest meter
narrow
    n. AO dynamic compression plate
    n. Deaver retractor
    n. elevator
    n. gauze roll
    n. lens
    n. washer
narrow-base quad cane
narrow-bite bone rongeur
NarrowFlex intra-aortic balloon catheter
nasal
    n. alligator forceps
    n. aspirator
    n. bivalve speculum
    n. bone forceps
    n. cartilage-holding forceps
    n. catheter
    n. chisel
    n. curette
    n. dilator
    n. dissector
    n. dorsal implant
    n. endoscopic telescope
    n. gouge
    n. hump-cutting forceps
    n. insertion forceps
    n. irrigator
    n. knife
    n. knife blade
    n. lower lateral forceps
    n. mallet
    n. needle holder forceps
    n. osteotome
    n. pack
    n. packing
    n. polyp forceps
    n. polyp hook
    n. probe
    n. prongs
    n. punch
    n. rasp
    n. retractor
    n. saw
    n. saw blade

n. scissors
n. septal forceps
n. snare
n. snare cannula
n. snare wire
n. snare wire carrier
n. splint
n. suction cup
n. suction tube
n. suture needle
n. tampon
n. tamponade
n. tampon sponge
n. tenaculum
n. trumpet
nasal-cutting forceps
nasal-dressing forceps
nasal-packing forceps
nasal-tip dressing
Nasa-Spec nasal speculum
Nash needle
Nashold
N. biopsy needle
N. TC electrode
nasobiliary
n. catheter
n. drain
n. tube
nasocystic
n. catheter
n. drain
n. drainage tube
nasoendoscope
Hirschman n.
nasoendotracheal tube
nasoenteric
n. feeding tube
nasofrontal
n. osteotome
n. suture
nasogastric
n. feeding tube
nasoileal tube
nasojejunal tube
nasolacrimal duct probe
nasolaryngopharyngoscope
flexible, steerable n.
nasolaryngoscope
Machida n.
nasomaxillary balloon
nasometer
nasopancreatic catheter
nasopharyngeal
n. biopsy forceps
n. fiberscope
n. retractor
n. speculum
nasopharyngolaryngofiberscope
Pentax n.
nasopharyngolaryngoscope
nasopharyngoscope
Broyles n.
flexible n.
Holmes n.
Meltzer n.

National n.
Smith & Nephew ENT n.
nasostat
Gottschalk n.
Naso-Tamp nasal packing sponge
nasotracheal
n. catheter
n. tube
nasovesicular catheter
Natchez Mobil-Trac system
Nathan pacemaker
National
N. all-metric transilluminator
N. cautery
N. cautery electrode
N. coagulator
N. ear speculum
N. electricator
N. general purpose cystoscope
N. Graves vaginal speculum
N. nasopharyngoscope
N. opal-glass transilluminator
N. proctoscope
natural
n. pacemaker
N. Profile abutment system
n. suture
NaturaLase
N. erbium laser
N. Er:YAG laser
natural-feel breast prosthesis
Natural-Hip
N.-H. prosthesis
N.-H. titanium hip stem
Natural-Knee II system
Natural-Lok
N.-L. acetabular cup
N.-L. acetabular cup prosthesis
Natvig wire-twister forceps
Naugh os calcis apparatus
Naugle orbitometer exophthalmometer
Nauth traction device
Navarre interventional radiology device
navicular screw
Navigator flexible endoscope
Navius stent
Navratil
N. retractor
N. stirrups
Nazorcap capnographic respiratory monitor
NBIH catheter
NC
NC Bandit catheter
NC Big Ranger OTW balloon catheter
NC Cobra balloon
NCC Hi-Lo Jet endotracheal tube
NC-stat nerve conduction system
NDM
N. adhesive wound dressing
N. Power-Point electrosurgical generator
NDSB occlusion balloon catheter

N

Nd:YAG
    neodymium:YAG laser
    neodymium:yttrium-aluminum-garnet
      Nd:YAG laser system
      Nd:YAG module
Nd:YLF laser
Neal
    N. catheter
    N. catheter trocar
    N. fallopian cannula
    N. insufflator
near-infrared
    n.-i. electronic endoscope
    n.-i. spectroscope
Nearly Me breast form
Nebauer
    N. ophthalmoendoscope
    N. ophthalmoscope
NEB total hip prosthesis
Nebuhaler inhaler
nebulization ventilator
nebulizer
    Acorn II n.
    AeroSonic personal ultrasonic n.
    AeroTech II n.
    air-powered n.
    bulb-operated n.
    Centimist n.
    Compu-Neb ultrasonic n.
    Dench n.
    DeVilbiss Pulmo-Aide n.
    Dura-Neb 2000 portable n.
    Emerson-Segal Medimizer
     demand n.
    Fisons n.
    G5 Mist-Ease n.
    hand-held n.
    Hudson T Up-Draft II disposable n.
    Incenti-neb n.
    jet n.
    John Bunn Mini-Mist n.
    Kidde n.
    Marquest Respirgard II n.
    medicinal n.
    Medi-Mist n.
    Metermatic nasal n.
    Micro-Mist disposable n.
    MicroSeal n.
    Microstat ultrasonic n.
    MiniHEART n.
    Mini-Neb n.
    Mistogen n.
    Misty-Neb n.
    Omron compressor n.
    penicillin n.
    PermaNeb n.
    Pulmo-Aide n.
    PulmoMate n.
    Pulmosonic ultrasonic n.
    Raindrop medication n.
    Respirgard II n.
    Schuco 2000 n.
    Selrodo n.
    Shuco-Myst n.
    side-arm n.
    small volume n.
    spinning disk n.
    Tote-A-Neb n.
    Twin Jet n.
    Ultra-Neb n.
    ultrasonic n.
    updraft n.
Necelon surgical gloves
neck
    n. rest
    n. roll
    n. support
neckband
    Zipper Medical tracheostomy
     tube n.
Neckcare pillow
Neck-Hugger cervical support pillow
Neck-Roll aromatherapy hot/cold pack
Necktrac traction device
neck-wrap halter
Nec Loc cervical collar
needle
    Abrams biopsy n.
    abscission n.
    Accucore II biopsy n.
    Accuject dental n.
    Ackerman n.
    Acland n.
    ACS n.
    Acumaster acupuncture n.
    Adair-Veress n.
    Addix n.
    Adson aneurysm n.
    Adson-Murphy trocar point n.
    Adson scalp n.
    Adson suture n.
    advancement n.
    Agnew tattooing n.
    Agrikola tattooing n.
    air aspirator n.
    Albarran-Reverdin n.
    Alcon CU-15 4-mil n.
    Alcon irrigating n.
    Alcon reverse cutting n.
    Alcon spatula n.
    Alcon taper-cut n.
    Alcon taper-point n.
    Aldrete n.
    Alexander tonsil n.
    Alexander tonsillar n.
    Altmann n.
    AMC n.
    Amersham CDCS A-type n.
    Amplatz angiography n.
    Amsler aqueous transplant n.
    Anchor surgical n.
    aneurysm n.
    angiography n.
    angular n.
    antral trocar n.
    antrum-exploring n.
    aortic root perfusion n.
    aortography n.
    aqueous transplant n.
    Arkan sharpening-stone n.

Arrow-Fischell EVAN n.
arterial n.
arteriography n.
ASAP channel cut automated
  biopsy n.
ASAP prostate biopsy n.
aspirating n.
aspiration biopsy n.
Atkinson retrobulbar n.
Atkinson single-bevel blunt-tip n.
Atkinson tip peribulbar n.
Atraloc n.
atraumatic n.
Austin n.
AV fistula n.
Babcock n.
Backlund biopsy n.
Ballade n.
Barbara n.
Bard biopsy n.
Bard Biopty cut n.
Barker n.
Barraquer n.
Barraquer-Vogt n.
Barrett hebosteotomy n.
Bauer Temno biopsy n.
BD bone marrow biopsy n.
BD Safety-Gard n.
BD SafetyGlide shielding
  hypodermic n.
Beath n.
Becton Dickinson Teflon-sheathed n.
Bengash n.
bent blunt n.
Berbecker n.
Bergeret-Reverdin n.
Berges-Reverdin n.
Bergström n.
beveled thin-walled n.
Beyer paracentesis n.
bicurved n.
Biegelseisen n.
Bier lumbar puncture n.
Bierman n.
biopsy n.
Biopty cut biopsy n.
Biosearch n.
bipolar n.
Birtcher electrosurgical n.
Black-Decker n.
Blackmon n.
Blair-Brown n.
bleeding n.
blunt n.
blunt-end sialogram n.
bone marrow biopsy n.
Bonney n.
boomerang bladder n.
Bovie n.
Bowman cataract n.
Bowman iris n.
Bowman stop n.
brain biopsy n.
Braun n.

breast localization n.
BRK-series transseptal n.
Brockenbrough curved n.
Brockenbrough transseptal n.
Brophy n.
Brophy-Deschamps n.
Brown cleft palate n.
Brown-Sanders fascial n.
Brown staphylorrhaphy n.
Brughleman n.
Brunner ligature n.
Buerger prostatic n.
Buncke quartz n.
Bunnell tendon n.
Burr butterfly n.
butterfly n.
BV2 n.
Calhoun n.
Calhoun-Hagler lens n.
Calhoun-Merz n.
Campbell ventricular n.
cardioplegic n.
Cardiopoint cardiac surgery n.
Carlens n.
carotid angiogram n.
Carpule n.
Carroll n.
Castroviejo vitreous-aspirating n.
cataract n.
cataract-aspirating n.
catgut n.
catheter n.
n. catheter jejunostomy
caudal n.
CD-5 n.
CE-24 n.
cerebral angiography n.
cervical suture n.
cesium n.
Charles flute n.
Charles vacuuming n.
Charlton antral n.
Chiba biopsy n.
Chiba eye n.
Chiba transhepatic
  cholangiography n.
Child-Phillips intestinal plication n.
Cibis ski n.
CIF n.
Clagett n.
Clas von Eichen n.
Cleasby spatulated n.
cleft palate n.
Cloquet n.
coaxial sheath cut-biopsy n.
Cobb-Ragde n.
Cobe AV fistular n.
Colapinto transjugular n.
Colorado microdissection n.
Colts cutting n.
Colver tonsillar n.
concentric n.
Concept Multi-Liner lining n.
Concept suturing n.
cone biopsy n.

N

needle *(continued)*

Cone ventricular n.
Conrad-Crosby bone marrow biopsy n.
Continental n.
Control Release pop-off n.
conventional n.
Cook endomyocardial n.
Cook Longdwel n.
Cook percutaneous entry n.
Cooley aortic vent n.
Cooley ventricular n.
Cooper chemopallidectomy n.
Cooper ligature n.
Cooper pallidectomy n.
CooperVision irrigating n.
CooperVision spatulated n.
Cope pleural biopsy n.
Cope thoracentesis n.
copper-clad steel n.
Core CO$_2$ insufflation n.
corneal suture n.
Corson n.
Costen iris n.
couching n.
Cournand arterial n.
Cournand arteriography n.
Cournand-Grino angiography n.
Cournand-Potts n.
Craig biopsy n.
Crawford fascial n.
Crosby biopsy n.
Crown n.
C-type acupuncture n.
CU-8 n.
Culp biopsy n.
Curran knife n.
Curry cerebral n.
curved suture n.
curved transjugular n.
CUSALap ultrasonic accessory n.
Cushing ventricular n.
cut biopsy n.
cut taper n.
cutting n.
cyclodiathermy n.
dacryocystorhinostomy n.
Daily cataract n.
Daiwa dental n.
Damshek n.
Dandy-Cairns brain n.
Dandy-Cairns ventricular n.
Dandy ventricular n.
Dattner n.
Davis knife n.
Davis tonsillar n.
Dean antral n.
Dean iris n.
Dean knife n.
Dean-Senturia n.
DeBakey n.
debridement n.
Dees renal n.
Dees suture n.

Deknatel K-n.
Delbet-Reverdin n.
Denis Browne cleft palate n.
DePuy-Weiss tonsillar n.
D'Errico ventricular n.
Deschamps ligature n.
Deschamps-Navratil ligature n.
desiccation n.
desiccation-fulguration n.
Desmarres paracentesis n.
Devonshire n.
diamond-point suture n.
Diamond SharpPoint n.
diathermal n.
diathermic precut n.
Dieckmann intraosseous n.
Dingman malleable passing n.
discission n.
diskogram n.
diskographic n.
disposable acupuncture n.
disposable aspiration n.
disposable biopsy n.
disposable injection n.
disposable suturing n.
Dispos-A-Ture single-use surgical n.
n. dissector
Dix n.
DLP cardioplegic n.
DN acupuncture n.
docking n.
Docktor n.
Dorsey n.
Dos Santos lumbar aortography n.
double-barreled n.
double-hub emulsifying n.
double-lumen n.
double-tipped center-threading n.
double-webbed n.
Douglas suture n.
Doyen n.
dragonhead n.
Drapier n.
Drews cataract n.
Drews lavage n.
n. driver
DS-9 n.
D-Tach removable n.
Duff debridement n.
dumbbell n.
Dupuy-Dutemps n.
Dupuy-Weiss tonsillar n.
dural n.
Durham n.
Durrani dorsal vein complex ligation n.
DuVries n.
Dyonics n.
East-Grinstead n.
Echo-Coat ultrasound biopsy n.
echogenic n.
egress n.
EJ bone marrow biopsy n.
n. electrode
Electrodes n.

electrosurgical n.
Ellis foreign body n.
Elschnig extrusion n.
Emmet n.
Emmet-Murphy n.
Empire n.
Endopath Ultra Veress n.
n. endosteal implant
Entree disposable CO_2
  insufflation n.
epilation n.
Epstein n.
Erosa disposable hypodermic n.
Espocan combined spinal/epidural n.
Estridge ventricular n.
Ethalloy TruTaper cardiovascular n.
Ethicon BV-75-3 n.
Ethicon ST-4 straight taper-point n.
Ethicon TG Plus n.
Ethicon TGW n.
Ethiguard n.
Euro-Med FNA-21 aspiration n.
eXcel-DR disposable/reusable Glasser
  laparoscopic n.
eXcel-DR pneumothorax n.
exploring n.
extended round n.
ExtraSafe butterfly infusion n.
extrusion n.
eyed suture n.
eyeless atraumatic suture n.
E-Z-EM cut biopsy n.
Falk n.
Farah cystoscopic n.
fascial n.
Federspiel n.
Feild-Lee biopsy n.
Fein n.
Fergie n.
Ferguson round-body n.
Ferguson suture n.
Ferris disposable bone marrow
  aspiration n.
filiform steel n.
filter n.
fine intestinal n.
Finochietto n.
Fischer pneumothoracic n.
Fisher eye n.
fishhook n.
fistula n.
flat spatula n.
flexible aspiration n.
flexible biopsy n.
flexible injection n.
Floyd pneumothorax n.
flute n.
Flynt aortography n.
Foltz n.
n. forceps
foreign body n.
four-sided cutting n.
Frackelton fascial n.
Framer tendon-passing n.
Francke n.

Frankfeldt hemorrhoidal n.
Franklin liver puncture n.
Franklin-Silverman prostatic
  biopsy n.
Franseen liver biopsy n.
Frazier ventricular n.
Frederick pneumothoracic n.
Frederick pneumothorax n.
French-eye n.
French spring-eye n.
Fritz vitreous transplant n.
front wall n.
full-intensity n.
27G n.
Gallie fascial n.
Gallini bone marrow aspiration n.
GAN-19 n.
ganglion injection n.
Gardner n.
gastrointestinal n.
general closure n.
Geuder corneal n.
Geuder keratoplasty n.
Gill n.
Gillmore n.
GIP/Medi-Globe prototype n.
Girard anterior chamber n.
Girard cataract-aspirating n.
Girard phacofragmatome n.
Girard-Swan n.
gold n.
Goldbacher rectal n.
Goldmann knife n.
Gordh n.
Gorsch n.
Graefe iris n.
GraNee n.
Grantham lobotomy n.
Greene n.
Greenfield n.
Green-Gould n.
Greenwald n.
Grice suture n.
Grieshaber corneal n.
Grieshaber iris n.
Grieshaber ophthalmic n.
Gripper n.
GS-9 n.
Guest n.
Gynex extended-reach n.
Haab knife n.
Hagedorn operation suture n.
half-intensity n.
Halle septal n.
Halsey n.
hammer-type acupuncture n.
harelip n.
Harken heart n.
Harvard n.
Haverhill n.
Hawkeye suture n.
Hawkins-Akins n.
Hawkins breast localization n.
Hearn n.
heart n.

N

needle *(continued)*
    Hegar n.
    Hegar-Baumgartner n.
    Hemoject n.
    hemorrhoidal n.
    Henton suture n.
    Henton tonsillar n.
    heparin-flushing n.
    Hessburg lacrimal n.
    Hey-Groves n.
    Heyner double n.
    high-risk n.
    Hingson-Edwards n.
    Hingson-Ferguson n.
    Hobbs n.
    Hoen ventricular n.
    n. holder
    n. holder clamp
    Holinger n.
    hollow n.
    Homer localizaton n.
    Homerlok n.
    hooked n.
    hookwire n.
    Hosford-Hicks n.
    Hourin tonsillar n.
    House-Barbara shattering n.
    House-Rosen n.
    House stapes n.
    Howard Jones n.
    Howell biliary aspiration n.
    Howell biopsy aspiration n.
    Huber point n.
    Hunstad infusion n.
    Hunt n.
    Hurd suture n.
    Hustead epidural n.
    Hutchins biopsy n.
    n. hydrophone
    hypodermic n.
    Hypospray jet injection n.
    Icofly infusion n.
    Ilg n.
    Iliff-Wright fascia n.
    Illinois n.
    illuminated suction n.
    Impex aspiration & injection n.
    Indian club n.
    Infusaid n.
    Ingersoll tonsillar n.
    injection n.
    insulated electrode n.
    internal nucleus hydrodelineation n.
    intestinal plication n.
    intraosseous n.
    intravenous n.
    Iocare titanium n.
    IOLAB irrigating n.
    IOLAB taper-cut n.
    IOLAB taper-point n.
    IOLAB titanium n.
    iridium n.
    iris n.
    irrigating-positioning n.

    Ito n.
    IV n.
    J n.
    Jalaguier-Reverdin n.
    Jameson strabismus n.
    Jamshidi adult n.
    Jamshidi-Kormed bone marrow biopsy n.
    Jamshidi liver biopsy n.
    Jelco n.
    JMS injection n.
    Jonesco wire suture n.
    Jordan n.
    Kader fishhook n.
    Kall modification of Silverman n.
    Kalt corneal n.
    Kalt eye n.
    Kalt vein n.
    Kangnian acupuncture n.
    Kaplan tracheostomy n.
    Kara cataract n.
    Karras angiography n.
    Keith abdominal n.
    Kelly intestinal n.
    Kelman n.
    KeyMed disposable variceal injection n.
    kidney suturing n.
    King suture n.
    Klatskin liver biopsy n.
    Klein infiltration n.
    Klima-Rosegger sternal n.
    Knapp iris knife n.
    Knight biopsy n.
    Kobak n.
    Koch nucleus hydrolysis n.
    Kohn n.
    Koontz hernia n.
    Kopan breast lesion localization n.
    Kormed disposable liver biopsy n.
    Kratz diamond-dusted n.
    Kronecker aneurysm n.
    lacrimal n.
    Lagleyze n.
    Lahey n.
    Laminex n.
    Lane cleft palate n.
    Lane suturing n.
    Lapides n.
    Laredo-Bard n.
    large-bore slotted aspirating n.
    Lee n.
    Lee & Westcott n.
    Leighton n.
    Lemmon n.
    L'Esperance n.
    Lewicky n.
    Lewis Pair-Pak n.
    Lewy-Holinger Teflon injection n.
    Lewy-Rubin Teflon glycerine-mixture injection n.
    Lewy Teflon glycerine-mixture injection n.
    Lichtwicz antral n.
    Lichtwicz-Bier antral n.

ligature n.
Lindeman transfusion n.
Linton-Blakemore n.
Lipschwitz n.
List n.
Litvak-Pereyra ligature n.
liver biopsy n.
lobotomy n.
lock n.
long n.
Longdwel catheter n.
Look retrobulbar n.
Loopuyt n.
Lo-Trau side-cutting n.
Lowell pleural n.
Lowette n.
Lowette-Verner n.
Lowsley ribbon-gut n.
LR n.
Luer n.
Luer-Lok n.
Lukens n.
lumbar aortography n.
lumbar puncture n.
Lundy fascial n.
Lundy-Irving caudal n.
Luongo n.
LX n.
Madayag biopsy n.
Maddox caudal n.
Magielski n.
Mahurkar fistular n.
malleable passing n.
Maltz n.
Maltzman n.
Mammalok localization n.
Manan cutting n.
Mantoux n.
March laser sclerostomy n.
Marion-Reverdin n.
Markham biopsy n.
Martin uterine n.
Marx n.
Mason-School aspirating n.
Masson fascial n.
Mathieu n.
Maumenee vitreous-aspirating n.
Mayo catgut n.
Mayo intestinal n.
Mayo trocar n.
Mayo trocar-point n.
McCaslin n.
McCurdy staphylorrhaphy n.
McDowell n.
McGee prosthesis n.
McGhan plastic surgical n.
McGowan n.
McGregor n.
McIntyre I&A n.
McIntyre irrigation/aspiration n.
mediastinoscopy aspirating n.
Medicut intravenous n.
Medisystems fistular n.
Menghini liver biopsy n.
meniscal repair n.

Mentor prostate biopsy n.
metal n.
metallic frontal n.
Metcoff pediatric biopsy n.
Meyer cyclodiathermy n.
Mick afterloading n.
MicroFlow phacoemulsification n.
Microlet electrode n.
micron n.
micropoint n.
micropuncture introducer n.
micro round-tip n.
Microvasive sclerotherapy n.
Millet n.
milliner's n.
Mixter ventricular n.
Mizzy n.
MO n.
modified CIF n.
modified spatula n.
Monopty n.
Morrow-Brown n.
Moss T-anchor n.
MPL dental n.
MPL Hypo intraosseous n.
Mueller n.
Multi-Pro 2000 biopsy n.
Murphy intestinal n.
myelography n.
Myelo-Nate n.
Nager palatal n.
Nager tonsillar n.
Nagielski n.
Namic localization n.
nasal suture n.
Nash n.
Nashold biopsy n.
Nelson ligature n.
neurography n.
neurosurgical suture n.
Neville ascending aortic air vent n.
Newman rectal injection n.
New oral n.
Nichols-Deschamps-Navratil
  ligature n.
Noci stimuli n.
NoKor n.
noncoring Huber n.
noncutting suture n.
nonferromagnetic n.
Nordenstrom Rotex II biopsy n.
nucleus hydrolysis n.
Oaks double n.
O'Brien airway n.
obstetrical block anesthesia n.
Ochsner n.
Oldfield n.
olive-tipped n.
Olympus NM-K-series
  sclerotherapy n.
Olympus NM-L-series n.
Olympus reusable oval cup forceps
  with n.
OmniTip side-firing laser n.
Op-Pneu laparoscopy n.

N

needle *(continued)*

optical n.
Optivis Surgalloy n.
oral n.
Osgood n.
Osterballe precision n.
Ostycut bone biopsy n.
Overholt rib n.
Pace ventricular n.
Page n.
Palmer-Drapier n.
palpating n.
Pannett n.
Paparella straight n.
paracentesis n.
paracervical nerve block n.
paraPRO n.
Parhad n.
Parhad-Poppen n.
Parker n.
Parker-Pearson n.
Payr vein n.
PC-7 n.
pediatric biopsy n.
Pencan spinal n.
Penfield biopsy n.
Pentax prototype n.
PercuCut biopsy n.
PercuCut cut-biopsy n.
PercuGuide n.
percutaneous cutting n.
Pereyra n.
peribulbar n.
pericardiocentesis n.
permanent n.
Permark micropigmentation n.
PermaSharp suture and n.
Pharmaseal n.
pilot n.
Pischel n.
Pitkin n.
plain eye n.
pleural biopsy n.
plication n.
Plum-Blossom acumpuncture n.
Pneumo-Matic insufflation n.
Pneumo-Needle n.
pneumoperitoneum n.
pneumothoracic injection n.
n. point suture passer/incision closure guide
Politzer paracentesis n.
polypropylene n.
polytef-sheathed n.
pop-off n.
Poppen ventricular n.
positioning n.
postmortem suture n.
Potocky n.
Potter n.
Potts n.
Potts-Cournand angiography n.
PrecisionGlide n.
precision lancet cutting n.

Presbyterian Hospital ventricular n.
Pricker n.
n. probe
probe n.
ProBloc insulated regional block n.
Promex biopsy n.
prostatic biopsy n.
Protect.Point n.
PS-2 n.
pudendal block anesthesia n.
Pulec n.
puncture n.
puncture-tip n.
Punctur-Guard n.
Quantico n.
quartz n.
Quincke-Babcock n.
Quincke-point spinal n.
Quincke spinal n.
radium ^{226}Ra n.
Radpour n.
Ranfac soft-tissue n.
Rashkind septostomy n.
razor-tip n.
RCB biopsy n.
rectal injection n.
renal n.
retrobulbar n.
Retter aneurysm n.
Reverdin suture n.
reverse-cutting n.
Rhoton straight point n.
rib n.
ribbon gut n.
Rica aneurysm n.
Rica cerebral angiography puncture n.
Rica suturing n.
Rider-Moeller n.
Riedel corneal n.
Riley arterial n.
Ring drainage catheter n.
Riza-Ribe n.
Robb n.
Roberts n.
Robinson-Smith n.
Rochester aortic vent n.
Rochester-Meeker n.
Rolf lance n.
root n.
Rosen n.
Rosenthal aspiration n.
Roser n.
Ross n.
Rotex II biopsy n.
round body n.
Rubin n.
Rubin-Arnold n.
Ruskin antral trocar n.
Ruskin sphenopalatine ganglion n.
Rutner biopsy n.
Rycroft n.
Sabreloc spatula n.
Sachs n.
SafeTap tapered spinal n.

Safety AV fistula n.
Sahli n.
Salah sternal puncture n.
SampleMaster biopsy n.
Sanders-Brown n.
Sanders-Brown-Shaw aneurysm n.
Sarot n.
Sato cataract n.
Saunders cataract n.
Saunders-Paparella n.
Savariaud-Reverdin n.
SC-1 n.
Scabbard n.
scalpene n.
scalp vein n.
Schanz n.
Schecter-Bryant aortic vent n.
Scheer n.
Scheie cataract-aspirating n.
Schmieden n.
Schmieden-Dick n.
Schuknecht n.
Schutt n.
scleral spatula n.
sclerostomy n.
sclerotherapy n.
Scoville ventricular n.
screw-tipped intraosseous n.
Sedan-Nashold n.
Seirin acupuncture n.
Seldinger arterial n.
Seldinger gastrostomy n.
self-aspirating cut-biopsy n.
septal n.
Septoject n.
Seraflo AV fistular n.
seton n.
Seven-Star acupuncture n.
Shambaugh palpating n.
Sharpoint Ultra-Guide ophthalmic n.
shattering n.
Sheldon-Spatz vertebral
  arteriogram n.
Sheldon-Swann n.
Shirodkar aneurysm n.
Shirodkar cervical n.
short n.
sialography n.
side-cutting spatulated n.
side-flattened n.
sidewall holed n.
silver n.
Silverman biopsy n.
Silverman-Boeker n.
Simcoe anterior chamber
  receiving n.
Simcoe II PC aspirating n.
Simcoe irrigating-positioning n.
Simcoe suture n.
Simmonds cricothyrotomy n.
Sims abdominal n.
Singer n.
SITE I&A n.
SITE macrobore plus n.
SITE phaco I&A n.

ski n.
Skinny Chiba n.
Sklar ligature n.
slotted n.
Sluder n.
small-bore n.
small-caliber n.
SmallPort n.
SmartNeedle n.
SMIC suture n.
Smiley-Williams arteriography n.
Solitaire n.
SonoVu US aspiration n.
n. spatula
spatula split n.
spatulated half-circle n.
sphenopalatine ganglion n.
spinal n.
Spinelli biopsy n.
n. spoon
spoon n.
spring-eye n.
spring-hook wire n.
Sprotte epidural n.
Sprotte spinal n.
spud n.
n. spud
stab n.
Stallerpointe n.
Stamey n.
standard n.
stapes n.
staphylorrhaphy n.
steel-winged butterfly n.
Steis bone marrow transplant n.
StereoGuide n.
stereotactic breast biopsy n.
sternal puncture n.
Stifcore transbronchial aspiration n.
Stille-Mayo-Hegar n.
Stille-Seldinger n.
Stimuplex block n.
Stocker cyclodiathermy puncture n.
stop n.
Storz aspiration biopsy n.
Storz flexible injection n.
strabismus n.
straight-point n.
straight suturing n.
Strasbourg-Fairfax in vitro
  fertilization n.
Straus curved retrobulbar n.
Sturmdorf cervical n.
Sturmdorf pedicle n.
Stylus suture n.
Subco n.
subconjunctival n.
suction biopsy n.
Sudan n.
Sulze diamond-point n.
Sure-Cut biopsy n.
Suresharp blood collecting n.
Suresharp dental n.
Sur-Fast n.
Surgicraft suture n.

N

needle (*continued*)
    Surgimedics TMP air aspirator n.
    Surgineedle pneumoperitoneum n.
    Sutton biopsy n.
    suturing n.
    swaged n.
    swaged-on n.
    Swan n.
    Swan knife-n.
    Swedgeon already-threaded n.
    Symmonds n.
    Szabo-Berci n.
    taper n.
    Tapercut n.
    tapered n.
    taper-point suture n.
    tattooing n.
    Tauber n.
    tax double n.
    Teflon-coated hollow-bore n.
    Teflon-covered n.
    Teflon glycerine-mixture injection n.
    Tek-Pro n.
    TEMNO biopsy n.
    tendon n.
    Terry-Mayo n.
    Terumo AV fistula n.
    Terumo dental n.
    Terumo hypodermic n.
    Tew n.
    TG140 n.
    thermistor n.
    n. thermocouple
    thin acupuncture n.
    thin-walled n.
    Thomas n.
    thoracentesis n.
    Thornton n.
    threaded eye n.
    through-the-scope injection n.
    Ticsay transpubic n.
    tie-on n.
    n. tip catheter
    tissue desiccation n.
    titanium alloy n.
    Titus venoclysis n.
    Tocantins bone marrow biopsy n.
    Todd eye cautery n.
    tonsillar suture n.
    Torrington French spring n.
    transaxillary n.
    translocation n.
    transpubic n.
    Travenol biopsy n.
    Travert n.
    n. trephination system
    triple-lumen n.
    trocar n.
    Troutman n.
    Tru-Cut biopsy n.
    Trupp ventricular n.
    Tru Taper Ethalloy n.
    TT-3 n.
    tungsten microdissection n.

    Tuohy lumbar aortography n.
    Tuohy spinal n.
    Turkel liver biopsy n.
    Turkel sternal n.
    Turner biopsy n.
    Turner-Warwick urethroplasty n.
    Tworek bone marrow-aspirating n.
    Ultra-Core biopsy n.
    ultrasonic cataract-removal lancet n
    Ultra-vue amniocentesis n.
    UMI n.
    University of Illinois biopsy n.
    University of Illinois marrow n.
    University of Illinois sternal
      puncture n.
    Updegraff cleft palate n.
    Updegraff staphylorrhaphy n.
    urethroplasty n.
    uterine n.
    Vacutainer n.
    vacuuming n.
    Variject n.
    Vastack n.
    Veenema-Gusberg prostatic biopsy n
    Veirs n.
    Venaflo n.
    Venflon n.
    venipuncture n.
    venous n.
    venting aortic Bengash n.
    ventricular n.
    Verbrugge n.
    Veress-Frangenheim n.
    Veress pneumoperitoneum n.
    Veress spring-loaded laparoscopic n.
    Vicat n.
    Viers n.
    Viking n.
    Vim n.
    Vim-Silverman n.
    Vim-Silverman biopsy n.
    Virginia n.
    Visi-Black surgical n.
    Visitec retrobulbar n.
    vitreous-aspirating n.
    vitreous transplant n.
    V. Mueller paracervical nerve
      block n.
    V. Mueller pudendal nerve block n.
    Vogt-Barraquer corneal n.
    von Graefe knife n.
    Voorhees n.
    Walker tonsillar n.
    Wang n.
    Wangensteen intestinal n.
    Wannagat injection n.
    Ward French n.
    Ward French-eye n.
    Waterfield n.
    Watson-Williams n.
    wedge-line n.
    Weeks n.
    Weiss n.
    Welsh olive-tipped n.
    Wergeland double n.

Wertheim-Navratil n.
Westcott biopsy n.
Westerman-Jansen n.
whirlybird n.
Whitacre spinal n.
Wiener eye n.
Williams cystoscopic n.
Williamson biopsy n.
Wilson-Cook electrode n.
winged steel n.
Wolf antral n.
Wood aortography n.
Wooten eye n.
Worst n.
Wright-Crawford n.
Wright fascia n.
Wright ophthalmic n.
Wright ptosis n.
Yale Luer-Lok n.
Yang n.
Yankauer septal n.
Yankauer suture n.
Zavala lung biopsy n.
Ziegler iris n.
Zoellner n.
Needle-Ease device
needleholder, needle holder (*See* holder)
needle-holder forceps
needle-knife
    n.-k. fistulotome
    n.-k. papillotome
    n.-k. wire
Needle-Less Suture
needle-nose
    n.-n. pliers
    n.-n. rongeur
    n.-n. vise-grip pliers
needlepoint
    n. cautery
    n. electrocautery
Needle-Pro needle protection device
needlescope device
Needlescoper endoscope
needle-tipped sphincterotome
Neer
    N. I, II shoulder prosthesis
    N. II shoulder system
    N. II total knee system
    N. II total shoulder system implant
Neesone root canal depth indicator
Neff
    N. femorotibial nail system
    N. meniscal knife
    N. percutaneous access set
negative
    n. eyepiece
    n. pressure device
Negus
    N. bronchoscope
    N. laryngoscope
    N. mouthgag
    N. pusher
    N. telescope
    N. tonsillar forceps
Negus-Broyles bronchoscope

Negus-Green forceps
Nehb D lead
Neider valvulotome
Neil-Moore
    N.-M. meatotomy electrode
    N.-M. perforator drill
Neiman nasal splint
Neisser syringe
Neitz CT-R cataract camera
Neivert
    N. chisel
    N. dissector
    N. double-ended retractor
    N. knife guide
    N. nasal polyp hook
    N. needle holder
    N. osteotome
    N. rocking gouge
    N. tonsillar knife
Neivert-Anderson osteotome
Neivert-Eves
    N.-E. tonsillar snare
    N.-E. tonsillar wire
Nek-L-O
    N.-L-O hot & cold pillow
    N.-L-O orthopaedic support/comfort
    pillow
Nélaton
    N. bullet probe
    N. rubber tube drain
    N. urethral catheter
Nellcor
    N. Durasensor adult oxygen
    transducer
    N. FS-series oximeter sensor
    N. N-2500 capnograph
    N. N-499 fetal oxygen saturation
    monitor
    N. N-400/FS system
    N. N10 ETCO$_2$/SpO$_2$ monitor
    N. N-series pulse oximeter
    N. Symphony blood pressure
    monitoring system
    N. Symphony N-3100 noninvasive
    blood pressure monitor
    N. Symphony N-3000 pulse
    oximeter
Nelson
    N. empyema trocar
    N. ligature needle
    N. line keeper
    N. lobectomy scissors
    N. lung-dissecting scissors
    N. lung forceps
    N. rib spreader
    N. rib stripper
    N. self-retaining rib retractor
    N. thoracic trocar
    N. tissue forceps
Nelson-Bethune shears
Nelson-Martin forceps
Nelson-Metzenbaum scissors
Nelson-Patterson empyema trocar
Nelson-Roberts stripper
Nelson-Vital dissecting scissors

N

Nemdi tweezer epilation device
NeoControl pelvic floor therapy system
NeoDerm dressing
NeoDura matrix
neodymium-doped yttrium-aluminum-
garnet laser (Nd:YAG laser)
neodymium laser
neodymium:YAG laser (Nd:YAG)
neodymium:yttrium-aluminum-garnet
(Nd:YAG)
    n.-a.-g. laser (Nd:YAG laser)
    n.-a.-g. laser system
neodymium:yttrium-lithium-fluoride
photodisruptive laser
Neo-Fit
    N.-F. neonatal endotracheal tube
     grip
    N.-F. neonatal endotracheal tube
     holder
Neoflex bendable knife
Neoguard percussor
NeoKnife
    N. cautery
    N. electrosurgical instrument
Neolens lens
Neolyte laser indirect ophthalmoscope
Neomed electrocautery
neonatal
    n. internal jugular puncture kit
    n. monitor
    n. sandbag
    n. scissors
    n. sternal retractor
    n. vascular clamp
    n. vascular forceps
    N. Y TrachCare catheter
NeoNaze nasal function restoration
device
Neoplex catheter
Neoplush foam
neoprene
    n. ankle support
    n. back support
    n. dressing
    n. elbow sleeve
    n. gloves
    n. hinged-knee brace
    n. Osgood-Schlatter knee brace
    n. wrist brace
    n. wrist orthosis
    n. wrist strap
NeoProbe
    N. gamma detection probe
    N. portable radioisotope detector
    N. radioactivity detector
    N. 1000 radioisotope detection
     system
Neo-Sert
    N.-S. umbilical vessel catheter
    N.-S. umbilical vessel catheter
     insertion set
Neos M pacemaker
Neosonic
    N. piezo ultrasonic unit

N. (P-5) SPM super powered mini
    retroprep/endo system
Neosono MC apex locator
neosphincter
    Acticon n.
Neo-Therm neonatal skin temperature
probe
Neo-trak 515A neonatal monitor
Neotrend system
Neotrode II neonatal electrode
NeoVO$_2$R volume control resuscitator
Neovision micro mirror
nephelometer
nephrolithotomy forceps
NephroMax catheter set
nephroscope
    Cabot n.
    Storz n.
Nephross dialyzer
nephrostomy
    n. catheter
    n. clamp
    n. tube
nerve
    N. Block Infusion Kit
    n. cuff
    n. fiber analyzer
    N. Fiber Analyzer laser
     ophthalmoscope
    n. holder
    n. pull hook
    n. root laminectomy dissector
    n. root retractor
    n. separator spatula
    n. stimulator
nerve-approximating clamp
nerve-integrity monitor
NervePace
    N. nerve conduction monitor
    N. nerve conduction testing machine
Nesbit
    N. cystoscope
    N. electrode
    N. electrotome
    N. hemostatic bag
    N. removable partial denture
    N. resectoscope
    N. tonsillar snare
nested
    n. step stool
    n. trocar
Nestor guiding catheter
net
    Jahnke-Barron heart support n.
    Roth endoscopy retrieval n.
    Roth polyp retrieval n.
    Tubegauz elastic n.
    ureteric retrieval n.
Netra intravascular ultrasound
Netterville double-ended elevator
Nettleship
    N. canaliculus dilator
    N. iris repositor
Nettleship-Wilder lacrimal dilator

Neubauer
    N. foreign body forceps
    N. hemocytometer
    N. lancet cannula
    N. vitreous micro-extractor forceps
Neubeiser adjustable forearm splint
Neuber bone tube
Neubuser tube-seizing forceps
Neufeld
    N. apparatus
    N. cast
    N. device
    N. driver
    N. femoral nail plate
    N. nail
    N. pin
    N. screw
    N. traction
    N. tractor
NeuFlex metacarpophalangeal joint implant
Neuhann
    N. cystitome
    N. cystotome
Neumann
    N. calipers block
    N. depth gauge
    N. double corneal marker
    N. razor blade fragment holder
    N. scissors
Neumann-Shepard corneal marker
Neurairtome drill
neural
    n. dissector
    n. prosthesis
NEURAY
    N. neurosurgical patty
    N. neurosurgical strip
Neuro
    N. N-50 lesion generator
    N. Stim 2000 Mk_1 stimulator
    N. Vasx
Neuro-Aide testing device
NeuroAvitene applicator
NeuroCom balance master
NeuroControl Freehand implant
NeuroCybernetic
    N. prosthesis
    N. prosthesis system
NeuroDrape surgical drape
neuroendoscope
    Chavantes-Zamorano n.
    Neuroview n.
Neurogard TCD system
neurography needle
Neuroguard transcranial Doppler
Neuroguide
    N. camera-processor
    N. interoperative viewing system
    N. monitor
    N. optical handpiece
    N. peel-away catheter introducer
    N. suction-irrigation adapter
    N. Visicath viewing catheter
Neurolase microsurgical CO_2 laser

NeuroLink II EEG data acquisition system
Neurolite SPECT scan
neurological
    N. Institute periosteal elevator
    n. percussion hammer
    n. percussor
    n. sponge
    n. tuning fork
Neuromed Octrode implantable pain management device
Neuromeet
    N. nerve approximator
    N. soft tissue approximator
neurometer device
Neuromod TENS unit
neuromuscular
    n. electrical stimulator (NMES)
    n. III stimulator
Neuropak 8 system
Neuropath biofeedback device
neuropatty
Neuropedic
    N. multidensity mattress
    N. neurolon mattress
Neuroperfusion pump
neuroprobe pain management system
Neuro-Pulse
    N.-P. nerve locator-stimulator
    N.-P. TENS unit
NeuroScan 3D imager
NeuroSector
    N. ultrasound
    N. ultrasound system
Neurosign 100 nerve monitor
NeuroStation frameless system
Neurostat Mark II cryoanalgesia system
NeuroStim TENS unit
neurostimulator
    Biotens n.
    Grass n.
    Jobstens n.
    percutaneous epidural n. (PENS)
    Staodyne EMS+2 n.
neurosurgical
    n. bur
    n. cottonoid
    n. dissector
    n. dressing forceps
    n. head holder
    n. headrest
    n. ligature forceps
    n. needle holder
    n. pledget
    n. scissors
    n. suction forceps
    n. suture
    n. suture needle
    n. tissue forceps
neurosuture
Neurotips
neurotome
    Bradford enucleation n.
Neurotone biofeedback device

N

Neuro-Trace
   N.-T. instrument
**Neurotrend continuous multiparameter
   system**
neurovascular
   n. forceps
   n. scissors
Neuroview
   N. integrated visualization system
   N. neuroendoscope
neurSector scanner
neutral
   n. density filter
   n. electrode
   n. hook
   n. position splint
neutralizer
   Glutex glutaraldehyde n.
Neutrocim dental cement
neutron therapy machine
Neuwirth-Palmer forceps
Nevada gonioscope
Neville
   N. ascending aortic air vent needle
   N. stent
   N. tracheal reconstruction prosthesis
   N. tracheobronchial prosthesis
Neville-Barnes forceps
Nevins
   N. dressing forceps
   N. tissue forceps
Nevyas
   N. double sharp cystitome
   N. drape retractor
   N. lens forceps
new
   N. Beginnings GelShapes silicone
   gel sheeting
   N. Beginnings topical gel sheeting
   N. biopsy forceps
   N. England Baptist acetabular cup
   N. England scoliosis brace
   N. Glucorder analyzer
   N. Jersey hemiarthroplasty prosthesis
   N. Jersey-LCS shoulder prosthesis
   N. Jersey-LCS total knee prosthesis
   N. Luer-type speaking tube
   N. Mind Set toe splint
   N. oral needle
   N. Orleans corneal cutting block
   N. Orleans endarterectomy stripper
   N. Orleans endarterectomy stripper
   set
   N. Orleans Eye & Ear fixation
   forceps
   N. Orleans lens
   N. Orleans lens loupe
   N. Orleans needle holder
   N. Skimmer blade
   N. speaking tube
   N. suture scissors
   N. tenaculum
   N. tissue forceps
   N. tracheal retractor
   N. tracheostomy hook

   N. tracheotomy hook
   N. ultra-thick powder-free latex
   surgical glove
   N. Vision magnification system
   N. Weavenit Dacron prosthesis
   N. Yorker guidewire
   N. York erysiphake
   N. York Eye and Ear cannula
   N. York Eye and Ear Hospital
   fixation forceps
   N. York glass suction tube
   N. York Hospital electrode
   N. York Hospital retractor
   N. York Orthopedic front-opening
   orthosis
   N. York University insert
   N. York University insert for
   orthosis
newborn eyelid retractor
Newell
   N. lid retractor
   N. nucleus hook
new happy bur
Newhart-Casselberry snare
Newhart hook
Newhart-Smith cup
Newington orthosis
Newkirk mouthgag
New-Lambotte osteotome
NewLife
   N. oxygen concentrator
   N. therapeutic mattress
   N. therapeutic surface
Newman
   N. proctoscope
   N. rectal injection needle
   N. tenaculum
   N. toenail plate
   N. uterine knife
   N. uterine tenaculum forceps
Newport
   N. cartilage gouge
   N. collar
   N. MC hip orthosis
   N. medical instrument
   N. total hip orthosis
   N. total hip orthosis system
   N. ventilator
Newsom side port nucleus cracker
Newton LLT guidewire
Newton-Morgan retractor
Newvicon
   N. camera tube
   N. vacuum chamber pickup tube
NewVues lens
Nexacryl tissue adhesive
Nexerciser Plus exercise system
NexGen
   N. complete knee replacement
   N. complete knee system
   N. knee component
   N. knee implant
   N. offset stem extension
NexStent carotid stent

Nextep
- N. Contour lower-leg walker
- N. knee brace
- N. Silhouette lower-leg walker

Nexus
- N. hip prosthesis
- N. implant
- N. 2 linear ablation catheter
- N. wheelchair seating system

Ney articulator

Nezhat
- N. irrigation tubing
- N. irrigator

Nezhat-Dorsey
- N.-D. suction-irrigator
- N.-D. trumpet valve
- N.-D. Trumpet Valve hydrodissector

NG
- NG feeding tube
- NG strip nasal tube fastener

NHS-activated HiTrap affinity column
Niagara temporary dialysis catheter
Niamtu
- N. video imaging
- N. video imaging system

nibbler
- N. laparoscopic probe
- Schultz anterior capsule n.

Niblitt dissector
Nicati foreign body spud
N'ice
- N. Stretch night splint
- N. Stretch night splint suspension system with Sealed Ice

Nichamin
- N. fixation ring
- N. hydrodissection cannula
- N. laser-assisted intrastromal keratomileusis (LASIK) irrigating cannula
- N. quick chopper
- N. triple chopper
- N. vertical chopper

Niche knife
Nichols
- N. aortic clamp
- N. infundibulectomy rongeur
- N. nasal siphon

Nichols-Deschamps-Navratil ligature needle
Nichols-Jehle coronary multihead catheter
Nickell cystoscope adapter
Nickelplast blank
nickel-titanium file
Nickerson Biggy vial
Nicola
- N. forceps
- N. gouge
- N. microforceps
- N. pituitary rongeur
- N. rasp
- N. raspatory
- N. tendon clamp

Nicolet
- N. Compass electromyography instrument
- N. Elite obstetrical Doppler
- N. Nerve Integrity Monitor (NIM-2)
- N. NMR spectrometer
- N. Pathfinder I recording device
- N. SM-300 stimulator
- N. Viking IIe EMG
- N. Viking II electrophysiologic system

Nicolet/EME Muller and Moll probe fixation device
Nicoll
- N. bone graft
- N. plate
- N. tendon prosthesis

Nidek
- N. AR-2000 objective automatic refractor
- N. 3Dx stereodisk camera
- N. EC-1000, -5000 excimer laser
- N. EchoScan
- N. EC-5000 refractive laser system
- N. Laser System laser
- N. MK-2000 keratome system

Niebauer
- N. finger-joint replacement prosthesis
- N. implant
- N. trapezium replacement prosthesis

Niebauer-Cutter implant
Niedner
- N. anastomosis clamp
- N. commissurotomy knife
- N. dissecting forceps
- N. pulmonic clamp

night
- n. drainage bag
- n. drain bottle
- N. Owl Pocket polygraph
- N. Preservers underpad

NightBird nasal CPAP
Nightimer carpal tunnel support
Nightingale examining lamp
NIH
- NIH cardiomarker catheter
- NIH Image 1.54 catheter
- NIH left ventriculography catheter
- NIH marking catheter
- NIH mitral valve forceps

Nihon tocodynamometer
Nikon
- N. aspheric lens
- N. FS-3 photo slit lamp Biomicroscope
- N. microprocessor-controlled camera
- N. Retinomax K-Plus autorefractor
- N. Retinopan fundus camera
- N. SMZ 2T magnifying lens
- N. zoom photo slit lamp

Nilsson-Stille abortion suction tube
Nilsson suction tube
NIM-2
- Nicolet Nerve Integrity Monitor

N

Nimbus
    N. Hemopump
    N. Hemopump cardiac assist device
Niplette device
nipper
    anterior crurotomy n.
    cuticle n.
    Dieter n.
    Dieter-House n.
    English anvil nail n.
    Hough anterior crurotomy n.
    House-Dieter malleus n.
    House malleus n.
    Lempert malleus n.
    malleus n.
    Miltex nail n.
    nail n.
    n. nail drill
    Rica malleus head n.
    SMIC malleus head n.
    Tabb crural n.
    Turnbull nail n.
    Wister n.
nipple
    Duckey n.
    Kock n.
    McGovern n.
NIR
    NIR ON Ranger balloon expandable stent
    NIR Primo balloon expandable stent
    NIR with SOX over-the-wire coronary stent
Niro
    N. arch bar
    N. bone-cutting forceps
    N. wire-twister forceps
    N. wire-twisting forceps
NIROYAL Advance balloon expandable stent
NIRstent stent
Nirvana pressure-reducing mattress
Nisbet
    N. eye forceps
    N. fixation forceps
Nishimoto Sangyo scanner
Nishizaki-Wakabayashi suction tube
Nissen
    N. cystic forceps
    N. gall duct forceps
    N. hassux forceps
    N. rib spreader
    N. suture
Nite Train-R enuresis conditioning device
nitinol
    n. guidewire
    n. K-file
    n. mesh-covered frame
    n. mesh stent
    n. self-expanding coil stent
    n. shape-memory alloy wire
    n. subglottic stenosis stent
    n. thermal memory stent

Ni-Ti Shape Memory alloy compression stapler
Nitra lamp
nitrile gloves
nitrogen-phosphorus detector
nitroglycerin transdermal patch
Nitrospray Plus cryosurgical device
Nitro wheelchair
NK dental capsule
NL3 guider
NMES
    neuromuscular electrical stimulator
NMR
    NMR LipoProfile device
    NMR spectrometer
No
    No Bounce mallet
    No Pour Pak suction catheter kit
    No Sting barrier film
Nobel Biocare implant
Nobelpharma
    N. gold prosthetic retaining screw
    N. implant
    N. implant system
Nobetec dental cement
Nobis aortic occluder
Noble
    N. iris forceps
    N. scissors
Noblock retractor
Noci stimuli needle
Nocito implant
N_2O cryosurgical unit
nocturnal penile tumescence monitor
Nogenol dental cement
NoHands foot-operated computer mouse system
Noiles
    N. posterior stabilized knee
    N. posterior stabilized knee prosthesis
    N. rotating hinge knee
    N. rotating-hinge knee mechanism
    N. rotating-hinge total knee prosthesis
noise
    n. level monitor
    n. reduction device
NoKor needle
Nokrome bifocal lens
Noland-Budd cervical curette
Nolan system collimator mounted contact shield
No-Lok compression screw
Nomad-LE EMG
nomogram
    Casebeer-Lindstrom n.
Nomos
    N. multiprogrammable R-wave inhibited demand pacemaker
    N. stereotactic system
nonabsorbable
    n. surgical suture
nonadherent foam
nonadhering dressing

nonadhesive dressing
non-arcon articulator
noncannulated nail
non-child-resistant container
noncompetitive pacemaker
noncompliant balloon
nonconductive guidewire
noncontact tonometer
noncoring Huber needle
noncrushing
    n. anterior resection clamp
    n. bowel clamp
    n. common duct forceps
    n. gastroenterostomy clamp
    n. gastrointestinal clamp
    n. intestinal clamp
    n. intestinal forceps
    n. liver-holding clamp
    n. pickup forceps
    n. tissue-holding forceps
    n. vascular clamp
noncutting
    n. suture needle
nondetachable
    n. endovascular balloon
    n. occlusive balloon
    n. silicone balloon catheter
nonenclosed magnet
nonfenestrated
    n. forceps
    n. Moore-type femoral stem
nonferromagnetic
    n. clip
    n. MR-compatible frame
    n. needle
    n. positioning device
nonflotation catheter
nonflow-directed catheter
nonhinged knee prosthesis
Nonin Onyx pulse oximeter
nonintegrated
    n. transvenous defibrillation lead
    n. tripolar lead
noninterfering separator
noninvasive
    n. continuous cardiac output monitor
    n. paddle
    n. temporary pacemaker
nonlatex dental dam
nonmagnetic
    n. dressing forceps
    n. tissue forceps
nonmedullated nerve fiber
nonocclusive dressing
nonperforating
    n. towel clamp
    n. towel forceps
nonpneumatic tourniquet
nonporous-coated endoprosthesis
nonrebreathing
    n. mask
    n. valve
nonrigid endoscope
nonslipping forceps

nonthoracotomy
    n. defibrillation lead system
    n. lead implantable cardioverter-defibrillator
    n. system antitachycardia device
nontoothed forceps
nontraumatizing
    n. catheter
    n. visceral forceps
nonweightbearing brace
nonwoven sponge
Noon
    N. AV fistular clamp
    N. AV fistular tunneler
    N. modified vascular access tunneler
noose
    Dormia n.
NoProfile
    N. balloon
    N. balloon catheter
Norco ulnar deviation support
Norcross periosteal elevator
Nordan-Colibri forceps
Nordan tying forceps
Nordenstrom
    N. Rotex II biopsy needle
Nordent
    N. amalgam condenser
    N. bone chisel
    N. bone curette
    N. bone file
    N. burnisher
    N. carver
    N. excavator
    N. explorer
    N. filling instrument
    N. hatchet
    N. hoe
    N. margin trimmer
    N. oral surgery elevator
    N. periodontic knife
    N. scaler
Nordent-Ochsenbein periodontic chisel
NordiCare
    N. Back Therapy system
    N. Enabler exerciser
    N. Strider exerciser
NordicTrack ski exerciser
Nordin-Ruiz trapezoidal marker
Nord orthodontic plate
Nordotrack motion EMG
Norelco
    N. allergen reducer
    N. mucotome
Norfolk intrauterine aspiration catheter
Norian
    N. Skeletal Repair System cancellous bone cement
    N. SRS cement
Norland
    N. bone densitometry
    N. digital oscilloscope
    N. pQCT XCT2000 scanner
    N. XR26 bone densitometer

N

Norman
 N. tibial bolt
 N. tibial pin
Normlgel protective wound dressing
Norm testing and rehabilitation system
Norport pump
Norrbacka bone elevator
Norrbacka-Stille lever
Norris
 N. button
 N. sponge forceps
 N. tip magnet
Nortech SLED electrode
Northbent suture scissors
Northgate SD-3 dual-purpose lithotriptor
North-South retractor
Northville brace
Norton
 N. adjustable cup reamer
 N. ball reamer
 N. endotracheal tube
 N. flow-directed Swan-Ganz
  thermodilution catheter
Norwegian system
Norwood
 N. forceps
 N. rectal snare
nose
 n. clip
 n. cone
 n. guard splint
nosecone
 CEM handswitching n.
Nosik transorbital leukotome
nostril thermistor
notcher device
notch filter
notchplasty blade
no-tie stretch lace
Noto
 N. dressing forceps
 N. ovum forceps
 N. polypus forceps
 N. sponge forceps
No-Touch delivery and mounting system
Nott-Gutmann vaginal speculum
Nottingham
 N. introducer
 N. One-Step tapered dilator
 N. ureteral dilator
Nott vaginal speculum
Nounton blade
Nourse bladder syringe
Nouvisage
 N. Deep Hydration body patch
 N. Deep Hydration glove
 N. Deep Hydration neck patch
Nova
 N. Aid lens
 N. Celltrak 12 hematology analyzer
 N. Curve lens
 N. II machine
 N. II pacemaker
 N. jaw hook
 N. Microsonics Image Vue system

 N. MR pacemaker
 N. Soft II lens
 N. thermodilution catheter
NovaBone
NovaBone-C/M
NovaCath multilumen infusion catheter
Novack special extraction set
Novacor
 N. DIASYS left ventricular assist
  device
 N. DIASYS left ventricular assist
  system
Novaflex intraocular lens
NovaGel silicone gel sheeting
Novagold mammary implant
Novak
 N. biopsy curette
 N. fixation forceps
 N. uterine curette
Novak-Schoeckaert endometrial curette
NovaLine Litho-S DUV excimer laser
Novametrix
 N. combination O_2/CO_2 sensor
 N. pulse oximeter
NovaPulse
 N. CO_2 laser
 N. laser system
Novar oral illuminator
Novascan scanning headpiece laser
Novastent stent
Novatec LightBlade laser
Novex wedged wheelchair cushion
Novo-10a CBF measuring device
NovolinPen device
Novoste catheter
Novus
 N. hydrocephalic valve
 N. LC threaded interbody fusion
  cage
 N. Medical image card
 N. mini valve
 N. Omni 2000 photocoagulator
 N. 2000 ophthalmoscope
 N. Verdi diode-pumped green
  photocoagulator
NOxBOX II monitor
Noyes
 N. chalazion punch
 N. ear forceps
 N. iridectomy scissors
 N. iris scissors
 N. nasal-dressing forceps
 N. nasal forceps
 N. rongeur
 N. speculum
Noyes-Shambaugh scissors
NP-3S auto chart projector
NPB-295 pulse oximeter
NS2000 bipolar generator system
N-Terface
 N.-T. contact-layer wound dressing
Nu
 Nu Gauze dressing
 Nu Gauze sponge

Nu-Brede packing and debridement sponge
nubular blade
nuclear
    n. magnetic resonance spectroscopy
    n. probe
nuclear-powered pacemaker
Nucleotome
    N. Endoflex
    N. Endoflex instrument
    N. Flex II
    N. Flex II cutting probe
    N. Micro I probe
Nucletron
    N. applicator
    N. MicroSelectron/LDR remote afterloader
    N. simulator
nucleus
    N. 22 cochlear implant
    n. cracker
    n. delivery cannula
    n. delivery loop
    n. delivery loupe
    n. erysiphake
    n. expressor
    n. hydrolysis needle
    N. multichannel cochlear implant
    n. removal loop
    n. removal loupe
    n. rotator
    n. spatula
Nu-Comfort colostomy appliance
Nu-Derm foam island dressing
Nu-Form truss
Nu-Gel clear hydrogel wound dressing
Nugent
    N. erysiphake
    N. fixation forceps
    N. iris hook
    N. rectus forceps
    N. soft cataract aspirator
    N. superior rectus forceps
    N. utility forceps
Nugent-Gradle
    N.-G. stitch scissors
Nugent-Green-Dimitry erysiphake
Nugowski forceps
Nu-Hope
    N.-H. adhesive
    N.-H. adhesive waterproof skin barrier
    N.-H. drainable one-piece pouch
    N.-H. hole cutter
    N.-H. Neonatal and Premee Pouches
    N.-H. pouch cover
    N.-H. skin barrier strip
    N.-H. tubing
    N.-H. urinary pouch
    N.-H. urine collection bottle
Nu-Knit
    N.-K. absorbable hemostat
    Surgicel N.-K.
NuKo knee orthosis

Numed
    N. intracoronary Doppler catheter
NuMED single balloon
Nunc cryotube
Nunez
    N. aortic clamp
    N. auricular clamp
    N. sternal approximator
    N. ventricular ventilation tube
Nunez-Nunez mitral stenosis knife
Nuport PEG tube
Nurolon suture
Nussbaum
    N. bracelet
    N. intestinal clamp
    N. intestinal forceps
NuStep
    N. exerciser
    N. total body recumbent stepper
nut
    n. alignment guide
    Close Encounter n.
    Kirschner traction bow n.
    locking n.
    nylon n.
    sleeved n.
    Stable-Lok n.
Nu-Thor thoracostomy device
Nu-Tip
    N.-T. disposable scissor tip
    N.-T. laparoscopic scissors
NutraCol hydrocolloid wound dressing
NutraDress zinc-saline dressing
NutraFil hydrophilic B dressing
NutraGauze hydrophilic wound dressing
Nu-Trake
    N.-T. cricothyrotomy device
    N.-T. Weiss emergency airway system
NutraShield perineal protectant
NutraStat calcium alginate wound dressing
NutraVue hydrogel dressing
Nutricath catheter
Nutromat Pad S feeding pump
Nuttall retractor
Nuva-Lite ultraviolet activator
Nuvaseal resin
Nuva-Tach resin
Nuvistor electronic tonometer
Nuvita lens
Nu-Vois artificial larynx
Nuvolase 660 laser system
NuVue lens
Nuwave transcutaneous electrical nerve stimulator
Nuway in-the-ear hearing aid
Nu-wrap roll dressing
Nyboer esophageal electrode
Nycore
    N. angiography pigtail catheter
    N. cardiac device
Nyhus-Nelson
    N.-N. gastric decompression tube
    N.-N. jejunal feeding tube

N

Nyhus-Potts intestinal forceps
Nylatex
    N. strap
    N. wrap
Nylex II Convoluted innerspring
Nylok
    N. bolt
    N. self-locking nail
nylon
    n. face mallet
    n. head mallet
    n. loop
    n. monofilament suture
    n. nut
    n. retention suture
    Rica n.
    n. scrub brush
    n. surgical sack
    n. 66 suture

nystagmus
    n. bulb
    n. glasses
Nystar Plus electronystagmogram
Nystroem
    N. abdominal suction tube
    N. hip nail
    N. nail driver
    N. retractor
    N. tumor forceps
Nystroem-Stille
    N.-S. driver
    N.-S. hip nail
    N.-S. retractor
Nytone enuretic control unit
NYU-Hosmer electric elbow and prehension actuator

O₂
O₂ Boot
O₂ disposable boot device
OA knee brace
Oaks
O. double needle
O. double straight cannula
Oasis
O. collagen plug
O. feather microscalpel
O. sheet introducer system
O. thrombectomy system
O. wound dressing
OAsys brace
OB-10 Comfort bite block
O'Beirne sphincter tube
Oberhill
O. obstetrical forceps
O. self-retaining retractor
Ober tendon passer
Oberto mouth prop
obese
o. support
o. walker
OB Gees maternity orthotic
OB/GYN chair
objective lens
oblique
o. bandage
o. muscle hook
o. prism
o. prism device
oblique-forward-viewing instrument
oblique-viewing
o.-v. echoendoscope
o.-v. endoscope
O'Brien
O. airway needle
O. fixation forceps
O. foreign body spud
O. marker
O. phrenic retractor
O. rib hook
O. rib retractor
O. rongeur
O. spatula
O. stitch scissors
O. suture scissors
O. tissue forceps
O'Brien-Elschnig forceps
O'Brien-Mayo scissors
O'Brien-Storz microhemostat
Obstbaum
O. lens spatula
O. synechia spatula
obstetrical
o. block anesthesia needle
o. decapitating embryotome
o. decapitating hook
o. forceps
o. retractor
o. spoon

obstructed shunt tube
Obtura II gutta percha system
obturator
Alcock o.
Alcock-Timberlake o.
o. appliance
blunt o.
blunt-tipped o.
cannulated o.
coagulating suction cannula o.
concave o.
convex o.
Cripps o.
distending o.
double-catheterizing sheath and o.
Ellik-Shaw o.
Endopath Optiview laparoscopic o.
Endotrac o.
Fitch o.
Frazier suction tube o.
Hemaflex PTCA sheath with o.
Hemaquet PTCA sheath with o.
Keene o.
LaparoSAC o.
Leusch atraumatic o.
Moria o.
Optiview optical surgical o.
palatal o.
Rumel tourniquet-eyed o.
sheath and o.
suction tube o.
Thal-Mantel o.
Thermafil Plus o.
Timberlake o.
tourniquet-eyed o.
ureteral catheter o.
visual o.
OBUS back support
Obwegeser
O. awl
O. channel retractor
O. orthognathic surgery instruments
O. periosteal retractor
O. splitting chisel
Obwegeser-Dalpont internal screw fixation
OCCI DISH pressure relief head cushion
occluder
air inflatable vessel o. clamp
Amplatzer septal o.
aortic o.
ASDOS umbrella o.
Bard clamshell septal o.
black/white o.
Brockenbrough curved-tip o.
CardioSeal septal o.
catheter tip o.
clip-on/tie-on o.
eye o.
Goffman o.
Halberg trial clip o.

occluder *(continued)*
    Heifitz carotid o.
    Kean-M-4 o.
    long o.
    lorgnette o.
    Maddox rod o.
    Microvena Das Angel Wings o.
    modified Rashkind PDA o.
    multiple-pin hole o.
    Nobis aortic o.
    Pediatric Cardiology Devices Sideris
      Buttoned device o.
    PFO-Star o.
    pinhole o.
    Pram combination o.
    radiolucent plastic o.
    Rashkind double-disk umbrella o.
    red lens o.
    Rumison side port fixation o.
    short o.
    single o.
    square-shaped o.
occluding
    o. clamp
    o. forceps
    o. fracture frame
occlusal rest bar
occlusion
    o. balloon
    o. catheter
    o. coil
occlusive
    o. balloon
    o. collodion dressing
    o. moisture-retentive dressing
    o. semipermeable dressing
occlusor
    Elastoplast eye o.
Ochsner
    O. aortic clamp
    O. arterial clamp
    O. arterial forceps
    O. ball-tipped scissors
    O. cartilage forceps
    O. diamond-edged scissors
    O. flexible spiral gallstone probe
    O. gallbladder trocar
    O. gallbladder tube
    O. gall duct probe
    O. gallstone probe
    O. hemostat
    O. hemostatic forceps
    O. hook
    O. malleable retractor
    O. needle
    O. ribbon retractor
    O. ring
    O. scissors
    O. spiral probe
    O. thoracic clamp
    O. thoracic trocar
    O. tissue/cartilage forceps
    O. tissue forceps
    O. vascular retractor
    O. wire twister
Ochsner-DeBakey spur crusher
Ochsner-Dixon arterial forceps
Ochsner-Favaloro self-retaining retractor
Ochsner-Fenger gallstone probe
Ockerblad
    O. forceps
    O. kidney clamp
    O. vessel clamp
OCL
    OCL Splint Roll Contour splinting
      system
    OCL volar splint
Ocoee scalp cleansing unit
O'Connor
    O. abdominal retractor
    O. biopsy forceps
    O. double-edged curette
    O. drape
    O. eye forceps
    O. finger cup
    O. flat tenotomy hook
    O. grasping forceps
    O. hook punch
    O. iris forceps
    O. lid clamp
    O. lid forceps
    O. marker
    O. muscle hook
    O. operating arthroscope
    O. rectal finger cot
    O. scleral depressor
    O. sheath
    O. sponge forceps
    O. vaginal retractor
O'Connor-Elschnig fixation forceps
O'Connor-O'Sullivan
    O.-O. abdominal retractor
    O.-O. self-retaining vaginal retractor
octagon roll
Octa-Hex implant
octapolar
    o. catheter
    o. lead
OCT compound
Octopus
    O. 101, 201 bowl perimeter
    O. holder
    O. 1-2-3 perimeter
    O. retractor
OctreoScan
    O. scanner
    O. system
Ocu-Guard ophthalmic wrap
Oculab Tono-Pen
Oculaid lens
ocular
    o. cautery
    o. cup
    o. Gamboscope lens
    o. Gamboscope loupe
    o. hypertension indicator
    o. marker

o. pressure reducer
o. prosthesis
Oculex drug delivery system
OcuLight
O. GLx green laser photocoagulator
O. SLx ophthalmic laser
oculocerebrovasculometer
oculocutaneous laser
oculogyric stimulator
Oculo-Plastik ePTFE ocular implant
oculoplasty corneal protector
oculoplethysmograph
Oculus
O. lens loop
O. trial frame
Ocuscan
Sonometric O.
O. 400 transducer
Ocutech Vision Enhancing system
ocutome
Berkeley Bioengineering o.
CooperVision o.
disposable o.
O. II fragmentation system
O'Malley o.
o. probe
STOO Series Ten Thousand o.
O. vitrectomy unit
o. vitrector
o. vitreous blade
ODAM defibrillator
Odelca camera unit
O'Dell spicule forceps
Odgen plate
Odland ankle prosthesis
Odman-Ledin catheter
O'Donoghue
O. cartilage feeler
O. cystourethroscope
O. dressing
O. knee splint
O. probe
O. stirrup splint
O. suture passer
odontoid peg-grasping forceps
Odontometer electronic apex locator
odor absorbent dressing
O'Dwyer tube
Odyssey phacoemulsification system
OEC
OEC Dual-Op barrel/plate
component
OEC lag screw component with
keyway
OEC Mini 6600 imaging system
OEC Series 9600 cardiac system
OEC-Diasonics
O.-D. 9400 fluoroscopy C-arm
system
O.-D. mobile C-arm image
intensifier
**OEC-Kuntscher Interlocking Pathfinder
nail**

OEM
OEM 503 humidifier
OEM Venturi MixOMask mask
Oertli wire lid retractor
Oesch hook
OES 4000 resectoscope
**Oettingen abdominal self-retaining
retractor**
office diagnostic rechargeable otoscope
off-pump coronary artery bypass
offset
o. cane
o. hand retractor
o. hinge
o. modified prosthesis
o. operating laparoscope
o. suspension feeder
O'Gawa
O. cataract-aspirating cannula
O. irrigating cannula
O. needle holder
O. suture-fixation forceps
O. suture forceps
O. two-way I&A cannula
O. tying forceps
O'Gawa-Castroviejo tying forceps
Ogden
O. Anchor soft tissue device
O. plate system
O. soft tissue to bone anchor
O. tissue reattachment mini system
Ogden-Senturia eustachian inflator
Ogee acetabular component
Ogura
O. cartilage forceps
O. nasal saw
O. tissue
O. tissue forceps
O'Hanlon
O. forceps
O. intestinal clamp
O'Hanlon-Poole suction tube
O'Hara forceps
O'Harris-Petruso cup
Ohio
O. bed
O. Bubble humidifier
O. critical care ventilator
O. Hope resuscitator
O. Nuclear Delta scanner
O. pressure infuser
O. safety trap overflow bottle
O. Vortex respiration monitor
O. warmer
Ohl periosteal elevator
Ohmeda
O. Care-Plus incubator
O. 9000 computer-cotrolled infusion
pump
O. continuous-vacuum regulator
O. hand-held oximeter
O. intermittent suction unit
O. probe
O. pulse oximeter
O. Rascal II Raman spectroscope

O

Ohmeda *(continued)*
    O. 5250 respiratory gas monitor
    O. Sevotec 5 vaporizer
    O. thoracic suction regulator
OIC emergency oxygen inhalator
oiled
    o. silk dressing
    o. silk suture
OIS image digitizing system
OIU cold knife
Oklahoma
    O. ankle joint
    O. ankle joint orthosis
    O. ankle prosthesis
    O. City cable
    O. iris wire retractor
Okmian microneedle holder
Okonek-Yasargil tumor fork
Olbert
    O. balloon
    O. balloon dilator
    O. NoProfile balloon dilatation catheter
old
    O. Martin bipolar cable
    o. smoothie bur
Oldberg
    O. brain retractor
    O. dissector
    O. elevator
    O. intervertebral disk forceps
    O. intervertebral disk rongeur
    O. laminectomy rongeur
    O. pituitary rongeur
    O. pituitary rongeur forceps
    O. straight retractor
Oldfield needle
Olerud
    O. internal fixator
    O. PSF fixation system
    O. PSF rod
    O. PSF screw
Oliair
    O. articulator
    O. mouth mirror
oligonucleotide probe
olivary catheter
olive
    Eder-Puestow metal o.
    Gergoyie o.
    Gergoyie-Guggenheim o.
    interchangeable vein stripper o.
    o. ring
    Savary-Gilliard metal o.
    o. wire
Olivecrona
    O. aneurysm clamp
    O. aneurysm forceps
    O. angular scissors
    O. brain spatula
    O. brain spoon
    O. clip applier
    O. clip-applying and removing forceps

    O. conchotome
    O. dissector
    O. dural scissors
    O. endaural rongeur
    O. guillotine scissors
    O. rongeur forceps
    O. silver clip
    O. trigeminal knife
    O. wire saw
Olivecrona-Gigli wire saw
Olivecrona-Stille dissector
Olivecrona-Toennis clip-applying forceps
Olivella-Garrigosa photocoagulator
Oliver scalp retractor
olive-tipped, olive-tip
    o.-t. bougie
    o.-t. cannula
    o.-t. catheter
    o.-t. dilator
    o.-t. irrigator
    o.-t. monopolar electrosurgical dissector
    o.-t. needle
    Welsh flat o.-t.
Olivier-Bertrand-Tipal frame
Olk
    O. membrane peeler
    O. membrane peeler knife
    O. retinal spatula
    O. vitreoretinal pick
    O. vitreoretinal spatula
Ollier
    O. graft
    O. rake retractor
    O. raspatory
Ollier-Thiersch
    O.-T. graft
    O.-T. implant
Olsen
    O. bayonet monopolar forceps
    O. cholangiogram clamp
    O. self-retaining Laparostat
Olsen-Hegar needle holder
Olshevsky tube
Olson phaco chopper
Olyco
    O. articulator
    O. mouth mirror
Olympia
    O. articulator
    O. mouth mirror
    O. Vacpac support
    O. Vacpac support device
Olympic
    O. needle holder
    O. Neostraint immobilizer
Olympus
    O. alligator-jaw endoscopic forceps
    O. angioscope
    O. automatic reprocessor
    O. basket-type endoscopic forceps
    O. BHT-2 microscope
    O. CBK fluorescence microscope
    O. CD-20Z heater probe

O. CD-Z-series heat probe thermocoagulator
O. CF-20 fibercolonoscope
O. CF-HM-series magnifying colonoscope
O. CF-L-series flexible sigmoidoscope
O. CF-MB-series colonoscope
O. CF-OSF-series flexible sigmoidoscope
O. CF-PL-series colonoscope
O. CF-P-series colonoscope
O. CF-series colonofiberscope
O. CF-series colonoscope
O. CF-series flexible sigmoidoscope
O. CF-T-series colonoscope
O. CF-UM3 colonoscope
O. CF-UM3 flexible echocolonoscope
O. CF-UM-series echoendoscope
O. CF-UM20 ultrasonic endoscope
O. CF-VL-series colonoscope
O. CF-200Z colonoscope
O. CG-P-series colonofiberscope
O. CHF-P-series choledochoscope
O. CHF-Q10 cholangioscope
O. CHF-series choledochoscope
O. clip-fixing device
O. CLV-series fiberoptic system
O. CLV-U 20 endoscopic halogen light source
O. continuous-flow resectoscope
O. CV-series colonoscope
O. CV-series endoscope
O. CYF-series OES cystofiberscope
O. diagnostic laparoscope
O. disposable cannula
O. disposable trocar
O. duodenofiberscope
O. endocamera
O. endoscopic ultrasound scanner
O. Endo-Therapy disposable biopsy forceps
O. ENF-P2 scope
O. ENF-P-series laryngoscope
O. esophagofiberscope
O. esophagoscope
O. EU-M-series endosonography image processor
O. Europe ETD automated endoscope washer
O. EUS-20 endoscopic ultrasound
O. EU-series endoscope
O. EUS-series endoscope
O. EVIS color computer chip system
O. EVIS Q-series endoscope
O. EVIS-series endoscope
O. EVIS video colonoscope
O. EW-series fiberoptic duodenoscope
O. FB-series biopsy forceps
O. FG-series forceps
O. fiberoptic bronchoscope
O. fiberoptic cystoscope

O. fiberoptic scope
O. fiberoptic sigmoidoscope
O. flexible hysterofiberscope
O. forward-viewing endoscope
O. FS-K-series endoscopic suture-cutting forceps
O. FS-series endoscopic suture-cutting forceps
O. gastrocamera
O. gastrostomy
O. GF-series echoendoscope
O. GF-series gastroscope
O. GF-UM-series echoendoscope
O. GF-UM-series endoscope
O. GF UM3 system
O. GF UM20 system
O. GIF-EUM-series echoendoscope
O. GIF-HM-series endoscope
O. GIF-J-series endoscope
O. GIF-K-series gastroscope
O. GIFK-XQ-series endoscope
O. GIF Q30 fiberscope
O. GIF-Q-series endoscope
O. GIF-series double-channel therapeutic videoendoscope
O. GIF-series duodenoscope
O. GIF-series echoendoscope
O. GIF-series gastroscope
O. GIF-series videoendoscope
O. GIF-SQ-series videoendoscope
O. GIF-1T10 echoendoscope
O. GIF-T-series endoscope
O. GIF-T-series videoendoscope
O. GIF-XP-series endoscope
O. GIF-XQ-series flexible gastroscope
O. GIF-XV-series endoscope
O. GIX-XQ-series videoendoscope
O. grasping rat-tooth forceps
O. GTF-series gastroscope
O. heat probe
O. hot biopsy forceps
O. HX-21L detachable mini-loop
O. hysteroscope
O. JF-series video duodenoscope
O. JF-T-series endoscope
O. JF-TV-series endoscope
O. JF-UM20 echoendoscope
O. JF-V-series endoscope
O. JF-V-series video duodenoscope
O. JT-series video duodenoscope
O. light source connector
O. 13 L injector
O. magnetic extractor forceps
O. MAJ363 FNA needle system
O. neonatal cystoscope
O. NM-K-series sclerotherapy needle
O. NM-L-series needle
O. N-series ultrathin endoscope
O. OES fiberscope
O. OES-series gastroscope
O. OM-1 endoscopic camera
O. OM-1 reflex camera
O. One-Step Button gastrostomy tube

Olympus *(continued)*
- O. operating camera
- O. operating laparoscope
- O. OSF scope
- O. OSP fluorescence measuring system
- O. OTV-S-series miniature camera
- O. PCF-series pediatric colonoscope
- O. pelican-type endoscopic forceps
- O. PJF-series pediatric duodenoscope
- O. PJF-series pediatric endoscope
- O. P-series endoscope
- O. PW-1L wash catheter
- O. Q-series endoscope
- O. rat-tooth endoscopic forceps
- O. resectoscope loop
- O. reusable oval cup forceps
- O. reusable oval cup forceps with needle
- O. SD-5L semicircular snare
- O. shark-tooth endoscopic forceps
- O. side-viewing endoscope
- O. SIF-M-series video enteroscope
- O. SIF-series video enteroscope
- O. SIF-SW-series video enteroscope
- O. SIF 100 video push endoscope
- O. SP-series image analyzer
- O. SSIF-series video enteroscope
- O. stone retrieval basket
- O. TJF-series endoscope
- O. tripod-type endoscopic forceps
- O. 2T-2000 twin-channel therapeutic gastroscope
- O. UES-series snare cautery device
- O. ultrasonic esophagoprobe
- O. ultrathin balloon-fitted ultrasound probe
- O. UM-R-series miniature ultrasonic probe
- O. UM-series echoendoscope
- O. UM-series endoscope
- O. UM-W-series endoscopic probe
- O. UM-1W transendoscopic ultrasound probe
- O. URF-P2 translaparoscopic choledochofiberscope
- O. URF type P2 flexible ureteroscope
- O. video duodenoscope
- O. video urology procedure system
- O. V-series endoscope
- O. VU-M2 endoscope
- O. VU-M-series echoendoscope
- O. VU-series echoendoscope
- O. W-shaped endoscopic forceps
- O. XCF-series endoscope
- O. XCF-XK-series endoscope
- O. XIF-series echoendoscope
- O. XIF-UM-series echoendoscope
- O. XJF-UM20 echoduodenoscope
- O. XK-10 endoscope
- O. XK-series oblique-viewing flexible fiberscope
- O. XMP-U2 catheter echoprobe
- O. XP-series endoscope
- O. XQ-series endoscope
- O. XSIF-series video enteroscope

Olympus II PTCA dilatation catheter

OM
- OM 2000 operating microscope
- OM 4 ophthalmometer

O'Malley
- O. jaw fracture splint
- O. ocutome
- O. self-adhering lens implant
- O. vitrector

O'Malley-Heintz
- O.-H. infusion cannula
- O.-H. vitreous cutter

O'Malley-Pearce-Luma lens
O'Malley-Skia transilluminator
Ombrédanne
- O. forceps
- O. mallet

Omed
- O. bulldog vascular clamp
- O. vented instrument guard

Omega
- O. compression hip screw
- O. 5600 noninvasive blood pressure monitor
- O. Plus compression hip system
- O. splinting material

Omega-NV balloon
OmegaPort access port
Omegascope OM2/070 flexible microendoscope
omental plug
Omiderm transparent adhesive film dressing
Ommaya
- O. cerebrospinal fluid (CSF) reservoir
- O. intraventricular reservoir system
- O. reservoir device
- O. reservoir implant material
- O. reservoir prosthesis
- O. reservoir transensor
- O. retromastoid reservoir
- O. shunt
- O. side-port flat-bottomed reservoir
- O. spinal fluid reservoir
- O. suboccipital reservoir
- O. ventricular reservoir
- O. ventricular tube

Omni
- O. Bloc bite blocks
- O. catheter
- O. infant heel warmer
- O. knee brace
- O. laser tip
- O. 2 microscope
- O. press
- O. pretibial buttress
- O. retractor
- O. SST balloon

Omni-Atricor pacemaker

Omnicarbon
O. heart valve prosthesis
O. prosthetic heart valve
OmniCath atherectomy catheter
Omnicor pacemaker
Omni-Ectocor pacemaker
Omnifit
O. acetabular cup
O. HA femoral component
O. HA hip stem
O. HA hip stem prosthesis
O. HA hip system
O. intraocular lens
O. knee prosthesis
O. Plus
O. Plus enhanced offset cemented hip system
O. Plus hip system
Omnifit-C
Osteonics O.-C.
Omniflex
O. balloon
O. balloon catheter
O. head
O. impression material
Omni-Flexor
O.-F. device
O.-F. wrist exerciser
Omni-Flow
O.-F. 4000 Plus
O.-F. 4000 Plus medication management system
Omni-LapoTract support system
Omniloc
O. dental implant
O. dental system
OmniMed argon-fluoride excimer laser
OmniMedia XRS scanner
Omni-Orthocor pacemaker
Omni-Park speculum
OmniPhase penile prosthesis
OmniPulse holmium laser
OmniPulse-MAX holmium laser
Omniscience
O. single-leaflet cardiac valve prosthesis
O. tilting-disk valve
O. tilting-disk valve prosthesis
O. valve device
Omnisil putty
Omni-Stanicor pacemaker
OmniStent stent
Omni-Theta pacemaker
OmniTip side-firing laser needle
Omnitone hearing aid
Omni-Tract vaginal retractor
Omni-Ventricor pacemaker
Omron
O. compressor nebulizer
O. Hem-601 automatic digital wrist blood pressure monitor
Omron/Marshall 97 automatic oscillometric digital blood pressure Monitor

On2 lateral transfer device
On-Command catheter
Oncor ApopTaq Kit
on-demand analgesia computer
One
O. Action Stent Introduction System
O. Time dressing kit
O. Time sharp debridement tray
O. Touch Basic
O. Touch basic glucometer
O. Touch blood glucose monitor
O. Touch II hospital blood glucose monitoring system
ONE Disposable microkeratome
one-hand speculum
one-hole angiographic catheter
one-horn bridge
O'Neill
O. cardiac clamp
O. cardiac surgical scissors
one-piece
o.-p. plate haptic silicone intraocular lens
o.-p. shunt with reservoir
One-Time disposable skin stapler
One-Touch
O.-T. blood glucose meter
O.-T. electrolysis unit
Ong capsulotomy scissors
Onik-Cohen percutaneous access catheter
onlay implant
OnLine ABG monitoring system
Ono
O. laryngobronchoscope atomizer
O. loupe for endoscope
On-Q
O.-Q. pain management system
O.-Q. pump
Ontrak
Abuscreen O.
On-X-mechanical bi-leaflet prosthetic heart valve
Onyx finger pulse oximeter
Onyx-R NiTi file
Opaca-Garcea ureteral catheter
opaque
ACTIVE LIFE one-piece drainable o.
ACTIVE LIFE one-piece precut closed-end o.
o. myringotomy tube
o. wire suture
Opdima digital mammography system
open
o. C-D hook
o. electrocautery snare
o. face mask
o. lens
o. magnet
o. sphincterotome
open-celled foam
open-end aspirating tube
open-ended ureteral catheter
open-heeled Unna boot

open-loop
o.-l. insulin delivery system
o.-l. intraocular lens
OpenPACS system
open-side vaginal speculum
open-tube rigid bronchoscope
OPERA
OPERA Star morcellator
OPERA Star resectoscope
OPERA Star SL hysteroscope
OPERA system
operating
o. loupe
o. microscope
o. platform
operative explorer
OPG-Gee instrument
Ophtec
O. Co. lens
O. occlusion implant
Ophthalas
O. argon/krypton laser
O. krypton laser
ophthalmic
o. blade
o. calipers
o. cautery electrode
o. cup
o. electrocautery
o. endoscope
o. hook
o. laser microendoscope
o. pick
o. sable brush
o. sponge
ophthalmodynamometer
Bailliart o.
dial-type o.
Reichert o.
ophthalmoendoscope
Nebauer o.
Zylik o.
ophthalmometer
American Optical o.
Haag-Streit o.
Hertel o.
Javal o.
OM 4 o.
ophthalmoplethysmograph
ophthalmoscope
Alcon indirect o.
Bailliart o.
binocular indirect o. with SPF
o. camera
confocal laser scanning o.
confocal scanning laser o.
cordless monocular indirect o.
Doran pattern stimulator o.
Exeter o.
Fisons indirect binocular o.
Friedenwald o.
Ful-Vue o.
Grafco o.
Gullstrand o.
Halberg indirect o.

halogen coaxial o.
Helmholtz o.
Highlight spectral indirect o.
indirect laser o.
Keeler o.
Loring o.
Mascot indirect o.
May o.
Mentor Exeter o.
metric o.
MK IV o.
monocular indirect o.
Morton o.
Nebauer o.
Neolyte laser indirect o.
Nerve Fiber Analyzer laser o.
Novus 2000 o.
Panoramic 200 nonmydriatic o.
polarizing o.
Polle pod attachment for o.
Propper binocular indirect o.
Propper-Heine o.
Reichert binocular indirect o.
Reichert Ful-Vue binocular o.
Rodenstock scanning laser o.
scanner laser o.
scanning laser o.
Schepens o.
Schepens-Pomerantzeff o.
Schultz-Crock binocular o.
TopSS scanning laser o.
Vantage o.
visuscope o.
Welch Allyn o.
Zeiss o.
Ophthalon suture
ophthalsonic pachymeter
Ophthascan
Alcon-Biophysic O.
Ophthasonic Ultrasonic Biometer
Ophthimus High-Pass Resolution perimeter
Opiela brace
OpMi
O. colposcope
O. microscopic drape
O. PRO magis surgical microscope
O. VISU 200 microscope
Opmilas
O. CO_2 multipurpose laser
O. 144 Plus laser system
O. 144 surgical laser
Opotow filling material
Oppenheim
O. brace
O. spring wire splint
Oppenheimer
O. knuckle-bender splint
O. spring wire splint
Op-Pneu
O.-P. insufflator
O.-P. laparoscopy needle
Oppociser
O. exercise device
O. hand exerciser

opponens splint
opposed loop-pair quadrature magnetic resonance coil
Opraflex
    O. dressing
    O. incise drape
Opsis DistalCam video system
OpSite
    O. drape
    O. Flexifix transparent film dressing
    O. Flexigrid dressing
    O. occlusive dressing
    O. PLUS dressing
    O. wound dressing
Opta 5 catheter
Optelec Passport magnifier
Op-Temp
    O.-T. cautery
    O.-T. disposable electrocautery
Optetrak total knee replacement system
Opthascan
    O. Mini-A scan
    O. Mini-A scanner
Opticaid lens loupe
optical
    o. aspirating curette
    o. biopsy forceps
    O. catheter
    o. digitizer
    o. Doppler velocimeter
    o. esophagoscope
    o. laryngoscope
    o. multichannel analyzer system
    o. needle
    o. pachymeter
    o. pedobarograph
    O. Radiation intraocular lens
    o. ureterotome
optically transparent electrode
Opticath oximeter catheter
OptiChamber drug holding device
optic implant
optics
    Boutin o.
    confocal o.
    o. cup
    mirror-based reflective o.
    SinuScope rigid rod lens o.
2-Optifit toric lens
Opti-Fix
    O.-F. acetabular cup
    O.-F. femoral component
    O.-F. total hip system
Optiflex intraocular lens
Opti-Flow permanent dialysis catheter
Opti-Gard eye protector
OptiHaler drug delivery system
Optilume prostate balloon dilator
Optima
    O. contact lens
    O. diamond knife
    O. I MPI pacemaker
    O. MPT-series III pacemaker
    O. pulse generator
    O. SPT pacemaker

OptiMax
    O. immunostaining system
    O. Supreme pressure-reduction mattress
Optimed glaucoma pressure regulator
Optimum blade
Option Orthotic Series
Optiphot-2UD microscope
Optiplanimat automated unit
Optipore
    O. scrub sponge
    O. wound-cleaning sponge
Opti 1 portable pH/blood gas analyzer
Optipost
    Brasseler O.
Opti-Pure
    O.-P. system
Optique microscope
Opti-Qvue Mixed Venous Saturation/CCO pulmonary artery catheter system
OptiScan 2000
Optiscope
    O. angioscope
    O. catheter
Optisson contrast material
Optistar MR contrast delivery system
Optiva catheter
Optiview
    O. optical surgical obturator
    O. trocar
Optivis Surgalloy needle
Opti-Vue plastic barrel
Opti-Vu lens
optode
    fluorescent o.
optoelectric measuring apparatus
Optokinetic stimulator
optometer
    infrared o.
    laser o.
OptoTrak motion-analysis system
Opt-Visor
    O.-V. lens
    O.-V. loupe
Opus pacemaker
OR-340 imaging system
Oracle
    O. Focus PTCA catheter
    O. Focus ultrasound imaging catheter
    O. intravascular ultrasound catheter
    O. Megasonics catheter
    O. Micro intravascular ultrasound catheter
    O. Micro Plus
    O. Micro Plus PTCA catheter
Ora-Gard disposable intraoral bite block
oral
    o. endoscope
    o. endotracheal tube
    o. esophageal stethoscope
    o. esophageal tube
    o. forceps
    o. implant

oral *(continued)*
    o. needle
    o. pharyngeal airway
    O. Scan computer imaging system
    O. Scan video imaging system
    o. screw
    o. screw mouthgag
    o. screw tongue depressor
    o. speculum mouthgag
    o. surgery handpiece
    o. temperature device
    O. Video Scope
Oral-B soft foam interdental brush
Oral-Cath catheter
Orandi knife
orange dye laser
Orascoptic
    O. acuity system
    O. fiberoptic headlight
    O. loupe extension
OraSure
    O. HIVG-1 collection device
    O. HIV-1 oral specimen collection device
    O. salivary collection device
Oratek
    O. chisel
    O. device
    O. thermal shrinking probe
Orban curette
orbicular retractor
Orbis-Sigma cerebrospinal fluid shunt valve
orbital
    o. compressor
    o. depressor
    o. floor implant
    o. floor prosthesis
    o. retractor
    O. shoulder stabilizer brace
Orbit blade
Orbiter treadmill
Orbix x-ray unit
Orbscan pachymeter
Orca surgical blade
ORC-B Ranfac cholangiographic catheter
orchidometer
    punched-out o.
    Test-Size o.
ORC posterior chamber intraocular lens
Oregon
    O. prosthesis
    O. tunneler
O'Reilly esophageal retractor
Orentreich punch
Oreopoulos-Zellerman catheter
Oretorp retractable knife
Orfit
    O. mask
    O. splint
Orfizip
    O. body jacket
    O. casting system
    O. knee cast

Organdi blade
organic
    o. dental cement
    o. liquid scintillator
organizer
    Hunt o.
    Suture VesiBand o.
Organon percutaneous E2 implant
Origin
    O. PDB 1000 balloon
    O. trocar
original
    O. Jacknobber II muscle-massage device
    o. Sweet eye magnet
O-ring attachments
OR 340 Intraoperative ultrasound
Orion
    O. anterior cervical plate
    O. balloon
    O. continence system
    O. device
    O. inhaler
    O. lumbar support
    O. model AE 940 ion analyzer
    O. pacemaker
    O. plate and screw
Oris pin
Orlando
    O. hip-knee-ankle-foot orthosis
    O. tibial plateau fracture bracing system
OrlandoTPFx bracing system
ORLAU
    ORLAU swivel walker
    ORLAU swivel walker orthosis
Orley retractor
Orlon vascular prosthesis
Orlowski stent
Ormco
    O. appliance
    O. band scissors
    O. band setter
    O. ligature director
    O. orthodontic arch-expander
    O. orthodontic hemostat
    O. orthodontic pliers
    O. pin
    O. preformed band
    O. wire bracket
oroendotracheal tube
oroesophageal overtube
orogastric
    o. Ewald tube
oropharyngeal pack
orotome
    Steinhauser o.
orotracheal tube
Orozco plate
Orr
    O. automatic reprocessor
    O. gall duct forceps
Orr-Buck extension tractor
Orthair oscillating saw
Orthairtome II drill

Orthawear antiembolism stockings
Orth-evac autotransfusion system
Orthex
   O. cannulated titanium bone screw
   O. reliever insole
   O. Relievers shoe insert
Orthicon camera
Orthion traction machine
ortho
   O. All-Flex diaphragm
   O. Cytofluorograf 50-H flow
     cytometer
   O. diaphragm kit
   o. disk
   O. Dx electromedical stimulator
   O. System 20 flow cytometer
   O. Tech performer knee brace
Ortho-Arch II orthotic
Ortho-Athrex instrument
Orthoband traction band
Ortho-Biotic recliner
OrthoBlend powered bone mill
OrthoBone pillow
Ortho-Cel pad
Orthoceph x-ray unit
Orthocomp cement
Orthocor II pacemaker
Orthoderm
   O. consummate air therapy bed
   O. convertible
   O. convertible II
   O. convertible mattress
Orthodoc presurgical planning system
orthodontic
   o. aligner
   o. appliance
   o. band
   o. band driver
   o. band setter
   o. base plate
   o. bracket
   o. cement
   o. impression tray
   o. resin
OrthoDyn
   O. bone substitute
   O. bone substitute material
Orthofix
   O. Cervical-Stim stimulator
   O. external fixation device
   O. intramedullary nail
   O. lengthening device
   O. M-100 distractor
   O. monolateral femoral external
     fixator
   O. pin
   O. prosthesis
   O. screw
Orthoflex
   O. dressing
   O. elastic plaster bandage
Ortho-Foam elbow/heel pad
OrthoFrame external fixation
Orthofuse implantable growth stimulator
OrthoGel liner

OrthoGen bone growth stimulator
Orthoglass splint material
orthogonal
   o. film
   o. laser
   o. radiofrequency coil
Ortho-Grip silicone rubber handle
Ortho-Ice
   O.-I. Multipaks pack
   O.-I. Multipaks system
Ortho-Jel impression material
Orthokinetics travel chair
Ortho-last splint
Ortholav
   O. irrigation and suction device
   O. pulsed irrigator
   O. suction
Ortholen sheet
Ortholoc
   O. Advantim revision knee system
   O. Advantim total knee system
   O. prosthesis
OrthoLogic bone growth stimulator
Orthomatrix binder
Orthomedics
   O. brace
   O. Stretch and Heel splint
Ortho-mesh
Orthomet
   O. Axiom total knee system
   O. Perfecta total hip system
Orthomite
   O. II adhesive
   O. resin
Ortho-Mold
   O.-M. spinal brace
   O.-M. splint
OrthoNail intramedullary fixation device
orthopaedic (*var. of* orthopedic)
OrthoPak
   O. bone growth stimulator system
   O. II bone growth stimulator
Ortho-Pal body support
Orthopantomograph-3
Orthopantomograph-series panoramic x-
   ray machine
orthopedic, orthopaedic
   o. bone file
   o. broach
   o. bur
   o. chisel
   o. curette
   o. cutting instrument
   o. depth gauge
   o. dynamometer
   o. elevator
   o. fixation device
   o. forceps
   o. goniometer
   o. gouge
   o. hammer
   o. hemostat
   o. impactor
   o. knife
   o. osteotome

O

orthopedic *(continued)*
  o. pin
  o. plate
  o. positioning seat
  o. rasp
  o. reamer
  o. rod
  o. rongeur
  o. scissors
  o. screw
  o. staple
  o. stockinette
  o. strap clavicle splint
  o. surgical pliers
  o. surgical stripper
  o. Universal drill

Orthopedic Systems Inc. (OSI)
Orthoplast
  O. dressing
  O. fracture brace
  O. isoprene splint
  O. jacket
  O. slipper cast

Orthoptic
  O. eye patch
  O. Therapy amblyoscope

Orthoralix
  Philips O.

Ortho-Rater
orthorhythmic pacemaker
orthoscopic lens
Orthoset
  O. cement
  O. radiopaque bone cement adhesive

orthosis
  adjustable advanced reciprocating gait o.
  A-frame o.
  Aliplast custom molded foot o.
  ankle o. (AO)
  ankle-foot o. (AFO)
  Aspen cervical thoracic o.
  balance padding o.
  bar-and-shoe o.
  Bauerfeind Malleolic ankle o.
  Beaufort seating o.
  Bebax o.
  BFO o.
  Biothotic foot o.
  BODI Dynamic o.
  BODI knee extension o.
  Boston post-op hip o.
  cable-twister o.
  calcaneal spur cookie o.
  Caligamed ankle o.
  Canadian knee o.
  cervical o. (CO)
  cervical thoracic o.
  cervicothoracic o.
  Comfy Elbow o.
  Comfy Knee o.
  Controller Shoulder O.
  copolymer ankle-foot o.

Craig-Scott o.
cruciform anterior spinal hyperextension o.
Daytona cervical o.
Dermoplast-Plastazote o.
Diabetic D-Sole foot o.
dial-lock o.
dual-photon electrospinal o.
Dynamic elbow o.
Dynamic knee o.
Dynamic wrist o.
elbow-wrist-hand o. (EWHO)
Engen palmar finger o.
external o.
E-Z arm abduction o.
FirmFlex custom o.
Flex Foam o.
Foot Levelers o.
Frejka o.
gator plastic o.
Gillette joint o.
Gillette modification of ankle-foot o.
GunSlinger shoulder o.
G/W Heel Lift, Inc. o.
hallux valgus o.
halo cervical o.
halo-vest o.
Heel Spur Special o.
hindfoot o.
hip guidance o.
hip-knee o.
hip-knee-ankle o.
Hosmer voluntary control (VC4) four-bar knee o.
Hyperex thoracic o.
inflatable thoracic lumbosacral o.
ipos heel relief o.
J-24 cervical o.
J-45 contraflexion o.
Jewett-Benjamin cervical o.
Jewett contraflexion o.
Jewett post-fusion o.
Jewett thoracolumbosacral o.
J-35 hyperextension o.
Johnson cervical thoracic o.
Johnson Kydex chairback o.
Johnson total hip stabilization o.
Jousto dropfoot splint, skid o.
J-55 postfusion o.
Kallassy o.
Kid-Dee-Lite o.
knee-ankle o.
knee-ankle-foot o.
knee extension o.
knee-foot-ankle o.
Knight-Taylor and Williams spinal o.
L.A. cervical o.
leather o.
Levy & Rappel foot o.
Ligamentus Ankle o.
L'Nard long opponens hand and wrist o.
L'Nard Multi-Podus o.

L'Nard thoracolumbosacral o.
LSU reciprocation-gait o.
lumbar o.
lumbosacral o.
Lynco foot o.
Malibu cervical o.
Malleoloc anatomic ankle o.
Maple Leaf o.
Marlin cervical o.
MCF shoulder o.
medical ankle o.
metal hybrid o.
Meyer cervical o.
Milwaukee scoliosis o.
Minerva o.
molded ankle-foot o.
MultiBoot o.
neoprene wrist o.
Newington o.
Newport MC hip o.
Newport total hip o.
New York Orthopedic front-
   opening o.
New York University insert for o.
NuKo knee o.
Oklahoma ankle joint o.
Orlando hip-knee-ankle-foot o.
ORLAU swivel walker o.
patellar tendon weightbearing
   brace o.
pediatric pressure relief ankle
   foot o.
pelvic stabilization o.
Perlstein o.
Phelps o.
plastic o.
polypropylene glycol ankle-foot o.
polypropylene glycol
   thoracolumbosacral orthosis
posterior leaf-spring ankle-foot o.
pressure relief ankle foot o.
Profile Sitting O.
Pro-glide o.
Progressive ankle o.
PSA thermoplastic o.
Pucci pediatrics hand o.
Pucci rehab knee o.
Rancho Los Amigos o.
Rebel knee o.
reciprocating gait o.
resting o.
Rochester hip-knee-ankle-foot o.
Scott-Craig o.
Scottish Rite hip o.
Seattle o.
Select joint o.
semirigid polypropylene ankle-
   foot o.
Shaeffer rigid o.
shoulder o.
shoulder-elbow-wrist-hand o.
single-photon electrospinal o.
Slim Option shoe o.
Sof Gel HeelCup o.
SOLEutions custom o.

SOMI o.
SportsFit thumb o.
Sport-Stirrup o.
standing frame o.
sternooccipital-mandibular
   immobilization o.
supracondylar knee-ankle o.
supramalleolar o.
Swede-O-Universal o.
Taylor thoracolumbosacral o.
Thera-Pos elbow o.
Thera-Pos knee o.
Therapy Carrot Finger O.
Thera-Soft hand/wrist o.
Theratotic firm foot o.
Theratotic soft foot o.
Thomas collar cervical o.
Thomas heel o.
thoracolumbar spinal o.
thoracolumbar standing o.
thoracolumbosacral spinal o.
tone-reducing ankle-foot o.
Toronto parapodium o.
total contact bivalve ankle-foot o.
TPE ankle-foot o.
TPE biomechanical foot o.
TRAFO o.
Transpire wrist o.
turnbuckle wrist o.
Ultrabrace o.
VAPC dorsiflexion assist o.
Vari-Duct hip and knee o.
Viscoheel K, N o.
Viscoheel SofSpot o.
weight-relieving o.
Williams o.
wrist-driven prehension o.

Orthosleep pillow
OrthoSorb
   O. absorbable pin
   O. pin fixation
   O. pin nail
Orthostar surgical table
**Orthotec pressurized fluid irrigation
   system**
orthotic (*See also* orthosis)
   Amfit o.'s
   ankle-foot o.
   o. attachment implant
   BIOflex penile o.
   Biofoot o.
   Biothotic o.
   Blue Line o.
   CLC o.
   o. coiled spring twister
   cork, leather, and elastic o.
   custom-healing o.
   DesignLine o.
   o. device
   Diab-A-Thotics o.
   DressFlex o.
   DSIS o.
   D-Soles o.
   Duraleve custom molded foot o.
   FirmFlex custom o.

C

orthotic *(continued)*
>   FlexiSport o.
>   Foot Levelers custom o.
>   functional o.
>   Golden Comfort o.
>   Golden Fitness o.
>   Healthflex o.
>   Kinetic Wedge o.
>   Ligamentus Ankle ankle o.
>   Lyte Fit o.
>   Magnathotics o.
>   Mayer o.
>   MBS snap-on o.
>   M-Pact flexible o.
>   OB Gees maternity o.
>   Ortho-Arch II o.
>   OrthoVise o.
>   ParFlex Plus o.
>   Plastizote o.
>   o. plate
>   Polydor Preforms o.
>   PRAFO adjustable o.
>   ProLite Plus runner's o.
>   Pucci Air o.
>   Rediform o.
>   Rohadur-Polydor o.
>   Rohadur-Schaefer o.
>   Rohadur-Whitman o.
>   Sandalthotics postural support o.
>   Slimthetics o.
>   Soft Super Sport o.
>   Soft Support Preforms o.
>   soft-tissue Super Sport o.
>   SOLEutions o.
>   Sport Preforms o.
>   Stratos o.
>   Superform Contours o.
>   Supralen cradle o.
>   Supralen Schaefer o.
>   Swiss Balance o.
>   Thermo HK/Rohadur o.
>   Thermo HK/Tepefom o.
>   Thinline uncovered o.
>   UCOheal o.
>   UCOlite o.
>   XO-soft-sole o.

orthotopic
>   o. biventricular artificial heart
>   o. univentricular artificial heart

Ortho-Trac adhesive skin traction bandage
Orthotron exerciser
Ortho-Turn transfer aid
Ortho-Vent bandage
OrthoVise
>   O. orthopaedic instrument
>   O. orthotic

OrthoWedge healing shoe
Ortho-Wick foam liner
Ortho-Yomy facebow
Orton enamel cleaver
Ortved stone dislodger
OS-5/Plus 2 knee brace

Osada
>   O. Beaver-XL handpiece unit
>   O. saw
>   O. XL-S30 electric handpiece system

Osbon pressure-point tension ring
Osborne
>   O. goniometer
>   O. osteotomy plate
>   O. punch

OSCAR ultrasonic bone cement removal system
Osciflator balloon inflation syringe
oscillating
>   o. grid
>   o. saw

oscillator
>   Hayek o.

OscilloMate 930 blood pressure measurement system
oscillometric blood pressure cuff
oscilloscope
>   cathode ray o.
>   Norland digital o.
>   single-channel electromyograph o.
>   single-channel nonfade o.
>   Tektronix digital o.

Oscor
>   O. atrial lead
>   O. pacemaker
>   O. pacing leads

Osgood needle
Oshar-Neumann 8-line corneal marker
O'Shaughnessy
>   O. arterial forceps
>   O. clamp
>   O. pince

O'Shea lens
Osher
>   O. air-bubble removal cannula
>   O. bipolar coaptation forceps
>   O. capsular forceps
>   O. conjunctival forceps
>   O. corneal scissors
>   O. diamond knife
>   O. foreign body forceps
>   O. globe rotator
>   O. haptic forceps
>   O. internal calipers
>   O. iris retractor
>   O. irrigating implant hook
>   O. lens-vacuuming cannula
>   O. lid retractor
>   O. malleable microspatula
>   O. micrometer cataract knife
>   O. needle holder
>   O. nucleus lens manipulator
>   O. nucleus stab expressor
>   O. pan-fundus lens
>   O. superior rectus forceps
>   O. surgical keratometer
>   O. surgical posterior pole lens

Osher-Fresnel intraocular lens
Oshukova collapsible bougie guide

OSI
  Orthopedic Systems Inc.
    OSI arthroscopic well-leg leg holder
    OSI extremity elevator
    OSI modular table system
    OSI Well Leg Support
OSM2 in vitro oximeter
Osmette osmometer
OsmoCyte
    O. island wound care dressing
    O. PCA pillow wound dressing
    O. pillow
osmometer
    freezing point o.
    Model 5500 vapor pressure o.
    Osmette o.
OSMO reverse-osmosis unit
osmotic minipump
OSM3 Radiometer
OsseoCare
    O. drill
    O. drilling equipment
    O. machine
Osseodent
    O. dental implant
    O. surgical drill
Osseofix implant system
osseointegrated oral implant
Osseotite two-stage procedure implant
osseous
    o. coagulum trap
    O. Coagulum Trap collecting
      system
    o. implant
    o. pin
ossicle
    Tutoplast auditory o.
ossicle-holding
    o.-h. clamp
    o.-h. forceps
ossicular chain replacement prosthesis
Ossoff-Karlan
    O.-K. laser forceps
    O.-K. laser laryngoscope
    O.-K. laser suction tube
    O.-K. microlaryngeal laser probe
Ossoff-Karlan-Dedo laryngoscope
Ossoff-Karlan-Jako laryngoscope
Ossoff-Karlen laryngoscope
Ossoff-Sisson surgical stent
Ostalloy 202 alloy
Ostby dam frame
OsteoAnalyzer
    O. densitometer
    O. device
OsteoArthritic knee brace
osteoarticular allograft
Osteobond
    O. copolymer bone cement
    O. vacuum mixing system
OsteoCap hip prosthesis
osteochondral autograft transfer system
Osteo-Clage cable system
osteoclast
    Collin o.

    Phelps-Gocht o.
    Rizzoli o.
osteodistractor
    Ace/Normed o.'s
OsteoGen
    O. bone graft
    O. bone grafting material
    O. HA dental implant
    O. implantable stimulator
Osteogenics
    O. BoneSource synthetic bone
      replacement
    O. BoneSource synthetic bone
      replacement material
**Osteogen resorbable osteogenic bone-
  filling implant**
OsteoGraf
    O. binder
    O. bone grafting material
OsteoGraf/D bone grafting material
OsteoGraf/LD bone grafting material
OsteoGraf/N
OsteoGraf/N-Block grafting material
Osteoguide
OsteoHarvester bone harvester
Osteolock
    O. HA femoral component
    O. hip prosthesis
    O. NP acetabular component
Osteo-Lock endodontic stabilization kit
**Osteomeasure computer-assisted image
  analyzer**
osteomeatal stent
Osteomed screw
osteomicrotome
    Tessier o.
Osteomin
    O. demineralized bone
    O. freeze dried bone
    O. Thermo-Ashed bone powder
    O. Thermo-Ashed bone powder
      Pulvograft
Osteon
    O. bur
    O. drill
Osteonics
    O. acetabular dome hole plug
    O. jig
    O. Omnifit-C
    O. Omnifit-HA component
    O. Omnifit-HA hip stem
    O. prosthesis
    O. reamer
    O. Scorpio insert
    O. Scorpio posterior cruciate
      retaining total knee system
    O. spinal system
Osteonics-HA coated femoral implant
Osteopatch
osteophyte elevator
osteoplastic flap clamp
Osteoplate implant
OsteoPower
    O. drilling and cutting machine

OsteoSet
O. bone filler
O. bone graft substitute
OsteoStat
O. disposable power tool
O. single-use power surgical equipment
OsteoStim
O. apparatus
O. implantable bone grown stimulator
osteotome
Albee o.
Alexander perforating o.
Anderson-Neivert o.
API o.
Army o.
Barsky nasal o.
bayonet o.
Blount scoliosis o.
Bowen o.
Box o.
Buck o.
Burton o.
Campbell o.
Carroll o.
Carroll-Legg o.
Carroll-Smith-Petersen o.
Chermel o.
Cherry o.
Cinelli o.
Clayton o.
Cloward spinal fusion o.
Cobb o.
Codman o.
Converse o.
Cook o.
Cottle crossbar chisel o.
Crane o.
Cross o.
curved o.
Dautrey o.
Dawson-Yuhl o.
Dingman o.
Epstein o.
flexible blade o.
Fomon o.
Frazier o.
French-pattern o.
Furnas bayonet o.
guarded o.
Hardt-Delima o.
Hendel guided o.
hexagonal handle o.
Hibbs o.
Hohmann o.
Hoke o.
Houston nasal o.
Howorth o.
Jarit hand surgery o.
Kazanjian action-type o.
lacrimal o.
Lahey Clinic thin o.
Lambotte o.
Lambotte-Henderson o.

lateral o.
Legg o.
Leinbach o.
Lexer o.
MacGregor o.
Manchester nasal o.
manual o.
Mathews o.
maxillofacial o.
Mayfield bayonet o.
McCollough o.
Meyerding o.
MGH o.
Micro-Aire o.
Miner o.
mini-Lambotte o.
mini-Lexer o.
Mitchell o.
Moberg o.
Moe o.
Moore o.
Murphy o.
nasal o.
nasofrontal o.
Neivert o.
Neivert-Anderson o.
New-Lambotte o.
orthopedic o.
osteotome o.
Padgett o.
Parkes lateral osteotomy o.
Parkes-Quisling o.
Peck o.
Quisling-Parkes o.
Read o.
Rhoton o.
Richards-Hibbs o.
Rish o.
Ristow o.
Rowland o.
Rubin nasofrontal o.
Sheehan o.
Silver nasal o.
sinus lift o.
slotting-bur o.
Smith-Petersen curved o.
Smith-Petersen straight o.
Stille o.
Stille-Stiwer o.
straight o.
Swanson o.
Tardy o.
Tessier o.
Ultra-Cut Hoke o.
Ultra-Cut Smith-Petersen o.
U. S. Army o.
Ward nasal o.
osteotomy pin
OsteoView
O. desktop hand x-ray system
O. device
Digital O.
O. digital bone densitometer
O. 2000 digital imaging system
Osteovit bone matrix

Osterballe precision needle
Ostic plaster dressing
ostium seeker
ostomy
  o. appliance
  o. bag
  O. Shadow Buddy
Ostreg spinal marker system
ostrum
  o. antral punch
  o. punch forceps
Ostrup vascularized rib graft
Ostycut bone biopsy needle
O'Sullivan
  O. self-retaining abdominal retractor
  O. vaginal retractor
O'Sullivan-O'Connor
  O.-O. self-retaining abdominal retractor
  O.-O. vaginal retractor
  O.-O. vaginal speculum
Oswestry-O'Brien spinal stapler
Osypka
  O. atrial lead
  O. Cereblate electrode
Otis
  O. anoscope
  O. bougie à boule
  O. bougie à boule dilator
  O. ureterotome
  O. urethral sound
  O. urethrotome
Oti Vac lighted suction unit
otoabrader
  Dingman o.
  Elsie-Brown o.
Otocap
  O. myringotomy blade
  O. myringotomy scalpel
OtoLam laser
otologic
  o. cup forceps
  o. scissors
OtoScan
  O. device
  O. ear aeration system
otoscope
  acoustic o.
  Advanced beta 200 o.
  Alpha fiberoptic pocket o.
  Bruening pneumatic o.
  Brunton o.
  Earscope o.
  fiberoptic o.
  Grafco o.
  Halogen o.
  Micro-Halogen o.
  Microtek Heine o.
  Mini-Fibralux pocket o.
  Minilux pocket o.
  office diagnostic rechargeable o.
  pneumatic o.
  Politzer air-bag o.
  Rica pneumatic o.
  Riester o.

  Siegel pneumatic o.
  Siegle o.
  SMIC pneumatic o.
  StarMed video o.
  surgical o.
  Toynbee o.
  video o.
  Welch Allyn dual-purpose o.
  Welch Allyn operating o.
  Wullstein ototympanoscope o.
Ototemp 3000 thermometer
ototome
  o. irrigation kit
  o. otological drill
Otovent autoinflation kit
Oto-Wick
  Pope O.-W.
Ottenheimer common duct dilator
Ott insufflator filter tubing
Ott-Mayo channel sampling kit
Otto
  O. Bock 1A30 Greissinger Plus foot
  O. Bock 1D25 Dynamic Plus foot
  O. Bock Greissinger Plus foot prosthesis
  O. Bock modular rotary hydraulic knee
  O. Bock Safety constant-friction knee
  O. Bock system electric hands
  O. Bock system electric hands prosthesis
  O. tissue forceps
Ottoback
  O. 3R65 children's hydraulic knee joint
  O. 3R45 modular knee joint
Oudin resonator
Oughterson forceps
Oulu neuronavigator system
OutBound syringe
Outerbridge uterine dilator
outflow cannula
outlet
  o. cannula
  o. forceps
output
  o. device
  o. signal processor
outrigger
  o. splint
  o. wire
OV-1 surgical keratometer
oval
  o. cup erysiphake
  o. cup forceps
  o. cutting bur
  o. esophagoscope
  o. eye
  o. optical zone marker
  o. piston gauge
  o. snare
  o. speculum
oval-open esophagoscope

oval-window
    o.-w. curette
    o.-w. excavator
    o.-w. hook
    o.-w. pick
    o.-w. piston evacuator
ovary forceps
Ovation
    O. falloposcopy system
    O. in-the-ear hearing aid
oven
    Coltene o.
    Thermoprep heating o.
over-bed table
overcouch tube
overdenture
    bar-supported o.
    implant-supported o.
    mandibular o.
    removable partial o.
overhead
    o. fracture frame
    o. frame trapeze
    o. light
Overholt
    O. clip-applying forceps
    O. dissecting forceps
    O. periosteal elevator
    O. rib needle
    O. rib raspatory
    O. rib spreader
Overholt-Finochietto rib spreader
Overholt-Geissendörfer arterial forceps
Overholt-Jackson bronchoscope
Overholt-Mixter dissecting forceps
overlapping pincer
overlay
    Airdance alternating o.
    AIR3787 static air mattress o.
    ALAMO alternating low-air-loss
        mattress o.
    Bi-Wave mattress o.
    Bodyline sleeper mattress o.
    BodyWrap premium o.
    DeRoyal mattress o.'s
    DU4072 Static air mattress o.
    First Step select low-air o.
    HYDRO-EASE II gel flotation
        mattress o.
    HYDRO-EASE I water flotation
        mattress o.
    IRIS 10,000 o.
    LA4072 low-air-loss o.
    o. mattress
    MIP anatomic o.
    PAL pump for air mattress o.
    Recovercare NPO non-powdered o.
    Recovercare system 1, 2 alternating
        pressure o.
    RIK fluid o.
    Stage IV crib o.
    Stimulite honeycomb mattress o.
    System 2000 alternating pressure
        pump & pad o.
    Tempur-Med hospital o.

    Topper mattress o.
    Ultraform mattress o.
    Vari-Zone variable density
        convoluted mattress o.
    x-ray o.
oversensing pacemaker
over-shoulder strap
Overstreet polyp forceps
over-the-door traction unit
over-the-endoscope Witzel dilator
over-the-guidewire esophageal dilator
over-the-needle
    o.-t.-n. infusion catheter
over-the-wire
    o.-t.-w. pacing lead
    o.-t.-w. probe
    o.-t.-w. PTCA balloon catheter
overtube
    flexible endoscopic o.
    Mill-Rose flexible endoscopic o.
    oroesophageal o.
    split o.
    Steigmann-Goff endoscopic
        ligature o.
    Williams varices injection o.
over-tying wire
Oves cervical cup
ovoid
    Delclos o.
    Fleming o.
    Fletcher-Suit tandem and o.
    Hankins lucite o.
    Hockin lucite o.
    Manchester o.
    tandem and o.
ovum
    o. curette
    o. forceps
OvuStick
Owatusi double catheter
Owen
    O. balloon
    O. cloth dressing
    O. gauze dressing
    O. hemostatic bag
    O. Lo-Profile dilation catheter
    O. nonadherent surgical dressing
Owens silk
oxalate system
Oxford
    O. fixator
    O. magnet
    O. Medilog frequency-modulated
        recorder
    O. miniature vaporizer inhaler
    O. nonkinking cuffed tube
    O. prosthesis
    O. 2-T large-bore imaging system
        scanner
    O. uncompartmental device
OxiFirst fetal monitoring system
OxiFlow meter
OxiLink oximetry probe cover
oximeter
    Accusat pulse o.

American Optical o.
Armstrong hand-held pulse o.
BCI 3301 hand-held pulse o.
BI-OX III ear o.
Cricket recording pulse o.
Criticare pulse o.
Critikon o.
Datascope 300 pulse o.
Datex model CH-S-23 pulse o.
Dinamap monitor/Oxytrak pulse o.
ear o.
FingerPrint o.
Healthdyne pulse o.
Hewlett-Packard ear o.
INVOS 3100 cerebral o.
INVOS transcranial cerebral o.
Masimo SET pulse o.
MiniOX V pulse o.
MRL o.
Nellcor N-series pulse o.
Nellcor Symphony N-3000 pulse o.
Nonin Onyx pulse o.
Novametrix pulse o.
NPB-295 pulse o.
Ohmeda hand-held o.
Ohmeda pulse o.
Onyx finger pulse o.
OSM2 in vitro o.
Oximetrix 3 o.
OxiScan pulse o.
Oxypleth pulse o.
Oxyrak pulse o.
OxyShuttle pulse o.
OxyTemp hand-held pulse o.
Oxytrak pulse o.
pulse o.
Satellite Plus pulse o.
Somanetics INVOS 3100 cerebral o.
SpaceLabs pulse o.
SpO$_2$-5001 o.
SpotCheck+ handheld pulse o.
tissue reflectance o.
oximetric catheter
Oximetrix
O. 3 oximeter
O. 3 system
oximetry
o. catheter
o. sensor
Oxiport blade
OxiScan pulse oximeter
Oxisensor
O. fetal oxygen saturation monitor
O. II adult adhesive sensor
O. oxygen transducer
Oxycel
O. dressing
O. gauze
Oxycure topical oxygen system
Oxydome oxygen therapy system

oxygen
o. analyzer
o. mask
o. saturation meter
o. supply line
o. tank
o. tent
oxygenator
Bentley o.
bubble o.
Capiox-E bypass system o.
Capiox hollow flow o.
Cobe CML o.
Cobe Optima hollow-fiber
membrane o.
DeBakey heart pump o.
Digi-Dyne cardiopulmonary
bypass o.
disk o.
extracorporeal membrane o. (ECMO)
extracorporeal pump o.
Gambro o.
High Flex D 700 S bubble o.
Lilliput neonatal o.
Maxima Plus plasma resistant
fiber o.
membrane o.
Monolyth o.
Oxyhood o.
Sarns membrane o.
Shiley o.
SpiralGold o.
Oxyguard
O. mouth block
O. oxygenating mouthguard
Oxy-Holter
Oxyhood
O. oxygenator
O. oxygen hood
O. pressurizer
oxylate dentin bonding system
**Oxylator EM-100 emergency resuscitation
device**
OxyLead interconnect cable
Oxylite
Oxymax
Oxymizer device
Oxypleth pulse oximeter
Oxypod oxygen hood
Oxy-Quik Mark IV oxygen inhalator
oxyquinoline dressing
Oxyrak pulse oximeter
OxyShuttle pulse oximeter
OxyTemp hand-held pulse oximeter
OxyTip sensor
Oxytrak pulse oximeter
**Oxy-Ultra-Lite ambulatory oxygen
systems**
Oyloidin suture
oyster splint

PA

PA 120 Osypka radiofrequency
probe
PA portal
PA Watch position-monitoring
catheter

PaBA anchor

pace

p. card
P. hysterectomy knife
P. periosteal elevator
P. Plus System scanner
P. ventricular needle

**Paceart complete pacemaker testing
system**

pacemaker

AA1 single-chamber p.
Accufix p.
Acculith p.
Activitrax single-chamber
responsive p.
Activitrax variable-rate p.
activity-guided p.
activity-sensing p.
Actros p.
AEC p.
Aequitron p.
AICD p.
AID-B p.
Alcatel p.
American Optical Cardiocare p.
American Optical R-inhibited p.
Amtech-Killeen p.
antitachycardia p.
AOO p.
Arco atomic p.
Arco lithium p.
artificial p.
Arzco p.
Astra p.
ASVIP p.
asynchronous mode p.
asynchronous ventricular VOO p.
atrial demand-inhibited p.
atrial demand-triggered p.
atrial-synchronous ventricular-
inhibited p. (ASVIP)
atrial synchronous ventricular-
inhibited p.
atrial tracking p.
atrial triggered ventricular-
inhibited p.
Atricor Cordis p.
atrioventricular junctional p.
atrioventricular sequential demand p.
Aurora dual-chamber p.
Autima II dual-chamber cardiac p.
automated external defibrillator p.
(AEDP)
Avius sequential p.
AV junctional p.
AV sequential demand p.

AV synchronous p.
Axios p.
Basix p.
Betacel-Biotronik p.
bifocal demand DVI p.
Biorate p.
Biotronik demand p.
bipolar p.
bladder p.
breathing p.
burst p.
Byrel SX p.
Byrel SX/Versatrax p.
cardiac p.
Cardio-Control p.
Cardio-Pace Medical Durapulse p.
p. catheter
Chardack-Greatbatch p.
Chardack Medtronic p.
Chorus DDD p.
Chorus RM rate-responsive dual-
chamber p.
Chronocor IV external p.
Chronos p.
cilium p.
Circadia dual-chamber rate-
adaptive p.
Classix p.
Command PS p.
committed mode p.
Cook p.
Coratomic R-wave inhibited p.
Cordis Atricor p.
Cordis Chronocor IV p.
Cordis Ectocor p.
Cordis fixed-rate p.
Cordis Gemini cardiac p.
Cordis Multicor p.
Cordis Omni Stanicor Theta
transvenous p.
Cordis Sequicor cardiac p.
Cordis Stanicor unipolar
ventricular p.
Cordis Synchrocor p.
Cordis Ventricor p.
Cortomic p.
Cosmos 283 DDD p.
Cosmos II DDD p.
Cosmos pulse-generator p.
CPI Astra p.
CPI DDD p.
CPI Maxilith p.
CPI Microthin DI, DII lithium-
powered programmable p.
CPI Minilith p.
CPI Ultra II p.
CPI Vigor p.
CPI Vista-T p.
cross-talk p.
Cyberlith demand p.
Cybertach automatic-burst atrial p.

P

pacemaker *(continued)*

Daig ESI-II or DSI-III screw-in lead p.
Dart p.
Dash single-chamber rate-adaptic p.
DDD p.
DDI mode p.
Delta TRS p.
demand cardiac p.
Devices, Ltd. p.
Dialog p.
Diplos M 5 p.
Discovery DDDR p.
Dromos p.
dual-chamber AV sequential p.
dual-chamber Medtronic.Kappa p.
dual-pass p.
Durapulse p.
DVI p.
ECT p.
Ectocor p.
ectopic atrial p.
Ela Chorus DDD p.
Elecath p.
electric cardiac p.
p. electrode
Electrodyne p.
electronic p.
Elema p.
Elema-Schonander p.
Elevath p.
Elgiloy lead-tip p.
Elite dual-chamber rate-responsive p.
Encor p.
endocardial bipolar p.
Enertrax p.
epicardial p.
Ergos O_2 dual-chamber rate-responsive p.
escape p.
external asynchronous p.
external demand p.
external-internal p.
externally-controlled noninvasive programmed stimulation p.
external transthoracic p.
Fast-Pass lead p.
fixed-rate asynchronous atrial p.
fixed-rate asynchronous ventricular p.
fully-automatic atrioventricular Universal dual-channel p.
Galaxy p.
GE p.
Gemini DDD p.
General Electric p.
Genisis dual-chamber p.
Guardian p.
Guidant CRM p.
heart p.
hermetically-sealed p.
implantable p.
implanted p.
Intermedics atrial antitachycardia p.

Intermedics Cyberlith X multiprogrammable p.
Intermedics lithium-powered p.
Intermedics Marathon dual-chamber rate-responsive p.
Intermedics Quantum unipolar p.
Intermedics Stride p.
Intermedics Thinlith II p.
Intertach p.
isotopic pulse generator p.
junctional p.
Kalos p.
Kantrowitz p.
Kelvin Sensor p.
Lambda Omni Stanicor p.
latent p.
Laurens-Alcatel nuclear powered p.
Legend p.
Leios p.
Leptos p.
Leukos p.
Lillehei p.
lithium p.
lithium-powered p.
Maestro implantable cardiac p.
Malith p.
Mallory RM-1 cell p.
malsensing p.
Maxilith p.
Medcor p.
Medtel p.
Medtronic Activitrax rate-responsive unipolar ventricular p.
Medtronic-Alcatel p.
Medtronic bipolar p.
Medtronic-Byrel-SX p.
Medtronic Chardack p.
Medtronic corkscrew electrode p.
Medtronic demand p.
Medtronic Elite II p.
Medtronic external/internal p.
Medtronic.Kappa 400 p.
Medtronic-Laurens-Alcatel p.
Medtronic Minix p.
Medtronic Pacette p.
Medtronic RF 5998 p.
Medtronic SP 502 p.
Medtronic SPO p.
Medtronic Symbios p.
Medtronic temporary p.
Medtronic Thera "i-series" cardiac p.
Medtronic-Zyrel p.
Mentor bladder p.
mercury cell-powered p.
Meridian p.
Meta DDDR p.
Meta II p.
Meta MV cardiac p.
Meta rate-responsive p.
Microlith P p.
Micro Minix p.
Microthin P2 p.
Mikros p.
Minilith p.

Minix p.
Minuet DDD p.
Multicor Gamma p.
Multicor II cardiac p.
Multilith p.
multiprogrammable p.
Nanos 1 p.
Nathan p.
natural p.
Neos M p.
Nomos multiprogrammable R-wave
  inhibited demand p.
noncompetitive p.
noninvasive temporary p.
Nova II p.
Nova MR p.
nuclear-powered p.
Omni-Atricor p.
Omnicor p.
Omni-Ectocor p.
Omni-Orthocor p.
Omni-Stanicor p.
Omni-Theta p.
Omni-Ventricor p.
Optima I MPI p.
Optima MPT-series III p.
Optima SPT p.
Opus p.
Orion p.
Orthocor II p.
orthorhythmic p.
Oscor p.
oversensing p.
Pacesetter ADDVENT 2060 LR p.
Pacesetter Synchrony p.
Pacette p.
Paragon p.
PASAR tachycardia reversion p.
PASYS p.
PDx pacing and diagnostic p.
permanent myocardial p.
permanent rate-responsive p.
permanent transvenous p.
permanent transvenous demand p.
  (PTDP)
permanent ventricular p.
Permathane Pacesetter lead p.
Phoenix 2 p.
Phoenix single-chamber p.
Phymos 3D p.
physiologic p.
Pinnacle p.
PolyFlex implantable pacing lead p.
Precept DR p.
Prima p.
Prism-CL p.
Programalith AV p.
Programalith II, III p.
programmable p.
Programmer III p.
Prolith p.
Prolog p.
Pulsar DDD p.
Pulsar NI implantable p.
P-wave-triggered ventricular p.

Q-T interval sensing p.
Quantum p.
radiofrequency p.
rate-modulated p.
rate-responsive p.
Reflex p.
Relay cardiac p.
rescuing p.
respiratory-dependent p.
reversion p.
RS4 p.
R-synchronous VVT p.
Schaldach electrode p.
Schuletz p.
screw-in lead p.
Seecor p.
Sensolog II, III p.
sensor-based single-chamber p.
Sensor Kelvin p.
Sequicor II, III p.
Shaldach p.
shifting p.
Siemens-Elema multiprogrammable p.
Siemens-Pacesetter p.
single-chamber p.
single-pass p.
sinus node p.
Sohes p.
Solar p.
Solis p.
Solus p.
Sorin p.
Spectraflex p.
Spectrax bipolar p.
Spectrax programmable Medtronic p.
Spectrax SX, SX-HT, SXT, VL,
  VM, VS p.
standby p.
Stanicor Gamma p.
Stanicor Lambda demand p.
Starr-Edwards p.
Starr-Edwards hermetically-sealed p.
Stride cardiac p.
Swing DR1 DDDR p.
Symbios p.
synchronous burst p.
synchronous mode p.
Synchrony I, II p.
Synergyst DDD p.
Synergyst II p.
Syticon 5950 bipolar demand p.
tachycardia-terminating p.
Tachylog p.
Telectronics p.
temperature-sensing p.
temporary transvenous p.
Thera-SR p.
Thermos p.
Thinlith II p.
tined lead p.
transcutaneous p.
transmural antitachycardia p.
transpericardial p.
transthoracic p.
transvenous ventricular demand p.

P

pacemaker *(continued)*
Trilogy DC+ p.
Trilogy SR+ single-chamber p.
Trios M p.
Triumph VR p.
Ultra p.
Unilith p.
unipolar atrial p.
unipolar atrioventricular p.
unipolar sequential p.
Unity-C cardiac p.
Unity VDDR p.
USCI Vario permanent p.
variable rate p.
Ventak AICD p.
Ventak ECD p.
Ventak PRx p.
Ventricor p.
ventricular asynchronous p.
ventricular demand p.
ventricular demand-inhibited p.
ventricular demand-triggered p.
ventricular-suppressed p.
ventricular-triggered p.
Versatrax cardiac p.
Versatrax II p.
Vicor p.
Vigor DDDR p.
Vista p.
Vitatrax II p.
Vitatron Diamond p.
Vitatron Diamond II p.
Vivalith-10 p.
Vivatron p.
VVD mode p.
VVI/AAI p.
VVI bipolar Programalith p.
VVIR single-chamber rate-
adaptive p.
VVI single-chamber p.
VVT p.
wandering atrial p.
Xyrel p.
Zitron p.
Zoll NTP noninvasive p.

pacemeter
Haag-Streit p.
Mishima-Hedbys attachment p.

Paceport catheter

Pace-Potts forceps

pacer
Intertach II p.
PolySafe p.

pacer-cardioverter-defibrillator
Jewel p.-c.-d.

pacer-cardioverter defibrillator (PCD)

Pacesetter
P. ADDVENT 2060 LR pacemaker
P. Affinity SR generator
P. knee brace
P. Synchrony III pulse generator
P. Synchrony pacemaker
P. Tendril DX pacing lead
P. Trilogy DR+ pulse generator

Pacette pacemaker

**Pacewedge dual-pressure bipolar pacing
catheter**

PachKnife
Corneo-Gage P.

Pach-Pen
P.-P. corneal thickness measurer
P.-P. XL pachymeter
P.-P. XL tonometer

pachymeter, pachometer
Advent p.
Compuscan-P p.
corneal p.
ophthalsonic p.
optical p.
Orbscan p.
Pach-Pen XL p.
Packo pars plana cannula p.
Sonogage ultrasound p.
Villasensor ultrasonic p.

Pachymetric P55 analyzer

Pacific
P. Coast flexible laminar bone stri
P. Coast hearing aid

Pacifico
P. cannula
P. catheter

pacing
p. catheter
p. esophageal stethoscope
p. wire
p. wire electrode

pack
Back-Ease aromatherapy hot/cold p.
Barrier laparoscopy LAVH p.
Barrier phaco extracapsular p.
Baxter personal Von-Loc ice p.
BodyIce cold p.
Cipro cystitis p.
CLO Recirculating Slim P.
Coldhot p.
Colpacs p.
cool p.
Cool Comfort cold p.
CP2 inflatable cold p.
DynaHeat hot p.
Endo Clip ML/Surgiport System p.
ErgoForm contoured cold p.
Flents breast comfort p.
gauze p.
gel p.
Glacier P.
Hodrocollator gel p.
hot moist p.
hot wet p.
hydrocollator p.
Hydrocollator steam p.
I.C.E. Down cold p.
instant cold p.
Jack Frost hot/cold p.
K p.
Kennedy sinus p.
Kirkland periodontal p.
Kold Kompress cold p.
Kool Kit cold therapy p.

koolPAK p.
Med-Wick nasal p.
Mikulicz p.
M-Zole 7 Dual P.
nasal p.
Neck-Roll aromatherapy hot/cold p.
oropharyngeal p.
Ortho-Ice Multipaks p.
PCA periodontal p.
Peri-Cold p.
Peri-Gel p.
Peri-Warm p.
Polar P.
Promise pad and pant trial p.
Rhino Rocket nasal p.
Slik-Pak non-stick nasal p.
Softouch Cold/Hot P.
Speedi-Pak sinus p.
Super Pak posterior nasal p.
TheraBeads microwaveable moist
heat p.
Thera-Med cold p.
Thermophore hot p.
Unna-Flex PLUS Venous ulcer
convenience p.
Whitehall Glacier P.

Packard
P. Auto-Gamma 5650 analyzer
P. intraocular lens
P. radioimmunoassay system

packed bead

packer
Allport gauze p.
Angell gauze p.
August automatic gauze p.
Balshi p.
Bernay uterine gauze p.
dental amalgam p.
gauze p.
Jewett bone chip p.
Kitchen postpartum gauze p.
Lorenz gauze p.
P. mosquito forceps
Ralks nasal gauze p.
Torpin automatic uterine gauze p.
P. tunnel silicone sponge
P. Wick extrusion handpiece
Woodson p.

Packiam retractor

packing
p. forceps
Kaltostat hydrofiber wound p.
Merocel epistaxis p.
Merogel nasal p.
nasal p.
Rhino Rocket nasal p.
SinuSeal nasal p.
p. strip
Weimert epistaxis p.

Pac-Kit Army-type tourniquet

Packo
P. pars plana cannula
P. pars plana cannula pachymeter

pad
Action OR p.

AirLITE support p.
Air-O-Pad p.
Akton p.
Aquaflex ultrasound gel p.
balance p.
Bauerfeind silicone heel p.
BDP p.
Bovie grounding p.
buttress p.
Cairpad incontinence p.
CarraGauze hydrogel wound
dressing p.
C.B.T. conductive stretcher p.
C.B.T. nonconductive stretcher p.
C.B.T. Siderail bumper p.
Charnley foam suture p.
Chaston eye p.
Cliniguard p.
cloverleaf met foot p.
cold p.
CONFORM II w/heel-ease Nature
Sleep pressure p.
Convoluted mattress p.
CP2 Inflat-A-Wrap cold p.
Curity ABD p.
dancer p.
digitizing p.
Dignity Plus briefmates p.
disposable electrode p.
EK-19 p.
Elasto-gel cushions/pressure p.'s
electrode p.
p. electrode
Elta derma sterile impregnated
hydrogel gauze p.
Envisan dextranomer p.
ESU dispersive p.
Etch-Master felt p.
Expansion control WAFFLE
mattress p.
eye p.
E-Z hold adhesive catheter tube
holder p.
flotation gel p.
fluid control trauma p.
gel p.
gelatin sponge p.
Gelfoam p.
Hapad longitudinal metatarsal
arch p.
heat p.
HK p.
horseshoe heel p.
horseshoe-shaped p.
hot p.
HubGuard IV cushion p.
Hydrocollator p.
hydropolymer p.
Iceman cold therapy p.
ImPad inflation p.
Impress Softpatch urinary p.
instrument stabilizer p.
Intersorb absorptive burn p.
Iodoflex solid gel p.
J p.

P

pad *(continued)*
  Johnson & Johnson non-stick p.'s
  K p.
  Kerlix cast p.
  KINS soaker p.
  lap p.
  LePad breast exam training p.
  Littmann defibrillation p.
  magnetic mat p.
  Mayfield pediatric horseshoe p.
  Medical genuine sheepskin p.
  Microcell alternating pressure p.
  Mikulicz p.
  3M Tegaderm transparent dressing
    with absorbent p.
  Ortho-Cel p.
  Ortho-Foam elbow/heel p.
  Pedifix hammertoe p.
  Pen/Alps distal p.
  Presence bladder control p.
  Pre-Vent boot style stirrup p.
  Pre-Vent knee crutch p.
  Pre-Vent OR table p.
  Pro-Ophtha eye p.
  Pro Peak decubitus p.
  Protouch p.
  Provide incontinence p.
  Ray-Tec x-ray detectable lap p.
  regular Trimshield p.
  Relton frame p.
  Roho Dry Flotation wheelchair p.
  Roho heel p.
  Scholl p.
  second skin p.
  sensor p.
  Signa P.
  Silipos digital p.
  SlimLine peach sheet care p.
  Sof-Rol cast p.
  SofSeat pressure relief p.
  Softeze self-adhering foam p.
  Sof-Wick lap p.
  SomaSensor p.
  Spectra p.
  Staph-Chek p.
  Steri-Pad gauze p.
  Stimulite honeycomb seating p.
  Super Eidersoft bed p.
  Super-Plus Trimshield p.
  Sure Sport p.
  table heating p.
  Telfa adhesive p.'s
  Tempur-Med lumbar p.
  Tempur-Med O.R. table p.
  Tempur-Med stretch p.
  Tempur-Med x-ray table p.
  TenderCloud pressure p.
  Tendersorb ABD p.
  TENS p.
  T-Foam bed p.
  Thermapad p.
  Thermophore moist heat p.
  TopiFoam gel-backed self-adhering
    foam p.

  UltraEase ultrasound p.
  ultrasound p.
  Vac-Pak P.
  ventilated incontinence p.
  wheelchair p.
  Zell p.
  ZeroG pressure relief p.
  Zimfoam p.
padded
  p. aluminum splint
  p. board splint
  p. clamp
  p. plywood splint
padding
  cast p.
  Delta-Rol cast p.
  Dyna-Flex Layer One p.
  Kerlix cast p.
  moleskin p.
  Molestick p.
  pressure relief p.
  Profex cast p.
  Protouch orthopaedic p.
  QuickStick p.
  Reston p.
  Sifoam p.
  Softexe non-adherent sub-bandage p.
  splint p.
  SurePress absorbent p.
  Thero-Skin gel p.
paddle
  compression p.
  noninvasive p.
  Rosen nucleus p.
  spot-compression p.
Padgett
  P. baseline pinch gauge
  P. dermatome blade
  P. electrodermatome
  P. endoscope
  P. hydraulic hand dynamometer
  P. implant
  P. manual dermatome
  P. mesh skin graft
  P. osteotome
  P. prosthesis
  P. shark-mouth cannula
Padgett-Concorde suction cannula
Padgett-Hood dermatome
PadKit sample collection system
Padua bladder urinary pouch
Page
  P. needle
  P. tonsillar forceps
  P. tonsillar knife
Pagenstecher
  P. lens scoop
  P. linen thread suture
Paine carpal tunnel retinaculotome
pain threshold gauge
Pajot decapitating hook
pak
  Akorn P.
  Hedges Corneal Wetting P.

SCD MaleFactor P.
tissue-wetting p.

PAL
h Diasole insole
h pump for air mattress overlay

Palacos
P. cement adhesive
P. radiopaque bone cement

Paladon
P. graft
P. implant material
P. prosthesis

palatal
p. bar
p. lifting device
p. obturator
p. prosthesis

palate
p. hook
p. retractor

palate-free activator
palate-type mouthgag
palatorrhaphy elevator
Palco enuretic alarm system
Palex
P. colostomy irrigation starter set
P. expansion screw

Palfique Estelite tooth shade resin material
Palfyn suture
Pall
P. Biomedical heat- and moisture-exchanging filter
P. ELD-96 Set Saver filter
P. leukocyte removal filter
P. leukogard-6 arterial line
P. transfusion filter

pallesthesiometer
Pallin
P. lens spatula
P. spring-assisted syringe

palmar
p. clip
p. plate
p. splint
p. swab kit

Palmaz
P. arterial stent
P. balloon-expandable iliac stent
P. biliary stent
P. Corinthian transhepatic biliary stent
P. vascular stent

Palmaz-Schatz
P.-S. balloon-expandable stent
P.-S. biliary stent
P.-S. coronary stent
P.-S. Crown balloon-expandable stent

PalmCups percussor
Palmer
P. biopsy forceps
P. bone nail
P. cruciate ligament guide
P. cutting forceps

P. grasping forceps
P. lens
P. ovarian biopsy forceps
P. uterine dilator

Palmer-Buono contact lens
Palmer-Drapier
P.-D. forceps
P.-D. needle

palm guard
PalmVue
P. ECG*stat*
P. system

Palomar E2000 laser
palpating needle
palpation probe
palpator
blunt p.
Farrior blunt p.

Palumbo
P. ankle stabilizer
P. dynamic patellar brace
P. patella tracker
P. stabilizing knee brace

Panacryl suture
Panalok
P. absorbable anchor
P. absorbable suture
P. RC QuickAnchor Plus suture anchor

Panasol II home phototherapy system
Panasonic
P. hearing aid
P. hearing aid battery

pancake MRI magnet
panchamber UV lens
Pancoast suture
pancreatic
p. duct stent
p. endoprosthesis

pancreatoscope
ultra-thin p.

Pancretec pump
Panda
P. gastrostomy tube
P. nasoenteric feeding tube
P. NCJ kit

Panelipse panoramic x-ray machine
panendoscope
cap-fitted p.
p. electrode
flexible forward-viewing p.
Foroblique p.
LoPresti p.
McC p.
McCarthy p.
Stern-McCarthry p.
Storz p.
Wolf rigid p.

Panex-E (Panoral) panoramic x-ray machine
panfundoscope
Rodenstock p.

Pang
P. biopsy forceps
P. nasopharyngeal forceps

P

Panje
P. implant
P. tube
P. voice button
P. voice prosthesis
Panje-Shagets tracheoesophageal fistula forceps
Pannett needle
panning dish
Pannu II intraocular lens
Pannu-Kratz-Barraquer speculum
PanoGauze
P. dressing
P. hydrogel-impregnated gauze
Panomat infusion pump
Panoplex hydrogel wound dressing
Panoramic
P. 200 nonmydriatic ophthalmoscope
P. 200 Ultra-Widefield ophthalmic imaging device
panoramic loupe
Panorex panoramic x-ray machine
PanoView
P. arthroscopic system
P. Optics lens
P. rod-lens ureteroscope
pant, pl. **pants**
Conveen net p.
Dignity easy access p.
Dignity Plus briefmates stretch mesh p.
Dignity Plus regular p.
Endo pants
Feeln' Sure p.
First Quality pad insert and p.
Free & Active incontinence p.
KINS pull-on waterproof p.
Lady & Sir dignity plus p.
MAST pants
Promise washable knit p.
reusable incontinence p.
Safe & Dry p.
Sani-Garm waterproof p.
Soft & Silent diaper p.
pantaloon brace
Panther catheter
pantoscope
Keeler p.
pants (pl. of pant)
Panzer gallbladder scissors
Papanicolaou smear tray
Paparella
P. angled-ring curette
P. canal knife
P. catheter
P. duckbill elevator
P. fenestrometer
P. footplate pick
P. incudostapedial joint knife
P. mastoid curette
P. middle ear instrument
P. monkey-head holder
P. myringotomy tube
P. probe
P. rasp calipers

P. self-retaining retractor
P. sickle knife
P. stapes curette
P. straight needle
P. tissue press
P. type II ventilation tube
P. wire-cutting scissors
Paparella-Frazier suction tube
Paparella-Hough excavator
Paparella-House
P.-H. curette
P.-H. knife
Paparella-Weitlaner retractor
paper
p. drape
filter p.
Papercuff disposable blood pressure cuff
Papette cervical collector
papilla drain
papilloma forceps
papillotome
30-30 p.
Accuratome precurved p.
Apollo 3 triple-lumen p.
Bard Companion p.
Bilisystem wire-guided p.
Cremer-Ikeda p.
double-lumen tapered-tip p.
dual-lumen p.
Erlangen p.
Frimberger-Karpiel 12 o'clock p.
Howell rotatable BII p.
Huibregtse-Katon p.
Microvasive p.
needle-knife p.
Piggyback needle-knife p.
precut p.
ProForma double-lumen p.
shark fin p.
Swenson p.
Wilson-Cook p.
Wiltek p.
wire-guided p.
Zimmon p.
papillotome/sphincterotome
Soehendra BII p./s.
Soehendra Precut p./s.
Swenson wire-guided p./s.
Papineau bone graft
PapNet
P. automated cervical cystology system
P. reader
papoose
p. board
p. board restraint
Pap-Perfect supply system
Pap Plus speculoscopy
Paquelin cautery
PAR
Parabath paraffin heat treatment system
paracentesis
p. knife
p. needle
paracervical nerve block needle

parachute
P. stone retrieval device
p. therapy
Paracine dressing
Paradentine dental restorative material
Paradigm ocular blood flow analyzer
paraffin
p. block
p. dressing
p. gauze
p. graft
p. implant
p. implant material
p. mitt
Parafil wax
ParaGard
P. intrauterine device
P. T380 copper IUD
Paragon
P. amalgam
P. ambulatory pump
P. Champion stent
P. Complete implant
P. coronary stent
P. infuser
P. laser
P. nitinol stent
P. pacemaker
P. single-stage dental implant
system
parallel
p. flow dialyzer
p. pin kit
p. plate dialyzer
parallel-hole medium sensitivity collimator
parallel-loop electrode
parallel-plate flow chamber
paramagnetic microsphere
Parama pulse wave generator
ParaMax
P. ACL guide system
P. angled driver
parametrium
p. clamp
p. forceps
Paramount 3-Way press bench
paranasal sinus shaver system
Parapost bur
paraPRO needle
Parascan scanning device
Parasmillie knife
Parastep I system
Paratrend
P. 7 continuous blood gas monitor
P. 7 fiberoptic PCO_2 sensor
P. 7 intravenous blood gas
monitoring system
P. 7+ sensor
PAR-C-Scan videokeratoscope
Parel-Crock vitreous cutter
Paré suture
ParFlex Plus orthotic
parfocal defraction lens
Parhad needle

Parhad-Poppen needle
Parham
P. band
P. support
Parham-Martin
P.-M. band
P.-M. bone-holding clamp
P.-M. fracture apparatus
P.-M. fracture device
parietal shunt
Parietex composite mesh
Paris
P. manual therapy table
plaster of P.
P. system
Paritene mesh graft
Park
P. blade
P. blade septostomy catheter
P. eye speculum
P. irrigating cannula
P. lens implantation forceps
P. Medical Systems scanner
P. rectal spreader
Parker
P. clamp
P. double-ended retractor
P. fixation forceps
P. micropump insulin infuser
P. needle
P. serrated discission knife
P. tenotomy knife
P. thumb retractor
P. tube
Parker-Bard
P.-B. blade
P.-B. handle
Parker-Glassman intestinal clamp set
Parker-Heath
P.-H. anterior chamber syringe
P.-H. cautery
P.-H. electrocautery
P.-H. piggyback
P.-H. piggyback probe
Parker-Kerr
P.-K. basting suture
P.-K. forceps
P.-K. intestinal clamp
Parker-Mott double-ended retractor
Parker-Pearson needle
Parkes
P. hump gouge
P. lateral osteotomy osteotome
P. nasal rasp
P. nasal retractor
Parkes-Quisling osteotome
Park-Guyton-Callahan eye speculum
Park-Guyton eye speculum
Park-Guyton-Maumenee speculum
Parkinson headholder
Park-Maumenee speculum
Park-O-Tron drill system
Parks
P. anal retractor
P. anal speculum

P

Parks *(continued)*
  P. bidirectional Doppler flowmeter
  P. ileoanal reservoir
  P. ileostomy pouch
Parma band
paronychia bur
parotidectomy retractor
parquetry set
Parr closed-irrigation system
parrot-beak basket
Par scissors
Parsonnet
  P. aortic clamp
  P. coronary probe
  P. dilator
  P. epicardial retractor
  P. pulse generator pouch
partial
  p. lower denture
  p. ossicular replacement prosthesis
  (PORP)
  p. rebreathing mask
  p. upper denture
partially-implantable catheter
partially-threaded pin
partial-occlusion
  p.-o. clamp
  p.-o. forceps
  p.-o. inferior vena cava clip
Partipilo clamp
Partnership
  P. implant
  P. instrument
  P. system
Partsch
  P. bone chisel
  P. bone gouge
P.A.S.
  P.A.S. Port Fluoro-Free
  P.A.S. Port Fluoro-Free catheter
  P.A.S. Port Fluoro-Free peripheral
  access system
PASAR tachycardia reversion pacemaker
Pasqualini implant
Passage
  P. balloon dilation catheter
  P. exchange balloon
Passager
  P. device
  P. endoprosthesis
  P. introducing sheath
  P. stent
Passarelli one-pass capsulorrhexis forceps
Passavant
  P. bar
  P. cushion
passer
  Arans pulley p.
  Batzdorf cervical wire p.
  Brand tendon p.
  Bunnell tendon p.
  Cappio suture p.
  Carroll tendon p.
  Carter-Thomason suture p.

Charnley wire p.
Concept ACL/PCL graft p.
Concept 2-pin p.
Crile wire p.
DeMayo suture p.
dermis-fat p.
Dingman wire p.
Ferszt ligature p.
Framer tendon p.
Furlow cylinder p.
Gallie tendon p.
Garrett vein p.
Gore suture p.
Hewson ligature p.
Hewson suture p.
Hoefflin suture p.
Holter distal catheter p.
Incavo wire p.
Joplin tendon p.
Lahey ligature p.
ligature p.
Malis ligature p.
MetraPass suture p.
Ober tendon p.
O'Donoghue suture p.
Protect-a-Pass suture p.
pulley p.
Shuttle-Relay suture p.
suture p.
tendon p.
Uni-Shunt catheter p.
Wedeen wire p.
wire p.
Withers tendon p.
Yankauer ligature p.
passing forceps
passive
  p. cutaneous anaphylaxis
  p. motion device
  p. track detector
passively shimmed superconducting magnet
passover humidifier
Passow chisel
Passport
  P. Balloon-on-a-Wire dilatation
  catheter
  P. bedside monitor
  P. instrumentation
Passy-Muir tracheostomy speaking valve
paste filler
Pastegraft
  Dembone demineralized cortical
  powder P.
Pasteur pipette
PASYS
  PASYS pacemaker
  PASYS single-chamber cardiac
  pacing system
patch
  Carrel p.
  Dacron intracardiac p.
  defibrillation p.
  Donaldson eye p.
  p. dressing

Dura-Guard p.
epicardial defibrillator p.
eye p.
p. eye
FTO eye p.
full-time occlusion eye p.
glue p.
Gore-Tex cardiovascular p.
Gore-Tex soft tissue p.
p. graft
p. implant
Ionescu-Shiley pericardial p.
Kper Knit p.
Kugel hernia p.
Lyrelle p.
Miniguard adhesive p.
monocular p.
nitroglycerin transdermal p.
Nouvisage Deep Hydration body p.
Nouvisage Deep Hydration neck p.
Orthoptic eye p.
polypropylene intracardiac p.
polytef soft tissue p.
Prolene Hernia system onlay p.
Prolene Hernia system underlay p.
Pro-Ophtha eye p.
RapiSeal p.
Rutkow sutureless plug and p.
Snugfit eye p.
Stat-padz defibrillator p.
Tanne corneal p.
Teflon intracardiac p.
Testoderm p.
Tissue-Guard bovine pericardial p.
Torpedo eye p.
Vascu-Guard peripheral vascular p.
wicking glue p.
patcher
Kartush tympanic membrane p.
Xomed Kartush tympanic
membrane p.
patch-graft
Dacron onlay p.-g.
Patel intraocular magnet
patella
p. bone saw
p. tracker
patellar
p. aligner
p. band
P. Band knee protector
p. button
p. cement clamp
p. drill guide
p. planer bushing
p. reamer guide
p. resection guide
p. shaft reamer
p. tendon-bearing
p. tendon-bearing below-knee
prosthesis
p. tendon weightbearing brace
orthosis
patella-resurfacing implant

patent
p. ductus clamp
p. ductus forceps
p. ductus retractor
p. stent
Paterson
P. brain clip forceps
P. laryngeal cannula
P. laryngeal forceps
P. long-shank brain clip
Pathfinder
P. catheter
P. exchange guidewire
P. microcatheter system
P. wire
pathometer attachment
patient
ARTMA virtual p. (AVP)
p. dose monitor
p. self-administration device
patient-controlled
p.-c. analgesia (PCA)
p.-c. anesthesia pump
PatientGuard underpad
patient-matched implant
patient-operated selector mechanism
Patil stereotactic system I, II
Patil-Syracuse mask
Paton
P. anterior chamber lens implant
forceps
P. capsular forceps
P. corneal dissector
P. corneal knife
P. corneal transplant forceps
P. double spatula
P. extra-delicate forceps
P. eye needle holder
P. eye shield
P. see-through corneal trephine
P. single spatula
P. suturing forceps
P. transplant spatula
P. tying/stitch removal forceps
Paton-Berens mules
Patrick drill
Patten-Bottom-Perthes brace
pattern
breast reduction p.
Collimator plugging p.
Harrington-Flocks multiple p.
p. matching card
p. trephine
p. umbilical scissors
Patterson
P. bronchoscopic forceps
P. empyema trocar
P. specimen forceps
Patterson-Nelson empyema trocar
Patton
P. bur
P. cannula
P. esophageal dilator
P. septal speculum
PattStrap knee support

patty
    Cellolite p.
    Codman surgical p.
    cottonoid p.
    NEURAY neurosurgical p.
Paufique
    P. blade
    P. corneal knife
    P. corneal trephine
    P. graft knife
    P. keratoplasty knife
    P. suturing forceps
Paufique-Duredge knife
Paul
    P. condom bag
    P. hemostatic bag
    P. intestinal drainage tube
    P. lacrimal sac retractor
    P. tendon hook
Paul-Mixter tube
Paulson
    P. infertility microtissue forceps
    P. infertility microtying forceps
    P. knee retractor
Paulus
    P. chin plate
    P. midfacial plate
    P. trocar system
Pautler infusion cannula
Pauwels fracture forceps
Pavenik monodisk device
Pavlik
    P. harness
    P. harness splint
Pavlo-Colibri corneal forceps
paws
    Medevice surgical p.
    Sil-Med instrument p.
Payne-Ochsner arterial forceps
Payne-Péan arterial forceps
Payne-Rankin arterial forceps
Payne retractor
Payr
    P. abdominal retractor
    P. gastrointestinal clamp
    P. grooved director
    P. probe
    P. pylorus clamp
    P. pylorus forceps
    P. resection clamp
    P. stomach clamp
    P. vein needle
Payr-Schmieden probe
PB-FOxS pediatric femoral sensor kit
PBI
    PBI Medical copper vapor laser
    PBI MultiLase D copper vapor laser
PBII blue loop lens
PC
    PC EDO ophthalmic office laser
    PC EEA stapler
    PC Performer knee
    PC Performer knee prosthesis
    PC shunt

PC-1000 panoramic x-ray machine
PC-7 needle
PCA
    patient-controlled analgesia
    porous-coated anatomic
        PCA acetabular cup
        PCA E-Series hip replacement
        PCA hip component
        PCA infuser
        PCA modular total knee
        PCA modular total knee system
        PCA periodontal pack
        PCA pump
        PCA revision total knee
        PCA total hip
        PCA total hip stem
        PCA unicompartmental knee
PCA-plus infusion device
PCD
    pacer-cardioverter defibrillator
    peritoneal dialysis catheter
    programmable cardioverter-defibrillator
    Jewel PCD
        PCD Transvene implantable cardioverter-defibrillator
        PCD Transvene implantable cardioverter-defibrillator system
PC-IOL lens
PCL-oriented placement marking hook
PD
    PD copper band
    PD crown post
    PD 2000 defibrillator
    PD dental wax
    PD excavator
    PD orthodontic wire
    PD polishing strip
    PD preformed crown
    PD reamer
    PD root canal post
    PD SS matrix band
PD-10 disposable Sephadex G-25 column
P.D. Access with Peel-Away needle introducer
PDA umbrella
PDB
    PDB preperitoneal distention balloon
    PDB preperitoneal distention balloon system
pDEXA x-ray peripheral bone densitometer
PDL intraligamentary syringe
PDS
    polydioxanone suture
    PDS II Endoloop suture
    PDS Vicryl suture
PDT
    PDT guidewire
PDx pacing and diagnostic pacemaker
PE
    PE LITE material
    PE Plus II balloon dilatation catheter
    PE Plus II peripheral balloon catheter

Peabody splint
Peacekeeper cannula
peacock dressing
peak
    P. anterior compression plate system
    P. fixation system
    p. flow meter
    p. flow whistle
    P. gait module
peakometer
Peakometer urinary flow-rate meter
Péan
    P. arterial forceps
    P. hemostatic clamp
    P. hemostatic forceps
    P. hysterectomy clamp
    P. hysterectomy forceps
    P. intestinal clamp
    P. intestinal forceps
    P. scissors
    P. sponge forceps
    P. vessel clamp
peanut
    p. dissector
    p. eye implant
    P. Secto dissector
    p. sponge
    p. sponge-holding forceps
peanut-fenestrated forceps
peanut-grasping forceps
peapod
    p. bead-type forceps
    p. chisel
    p. intervertebral disk forceps
    p. intervertebral disk rongeur
    upbiting p.
Pearce
    P. coaxial I&A cannula
    P. eye speculum
    P. intraocular glide
    P. nucleus hydrodissector
    P. posterior chamber intraocular
      lens
    P. Tripod cataract lens
    P. Tripod intraocular lens
    P. vaulted-Y lens implant
Pearce-Keates bifocal intraocular lens
Pearce-Knolle irrigating lens loop
PEARL
    physiologic endometrial ablation/resection
      loop
Pearlcast polymer plaster bandage
Pearlon impression material
Pearman
    P. penile implant material
    P. penile prosthesis
    P. transurethral hemostatic bag
Pearsall
    P. Chinese twisted suture
    P. silk suture
pear-shaped
    p.-s. bur
    p.-s. extension tube
    p.-s. fluted bag
    p.-s. nerve hook

Pearson
    P. attachment to Thomas frame
    P. chisel
    P. flexed-knee apparatus
Pease
    P. bone drill
    P. reamer
Pease-Thomson traction bow
PEC
    P. modular total knee system
    P. total hip system
Peck
    P. chisel
    P. inlay wax
    P. osteotome
    P. rake retractor
Peck-Joseph scissors
pectoral catheter
pectoralis muscle implant
Peczon
    P. I&A cannula
    P. I&A unit
    P. I&A vectis
pedal exerciser
pedal-mode ergometer
Pedar
    P. in-shoe measurement system
    P. pressure measurement system
Pederson vaginal speculum
pedestal
    IMP surgical leg p.
    p. massage table
    surgical leg p.
Pedi Asta frameless air support therapy
Pedia-Trake tube
pediatric
    p. abdominal retractor
    p. balloon catheter
    p. biopsy needle
    p. biplane TEE probe
    p. bridge
    p. bulldog clamp
    P. Cardiology Devices Sideris
      Buttoned device occluder
    p. C-D hook
    p. circle
    p. circle system
    p. Cotrel-Dubousset rod
    p. drainable pouch
    p. endoscope
    p. esophagoscope
    p. Foley catheter
    p. forceps
    p. gastroscope
    p. Hendren retractor blade
    p. Karickhoff laser lens
    p. lid speculum
    p. mastoid retractor blade
    P. Nutrition Surveillance System
    p. perineal retractor ring
    p. pigtail catheter
    p. PRAFO brace
    p. pressure relief ankle foot
      orthosis
    p. Racine adapter

P

pediatric *(continued)*
    p. rectal dilator
    p. retractor adjustable arm
    p. retractor malleable wire hand
    p. sandbag
    p. self-retaining retractor
    p. speculum
    p. telescope
    p. three-mirror laser lens
    p. transfer pouch
    p. TSRH hook
    p. urostomy pouch
Pedicath catheter
pedicle
    p. C-D hook
    p. clamp
    p. connector
    p. finder
    p. forceps
    p. hook
    p. implant
    p. plate
    p. screw
    p. screw construct
    p. sounder
Pedic sponge
Pedi-Cushions cushion
Pedifix hammertoe pad
PediKair pediatric low-air-loss bed
Pedilen polyurethane foam
Pediplast
    P. cushion
    P. moldable footcare compound
pedobarograph
    Biokinetics p.
    EMED-SF p.
    optical p.
pedometer
Pedors orthopaedic shoe
Peel-Away
    P.-A. introducer set
peel-away
    p.-a. banana catheter
    p.-a. introducer
    p.-a. sheath
peeler
    membrane p.
    Olk membrane p.
Peeler-Cutter vitrector
peel-off catheter
Peel Pak bag
Peep
    P. valve
    P. ventilator
Peep-Keep II adapter
Peers towel clamp
Peeso reamer
Peet
    P. lighted splanchnic retractor
    P. mosquito forceps
    P. nasal rasp
    P. splinter forceps
Pee Wee low-profile gastrostomy tube

PEG
    percutaneous endoscopic gastrostomy
    PEG bumper
    Gauderer-Ponsky PEG
    Ponsky-Gauderer type PEG
    Sandoz Caluso PEG
    PEG self-adhesive elastic dressing
    PEG tube
peg
    anchoring p.
    p. board lateral positioning device
    epithelial rete p.
    fiber-metal p.
    p. flap
    glenoid alignment p.
    Harrison-Nicolle polypropylene p.
    Kinemax removable fixation p.
    locking p.
    rete p.
    stringing p.
Pegasus
    P. Airwave pressure relief system
    P. Nd:YAG surgical laser
pegged tibial prosthesis
Peiper-Beyer bone rongeur
pelican biopsy forceps
Pelkmann
    P. foreign body forceps
    P. gallstone forceps
    P. sponge forceps
    P. uterine forceps
Pelle Peel microdermabrader
Pelli-Robson letter chart
Pelorus
    P. stereotactic frame
    P. surgical system
Pelosi
    P. fibrotome
    P. illuminator
    P. uterine manipulator
pelvic
    p. bench
    p. block
    p. clamp
    p. floor therapy system
    P. Organ Prolapse-Quantified system
    p. phased-array coil
    p. reconstruction kit
    p. reduction forceps
    p. snare
    p. stabilization orthosis
    p. tissue forceps
    p. traction belt
pelvimeter
    Baudelocque p.
    Briesky p.
    Collin p.
    Collyer p.
    DeLee p.
    DeLee-Breisky p.
    Douglas measuring plate p.
    Hanley-McDermott p.
    Martin p.
    Rica p.
    Schneider p.

Thole p.
Thomas p.
Thoms p.
Williams internal p.
Pemberton
P. forceps
P. retractor
P. sigmoid clamp
P. spur-crushing clamp
Pemco
P. cannula
P. prosthetic valve
P. retractor
pen
EpiE-Z P.
EpiE-Z P.-Jr
Genotropin p.
gentian violet marking p.
hydrophobic barrier p.
ImmEdge P.
Intron A multidose p.
ITO laser p.
light p.
marking p.
Pilot Spotlighter p.
p. pump insulin infuser
red-beam laser p.
Rhein reusable cautery p.
skin marking p.
Skin Skribe p.
STA-Pen writer p.
surgical marking p.
Viomedex surgical marking p.
Pen/Alps distal pad
Penberthy double-action aspirator
Pencan spinal needle
pencil
cataract p.
p. cautery
Cheshire electrosurgical p.
p. Doppler probe
p. drain
electrosurgical p.
glaucoma p.
MegaDyne electrocautery p.
retinal detachment p.
straight bipolar p.
Valleylab p.
vitreous p.
Wallach cryosurgical p.
Weck electrosurgery p.
pencil-grip instrument
pencil-handled laryngoscope
pencil-tip
p.-t. cautery
p.-t. drill
pencil-tipped
p.-t. drill
p.-t. electrode
Penco Walker Sleds
Pendoppler ultrasonic fetal heart detector
Pendula cast cutter
pendulum scalpel
penetrating drill

penetrometer
Benoist p.
Penfield
P. biopsy needle
P. dissector
P. retractor
P. silver clip
P. watchmaker suture forceps
penicillin nebulizer
penile
p. biothesiometer
p. clamp
p. Doppler
p. implant
Peninject 2.25 injector
penlight
Heine p.
LICO disposable p.
Welch Allyn halogen p.
Penlon
P. infant resuscitator
P. vaporizer
Penn
P. finger drill
P. pouch
P. State total artificial heart
P. State ventricular assist device
P. swivel hook
P. tuning fork
Penn-Anderson
P.-A. scleral fixation forceps
pennate suction catheter
Pennig
P. dynamic wrist fixator
P. minifixator
P. minifixator device
Pennine
P. leg bag
P. Nélaton catheter
Pennine-O'Neil urinary catheter introducer
Pennington
P. clamp
P. hemorrhoidal forceps
P. hemostatic forceps
P. rectal speculum
P. septal dissector
P. septal elevator
P. tissue forceps
P. tissue-grasping forceps
Pennybacker rongeur
Pen-Probe instrument
PenRad mammography clinical reporting system
Penrose
P. sump drain
P. tube
PENS
percutaneous epidural neurostimulator
PENSIL catheter Penn State Intravascular Lung catheter
PentaCath catheter
Pentalumen catheter
PentaPace QRS catheter

P

Pentax
> P. bronchofiberscope
> P. bronchoscope
> P. choledochocystonephrofiberscope
> P. duodenoscope
> P. EC-series video endoscope
> P. EG-series video endoscope
> P. EG-series videoendoscope
> P. EG-2900 videogastroscope
> P. EndoNet
> P. EndoNet digital endoscope
> P. EUP-EC-series ultrasound gastroscope
> P. FC-series colonoscope
> P. FD-series duodenofiberscope
> P. FD-series video endoscope
> P. FG-series ultrasound endoscope
> P. FG-series ultrasound gastrofiberscope
> P. FG-series video endoscope
> P. FG-36UX linear scanning echoendoscope
> P. fiberscope
> P. flexible endoscope
> P. flexible sigmoidoscope
> P. FS-series fiberoptic sigmoidoscope
> P. light source connector
> P. lithotriptor
> P. nasopharyngolaryngofiberscope
> P. prototype needle
> P. side-viewing endoscope
> P. sigmoidofiberscope
> P. Spotmatic camera
> P. VSB-P2900 pediatric colonoscope
> P. VSB-P-series enteroscope

Pentax-Hitachi FG32UA endosonographic system
Penthrane analgizer
pentose phosphate shunt
PEP mask
Perative enteral feeding container
Per-C-Cath catheter
Perception scanner
Percival gastric balloon
Perclose
> P. PVS device
> P. suture device
> P. vascular closure device

Perclose/Prostar device
Percoll
> P. bead
> P. filter

Percor
> P. dilator
> P. dual-lumen (DL) intra-aortic balloon catheter

Percor-Stat-DL catheter
Percor-Stat intra-aortic balloon
PercuCut
> P. biopsy needle
> P. cut-biopsy needle

Percufix catheter cuff kit
Percuflex
> P. Amsterdam stent
> P. biliary stent
> P. endopyelotomy stent
> P. flexible biliary stent
> P. nephrostomy catheter
> P. Plus ureteral stent

PercuGuide needle
percussion hammer
percussor
> cup palm manual p.
> English hospital reflex p.
> G5 Flimm Fighter p.
> G5 Neocussor p.
> McGill neurological p.
> mechanical p.
> Neoguard p.
> neurological p.
> PalmCups p.

Percu-Stay catheter fastener
PercuSurge recovery system device
percutaneous
> p. access kit
> p. atherectomy device
> p. brachial sheath
> p. cardiopulmonary bypass support
> p. catheter introducer kit
> p. central venous catheter
> p. cutting needle
> p. discoscope
> p. diskoscope
> p. dorsal column stimulator implant
> p. drainage catheter
> p. endoscopic gastrostomy (PEG)
> p. endoscopic gastrostomy tube
> p. endoscopic jejunostomy
> p. epidural electrode
> p. epidural nerve stimulator
> p. epidural neurostimulator (PENS)
> p. intra-aortic balloon counterpulsation catheter
> p. K-wire
> p. nephrostomy Malecot catheter
> p. nephrostomy tube
> p. pencil Doppler probe
> p. pin
> p. rotational thrombectomy catheter
> p. spinal endoscope
> p. stick
> P. Stoller Afferent Nerve Stimulation (PerQ Sans) system
> p. thecoperitoneal shunt
> p. transhepatic biliary drainage catheter
> p. transhepatic pigtail catheter
> p. transluminal coronary angioplasty catheter
> p. ultrasonic lithotriptor
> p. ureteral stent
> p. vascular surgery

Percy
> P. amputating saw
> P. amputation retractor
> P. bone retractor
> P. clamp
> P. intestinal forceps

P. plate
P. tissue forceps
Percy-Wolfson
P.-W. gallbladder forceps
P.-W. gallbladder retractor
PerDUCER pericardial access device
Perdue
P. hemostat
P. tonsillar hemostat forceps
Pereyra
P. ligature cannula
P. needle
P. needle driver
Perez-Castro forceps
Perfecta
P. femoral stem
P. hip prosthesis
P. Interseal total hip system
Per-fit percutaneous tracheostomy kit
PerFix
P. hernia plug
P. Marlex mesh plug
PerFixation
P. screw
P. system
Perflex
P. stainless steel stent and delivery
system bilary stent
P. stainless steel stent and delivery
system biliary system
perforating
p. bur
p. twist drill
perforation rasp
perforator
Aesculap skull p.
Amnihook amniotic membrane p.
Anspach cranial p.
antral p.
Baylor amniotic p.
Bishop antral p.
Boyd p.
Codman disposable p.
cranial p.
Cushing cranial p.
DeLee-Perce membrane p.
D'Errico p.
Dodd p.
p. drill
Heifitz skull p.
Hillis p.
Joseph antral p.
Kalinowski p.
Lasette laser finger p.
Lempert p.
membrane p.
Politzer ear p.
powered automatic skull p.
Royce tympanum p.
Smellie obstetrical p.
Smith p.
spondylophyte annular dissector p.
Stein membrane p.
Thornwald antral p.
tympanum p.

Wellaminski antral p.
Williams p.
Performa
P. Acoustic Imaging system
P. diagnostic ultrasound imaging
system
P. ultrasound
Performance
P. knee prosthesis
P. modular total knee system
P. unicompartmental knee system
performer ultralight knee brace
Perf-Plate cranial plate
perfusion
p. balloon catheter
p. cannula
p. monitor
p. O ring
perfusor
Belsey p.
periapical curette
periaqueductal gray electrode
periareolar retractor
peribulbar needle
pericarbon bioprosthesis
pericardial snare
pericardiocentesis needle
pericardiotomy scissors
Peri-Cold pack
Peri-Comfort seating cushion
pericortical clamp
Peries medicated hygienic wipe dressing
Periflow
P. peripheral balloon angioplasty-
infusion catheter
Periflux
P. 3 laser-Doppler flowmetry
P. PF 1 D blood-flow meter
Peri-Gel pack
Peri-Guard
P.-G. vascular graft
P.-G. vascular graft guard
perilimbal suction
perimeter
automated hemisphere p.
Brombach p.
Canon p.
Cilco p.
CooperVision imaging p.
Digilab p.
Ferree-Rand p.
Goldmann p.
Henson CFS 2000 p.
Humphrey p.
Interzeag bowl p.
Medmont M600 p.
Octopus 1-2-3 p.
Octopus 101, 201 bowl p.
Ophthimus High-Pass Resolution p.
Peritest p.
Schweigger hand p.
Perimount RSR pericardial bioprosthesis
perineal
p. bandage
p. prostatectomy retractor

P

perineal *(continued)*
 p. self-retaining retractor
 p. surgical apron
perineometer
 Gynos p.
 Kegel p.
 Peritron p.
Perio
 P. Pik irrigator
 P. Temp dental probe
periodontal
 p. probe
 p. prosthesis
periodontometer, periodontimeter
 Mühlemann p.
PerioGlas
 P. material
 P. synthetic bone graft
periosteal
 p. elevator
 p. raspatory
 p. spicule sweeper
periosteotome
 Alexander costal p.
 Alexander-Farabeuf costal p.
 Ballenger p.
 Brophy p.
 Brown p.
 costal p.
 Dean p.
 Ferris Smith-Lyman p.
 Fomon p.
 Freer p.
 Jansen p.
 Joseph p.
 Moorehead p.
 Potts p.
 Speer p.
 Vaughan p.
 West-Beck p.
Periotemp system
Periotest
 P. implant
 P. Implant Innovations gold screw
 P. system
PerioWise probe
peripheral
 P. AngioJet system
 p. atherectomy catheter
 p. atherectomy system
 p. blood vessel forceps
 p. indwelling intermediate infusion device
 p. interface adapter
 p. iridectomy forceps
 p. long-line catheter
 p. nerve glove
 p. vascular clamp
 p. vascular forceps
 p. vascular retractor
peripherally
 p. inserted catheter
 p. inserted central catheter (PICC)
 p. inserted central catheter line

 p. inserted central venous catheter (PICVC)
periscopic spectacles
Peri-Strips
 P.-S. Dry
Peritest perimeter
peritoneal
 p. button
 p. clamp
 p. dialysis catheter (PCD)
 p. forceps
 p. reflux control catheter
peritoneojugular shunt
peritoneoscope
 Menghini-Wildhirt p.
peritoneovenous shunt
Peritronics Medical Inc. fetal monitoring system
Peritron perineometer
periumbilical port
Peri-Warm pack
Perkin-Elmer model 5000 atomic absorption spectrophotometer
Perkins
 P. applanation tonometer
 P. elevator
 P. otologic retractor
 P. split-weight tractor
 P. traction
Per-Lee
 P.-L. equalizing tube
 P.-L. myringotomy tube
 P.-L. ventilation tube
Perlon suture
Perlstein
 P. brace
 P. joint
 P. orthosis
Permacol mesh
Perma-Cryl denture base material
Perma-Flow coronary bypass graft
Perma-Hand
 P.-H. braided silk suture
Permalens lens
Permalock
 Weber P.
Permalume polyurethane
PermaMesh
 P. hydroxyapatite woven sheet matrix
 P. material
Perman cartilage forceps
PermaNeb nebulizer
permanent
 p. cardiac pacing lead
 p. myocardial pacemaker
 p. needle
 p. rate-responsive pacemaker
 p. silicone catheter
 p. transvenous demand pacemaker (PTDP)
 p. transvenous pacemaker
 p. ventricular pacemaker
Perman-Stille abdominal retractor

PermaRidge
P. delivery syringe
Permark
P. Enhancer III pigmenting unit
P. micropigmentation needle
P. micropigmentation system
Perma-Seal dialysis access graft
PermaSharp
P. PGA suture
P. suture and needle
PermaSoft reline material
Permathane
P. lead
P. Pacesetter lead pacemaker
Permatone denture material
PermCath
P. dual-lumen catheter
permucosal implant system
Perneczky aneurysm clip
Perone
P. laser-assisted intrastromal
keratomileusis (LASIK) marker
P. LASIK flap forceps
peroral
p. gastroscope
p. pancreatoscope system
Per-Q-Cath CVP catheter
Perras mammary prosthesis
Perras-Papillon breast prosthesis
Perritt
P. fixation forceps
P. lens forceps
Perry
P. forceps
P. ileostomy bag
P. latex Penrose drainage tubing
P. Noz-Stop kit
P. ostomy irrigator
P. pediatric Foley latex catheter
P. sensor
PerryAnal/PerryVaginal EMG sensor
Perry-Foley catheter
PerryMeter anal EMG sensor
Personal
P. Best peak flowmeter
P. Catheter 100% silicone
intermittent catheter
P. Heart Device
Persona monitoring kit
Personna
P. Plus disposable Teflon scalpel
P. prep blades
P. surgical blade
Perspective
P. chest imaging system
P. dental imaging system
perspex
p. block
P. button
P. CQ intraocular lens
P. CQ-Shearing-Simcoe-Sinskey lens
P. rod
P. tube
Per-Stat-DL catheter

Perthes
P. reamer
P. sling
Pertrach percutaneous tracheostomy tube
pervenous catheter
PE-series implantable pronged unipolar electrode
pessary
Albert-Smith p.
Biswas Silastic vaginal p.
bladder neck support p.
Blair modification of Gellhorn p.
blue ring p.
Chambers doughnut p.
Chambers intrauterine p.
cube p.
cup p.
diaphragm p.
doughnut p.
Dumas p.
Dumontpallier p.
Dutch p.
Emmet-Gellhorn p.
Findley folding p.
Gariel p.
Gehrung p.
Gellhorn p.
globe prolapsus p.
Gold p.
Gynefold prolapse p.
Gynefold retrodisplacement p.
Hodge p.
hollow lucite p.
intrauterine p.
lever p.
Maydl p.
Mayer p.
Menge p.
Milex p.
Plexiglas Gellhorn p.
Prentif p.
Prochownik p.
prolapsus p.
red p.
retroversion p.
ring p.
safety p.
Smith-Hodge p.
Smith retroversion p.
stem p.
Thomas p.
Vimule p.
White foam p.
Wylie stem p.
Zwanck radium p.
Pess lid everter
PET
PET balloon
PET balloon Simpson atherectomy
device
petaling the cast
Petanguy-McIndoe gouge
Peter-Bishop forceps
Petersen rectal bag

Peterson
P. cervical collar
P. nail
P. skeletal traction bow
Peters tissue forceps
Petit
P. facial mask
P. tourniquet
PETite scanner
Petralit dental cement
Petri dish
petrolatum
p. gauze
p. gauze dressing
Pettigrove
P. laser-assisted intrastromal keratomileusis set
P. LASIK set
Peyman
P. intraocular forceps
P. special optics for low vision lens
P. vitrectomy unit
P. vitrector
P. vitreophage unit
P. vitreous-grasping forceps
P. vitreous scissors
P. wide-field lens
Peyman-Green
P.-G. vitrectomy lens
P.-G. vitreous forceps
Peyman-Tennant-Green lens
Peyton brain spatula
Pezzer
P. drain
P. mushroom-tipped catheter
P. self-retaining urethral catheter
P. suprapubic cystostomy catheter
PF
PF Lee pediatric goniolens
PF night splint
PF Universal solder
PF-8P peroral pancreatoscope system
Pfau
P. atticus sphenoidal punch
P. polyp forceps
PFC
PFC component
PFC Sigma total knee system
PFC total hip replacement system
Pfeifer catheter
Pfeiffer-Grobety activator
Pfeiffer mechanical dosing pump
Pfister-Schwartz
P.-S. basket forceps
P.-S. sheath
P.-S. stone basket
P.-S. stone dislodger
P.-S. stone retriever
Pfister stone basket
Pfizer scanner
PFO-Star occluder
PGK (Panos G. Koutrouvelis, M.D.) stereotactic device

Phaco
P. Commander phacoemulsification system
P. Emulsifier Cavitron unit
Phaco-4 diamond step knife
phacoblade
Myocure p.
phacodialysis spatula
phacoemulsification
p. cautery
p. handpiece
phacoemulsificator
Phaco-Emulsifier
Cavitron P.-E.
Kelman P.-E.
MVS P.-E.
PhacoFlex
P. II foldable intraocular lens implant
P. II intraocular lens
Phacojack phaco system
Phakic 6 lens
phakofragmatome
Girard p.
phalangeal
p. broach
p. clamp
p. forceps
Phaneuf
P. arterial forceps
P. clamp
P. hysterectomy forceps
P. peritoneal forceps
P. uterine artery forceps
P. uterine artery scissors
P. vaginal forceps
phantom
P. cardiac guidewire
p. clamp
Compass stereotactic p.
p. frame
Imatron CT bone mineral p.
P. interference screw
P. nasal mask
three-dimensional SPECT p.
P. V Plus balloon dilatation catheter
Pharmacia
P. corneal trephine
P. Intermedics
P. Intermedics ophthalmics intraocular lens
P. lancet
P. Visco J-loop lens
Pharmaseal
P. catheter
P. closed drain
P. disposable cervical dilator
P. disposable uterine sound
P. needle
PharmChek sweat patch drug detection system
Pharmex disposable catheter

pharyngeal
    p. airway
    p. retractor
pharyngometer
    EccoVision acoustic p.
pharyngoscope
    Hays p.
    Proud-Beck p.
pharyngotympanic tube
Phase-A-Caps alloy
Phaseafill dental composite
Phasealloy alloy
phased
    p. array sector transducer
    p. array ultrasonographic device
phased-array
    p.-a. body-coil MR imaging
    p.-a. color-flow ultrasound system
    p.-a. torso coil
phase-difference haloscope
phase-sensitive detector
Phazet lancet
Pheifer-Young retractor
Phelan vein stripper
Phelps
    P. brace
    P. orthosis
    P. splint
Phelps-Gocht osteoclast
PHEMA core-and-skirt keratoprosthesis
Phemister
    P. biopsy trephine
    P. brace
    P. onlay bone graft
    P. punch
    P. raspatory
    P. raspatory elevator
    P. reamer
    P. splint
Phenol EZ swab
Philadelphia
    P. cervical collar
    P. collar cervical traction
Philips
    P. Angiodiagnostics 96 apparatus
    P. CM 12 electron microscope
    P. DVI 1 system
    P. Easyguide navigation system
    P. Gyroscan
    P. Gyroscan ACS scanner
    P. Gyroscan NT-series scanner
    P. Gyroscan S5 scanner
    P. Gyroscan T5 scanner
    P. linear accelerator
    P. Orthoralix
    P. SensorTouch temple thermometer
    P. small-bore system scanner
    P. spiral CT scanner
    P. toe force gauge
    P. Tomoscan SR 6000 CT scanner
    P. T-60 tomoscanner
    P. ultrasound machine
Phillips
    P. dilator
    P. fixation forceps

    P. recessed-head screw
    P. rectal clamp
    P. screwdriver
    P. swan neck forceps
    P. urethral catheter
    P. urethral whip bougie
    P. urologic catheter
Philly bolt
phimosis forceps
Phinformer portable recorder
Phipps forceps
phlebograph
    impedance p.
Phoenix
    P. ancillary valve
    P. Anti-Blok ventricular catheter
    P. cruciform valve
    P. fifth ventricle system
    P. outrigger splint
    P. 2 pacemaker
    P. POWERLOFT series I, II
        alternating air flotation
    P. single-chamber pacemaker
    P. total artificial heart
    P. total hip prosthesis
phone
    Picasso telemedicine p.
phonologic acquisition device
phonometer
    Tektronix digital p.
**Phoresor II iontophoretic drug delivery
    system**
phorometer
phoro-optometer
phoroptor
    A-O minus cylinder P.
    A-O plus cylinder P.
PhosphorImager system
photic-evoked response stimulator
photocatalytic air filtration system
photocoagulator
    American Optical p.
    argon laser p.
    Coherent p.
    Coherent argon laser p.
    Ialo p.
    infrared ray p.
    IOLAB I&A p.
    Mira p.
    Novus Omni 2000 p.
    Novus Verdi diode-pumped green p.
    OcuLight GLx green laser p.
    Olivella-Garrigosa p.
    sapphire crystal infrared p.
    Ultima 2000 p.
    xenon arc p.
    Zeiss xenon arc p.
photoculdoscope
    Decker p.
PhotoDerm
    P. bright light delivery system
    P. MultiLight system
    P. PL handpiece
    P. PL, VL pulsed light device
    P. VL/PL hair removal system

P

photodisrupting laser
photoelectric multiplier tube
PhotoFix alpha pericardial bioprosthesis
photogastroscope
    Krentz p.
PhotoGenica
    P. LPIR with TKS laser
    P. T^{10} laser
    P. T laser system
    P. T^{10} tattoo removal system
    P. V laser
    P. VLS pulsed dye laser
photogrammeter
    Raster p.
photoionization detector
photo-kerato attachment
photokeratoscope
    Allergan-Humphrey p.
    AMO p.
    CooperVision refractive surgery p.
    Corneascope nine-ring p.
    Tomey TMS-1 p.
photokeratoscopy
    digital subtraction p.
photolaparoscope
    Lent p.
    Wolf p.
photometer
    Förster p.
    HemoCue hemoglobin p.
    Kowa laser flare-cell p.
    reflectance p.
    TUR-Cue p.
photomultiplier
    EMI 9813B p.
    p. tube
Photon
    P. laser
    P. LaserPhacolysis Probe
    P. Ocular Surgery system
    P. Radiosurgery system
photon-activated drug delivery system
photonic
    p. radiosurgical system
    P. stadiometer
Photopic Imaging ultrasound system
PhotoPoint laser
photoptometer
    Förster p.
Phototome system
phototube output circuit
photovaporizing laser
photovolt pH meter
pH probe
phrenicectomy forceps
phrenic retractor
pH-sensitive radiotelemetry capsule
Phymos 3D pacemaker
Phynox
    P. cobalt alloy clip
    P. cobalt alloy clip material
Physio-Control Lifestat
  sphygmomanometer
PhysioGymnic exercise ball

physiologic
    p. endometrial ablation/resection
      loop (PEARL)
    p. pacemaker
Physio-Roll-R-Cise exerciser
Physio-Roll VisuaLiser exercise ball
Physios CTM 01 cardiac transplant
  monitoring system
Physio-Stim Lite bone growth stimulator
Phystan implant
piano-style guidewire stent
piano-wire
    p.-w. dorsiflexion brace
    p.-w. staff
PIBC catheter
Picasso telemedicine phone
PICC
    peripherally inserted central catheter
    Arrow PICC
    PICC line
Piccolino
    P. balloon
    P. Monorail balloon device
    P. Monorail catheter
pick
    anterior footplate p.
    Austin p.
    Bellucci p.
    Burch fixation p.
    Burch ophthalmic p.
    P. chisel
    Cooley p.
    Crabtree dissector p.
    Crane dental p.
    dental p.
    Desmarres fixation p.
    double-ended root tip dental p.
    Farrior anterior footplate p.
    Farrior oval-window p.
    Farrior posterior footplate p.
    fiberoptic p.
    fixation p.
    footplate p.
    P. and Go monitor
    Guilford-Wright footplate p.
    Guilford-Wright stapes p.
    Hayden footplate p.
    Hoffmann scleral fixation p.
    Hough stapedectomy footplate p.
    House-Barbara p.
    House-Crabtree dissector p.
    House obtuse p.
    House oval-window p.
    House strut p.
    p. knife
    Kos p.
    light pipe p.
    McGee footplate p.
    Michel p.
    microsurgical ear p.
    Olk vitreoretinal p.
    ophthalmic p.
    oval-window p.
    Paparella footplate p.
    posterior footplate p.

Rhein p.
Rice p.
right-angle p.
Rosen p.
Saunders-Paparella p.
Scheer p.
Schuknecht p.
scleral p.
Shea p.
Sinskey p.
slightly-curved ear p.
stapedectomy footplate p.
stapes p.
strut p.
Tabb knife p.
Trent p.
Wells scleral suture p.
Wilder p.
Wright-Guilford footplate p.
Wright-Guilford stapes p.

Picker
P. camera
P. CS, CT, MR scanner
P. Dyna Mo collimator
P. PQ helical CT scanner
P. PQ spiral CT scanner
P. Synerview 600 scanner
P. system
P. Vista HPQ MRI scanner
P. Vista MagnaScanner scanner

picket
P. Fence fiducial localization stereotactic system
p. fence guide
P. Fence leg positioner

Pickett scissors
Pickford-Nicholson
P.-N. analmoscope
P.-N. anomaloscope

Pickrell
P. hook
P. retractor

pickup
Adson p.
DeBakey p.
p. noncrushing forceps
rat-tooth p.
Shoch foreign body p.
p. spatula suture
toothed p.
p. tube

Pico-ST II low-profile balloon catheter
Picot
P. vaginal retractor
P. vaginal speculum

Picotip
Endotak P.

picture
p. archival communication system
P. Archiving and Communications System

picture-in-picture monitor
PICVC
peripherally inserted central venous catheter

Pidcock
P. nail
P. pin

PI disposable stapler
Pie
P. Medical CAAS II analysis system
P. Medical ultrasound
P. Medical ultrasound system

Piedmont all-cotton elastic dressing
Pierce
P. antral trocar
P. antrum wash tube
P. attic cannula
P. cheek retractor
P. coaxial I&A cannula
P. cryptotome
P. elevator
P. I&A unit
P. I&A vectis
P. irrigating vectis
P. nasal cup
P. rongeur
P. submucous dissector

Pierce-Donachy Thoratec ventricular assist device
Pierce-Kyle trocar
Pierse
P. corneal Colibri-type forceps
P. eye speculum
P. fixation forceps
P. tip forceps

Pierse-Colibri corneal utility forceps
Pierse-Hoskins forceps
piesimeter
Hales p.

piezoelectric
p. accelerometer
p. crystal
p. shock wave lithotriptor
p. transducer

piezoelectrical stimulator
Piezolith (2300 and 2500 model) lithotriptor
piezo-resistive transducer
Piffard
P. dermal curette
P. placental curette

Pigg-O-Stat
P.-O.-S. immobilization device
P.-O.-S. x-ray chair

piggyback
p. contact lens
p. implant
P. needle-knife papillotome
Parker-Heath p.
p. probe

Pigott forceps
pigskin graft
pigtail
p. biliary stent
p. catheter
p. endoprosthesis
p. nephrostomy drain
p. nephrostomy tube

P

pigtail *(continued)*
    p. probe
    p. tendon stripper
Pik
    Grossan nasal irrigator tip with
       Water P.
    P. Stick Reacher
Pike jawed forceps
Pilcher
    P. catheter
    P. suprapubic hemostatic bag
pile clamp
pillar
    p. forceps
    p. retractor
pillar-and-post microsurgical retractor
pillar-grasping forceps
pill counter
Pillet hand prosthesis
Pilliar total hip replacement
Pilling
    P. bronchoscope
    P. collector
    P. dilator
    P. duralite tube
    P. Excalibur gauge
    P. fiberoptic illuminator
    P. forceps
    P. gouge
    P. laryngofissure shears
    P. microanastomosis clamp
    P. needle holder
    P. pediatric clamp
    P. retractor
Pilling-Favaloro retractor
Pilling-Hartmann speculum
Pilling-Liston bone utility forceps
Pilling-Negus clamp-on aspirator
Pilling-Ruskin rongeur
Pilling-Wolvek sternal approximator
Pillo-Boot Lower leg positioning device
Pillo-Pedic
    P.-P. cervical traction pillow
Pillo Pro dressing
Pillo-Pump alternating pressure system
pillow
    abduction p.
    air p.
    Bedge p.
    Body buddy-body p.
    Capello slim-line abduction p.
    Carter p.
    cervical sleep p.
    Crescent memory p.
    Crescent-Pillo p.
    Dream P.
    Flip-Flop p.
    foot p.
    FossFill Health P.
    Frejka hip p.
    Heart p.
    heel p.
    Hugg-L-O p.
    IMP-Capello slimline abduction p.

    Knee Pillo p.
    Max-Relax p.
    Mediflow waterbase p.
    Neckcare p.
    Neck-Hugger cervical support p.
    Nek-L-O hot & cold p.
    Nek-L-O orthopaedic
       support/comfort p.
    OrthoBone p.
    Orthosleep p.
    OsmoCyte p.
    Pillo-Pedic cervical traction p.
    positioning p.
    Pron p.
    Richard p.
    Rubens p.
    Sand-Eze EGD p.
    shoulder abduction p.
    Softeze water p.
    Tempur-Med p.
    Tempur-Pedic pressure relieving
       Swedish p.
    T-Foam p.
    Theracloud p.
    Therapeutica sleeping p.
    TherArc p.
    Therasleep cervical p.
    Tri-Core cervical support p.
    vacuum p.
    Wal-Pil-O neck p.
Pillow perfect zipper cover
pillow-shaped balloon
Pil-O-Splint wrist splint
pilot
    P. audiometer
    p. bur
    p. drill
    p. needle
    P. point screw
    P. Spotlighter pen
    P. suturing guide
Pilotip
    P. catheter
    P. catheter guide
pin
    Ace p.
    Apex p.
    Arthrex zebra p.
    ARUM Colles fixation p.
    ASIF screw p.
    Asnis p.
    Austin Moore p.
    p. ball system
    Barr p.
    beaded hip p.
    Beath p.
    Belos compression p.
    bevel-point Rush p.
    Biofix system p.
    biphasic p.
    Böhler p.
    Böhler-Knowles hip p.
    Böhler-Steinmann p.
    Bohlman p.
    breakaway p.

Breck p.
calibrated p.
Canakis beaded hip p.
cancellous p.
Caspar distraction p.
Charnley p.
p. chuck
cloverleaf p.
Co-Cr-Mo p.
Compere threaded p.
Conley p.
cortical p.
Craig p.
p. crimper
Crowe pilot point on Steinmann p.
Crowe-tip p.
Crutchfield skull-tip p.
Davis p.
Delitala T-p.
deluxe FIN p.
Denham p.
derotational p.
Deyerle p.
distraction p.
distractor p.
duodenal p.
Ender p.
endodontic p.
Fahey p.
Fahey-Compere p.
femoral guide p.
Fisher half p.
fixation p.
friction lock p.
Furness-Clute p.
Getz root canal p.
Gingrass-Messer p.
Gouffon hip p.
p. guard
p. guide
Hagie p.
Hahnenkratt root canal p.
Hansen-Street p.
Hatcher p.
Haynes p.
p. headholder
p. headrest
Hegge p.
Hessel-Nystrom p.
Hewson breakaway p.
hexhead p.
Hoffmann apex fixation p.
Hoffmann transfixion p.
p. holder
hook-end intramedullary p.
p. implant
Intraflex intramedullary p.
intramedullary p.
Jones p.
Jurgan p.
Kirschner wire p.
Knowles hip p.
Kronendonk p.
Kronfeld p.
Küntscher femur guide p.

lateral guide p.
LIH hook p.
Link-Plus retention p.
Lottes p.
Marble bone p.
Markley retention p.
Mayfield disposable skull p.
Mayfield skull clamp p.
McBride p.
mechanic's p.
medullary p.
metal p.
Modny p.
Moore fixation p.
Moule screw p.
Mt. Sinai skull clamp p.
Neufeld p.
Norman tibial p.
Oris p.
Ormco p.
Orthofix p.
orthopedic p.
OrthoSorb absorbable p.
osseous p.
osteotomy p.
partially-threaded p.
percutaneous p.
Pidcock p.
Pischel p.
Pugh hip p.
rasp p.
resorbable polydioxanone p.
restorative p.
ReUnite orthopedic p.
revolving Ge-68 p.
Rhinelander p.
Rica wire guide p.
Riordan p.
Rissler p.
Rissler-Stille p.
Roger Anderson p.
Rush intramedullary fixation p.
safety p.
Safir p.
Sage p.
Scand p.
Schanz p.
Schneider self-broaching p.
Schweitzer p.
self-broaching p.
self-tapering p.
Shantz p.
Shriners Hospital p.
skeletal p.
Smillie p.
Smith-Petersen fracture p.
SMo Moore p.
smooth p.
Snap fixation p.
spring p.
sprue p.
stabilizing guide p.
Stader p.
Steinmann calibrated p.
Steinmann fixation p.

pin *(continued)*
    Street p.
    strut-type p.
    Surgin hemorrhage occluder p.
    p. suture
    Synthes guide p.
    tapered p.
    threaded guide p.
    tibial guide p.
    titanium half p.
    torlone fixation p.
    trochanteric p.
    Turner p.
    tutoFix cortical p.
    union broach retention p.
    Venable-Stuck fracture p.
    p. vise
    von Saal medullary p.
    Walker hollow quill p.
    Watanabe p.
    Watson-Jones guide p.
    Webb p.
    p. wheel
    Zimfoam p.
    Zimmer p.
Pinard
    P. fetal stethoscope
    P. fetoscope
pin-bending forceps
pince
    O'Shaughnessy p.
pincer
    overlapping p.
pinch
    p. forceps
    p. gauge
    P. Gauge and Jackson Strength
    Evaluation System
    p. tree
pinchcock clamp
pinchometer
    Prestop p.
pin-deburring die
pineapple bur
Pineda LASIK Flap Iron
pinhole
    p. camera
    p. collimator
    p. occluder
pin-index safety system
pinion
    p. headholder
    p. headrest
pink
    p. dressing
    p. twisted cotton suture
Pinkerton balloon catheter
Pinky ball
Pinnacle
    P. contact Nd:YAG fiber
    P. introducer sheath
    P. pacemaker

P. 3 radiation therapy planning
    system
    P. reusable underpad
Pinn.ACL guide system
Pinpoint stereotactic arm
pin-seating forceps
pins and plaster
Pinto
    P. dissector tip
    P. distractor
    P. superficial dissection cannula
pin-to-bar clamp
pinwheel
    Clean-Wheel disposable
    neurological p.
    Grafco p.
    Safe-T-Wheel p.
    p. sensation gauge
    P. system
    Taylor p.
    Wartenberg p.
Pio root canal depth indicator
PIP/DIP strap
pipe
    P. check kit PAD device
    endoscopic washing p.
    fiberoptic light p.
    light p.
    Mauch double-sheathed plastic
    wash p.
    Storz disposable fiberoptic light p.
    p. tree
Pipelle
    P. endometrial curette
    P. endometrial suction catheter
Pipelle-deCornier endometrial curette
Piper
    P. lateral wall retractor
    P. obstetrical forceps
Pipet Curet
pipette
    light p.
    Pasteur p.
    Unopette p.
    Wallace p.
Piranha uteroscopic biopsy forceps
Pirquet tongue depressor
Pisces
    P. electrode
    P. implant
    P. spinal cord stimulation device
    P. spinal cord stimulation system
Pischel
    P. electrode
    P. micropin
    P. micropin forceps
    P. needle
    P. pin
    P. scleral ruler
Pistofidis cervical biopsy forceps
pistol-grip
    p.-g. hand drill
    p.-g. instrument
piston
    Austin p.

Causse p.
Guilford-Wright Teflon wire p.
House p.
McGee platinum/stainless steel p.
MTS electrohydraulic p.
p. stapes prosthesis
Teflon p.
p. wire
Pitanguy forceps
Pitha
P. foreign body forceps
P. urethral forceps
Pitkin
P. dermatome
P. needle
P. syringe
Pitot tube
Pittman needle holder
Pittsburgh triangular frame
Pitt talking tracheostomy tube
pituitary
p. curette
p. forceps
p. rongeur
p. spoon
pivot
p. aneurysm clip
P. balloon
p. clip applier
P. fixed-wire balloon catheter
p. lock
p. microanastomosis approximator
pivoting
p. surgical arm board
p. table
Pixi bone densitometer
Pixie minilaparoscope
Pixsys
P. FlashPoint camera
P. FlashPoint digitizer
PKS-25 apparatus stapler
placement forceps
placental
p. clamp
p. curette
placenta previa forceps
Placer guidewire
Placido
P. da Costa disk
P. disk
P. keratoscope
P. 25-ring cone
Placido-disk videokeratoscopy system
placido ring
plagiocephaly
p. headband
p. helmet
plain
p. catgut suture
p. collagen suture
p. ear hook
p. ear spoon
p. eye needle
p. forceps
p. gauze

p. gut suture
p. rib shears
p. rotary scissors
p. screwdriver
p. vesical trocar
p. wire speculum
plain-end grooved director
plain-line articulator
plain-pattern plate
Plak-Vac oral suction brush
planar
p. blade
p. circular coil
p. I mesh implant
Planarm Haag Streit attachment
planer
calcar p.
Rubin bone p.
Rubin cartilage p.
Plange spud
planimeter
plano
p. lens
p. T-bandage
planoconcave lens
planoconvex
p. eye implant
p. lens
p. nonridge lens
planoconvex-shaped disk
Planostretch stockings
plantar fasciitis night splint
plaque-cracker
LeVeen p.-c.
plaque retriever
plasma
p. clot diffusion chamber
p. prothrombin conversion
accelerator
p. scalpel
p. TFE vascular graft
plasmapheresis through a Prosorba column
PlasmaPlex bottle
Plastalume
P. bulb-ended splint
P. straight splint
plaster
p. bandage
below-knee walking p.
Hapset hydroxyapatite bone graft p.
p. knife
long leg p.
p. pants dressing
p. of Paris
pins and p.
p. saw
p. shears
p. spatula
p. splint
p. spreader
plaster-of-Paris (POP)
p.-o.-P. bandage (POP bandage)
p.-o.-P. cast
p.-o.-P. dressing

P

615

plaster-of-Paris *(continued)*
    p.-o.-P. jacket
    p.-o.-P. splint
Plastibell
    P. circumcision clamp
    P. circumcision device
    P. compression instrument
plastic
    p. bracket
    p. cannula
    p. collar
    p. connector
    p. corneal protector
    p. curette
    p. disposable irrigating vectis
    p. drape
    p. dressing
    p. end caps
    p. endoprosthesis
    p. endosurgical system
    p. eye shield
    p. femoral plug
    p. forceps
    p. mouth guard
    p. orthosis
    p. prism
    p. scalp clip
    p. sewing ring
    p. sphere eye implant
    p. stent
    p. strip
    p. surgery scissors
    p. suture
    p. Tiemann catheter
    p. utility scissors
    p. wax material
PlastiCast adjustable joint cast system
plastic-cuffed tracheostomy tube
Plasticeph cephalometer
Plasticor prosthesis
Plasti-Pore ossicular replacement prosthesis
Plastiport TORP
Plastizote
    P. arch support
    P. cervical collar
    P. foot bed
    P. orthotic
    P. orthotic device
    P. shoe
Plastodent
    P. dental impression adhesive
    P. wax
Plast-O-Fit
    P.-O.-F. thermoplastic bandage
    P.-O.-F. thermoplastic bandage system
plate
    absorbable p.
    acetabular reconstruction p.
    Alta channel bone p.
    Alta condylar buttress p.
    Alta distal fracture p.
    Alta femoral p.

Alta supracondylar bone p.
Anchor p.
AO dynamic compression p.
AO reconstruction p.
ASIF broad dynamic compression bone p.
ASIF T p.
Association for the Study of Internal Fixation (ASIF) p.
Babcock p.
Badgley p.
Bagby compression p.
Balser hook p.
base p.
Batchelor p.
p. bender
Berke-Jaeger lid p.
Bimler elastic p.
biodegradable p.
Blackstone anterior cervical p.
Blair talar body fusion blade p.
Blair tibiotalar arthrodesis blade p.
Blanchard traction device blade p.
blood agar p.
Blount blade p.
bone flap fixation p.
Bosworth spline p.
broad AO dynamic compression p.
Brophy p.
buccal cortical p.
butterfly-shaped monoblock vertebral p.
buttress p.
buttress-type p.
Capener nail p.
CAPIS compression p.
CAPIS reconstruction p.
Caspar anterior cervical p.
Caspar trapezoidal p.
cervical p.
CHS supracondylar bone p.
coaptation p.
cobra-head p.
Coffin p.
compression p.
Concise side p.
condylar lag screw p.
connecting p.
contoured anterior spinal p.
cortical oral p.
craniocervical p.
craniomaxillofacial p.
Crockard midfacial osteotomy retractor p.
C-shaped p.
p. cutter
Danek cervical fusion p.
deck p.
depth p.
Deyerle bone graft p.
3D-flat Lactosorb p.
double-angled blade p.
double-H p.
Doughty tongue p.
Driessen hinged p.

Dupont distal humeral p.
Dwyer-Hall p.
Dynamic Bridging p.
dynamic compression p.
eccentric dynamic compression p.
Eggers bone p.
Elliot knee p.
Elliott blade p.
Ellis buttress p.
end p.
fenestrated compression p.
finger p.
Foley p.
four-hole anteromedial Alta
  straight p.
four-hole side p.
Fresnel zone p.
fusion p.
gait p.
Gallannaugh bone p.
Galveston p.
Gambro Liendia p.
Geibel blade p.
Gelfilm p.
genial advancement p.
Goidnich bone p.
Haid cervical p.
Haid Universal bone p.
half-circle p.
Hansen-Street anchor p.
Hardy-Rand-Rittler p.
Harlow p.
Harm posterior cervical p.
Harris p.
Hawley bite p.
Hicks lugged p.
Hoen skull p.
Hospidex microtiter p.
H-shaped p.
Hubbard p.
impactor p.
inner lip p.
interfragmentary p.
Ishihara pseudoisochromatic p.
isochromatic p.
Jaeger metal lid p.
Jewett double-angled osteotomy p.
Jewett nail p.
Jewett slotted p.
Kessel osteotomy p.
keyed supracondylar p.
Kingsley orthodontic p.
Kleer base p.
Laing osteotomy p.
Lane fracture p.
Lawson-Thornton p.
L-buttress p.
lead p.
Leibinger 3-D bone p.
Leibinger Micro Plus p.
Leibinger mini Würzburg p.
Leibinger Würzburg p.
Letournel acetabular fracture
  bone p.
lid p.

limited-contact dynamic
  compression p.
lingual cortical p.
locking reconstruction p.
long-span rigid p.
Lorenz titanium screws and p.
low-contact dynamic compression p.
low-contact stress p.
low profile p.
L-plate p.
L-shaped p.
Luer reconstruction p.
Luhr fixation p.
Luhr mandibular p.
Luhr MCS bone p.
Luhr microbone p.
Luhr microfixation cranial p.
Luhr minifixation bone p.
Luhr pan p.
Luhr Vitallium micromesh p.
Lundholm p.
Luque II p.
Lynch mucosa separator p.
mandibular bridging p.
mandibular staple bone p.
Massie II p.
Maxisorb test p.
May anatomical bone p.
McBride p.
McDonald bone p.
McLaughlin hip p.
Medoff sliding femoral p.
Medoff sliding fracture p.
metal reconstruction p.
Meurig Williams spinal fusion p.
micro-adaption p.
Milch resection p.
Mini Orbita p.
Moberg bone p.
modified Grace p.
Moe intertrochanteric p.
Moore blade p.
Moore-Blount p.
Moore sliding nail p.
Morscher anterior cervical p.
Morscher titanium cervical p.
mouthgag tooth p.
mucosal separator p.
Mueller-Hinton-supplemented agar p.
multipoint contact p.
nail p.
narrow AO dynamic compression p.
Neufeld femoral nail p.
Newman toenail p.
Nicoll p.
Nord orthodontic p.
Odgen p.
Orion anterior cervical p.
Orozco p.
orthodontic base p.
orthopedic p.
orthotic p.
Osborne osteotomy p.
palmar p.
Paulus chin p.

P

plate · plating

plate *(continued)*
Paulus midfacial p.
pedicle p.
Percy p.
Perf-Plate cranial p.
plain-pattern p.
polydioxanone p.
PolyMedics p.
Profil-O-Plastic preshaped chin p.
Profil-O-Plastic preshaped
midfacial p.
pseudoisochromatic p.
reconstruction p.
resorbable p.
Rhinelander p.
Richards-Hirschhorn p.
Richards sideplate p.
Robin orthodontic p.
Rohadur gait p.
round hole p.
Roy-Camille p.
RSDCP p.
safety p.
Schwartz p.
Schweitzer spring p.
semitubular blade p.
Senn bone p.
serpentine bone p.
seven-hole p.
Sherman bone p.
side p., sideplate
Silastic p.
six-hole mandibular p.
Skirrow agar p.
skull p.
slotted bone p.
Smith-Petersen bone p.
Smith-Petersen intertrochanteric p.
SMo p.
snap-on inserter p.
spring p.
stabilization p.
Stahl calipers p.
stainless steel AO p.
staple bone p.
Steffee pedicle p.
Steffee screw p.
Steinhauser p.
Storz p.
superior border p.
supracondylar p.
symmetrical sacral p.
symmetrical thoracic vertebral p.
Synthes AO reconstruction p.
Synthes dorsal distal radius p.
Synthes maxillofacial locking
reconstruction p.
Synthes maxillofacial titanium p.
Synthes stainless steel
minifragment p.
Synthes titanium minifragment p.
Tacoma sacral p.
tantalum p.
T-buttress p.
Teflon p.
Temple University p.
tendon p.
thoracolumbosacral p.
Thornton p.
THORP-type mandibular
reconstruction p.
three-hole p.
tibial p.
TiMesh orthognathic strap p.
titanium AO p.
titanium hollow osseointegrating
reconstruction p.
titanium hollow-screw
osseointegrating reconstruction p.
toe p.
tongue p.
Townsend-Gilfillan p.
trochanteric p.
T-shaped AO p.
tubular p.
Tupman osteotomy p.
two-hole p.
Universal bone p.
V-blade p.
Venable bone p.
Vitallium Elliott knee p.
Vitallium Hicks radius p.
Vitallium Wainwright blade p.
Vitallium Walldius mechanical
knee p.
V-type intertrochanteric p.
Wenger slotted p.
Whitman p.
Wilson spinal fusion p.
Wright knee p.
Würzburg p.
Y-bone p.
Z-plate p.
Zuelzer hook p.
plate-holding forceps
platelet-shaped knife
plate-spacer washer
platform
Aspen ultrasound p.
BYR-300 imaging and
illumination p.
Cemax PACS p.
p. forceps
Ladarvision P.
Midline Hi-Lo Mat P.
operating p.
positioning p.
PSI-TEC aspiration/irrigation p.
StealthStation treatment guidance p.
TomTec echo p.
Platina
P. clip lens
P. intraocular lens implant
plating
Caspar p.
eccentric dynamic compression p.
Gotfried percutaneous
compression p.

618

Leibinger p.
variable spinal p.

platinum
p. blade meatotomy electrode
p. embolization coil
p. eyelid implant
p. microcoil
p. oxygen electrode
P. Plus guidewire
p. probe spatula
p. stationary table
p. wire

platinum-Dacron microcoil
Platorit investment material
platysma inerlocking suture sling
Playfair uterine caustic applicator
Pleatman
P. pouch
P. sac

pledget
cotton p.
cottonoid p.
Dacron p.
p. dressing
felt p.
Gelfoam p.
Meadox Teflon felt p.
neurosurgical p.
polypropylene p.
p. sponge
p. suture
Teflon p.

pledgeted
p. Ethibond suture
p. mattress suture

PlegiaGuard
P. safety device

Plenk-Matson raspatory
Plester retractor
plethysmograph
air p.
face-out, whole-body p.
jerkin p.
Medgraphics body p.
mercury-in-rubber strain gauge p.
Respitrace inductive p.
RIP p.
venous p.

pleural
p. biopsy needle
p. biopsy needle shears
p. biopsy punch
p. dissector
p. tube

Pleura-Stay
pleurectomy forceps
Pleur-evac
P.-e. autotransfusion system
P.-e. chest catheter
P.-e. device
P.-e. suction
P.-e. suction tube

pleurx catheter
Plexidure insole

Plexiglas
P. base
P. eye implant
P. Gellhorn pessary
P. graft
P. jig
P. radiographic ruler
P. spacer
P. tissue equivalency block

PlexiPulse
P. compression device

Pley
P. capsular forceps
P. extracapsular forceps

PLI-100 pico-injector pipette system
plication needle
pliers
Allen root p.
Beck p.
Becker-Parkin p.
bending p.
Berbecker p.
College p.
crown-crimping p.
debonding p.
dental p.
extraction p.
fisherman's p.
heavy-duty p. with side-cutter
Jacob-Swan goniotomy p.
Jelenko p.
K-Y p.
ligature-locking p.
Luhr Microfixation System p.
Mathieu p.
needle-nose p.
needle-nose vise-grip p.
Ormco orthodontic p.
orthopedic surgical p.
Power Grip p.
Reill wire-cutting p.
Risley p.
root p.
Schwarz arrow-forming p.
slip-joint p.
SMIC p.
Sontec p.
square-end p.
Stille flat p.
threader rod holder p.
vise-grip p.

Plondke uterine forceps
plug
Air-Lon decannulation p.
Alcock catheter p.
Avina female urethral p.
Berkeley Bioengineering brass
scleral p.
Biomet p.
Bio-Plug canal p.
bone femoral p.
brass scleral p.
Buck p.
Catamaran swim p.
catheter p.

P

plug *(continued)*
    collagen p.
    Coloplast one-piece conseal p.
    Coloplast two-piece conseal p.
    Concept bone tunnel p.
    Corner p.
    Counsellor p.
    p. cutter
    Dittrich p.
    Doc's ear p.
    Dohlman p.
    dome hole p.
    EaglePlug tapered-shaft punctum p.
    EagleVision Freeman punctum p.
    Exeter intramedullary bone p.
    femoral p.
    Freeman punctum p.
    gastrostomy p.
    glass vaginal p.
    Herniamesh surgical p.
    Herrick lacrimal p.
    Insta-Putty silicone ear p.
    intramedullary canal p.
    Isberg scleral p.
    Johnston gastrostomy p.
    Kirschner femoral canal p.
    Luer-Lok male adapter p.
    Mack ear p.
    methyl methacrylate cranioplastic p.
    Micro punctum p.
    Oasis collagen p.
    omental p.
    Osteonics acetabular dome hole p.
    PerFix hernia p.
    PerFix Marlex mesh p.
    plastic femoral p.
    polypropylene p.
    punctum p.
    Reich-Nechtow p.
    R-Med p.
    scleral p.
    sealing window p.
    Seidel p.
    Shiley decannulation p.
    Sims vaginal p.
    Super punctum p.
    tapered-shaft punctum p.
    TearSaver punctum p.
    Teflon p.
    Umbrella punctum p.
    Woodson p.
plug-finishing bur
plugger
    amalgam p.
    Bredall amalgam p.
    endodontic p.
    Mity p.
    Schilder p.
    serrated amalgam p.
    SMIC root canal p.
plugging instrument
plumbeous zirconate titanate tip
Plum-Blossom acupuncture needle
Plume-Away evacuator

PlumeSafe Whisper 602 smoke evacuation system
Plumicon camera tube
Plummer
    P. bag
    P. modified bougie
    P. water-filled pneumatic esophageal dilator
Plummer-Vinson
    P.-V. apparatus
    P.-V. esophageal dilator
    P.-V. radium esophageal applicator
plunger
    dome p.
plunger-type femoral pressurizer
plus
    Bio Gard P.
    BIS Sensor P.
    BSS P.
    Candela MiniScope P.
    Cytobrush P.
    DPS P.
    Dualer P.
    Hydra Vision P.
    Hydro P.
    Laserprobe-PLR P.
    Lithostar P.
    Omnifit P.
    Omni-Flow 4000 P.
    Oracle Micro P.
    Pneu Care P.
    p. power lens
    Richards Solcotrans P.
    Siemens Lithostar P.
    Siemens Somatom P.
    Sonicare P.
    Steri-Cuff P.
    Suture Strip P.
    Synergy P.
Plyoback Rebounder
PlyoSled exerciser
Plystan
    P. graft
    P. prosthesis
PMI implant
PMMA
    polymethyl methacrylate
    PMMA centering sleeve
    PMMA centralizer
    PMMA haptic
    PMMA hard contact lens
    PMMA implant
    PMMA intraocular lens
PMT
    PMT AccuSpan tissue expander
    PMT Cortac cortical electrode
    PMT Depthalon depth electrode
    PMT halo brace
    PMT InVac in-line suction control device
    PMT MacroVac suction-irrigator
    PMT MicroVac suction device
    PMT robotic fulcrumless tomographic system

Pneu
P. Care ICU dynamic low-air-loss bed
P. Care Pedibed dynamic pediatric low-air-loss bed
P. Care Plus
P. Knee brace

pneumatic
p. ankle tourniquet
p. antiembolic stockings
p. bag
p. balloon catheter
p. balloon dilator
p. 4-bar linkage knee
p. chair lift
p. compression boot
p. compression stockings
p. cuff
p. garment
p. microscope
p. otoscope
p. tonometer
p. walker

pneumatometer
Semm CO_2 p.

pneumatonograph

pneumatonometer
Digibind p.
Micro One p.
Modular One p.

pneumoballistic lithotriptor

pneumodissection

pneumodissector
laparoscopic p.

pneumohydraulic capillary infusion system

Pneumo-Matic insufflation needle

Pneumomat laparoscopic insufflator

Pneumo-Needle needle

pneumoperitoneum needle

pneumo sleeve

pneumostatic dilator

Pneumotach

pneumotachograph
Fleish No. 2 p.
Gould Godard p.

pneumotachometer
Collins SurveyTach p.
hot-wire p.
MicroTach p.
Rudolph linear p.

pneumothoracic
p. apparatus
p. injection needle

pneumotome
Wappler p.

pneumotonometer

Pneumotron ventilator

Pneumo-Wrap

pneuPAC
p. resuscitator
p. ventilator

Pneu-Scale frameless air support therapy

Pneu-trac cervical collar

POC
POC balloon
POC Bandit catheter

Pocket-Dop
P.-D. blood-flow detector
P.-D. fetal heart rate monitor
P.-D. fetal stethoscope
P.-D. II

Pockethaler
Vancenase P.

Pocketpeak peak flowmeter

pocket probe

PodoSpray nail drill system

Pogon chair

Poh mouth mirror

point
Crowe pilot p.
drill p.
p. electrode
Excell polishing p.
p. forceps
G-C "SMOOTH CUT" diamond p.
gutta-percha p.
Mathews drill p.
powered automatic stopping drill p.
Raney-Crutchfield drill p.
p. resolved spectroscopy
self-stopping drill p.
Starlite p.
Universal drill p.
William Dixon Cratex p.

pointed
p. awl
p. cone bur

pointed-tip electrode

pointer
Baton laser p.
LaserMed laser p.
metallic p.

Pointer one-piece all-PMMA intraocular lens

Point-of-care analysis

point-of-reduction clamp

point-search instrument

Polack keratoscope

Polar
P. Bair forced-air active cooling device
P. Care 500 cryotherapy device
P. coordinate system
P. Pack
P. Vantage XL heart rate monitor
P. wrist monitor

polarimeter
confocal scanning laser p.
scanning laser p.

Polaris
P. adjustable spinal cage implant
P. cage
P. electrode
P. laparoscope
P. LE catheter
P. Mansfield/Webster deflectable tip
P. 1.32 Nd:YAG laser
P. reusable cutter

P

Polaris *(continued)*
  P. reusable dissector
  P. reusable forceps
  P. reusable grasper
  P. reusable laparoscopic instrument
  P. steerable diagnostic catheter
polarizing ophthalmoscope
Polar-Mate
  P.-M. bipolar coagulator
  P.-M. bipolar microcoagulator
polarographic needle electrode
Polaroid
  P. CB-100 camera
  P. HealthCam system
  P. instant endocamera
  P. vectograph slide
Polaron sputter coater
Polarus
  P. humeral rod
  P. Plus humeral fixation system
  P. positional humeral fixation
    system
Polavision Land camera for endoscopy
Polcyn elevator
pole
  walking p.
Polhemus
  P. 3 digitizer
  P. 3 digitizer scanner
  P. 3Space digitizer
Poliak eye retractor
poliglecaprone 25 suture
polio laryngoscope
Polisar-Lyons
  P.-L. adapted tracheal tube
  P.-L. tracheal tube
polisher
  Anis ball reverse-curvature
    capsular p.
  Anis disk capsular p.
  Bechert capsular p.
  Buedding squeegee cortex extractor
    and p.
  capsular p.
  capsule p.
  Drews capsular p.
  Freeman capsular p.
  Gill-Welsh capsular p.
  Holladay posterior capsular p.
  Jensen capsular p.
  Knolle capsular p.
  Knolle capsule p.
  Kraff capsular p.
  Kratz p.
  Kratz-Jensen p.
  Look capsular p.
  Tennessee capsular p.
  Terry silicone capsular p.
  Torchia capsular p.
  Yaghouti LASIK P.
polishing
  p. brush
  p. bur
  p. strip

Politzer
  P. air bag
  P. air-bag otoscope
  P. air syringe
  P. angular ear knife
  P. ear perforator
  P. ear speculum
  P. paracentesis needle
Politzer-Ralks knife
Polk
  P. finger goniometer
  P. placental forceps
  P. sponge forceps
Polle pod attachment for
  ophthalmoscope
Polley-Bickel trephine
Pollock
  P. double corneal forceps
  P. punch
  P. sweetheart periosteal elevator
  P. wimp wire impactor
  P. zygoma elevator
Pollock-Dingman elevator
polly power grip
pollywog
Polmedco endotracheal tube cuff
Polokoff rasp
Poloxamer 407 barrier material
POLY
  P. balloon catheter
Poly
  P. CS device
  P. Surgiclip absorbable clip
polyamide
  p. mesh
  p. suture
polyanhydride biodegradable polymer
  wafer
polyaxial cervical screw
polybutester suture
polycarboxylate cement
Poly-Cath catheter
polycationic histochemical probe
Polycel bone composite prosthesis
polycentric knee prosthesis
Polydek suture
Polyderm
  P. border with Covaderm tape
  P. foam wound dressing
Poly-Dial insert
polydioxanone
  p. plate
  p. sheet
  p. suture (PDS)
Polydor Preforms orthotic
polyene thread
polyester
  p. fiber suture
polyether implant material
polyethylene
  ArCom compression-molded p.
  ArCom processed p.
  p. cannula
  carbon fiber-reinforced p.
  p. collar button

p. drain
extruded bar p.
p. foam
p. glycol
p. graft
high density p.
p. implant material
p. intravenous catheter
p. liner
p. liner implant component
porous p.
p. retractor tape
p. seat heart valve
p. socket
p. sphere implant
p. stent
p. strut
p. suture
p. talar prosthesis
p. terephthalate balloon
p. T-tube
p. tube
p. tubing
polyethylene-faced
p.-f. driver
p.-f. mallet
polyfilament suture
PolyFlex
P. implantable pacing lead
pacemaker
P. traction dressing
Polyfloat system II mattress replacement
Polyflux hemodialyzer
Polyform splint
polygalactic acid suture
PolyGIA stapling device
polyglactin
p. mesh
p. 910 suture
polyglecaprone 25 suture
polyglycolate suture
polyglycolic
p. acid suture
p. mesh
polyglycolide implant
polyglyconate suture
polygoniometer
polygon mirror
polygraph
Gould p.
Mackenzie p.
Night Owl Pocket p.
polylactic acid arrow
polylactide
p. absorbable screw
p. implant
Polylite quilted underpad
poly-L-lysine-coated glass slide
Poly-Lock bonding
PolyMedics plate
Polymed splint
PolyMem
P. adhesive surgical wound dressing
P. foam wound dressing

polymer
Bioplastique p.
HTR p.
Hydrolene p.
Hylamer orthopaedic bearing p.
P.Q. viscoelastic p.
superabsorbent p.
p. tooth replica implant
polymer-coated, drug-eluting stent
PolymerFriction total knee
polymeric
p. biomaterial
p. endoluminal paving stent
polymethyl
p. methacrylate (PMMA)
p. methacrylate bone cement
p. methacrylate ear splint
p. methacrylate implant
polymethyl
polyolefin copolymer balloon
polypectomy snare
polyp forceps
polyphase generator
Poly-Plus Dacron vascular graft
Polyprep centrifuge
polypropylene
p. button
p. button suture
p. glycol ankle-foot orthosis
p. glycol thoracolumbosacral orthosis
p. hand brush
p. intracardiac patch
p. intraocular lens
p. mesh
p. needle
p. pledget
p. plug
polypus forceps
Polyrox Fractal active fixation lead
PolySafe pacer
Polysil-Foley catheter
Polyskin
P. II dressing
polysomnograph
p. electroencephalograph 20-channel
EEG recorder
Sleepscan p.
Polysorb
P. absorbable staple
P. heel cup
P. liner
P. 55 stapler
P. suture
Polystan
P. cardiotomy reservoir
P. implant
P. perfusion cannula
P. venous return catheter
Polystim electrode
polysulfone
p. dialyzer
p. membrane
PolyTech nonlatex self-adhering urinary external catheter
Polytec LaseAway Q-switched ruby laser

polytef-sheathed needle
polytef soft tissue patch
polytetraflouroethylene-covered stent
polytetrafluoroethylene (PTFE)
    expanded p. (EPTFE)
    p. (PTFE) implant
    p. (PTFE) mesh
    p. (PTFE) prosthesis
    p. (PTFE) stent graft
    p. sock
polytome
    p. instrument
    Massiot p.
Polytrac
    P. Gomez retractor
PolyTrach dressing
Polytron PT 3000 homogenizer
polyurethane
    p. bandage
    p. graft
    p. implant material
    p. nasoenteric catheter
    Permalume p.
    p. stent
polyurethane-coated silicone breast implant
polyvinyl
    p. alcohol foam
    p. alcohol splint
    p. alcohol sponge
    p. bougie
    p. catheter
    p. chloride balloon
    p. chloride endotracheal tube
    p. curette
    p. dilator
    p. drain
    p. graft
    p. implant material
    p. prosthesis
    p. sponge implant
    p. tubing
polyvinylsiloxane putty
Polyviolene polyester suture material
PolyWic
    P. dressing
    P. wound filling material
POMARD anthropomorphic measurement reference chart
Pomeranz
    P. aortic clamp
    P. hiatal hernia retractor
Pomeroy ear syringe
pommel cushion
POMS 20/50 oxygen conservation device
poncho restraint
Ponseti splint
Ponsky
    P. Endo-Sock specimen retrieval bag
    P. PEG tube
    P. Pull
Ponsky-Gauderer
    P.-G. PEG tube
    P.-G. type PEG

pontoon spica cast
pool
    AquaMotion p.
    Endless Pool physical therapy p.
    SwimEx p.
Poole
    P. abdominal suction tube
    P. trocar
Pool-Pfeiffer self-locking clip
POP
    plaster-of-Paris
    POP bandage
Pope
    P. halo dressing
    P. Oto-Wick
    P. rectal knife
    P. wick
popliteal retractor
pop-off
    p.-o. needle
    p.-o. suture
    p.-o. valve
"pop-on" self-adhering male external catheter
Poppen
    P. aortic clamp
    P. electrosurgical coagulator
    P. Gigli-saw guide
    P. intervertebral disk forceps
    P. intervertebral disk rongeur
    P. laminectomy rongeur
    P. monopolar cautery cord
    P. periosteal elevator
    P. pituitary rongeur
    P. Ridge Sensitometer
    P. suction tube
    P. sympathectomy scissors
    P. ventricular needle
Poppen-Blalock carotid artery clamp
Poppen-Blalock-Salibi carotid clamp
Poppen-Gelpi laminectomy self-retaining retractor
Poppers tonsillar guillotine
poppet
    ball p.
    barium-impregnated p.
    prosthetic p.
pop rivet
Poracryl resin
porcine
    p. bioprosthesis
    p. graft
    p. heart valve
    p. prosthesis
Porex
    P. drainage system
    P. Medpor implant
    P. nerve locator
    P. paranasal implant
    P. PHA implant
Porges
    P. Neoflex dilator
    P. stone dislodger
Pori and Rowe EEG receiver
Porites coral material

Porocoat
> P. coating
> P. material

Porocool prosthesis

Porolon sponge

Poron
> P. cellular urethane
> P. 400 insole

Poroplastic splint

porous
> p. coating
> p. hydroxyapatite sphere
> p. metallic stent
> p. polyethylene
> p. polyethylene implant

porous-coated
> p.-c. anatomic (PCA)
> p.-c. anatomic knee prosthesis

Porovin dental resin

PORP
> partial ossicular replacement prosthesis
> Richards hydroxyapatite PORP

port
> A-Port implantable p.
> Berkeley Bioengineering infusion terminal p.
> butterfly needle infusion p.
> Celsite brachial p.
> Celsite implanted p.
> Celsite pediatric p.
> Cordis multipurpose access p.
> endoscopic access p.
> endoscopic threaded imaging p.
> EndoTIP imaging p.
> Gill-Welsh guillotine p.
> Hassan-type p.
> Hasson blunt p.
> implantable infusion p.
> Infuse-a-Port p.
> infusion p.
> low-profile, port implantable p.
> Luer-Lok p.
> lumbar p.
> OmegaPort access p.
> periumbilical p.
> p. protector
> Quinton Q-Port vascular access p.
> single p.
> tangential p.
> Thora-Port p.
> Titanium VasPort p.
> treatment p.
> Universal catheter access p.
> Vasport access p.
> venous access p.
> Visiport p.
> Vortex Clear-Flow p.

portable
> p. blood irradiator
> p. insulin dosage-regulating apparatus
> p. insulin infusion pump
> p. respirator
> p. suction aspirator

> P. Topical Hyperbaric Oxygen Extremity Chamber
> p. topical hyperbaric oxygen extremity chamber

Port-A-Cath
> P.-A.-C. device
> P.-A.-C. implantable catheter
> P.-A.-C. implantable catheter system

portacaval
> p. H graft
> p. shunt

Port-Access
> St. Jude Medical P.-A.

Portadial kidney machine

Port-A-FEESST case

PortaFlo urine collection system

portal
> AP p.
> p. cannula
> p. catheter
> fixed-beam p.
> integrated sideport access p.
> PA p.
> P. Pro 2 treatment chair

portal-phased spiral CT scan

Porta-Lung noninvasive extrathoracic ventilator

PortalVision radiation oncology system

Porta Pulse 3 portable defibrillator

Portaray dental x-ray unit

Porta-Resp monitor

Portazam portable exam chair

Porter duodenal forceps

Porter-Kolpe biliary biopsy set

Porter-O-Surgical cutter

Portex
> P. bacterial filter
> P. Blue Line tracheostomy tube
> P. chorionic villus sampling catheter
> P. nasopharyngeal airway
> P. Neo-Vac meconium suction device
> P. nylon cannula
> P. Per-fit tracheostomy kit
> P. Per-Fit tracheostomy tube
> P. preformed blue line tracheal tube
> P. Soft-Seal cuff system
> P. SS endotracheal tube cuff
> P. Thermo-Vent heat and moisture device
> P. ThermoVent heat and moisture exchanger
> P. XL endotracheal tube cuff

Portex-Gibbon catheter

Portmann
> P. drill
> P. retractor
> P. speculum holder

Portnoy
> P. DPV device
> P. multiflanged catheter
> P. ventricular cannula
> P. ventricular catheter

portogram
> SMA p.

P

portography
 arterial p.
Porto-lift
portosystemic shunt
Porto-Vac
 P.-V. catheter
 P.-V. suction tube
PortSaver PercLoop device
Porzett splint
Posada-Vasco orbital retractor
Posey
 P. bar kit
 P. bed cradle
 P. below-the-knee castbelt
 P. belt
 P. drop seat
 P. grip
 P. Palm Cone
 P. restraint
 P. SkinSleeves
 P. sling
 P. snare
Posicam
 P. HZ PET scanner
Posilok instrument holder
Posi-Stop drill
Positex knee wedge
positional feedback stimulation trainer
positioner
 Assistant Free Stulberg leg p.
 Bareskin knee p.
 beach chair p.
 body p.
 BodyCushion p.
 Body Wrap foam p.
 CAS-8000V general angiography p.
 Cook stent p.
 Craniad cup p.
 cup p.
 eggcrate p.
 Foot Waffle p.
 Grasshopper p.
 Hold-and-Hold p.
 IMP Universal lateral p.
 Kirschenbaum foot p.
 knee p.
 lateral p.
 leg p.
 p. luer
 Mark II Stulberg hip p.
 Mark II Wixson hip p.
 MB&J knee p.
 McCaffrey p.
 McConnell shoulder p.
 McGuire pelvic p.
 Medline p.
 Miller bracket p.
 Montreal p.
 Picket Fence leg p.
 Prep-Assist p.
 Profex arthroscopic leg p.
 ProForm p.
 Schlein shoulder p.
 shoulder abduction p.
 Stulberg hip p.

 Stulberg Mark II leg p.
 SurgAssist leg p.
 Ther-A-Shapes p.
 TMJ head p.
 Vac-Pac p.
 Wixson hip p.
 Zimfoam pad and patient p.
positioning
 p. needle
 p. pillow
 p. platform
position-sensing catheter
positive
 p. end-expiratory pressure
 p. expiratory pressure
 p. eyepiece
Positrap
 P. mini-retrieval basket
 P. retriever
Positrol
 P. cardiac device
 P. II Bernstein catheter
 P. USCI catheter
positron
 p. emission tomography balloon
 (PET balloon)
 p. scintillation camera
Posner
 P. diagnostic gonioprism
 P. diagnostic lens
 P. slit lamp
 P. surgical gonioprism
post
 Caspar retraction p.
 P. forceps
 Hahnenkratt root canal p.
 PD crown p.
 PD root canal p.
 Prep-Tite p.
 Stalite root canal p.
 surgical instrument p.
 transosseous p.
 P. washing cannula
postauricular
 p. ear dressing
 p. hearing aid
 p. retractor
posterior
 p. capsule scrubber
 p. chamber intraocular lens
 p. chamber lens implant
 p. convex intraocular lens
 p. distraction instrumentation
 p. footplate pick
 p. forceps
 p. fossa retractor
 p. hook-rod spinal instrumentation
 p. leaf-spring ankle-foot orthosis
 p. neck surface coil
 p. reduction device
 p. rod system
 p. thigh bar
 p. urethral retractor
postgadolinium scan
Post-Harrington erysiphake

postmortem suture needle
postnasal
- p. balloon
- p. balloon tamponade
- p. dressing
- p. sponge forceps

postoperative
- p. flexor tendon traction brace
- p. mammary support
- p. shoe

postpyloric feeding tube
post-TUR irrigation clamp
Posture
- P. Curve lumbar cushion
- P. Pump Lordoticiser
- P. Pump Spine Trainer
- P. S'port
- P. Wedge seat cushion

post-urethroplasty review speculum
Pos-T-Vac vacuum erection device
Potain
- P. apparatus
- P. aspirating trocar
- P. aspirator

potassium titanyl phosphate laser
potential acuity meter
potentiometer
- linear p.

Potocky needle
Potta coarctation forceps
Potter
- P. modified knife
- P. needle
- P. sickle knife
- P. sponge forceps
- P. tonsillar forceps

Potter-Bucky diaphragm
Potter-Elvehjem homogenizer
Potts
- P. aortic clamp
- P. bronchial forceps
- P. bulldog forceps
- P. cardiovascular clamp
- P. coarctation clamp
- P. coarctation forceps
- P. dental elevator
- P. dissector
- P. divisional clamp
- P. expansile dilator
- P. expansile knife
- P. expansile valvulotome
- P. fixation forceps
- P. infant rib shears
- P. intestinal forceps
- P. ligature
- P. needle
- P. patent ductus clamp
- P. patent ductus forceps
- P. periosteotome
- P. pulmonic clamp
- P. shunt
- P. splint
- P. tenaculum
- P. tenotomy scissors

- P. thumb forceps
- P. vascular scissors

Potts-Cournand angiography needle
Potts-DeBakey clamp
Potts-DeMartel gall duct scissors
Potts-Nevins dressing forceps
Potts-Niedner aortic clamp
Potts-Riker
- P.-R. dilator
- P.-R. valvulotome

Potts-Satinsky clamp
Potts-Smith
- P.-S. aortic clamp
- P.-S. arterial scissors
- P.-S. bipolar forceps
- P.-S. dissecting scissors
- P.-S. dressing forceps
- P.-S. monopolar forceps
- P.-S. needle holder
- P.-S. pulmonic clamp
- P.-S. reverse scissors
- P.-S. tissue forceps

Potts-Yasargil scissors
pouch
- Atlantic "O-Dor-Less" P.'s
- Bard closed-end adhesive p.
- Bard drainage adhesive p.
- Bard security p.
- bladder replacement urinary p.
- Bongort Lifestyles Closed-End P.'s
- Bongort Max-E-Pouch p.
- Bongort one-piece drainable p.
- Bongort one-piece ostomy p.
- Bongort urinary diversion p.
- Cardio-Cool myocardial protection p.
- CenterPointLock two-piece ostomy system: closed p.
- CenterPointLock two-piece ostomy system: drainable p.
- Coloplast one-piece post-op drainable p.
- Coloplast one-piece small drainable p.
- Coloplast one-piece standard drainable p.
- Coloplast two-piece small drainable p.
- Coloplast two-piece small urostomy p.
- ConvaTec ostomy p.
- ConvaTec urostomy p.
- Dansac Combi Colo F one-piece p.
- Dansac Contour 1 mini one-piece p.
- Dansac Contour 1 oval one-piece p.
- Dansac standard F one-piece p.
- Dennis Brown p.
- Durahesive Wafer p.
- female urinary p.
- FirstChoice closed p.
- FirstChoice post-operative drainable p.
- FirstChoice urostomy p.
- Florida urinary p.

P

pouch (*continued*)
    Guardian two-piece ostomy system: closed p.
    Guardian two-piece ostomy system: drainable p.
    Guardian two-piece ostomy system: urostomy p.
    HolliGard seal closed stoma p.
    Hollister First Choice p.
    Hunt-Lawrence p.
    Kataya seal closed stoma p.
    Le Bag urinary p.
    Lo-Profile urostomy p.
    Mainz p.
    ManHood absorbent p.
    Mansson urinary p.
    Marlen's Ultra one-piece p.
    Marsupial p.
    Mentor absorbent p.
    Nu-Hope drainable one-piece p.
    Nu-Hope Neonatal and Premee P.'s
    Nu-Hope urinary p.
    Padua bladder urinary p.
    Parks ileostomy p.
    Parsonnet pulse generator p.
    pediatric drainable p.
    pediatric transfer p.
    pediatric urostomy p.
    Penn p.
    Pleatman p.
    Preemie p.
    Premier drainable p.
    Premier urostomy p.
    Premium closed p.
    Premium drainable p.
    Q-T's p.
    Reality vaginal p.
    retracted penis p.
    Rowland p.
    Sheer Plus p.
    Squibb urostomy p.
    Studer p.
    Sur-Fit flexible and drainable p.
    Sur-Fit Natura p.
    Sur-Fit urostomy p.
    Sur-Fit wafer and drainable p.
    Tena p.
    Tenador male p.
    Torbot Plastic p.
    Torbot Rubber p.
    p.-type sling

Pouchkins
    P. pediatric ostomy belt
    P. pediatric ostomy system
Pousson pigtail catheter
Poutasse
    P. renal artery clamp
    P. renal artery forceps
powder
    p. blower
    p. board
    Cel Touch white indicator p.
    Chronicure protein hydrolysate p.
    Comfeel p.
    Dembone demineralized cortical p.
    demineralized cortical bone p.
    Denpac porcelain p.
    Francer porcelain p.
    hyCURE wound care p.
    Osteomin Thermo-Ashed bone p.
    Royl-Derm protectant p.
    Stomahesive p.
    Tru-Stain acrylic p.
    Vitadur-N porcelain p.
Powell wand
power
    p. adapter
    p. amplifier
    P. Anthro shoe
    P. cannula
    p. Doppler
    P. Doppler ultrasound
    p. drill
    P. Grip pliers
    p. injector
    p. peak filter
    P. Play knee brace
    P. Pogo stationary exerciser
    p. rasp
    p. router
    P. Trainer cycle
    P. Web hand exerciser
    p. wheelchair
PowerBelt lower back and abdominal support belt
PowerCut drill blade
powered
    p. automatic skull perforator
    p. automatic stopping drill point
Powerflex
    P. CMP exerciser
    P. tape
Powerforma surgical drill
PowerGrip
    P. stent
    P. stent delivery system
Powerheart automatic external cardioverter-defibrillator
Powermatic table
POWERPoint orthotic shoe insert
PowerProxi Sonic interdental toothbrush system
PowerStar bipolar scissors
PowerTilt
    HiLo P.
PowerVision ultrasound
Pozzi
    P. tenaculum
    P. tenaculum forceps
PPG probe
PPT
    PPT insole system
    PPT MXL soft molded insole
    PPT Plastazote insole
    PPT RX firm molded insole
    PPT sheet
pQCT microscanner
P.Q. viscoelastic polymer
Praeger iris hook

PRAFO
  PRAFO adjustable orthotic
  PRAFO KAFO attachment
Pram combination occluder
Pratt
  P. anoscope
  P. antral curette
  P. bivalve retractor
  P. bivalve speculum
  P. crypt hook
  P. cystic hook
  P. ethmoid curette
  P. hemostatic forceps
  P. nasal curette
  P. proctoscope
  P. rectal dilator
  P. rectal director
  P. rectal hook
  P. rectal probe
  P. rectal scissors
  P. rectal speculum
  P. tenaculum
  P. tissue forceps
  P. T-shaped hemostatic forceps
  P. urethral sound
  P. uterine dilator
  P. vulsellum forceps
Pratt-Smith hemostatic forceps
preamplifier
  ARZCO p.
Preceder interventional guidewire
Precept DR pacemaker
prechopper
  Akahoshi phaco p.
President stem
precise
  P. anastomotic coupler
  P. disposable skin stapler
  p. lesion measuring device
precision
  P. Cosmet lens
  P. hip system
  p. lancet cutting needle
  P. Osteolock femoral component
  P. Osteolock femoral component system
  P. Osteolock femoral prosthesis
  P. Osteolock hip prosthesis
  P. Osteolock stem
  P. Osteolock total hip
  P. QID glucose monitoring system
  P. refractor
  P. Strata hip system
  P. tack instrument
Precision-Cosmet intraocular lens implant
PrecisionGlide needle
Pre-Cision miniature and microminiature scalpel
Preci-Slot dental attachment
Precisor Direct Bite biopsy forceps
Preci-Vertix kit
PreClean soak system
preclotted graft
Preclude
  P. dura substitute prosthesis

  P. IMA sleeve
  P. pericardial membrane
  P. peritoneal membrane
  P. spinal membrane
Precoat Plus femoral prosthesis
precollagenous filamentous material
precompression jig
precontoured unit rod
precordial stethoscope
precut papillotome
Predator balloon catheter
Preefer eye speculum
Preemie pouch
preformed
  p. clasp
  p. Cordis catheter
  p. polyvinyl chloride endotracheal tube
Premier
  P. drainable mini-pouch
  P. drainable pouch
  P. I&A unit
  P. pincore latex cushion
  P. urostomy pouch
Premiere vitreous cutter
Premium
  P. CEEA circular stapler
  P. CEEA circular stapling device
  P. closed pouch
  P. DEEA circular stapling device
  P. drainable pouch
  P. Plus CEEA disposable stapler
  P. Poly CS-57 stapler
PREMIX-SLIP premixed instrument milk lubricant and rust inhibitor
Premo guidewire
premounted stent
Prentif pessary
Prentiss forceps
Prenyl jacket
preparation
  ThinPrep cytologic p.
Prep-Assist
  P.-A. legholder
  P.-A. positioner
Preperitioneal distension balloon
Prep-IM hip bone preparation kit
preplaced suture
Preposition ColorCards
Preptic dressing
Prep-Tite post
prepuce forceps
presbyopia glasses
Presbyterian
  P. Hospital forceps
  P. Hospital occluding clamp
  P. Hospital staphylorrhaphy elevator
  P. Hospital T-clamp
  P. Hospital tubing clamp
  P. Hospital ventricular needle
Prescriptor hearing aid
Presence bladder control pad
preshaped catheter
Preshaw clamp
presphenoethmoid suture

P

press · Prima

press
Cali-Press graft p.
CamStar power leg p.
fascial p.
House Gelfoam p.
Omni p.
Paparella tissue p.
p. plate needle holder
Sheehy fascial p.
tissue p.
tissue graft p.
press-button chuck
Press-Fit
P.-F. collared femoral stem P.-F.
P.-F. condylar component
P.-F. condylar total knee
P.-F. femoral component
P.-F. implant
P.-F. prosthesis
P.-F. stem
P.-F. total condylar knee system
Press-Mate model 8800T blood pressure monitor
Presso cardiac device
Presso-Elastic dressing
pressometer
Jarcho p.
press-on prism
Pressoplast compression dressing
Pressore wrapping pressure monitor
Presso-Superior dressing
PressPak dispenser
PresSsion pneumatic garment
pressure
Alladin InfantFlow nasal continuous positive air p.
p. bandage
p. cuff
p. earring
p. equalization tube
p. equalizing tube
p. forceps
p. gauge
p. glove
P. Guard guidewire
P. Guard II
p. injector
p. length loop
p. patch dressing
p. phosphene tonometer
positive end-expiratory p.
positive expiratory p.
p. relief ankle foot orthosis
p. relief padding
p. relief shoe
p. ring
P. Sentinel reamer
sequential p.
p. shield
p. sling
p. sore status tool
p. transducer
p. transducer-monitor system
p. ventilator
pressure-cycled ventilator

PressureEasy cuff inflation device
Pressurefuse automatic constant pressure device
PressureGuard
P. IV alternating pressure mattress
P. Select patient adjustable pressure management system
pressure-point tension ring
pressure-preset ventilator
pressure-producing earring
pressure-relief cushion
PressureSense monitor
Pressure-Specified Sensory Device
pressurizer
Oxyhood p.
plunger-type femoral p.
Pressurometer blood pressure monitor
Presto
P. cardiac device
P. spirometry system
Presto-Flash spirometry system
Preston
P. ligamentum flavum forceps
P. overhead pulley
P. pinch gauge
P. Traveler CPM exerciser
Preston-Hopkins ligator
Prestop pinchometer
pretapped Synthes lag screw
pretarget filtration system
Pre-Vent
P.-V. boot style stirrup pad
P.-V. elbow protector
P.-V. heel protector
P.-V. knee crutch pad
P.-V. OR table pad
P.-V. ulnar nerve protector
PreVENT Anti-Reflux filter
Preventix modular mattress replacement system
Prevent Plus boys training brief
preVent Pneumotach flowmeter
Prevue system
P.R. heat moldable insert
Pribram suction tube
Price
P. corneal punch
P. corneal transplant system
P. Donor Cornea Punch set
P. muscle clamp
P. radial marker
Price-Thomas
P.-T. bronchial clamp
P.-T. bronchial forceps
P.-T. rib stripper
Pricker needle
Priessnitz
P. bandage
P. dressing
Priestley-Smith retinoscope
Priestly catheter
Priest wasp-waist laryngostat
Prima
P. KTP/532 laser
P. Laser catheter

P. laser guide wire
P. pacemaker
P. Series LEEP speculum
P. Series specula
P. Total Occlusion device
Primaderm foam dressing
Primallor alloy
Primapore tape and gauze wound dressing
primary
p. clip
p. trimming bur
Primbs-Circon indirect video ophthalmoscope system
Primbs suturing forceps
Prime balloon
Primer
P. compression dressing
P. compression wrap
P. flexible Unna boot
P. modified Unna boot
PrimeTime
P. disposable underpad
P. Plus adult disposable brief
primordial catheter tube
Primus prostate machine
Prince
P. advancement forceps
P. dissecting scissors
P. electrocautery
P. eye cautery
P. muscle clamp
P. muscle forceps
P. rongeur
P. tonsillar scissors
P. trachoma forceps
Prince-Potts scissors
Pringle clamp
Printz aspirator
prism
Allen-Thorpe gonioscopic p.
bar p.
base-down p.
Becker gonioscopic p.
Berens p.
DermaGard p.
diopter p.
Drews inclined p.
Fresnel p.
Goldmann contact lens p.
gonioscopic p.
hand-held rotary p.
Jacob-Swan gonioscopic p.
Keeler p.
p. loupe
Maddox p.
oblique p.
plastic p.
press-on p.
Risley rotary p.
scanning p.
square p.
P. 2000XP gamma camera
Prisma digital hearing aid

prismatic
p. contact lens
p. gonioscopic lens
p. goniotomy lens
p. spectacles
Prism-CL pacemaker
Pritchard
P. cannula
P. elevator
P. syringe
P. total elbow prosthesis
Pritikin scleral punch
Prizm
P. Electro-Mesh Sock electrode
P. Electro-Mesh Z-Stim-II stimulator
Pro
P. Balance Master
P. Peak decubitus pad
P. Pulse irrigator
P. Relief gel/foam wheelchair cushion
P. traction table
Pro-8 ankle brace
ProAdvantage knee prosthesis
ProAire portable rotation system
Pro-Bal protected balloon-tipped catheter
probe
acoustic impedance p.
ADD side-directed p.
Alcon vitrectomy p.
Aloka MP-PN ultrasound p.
Amoils p.
Amussat p.
Ando motor-driven p.
AnEber p.
Anel lacrimal p.
AngeLase combined mapping-laser p.
angled p.
Arbuckle sinus p.
Arndorfer esophageal motility p.
Aspir-Vac p.
back-stop laser p.
Bakes p.
Balectrode pacing p.
p. balloon catheter
P. balloon-on-a dilatation system
Bard p.
Barr fistular p.
Barr rectal p.
Becker p.
Beckman p.
Benger p.
Bermen-Werner p.
Beyer pigtail p.
BICAP bipolar hemostasis p.
BiLAP bipolar laparoscopic p.
biliary balloon p.
biometry p.
biopsy p.
biplane intracavitary p.
biplane sector p.
Bipolar Circumactive P. (BICAP, BiCAP)
Bipolar EndoStasis p.

probe *(continued)*
  bipolar hemostasis p.
  Birtcher electrocautery p.
  blind endosonography p.
  blood-flow p.
  blunt lacrimal p.
  blunt-tip p.
  Bodian lacrimal pigtail p.
  Bodian minilacrimal p.
  Bowman lacrimal p.
  Brackett dental p.
  brain p.
  Brenner rectal p.
  Bresgen frontal sinus p.
  Brock p.
  Brodie fistular p.
  bronchoscopic p.
  Bruel & Kjaer transvaginal
    ultrasound p.
  Brunner p.
  Brymill cryosurgical p.
  Buck ear p.
  Buie fistula p.
  bullet p.
  Bunnell dissecting p.
  Bunnell forwarding p.
  calibrated p.
  canaliculus p.
  CAPDH p.
  cardiac p.
  Castroviejo lacrimal sac p.
  cataract p.
  catheter-based ultrasound p.
  catheter ultrasound p.
  cDNA p.
  Chandler V-pacing p.
  Cherry brain p.
  chrome p. with eye
  Circon-ACMI electrohydraulic
    lithotriptor p.
  Clinitex Charles
    endophotocoagulator p.
  coagulation p.
  Coakley nasal p.
  Cody magnetic p.
  CO_2 laser p.
  common duct p.
  conical p.
  Contact Laser bullet p.
  Contact Laser chisel p.
  Contact Laser conical p.
  Contact Laser convex p.
  Contact Laser flat p.
  Contact Laser interstitial p.
  Contact Laser round p.
  continuously perfused p.
  convex p.
  coronary artery p.
  Corson needle electrosurgical p.
  Crawford canaliculus p.
  Criticare sensor p.
  cross-sectional anal sphincter p.
  cryogenic p.
  cryopexy p.

  cryotherapy p.
  C-Trak handheld gamma p.
  curved retinal p.
  Dandy p.
  Desjardins gallstone p.
  dilating p.
  dilator p.
  p. dilator
  disposable p.
  dissecting p.
  dissection p.
  Dix spud p.
  Dobbhoff bipolar coagulation p.
  Dodick photolysis p.
  Doppler flow echocardiographic p.
  Doppler four-beam laser p.
  Doppler ultrasonic p.
  dot-plotted p.
  double-ended chrome p.
  double-ended nickelene p.
  double-ended silver p.
  drum p.
  Dymer excimer delivery p.
  ear p.
  Earle rectal p.
  echo p.
  echocardiographic p.
  electric p.
  electrohydraulic lithotripsy p.
  electrohydraulic lithotriptor p.
  electromagnetic flow p.
  electromagnetic focusing field p.
  electrosurgical monopolar spatula p.
  Ellis foreign body spud p.
  Ellis foreign body spud needle p.
  Emmet uterine p.
  end-fire transrectal p.
  endocavitary p.
  Endocavity V33W p.
  endocervical p.
  endolaser p.
  Endopath needle tip
    electrosurgery p.
  Endo-P-Probe endorectal p.
  endoscopic BICAP p.
  endoscopic heat p.
  EndoSound ultrasound p.
  EndoStasis p.
  Endotrac p.
  Envision endocavity p.
  Esmarch tin bullet p.
  Esmarch p. with Myrtle leaf end
  esophageal temperature p.
  eustachian p.
  extended sector ultrasonic p.
  eye p.
  Fenger gall duct p.
  Fenger spiral gallstone p.
  Ferguson esophageal p.
  fiberoptic p.
  FIDUS p.
  filiform bougie p.
  Fish antral p.
  Fish sinus p.
  fistula p.

flexible endosonography p.
flow p.
Fluhrer bullet p.
Fluhrer rectal p.
fluorescent p.
fluoroptic thermometry p.
Fogarty biliary balloon p.
foreign body p.
four-beam laser Doppler p.
fragmentation p.
Fränkel sinus p.
free-spinning p.
French lacrimal p.
Fresgen frontal sinus p.
Frigitronics freeze-thaw cryopexy p.
frontal sinus p.
Gabor p.
Gallagher bipolar mapping p.
gall duct p.
gallstone p.
galvanic p.
gamma p.
gamma-detecting p.
Gant rectal p.
gear shift pedicle p.
Geldmacher tendon-passing p.
general p.
Gillquist-Oretorp-Stille p.
Gilmore p.
Girard Fragmatome p.
Girdner p.
Gold p.
Goldman-Fox p.
G3PDH cDNA p.
Gross p.
Hagar p.
hand-held exploring electrode p.
hand-held mapping p.
Harms trabeculotomy p.
Hayden p.
heater p.
Heller p.
Henning-Keinkel stomach p.
Hertzog pliable p.
Hewlett-Packard biplane 5-MHz p.
Hewlett-Packard omniplane 5-
  MHz p.
high-frequency miniature p.
high-resolution p.
Hitachi convex-convex biplane p.
Hitachi convex ultrasound p.
Hitachi fingertip ultrasound p.
Hitachi linear ultrasound p.
Hitachi transrectal ultrasound p.
Hitachi transvaginal ultrasound p.
hockey-stick electrosurgical p.
Hoffrel transesophageal p.
Hotz ear p.
24-hour esophageal pH p.
Huber p.
Ilg p.
Iliff lacrimal p.
illuminated p.
Injectate p.
injection gold p.

IntraDop p.
intraductal ultrasound p.
intraluminal p.
intraoperative ultrasonic p.
irrigating p.
Jacobson blood vessel p.
Jacobson vas deferens p.
Jako laryngeal p.
Jannetta p.
Jansen-Newhart mastoid p.
J-hook electrosurgical p.
Jobson-Horne p.
Josephberg p.
Kalk palpitation p.
Kartch pigtail p.
Keeler-Amoils curved cataract p.
Keeler-Amoils glaucoma p.
Keeler-Amoils long-shank retinal p.
Keeler-Amoils-Machemer retinal p.
Keeler-Amoils microcurved
  cataract p.
Keeler-Amoils ophthalmic long-
  shank p.
Keeler-Amoils ophthalmic Machemer
  retinal p.
Keeler-Amoils ophthalmic straight
  cataract p.
Keeler-Amoils ophthalmic
  vitreous p.
Kennerdell-Maroon p.
Killian p.
Kirschner guiding p.
Kistner p.
Kleinsasser p.
Knapp iris p.
Kocher p.
Koenig p.
Kron bile duct p.
Kry-Med 300 p.
KTP laser p.
lacrimal duct p.
lacrimal intubation p.
laparoscopic Doppler p.
large-bore heat p.
Larry rectal p.
laryngeal p.
laser p.
laser-Doppler flowmetry p.
laser-Doppler Periflux PF-3 p.
Laserflow Doppler p.
Lente silver nitrate p.
L-hook electrosurgical p.
Liebreich p.
light monitoring p.
Lilienthal p.
Lillie frontal sinus p.
Linde cryogenic p.
lithotriptor p.
localizing p.
Lockhart-Mummery p.
Lucae ear p.
magnetic eye p.
magnetometer p.
malleable p.
MAMTAT p.

P

probe (*continued*)
    Manhattan Eye & Ear p.
    Mannis suture p.
    Martin uterine fistula p.
    mastoid p.
    Max-I-Probe irrigation p.
    Mayo common duct p.
    Mayo kidney stone p.
    Mayo uterine p.
    McKesson mouth p.
    Meadox Surgimed Doppler p.
    mechanical rotating p.
    Medi-Tech bipolar p.
    Medrad Mrinnervu endorectal
      colon p.
    Meerschaum p.
    meniscectomy p.
    Merit-B periodontal p.
    MEVA p.
    microballoon p.
    microlaryngeal laser p.
    micromultiplane transesophageal
      echocardiographic p.
    MicroSmooth p.
    Microvit p.
    miniature p.
    miniaturized ultrasound catheter p.
    Mixter common duct p.
    Mixter Dilaprobe p.
    Mixter dilating p.
    Mixter gall duct p.
    Mixter irrigating p.
    Modulap p.
    monitoring p.
    Moynihan bile duct p.
    Moynihan gallstone p.
    Mui Scientific 6-channel esophageal
      pressure p.
    Muldoon lacrimal p.
    multielectrode p.
    multilumen p.
    multiplane intracavitary p.
    Myrtle leaf p.
    Nabors p.
    nasal p.
    nasolacrimal duct p.
    needle p.
    p. needle
    Nélaton bullet p.
    NeoProbe gamma detection p.
    Neo-Therm neonatal skin
      temperature p.
    Nibbler laparoscopic p.
    nuclear p.
    Nucleotome Flex II cutting p.
    Nucleotome Micro I p.
    Ochsner-Fenger gallstone p.
    Ochsner flexible spiral gallstone p.
    Ochsner gall duct p.
    Ochsner gallstone p.
    Ochsner spiral p.
    ocutome p.
    O'Donoghue p.
    Ohmeda p.

    oligonucleotide p.
    Olympus CD-20Z heater p.
    Olympus heat p.
    Olympus ultrathin balloon-fitted
      ultrasound p.
    Olympus UM-R-series miniature
      ultrasonic p.
    Olympus UM-W-series
      endoscopic p.
    Olympus UM-1W transendoscopic
      ultrasound p.
    Oratek thermal shrinking p.
    Ossoff-Karlan microlaryngeal
      laser p.
    over-the-wire p.
    palpation p.
    PA 120 Osypka radiofrequency p.
    Paparella p.
    Parker-Heath piggyback p.
    Parsonnet coronary p.
    Payr p.
    Payr-Schmieden p.
    pediatric biplane TEE p.
    pencil Doppler p.
    percutaneous pencil Doppler p.
    periodontal p.
    Perio Temp dental p.
    PerioWise p.
    pH p.
    Photon LaserPhacolysis P.
    piggyback p.
    pigtail p.
    pocket p.
    p. point scissors
    polycationic histochemical p.
    PPG p.
    Pratt rectal p.
    Probex p.
    pulpal microdialysis p.
    quartz fiberoptic p.
    Quickert-Dryden lacrimal p.
    Quickert lacrimal p.
    Radiometer p.
    rectal p.
    Reddick-Saye Lav-1 I&A p.
    Reddick-Saye Lav-1 irrigating and
      aspirating p.
    reflectance spectrophotometric p.
    reverse-cutting p.
    reverse-cutting meniscal p.
    Rica ear p.
    Richards p.
    right-angle blunt p.
    rigid endosonography p.
    Ritleng p.
    RNA p.
    Robicsek vascular p.
    Rockey dilating p.
    Rohrschneider p.
    Rolf lacrimal p.
    Rollet lacrimal p.
    Rosen ear p.
    Rosen endaural p.
    Rubinstein p.
    salpingeal p.

Sandhill p.
Sarns temperature p.
Schmieden p.
scissors p.
Sheer p.
p. shield
Shirodkar p.
side-hole cannulated p.
Siemens linear p.
Siemens vaginal p.
silver p.
Silverstein stimulator p.
Simpson sterling lacrimal p.
Sims uterine p.
simultaneous thermal diffusion blood flow and pressure p.
sinus p.
Skillern sphenoidal p.
SMIC periodontal abscess p.
SmokEvac electrosurgical p.
Softflo fiber optic p.
Sonablate transrectal p.
Sonocath ultrasound p.
p. spatula
spatula electrosurgical p.
spear-ended chrome p.
spear-pointed nickelene p.
Spectraprobe-Max p.
Spencer labyrinth exploration p.
sphenoidal p.
Spiesman fistular p.
SpineStat side-directed diskectomy p.
spinning p.
spiral p.
Stacke p.
standard hook electrosurgical p.
Storz-Bowman lacrimal p.
Storz pigtail p.
straight retinal p.
suction p.
Surgiflex WAVE XP suction/irrigation p.
Swiss Lithoclast pneumatic lithotripsy p.
tactile p.
Teflon p.
telephone p.
temperature p.
Theobald sinus p.
thermistor p.
through-the-scope catheter p.
tin-bullet p.
trabeculotomy p.
transcranial Doppler p.
transesophageal echocardiography p.
Transonic flow p.
transrectal p.
TrueVision transvaginal p.
truncated NMR p.
Tufcote epilation p.
tulip p.
tumor p.
ultrasonic p.
ultrasound catheter p.
Universal vaginal p.

Urrets-Zavalia p.
USCI p.
uterine p.
vacuum intrauterine p.
Valliex uterine p.
Vasamedics PR-434 implantable prism laser p.
Versadopp Doppler p.
vertebrated p.
Vibrodilator p.
ViraType p.
vitrector p.
V33W high-density endocavity p.
Vygantas-Wilder retinal drainage p.
Wasko common duct p.
water p.
Weaver sinus p.
Welch Allyn rectal p.
Werb right-angle p.
whalebone eustachian p.
whirlybird p.
Williams lacrimal p.
wire p.
Woodson p.
Worst p.
Worst double-ended pigtail p.
Xomed rectal p.
Yankauer salpingeal p.
Yellow Springs p.
Yeoman p.
YSI Foley p.
YSI neonatal temperature p.
Ziegler lacrimal p.
Ziegler needle p.
probe-ended grooved director
PROBE-SV spectrometer
Probex probe
probing sheath exchange catheter
ProBloc insulated regional block needle
ProBond dentin bonding agent
Procath electrophysiology catheter
procedure drape
Procera system
processed carbon implant
processor
array p.
Cobe 2991 cell p.
ESPrit ear level speech p.
Hope p.
Miles V.I.P. 300 vacuum infiltration p.
Mini speech p.
Olympus EU-M-series endosonography image p.
output signal p.
Procomat small-tank semiautomatic p.
real-time video p.
Terumo Steri-Cell p.
ThinPrep p.
video p.
wearable speech p.
Prochownik pessary
Pro-Clude transparent wound dressing

Procomat small-tank semiautomatic
processor
Pro-Comelastic abdominal belt
Procomp pelvic muscle reeducation
equipment
PRO/Covers ultrasound probe sheath
ProCross
    P. Rely balloon
    P. Rely over-the-wire balloon
    catheter
proctological
    p. ball electrode
    p. cotton carrier
    p. grasping forceps
    p. polyp forceps
Proctor
    P. cheek retractor
    P. laryngopharyngoscope
    P. laryngostat
    P. mucosal elevator
    P. phrenectomy forceps
    P. phrenicectomy forceps
    P. suction tube
Proctor-Bruce mastoid searcher
Proctor-Hellens laryngostat
Proctor-Livingston endoprosthesis
proctoscope
    ACMI p.
    Bacon p.
    Boehm p.
    Fansler p.
    Gabriel p.
    Goldbacher p.
    Hirschman p.
    Hirschman-Martin p.
    Kelly p.
    Lieberman p.
    Montague p.
    Morgan p.
    Morgan-Boehm p.
    National p.
    Newman p.
    Pratt p.
    Pruitt p.
    Salvati p.
    Sims p.
    Tuttle p.
    Vernon-David p.
    Welch Allyn p.
    Yeoman p.
proctoscopic
    p. fulguration electrode
proctosigmoidoscope
    ACMI fiberoptic p.
    fiberoptic p.
ProCyte transparent adhesive film
dressing
Prodigy lens inserter
ProDynamic monitor
Proetz
    P. mouthgag
    P. syringe
    P. tongue depressor
Proetz-Jansen mouthgag

Profex
    P. arthroscopic leg positioner
    P. arthroscopic tourniquet
    P. cast padding
    P. finger cot
ProFile
    P. file
    P. orifice shaper
    P. variable taper rotary instruments
Profile
    P. hip prosthesis
    P. mammography system
    P. pediatric polypectomy snare
    P. Plus balloon dilatation catheter
    P. Sitting Orthosis
    P. total hip system
profilometer
    Cottle p.
    laryngoscope p.
    Straith p.
Profil-O-Plastic
    P.-O.-P. preshaped chin plate
    P.-O.-P. preshaped midfacial plate
ProFinesse II ultrasonic handpiece
Profix
    P. confirming tibial insert
    P. metaphyseal tibial stem
    P. nonporous tibial base
    P. porous femoral component
    P. total knee replacement system
proflavin wool dressing
Proflex
    P. dilatation catheter
ProFlex wrist support
ProFlo vascular compression therapy
Pro-Flo XT catheter
Profore
    P. bandage system
    P. four-layer bandage
    P. four-layer wound dressing
    P. wound contact layer
ProForm
    P. maxim pressure reduction
    mattress
    P. maxim-VE pressure reduction
    mattress
    P. positioner
    P. strata
ProForma
    P. cannula
    P. double-lumen papillotome
Progestasert intrauterine device
Pro-glide
    P.-g. orthosis
    P.-g. splint
Prograft Exluder bifurcated endograft
Programalith
    P. AV pacemaker
    P. II, III pacemaker
    P. III pulse generator
programmable
    p. cardioverter-defibrillator (PCD)
    p. pacemaker
    p. pulse generator
    p. pump

p. valve
p. VariGrip II prosthetic control system

programmer
P. III pacemaker
p. wand

progressive
P. ankle orthosis
p. dilators
P. palm guard

projector
acuity visual p.
fiberoptic light p.
Marco chart p.
NP-3S auto chart p.
Tagarno 3SD cine p.
Tagarno 3SD cineangiography p.
Topcon chart p.

Project Research Ophthalmic specular microscope
Pro-Koester wide-field SCM microscope
Prokop intraocular lens
Prolapse coil
prolapser
Stone lens nucleus p.

prolapsus pessary
Prolase
P. fiber
P. II
P. II lateral firing Nd:YAG laser

Prolene
P. Hernia system
P. Hernia system connector
P. Hernia system onlay patch
P. Hernia system underlay patch
P. mesh
P. mesh sheet
P. mesh silo
P. polypropylene suture
P. stitch

ProLine endoscopic instrument
ProLite Plus runner's orthotic
Prolith pacemaker
Prolog pacemaker
PROloop
P. instrument

Promag 2.2 biopsy gun
Promedica video carts
Promex biopsy needle
Promise
P. brief
P. pad and pant system
P. pad and pant trial pack
P. washable knit pant

Promoe enteral feeding container
pronation spring-control device
pronator drill
prone cranial support device
Pronex pneumatic device
pronged retractor
prongs
nasal p.

Pronova suture
Pron-Pillo head positioning device

Pron pillow
Pronto cement
Pro-Op frameless air support therapy
Pro-Ophtha
P.-O. absorbent stick sponge
P.-O. drape
P.-O. dressing
P.-O. eye pad
P.-O. eye patch
P.-O. stick
P.-O. type-K, -S shield

ProOsteon
P. implant 500 coralline hydroxyapatite bone void filler
P. implant graft material
P. synthetic bone implant

prop
Moult mouth p.
Oberto mouth p.

Propaq Encore vital signs monitor
Pro/Pel
P. cannulated interference screw
P. coating
P. coating cardiac device
Hi-Torque Floppy with P.

Proplast
P. graft
P. HA
P. I, II porous implant material
P. preformed facial implant
P. prosthesis
P. TORP

Proplast-Teflon disk implant
Pro-Post system
Propper
P. binocular indirect ophthalmoscope
P. retinoscope

Propper-Heine ophthalmoscope
Prop'r Toes hammer toe cushion
propylene dressing
PRO-Q skin protectant
ProROM walker
Proscan ultrasound imaging system
Proscope anoscope
Pro-series frameless air support therapy
ProSeries laparoscopic laser system
proserum prothrombin conversion accelerator
Proshield
P. collagen corneal shield
P. Plus skin protectant

ProShifter ACL sports brace
Prosorba column
Prospec disposable speculum
ProSpeed CT scanner
ProstaCoil self-expanding stent
Prostakath urethral stent
Prostalac total hip prosthesis
Prostalase
P. laser
P. laser system

Prostaprobe catheter
Prostar
P. Plus percutaneous closure device

Prostar *(continued)*
    P. XL hemostatic puncture closure device
    P. XL percutaneous closure device
ProstaScint system
Prostasert
prostatectomy
    p. bag
    p. forceps
Prostathermer prostatic hyperthermia system
prostatic
    p. aluminum electrode
    p. biopsy needle
    p. bridge catheter
    p. dissector
    p. driver
    p. lobe forceps
    p. needle holder
    p. retractor
    p. stent
    p. tractor
Prostatron transurethral thermotherapy device
prosthesis
    acrylic bar p.
    AcuMatch M Series modular femoral hip p.
    Airprene hinged knee p.
    Allen-Brown p.
    Allurion foot p.
    Alumina cemented total hip p.
    Ambicor inflatable p.
    Ambicor penile p.
    American Heyer-Schulte chin p.
    American Heyer-Schulte-Hinderer malar p.
    American Heyer-Schulte mammary p.
    American Heyer-Schulte-Radovan tissue expander p.
    American Heyer-Schulte rhinoplasty p.
    American Heyer-Schulte testicular p.
    American Medical Systems penile p.
    AML total hip p.
    AMS Ambicore penile p.
    AMS 700CX-series penile p.
    AMS Hydroflex penile p.
    AMS M-series malleable penile p.
    Amsterdam-type p.
    AMS Ultrex penile p.
    Anatomic Precoat hip p.
    Anderson columellar p.
    Angelchik antireflux p.
    antibiotic-loaded acrylic cement total joint p.
    Apollo hip p.
    Apollo knee p.
    Arion rod eye p.
    arterial graft p.
    articulated chin p.
    Ashley breast p.

    Atkinson p.
    Attenborough total knee p.
    Aufranc-Turner hip p.
    auricular p.
    Austin Moore hip p.
    Balance hip p.
    ball-and-cage p.
    ball-and-socket ankle p.
    ball valve p.
    Bankart shoulder p.
    Barnard mitral valve p.
    Bateman finger p.
    Bateman UPF II shoulder p.
    Baxter mechanical valve p.
    Beall mitral valve p.
    Bechtol p.
    Becker breast p.
    Becker hand p.
    Becker tissue expander p.
    Beck-Steffee total ankle p.
    below-knee prosthesis (*var. of* BK p.)
    Bentall cardiovascular p.
    Bi-Angular shoulder p.
    BIAS p.
    bicondylar ankle p.
    bifurcated seamless p.
    Bi-Metric hip p.
    Bi-Metric Interlok femoral p.
    Bi-Metric porous primary femoral p.
    Bingham knee p.
    Bio-Chromatic hand p.
    Bioclad with pegs reinforced acetabular p.
    Bioglass p.
    Bio-Groove acetabular p.
    Bio-Groove Macrobond HA femoral p.
    Biolox ball head p.
    Biomet AGC knee p.
    Biomet hip p.
    Biometric p.
    Biomet total toe p.
    Bionic ear p.
    Bionit vascular p.
    bisque-baked p.
    Bivona-Colorado dummy p.
    Bivona-Colorado voice p.
    Bivona Duckbill voice p.
    Bivona Ultra Low voice p.
    Björk p.
    Björk-Shiley aortic valve p.
    Björk-Shiley convexoconcave 60-degree valve p.
    Björk-Shiley floating disk p.
    BK p., below-knee prosthesis
    bladder-neck support p.
    Blauth knee p.
    Blom-Singer indwelling low-pressure voice p.
    Blom-Singer tracheoesophageal p.
    Bock knee p.
    Bograb Universal offset ossicular p.
    bovine collagen material p.
    Braunwald-Cutter ball valve p.

Buchholz hip p.
Buechel-Pappas total ankle p.
Byars mandibular p.
Caffinière p.
caged ball valve p.
calcar replacement femoral p.
Callender technique hip p.
Calnan-Nicoll synthetic joint p.
camouflage p.
Canadian hip disarticulation p.
Capetown aortic valve p.
CarboMedics cardiac valve p.
Carbon Copy HP foot p.
Carbon Copy II foot p.
Carbon Copy II lightweight p.
Cardona keratoprosthesis p.
Carpentier annuloplasty ring p.
Carpentier-Edwards aortic valve p.
Carpentier-Edwards glutaraldehyde-
  preserved porcine xenograft p.
Carpentier-Rhone-Poulenc mitral
  ring p.
Carrion penile p.
Cartwright heart p.
Cartwright valve p.
Cathcart orthocentric hip p.
CDH Precoat Plus hip p.
Celestin endoesophageal p.
Centralign Precoat hip p.
ceramic ossicular p.
Ceramion p.
Ceravital incus replacement p. ·
CFS hip p.
Charnley acetabular cup p.
Charnley cemented hip p.
Charnley-Hastings p.
Charnley hip p.
Charnley knee p.
Charnley-Mueller hip p.
Charnley total hip p.
Chopart partial foot p.
Choyce MK II keratoprosthesis p.
Cintor knee p.
Cirrus foot p.
clamshell p.
cleft palate p.
Cloutier unconstrained knee p.
cobalt-chromium alloy p.
Co-Cr-Mo p.
Co-Cr-W-Ni alloy p.
collar p.
College Park TruStep foot p.
combination gel and inflatable
  mammary p.
Conley mandibular p.
constrained hinged knee p.
constrained nonhinged knee p.
Cooley-Bloodwell mitral valve p.
Cooley Dacron p.
Coonrad-Morrey total elbow p.
C-2 OsteoCap hip p.
crimped Dacron p.
crimped-wire p.
Cronin Silastic mammary p.
Cross-Jones disk valve p.

cruciate-retaining p.
cruciate-sacrificing p.
Crutchfield tongs p.
CSF p.
CUI artificial breast p.
CUI chin p.
CUI eye sphere p.
CUI gel mammary p.
CUI nasal p.
CUI saline mammary p.
CUI tendon p.
CUI testicular p.
custom total alloplastic TMJ
  reconstruction p.
Cutter aortic valve p.
Cutter-Smeloff aortic valve p.
Cutter-Smeloff cardiac valve p.
cylinder penile distendible p.
cylinder penile nondistendible p.
Dacron arterial p.
Dacron bifurcation p.
Dacron vessel p.
Dallop-type fascial p.
DANA shoulder p.
Deane unconstrained knee p.
DeBakey ball-valve p.
DeBakey valve p.
DeBakey Vasculour-II vascular p.
Dee elbow p.
De La Caffinière
  trapeziometacarpal p.
DeLaura knee p.
DeLaura-Verner knee p.
Delrin biomaterial joint
  replacement p.
Deon hip p.
DePalma hip p.
DePuy hip p. with Scuderi head
Deune knee p.
De Vega p.
Dilamezinsert penile p.
Dimension-C femoral stem p.
Dimension hip p.
distal radioulnar joint p. (DRUJ
  prosthesis)
double-pigtail p.
DRUJ p.
    distal radioulnar joint prosthesis
dual-lock total hip p.
duckbill voice p.
Duocondylar knee p.
Duo-Lock hip p.
Duo-Patellar knee p.
Duracon p.
Dura-II positionable penile p.
DuraPhase inflatable penile p.
DuraPhase semirigid penile p.
Duromedics valve p.
DynaFlex penile p.
dynamic penile p.
ear pinna p.
ear piston p.
Eaton trapezium finger joint
  replacement p.
Edwards seamless p.

prosthesis (*continued*)

Edwards Teflon intracardiac patch p.
E-2 foot p.
Efteklar-Charnley hip p.
Ehmke ear p.
Eicher hip p.
ELP femoral p.
Endo hinged knee p.
Endo rotating knee joint p.
Endo sled p.
Engh porous metal hip p.
Englehardt femoral p.
English-McNab shoulder p.
Entegra p.
EPTFE graft p.
ERCP conventional p.
Eriksson knee p.
ESKA-Jonas silicone-silver penile p.
EsophaCoil p.
Esser p.
Estecar p.
Ethicon Polytef paste p.
Ethrone p.
Evolution hip p.
Ewald elbow p.
expandable p.
fascia lata p.
femorofemoral crossover p.
Fett carpal p.
p. fin
Finney Flexirod penile p.
Finn knee revision p.
FIRST knee p.
fixed expansion p.
fixed femoral head p.
Flatt finger p.
Flex-Foot p.
FLEX H/A total ossicular p.
Flexi-Flate I, II penile p.
Flexi-Rod penile p.
Fountain design p.
four-bar polycentric knee p.
Fox p.
Fox-Blazina p.
Fredricks mammary p.
Free-Flow system p.
Freeman modular total hip p.
Freeman-Samuelson knee p.
Freeman-Swanson knee p.
fully constrained tricompartmental knee p.
Gaffney ankle p.
Galante hip p.
gel-filled p.
gel-saline Surgitek mammary p.
Gemini hip system p.
Genesis knee p.
Geometric total knee p.
Georgiade breast p.
GFS Mark II inflatable penile p.
Gianturco p.
Gilbert p.
Gilfillan humeral p.

Giliberty acetabular p.
Gillette joint p.
Gillies p.
Girard keratoprosthesis p.
glass penile p.
glottic p.
Golaski-UMI vascular p.
golf tee-shaped polyvinyl p.
Goodhill p.
Gore-Tex knee p.
Gott-Daggett heart valve p.
Gott low-profile p.
Greissinger foot p.
Gripper acetabular cup p.
Groningen voice p.
Gruppe wire p.
GSB elbow p.
GSB knee p.
Guepar II hinged knee p.
Guilford-Wright p.
Gunston-Hult knee p.
Gunston polycentric knee p.
Gustilo knee p.
Haering esophageal p.
Hall-Kaster tilting-disk valve p.
Hamas upper limb p.
Hammersmith mitral valve p.
Hancock aortic valve p.
Hancock mitral valve p.
Hanger p.
Hanslik patellar p.
Harken p.
Harris cemented hip p.
Harris-Galante porous hip p.
Harris Micromini p.
Harrison interlocked mesh p.
Harris precoat p.
Hartley mammary p.
Haynes-Stellite implant metal p.
HD II total hip p.
Helanca seamless tube p.
Henschke-Mauch SNS lower limb p.
Herbert knee p.
heterograft p.
Hexcel total condylar p.
Heyer-Schulte breast p.
HG Multilock hip p.
Hinderer malar p.
hinged constrained knee p.
hinged great toe replacement p.
hinged implant p.
hinged-leaflet vascular p.
hinged total knee p.
hinge-knee p.
hingeless heart valve p.
hip disarticulation p.
Hittenberger p.
HKAFO p.
hollow sphere p.
homograft p.
Hosmer WALK p.
Hosmer weight-activated locking knee p.
House piston p.

House tantalum p.
House wire stapes p.
Howmedica Kinematic II knee p.
Howorth p.
Howse-Coventry hip p.
HPS II total hip p.
HSS total condylar knee p.
Hufnagel low-profile heart p.
Hunter tendon p.
hybrid p.
hydraulic knee unit p.
Hydroflex penile p.
Hydroxial hip p.
hydroxyapatite ossicular p.
I-beam hemiarthroplasty hip p.
Identifit hip p.
Image custom external breast p.
immediate postoperative p.
Impact modular porous p.
implant-borne p.
implant-supported fixed p.
Impra collagen-impregnated
  Dacron p.
incus replacement p.
Indong Oh p.
Infinity modular hip p.
inflatable mammary p.
inflatable Mentor penile p.
inflatable penile p.
Inronail fingernail p.
Inronail toenail p.
Insall-Burstein knee p.
Integral Interlok femoral p.
Integrity acetabular cup p.
Intermedics Natural-Knee knee p.
internal ear p.
Inter-Op acetabular p.
Introl bladder neck support p.
Ionescu-Shiley aortic valve p.
Iowa total hip p.
iridium p.
ischial weightbearing p.
isoelastic pelvic p.
Ivalon p.
Jenny mammary p.
Jewett p.
Jobst p.
Jonas penile p.
Jonathan Livingston Seagull
  patella p.
Joplin toe p.
Judet hip p.
KAFO p.
Kaster mitral valve p.
Kaufman III anti-incontinence p.
Kaufman male urinary
  incontinence p.
Kay-Shiley disk valve p.
Kay-Suzuki p.
K/B p.
KD chin p.
Keeler p.
Kessler p.
Kinematic II rotating-hinge total
  knee p.

Kinemax Plus knee p.
Kirschner total shoulder p.
KMC femoral stem p.
KMP femoral stem p.
KMW/PC femoral p.
knee-bearing p.
knitted p.
knitted Teflon p.
knitted vascular p.
Koenig MPJ p.
Krause-Wolfe p.
Lacey p.
Lagrange-Letoumel hip p.
Lanceford p.
Landers-Foulks p.
Lash-Loeffler penile p.
Lattimer Silastic testicular p.
Leadbetter-Politano ureteral
  implant p.
Leake Dacron mandible p.
Leeds-Keio ligament p.
Leinbach hip p.
Lewis expandable adjustable p.
Lezinski Flex-HA PORP ossicular
  chain p.
Lillehei-Cruz-Kaster valve p.
Lillehei-Kaster cardiac valve p.
Lillehei-Kaster mitral valve p.
Link cementless reconstruction
  hip p.
Link MP hip noncemented
  reconstruction p.
Lippman hip p.
Lippy modified p.
Liverpool knee p.
Lo Bak spinal support p.
locking p.
Longevity V-Lign hip p.
Lo-Por vascular graft p.
Lord total hip p.
Lorenz SMO p.
lower limb p.
low-pressure voice p.
low-profile p.
Lubinus knee p.
lunate p.
MacIntosh tibial plateau p.
MacNab-English shoulder p.
Macrofit hip p.
madreporic hip p.
Magnuson-Cromie p.
Magnuson valve p.
Magovern-Cromie p.
malleable p.
malleus-incus p.
Mallory-Head porous primary
  femoral p.
mammary p.
Mammatech breast p.
Mangat curvilinear chin p.
MAPF femoral stem p.
Marlex mesh p.
Marlex methyl methacrylate p.
Marmor modular knee p.
Master step foot p.

prosthesis *(continued)*
    Matchett-Brown p.
    Mathys p.
    Matrol femoral head p.
    maxillary p.
    Mayo semiconstrained elbow p.
    Mayo total ankle p.
    M-C p.
    McBride femoral p.
    McBride-Moore p.
    McCutchen SLT hip p.
    McGee ear piston p.
    McGehee elbow p.
    McGhan breast p.
    McKee-Farrar hip p.
    McKee femoral p.
    McKee totally constrained elbow p.
    McKeever patellar cap p.
    McNaught p.
    MCP finger joint p.
    Meadox-Cooley woven low-
      porosity p.
    Meadox woven velour p.
    Mecring acetabluar p.
    Medi-graft vascular p.
    Medoc-Celestin endoprosthesis p.
    Medtronic-Hall heart valve p.
    Medtronic-Hall tilting-disk valve p.
    Megasource penile p.
    Meme breast p.
    Mentor Alpha 1 inflatable penile p.
    Mentor breast p.
    Mentor GFS penile p.
    Mentor IPP penile p.
    Mentor malleable penile p.
    Mentor Mark II penile p.
    Mentor Self-Cath penile p.
    mesh stent p.
    metacarpophalangeal p.
    metal bucket-handle p.
    metal femoral head p.
    metal-on-metal articulating
      intervertebral disk p.
    Metasul hip p.
    Meyerding p.
    MGH knee p.
    MG II knee p.
    microcrimped p.
    Microknit vascular graft p.
    Microloc knee p.
    Microvel p.
    Miller-Galante hip p.
    Milliknit arterial p.
    Milliknit Dacron p.
    Milliknit vascular graft p.
    Minneapolis hip p.
    Mittlemeir ceramic hip p.
    modified Moore hip locking p.
    modular Austin Moore hip p.
    modular Iowa Precoat total hip p.
    modular total hip p.
    Monk hip p.
    monostrut cardiac valve p.
    Moon-Robinson stapes p.

    Moore femoral neck p.
    Moore hip p.
    Moretz p.
    Moseley glenoid rim p.
    Mueller-Charnley hip p.
    Mueller total hip p.
    Muhlberger orbital p.
    Mules p.
    Mulligan Silastic p.
    Murray knee p.
    myoelectric p.
    Naden-Rieth p.
    natural-feel breast p.
    Natural-Hip p.
    Natural-Lok acetabular cup p.
    NEB total hip p.
    Neer I, II shoulder p.
    neural p.
    NeuroCybernetic p.
    Neville tracheal reconstruction p.
    Neville tracheobronchial p.
    New Jersey hemiarthroplasty p.
    New Jersey-LCS shoulder p.
    New Jersey-LCS total knee p.
    New Weavenit Dacron p.
    Nexus hip p.
    Nicoll tendon p.
    Niebauer finger-joint replacement p.
    Niebauer trapezium replacement p.
    Noiles posterior stabilized knee p.
    Noiles rotating-hinge total knee p.
    nonhinged knee p.
    ocular p.
    Odland ankle p.
    offset modified p.
    Oklahoma ankle p.
    Ommaya reservoir p.
    Omnicarbon heart valve p.
    Omnifit HA hip stem p.
    Omnifit knee p.
    OmniPhase penile p.
    Omniscience single-leaflet cardiac
      valve p.
    Omniscience tilting-disk valve p.
    orbital floor p.
    Oregon p.
    Orlon vascular p.
    Orthofix p.
    Ortholoc p.
    ossicular chain replacement p.
    OsteoCap hip p.
    Osteolock hip p.
    Osteonics p.
    Otto Bock Greissinger Plus foot p.
    Otto Bock system electric hands p.
    Oxford p.
    Padgett p.
    Paladon p.
    palatal p.
    Panje voice p.
    partial ossicular replacement p.
      (PORP)
    patellar tendon-bearing below-
      knee p.
    PC Performer knee p.

Pearman penile p.
pegged tibial p.
Perfecta hip p.
Performance knee p.
periodontal p.
Perras mammary p.
Perras-Papillon breast p.
Phoenix total hip p.
Pillet hand p.
piston stapes p.
Plasticor p.
Plasti-Pore ossicular replacement p.
Plystan p.
Polycel bone composite p.
polycentric knee p.
polyethylene talar p.
polytetrafluoroethylene (PTFE) p.
polyvinyl p.
porcine p.
Porocool p.
porous-coated anatomic knee p.
Precision Osteolock femoral p.
Precision Osteolock hip p.
Preclude dura substitute p.
Precoat Plus femoral p.
Press-Fit p.
Pritchard total elbow p.
ProAdvantage knee p.
Profile hip p.
Proplast p.
Prostalac total hip p.
prosthetic antibiotic-loaded acrylic
  cement total joint p.
Protasul femoral p.
Protek p.
Proud septal p.
Provox voice p.
PTB cast p.
PTS p.
Quantum foot p.
RAM knee p.
Ranawat-Burstein hip p.
Rancho external fixation p.
Randelli shoulder p.
Rashkind double-disk occluder p.
Rastelli p.
Reese p.
Reverdin p.
Revive system penile p.
R-HAB lighter weight ankle p.
Richards hydroxyapatite PORP p.
Richards hydroxyapatite TORP p.
Richards maximum contact cruciate-
  sparing p.
Richards Zirconia femoral head p.
Ring hip p.
Ring knee p.
Robinson incus replacement p.
Robinson middle ear p.
Robinson-Moon-Lippy stapes p.
Robinson-Moon stapes p.
Robinson piston p.
Robinson stapes p.
Rochester HKAFO p.
Rock-Mulligan p.

Rose L-type nose bridge p.
Rosenfeld hip p.
Rosen inflatable urinary
  incontinence p.
rotating-hinge knee p.
Rothman Institute femoral p.
Ruddy stapes p.
SACH p.
sacral segmental nerve stimulation
  implantable neural p.
saddle p.
Safian design p.
Safian rhinoplasty p.
Saint George knee p.
Saint Jude p.
Sampson p.
Sauerbruch p.
Sauvage fabric graft p.
Sauvage filamentous p.
Savastano Hemi-Knee p.
Sbarbaro tibial p.
Scarborough p.
SCDT heart valve p.
Scheer Tef-wire p.
Schlein total elbow p.
Schlein trisurface ankle p.
Schuknecht Gelfoam wire p.
Schuknecht Teflon wire piston p.
Schuknecht Tef-Wire p.
Schurring ossicle cup p.
Scott AMS inflatable penile p.
Scuderi p.
Scurasil device p.
S-E p.
seamless p.
Seattle Foot p.
Select ankle p.
Select shoulder p.
self-articulating femoral p.
self-centering Universal hip p.
Sense-of-Feel p.
shaft p.
Shea polyethylene p.
Shea Teflon piston p.
Sheehan knee p.
Sheehy incus replacement p.
Shier knee p.
shoulder p.
Silastic ball spacer p.
Silastic chin p.
Silastic fimbrial p.
Silastic mammary p.
Silastic otoplasty p.
Silastic penile p.
Silastic sheeting keel p.
Silastic standard elastometer p.
Silastic testicular p.
Silflex intramedullary p.
silicone doughnut p.
silicone elastomer p.
silicone gel p.
silicone trapezium p.
Silima breast p.
Siloxane p.
Siltex Becker 50 breast p.

P

prosthesis *(continued)*
Singer-Blom ossicular p.
Singh speech system voice
  rehabilitation p.
single-axis ankle p.
Sinterlock implant metal p.
Sivash hip p.
SKI knee p.
Small-Carrion penile p.
Smeloff-Cutter ball-valve p.
Smith-Petersen hip cup p.
Smith total ankle p.
SMo p.
p. smooth wire
Snyder breast p.
solid-ankle, cushioned-heel foot p.
solid silicone orbital p.
Sorin mitral valve p.
Sparks mandrel p.
Spectron p.
Speed radius cap p.
spherocentric knee p.
Springlite lower limb p.
S-ROM femoral stem p.
S-ROM hip p.
stabilocondylar knee p.
Stanmore shoulder p.
stapedectomy p.
Starr ball heart p.
Starr-Edwards aortic valve p.
Starr-Edwards ball valve p.
Starr-Edwards mitral p.
STD+ titanium total hip p.
stemmed tibial p.
stentless porcine aortic valve p.
Stenzel rod p.
Stevens-Street elbow p.
St. George total elbow p.
St. Jude Medical p.
St. Jude mitral valve p.
Subrini penile p.
Sulzer p.
SuperCup acetabular cup p.
Supramid p.
Surgitek mammary p.
Surgitek penile p.
Sutter double-stem silicone
  implant p.
Sutter MCP finger joint p.
Sutter-Smeloff heart valve p.
Swanson finger joint p.
Swanson flexible hallux valgus p.
Swanson great toe p.
Swanson metacarpal p.
Swanson metatarsal p.
Swanson Silastic elbow p.
Swanson wrist p.
Syme amputation p.
Syme foot p.
Synatomic total knee p.
Taperloc femoral p.
TARA total hip p.
TCCK unconstrained knee p.
Techmedica p.

Teflon tri-leaflet p.
Teflon woven p.
Tef-wire p.
temporary p.
tendon p.
Tevdek p.
Thackray hip p.
Tharies hip replacement p.
Thiersch p.
T-28 hip p.
Thompson femoral head p.
Thompson femoral neck p.
Thompson hemiarthroplasty hip p.
threaded titanium acetabular p.
Thrust femoral p.
Ti-BAC II hip p.
tibial plateau p.
Ti/CoCr hip p.
Tilastin hip p.
tilting-disk aortic valve p.
titanium p.
Tivanium hip p.
TK Optimizer knee p.
TMJ fossa-eminence p.
toe p.
TORP ossicular p.
torque-type p.
total alloplastic TMJ
  reconstruction p.
total ossicular p.
total ossicular replacement p.
  (TORP)
Townley TARA p.
Townley total knee p.
trapeziometacarpal joint
  replacement p.
TR-28 hip p.
Triad p.
trial p.
triaxial semiconstrained elbow p.
Tricon-M cruciate-sparing p.
Tricon-M patellar p.
trileaflet p.
Trilicon external breast p.
Tri-Lock total hip p. with Porocoa
Tronzo p.
trunnion-bearing hip p.
TruStep foot p.
TTAP-ST acetabular p.
Turner p.
two-pronged stem finger p.
Tygon esophageal p.
UCBL p.
UCI p.
Ultraflex esophageal p.
Ultra Low resistance voice p.
Ultrec Plus penile p.
umbrella-type p.
unconstrained p.
unicondylar p.
Uni-Flate 1000 penile p.
Universal p.
upper extremity myoelectric p.
urinary incontinence p.
UroLume endourethral Wallstent p.

USCI bifurcated Vasculour II p.
USCI-DeBakey vascular p.
USCI Sauvage EXS side-limb p.
Usher Marlex mesh p.
Utah arm electronic p.
vaginal prolapse p.
Valls p.
valved voice p.
Vanghetti limb p.
Vascutek vascular p.
Viscoheel K, N p.
Viscoheel SofSpot p.
Vitallium allow cobalt-chrome p.
Vitallium Moore self-locking p.
Vivosil p.
Voltz wrist joint p.
Wada hingeless heart valve p.
Wagner resurface p.
Walldius Vitallium mechanical
 knee p.
Wallstent esophageal p.
Warsaw hip p.
Waugh p.
Wayfarer p.
Weaveknit vascular p.
Wehrs incus p.
Weller total hip joint p.
Wesolowski vascular p.
Wheeler p.
Whiteside p.
Wiles p.
Wilke boot p.
Wilson-Cook esophageal balloon p.
Wilson-Cook plastic p.
wire-fat ear p.
wire stapes p.
Wolf p.
woven-tube vascular graft p.
Wright knee p.
Xenophor femoral p.
Zimaloy femoral head p.
Zimmer Centralign Precoat hip p.
Zimmer shoulder p.
Zimmer tibial p.
Ziramic femoral head p.
Zirconia orthopaedic p.
Zweymuller-Alloclassic p.
Zweymuller hip p.

prosthetic
p. antibiotic-loaded acrylic cement
p. antibiotic-loaded acrylic cement
 total joint prosthesis
p. appliance
p. buttock contour
p. cup
p. device
p. foam
p. graft
p. heart valve
p. lens
p. poppet
p. socket
p. valve holder
p. valve sewing ring

ProStool

ProStretch
P. exerciser
ProSys
P. leg bag comfort strap
P. Samec D, self-adhering, nonlatex
 male external catheter, short
 sheath
P. Samec NL, self-adhering
 nonlatex male external catheter,
 normal length sheath
P. silicone sterile 2-way, 3-way
 Foley catheter
P. Urahesive system LA latex male
 external condom catheter with
 Urahesive strip
P. Urihesive system LA and system
Protasul femoral prosthesis
ProTech instrument protection tray
ProTect abutment
ProtectaCap cap
Protectaid contraceptive sponge
protectant
Lantiseptic skin p.
NutraShield perineal p.
PRO-Q skin p.
Proshield Plus skin p.
Protect-a-Pass suture passer
protected
p. bronchoscopic brush
p. knife handle
p. specimen microbiology brush
Protection
P. Plus belted undergarment
P. Plus brief
P. Plus disposable underpad
protective
p. bandage
p. dressing
p. glasses
p. mattress cover
protector
Adson dural p.
alar p.
Arroyo p.
Arruga p.
bite p.
Breast Implant P.
Buratto flap p.
Cast Gard cast p.
Cottle alar p.
Crouch corneal p.
dural p.
eggcrate p.
EpiFlex heel and elbow p.
eye p.
Genuine sheepskin elbow p.
Genuine sheepskin heel p.
p. guide
hearing p.
Heelbo decubitus p.
Heeler inflatable heel p.
HP1035 gel heel p.
Isovis wound p.
Joseph saw p.
Jurgan Pin Ball pin p.

protector *(continued)*
    KINS fitted mattress p.
    Kodel polyester elbow p.
    Lapwall wound p.
    Limb and elbow p.
    Meds eye p.
    P. meniscus suturing system
    M-F heel p.
    MouthGuard oral p.
    oculoplasty corneal p.
    Opti-Gard eye p.
    Patellar Band knee p.
    plastic corneal p.
    p. plus wire
    port p.
    Pre-Vent elbow p.
    Pre-Vent heel p.
    Pre-Vent ulnar nerve p.
    pulse ox p.
    Roho heel p.
    Seal-Tight cast p.
    Seraflo transducer p.
    ShowerSafe waterproof cast and
        bandage p.
    P. suturing device
    Terumo transducer p.
    The Heeler inflatable heel p.
    tissue p.
    Toes P.
    Ultra-Care heel/elbow p.
    X-tend back p.
Protecto splint
Protect.Point needle
Protégé
    P. Plus microscope
    P. 3010 syringe infusion pump
Protegen material
Protek
    P. joint implant
    P. prosthesis
Pro-Tex face shield
prothelen set
ProThotics insole
ProTime microcoagulation system
Protocult stool sampling device
protological biopsy forceps
proton
    p. MR spectroscopy
proton-density axial MR scan
proton-density-weighted MRI
ProTon portable tonometer
prototype cholangioscope
Protouch
    P. material
    P. orthopaedic padding
    P. pad
ProTouch resectoscope
ProTrac
    P. ACL tibial guide
    P. cruciate reconstruction
        measurement device
    P. system for knee surgery
protractor
    cephalometric p.

    Demariniff p.
    Dexterity P.
    Harrington p.
    triplanar p.
    Zimmer p.
protrusio
    p. cage
    p. shell
Pro-Turn frameless air support therapy
Proud
    P. adenoidectomy forceps
    P. fascia crusher
    P. infant turbinate speculum
    P. septal prosthesis
Proud-Beck pharyngoscope
Proud-White uvula retractor
Pro-Vent
    P.-V. ABG kit
    P.-V. arterial blood sampling kit
Provide
    P. incontinence pad
    P. underpad
Providence
    P. Hospital arterial forceps
    P. Hospital clamp
    P. Hospital hemostat
    P. scoliosis system
Provider
    P. 6000 ambulatory dual-channel
        infusion pump
    P. 5500 patient-controlled analgesia
        device
provisional liner
Provit filling material
Provocative sensitivity balloon
Provox
    P. tracheoesophageal speaking valve
    P. voice prosthesis
Prowler microcatheter
Proxiderm wound closure system
Proxi-Floss cleaning appliance
proximal
    p. cement spacer
    p. over-shoulder strap
Proximate
    P. disposable skin stapler
    P. flexible linear stapler
    P. linear cutter
Proximate-ILS curved intraluminal
    stapler
Proxi-Strip suture
Pruitt
    P. anoscope
    P. irrigation catheter
    P. occlusion catheter
    P. proctoscope
    P. vascular shunt
Pruitt-Inahara
    P.-I. balloon-tipped perfusion
        catheter
    P.-I. carotid shunt
    P.-I. vascular shunt
Pryor-Péan vaginal retractor
PS-2 needle
PSA thermoplastic orthosis

PSC pronation/spring control
pseudoisochromatic plate
PSI-TEC aspiration/irrigation platform
PS Medical Flow Control valve
psoas retractor
PSS Powered disposable skin stapler
PTB
    P. brace
    P. cast prosthesis
PTBD catheter
PTCA catheter
PTDP
    permanent transvenous demand pacemaker
pterygium
    p. knife
    p. scissors
pterygoid chisel
PTFE
    polytetrafluoroethylene
    PTFE Gore-Tex graft
    PTFE shunt
PTFE-containing implant
PTFE-covered Palmaz stent
ptosis
    p. clamp
    p. forceps
    p. knife
    p. scissors
    p. snare
PTS prosthesis
Pucci
    P. Air orthotic
    P. pediatrics hand orthosis
    P. rehab knee orthosis
    P. splint
Pucci-Seed
    P.-S. hook
    P.-S. spatula
Puck
    P. cutfilm changer
    P. film changer
Puddu
    P. drill guide
    P. tibial aimer
pudendal
    p. block anesthesia needle
    p. needle guide
Pudenz
    P. barium cardiac catheter
    P. connector
    P. flushing chamber
    P. flushing valve
    P. infant cardiac catheter
    P. peritoneal catheter
    P. reservoir
    P. tube
    P. valve-flushing shunt
    P. ventricular catheter
Pudenz-Heyer
    P.-H. clamp
    P.-H. vascular catheter
Pudenz-Schulte thecoperitoneal shunt
Puestow
    P. dilator
    P. guide wire

Puestow-Olander gastrointestinal tube
Pugh
    P. barrel component
    P. driver
    P. hip pin
    P. self-adjusting nail
    P. tractor
Puig
    P. Massana-Shiley annuloplasty ring
    P. Massana-Shiley annuloplasty
      valve
Puka chisel
Pulec needle
Pul-Ez
    P.-E. exerciser
    P.-E. shoulder pulley
pull
    p. knife
    Ponsky P.
    p. rasp
    p. screw
pull-apart introducer
puller
    MAGneedle p.
pulley
    p. passer
    Preston overhead p.
    Pul-Ez shoulder p.
    Range-Master p.
    shoulder p.
pull-out button
Pulmanex
Pulmo-Aide
    P.-A. nebulizer
    P.-A. Traveler
    P.-A. ventilator
PulmoMate nebulizer
Pulmo-Mist compressor
Pulmonair 40 bed
pulmonary
    p. arterial catheter
    p. arterial clamp
    p. arterial forceps
    p. arterial snare
    p. artery balloon pump
    p. artery catheter
    p. artery sling
    p. autograft valve
    p. balloon
    p. embolism clamp
    p. flotation catheter
    p. nodulectomy clamp
    p. retractor
    p. triple-lumen catheter
    p. vessel clamp
    p. vessel forceps
Pulmonex dynamic air therapy unit
pulmonic stenosis clamp
Pulmopak pump
Pulmosonic ultrasonic nebulizer
pulmowrap
pulp
    p. canal file
    p. chamber
pulpal microdialysis probe

P

Pulpdent cavity liner
pulped muscle dressing
Pulsair.5 oxygen portable unit
Pulsair tonometer
Pulsar
    P. DDD pacemaker
    P. Max sensor
    P. NI implantable pacemaker
    P. obstetrical two-channel TENS
    unit
pulsatile
    p. assist device
    p. jet lavage
pulsating low-air-loss bed
Pulsator
    P. anaerobic syringe
    P. dry heparin arterial blood gas
    kit
Pulsatron II hand-held nerve stimulator
Pulsavac
    P. III wound debridement system
    P. lavage
pulse
    p. lavage
    p. oximeter
    p. oximetry device
    p. ox protector
    p. spray catheter
    p. wave Doppler
pulsed
    p. angiolaser
    p. Doppler
    p. Doppler ultrasonic flowmeter
    p. Doppler ultrasound
    p. galvanic stimulator
    p. light
    p. metal vapor laser
    p. tunable dye laser
    p. ultrasonic velocity detector
    p. yellow dye laser
pulsed-range gated Doppler instrument
pulse-height analyzer
PulseMaster laser
Pulse-Pak infusion kit
PulseSpray
    P. injector
    P. pulsed infusion system
Pulsolith
    P. coumarin pulsed-dye laser
    P. laser lithotriptor
Pulsox-5
    Pulsoxymeter P.
Pulsoxymeter Pulsox-5
pulverizer
    Thermovac tissue p.
Pulvertaft suture
Pulvograft
    Dembone demineralized cortical
    powder P.
    Osteomin Thermo-Ashed bone
    powder P.
pumice stone
pump
    Abbott infusion p.
    ACAT 1 intraaortic balloon p.

Advanced Collection breast p.
ALZET continuous infusion
    osmotic p.
AMO HPF 500 p.
angle port p.
ankle rehab p.
aortic balloon p.
Asahi blood plasma p.
ASID Bonz PP infusion p.
Autosyringe p.
A-V Impulse foot p.
balloon p.
Bard cardiopulmonary support p.
Bard Infus-OR syringe-type
    infusion p.
Bard PCA p.
Bard TransAct intraaortic balloon
Barron p.
Basis breast p.
Baxter Flo-Gard 8200 volumetric
    infusion p.
Baxter PCA p.
Baxter volumetric infusion p.
Bio-Medicus centrifugal p.
Bio-Pump p.
blood p.
Bluemle p.
BVS p.
CADD-Plus intravenous infusion p.
CADD-TPN p.
cardiac balloon p.
Carrel-Lindbergh p.
centrifugal p.
Chicco breast p.
Chid breast p.
Clarus model 5169 peristaltic p.
Cobe double blood p.
Companion feeding p.
Compat enteral feeding p.
compression p.
computer-controlled infusion p.
Conjugate export p.
continuous subcutaneous insulin
    infusion p.
continuous-wave arthroscopy p.
Cordis Hakim p.
Cordis Secor implantable p.
Cormed ambulatory infusion p.
CPI90-100 insulin p.
CRS-series alternating overlay
    with p.
CTI infusion p.
Datascope system 90 intra-aortic
    balloon p.
Deltec-Pharmacia CADD p.
DeVilbiss suction p.
Disetronic infuser syringe p.
drug infusion p.
Dura-Neb portable nebulizer p.
ECMO p.
Egnell breast p.
elastomeric p.
Elmed peristaltic irrigation p.
Emerson p.
Entera-Flo enteral feeding p.

Enteroport feeding p.
extracorporeal p.
extremity p.
EZ hand p.
Felig insulin p.
Fenwal hemapheresis p.
flexible p.
Flexiflo enteral p.
Flexiflo feeding p.
Flocare 500 feeding p.
Flo-Gard p.
Flowtron DVT p.
Frenta Mat feeding p.
Frenta System II feeding p.
Gomco thoracic drainage p.
Grafco breast p.
Graseby anesthesia p.
Gynkotek p.
Hakim-Cordis p.
Harvard 2 dual-syringe p.
heart p.
HeartMate portable p.
hepatic artery infusion p.
Holter p.
H-TRON plus V100 insulin
  infusion p.
IMED Gemini PC-2 volumetric p.
IMED infusion p.
implantable osmotic p.
implanted infusion p.
Infumed p.
InfuO.R. drug delivery p.
Infusaid infusion p.
Infuse-a-Port p.
infusion p.
Intelliject p.
intermittent extremity p.
intraaortic balloon p. (IABP)
ion p.
Isoflow p.
IVAC volumetric infusion p.
Jobst athrombotic p.
Jobst extremity p.
KAAT II Plus intra-aortic
  balloon p.
Kangaroo feeding p.
Kendall McGaw Intelligent p.
Klein p.
KM-1 breast p.
Kontron intra-aortic balloon p.
Lactina Select breast p.
Lamis Autofuse infusion p.
left ventricular bypass p.
Life Care p.
Lifestream centrifugal p.
Lindbergh p.
Linvatec arthroscopic infusion p.
LVAS implantable p.
MagMag breast p.
Mary Jane breast p.
MasterFlex p.
Master Flow Pumpette p.
McGaw volumetric p.
McKinley EpM p.
Medela breast p.

Medela Dominant vacuum
  delivery p.
Medela manual breast p.
Medex Protege 3010 syringe
  infusion p.
Medfusion (1001, 2001) syringe
  infusion p.
Medtronic SynchroMed
  implantable p.
Microjet Quark portable p.
Miltex p.
MiniMed III infusion p.
Mistette nasal spray p.
Multipulse 1000 compression p.
Na-K exchange p.
Neuroperfusion p.
Norport p.
Nutromat Pad S feeding p.
Ohmeda 9000 computer-cotrolled
  infusion p.
On-Q p.
Pancretec p.
Panomat infusion p.
Paragon ambulatory p.
patient-controlled anesthesia p.
PCA p.
Pfeiffer mechanical dosing p.
portable insulin infusion p.
programmable p.
Protégé 3010 syringe infusion p.
Provider 6000 ambulatory dual-
  channel infusion p.
pulmonary artery balloon p.
Pulmopak p.
Pump In Style breast p.
Quantum enteral p.
rapid infusion p.
roller p.
roller head perfusion p.
Sage Instruments syringe p.
Salem p.
Sarns 7000 MDX p.
Sarns Siok II blood p.
Sartorius breast p.
sequential extremity p.
Servo p.
Shiley Infusaid p.
Sigma 6000+ infusion p.
Stat 2 Pumpette disposable IV p.
subcutaneous morphine p.
suction p.
sump p.
surgical suction p.
SurgiPeace analgesia p.
SynchroMed implantable p.
SynchroMed programmable p.
syringe p.
syringe-type infusion p.
System V irrigation p.
Talley p.
Thoratec p.
Tonkaflo p.
Travenol infusion p.
TurboStaltic p.
Unicare breast p.

pump *(continued)*
  P. Vac III
  P. Vac Plus system
  Verifuse ambulatory infusion p.
  Versaflow p.
  volumetric infusion p.
pumped dye laser
Pumpette
  Master Flow P.
  Stat 2 P.
Pump-It-Up
  P.-I.-U. pneumatic socket
  P.-I.-U. pneumatic socket volume
    management system
PumpPals shoe insoles
punch
  Abrams pleural biopsy p.
  Acufex rotary p.
  adenoid p.
  Adler attic ear p.
  Ainsworth p.
  Alexander antrostomy p.
  Anderson (Abrams modified)
    biopsy p.
  antral p.
  aortic p.
  baby Tischler biopsy p.
  backbiting bone p.
  Bailey p.
  Baker p.
  Barron donor corneal p.
  Baumgartner p.
  Berens corneoscleral p.
  Beyer atticus p.
  biopsy p.
  p. block
  bone hole p.
  Brock infundibular p.
  Brooks adenoidal p.
  Bruening p.
  Buerger p.
  Caspari suture p.
  Casselberry suture p.
  Casteyer prostatic p.
  Castroviejo corneoscleral p.
  Cault p.
  cervical p.
  Charnley femoral prosthesis neck p.
  cigar handle basket p.
  Citelli laminectomy p.
  Citelli-Meltzer atticus p.
  Cloward bone p.
  Cloward-Dowel p.
  Cloward-English p.
  Cloward-Harper cervical p.
  Cloward intervertebral p.
  Cloward square p.
  Cone bone p.
  Cone skull p.
  Cordes circular p.
  Cordes ethmoidal p.
  Cordes semicircular p.
  Cordes sphenoidal p.
  Cordes square p.

  Corgill bone p.
  corneal p.
  corneoscleral p.
  Cottingham p.
  cruciate p.
  cutaneous p.
  Davol canal wall p.
  Descemet membrane p.
  Deyerle p.
  disposable aortic rotating p.
  Dorsey cervical foraminal p.
  Dyonics suction p.
  DyoVac suction p.
  Ellison glenoid rim p.
  Entrease variable depth p.
  Eppendorf p.
  ethmoidal p.
  Ewald-Hensler arthroscopic p.
  Faraci p.
  Faraci-Skillern sphenoid p.
  Fehling TOP ejector p.
  Ferris Smith p.
  Ferris Smith-Kerrison p.
  finned-stem p.
  Flateau oval p.
  fluted stem p.
  p. forceps
  Frangenheim hook p.
  Frenckner-Stille p.
  Gass cervical p.
  Gass corneoscleral p.
  Gass scleral p.
  Gass sclerotomy p.
  Gelfoam p.
  Gellhorn uterine biopsy p.
  Gibbs eye p.
  Goldman cartilage p.
  Goosen vascular p.
  Gosteyer p.
  Graham-Kerrison p.
  Gruenwald nasal p.
  Grundelach p.
  p. guide
  Gusberg endocervical biopsy p.
  hair transplant p.
  Haitz canaliculus p.
  Hajek-Koffler reversible p.
  Hajek-Koffler sphenoidal p.
  Hajek-Skillern sphenoidal p.
  Hardy sellar p.
  Harper cervical laminectomy p.
  Hartmann biopsy p.
  Hartmann-Citelli ear p.
  Hartmann ear p.
  Hartmann nasal p.
  Hartmann tonsillar p.
  Hirsch hypophyseal p.
  Holth corneoscleral p.
  Holth-Rubin p.
  Holth scleral p.
  Holth sclerectomy p.
  Housepian sellar p.
  I-beam cement p.
  I-beam Press-Fit p.
  infundibular p.

Ingraham skull p.
Jackson p.
Jacobson vessel p.
Jansen-Middleton septal p.
Johnson-Kerrison p.
Joseph p.
Karolinska-Stille p.
Karp aortic p.
Kelly p.
Kelly-Descemet membrane p.
Kerrison bone p.
Kerrison-Jacoby p.
Kerrison laminectomy p.
Kerrison-Rhoton sellar p.
Keyes cutaneous biopsy p.
Keyes dermatologic p.
Keyes skin p.
Keyes vulvar p.
keyhole p.
King adenoidal p.
Klause antral p.
Klause-Carmody antral p.
Klein p.
Knighton-Kerrison p.
Koffler-Hajek sphenoidal p.
Krause angular oval p.
Lange antral p.
Lebsche sternal p.
Leksell p.
Lempert malleus p.
Lermoyez nasal p.
Lewis-Resnik p.
linear scissor p.
Lineback adenoidal p.
Lund-Dodick p.
Luntz-Dodick p.
MacKenty sphenoidal p.
Mauermayer stone p.
McGoey Vitallium p.
Meltzer adenoid p.
Meltzer tonsillar p.
Mendez-Schubert aortic p.
Merz aortic p.
MGM glenoidal p.
Miltex disposable biopsy p.
Mixter brain biopsy p.
modified sclerectomy p.
Mulligan cervical biopsy p.
Murphy p.
Myerson biting p.
Myles nasal p.
p. myringotomy system
nasal p.
Noyes chalazion p.
O'Connor hook p.
Orentreich p.
Osborne p.
ostrum antral p.
Pfau atticus sphenoidal p.
Phemister p.
pleural biopsy p.
Pollock p.
Price corneal p.
Pritikin scleral p.
Raney laminectomy p.

Rathke p.
Reaves p.
Rhoton sellar p.
Richter laminectomy p.
p. rongeur
Ronis adenoidal p.
Ronis tonsillar p.
Rothman-Gilbard corneal p.
Rowe glenoidal p.
Rubin-Holth sclerectomy p.
Sachs cervical p.
Scheicher laminectomy p.
Scheinmann biting p.
Schlesinger cervical p.
Schmeden tonsillar p.
Schnaudigel sclerotomy p.
Schubert uterine biopsy p.
scleral p.
sclerectomy p.
sclerotomy p.
Seiffert grasping p.
Seletz Universal Kerrison p.
sellar p.
side-biting ostrum p.
Skillern p.
skin p.
skull p.
Smeden tonsillar p.
Smillie nail p.
Smithuysen sphenoidal p.
Sokolowski antral p.
Sparks atrioseptal p.
Spencer oval p.
Spencer triangular adenoid p.
sphenoidal bone p.
Spies ethmoidal p.
Spurling-Kerrison laminectomy p.
Stammberger antral p.
Stevenson capsular p.
Storz corneoscleral p.
Storz intranasal antral p.
Stough p.
Struyken p.
suction p.
Swan corneoscleral p.
Sweet sternal p.
Takahashi ethmoidal p.
Takahashi nasal p.
Tanne corneal p.
Thompson p.
Thoms-Gaylor biopsy p.
Thomson adenoidal p.
Tischler cervical biopsy p.
Tischler-Morgan biopsy p.
Tomey trabeculectomy p.
tonsillar p.
TOP ejector p.
Townsend biopsy p.
p. trephine
Troutman p.
Turkel prostatic p.
uterine biopsy p.
Van Struyken nasal p.
Veenema-Gusberg prostatic p.
vessel p.

P

punch *(continued)*
    Wagner antral p.
    Walser corneoscleral p.
    Walton corneoscleral p.
    Walton-Schubert p.
    Watson-Williams ethmoidal p.
    Weck endoscopic suture p.
    Whitcomb-Kerrison laminectomy p.
    Wilde ethmoidal p.
    Wilde nasal p.
    Williams-Watson ethmoidal p.
    Wittner cervical biopsy p.
    Woolley tibia p.
    Yankauer p.
    Yankauer antral p.
    Yeoman biopsy p.
punched-out orchidometer
punctal
    p. dilator
    p. lens
punctate electrode
punctum
    p. dilator
    p. plug
puncture
    p. needle
    p. transducer
puncture-tip needle
Punctur-Guard
    P.-G. needle
    P.-G. Revolution safety needle
      holder
Puno-Winter-Byrd system
Puntenney tying forceps
Puntowicz arterial forceps
pupil
    p. dilator
    p. spreader/retractor forceps
pupillary membrane scissors
pupillograph
pupillometer
    Colvard p.
pupilloscope
Pura-Vario stent
Purcell self-retaining abdominal retractor
purifier
    Air Supply air p.
Puritan
    P. Bennett ETCO2 multigas
      analyzer
    P. Bubble-Jet
    P. swab
Puritan-Bennett
    P.-B. BiLevel Knight Star 335
      machine
    P.-B. 7250 metabolic monitor
    P.-B. ventilator
Purkinje image tracker
Purlon suture
Purstring disposable instrument
Pursuer CBD helical basket
Pursuit catheter
push
    p. cuff

    P. medical brace
    p. rasp
Push-Ease
    P.-E. Quad cuff
    P.-E. wheelchair glove
pusher
    Aker lens p.
    Arrequi KPL laparoscopic knot p.
    p. catheter
    Charnley femoral prosthesis p.
    chorda tympani p.
    Clarke-Reich knot p.
    De La Vega lens p.
    Endo-Assist endoscopic knot p.
    Fresnel lens p.
    Gazayerli knot p.
    heliX knot p.
    hemispherical p.
    hook p.
    Jacobson suture p.
    Jako knot p.
    knot p.
    lens p.
    Mangum knot p.
    Martin Surefit lens p.
    Mershon band p.
    metal-tipped stent p.
    MetraTie knot p.
    Negus p.
    Ranfac KPL laparoscopic knot p.
    Revo loop handle knot p.
    Shuletz p.
    Visitec lens p.
    p. wire
push/pull
    Ilg p.
    Kuglen p.
push-pull catheter
push-up block
Puth abduction splint
Put-In driver
Putnam evacuator catheter
Putterman
    P. levator resection clamp
    P. ptosis clamp
Putterman-Chaflin ocular asymmetry
    device
Putti
    P. arthroplasty gouge
    P. bone file
    P. bone rasp
    P. frame
    P. splint
Putti-Platt
    P.-P. director
    P.-P. instrumentation
putty
    AlloMatrix injectable p.
    Bishop p.
    Blue Brand therapy p.
    color-coded therapy p.
    DynaGraft p.
    Grafton moldable p.
    matrix Grafton p.
    Omnisil p.

polyvinylsiloxane p.
Thera-Plast p.
Thera-Putty exercise p.
PVA spear
PVB suture
PVC
    PVC drain
    PVC tubing
PV foam
P-wave-triggered ventricular pacemaker
**PWB transpedicular spine fixation
    system**
Pye cannula
pyeloureteral catheter
pylon
    Stratus impact reducing p.
pyloric stenosis dilator
pylorodilator
pylorus clamp
PyMaH
    P. nylon balanced bladder
    P. pre-gaged cuff
    P. Trimline sphygmomanometer
    system
Pynchol headband
Pynchon
    P. applicator

    P. cannula
    P. ear snare
    P. mouthgag
    P. nasal speculum
    P. suction tube
    P. tongue depressor
Pynchon-Lillie tongue depressor
pyoktanin catgut suture
Pyramesh cage
pyramid
    p. cannula
    p. Toomey tip
pyramidal
    p. electrode
    p. eye implant
Pyrex
    P. eye sphere
    P. T-tube
pyroglycolic acid suture
Pyrolyte ball-cage heart valve
Pyrost bone replacement
pyxigraphic
    p. device
    p. sampling capsule

QAD-1 sonography unit
Q-cath catheter
Q-catheter catheterization recording
system
QDR-1500, -2000 bone densitometer
QIAmp tissue kit
Qlicksmart blade removal system
Q-Maxx side-firing laser device
Q-Plex
    Q.-P. cardio-pulmonary exercise
    system
Q-prep system
Q-Ray bracelet
QSA dressing forceps
QS alexandrite laser
Q-Star
    Q-S. IV pressure-relief mattress
    Q-S. Voyager pressure-reduction
    mattress
Q-Stress treadmill
Q-switched
    Q.-s. alexandrite laser
    Q.-s. Er:YAG laser
    Q.-s. Nd:YAG laser
    Q.-s. neodymium:YAG laser
    Q.-s. neodymium:yttrium aluminum-
    garnet laser
    Q.-s. ruby laser
Q-Tee cleaning swab
Q-Tel Progressive CareMonitor
Q-T interval sensing pacemaker
Q-T's pouch
quad
    q. board
    Q. cutting tip
Quadcat wire
Quad-Lumen
    Q.-L. drain
    Q.-L. drain with radiopaque stripe
QuadPediatric fundus lens
QuadPolar
    Q. electrode
quad-ported laser-assisted intrastromal
    keratomileusis (LASIK) irrigating
    cannula
Quadracut ACL shaver system
Quadra-Flo infusion catheter
QuadraLase advanced surgical fiber
    system
Quadrant advanced shoulder brace
Quadra pipetting system
quadraplegic standing frame
quadrature
    q. cervical spine coil
    q. phase detector
    q. radiofrequency receiver coil
    q. surface coil MRI system
    q. surface coil system stem
    q. T/L surface coil
quadriceps boot
Quadrilite 6000 fiberoptic headlight

quadripolar
    q. cutting forceps
    q. electrode catheter
    q. 6-French diagnostic
    electrophysiology catheter
    q. pacing catheter
    q. steerable electrode catheter
    q. steerable mapping/ablation
    catheter
quadrisected minigraft dilator
Quadro dressing
Quadtro cushion
QualCare knee brace
QualCraft
    Q. ankle support
    Q. short elastic wrist support
    Q. splint
    Q. strap
Qualtex surgical drape
Quantec endodontic instrument
Quantico needle
Quanticor catheter
Quantimet 500 analyzing system
Quantrex Sweep 650 ultrasonic cleansing
    system
Quantum
    Q. biliary inflation device
    Q. enhancement knife
    Q. enteral pump
    Q. foot prosthesis
    Q. hearing aid
    Q. pacemaker
    Q. Ranger OTW balloon catheter
    Q. TTC biliary balloon
    Q. TTC biliary balloon dilator
QuantX color quantification tool
quarantine drain
Quartet system
quartz
    q. fiberoptic probe
    q. lamp
    q. needle
    q. rod
    q. transducer
quartz-glass container
Quartzo device
Queen Anne dressing
Quengel device
Quervain
    Q. abdominal retractor
    Q. cranial forceps
    Q. elevator
    Q. rib spreader
    Q. rongeur
Quervain-Sauerbruch retractor
Questek laser tube
Questus
    Q. Leading Edge arthroscopic
    grasper-cutter
    Q. Leading Edge sheathed
    arthroscopy knife

Quevedo
Q. conjunctival forceps
Q. fixation forceps
Q. suturing forceps
quick
Q. Bend flex clamp
q. catheter
q. connector
Q. CT9800 scanner
Q. Drain valve
QuickAnchor
Mitek Micro Q.
Mitek Mini Q.
Resolve Q.
Quickbox container
QuickCast
Q. splint
Q. wrist immobilizer
Quickert
Q. grooved director
Q. lacrimal probe
Q. suture
Quickert-Dryden lacrimal probe
Quicket tourniquet
QuickFlash arterial catheter
QuickFurl
Q. DL
Q. double-lumen balloon
Q. single-lumen balloon
Quickie
Q. Carbon wheelchair
Q. EX wheelchair
Q. GPS wheelchair
Q. GP Swing-Away wheelchair
Q. GPV wheelchair
Q. GP wheelchair
Q. Kidz wheelchair
Q. Recliner wheelchair
Q. Ti wheelchair
Quick-Lite lamp
Quicknet monitor interface
QuickRinse automated instrument rinse system
Quick-Sil
Q.-S. silicone system
Q.-S. starter kit
QuickSilver hydrophilic-coated guide wire
QuickStick padding

Quickswitch irrigation/aspiration ophthalmic device
Quiet interference screw
Quiet-Vac vacuum
Quik
Q. Connect fetal monitor
Q. splint
Quikcoff device
Quik-Temp thermometer
quill sheath
quilt
Thermacare q.
Quimby
Q. gum scissors
Q. implant system
Quincke
Q. spinal needle
Q. tube
Quincke-Babcock needle
Quincke-point spinal needle
Quinn holder
Quinones-Neubüser uterine-grasping forceps
Quinones uterine-grasping forceps
Quinton
Q. biopsy catheter
Q. central venous catheter
Q. dual-lumen catheter
Q. peritoneal catheter
Q. PermCath catheter
Q. Q-Port catheter
Q. Q-Port vascular access port
Q. Quik-Prep electrode
Q. suction biopsy instrument
Q. tube
Quinton-Mahurkar dual-lumen peritoneal catheter
Quinton-Scribner shunt
Quintron
Q. AlveoSampler
Q. Microlyzer 12 chromatograph
Quire
Q. foreign body forceps
Q. mechanical finger forceps
Q. mechanical finger snare
Quisling intranasal hammer
Quisling-Parkes osteotome
QUS-2 calcaneal ultrasonometer
Qwik-Clean dressing

RaAct NMES device
Raaf
    R. Cath vascular catheter
    R. dual-lumen catheter
    R. flexible lighted spatula
    R. forceps
Raaf-Oldberg
    R.-O. intervertebral disk forceps
    R.-O. rongeur
Rabbit mouthgag
Rabiner neurological hammer
Rabinov cannula
Racestyptine
    R. cord
    R. retraction ring
racetrack
    r. Microtron
    r. Microtron accelerator
rack
    Hausmann weight r.
    Jannetta sterilizing r.
    Luneau retinoscopy r.
RackBeta scintillation counter
Racz catheter
RAD40 sinus blade
RAD Airway laryngeal blade
Radcliff perineal retractor
RADenoid adenoidectomy blade
radial
    r. artery catheter
    r. iridotomy scissors
    R. Jaw bladder biopsy forceps
    R. Jaw hot biopsy forceps
    R. Jaw single-use biopsy forceps
    r. keratotomy knife
    r. keratotomy marker
    r. nerve glove
    r. sector scanning echoendoscope
    r. sponge
radiant
    r. heat device
    r. heat warmer
radiation
    r. beam monitor
    r. simulator
    r. therapy planning system
radiative hyperthermia device
RadiMedical fiberoptic pressure-monitoring wire
Radin-Rosenthal implant
radioactive stent
radiocarpal implant
Radiofocus
    R. catheter guidewire
    R. Glidewire
    R. Glidewire angiography catheter
    R. introducer B kit
radiofrequency
    r. ablator
    r. coil
    r. hot balloon

    r. needle electrode system
    r. pacemaker
radiofrequency-generated thermal balloon catheter
radio frequency generator
radiographic
    r. grid
    r. image processing system
    r. imaging system
radioimmunoassay kit
radioisotope
    r. camera
    r. capsule
    r. stent
radiologic portacaval shunt
radiolucent
    r. cranial pin headholder
    r. operating room table extension
    r. plastic occluder
    r. sound
    r. spine frame
    r. splint
RadioLucent wrist fixation system
Radiometer
    R. ABL 500 blood gas analyzer
    R. autotitrator
    OSM3 R.
    R. probe
    scanning R.
Radionics
    R. articulated arm system
    R. bipolar coagulation unit
    R. bipolar instrument
    R. CRW stereotactic head frame
    R. radiofrequency lesion generator
    R. stimulus generator
radionucleotide imaging
radionuclide carrier system
radiopaque
    r. calibrated catheter
    r. end marker
    r. ERCP catheter
    r. nitinol stent
    r. silastic catheter
    r. tantalum stent
radioscope
    Lombart r.
radiotranslucent rod
radium ^{226}**Ra needle**
Radius
    R. enteral feeding tube
    R. self-expanding stent
Radix anchor
Radix-Raney jacket
RadNet
    R. radiology information system
Radnoid microdebrider
Radovan
    R. breast implant
    R. tissue expander
    R. tissue expander tip

R

Radpour
R. irrigator
R. needle
Radpour-House
R.-H. suction irrigator
R.-H. suction tube
RadStat
RAE endotracheal tube
RAE-Flex tracheal tube
Ragnell
R. double-ended retractor
R. drain
R. undermining scissors
Ragnell-Davis double-ended retractor
rail
Railguard bed r.
railguard
RG7021 Inflatable bed r.
Railguard bed rail
railway catheter
Raimondi
R. hemostat
R. low-pressure shunt
R. peritoneal catheter
R. scalp hemostatic forceps
R. ventricular catheter
Rainbow
R. drill
R. envelope arm snare
R. fracture frame
R. vacuum
Raindrop medication nebulizer
Rainin
R. iris hook
R. lens hook
R. lens spatula
rake
5-prong r. blade
r. retractor
Ralks
R. bone drill
R. ear forceps
R. ear retractor
R. eye magnet
R. fingernail drill
R. mallet
R. nasal gauze packer
R. reversible knife
R. sinus applicator
R. splinter forceps
R. thoracic clamp
R. tuning fork
R. wire-cutting forceps
Ralks-Davis mouthgag
Ramel set
Ramirez
R. manipulator
R. periosteal elevator
R. shunt
R. Silastic cannula
R. winged catheter
Ramitec bite material
RAM knee prosthesis
Rampley sponge forceps
Rampton facebow

Ramsbotham decapitating hook
Ramsden eyepiece
Ramses
R. diaphragm
R. diaphragm introducer
Ramsey County pyoktanin catgut suture
Ramstedt
R. clamp
R. pyloric stenosis dilator
ramus
r. blade
r. blade implant
r. endosteal implant
r. stripper
Ranawat-Burstein
R.-B. hip prosthesis
R.-B. porous stem
R.-B. total hip system
Rancho
R. ankle foot control device
R. cube
R. Cube system
R. external fixation instrument
R. external fixation prosthesis
R. external fixation system
R. Los Amigos feeder
R. Los Amigos orthosis
R. Los Amigos splint
R. swivel hinge
Rand
R. bayonet ring curette
R. forceps
R. microballoon
Randall
R. endometrial biopsy curette
R. stone forceps
R. uterine curette
Randelli shoulder prosthesis
Rand-House suction tube
Rand-Malcolm cranial x-ray frame
Randolph
R. cyclodialysis cannula
R. irrigator
random-zero sphygmomanometer
Randot circle
Rand-Radpour suction tube
Rand-Wells pallidothalmomectomy guide
Raney
R. bone drill
R. cranial drill
R. dissector
R. flexion jacket brace
R. Gigli-saw guide
R. jacket
R. laminectomy punch
R. laminectomy retractor
R. laminectomy rongeur
R. perforator drill
R. periosteal elevator
R. rongeur forceps
R. scalp clip
R. scalp clip applier
R. scalp clip-applying forceps
R. spinal fusion curette
R. spring steel clip

R. stirrup-loop curette
R. straight coagulating forceps
Raney-Crutchfield
R.-C. drill point
R.-C. skull tongs
Ranfac
R. cannula
R. cholangiographic catheter
R. KPL laparoscopic knot pusher
R. soft-tissue needle
Range-Master pulley
range-of-motion brace
Ranger
R. OTW balloon catheter
Ranieri clamp
Rankin
R. anastomosis clamp
R. arterial forceps
R. hemostat
R. hemostatic forceps
R. intestinal clamp
R. prostatic retractor
R. prostatic tractor
R. stomach clamp
R. suture
Rankin-Crile forceps
Rankow forceps
Ransford loop
Ranzewski intestinal clamp
rapid
r. cuff inflator
r. exchange balloon catheter
r. exchange Flowtrack catheter
r. infusion pump
Rapide
R. wound suture
RapidFire multiple band ligator
Rapido
Rapido-mat
RapiSeal patch
Rappaport-Sprague stethoscope
Rappazzo
R. foreign body scissors
R. haptic scissors
R. intraocular foreign body forceps
R. intraocular lens
R. intraocular manipulator
R. iris hook
R. speculum
Rapp forceps
rare earth intraocular magnet
Rascal II anesthetic gas monitor
Rashkind
R. balloon
R. cardiac device
R. double-disk occluder prosthesis
R. double-disk umbrella occluder
R. double-umbrella device
R. hooked device
R. septostomy balloon catheter
R. septostomy needle
R. umbrella
Rasor blood pumping system
rasp (*See also* raspatory)
Aagesen disposable r.

Agris r.
antral r.
Arthrofile orthopaedic r.
Aufricht glabellar r.
Aufricht-Lipsett nasal r.
Aufricht nasal r.
Austin Moore r.
Bankart r.
Bardeleben r.
Barsky nasal r.
Bartholdson-Stenstrom r.
bell r.
Berne nasal r.
Bio-Modular humeral r.
Bio-Moore r.
Black r.
bone r.
Bowen r.
Brawley sinus r.
Bristow r.
Brown r.
Charnley r.
Cohen sinus r.
compound curved r.
Concept arthroscopy r.
Converse r.
convex r.
Cottle r.
Cottle-MacKenty r.
Cottle nasal r.
Dean r.
diamond r.
down-curved r.
Doyen costal r.
Doyen rib r.
ear r.
Eicher r.
Endotrac r.
Epstein bone r.
facet r.
Farabeuf bone r.
Farabeuf-Collin r.
Farrior r.
femoral r.
Filtzer interbody r.
Fischer nasal r.
Fomon nasal r.
Friedman r.
frontal sinus r.
Gallagher antral r.
Gam-Mer r.
Georgiade r.
glabellar r.
Gleason r.
Good antral r.
hand surgery r.
Herczel rib r.
Hylin r.
interbody fusion r.
Israel nasal r.
Joseph nasal r.
Kalinowski r.
Kalinowski-Verner r.
Kessler podiatry r.
Key r.

R

rasp *(continued)*
    Kleinert-Kutz r.
    Koenig r.
    Lamont nasal r.
    Leurs nasal r.
    Lewis nasal r.
    Lundsgaard r.
    Lundsgaard-Burch corneal r.
    Maliniac nasal r.
    Mallory-Head Interlok r.
    Maltz-Anderson nasal r.
    Maltz-Lipsett nasal r.
    Maltz nasal r.
    Matchett-Brown stem r.
    McCabe-Farrior r.
    McCabe perforation r.
    McCollough r.
    McGee oval-window r.
    McIndoe r.
    microbayonet r.
    Miller r.
    Moore stem r.
    nasal r.
    Nicola r.
    orthopedic r.
    Parkes nasal r.
    Peet nasal r.
    perforation r.
    r. pin
    Polokoff r.
    power r.
    pull r.
    push r.
    Putti bone r.
    Reidy r.
    Ringenberg r.
    Ritter r.
    Robb-Roberts rotary r.
    Rubin oblique r.
    Saunders-Paparella window r.
    Scheer oval window r.
    side-cutting r.
    snow plow r.
    Southworth r.
    Spratt nasofrontal r.
    Stenstrom r.
    straight r.
    Sullivan sinus r.
    surgical general r.
    Thompson frontal sinus r.
    Thompson stem r.
    triangular r.
    ulnar r.
    V. Mueller diamond r.
    Watson-Williams sinus r.
    Wiener antral r.
    Wiener nasal r.
    Wiener-Pierce antral r.
    Wiener Universal frontal sinus r.
    window r.
    Woodward antral r.
raspatory *(See also* rasp)
    Alexander rib r.
    Artmann r.

    Babcock r.
    Bacon periosteal r.
    Ballenger r.
    Barsky cleft palate r.
    Bastow r.
    Beck pericardial r.
    Bennett r.
    Berry rib r.
    bronchocele sound r.
    Brunner r.
    cleft palate r.
    Collin r.
    Converse r.
    Coryllos rib r.
    Cushing r.
    Davidson-Mathieu rib r.
    Davidson-Sauerbruch rib r.
    Dolley r.
    Doyen rib r.
    Edwards r.
    Edwards-Verner r.
    Farabeuf r.
    Farabeuf-Collin r.
    Farabeuf-Lambotte r.
    Farrior mushroom r.
    fishtail spatula r.
    French-pattern r.
    Friedrich r.
    Gam-Mer oblique r.
    Hein r.
    Herczel rib r.
    Hill nasal r.
    Hoen periosteal r.
    Hopkins Hospital periosteal r.
    Howarth nasal r.
    Jansen mastoid r.
    Joseph nasal r.
    Joseph periosteal r.
    Joseph-Verner r.
    Kirmisson periosteal r.
    Kleesattel r.
    Kocher r.
    Koenig r.
    Kokowicz r.
    Ladd r.
    Lambert-Berry rib r.
    Lambotte rib r.
    laminectomy r.
    Lane periosteal r.
    Langenbeck-O'Brien r.
    Langenbeck periosteal r.
    Lebsche r.
    Lewis periosteal r.
    Mannerfelt r.
    Mathieu r.
    Matson r.
    Matson-Alexander r.
    Matson-Plenk r.
    McGee r.
    McIndoe r.
    Moore r.
    Mott r.
    Nicola r.
    Ollier r.
    Overholt rib r.

periosteal r.
Phemister r.
Plenk-Matson r.
rib r.
Sauerbruch-Frey r.
Sayre periosteal r.
Scheuerlen r.
Schneider r.
Schneider-Sauerbruch r.
Sédillot r.
Semb rib r.
Sewall r.
Shuletz r.
Shuletz-Damian r.
skull r.
Stenstrom r.
Stille-Crafoord r.
Stille-Doyen r.
Stille-Edwards r.
Stillenberg r.
sympathetic r.
Trelat palate r.
Wiberg r.
Willauer r.
Williger r.
Yasargil r.
Zenker r.
Zoellner r.

Rastelli
R. conduit
R. graft
R. implant
R. prosthesis
Raster photogrammeter
ratchet
r. clamp
r. tourniquet
ratchet-type brace
rate-adaptive device
rate-modulated pacemaker
rate-responsive pacemaker
Rathke punch
Rath treatment table
Ratliff-Blake gallstone forceps
Ratliff-Mayo gallstone forceps
rat-tail catheter
rat-tooth
r.-t. forceps
r.-t. pickups
r.-t. rongeur
Rauchfuss
R. sling
R. sling splint
R. snare
Raulerson introducer syringe
Ravich
R. bougie
R. clamp
R. lithotriptoscope
R. lithotrite
R. needle holder
R. ureteral dilator
Ray
R. brain spatula
R. brain spoon

R. kidney stone forceps
R. nasal speculum
R. pituitary curette
R. rhizotomy electrode
R. RRE-TM thermistor electrode
R. TFC device
R. threaded fusion cage
Raylor
R. bone impactor
R. malleable retractor
Rayner-Choyce
R.-C. eye implant
R.-C. intraocular lens
Rayner lens
Rayopak
Raypaque resin
Ray-Parsons-Sunday staphylorrhaphy elevator
Rayport
R. dural knife
R. muscle clamp
Ray-Tec
R.-T. band
R.-T. dressing
R.-T. x-ray detectable lap pad
R.-T. x-ray detectable surgical sponge
Raz double-prong ligature carrier
Razi cannula introducer
razor
Bard-Parker r.
r. blade
r. bladebreaker
r. blade holder
r. blade knife
Castroviejo r.
Castroviejo oscillating r.
Credo r.
Detroit Receiving Hospital r.
Emir r.
r. scalpel
Weck-Prep orderly r.
razor-blade trephine
razor-tip needle
RB1 suture
RB face mask
R&B portable pneumothorax apparatus
RBS face mask
RC1, RC2 catheter
RC-2 fundus camera
RCB biopsy needle
reabsorbable suture
reach-and-pin forceps
reacher
Double Duty cane r.
E-Z R.
Pik Stick R.
ReAct NMES device
reactor
breeder r.
fast-breeder r.
Read
R. chisel
R. facial curette
R. forceps

Read (*continued*)
    R. gouge
    R. oral curette
    R. osteotome
    R. periosteal elevator
reader
    AutoPap r.
    Bio-kinetics r.
    Fisher microcapillary tube r.
    microtitration plate r.
    PapNet r.
Real-EaSE neck and shoulder relaxer
Reality vaginal pouch
Real scissors
real-time
    r.-t. B scanner
    r.-t. confocal scanning laser microscope
    r.-t. format converter
    r.-t. two-dimensional Doppler flow-imaging system
    r.-t. video processor
reamer
    acorn r.
    AMBI r.
    Anatomic/Intracone r.
    Aufranc finishing ball r.
    Aufranc finishing cup r.
    Aufranc offset r.
    Austin Moore bone r.
    r. awl
    bone r.
    r. bushing
    calcar r.
    canal r.
    cannulated four-flute r.
    chamfer r.
    Charnley deepening r.
    Charnley expanding r.
    Charnley taper r.
    Charnley trochanter r.
    r. clamp
    core r.
    debris-retaining acetabular r.
    Dentatus r.
    DePuy cannulated r.
    Duthie r.
    end-cutting r.
    endodontic r.
    expanding r.
    femoral shaft r.
    final-cut acetabular r.
    flexible r.
    flexible-wire bundle r.
    fluted r.
    Gray flexible intramedullary r.
    Green-Armytage r.
    Gruca hip r.
    Hall Versipower r.
    Harris brace-type r.
    Harris center-cutting acetabular r.
    Hewson-Richards r.
    humeral r.
    Indiana r.
    Intracone intramedullary r.
    intramedullary r.
    Jergensen r.
    Jergensen-Trinkle r.
    Jewett socket r.
    K r.
    Küntscher shaft r.
    Lorenz r.
    Lottes r.
    MacAusland finishing-ball r.
    MacAusland finishing-cup r.
    Mallory-Head Interlok r.
    Marin r.
    medullary canal r.
    Mira-Charnley r.
    Mira female trochanteric r.
    Mira femoral head r.
    Moore bone r.
    Murphy ball r.
    Norton adjustable cup r.
    Norton ball r.
    orthopedic r.
    Osteonics r.
    patellar shaft r.
    PD r.
    Pease r.
    Peeso r.
    Perthes r.
    Phemister r.
    Pressure Sentinel r.
    revision conical r.
    Rispi Micromega r.
    Rowe glenoidal r.
    Rush awl r.
    Schneider nail shaft r.
    shaft r.
    shelf r.
    Smith-Petersen hip r.
    Sovak r.
    spiral trochanteric r.
    spot face r.
    straight r.
    Sturmdorf cervical r.
    Swanson r.
    tapered r.
    T-handle r.
    Tinel tapered r.
reaming awl
rear-entry ACL drill guide
rear-tip extender
Reaves punch
Rebel knee orthosis
Rebounder
    Plyoback R.
rebreathing
    r. bag
    r. mask
Récamier uterine curette
receive-only circular surface coil
receiver
    Medtronic radiofrequency r.
    Pori and Rowe EEG r.
recessed balloon septostomy catheter
recession forceps

reciprocal
    r. ohm meter
    r. planing instrument
reciprocating
    r. gait orthosis
    r. power handpiece
    r. saw
Recklinghausen tonometer
recliner
    r. air chair
    Hydro Soothe r.
    Lumex Preferred Care r.
    Ortho-Biotic r.
reclining chair
Recon nail
reconstruction plate
recorder
    blood pressure r.
    cardiac output r.
    circadian event r.
    Del Mar Avionics three-channel r.
    Digitrapper EGG r.
    Dopcord r.
    Eigon CardioLoop r.
    Gould-Brush 481 eight-channel r.
    Gould ES 1000 r.
    graphic level r.
    HeartCard cardiac event r.
    Hellige electrocardiographic r.
    Honeywell r.
    intraocular tension r.
    Iriscorder r.
    King of Hearts event r.
    Leeds-Northrup Speedomax r.
    Marquette Holter r.
    MEDILOG 4000 ambulatory
      ECG r.
    MEDILOG ambulatory ECG r.
    MicroDigitrapper apnea r.
    Mingograf 82 r.
    Myoexorciser 1000 r.
    Narco Biosystems rectilinear r.
    Narco Physiograph-6B r.
    Oxford Medilog frequency-
      modulated r.
    Phinformer portable r.
    polysomnograph
      electroencephalograph 20-channel
      EEG r.
    Rectigraph-8K r.
    rectilinear r.
    Respitrace r.
    Reveal insertable loop r.
    Sandhill-800 TDS chart r.
    Sekomic SS-100F r.
    SNAP sleep r.
    Sony video r.
    Toshiba ERVF 1A video floppy r.
    video r.
recording electrode
Recovercare
    R. NPO non-powdered overlay
    R. system 1, 2 alternating pressure
      overlay

    R. System 3 low-air, loss-alternating
      pressure mattress
rectal
    r. balloon
    r. catheter
    r. cautery snare
    r. cautery wire
    r. clamp
    r. coil MRI
    r. curette
    r. dilator
    r. expander
    r. finger cot
    r. forceps
    r. hook
    r. hook retractor
    r. injection cannula
    r. injection needle
    r. multiplane transducer
    r. probe
    r. snare insulated stem
    r. snare stem brush
    r. speculum
    r. trocar
    r. tube
rectangle
    Harshill r.
    Luque r.
rectangular
    r. awl
    r. blade
    r. brain spatula
    r. tapper
    r. wire
rectifier
    full-wave r.
    silicon-controlled r.
    r. tube
Rectigraph-8K recorder
rectilinear recorder
rectoromanoscope
rectoscope
    Storz continuous-flow r.
rectosigmoidoscope
recumbent cycle
recurrent bandage
red
    R. Cross adhesive dressing
    r. laser
    r. lens occluder
    r. pessary
    R. Reflex Lens Systems lens
    R. Robinson catheter
    r. rubber catheter
    r. rubber endotracheal tube
    r. Witch bur
red-beam
    r.-b. laser
    r.-b. laser pen
Reddick cystic duct cholangiogram
catheter
Reddick-Saye
    R.-S. cannula
    R.-S. hydrosector
    R.-S. Lav-1 I&A probe

R

Reddick-Saye *(continued)*
R.-S. Lav-1 irrigating and aspirating probe
R.-S. screw
R.-S. screw catheter
R.-S. trocar
Redfield IRC 2100 infrared coagulator
red-free filter
Redi-Around finger splint
Redi Bur
Rediform orthotic
RediFurl
R. double-lumen balloon
R. single-lumen balloon
R. TaperSeal IAB catheter
RediGuard
R. catheter
R. IAB catheter
Redi-kit
LEEP R.-k.
Reditron refractometer
Redivac
R. suction drain
R. suction tube
Redi-Vu teleradiology system
Redo intestinal clamp
Redon drain
red-tip aspirator
reduced Snellen card
reducer
Cloward cervical dislocation r.
McCannel ocular pressure r.
Norelco allergen r.
ocular pressure r.
reducing fracture frame
reduction
r. instrument
r. ring
Redy
R. 2000 hemodialysis system
R. hemodialyzer
R. Sorbent dialysis system
Reebok
R. Slide system
R. Step system
Reece
R. orthopaedic shoe
R. osteotomy guide
R. PO shoe
Reed cast belt
Reeh stitch scissors
reel aspiration cannula
reentrant well chamber
Re-Entry Malecot catheter set
Rees
R. dermatome
R. face lift scissors
R. lighted retractor
Reese
R. advancement forceps
R. dermatome
R. dermatome blade
R. muscle forceps
R. prosthesis

R. ptosis knife
R. stimulator
Reese-Drum dermatome
reference
r. catheter
r. coordinate system
r. electrode
Refine fusion system
Refinity Coblation system
reflectance
r. photometer
r. spectrophotometer
r. spectrophotometric probe
r. TS-200 spectrum analyzer
Reflection
R. I, V, and FSO acetabular cup
R. liner
reflectometer
r. tuning unit
Reflec UV instant camera
reflex
R. articulating endoscopic cutter
R. gun
r. hammer
R. pacemaker
R. skin stapler
R. SuperSoft steerable guidewire
Re/Flex filter
ReFlexion implant system
ReFlex wand
Reformers
Stott R.
reform eye implant
refractionometer
Hartinger Coincidence r.
Zeiss vertex r.
refractometer
Abbe r.
AMO r.
Canon auto r.
Hoya HDR objective r.
Hoya MRM objective r.
meridional r.
Reditron r.
Speedy-1 Auto r.
Topcon RM-A2300 auto r.
refractor
Agrikola r.
Amoils r.
AR 1000 r.
ARK-Juno r.
automated r.
Barraquer-Krumeich-Swinger r.
Berens r.
Brawley r.
Bronson-Turtz r.
Campbell r.
Canon r.
Castallo r.
Castroviejo r.
Coburn r.
CooperVision Diagnostic Imaging r.
Desmarres r.
Elschnig r.
Ferris Smith-Sewall r.

R

Fink r.
Goldstein r.
Gradle r.
Graether r.
Green r.
Groenholm r.
Hartstein r.
Hillis r.
Humphrey automatic r.
Kirby r.
Knapp r.
Kronfeld r.
Kuglen r.
Leland r.
Marco ARK-2000 r.
McGannon r.
Mueller r.
Nidek AR-2000 objective
    automatic r.
Precision r.
Reichert r.
Remote Vision electronic r.
Retinomax 2 Auto R.
Rizzuti r.
Rollet r.
Schepens r.
SR-IV Programmed Subjective r.
Stevenson r.
Topcon r.
Ultramatic Rx Master Phoroptor r.
Wilmer r.
Regain home EMG trainer
Regal Acrylic/Stretch prosthetic sock
Regan-Lancaster dial
Regan low-contrast acuity chart
Regaud radium colpostat
Regency SR+ pulse generator
REGENTEX GBR-200 membrane
Regugauge suction regulator
regular Trimshield pad
regulator
high-flow r.
low-flow r.
Medela membrane r.
Ohmeda continuous-vacuum r.
Ohmeda thoracic suction r.
Optimed glaucoma pressure r.
Regugauge suction r.
Regu-Vac r.
suction Regugauge r.
Vacutron suction r.
Regulus frameless stereotactic system
Regu-Vac regulator
2+2 Rehab collar
Rehbein
R. infant abdominal retractor
R. internal steel strut
R. rib spreader
Rehfuss
R. duodenal tube
R. stomach tube
Rehne
R. abdominal retractor
R. skin graft knife

Reich curette
Reichert
R. antroscope
R. binocular indirect ophthalmoscope
R. camera
R. fiberoptic sigmoidoscope
R. flexible sigmoidoscope
R. Ful-Vue binocular
    ophthalmoscope
R. Ful-Vue spot retinoscope
R. lensometer
R. noncontact tonometer
R. ophthalmodynamometer
R. radius gauge
R. refractor
R. slit lamp
R. stereotaxic brain apparatus
R. stereotaxy system
R. Ultramatic Rx Master Phoroptor
    refracting instrument
**Reichert-Lenschek advanced logic
    lensometer**
Reichert-Mundinger
R.-M. stereotactic device
R.-M. stereotactic head frame
R.-M. stereotactic system
**Reichert-Mundinger-Fischer stereotactic
    frame**
Reichling corneal scissors
Reich-Nechtow
R.-N. arterial clamp
R.-N. cervical biopsy curette
R.-N. dilator
R.-N. hypogastric artery forceps
R.-N. hysterectomy forceps
R.-N. plug
Reid retinoscope
Reidy rasp
Reif catheter
Reill
R. forceps
R. needle holder
R. wire-cutting pliers
reimplanted electrode
Reinecke-Carroll lacrimal tube
Reiner
R. curette
R. ear syringe
R. plaster knife
R. rongeur
Reiner-Alexander ear syringe
Reiner-Beck tonsillar snare
Reiner-Knight ethmoid-cutting forceps
reinforced tracheostomy tube
Reinhart retractor
Reinhoff
R. arterial forceps
R. dissector
R. rib spreader
R. swan neck clamp
R. thoracic scissors
Reinhoff-Finochietto
R.-F. rib contractor
R.-F. rib spreader

Reipen
    R. cannula
    R. speculum
Reisinger lens-extracting forceps
ReJuveness
    R. pure silicone sheeting
    R. scar silicone sheet
Rekow system
Relat vaginal speculum
Relax-a-Cizor exerciser
relaxer
    Real-EaSE neck and shoulder r.
relaxograph
    Datex r.
relaxometer
    Bruker r.
    IBM field-cycling research r.
Relay
    R. cardiac pacemaker
    R. suture delivery system
release
    R. non-adhering dressing
    r. sleeve
Release-NF camera
Reliance
    R. CM femoral component
    R. device
    R. urinary control insert
    R. urinary control insert catheter
    R. urinary control stent
Relia-Vac drain
Relief Band device
reline material
reliner
    Brimms denture r.
    Coe-Rect denture r.
    Coe-Soft denture r.
    Hydro-Cast r.
    Simpa denture r.
    Super-Soft denture r.
Reliquet lithotrite
Relton frame pad
Relton-Hall spinal frame
Remac system
Rema-Exakt investment material
Rem-air 750 XL, XXL model
Remak band
Remaloy wire
Remanium
    R. alloy
    R. wire
Remedy
    R. colostomy appliance
    R. ileostomy appliance
Remine mastectomy skin flap retractor
remote
    r. control afterloading machine
    R. Vision electronic refractor
removable
    r. partial denture
    r. partial overdenture
removal mesh silo
Removatron epilator
Remove adhesive remover wipe

remover
    adhesive tape r.
    Atwood bridge r.
    Atwood crown r.
    Bailey foreign body r.
    Bard adhesive and barrier film r.
    Biomet Ultra-Drive cement r.
    Braithwaite clip r.
    clip r.
    Crown-A-Matic crown and bridge
    Damon-Julian ring r.
    DMV II contact lens r.
    Ferrolite crown r.
    foreign body r.
    frog cortex r.
    Macaluso stent r.
    Mead bridge r.
    Mead crown r.
    medical adhesive r.
    modular head r.
    Morrell crown r.
    Richwil bridge r.
    Richwil crown r.
    ring r.
    Schuknecht foreign body r.
    Tott ring r.
    Universal clip r.
    Wölfe-Böhler cast r.
REM PolyHesive II patient return electrode
Remy separator
Renaflo hollow fiber dialyzer
Renaissance
    R. crown system
    R. spirometry system
renal
    r. artery clamp
    r. artery forceps
    r. needle
    r. pedicle clamp
    r. sinus retractor
    r. sympathetic nerve activity recording electrode
    R. System HF250 filter
    R. systems dialyzer
Renalin dialyzer
Renata battery
Renatron
    R. dialyzer
    R. II dialyzer reprocessing system
Rendell-Baker Soucek mask
Renegade microcatheter
Renolux convertible car seat
renovascular stent
Renovist II injector
Rentrop infusion catheter
Reo Macrodex suture
REP Bands exercise band
Repela surgical gloves
Repel bioresorbable barrier film
reperfusion catheter
Replace
    R. implant system
    R. system tapered implant
replaceable blade

replacement
Biolox ceramic ball head for hip r.
Bi-Wave plus mattress r.
Calcitite bone r.
r. collection bag
Cosgrove mitral valve r.
Howmedica Centrax head r.
Kirschner Medical Dimension hip r.
Manchester knee r.
Mueller-type femoral head r.
NexGen complete knee r.
Osteogenics BoneSource synthetic
bone r.
PCA E-Series hip r.
Pilliar total hip r.
Polyfloat system II mattress r.
Pyrost bone r.
Stage IV mattress r.
temporary skin r.

replacer
Green iris r.
Smith-Fisher iris r.

replant splint
RepliCare Thin hydrocolloid dressing
replicator
Steers r.
Replica total hip replacement system
Repliderm dressing
Repliform graft
Replogle
R. catheter
R. tube
Re-Ply TENS electrode
repositioner
Wilson-Cook prosthesis r.
repositor
iris r.
Knapp iris r.
Koman-Nair iris r.
Nettleship iris r.

reprocessor
AER+ automatic endoscope r.
American Endoscopy automatic r.
automated endoscope r.
automatic endoscopic r.
Bard automatic r.
Custom Ultrasonic automatic r.
ECI automatic r.
KeyMed automatic r.
Lutz automatic r.
MediVators DSD-91P endoscope r.
Olympus automatic r.
Orr automatic r.
Steris automatic r.
Reprodent acrylic tooth material
Repro head halter
Resano
R. sigmoid forceps
R. thoracic scissors
ResCue Key
rescuing pacemaker
Research Medical straight multiple-holed
aortic cannula

resection
r. clamp
r. intestinal forceps
resector
Accu-Line distal femoral r.
Accu-Line tibial r.
Dyonics full-radius r.
Friedrich-Petz machine r.
full-radius r.
Gator r.
Stryker r.
XPS Striaightshot micro tissue r.
resectoscope
ACMI r.
r. adapter
Bard r.
Baumrucker r.
continuous-flow Wolfe r.
r. curette
Elite System rotating r.
Ellik r.
Foroblique microlens r.
Iglesias continuous-flow r.
Iglesias fiberoptic r.
Iglesias microlens r.
Kaplan r.
Mauermayer r.
McCarthy continuous-flow r.
McCarthy microlens r.
McCarthy miniature r.
McCarthy multiple r.
Nesbit r.
OES 4000 r.
Olympus continuous-flow r.
OPERA Star r.
ProTouch r.
Richard Wolf video r.
Scott rotating r.
r. sheath
specialized tissue-aspirating r.
Stern-McCarthy electrotome r.
Storz direct-view r.
Storz-Iglesias r.
Storz laser r.
Streak r.
Thompson direct full-vision r.
Timberlake obturator r.
USA Elite System GYN rotating
continuous-flow r.
Wappler r. with microlens optics
reservoir
Accu-Flo CSF r.
Braden flushing r.
Camey r.
Cardiometrics cardiotomy r.
cardiotomy r.
Cobe cardiotomy r.
contiguous spinal fluid r.
CSF r.
Denver r.
double bubble flushing r.
double-dome r.
r. face mask
flat bottom r.
flushing r.

reservoir *(continued)*
    Foltz flushing r.
    Hakim r.
    Heyer-Schulte Jackson-Pratt wound-drainage r.
    Heyer-Schulte-Ommaya CSF r.
    Heyer-Schulte wedge-suction r.
    H-H Rickham cerebrospinal fluid r.
    Holter-Rickham ventriculostomy r.
    Holter-Salmon-Rickham ventriculostomy r.
    Holter-Selker ventriculostomy r.
    Holter ventriculostomy r.
    ICV r.
    Intersept cardiotomy r.
    inverted U-pouch ileal r.
    Jackson-Pratt large-volume suction r.
    Jostra cardiotomy r.
    J-Vac bulb suction r.
    Kock ileal r.
    large-volume suction r.
    LeBag r.
    Mainz pouch urinary r.
    Molded Bulb closed wound drainage r.
    Ommaya cerebrospinal fluid (CSF) r.
    Ommaya retromastoid r.
    Ommaya side-port flat-bottomed r.
    Ommaya spinal fluid r.
    Ommaya suboccipital r.
    Ommaya ventricular r.
    Parks ileoanal r.
    Polystan cardiotomy r.
    Pudenz r.
    Resipump pump r.
    retromastoid Ommaya r.
    Rickham r.
    Salmon-Rickham ventriculostomy r.
    Sci-Med extracorporeal silicone rubber r.
    Selker ventriculostomy r.
    Shiley cardiotomy r.
    side-port flat-bottomed Ommaya r.
    suboccipital Ommaya r.
    UNI r.
    Uni-Shunt with elliptical r.
    William Harvey cardiotomy r.
    wound drainage r.

resin
    Aclec r.
    Astron r.
    Astron dental r.
    Bondeze r.
    Bowen r.
    Brilliant light-cured r.
    Celay Tech light curing r.
    r. cement
    Coe orthodontic r.
    Concise r.
    Dentalon R r.
    Dentsply r.
    diacrylate r.
    Directon r.

    Dynabond r.
    Effapoxy r.
    Endur r.
    Genie r.
    Ivocryl r.
    Lee orthodontic r.
    light-curing r.
    Myerson r.
    Nuvaseal r.
    Nuva-Tach r.
    orthodontic r.
    Orthomite r.
    Poracryl r.
    Porovin dental r.
    Raypaque r.
    Royale III denture r.
    Shur r.
    Solo-Tach r.
    r. sphere
    Technovit acrylic r.
    ultraviolet light-polymerized r.
    unfilled r.
    Vynacron r.
    Vynagel dental r.

Resipump pump reservoir
resistance wire heater
Resistex
    R. expiratory resistance exerciser
    R. PEP therapy device
resistive
    r. chair exercise kit
    r. exerciser
    r. exercise table
ResMed CPAP Sullivan III machine
Resnick
    R. button bipolar coagulator
    R. Tone Emitter I intraoral electrolarynx device
Resolve QuickAnchor
resonance generator
resonator
    birdcage r.
    bridged loop-gap r.
    Faraday shielded r.
    flexible surface-coil-type r.
    multicoupled loop-gap r.
    Oudin r.
resorbable
    r. copolymer PGA/PLLA-Lactosorb miniplate fixation system
    r. plate
    r. plate and screw
    r. polydioxanone pin
    r. thread clip applicator
ReSound
    R. CC4 hearing aid
    R. Digital 2000 hearing aid
    R. Digital 5000 hearing device
Respiradyne
respiration bronchoscope
respiratometer
    Collins r.
respirator *(See also* ventilator)
    Ambu r.
    BABYbird II r.

Bath r.
Bear 5 r.
Bennett r.
Bird Mark 8 r.
Bourns electronic adult r.
Bourns infant r.
Bragg-Paul r.
Breeze r.
cabinet r.
Clevedan positive pressure r.
cuirass r.
Dann r.
Drinker tank r.
Emerson cuirass r.
Engstrom r.
Gill I r.
Huxley r.
MA-1 r.
mechanical r.
mechanically assisted r.
Med-Neb r.
Merck r.
Monaghan r.
Morch r.
Morsch-Retec r.
Moynihan r.
portable r.
Sanders jet ventilation device r.
respiratory-dependent pacemaker
respiratory function monitor
Respirex incentive spirometer
Respirgard II nebulizer
respirometer
Dräger r.
Fraser Harlake r.
Haloscale r.
hot-wire r.
Wright r.
Respironics
R. BiPAP machine
R. CPAP machine
Respitrace
R. inductive plethysmograph
R. machine
R. recorder
Respond wire
Response cushion
Resposable Spacemaker surgical balloon dissector
Res-Q
R.-Q. ACD
R.-Q. ACD implantable cardioverter-defibrillator
R.-Q. AICD
R.-Q. arrhythmia control device
R.-Q. ICD generator
Res-Q-Vac emergency suction system
rest
Adson head r.
Cedar anesthesia face r.
Chan wrist r.
Chiroflow back r.
Core Hibak R.
Core Lobak R.
Core Sitback R.

face r.
foot r.
Krause arm r.
Mayfield head r.
Mouse Nest mouse r.
Muirhead pelvic r.
neck r.
SutureMate needle r.
Restcue
R. bed
R. CC dynamic air therapy unit
resting
r. foot sling
r. orthosis
Reston
R. foam wound dressing
R. hydrocolloid dressing
R. padding
R. polyurethane foam
R. sponge
Restoration
R. acetabular system
R. GAP acetabular cup
R. Secur-Fit X'tra acetabular shell
Restoration-HA hip system
restorative
Amelogen composite dental r.
r. pin
Restore
R. ACL guide system
R. alginate wound dressing
R. bone implant
R. CalciCare dressing
R. close tolerance dental implant system
R. Cx wound care dressing
R. dental implant
R. extra-thin dressing
R. hair replacement imaging
R. hydrocolloid dressing
R. hydrogel dressing
R. orthobiologic soft-tissue implant
R. Plus wound care dressing
R. threaded implant
restraint
Circumstraint r.
papoose board r.
poncho r.
Posey r.
vacuum-operated viscous r.
restrictor
Biostop G cement r.
Buck femoral cement r.
cement r.
Charnley cement r.
femoral canal r.
Resume electrode
Resurface laser resurfacing imaging
Resuscitaire neonatal resuscitation unit
resuscitation cart
resuscitator
ACD r.
Ambu infant r.
BagEasy disposable manual r.
bag-valve r.

resuscitator *(continued)*
DMR2 disposable manual r.
First Response manual r.
Fisher-Paykel RD1000 r.
heart-lung r.
High Oxygen PRM r.
Hope r.
Hudson Lifesaver r.
infant Ambu r.
Laerdal infant r.
Lifemask infant r.
NeoVO₂R volume control r.
Ohio Hope r.
Penlon infant r.
pneuPAC r.
Robertshaw bag r.
Safe Response manual r.
SureGrip manual r.

retainer
r. arch bar
r. closure
continuous bar r.
direct r.
extracoronal r.
Hahnenkratt r.
Hawley r.
indirect r.
r. insert
intracoronal r.
matrix r.
McNealey-Glassman visceral r.
Mectra Tissue Sample R.
r. ring
space r.
SurgiFish visceral r.
Thermoskin heat r.
Tofflemire r.
viscera r.

retaining
r. device
r. retractor

Retcam 120 digital camera

retention
r. bar
r. catheter
r. drill
r. ring
r. suture bolster
r. suture bridge

rete peg

retinaculotome
Paine carpal tunnel r.

retinal
r. detachment hook
r. detachment pencil
r. detachment syringe
r. diathermy electrode
r. ellipsometer
r. Gelfilm implant
r. probe sleeve

Retinomax
R. 2 Auto Refractor
R. cordless hand-held autorefractor
R. refractometry instrument

retinometer
Heine Lambda 100 r.

Retinopan 45 camera

retinoscope
Boilo r.
Copeland streak r.
electric r.
Ful-Vue spot r.
Ful-Vue streak r.
Keeler r.
Macula r.
Priestley-Smith r.
Propper r.
Reichert Ful-Vue spot r.
Reid r.
spot r.
Welch Allyn standard r.
Welch Allyn streak r.

retractable stylet

retracted penis pouch

retracting rod

retraction ring

retractor
Abadie self-retaining r.
abdominal ring r.
abdominal vascular r.
Ablaza aortic wall r.
Ablaza-Blanco cardiac valve r.
Abramson r.
Adams r.
Adamson r.
Adson-Beckman r.
Adson brain r.
Adson cerebellar r.
Adson splanchnic r.
Agrikola lacrimal sac r.
airgun r.
Airlift balloon r.
alar r.
Alden r.
Alexander r.
Alexander-Ballen orbital r.
Alexander-Matson r.
Alexian Hospital r.
Alfreck r.
Allen r.
Allis lung r.
Allison lung r.
Allport-Babcock r.
Allport-Gifford r.
Allport mastoid bayonet r.
Alm microsurgery r.
Alm self-retaining r.
Alter lip r.
aluminum cortex r.
Amenabar iris r.
American Heyer-Schulte brain r.
Amoils iris r.
amputation r.
anal r.
Anderson-Adson self-retaining r.
Anderson double-end r.
Andrews tracheal r.
angled decompression r.
angled iris r.

angled vein r.
Ankeney sternal r.
Ann Arbor phrenic r.
anterior prostatic r.
Anthony pillar r.
antral r.
AOR collateral ligament r.
aortic valve r.
Apfelbaum cerebellar r.
apicolysis r.
appendectomy r.
appendiceal r.
arch rake r.
Arem r.
Arem-Madden r.
arm r.
Army-Navy r.
Aronson esophageal r.
Aronson lateral sternomastoid r.
Arruga eye r.
Arruga globe r.
Ashley r.
Assistant Free r.
Aston nasal r.
Aston submental r.
atrial septal r.
Aufranc cobra r.
Aufranc femoral neck r.
Aufranc hip r.
Aufranc psoas r.
Aufranc push r.
Aufricht nasal r.
Austin dental r.
automatic skin r.
Auvard weighted vaginal r.
Azar iris r.
Babcock r.
baby Adson brain r.
baby Balfour r.
baby Collin abdominal r.
baby Roux r.
baby Senn-Miller r.
baby Weitlaner self-retaining r.
Backmann thyroid r.
Bacon cranial r.
Badgley laminectomy r.
Bahnson sternal r.
Bakelite r.
Balfour center-blade abdominal r.
Balfour pediatric abdominal r.
Balfour self-retaining r.
Balfour r. with fenestrated blade
Ballantine hemilaminectomy r.
Ballen-Alexander orbital r.
ball-type r.
Bankart rectal r.
Bankart shoulder r.
Barkan bident r.
Baron r.
Barraquer-Krumeich-Swinger r.
Barraquer lid r.
Barrett-Adson cerebellum r.
Barron r.
Barr self-retaining rectal r.
Barsky nasal r.

Bauer r.
Beardsley esophageal r.
Beatty pillar r.
Beaver r.
beaver-tail r.
Bechert-Kratz cannulated nucleus r.
Becker r.
Beckman-Adson laminectomy r.
Beckman-Eaton laminectomy r.
Beckman goiter r.
Beckman self-retaining r.
Beckman thyroid r.
Beckman-Weitlaner laminectomy r.
Bellfield wire r.
Bellman r.
Bellucci-Wullstein r.
Benedict r.
Beneventi self-retaining r.
Bennett bone r.
Bennett tibial r.
bent malleable r.
Berens esophageal r.
Berens lid r.
Berens mastectomy skin flap r.
Berens thyroid r.
Bergen r.
Bergman tracheal r.
Bergman wound r.
Berkeley r.
Berkeley-Bonney self-retaining
  abdominal r.
Berlind-Auvard r.
Berna infant abdominal r.
Bernay tracheal r.
Bernstein nasal r.
Bertin hip r.
Bethune phrenic r.
Bicek vaginal r.
bident r.
Biestek thyroid r.
bifid gallbladder r.
bifurcated r.
Biggs mammoplasty r.
biliary r.
Billroth ovarian r.
Billroth-Stille r.
Bishop r.
bivalved r.
Black r.
bladder r.
r. blade
Blair-Brown vacuum r.
Blair four-prong r.
Blakesley uvular r.
Blanco r.
Bland perineal r.
Blount double-prong r.
Blount hip r.
Blount knee r.
Blount single-prong r.
blunt rake r.
boardlike r.
Bodnar knee r.
Boley r.
bone r.

retractor *(continued)*
    Bookwalter-Balfour r.
    Bookwalter-Goulet r.
    Bookwalter-Harrington r.
    Bookwalter-Hill-Ferguson rectal r.
    Bookwalter-Kelly r.
    Bookwalter-Magrina vaginal r.
    Bookwalter ring r.
    Bookwalter-St. Mark deep pelvic r.
    Bose r.
    Bosworth nerve root r.
    bowel r.
    Boyd r.
    Boyes-Goodfellow hook r.
    Braastad costal arch r.
    brain silicone-coated r.
    Brantley-Turner vaginal r.
    Brawley scleral wound r.
    Breen r.
    Breisky-Navratil straight r.
    Breisky vaginal r.
    Brewster phrenic r.
    Briesky Navritrol r.
    Briggs r.
    Brinker hygienic tissue r.
    Bristow-Bankart humeral r.
    Bristow-Bankart soft tissue r.
    Brompton Hospital r.
    Bronson-Turtz iris r.
    Brophy tenaculum r.
    Brown-Burr modified Gillies r.
    Brown uvular r.
    Bruch mastoid r.
    Bruening r.
    Brunner r.
    Brunschwig visceral r.
    Bucy spinal cord r.
    Budde halo neurosurgical r.
    Budde halo ring r.
    Buie r.
    Buie-Smith anal r.
    bulb r.
    Bulnes-Sanchez r.
    Burford-Finochietto rib r.
    Burford rib r.
    Busenkell posterior hip r.
    Butler dental r.
    Butler pillar r.
    buttonhook nerve r.
    Bycroft-Brunswick thyroid r.
    Byford r.
    Cairns scalp r.
    Callahan r.
    Campbell lacrimal sac r.
    Campbell nerve root r.
    Campbell self-retaining r.
    Campbell suprapubic r.
    Canadian chest r.
    Cardillo r.
    cardiovascular r.
    Carlens-Stille tracheal r.
    Carlens tracheotomy r.
    Caroline finger r.
    Carroll-Bennett finger r.

    Carroll offset hand r.
    Carroll self-retaining spring r.
    Carten mitral valve r.
    Carter r.
    Caspar cervical r.
    Castallo eyelid r.
    Castaneda infant sternal r.
    Castroviejo adjustable r.
    Castroviejo lid r.
    cat's paw r.
    Cave knee r.
    cecostomy r.
    cerebellar r.
    cerebral r.
    cervical disk r.
    Cer-View lateral vaginal r.
    chalazion r.
    Chamberlain-Fries atraumatic r.
    Chandler knee r.
    Chandler laminectomy r.
    channel r.
    Charnley horizontal r.
    Charnley initial incision r.
    Charnley knee r.
    Charnley pin r.
    Charnley self-retaining r.
    Charnley standard stem r.
    Cheanvechai-Favaloro r.
    cheek r.
    Cherry laminectomy self-retaining r.
    Cherry S-shaped brain r.
    Cheyne r.
    Children's Hospital pediatric r.
    Chitten-Hill r.
    Christie gallbladder r.
    Cibis-Vaiser muscle r.
    claw r.
    Clayman lid r.
    Clevedent r.
    Cleveland IMA r.
    r. clip
    Cloward blade r.
    Cloward brain r.
    Cloward cervical r.
    Cloward-Cushing vein r.
    Cloward dural r.
    Cloward-Hoen laminectomy r.
    Cloward nerve root r.
    Cloward self-retaining r.
    Cloward tissue r.
    Cobb r.
    cobra-head r.
    Cocke large flap r.
    Cohen r.
    Cole duodenal r.
    Coleman r.
    collapsible tissue r.
    collar-button iris r.
    Collin abdominal r.
    Collin-Hartmann r.
    Collins-Mayo mastoid r.
    Collin sternal self-retaining r.
    Collis anterior cervical r.
    Collis posterior lumbar r.
    Collis-Taylor r.

R

Colonial r.
Colver tonsillar r.
Comyns-Berkeley r.
condylar neck r.
Cone laminectomy r.
Cone scalp r.
Cone self-retaining r.
contour scalp r.
Converse blade r.
Converse double-ended alar r.
Converse nasal r.
Conway lid r.
Cook rectal r.
Cooley aortic r.
Cooley atrial valve r.
Cooley carotid r.
Cooley femoral r.
Cooley-Merz sternal r.
Cooley-Merz sternum r.
Cooley mitral valve r.
Cooley MPC cardiovascular r.
Cooley neonatal sternal r.
Cooley rib r.
Cooley sternotomy r.
Cope double-ended r.
corner r.
corrugated forehead r.
cortex r.
Coryllos r.
Cosgrove mitral valve r.
costal arch r.
Costenbader r.
Coston-Trent iris r.
Cottle alar r.
Cottle four-prong r.
Cottle hook r.
Cottle-Joseph r.
Cottle nasal r.
Cottle-Neivert r.
Cottle pillar r.
Cottle pronged r.
Cottle sharp-prong r.
Cottle single-blade r.
Cottle soft palate r.
Cottle upper lateral exposing r.
Cottle weighted r.
Crafoord r.
Craig-Sheehan r.
cranial r.
crank frame r.
Crawford aortic r.
Crego periosteal r.
Crile thyroid double-ended r.
Crockard hard palate r.
Crockard pharyngeal r.
Crotti goiter r.
Crotti thyroid r.
Crowe-Davis mouth r.
Cushing aluminum r.
Cushing angled decompression r.
Cushing bivalve r.
Cushing brain r.
Cushing decompression r.
Cushing-Kocher r.
Cushing nerve r.

Cushing self-retaining r.
Cushing S-shaped r.
Cushing straight r.
Cushing subtemporal r.
Cushing vein r.
dacryocystorhinostomy r.
Dallas r.
Danek self-retaining r.
Danis r.
Darling popliteal r.
Darrach r.
Dautrey r.
David-Baker eyelid r.
Davidoff trigeminal r.
Davidson erector spinae r.
Davidson scapular r.
Davis brain r.
Davis double-ended r.
Davis pillar r.
Davis self-retaininig scalp r.
Deaver pediatric r.
DeBakey-Balfour r.
DeBakey chest r.
DeBakey-Cooley Deaver-type r.
Decker r.
decompressive r.
Dedo laser r.
deep abdominal r.
deep blunt rake r.
deep Deaver r.
DeLaginiere abdominal r.
Delaney phrenic r.
de la Plaza transconjunctival r.
DeLee corner r.
DeLee Universal r.
DeLee vaginal r.
DeLee vesical r.
DeMartel self-retaining brain r.
Denis Browne pediatric r.
Denis Browne ring r.
dental r.
Denver-Wells atrial r.
Denver-Wells sternal r.
DePuy r.
D'Errico-Adson r.
D'Errico nerve root r.
Desmarres cardiovascular r.
Desmarres lid r.
Desmarres valve r.
Desmarres vein r.
Deucher abdominal r.
Devine-Millard-Aufricht r.
Di-Main r.
Dingman flexible r.
Dingman Flexsteel r.
Dingman-Senn r.
Dingman zygoma hook r.
disposable iris r.
Dixon center-blade r.
Doane knee r.
Dockhorn r.
dog chain r.
Dohn-Carton brain r.
Dorsey nerve root r.
Dorton self-retaining r.

retractor *(continued)*
Dott r.
double-bent Hohmann acetabular r.
double-cobra r.
double-crank r.
double-ended r.
double-fishhook r.
Downing II laminectomy r.
Doyen child abdominal r.
Doyen vaginal r.
Dozier radiolucent Bennett r.
Drews iris r.
Drews-Rosenbaum iris r.
dual nerve root suction r.
Duane r.
dull r.
dull-pronged r.
Dumont r.
duodenal r.
dural suction r.
Duryea r.
Eastman vaginal r.
East-West soft tissue r.
Eccentric "Y" adjustable finger r.
Echols r.
Eddey parotid r.
Edinburgh brain r.
Effenberger r.
Elias lid r.
Eliasoph lid r.
Elite Farley r.
Elschnig lid r.
Emmet obstetrical r.
Emory EndoPlastic r.
endaural r.
Endoflex endoscopic r.
EndoRetract r.
Endotrac r.
Enker self-retaining brain r.
epicardial r.
epiglottis r.
erector spinae r.
ESI long, narrow mammoplasty r.
esophageal r.
examination r.
eXpose r.
externofrontal r.
extraoral sigmoid notch r.
eyelid r.
facelift r.
Falk vaginal r.
fan elevator r.
fan liver r.
Farabeuf double-ended r.
Farley Elite spinal r.
Farmingdale r.
Farr self-retaining r.
Farr spring r.
Farr wire r.
Fasanella double-ended iris r.
fat pad r.
Favaloro atrial r.
Favaloro self-retaining sternal r.
Federspiel cheek r.

Feldman lid r.
femoral neck r.
Ferguson r.
Ferguson-Moon rectal r.
Fernstroem bladder r.
Fernstroem-Stille r.
Ferris Smith orbital r.
Ferris Smith-Sewall orbital r.
fiberoptic r.
finger rake r.
Fink lacrimal r.
Finochietto-Geissendorfer rib r.
Finochietto hand r.
Finochietto infant rib r.
Finochietto laminectomy r.
Finsen r.
Fisch dural r.
Fisher double-ended r.
Fisher fenestrated lid r.
Fisher lid r.
Fisher-Nugent r.
Fisher tonsillar r.
five-prong rake blade r.
fixed ring r.
flexible translimbal iris r.
FlexPosure endoscopic r.
Flexsteel ribbon r.
Foerster abdominal r.
Fomon hook r.
Fomon nasal r.
force fulcrum r.
Ford-Deaver r.
Forker r.
Foss bifid gallbladder r.
Foss biliary r.
four-prong r.
Fowler self-retaining r.
Franklin malleable r.
Franz abdominal r.
Frater intracardiac r.
Frazier cerebral r.
Frazier-Fay r.
Frazier laminectomy r.
Frazier lighted r.
Freeman facelift r.
Freer dural r.
Freer skin r.
Freer submucous r.
Freiberg hip r.
Freiberg nerve root r.
Freidrich-Ferguson r.
French S-shaped brain r.
French-Stern-McCarthy r.
Friedman perineal r.
Friedman vaginal r.
Fritsch abdominal r.
Fujita snake r.
Fukuda humeral head r.
Fukushima r.
Fullerview flexible iris r.
Fulton r.
Gabarro r.
gallbladder r.
gallows-type r.
Gam-Mer medial esophageal r.

Gam-Mer occipital r.
Gant gallbladder r.
Garrett peripheral vascular r.
Garrigue vaginal r.
gastric resection r.
Gaubatz rib r.
Gauthier r.
Gazayerli endoscopic r.
Gazayerli-Mediflex r.
Geissendorfer rib r.
Gelpi abdominal r.
Gelpi-Lowrie r.
Gelpi perineal r.
Gelpi self-retaining r.
Gelpi vaginal r.
general r.
Gerbode sternal r.
Gerow-Harrington heart-shaped distal
  end r.
Ghazi rib r.
Gibson-Balfour abdominal r.
Gifford-Jansen mastoid r.
Gifford mastoid r.
Gifford scalp r.
Gillies single-hook skin r.
Gil-Vernet lumbotomy r.
Gil-Vernet renal sinus r.
Givner lid r.
Glaser laminectomy r.
Glass abdominal r.
Glenner vaginal r.
Goelet double-ended r.
goiter r.
Goldstein lacrimal sac r.
Goligher modification of the
  Berkeley-Bonney r.
Goligher sternal-lifting r.
Gomez gastric r.
Gooch mastoid r.
Good r.
Goodhill r.
Goodyear tonsillar r.
Gosset abdominal r.
Gosset appendectomy r.
Gosset self-retaininig r.
Gott malleable r.
Gradle eyelid r.
Graether r.
Grant gallbladder r.
Gray surgical r.
Greenberg-Sugita r.
Greenberg Universal r.
Green goiter r.
Green thyroid r.
Greenwald r.
Grice r.
Grieshaber-Balfour r.
Grieshaber flexible iris r.
Grieshaber self-retaining r.
Grieshaber spring wire r.
Groenholm lid r.
Gross iris r.
Gross patent ductus r.
Gross-Pomeranz-Watkins r.
Gross-Pomeranz-Watkins atrial r.

Gruenwald r.
Guilford-Wright meatal r.
Guthrie r.
Guttmann obstetrical r.
Guttmann vaginal r.
Guzman-Blanco epiglottic r.
Haight-Finochietto rib r.
Haight pulmonary r.
Haight rib r.
Hajek antral r.
Hajek lip r.
half-moon r.
halo r.
Hamburger-Brennan-Mahorner
  thyroid r.
Hamby brain r.
Hamby-Hibbs r.
hand r.
hand-held r.
hard palate r.
Hardy-Duddy vaginal r.
Hardy lip r.
Harken rib r.
Harrington bladder r.
Harrington Britetrac r.
Harrington-Deaver r.
Harrington-Pemberton
  sympathectomy r.
Harrington splanchnic r.
Harrington sympathectomy r.
Harrison chalazion r.
Hartstein irrigating iris r.
Hartzler rib r.
Haslinger palate r.
Haslinger uvular r.
Hasson r.
Haverfield hemilaminectomy r.
Haverfield-Scoville
  hemilaminectomy r.
Haynes r.
Hays finger r.
Hays hand r.
Heaney hysterectomy r.
Heaney-Simon hysterectomy r.
Heaney-Simon vaginal r.
Heaney vaginal r.
Hedblom rib r.
Heifitz r.
Heiss mastoid r.
Heiss soft tissue r.
Helfrick anal r.
Helveston "Great Big Barbie" r.
hemilaminectomy r.
Henderson self-retaining r.
Henley carotid r.
Henner endaural r.
Henner T-model endaural r.
Henning meniscal r.
Henrotin r.
hernia r.
Hertzler baby rib r.
Hess nerve root r.
Heyer-Schulte brain r.
Hibbs self-retaining laminectomy r.
Hill-Ferguson rectal r.

R

retractor *(continued)*

Hillis eyelid r.
Hill rectal r.
Himmelstein sternal r.
Hirschman r.
Hoen hemilaminectomy r.
Hoen scalp r.
Hohmann r.
Holman lung r.
Holscher nerve r.
Holzbach abdominal r.
Holzheimer mastoid r.
Holzheimer skin r.
Homan r.
hook r.
r. hook
Horgan r.
horizontal flexible bar r.
Hosel r.
House hand-held double-end r.
House-Urban middle fossa r.
Howorth toothed r.
Huang Universal arm r.
Hubbard r.
Hudson bone r.
humeral r.
Hunt bladder r.
Hupp tracheal r.
Hurd tonsillar pillar r.
Hurson flexible r.
Hutchinson iris r.
hysterectomy r.
IMA r.
incision r.
infant abdominal r.
infant eyelid r.
infant rib r.
Inge laminectomy r.
initial incision r.
intestinal occlusion r.
intracardiac r.
intradural r.
iris r.
Iron Intern r.
irrigating mushroom r.
Israel blunt rake r.
Jackson self-retaining goiter r.
Jackson tracheal r.
Jackson vaginal r.
Jacobson bladder r.
Jacobson goiter r.
Jaeger lid r.
Jaffe-Givner lid r.
Jaffe wire lid r.
Jako laser r.
Jannetta posterior fossa r.
Jansen-Gifford mastoid r.
Jansen mastoid r.
Jansen scalp r.
Jansen-Wagner mastoid r.
Jarit cross-action r.
Jarit-Deaver r.
Jarit P.E.E.R. r.
Jarit renal sinus r.

Jarit spring-wire r.
Jefferson self-retaining r.
Joe's hoe r.
Johns Hopkins gallbladder r.
Johnson cheek r.
Johnson hook r.
Johnson ventriculogram r.
Jones IMA epicardial r.
Jorgenson r.
Joseph skin hook r.
Joseph wound r.
Joystick r.
Judd-Allis intestinal r.
Judd-Mason bladder r.
Judd-Mason prostatic r.
Kalamarides dural r.
Kanavel-Senn r.
Kapp Surgical Instrument total knee r.
Karmody vascular spring r.
Kartush insulated r.
Kasdan r.
Kaufer type II r.
Kaufman type II r.
Keeler-Fison tissue r.
Keeler-Rodger iris r.
Keizer-Lancaster lid r.
Keizer lid r.
Kel r.
Kelly abdominal r.
Kelly-Sims vaginal r.
Kelman iris r.
Kennerdell-Maroon orbital r.
Kennerdell medial orbital r.
Kerrison r.
kidney r.
Killey molar r.
Killian-King goiter r.
Kilner nasal r.
Kilner skin hook r.
Kilpatrick r.
King-Hurd r.
King self-retaining goiter r.
Kirby lid r.
Kirchner r.
Kirkland r.
Kirklin atrial r.
Kirschenbaum r.
Kirschner abdominal r.
Kirschner-Balfour abdominal r.
Kitner r.
Kleinert-Kutz hook r.
Kleinert-Ragnell r.
Kleinsasser r.
Klemme appendectomy r.
Klemme gasserian ganglion r.
Klemme laminectomy r.
Kliners alar r.
Knapp lacrimal sac r.
knee r.
Knighton hemilaminectomy self-retaining r.
Kobayashi r.
Kocher bladder r.
Kocher blade r.

Kocher bone r.
Kocher-Crotti self-retaining goiter r.
Kocher gallbladder r.
Kocher-Langenbeck r.
Kocher self-retaining goiter r.
Kocher-Wagner r.
Koenig vein r.
Koerte r.
Koneg r.
Korte r.
Korte-Wagner r.
Kozlinski r.
Krasky r.
Kretschmer r.
Kristeller vaginal r.
Kronfeld eyelid r.
Krönlein-Berke r.
Kuda r.
Kuglen lens r.
Kuyper-Murphy sternal r.
Kwapis subcondylar r.
Lack tongue r.
lacrimal sac r.
Lahey Clinic nerve root r.
Lahey goiter r.
Lahey thyroid r.
laminectomy self-retaining r.
Landau vaginal r.
Landon narrow-bladed r.
Lane r.
Lange bone r.
Lange-Hohmann bone r.
Langenbeck-Cushing vein r.
Langenbeck-Green r.
Langenbeck-Mannerfelt r.
Langenbeck periosteal r.
Laplace liver r.
laryngeal r.
laryngofissure r.
lateral wall r.
Latrobe soft palate r.
Lawton-Balfour self-retaining r.
leaflet r.
Leasure tracheal r.
Leatherman trochanteric r.
Lee double-ended r.
Legen self-retaining r.
Legueu bladder r.
Legueu kidney r.
Lemmon self-retaining sternal r.
Lemole atrial valve self-retaining r.
Lemole mitral valve r.
Lempert r.
Lempert-Colver r.
LeVasseur-Merrill r.
Levinthal surgery r.
Levy articulating r.
Levy perineal r.
Lewis r.
Leyla self-retaining brain r.
Leyla-Yasargil self-retaining r.
lid r.
Liddicoat aortic valve r.
lighted r.
LightWare micro r.

Lilienthal-Sauerbruch r.
Lillehei r.
Lillie r.
Linton splanchnic r.
lip r.
Little r.
liver r.
Lockhart-Mummery r.
Lofberg thyroid r.
Logan lacrimal sac self-retaining r.
London narrow-bladed r.
Lone Star r.
long atraumatic r.
loop r.
Lorie cheek r.
Lothrop tonsillar r.
Lothrop uvular r.
Lovejoy r.
Love nasopharyngeal r.
Love nerve root r.
Love uvula r.
Lowman hand r.
Lowsley prostate r.
Luer double-ended tracheal r.
Luer S-shaped r.
Lukens double-ended tracheal r.
Lukens epiglottic r.
Lukens thymus r.
lumbar r.
lumbotomy r.
lung r.
Luongo hand r.
Luther-Peter r.
MacAusland-Kelly r.
MacAusland muscle r.
MacKay contour self-retaining r.
MacKool capsule r.
MacVicar double-end strabismus r.
Magrina-Bookwalter vaginal r.
Mahorner thyroid r.
Maison r.
Maliniac nasal r.
Malis cerebellar r.
Malis cerebral r.
malleable blade r.
malleable copper r.
malleable ribbon r.
malleable stainless steel r.
Maltz r.
mandibular body r.
Mannerfelt r.
Manning r.
manual r.
Markham-Meyerding
  hemilaminectomy r.
Mark II Chandler total knee r.
Mark II concave total knee r.
Mark II lateral collateral
  ligament r.
Mark II modular weighted r.
Mark II PCL r.
Mark II "S" total knee r.
Mark II Stubbs short-prong
  collateral ligament r.
Mark II wide PCL knee r.

retractor *(continued)*

Mark II "Z" knee r.
Markley r.
Martin abdominal r.
Martin cheek r.
Martin lip r.
Martin nerve root r.
Martin palate r.
Martin rectal hook r.
Martin vaginal r.
Mason-Judd bladder r.
Mason-Judd self-retaining r.
mastectomy skin flap r.
mastoid self-retaining r.
Mathieu double-ended r.
Matson-Mead apicolysis r.
Mattison-Upshaw r.
Mayfield r.
Mayo abdominal r.
Mayo-Adams appendectomy r.
Mayo-Adams self-retaining r.
Mayo-Collins appendectomy r.
Mayo-Collins double-ended r.
Mayo-Collins mastoid r.
Mayo-Lovelace abdominal r.
Mayo-Simpson r.
McBurney fenestrated r.
McBurney thyroid r.
McCabe antral r.
McCabe parotidectomy r.
McCabe posterior fossa r.
McCool capsule r.
McCullough externofrontal r.
McGannon iris r.
McGill r.
McIndoe r.
McNealey visceral r.
meat hook r.
Medicon rib r.
Mediflex Gazayerli r.
Meigs r.
Meller lacrimal sac r.
meniscal r.
Merrill-Levassier r.
metacarpal double-ended r.
metal bar r.
Meyer biliary r.
Meyerding-Deaver r.
Meyerding finger r.
Meyerding self-retaining laminectomy r.
microlumbar diskectomy r.
microsurgical r.
microvascular modified Alm r.
Middledorf r.
middle fossa r.
Middlesex-Pointe r.
Mikulicz abdominal r.
Mikulicz liver r.
Miles r.
Milex r.
Miller r.
Miller-Senn double-ended r.
Milligan self-retaining r.

Millin-Bacon bladder self-retaining
Millin-Bacon retropubic prostatectomy r.
Millin retropubic bladder r.
Millin self-retaining r.
Miltex r.
mini-Hohmann r.
Minnesota r.
Miskimon cerebellar self-retaining
mitral valve r.
Moberg r.
Moberg-Stille r.
Mollison self-retaining r.
Moon rectal r.
Moore bone r.
Moorehead cheek r.
Moorehead dental r.
Morris r.
Morrison-Hurd pillar r.
Morse modified Finochietto r.
Morse sternal r.
Morse valve r.
Mosher lifesaver r.
Mott double-ended r.
Mueller-Balfour self-retaining r.
Mueller lacrimal sac r.
Mufson-Cushing r.
Muldoon lid r.
multiprong rake r.
multipurpose r.
Munro self-retaining r.
Murless head r.
Murphy-Balfour r.
Murphy gallbladder r.
Murphy rake r.
Murtagh self-retaining infant scalp r.
Naclerio diaphragm r.
narrow Deaver r.
nasal r.
nasopharyngeal r.
Navratil r.
Neivert double-ended r.
Nelson self-retaining rib r.
neonatal sternal r.
nerve root r.
Nevyas drape r.
newborn eyelid r.
Newell lid r.
Newton-Morgan r.
New tracheal r.
New York Hospital r.
Noblock r.
North-South r.
Nuttall r.
Nystroem r.
Nystroem-Stille r.
Oberhill self-retaining r.
O'Brien phrenic r.
O'Brien rib r.
obstetrical r.
Obwegeser channel r.
Obwegeser periosteal r.
Ochsner-Favaloro self-retaining r.
Ochsner malleable r.

Ochsner ribbon r.
Ochsner vascular r.
O'Connor abdominal r.
O'Connor-O'Sullivan abdominal r.
O'Connor-O'Sullivan self-retaining
vaginal r.
O'Connor vaginal r.
Octopus r.
Oertli wire lid r.
Oettingen abdominal self-retaining r.
offset hand r.
Oklahoma iris wire r.
Oldberg brain r.
Oldberg straight r.
Oliver scalp r.
Ollier rake r.
Omni r.
Omni-Tract vaginal r.
orbicular r.
orbital r.
O'Reilly esophageal r.
Orley r.
Osher iris r.
Osher lid r.
O'Sullivan-O'Connor self-retaining
abdominal r.
O'Sullivan-O'Connor vaginal r.
O'Sullivan self-retaining
abdominal r.
O'Sullivan vaginal r.
r. oval sprocket frame
Packiam r.
palate r.
Paparella self-retaining r.
Paparella-Weitlaner r.
Parker double-ended r.
Parker-Mott double-ended r.
Parker thumb r.
Parkes nasal r.
Parks anal r.
parotidectomy r.
Parsonnet epicardial r.
patent ductus r.
Paul lacrimal sac r.
Paulson knee r.
Payne r.
Payr abdominal r.
Peck rake r.
pediatric abdominal r.
pediatric self-retaining r.
Peet lighted splanchnic r.
Pemberton r.
Pemco r.
Penfield r.
Percy amputation r.
Percy bone r.
Percy-Wolfson gallbladder r.
periareolar r.
perineal prostatectomy r.
perineal self-retaining r.
peripheral vascular r.
Perkins otologic r.
Perman-Stille abdominal r.
pharyngeal r.
Pheifer-Young r.

phrenic r.
Pickrell r.
Picot vaginal r.
Pierce cheek r.
pillar r.
pillar-and-post microsurgical r.
Pilling r.
Pilling-Favaloro r.
Piper lateral wall r.
Plester r.
Poliak eye r.
Polytrac Gomez r.
Pomeranz hiatal hernia r.
popliteal r.
Poppen-Gelpi laminectomy self-
retaining r.
Portmann r.
Posada-Vasco orbital r.
postauricular r.
posterior fossa r.
posterior urethral r.
Pratt bivalve r.
Proctor cheek r.
pronged r.
prostatic r.
Proud-White uvula r.
Pryor-Péan vaginal r.
psoas r.
pulmonary r.
Purcell self-retaining abdominal r.
Quervain abdominal r.
Quervain-Sauerbruch r.
Radcliff perineal r.
Ragnell-Davis double-ended r.
Ragnell double-ended r.
rake r.
Ralks ear r.
Raney laminectomy r.
Rankin prostatic r.
Raylor malleable r.
rectal hook r.
Rees lighted r.
Rehbein infant abdominal r.
Rehne abdominal r.
Reinhart r.
Remine mastectomy skin flap r.
renal sinus r.
retaining r.
retropubic prostatectomy r.
rib r.
ribbon malleable r.
Rica brain r.
Rica mastoid r.
Rica multipurpose r.
Rica posterior cranial fossa r.
Ricard abdominal r.
Rica scalp r.
Richards abdominal r.
Richardson abdominal r.
Richardson appendectomy r.
Richardson-Eastman double-ended r.
Richter vaginal r.
Rigby abdominal r.
Rigby appendectomy r.
Rigby bivalve r.

retractor *(continued)*
 Rigby rectal r.
 Rigby vaginal r.
 right-angle r.
 ring abdominal r.
 Rissler kidney r.
 Rizzo r.
 Rizzuti iris r.
 Roberts thumb r.
 Robin-Masse abdominal r.
 Robinson lung r.
 Rochester atrial septal r.
 Rochester colonial r.
 Rochester-Ferguson double-ended r.
 Rochester rake r.
 Rollet eye r.
 Rollet lacrimal sac r.
 Rollet lake r.
 Rollet skin r.
 Roos brachial plexus root r.
 Rose double-ended r.
 Rosenbaum-Drews iris r.
 Rosenbaum-Drews plastic r.
 Rosenbaum iris r.
 Rosenberg full-radius blade
  synovial r.
 Rosenberg-Sampson r.
 Rose tracheal r.
 Ross aortic valve r.
 Rotalok skin r.
 Rothon r.
 Roux double-ended r.
 Rowe boathook r.
 Rowe humeral head r.
 Rowe orbital floor r.
 Rowe scapular neck r.
 Rudolph trowel r.
 Rultract internal mammary artery r.
 Rumel r.
 Ryecroft r.
 Ryerson bone r.
 Sachs angled vein r.
 Sachs-Cushing r.
 Samb r.
 Sanchez-Bulnes lacrimal sac self-
  retaining r.
 Sato lid r.
 Sauerbruch r.
 Sauerbruch-Zukschwerdt rib r.
 Sawyer rectal r.
 Sayre r.
 scalp self-retaining r.
 Scanlan pediatric r.
 scapular r.
 Schepens orbital r.
 Schindler r.
 Schink metatarsal r.
 Schnitker scalp r.
 Schoenborn r.
 Scholten sternal r.
 Schuknecht postauricular self-
  retaining r.
 Schuknecht-Wullstein r.
 Schultz iris r.

 Schwartz laminectomy self-
  retaining r.
 scleral wound r.
 Scoville Britetrac r.
 Scoville cervical disk self-
  retaining r.
 Scoville-Haverfield laminectomy r.
 Scoville hemilaminectomy self-
  retaining r.
 Scoville laminectomy r.
 Scoville nerve root r.
 Scoville psoas muscle r.
 Scoville-Richter self-retaining r.
 Scoville self-retaining r.
 Segond abdominal r.
 Seldin dental r.
 Seletz-Gelpi self-retaining r.
 self-adhering lid r.
 self-retaining abdominal r.
 self-retaining brain r.
 self-retaining ring r.
 self-retaining skin r.
 self-retaining spring r.
 Sellor rib r.
 Semb lung r.
 Semb self-retaining r.
 Senn-Dingman double-ended r.
 Senn double-ended r.
 Senn-Green r.
 Senn-Kanavel double-ended r.
 Senn mastoid r.
 Senn-Miller r.
 Senn self-retaining r.
 Senturia r.
 serrated r.
 serrefine r.
 Sewall orbital r.
 Shambaugh endaural self-retaining r.
 sharp-pronged r.
 Shearer lip r.
 Sheehan r.
 Sheldon-Gosset self-retaining r.
 Sheldon hemilaminectomy self-
  retaining r.
 Sherwin self-retaining r.
 Sherwood r.
 short Heaney r.
 Shriners Hospital interlocking r.
 Shuletz-Paul rib r.
 Shurly tracheal r.
 sigmoid notch r.
 Silverstein lateral venous sinus r.
 Simon vaginal r.
 Sims double-ended r.
 Sims-Kelly vaginal r.
 Sims rectal r.
 Sims vaginal r.
 single-blade r.
 single-hook r.
 single-prong broad acetabular r.
 Sisson-Love r.
 Sisson spring r.
 Sistrunk band r.
 Sistrunk double-ended r.
 six-prong rake r.

skin flap r.
skin hook r.
skin self-retaining r.
Sloan goiter self-retaining r.
Sluder palate r.
Small rake r.
Small tissue r.
SMIC cheek r.
Smillie knee joint r.
Smith anal r.
Smith-Buie anal r.
Smith-Buie self-retaining rectal r.
Smith nerve root suction r.
Smith-Petersen capsular r.
Smith rectal self-retaining r.
Smith vaginal self-retaining r.
Smithwick r.
Snitman endaural self-retaining r.
Sofield r.
soft palate r.
soft tissue blade r.
Spacekeeper r.
Space-OR r.
spike r.
spinal cord r.
Spivey iris r.
splanchnic r.
spoon r.
spring r.
spring-loaded self-retaining r.
spring-wire r.
Spurling r.
S-shaped brain r.
Stack r.
Stamey dorsal vein apical r.
stay suture r.
Steiner-Auvard vaginal r.
stereotactic r.
sternal r.
sternotomy r.
Stevens lacrimal r.
Stevens muscle hook r.
Stevenson lacrimal sac r.
Stille-Broback knee r.
Stille cheek r.
Stille heart r.
Stiwer r.
St. Luke's r.
St. Mark's Hospital r.
St. Mark's lipped r.
St. Mark's pelvis r.
Stookey r.
Storer thoracoabdominal r.
Storz r.
straight r.
Strandell r.
Strandell-Stille r.
Strully nerve root r.
Stuck self-retaining laminectomy r.
Suarez r.
submucous r.
Sugita r.
suprapubic self-retaining r.
surgical r.
Sweeney posterior vaginal r.

Sweet amputation r.
sweetheart r.
Symmonds hysterectomy r.
sympathectomy r.
table-fixed r.
Tang r.
TARA retropubic r.
Taylor Britetrac r.
Taylor fiberoptic r.
Taylor spinal r.
T-bar r.
Tebbets ribbon r.
Teflon iris r.
Temple-Fay laminectomy r.
Tepas r.
Terino facial implant r.
Tew cranial r.
Tew spinal r.
Theis self-retaining rib r.
Theis vein r.
Thomas r.
Thoma tissue r.
Thompson r.
Thorlakson deep abdominal r.
Thorlakson multipurpose r.
Thornton iris r.
three-prong rake blade r.
thumb r.
Thurmond iris r.
thymus r.
thyroid r.
tibial r.
Tiko pliable iris r.
Tiko rake r.
Tillary double-ended r.
tissue r.
titanium wound r.
T-model endaural r.
Toennis r.
tongue r.
tonsillar pillar r.
toothed r.
Tower interchangeable r.
Tower rib r.
Tower spinal r.
tracheal r.
transconjunctival r.
transoral r.
Trent eye r.
trigeminal self-retaining r.
Tubinger self-retaining r.
Tucker-Levine vocal cord r.
Tuffier abdominal r.
Tuffier-Raney laminectomy r.
Tuffier rib r.
Tupper hand-holder and r.
Turner-Doyen r.
Turner-Warwick posterior urethral r.
Turner-Warwick prostate r.
two-prong rake r.
Tyrer nerve root r.
Tyrrell hook r.
Ullrich self-retaining laminectomy r.
Ullrich-St. Gallen self-retaining r.
umbrella r.

R

retractor *(continued)*
 Universal r.
 Upper Hands self-retaining r.
 upper-lateral exposing r.
 Urban r.
 USA r.
 U. S. Army double-ended r.
 U-shaped r.
 uvular r.
 Vacher self-retaining r.
 vacuum r.
 vaginal r.
 vagotomy r.
 Vail lid r.
 Vaiser-Cibis muscle r.
 Valin hemilaminectomy self-
  retaining r.
 Vasco-Posada orbital r.
 vascular spring r.
 Veenema retropubic self-retaining r.
 vein hook r.
 ventriculogram r.
 Verbrugge r.
 vertical self-retaining bone r.
 vesical r.
 vessel r.
 Viboch iliac graft r.
 Villalta r.
 Vinke r.
 Visitec iris r.
 V. Mueller-Balfour abdominal r.
 V. Mueller fiberoptic r.
 Volkmann finger r.
 Volkmann hand r.
 Volkmann pocket r.
 Volkmann rake r.
 Wachtenfeldt-Stille r.
 Walden-Aufricht nasal r.
 Walker gallbladder r.
 Walker lid r.
 Walter-Deaver r.
 Walter nasal r.
 Wangensteen r.
 W. D. Johnson epicardial r.
 Weary nerve root r.
 Webb r.
 Webb-Balfour self-retaining
  abdominal r.
 Webster abdominal r.
 Weder r.
 Weder-Solenberger pillar r.
 Weder-Solenberger tonsillar r.
 weighted posterior r.
 Weinberg "Joe's hoe" double-
  ended r.
 Weinberg vagotomy r.
 Weinstein horizontal r.
 Weinstein intestinal r.
 Weitlaner brain r.
 Weitlaner hinged r.
 Weitlaner microsurgery r.
 Weitlaner self-retaining r.
 Wellington Hospital vaginal r.
 Welsh iris r.

 Wesson perineal self-retaining r.
 Wesson vaginal r.
 Wexler abdominal r.
 Wexler-Balfour r.
 Wexler-Bantam r.
 Wexler deep-spreader blade
  abdominal r.
 Wexler large-frame abdominal r.
 Wexler lateral side-blade
  abdominal r.
 Wexler malleable-blade abdominal
 Wexler self-retaining r.
 Wexler Universal joint abdominal
 Wexler vaginal r.
 Wexler X-P large abdominal r.
 White-Lillie r.
 White-Proud uvular r.
 Wichman r.
 Wieder dental r.
 Wieder pillar r.
 Wieder-Solenberger pillar r.
 Wiet r.
 Wigderson ribbon r.
 Wilder scleral self-retaining r.
 Wilkes self-retaining r.
 Wilkinson abdominal r.
 Wilkinson-Deaver blade abdominal
 Wilkinson ring-frame abdominal r.
 Wilkinson self-retaining abdominal
 Willauer-Deaver r.
 Williams microlumbar r.
 Williams rod self-retaining r.
 Wills eye lacrimal r.
 Wilmer-Bagley r.
 Wilmer cryosurgical iris r.
 Wilmer iris r.
 Wilson r.
 Wiltse-Bankart r.
 Wiltse-Gelpi self-retaining r.
 Wiltse iliac r.
 Winsburg-White r.
 wiring r.
 Wise orbital r.
 Wolf meniscal r.
 Wolfson gallbladder r.
 Woodward r.
 Worrall deep r.
 Wort antral r.
 Wullstein self-retaining ear r.
 Wullstein-Weitlaner self-retaining r.
 Wylie renal vein r.
 Wylie splanchnic r.
 Yasargil r.
 Yasargil-Leyla brain r.
 Young anterior prostatic r.
 Young bifid r.
 Young bladder r.
 Young bulb r.
 Young lateral prostatic r.
 Young prostatic r.
 Yu-Holtgrewe prostatic r.
 Z r.
 Zalkind-Balfour center-blade r.
 Zalkind-Balfour self-retaining r.
 Zalkind lung r.

Zenker r.
Zimberg esophageal hiatal r.
Zylik-Michaels r.

retrieval
r. balloon
r. device
r. forceps
r. loop

retriever
basket r.
Brimfield magnetic r.
Carroll tendon r.
Entract stone r.
Golden R.
Kleinert-Kutz tendon r.
magnetic r.
Pfister-Schwartz stone r.
plaque r.
Positrap r.
snail-headed catheter r.
Soehendra stent r.
stone r.
three-pronged polyp r.
ureteral stone r.
Vantec loop r.
Warren-Wilder r.
Wilson-Cook ministent r.

retrobulbar needle
retroflexed cystoscopy sheath
retrograde
r. bougie
r. curette
r. electrode
r. femoral catheter
r. knife
r. meniscal blade
r. occlusion balloon catheter
r. valvulotome

retrograde-cutting hook-shaped knife
retromastoid Ommaya reservoir
Retromax endopyelotomy stent
retroperfusion catheter
retropubic prostatectomy retractor
retroreflective marker
Retroscan
retroscopic lens
retrospective
r. bronchoscopic telescope
retroversion pessary
Retrox Fractal active fixation lead
Retter aneurysm needle
return-flow
r.-f. cannula
r.-f. hemostatic catheter
r.-f. retention catheter
Retzius system
Reul
R. aortic clamp
R. coronary artery scissors
R. coronary forceps
ReUnite
R. hand fixation
R. orthopedic pin
R. orthopedic screw

R. resorbable orthopedic fixation system
R. VersaTile fixation
reusable
r. incontinence pant
r. laparoscopic electrode
r. Sorensen 2000 cc cannister
r. vein stripper
r. and washable adult pin-style diaper
r. and washable adult snap diaper
r. and washable underpad
Reuse Expanda-graft dermatome
Reuss table
Reuter
R. bobbin collar button
R. bobbin implant
R. bobbin ventilation tube
R. suprapubic trocar and cannula system
Reveal
R. insertable loop recorder
R. MLR+ camera
R. single lens reflex camera
Revelation
R. handpiece
R. hip system
Reverdin
R. abdominal spatula
R. graft
R. holder
R. implant
R. prosthesis
R. suture needle
reverse
r. adenotome
r. cystotome
r. intraocular lens
r. Kingsley splint
r. knuckle-bender splint
r. scissors
reverse-action hypophysectomy forceps
reverse-angle skid curette
reverse-bevel laryngoscope
reverse-curve
r.-c. adenoid curette
r.-c. clamp
reverse-cutting
r.-c. meniscal probe
r.-c. needle
r.-c. probe
r.-c. scissors
reversed arm leads
reverse-shape implant
reverse-threaded screw
reversible lid speculum
reversion pacemaker
revised
r. Salzburg lag screw system
r. Würzburg mandibular reconstruction system
ReVision
R. hip stem
R. nail
R. nail system

R

revision
 r. conical reamer
RevitaLase erbium cosmetic laser
Revitalizer Soft-Start nasal CPAP
Revivac catheter
Revive system penile prosthesis
Revo
 R. loop handle knot pusher
 R. retrievable cancellous screw
 R. suture anchor
Revolution lens
revolving Ge-68 pin
Revots vulsellum tenaculum
Rew-Wyly
 R.-W. blade
 R.-W. mouthgag
Rexton hearing aid
Reynolds
 R. dissecting clamp
 R. dissecting scissors
 R. infusion catheter
 R. Pathfinder 3 analyzer
 R. resection clamp
 R. skull traction tongs
 R. vascular clamp
Reynolds-Jameson vessel scissors
Reynold-Southwick H-graft portacaval
 shunt
Rezaian
 R. interbody external fixation device
Rezek forceps
Rezifilm dressing
Rezinian spinal fixator
Reziplast spray-on dressing
RF
 RF ablation system
 RF Ablatr ablation catheter
 RF balloon catheter
 RF Marinr catheter
 RF Performer catheter
RG7021 Inflatable bed railguard
R-HAB lighter weight ankle prosthesis
Rhein
 R. Advantage diamond knife
 R. capsulorhexis cystitome forceps
 R. clear corneal diamond knife
 R. 3-D trapezoid diamond blade
 R. fine foldable lens-insertion
  forceps
 R. pick
 R. reusable cautery pen
Rheinberg microscope
Rheinstaedter
 R. flushing curette
 R. uterine curette
Rheo Dopplex II
rheolytic catheter
Rhinelander
 R. clamp
 R. guide
 R. pin
 R. plate
Rhino
 R. Cruiser Pavlik harness
 R. Kicker Pavlik harness

 R. Rocket dressing
 R. Rocket nasal pack
 R. Rocket nasal packing
 R. Triangle hip abduction brace
rhinolaryngoscope
rhinolaryngostroboscopy system
rhinolarynx stroboscope
Rhinoline endoscopic sinus surgery
 system
rhinomanometer
 Storz r.
rhinometer
 Hood Laboratories Eccovision
  acoustic r.
 two-microphone acoustical r.
rhinoplasty
 r. diamond bur
 r. implant
rhinoscope
 Wolf-Post r.
 Wylie-Post r.
rhinoscopic mirror
Rhinotec shaver
Rhinotherm hyperthermia treatment
 system
rhodamine laser
Rhode Island Secto dissector
rhodium
 r. anode
 r. filter
Rhoton
 R. ball dissector
 R. bayonet needle holder
 R. bayonet scissors
 R. bipolar forceps
 R. blunt-ring curette
 R. cup forceps
 R. dural forceps
 R. elevator
 R. enucleator
 R. grasping forceps
 R. horizontal-ring curette
 R. loop curette
 R. microcup forceps
 R. microcurette
 R. microdissecting forceps
 R. microdissector
 R. microforceps
 R. microneedle holder
 R. microscissors
 R. microsurgical scissors
 R. microtying forceps
 R. microvascular forceps
 R. nerve hook
 R. osteotome
 R. pituitary curette
 R. 3-prong fork
 R. ring tumor forceps
 R. round dissector
 R. sellar punch
 R. spatula dissector
 R. spoon curette
 R. straight point needle
 R. tissue forceps
 R. transsphenoidal bipolar forceps

R. tying forceps
R. vertical ring curette
Rhoton-Adson
R.-A. dressing forceps
R.-A. tissue forceps
Rhoton-Cushing tissue forceps
Rhoton-Merz
R.-M. rotatable coupling head
R.-M. suction tube
Rhoton-Tew bipolar forceps
RhythmScan
rhytidectomy scissors
Riahl coronary compressor
rib
r. approximator
r. brad awl
r. contractor
r. drill
r. edge stripper
r. needle
r. raspatory
r. retractor
r. rongeur forceps
r. shears
r. spreader
Riba
R. electrical ureteral meatotome
R. electrourethrotome electrode
R. urethrotome
Riba-Valeira forceps
ribbed
r. hook
r. sterile tubing
Ribble
R. bandage
R. dressing
ribbon
r. arch appliance
r. blade
r. gauze dressing
r. gut needle
r. gut suture
r. malleable retractor
**RiboPrinter microbial characterization
system**
Rica
R. anesthetic laryngoscope
R. aneurysm needle
R. anterior commissure laryngoscope
R. arterial clamp
R. bone drill
R. bone hammer
R. bone mallet
R. bone rongeur
R. brain retractor
R. brain spatula
R. cerebral angiography puncture
needle
R. cerumen hook
R. clip-applying forceps
R. cotton carrier
R. cranial rongeur
R. cranioclast
R. cross-action towel clip
R. dermatome

R. ear curette
R. ear polypus scissors
R. ear probe
R. ear speculum
R. esophagoscopy set
R. eustachian catheter
R. forceps holder
R. hemostatic forceps
R. infant laryngoscope
R. laminectomy rongeur
R. lipoma curette
R. malleus head nipper
R. mastoid chisel
R. mastoid curette
R. mastoid gouge
R. mastoid retractor
R. mastoid rongeur
R. mastoid suction tube
R. microarterial clamp
R. multipurpose retractor
R. myringotome
R. nasal septal speculum
R. nylon
R. pelvimeter
R. pneumatic otoscope
R. posterior cranial fossa retractor
R. powder blower
R. scalp retractor
R. silver clip
R. skull perforator set
R. spinal rongeur
R. stem clamp
R. surgical catgut
R. suture clip
R. suturing needle
R. tracheostomy cannula
R. trigeminal knife
R. tuning fork
R. Universal trocar
R. uterine curette
R. uterine sound
R. vaginal speculum
R. vessel clamp
R. wire guide pin
R. wire saw
Rica-Adson forceps
Ricard abdominal retractor
Rice pick
Richard
R. Gruber speculum
R. pillow
R. Wolf arthroscope
R. Wolf laparoscopic trocar
R. Wolf Medical Instruments
diagnostic laparoscope
R. Wolf Medical Instruments
operating laparoscope
R. Wolf nasal epistaxis system
R. Wolf video resectoscope
Richard-Allan surgical ruler
Richards
R. abdominal retractor
R. bone clamp
R. bone curette
R. bone hook

Richards *(continued)*
- R. bone tap
- R. chisel
- R. classic compression hip screw
- R. Colles fracture frame
- R. combination mallet
- R. drape
- R. drill guide
- R. ethmoid curette
- R. fixation staple
- R. fixator system
- R. forceps
- R. headrest
- R. hip endoprosthesis system
- R. hydroxyapatite PORP
- R. hydroxyapatite PORP prosthesis
- R. hydroxyapatite TORP prosthesis
- R. lag screw compression device
- R. locking rod
- R. mastoid curette
- R. maximum contact cruciate-sparing prosthesis
- R. ministaple
- R. modular hip system
- R. Phillips screwdriver
- R. pistol-grip drill
- R. probe
- R. sideplate plate
- R. Solcotrans orthopaedic drainage-reinfusion system
- R. Solcotrans Plus
- R. Solcotrans Plus drainage system
- R. tamp
- R. tonsillar forceps
- R. wire twister
- R. Zirconia femoral head prosthesis

Richards-Andrews forceps
Richards-Cobb
- R.-C. spinal elevator
- R.-C. spinal gouge

Richards-Hibbs
- R.-H. chisel
- R.-H. gouge
- R.-H. osteotome

Richards-Hirschhorn plate
Richards-Lovejoy bone drill
Richards-Moeller pneumatic air-filled dilator
Richardson
- R. abdominal retractor
- R. appendectomy retractor
- R. periosteal elevator
- R. polyethylene tube introducer
- R. rod
- R. shaver

Richardson-Eastman double-ended retractor
Riches
- R. artery forceps
- R. bladder syringe
- R. diathermy forceps

Richet
- R. bandage
- R. dressing

Rich forceps
Richie brace
Rich-Mar 510 external ultrasound
Richmond
- R. bolt
- R. forceps
- R. subarachnoid screw
- R. subarachnoid screw sensor
- R. subarachnoid twist drill
- R. subarachnoid wrench

Richnau-Holmgren ear speculum
Richter
- R. bone drill
- R. forceps
- R. laminectomy punch
- R. scissors
- R. screwdriver
- R. vaginal retractor

Richter-Heath clip-removing forceps
Richwil
- R. bridge remover
- R. crown remover

Rickett facebow
Rickham
- R. cup
- R. reservoir
- R. reservoir shunt

rickshaw rehab exerciser
Riddle coagulator
Rider-Moeller
- R.-M. cardiac dilator
- R.-M. needle

ridge forceps
Ridley
- R. anterior chamber lens implant
- R. forceps
- R. Mark II lens implant

Ridlon
- R. plaster knife
- R. spreader

Ridpath ethmoid curette
Riecken PQ premium heel cup
Riecker-Kleinsasser laryngoscope
Riecker respiration bronchoscope
Riedel
- R. corneal needle

Riepe-Bard gastric balloon
Riester otoscope
Rife machine
Rigby
- R. abdominal retractor
- R. appendectomy retractor
- R. bivalve retractor
- R. rectal retractor
- R. vaginal retractor

Rigg cannula
RIGHT
- RIGHT 3200 Advantage ultrasound scanner

right
- R. Clip applier
- r. Judkins catheter
- R. Light examination light
- r. ventricular assist device (RVAD)

r. ventricular coil
r. ventricular wall device
right-angle
r.-a. bipolar cautery
r.-a. blunt probe
r.-a. booster clip
r.-a. chest catheter
r.-a. chest tube
r.-a. colon clamp
r.-a. curette
r.-a. drill
r.-a. electrode
r.-a. elevator
r.-a. erysiphake
r.-a. examining telescope
r.-a. forceps
r.-a. hook
r.-a. knife
r.-a. pick
r.-a. retractor
r.-a. scissors
r.-a. screwdriver
right-angled telescopic lens
right-handed corneal scissors
rigid
r. biopsy forceps
r. curette
r. endoscope
r. endosonography probe
r. external distraction system
r. gas-permeable contact lens
r. holding rod
r. internal fixation device
r. intranasal endoscope
r. intraocular lens
r. kidney stone forceps
r. pedicle screw
r. postoperative brace
r. sigmoidoscope
r. sound
r. ventriculoscope
Rigidometer
Digital Inflection R.
Rigiflator hand-held inflation/deflation device
Rigiflex
R. ABD balloon dilatation catheter
R. achalasia balloon
R. achalasia balloon dilator
R. biliary balloon dilatation catheter
R. esophageal TTS
R. OTW balloon dilatation catheter
R. TTS balloon
R. TTS balloon dilatation catheter
R. TTS balloon dilator
RigiScan
R. device
R. penile tumescence and rigidity monitor
RIGS system stem
RIJ catheter
RIK
RIK Defender prevention mattress
RIK fluid mattress
RIK fluid overlay
RIK foothugger
RIK FootHugger fluid heel boot
Riley
R. arterial needle
ring
r. abdominal retractor
Ace-Colles half r.
AnnuloFlex flexible annuloplasty r.
r. applicator
r. bayonet Rand curette
Bickel r.
R. biliary drainage catheter
r. biliary stent
biofragmentable anastomotic r.
blepharostat r.
Bloomberg SuperNumb anesthetic r.
Bonaccolto-Flieringa scleral r.
Bonaccolto scleral r.
Bookwalter retractor r.
Bookwalter segmented r.
Bookwalter vaginal retractor r.
Bores twist fixation r.
Brown-Roberts-Wells base r.
Budde halo r.
Burr corneal r.
Buzard-Thornton fixation r.
Carpentier r.
Carpentier-Edwards Physio annuloplasty r.
cataract mask r.
r. cataract mask eye shield
r. cataract mask shield
CBI stereotactic r.
centering r.
Charnley centering r.
r. clamp
r. clip
confidence r.
constriction r.
Cook continence r.
corneal r.
corneal transplant centering r.
Cosman-Roberts-Wells stereotactic r.
Crawford suture r.
r. cushion
r. cutter
double-flanged valve sewing r.
R. drainage catheter needle
Duran annuloplasty r.
elastic O r.
r. electrode
Estring estradiol vaginal r.
Estring silicone vaginal r.
Falope tubal sterilization r.
Fine crescent fixation r.
Fine-Thornton scleral fixation r.
fixation r.
Fleischer r.
Flieringa fixation r.
Flieringa-Kayser fixation r.
Flieringa-LeGrand fixation r.
Flieringa scleral r.
foam r.
r. forceps
Gimbel stabilizing r.

ring *(continued)*
   Girard scleral r.
   gold r.
   half r.
   head r.
   R. hip prosthesis
   Ilizarov r.
   Intacs intrastromal corneal r.
   intravaginal r.
   invalid r.
   Japanese erection r.
   Katena r.
   Kayser-Fleischer r.
   KeraVision Intacs intracorneal r.
   KF r.
   R. knee prosthesis
   knitted sewing r.
   Landers irrigating vitrectomy r.
   Landolt C r.
   laparotomy sponge r.
   r. lens expressor
   Lyon r.
   Magrina-Bookwalter vaginal
     retractor r.
   Martinez corneal transplant
     centering r.
   Martinez scleral centering r.
   Mayo perfusing "O" r.
   McKinney fixation r.
   McNeill-Goldmann blepharostat r.
   McNeill-Goldmann scleral r.
   Mertz keratoscopy r.
   metal sewing r.
   Moran-Karaya r.
   Moretsky LASIK hinge protector
     fixation r.
   Mose concentric r.
   Nakayama r.
   Nichamin fixation r.
   Ochsner r.
   olive r.
   Osbon pressure-point tension r.
   pediatric perineal retractor r.
   perfusion O r.
   r. pessary
   placido r.
   plastic sewing r.
   pressure r.
   pressure-point tension r.
   prosthetic valve sewing r.
   Puig Massana-Shiley annuloplasty r.
   Racestyptine retraction r.
   reduction r.
   r. remover
   retainer r.
   retention r.
   retraction r.
   r. retractor blade
   Schatzki r.
   scleral expander r.
   Sculptor annuloplasty r.
   Sculptor flexible annuloplasty r.
   sewing r.
   Silastic r.
   silicone elastomer r.
   sizing r.
   SJM Sequin annuloplasty r.
   SJM Tailor annuloplasty r.
   sponge r.
   St. Jude annuloplasty r.
   r. stripper
   Suarz continence r.
   suction r.
   suture r.
   symblepharon r.
   Tano r.
   tantalum "O" r.
   Thornton-Fine r.
   Thornton fixating r.
   Tolentino r.
   r. tongue blade
   Tru-Arc blood vessel r.
   Turner-Warwick adult retractor r.
   Turner-Warwick pediatric perineal
     retractor r.
   vacuum fixation r.
   Valtrac absorbable biofragmentable
     anastomosis r.
   V1 halo r.
   Villasenor-Navarro fixation r.
   Waldeyer r.
   Walsh pressure r.
   Wolf-Yoon r.
   Yoon tubal sterilization r.
   zipper r.
ring-curette
   Fukushima r.-c.
ring-cutting saw
Ring-Derlan TM biliary endoprosthesis
ringed formed forceps
Ringenberg
   R. electrode
   R. rasp
   R. stapedectomy forceps
ring-handled bulldog clamp
ring-jawed holding clamp
RingLoc
   R. acetabular series
   R. instrument
Ring-McLean
   R.-M. catheter
   R.-M. sump tube
ring-rotation forceps
ring-tip forceps
ring-type
   ring-type imaging system
   ring-type rigidity measuring device
Rinn
   R. XCP film holder
   R. XCP radiographic paralleling
     device
Rionet hearing aid
Riordan
   R. flexible silver cannula
   R. pin
rip-cord suture
RIP plethysmograph

Ripstein
  R. arterial forceps
  R. tissue forceps
Rish
  R. cartilage knife
  R. chisel
  R. osteotome
Risley
  R. pliers
  R. rotary prism
Rispi Micromega reamer
Risser
  R. cast table
  R. frame
  R. localizer
  R. localizer scoliosis cast
  R. turnbuckle cast
  R. wedging jacket
Risser-Cotrel body cast
Rissler
  R. kidney retractor
  R. mallet
  R. periosteal elevator
  R. pin
  R. vein sound
Rissler-Stille pin
Ristow osteotome
Ritch
  R. contact lens
  R. nylon suture laser lens
  R. trabeculoplasty laser lens
Ritchey nail starter
Ritchie
  R. catheter
  R. cleft palate tenaculum
  R. nail starter
Ritch-Krupin-Denver eye valve insertion forceps
RiteBite biopsy forceps
Ritleng probe
Ritter
  R. Bovie
  R. coagulator
  R. coagulator electrosurgical unit
  R. forceps
  R. meatal dilator
  R. rasp
  R. sound
  R. suprapubic suction drain
  R. suprapubic suction tube
Ritter-Bantam
  R.-B. Bovie coagulator
  R.-B. Bovie electrosurgical unit
Riva Rocci sphygmomanometer
Rivas vascular catheter
Riverbank Laboratories tuning fork
rivet
  r. gun
  pop r.
Riwomat respirator jet
Riza-Ribe needle
Rizzo
  R. dorsal implant
  R. retractor
Rizzoli osteoclast

Rizzuti
  R. double-prong forceps
  R. fixation forceps
  R. graft carrier spatula
  R. graft carrier spoon
  R. iris expressor
  R. iris retractor
  R. keratoplasty scissors
  R. lens expressor
  R. refractor
  R. scleral forceps
  R. superior rectus forceps
Rizzuti-Bonaccolto instruments
Rizzuti-Fleischer instruments
Rizzuti-Furness cornea-holding forceps
Rizzuti-Kayser-Fleischer instruments
Rizzuti-Lowe instruments
Rizzuti-Maxwell instruments
Rizzuti-McGuire corneal section scissors
Rizzuti-Soemmering instrument
Rizzuti-Spizziri cannula knife
Rizzuti-Verhoeff forceps
RK marker
r\LS red blood cell filtration system
RLS videostroboscopy system
R-Med
  R.-M. mini-retractor
  R.-M. plug
RNA probe
R-N clamp
Roach
  R. ball precision attachment
  R. clasp
Roadmapper
  FluoroPlus R.
Roadrunner
  R. PC guidewire
  R. wire
Roane bullet tip
Robb
  R. antral cannula
  R. needle
  R. tonsillar forceps
  R. tonsillar knife
Robbins
  R. Acrotorque hand engine
  R. automatic tourniquet
Robb-Roberts rotary rasp
Robert
  R. Jones bandage
  R. Jones bulky soft compressive dressing
  R. Jones splint
  R. nasal snare
Robertazzi nasopharyngeal airway
Roberts
  R. abdominal trocar
  R. applicator
  R. arterial forceps
  R. bronchial forceps
  R. dental implant
  R. episiotomy scissors
  R. esophageal speculum
  R. folding esophagoscope
  R. headrest

Roberts *(continued)*
  R. hemostatic forceps
  R. hip dissecting chisel
  R. needle
  R. oval esophagoscope
  R. oval speculum
  R. self-retaining laryngoscope
  R. thumb retractor
Roberts-Gill periosteal elevator
Robertshaw
  R. bag resuscitator
  R. tube
Roberts-Jesberg esophagoscope
Roberts-Nelson
  R.-N. lobectomy tourniquet
  R.-N. rib stripper
Robertson
  R. corneal trephine
  R. suprapubic drain
  R. tonsillar forceps
  R. tonsillar knife
Roberts-Singley
  R.-S. dressing forceps
  R.-S. thumb forceps
Robicsek vascular probe
Robin
  R. chalazion clamp
  R. orthodontic plate
Robinject needle injector
Robin-Masse abdominal retractor
Robinson
  R. artificial pneumothorax apparatus
  R. bag
  R. equalizing tube
  R. flap knife
  R. incus replacement prosthesis
  R. lung retractor
  R. middle ear prosthesis
  R. piston prosthesis
  R. pocket arthrometer
  R. stapes prosthesis
  R. stone basket
  R. stone dislodger
  R. strut
  R. urethral catheter
Robinson-Moon
  R.-M. prosthesis inserter
  R.-M. stapes prosthesis
Robinson-Moon-Lippy stapes prosthesis
Robinson-Smith
  R.-S. needle
  R.-S. tamp
Robles cutting point cannula
Robodoc
  Robodoc system
  R. robot
Roboprep G instrument
robot
  Aesop 2000, 3000 endoscopic stabilizer r.
  automated endoscopic system for optimal positioning surgical r.
  Long Beach stereotactic r.
  Minerva r.

  Robodoc r.
  R. Starr II camera
  Zeus r.
robotic-automated assist device
robotics-controlled stereotactic frame
Robotrac passive retraction system
Robson intestinal forceps
ROC
  ROC XS suture anchor
  ROC XS suture fastener
Rocabado posture gauge
Rochester
  R. aortic vent needle
  R. atrial septal retractor
  R. awl
  R. bone trephine
  R. bone trephine device
  R. colonial retractor
  R. dressing
  R. gallstone forceps
  R. harvest bone cutter
  R. hip-knee-ankle-foot orthosis
  R. HKAFO prosthesis
  R. hook clamp
  R. lamina elevator
  R. laminar dissector
  R. Medical self-adhering male external catheter
  R. Medical 100% silicone Foley catheter
  R. mitral stenosis knife
  R. needle holder
  R. oral tissue forceps
  R. rake retractor
  R. recipient bone cutter
  R. Russian tissue forceps
  R. scissors
  R. sigmoid clamp
  R. spinal elevator
  R. suction tube
  R. syringe
  R. tissue forceps
  R. tracheal tube
Rochester-Carmalt hysterectomy forceps
Rochester-Davis forceps
Rochester-Ewald tissue forceps
Rochester-Ferguson
  R.-F. double-ended retractor
  R.-F. scissors
Rochester-Harrington forceps
Rochester-Kocher clamp
Rochester-Meeker needle
Rochester-Mixter
  R.-M. arterial forceps
  R.-M. gall duct forceps
Rochester-Mueller forceps
Rochester-Ochsner
  R.-O. forceps
  R.-O. hemostat
  R.-O. scissors
Rochester-Péan
  R.-P. clamp
  R.-P. hemostat
  R.-P. hysterectomy forceps
Rochester-Rankin arterial forceps

Rochette bridge
Rock
    R. ankle exercise board
    R. endometrial suction curette
    R. & Roller exercise board
rocker
    r. board
    r. boot
    Carolina r.
    hematology r.
    r. knife
    Uniplane r.
rocker-bottom cast boot shoe
Rockert dilator
Rockey
    R. dilating probe
    R. endoscope
    R. forceps
    R. mediastinal cannula
    R. tracheal cannula
    R. vascular clamp
Rockey-Thompson catheter
Rock-Mulligan prosthesis
Rockwood shoulder screw
rocky boat exerciser
rod
    Alta CFX reconstruction r.
    Alta femoral intramedullary r.
    Alta humeral r.
    Alta intramedullary r.
    Alta reconstruction r.
    Alta tibial r.
    r. bender
    Bickel intramedullary r.
    Biofix absorbable r.
    Biofix fixation r.
    cloverleaf r.
    cold rolled r.
    colostomy r.
    compression r.
    condyle r.
    Cotrel-Dubousset pediatric r.
    r. cutter
    Danek r.
    degradable polyglycolide r.
    Delrin push r.
    Delta r.
    distraction r.
    double-L spinal r.
    dual square-ended Harrington r.
    Edwards-Levine r.
    Edwards Universal r.
    r. electrode
    enamel r.
    Ender r.
    Enneking r.
    Fixateur Interne r.
    flared spinal r.
    glass retracting r.
    Green-Armytage polythene r.
    Hamby r.
    Harrington dual square-ended r.
    Harris condylocephalic r.
    r. holder
    Hopkins r.

House measuring r.
Hunter tendon r.
impactor r.
impingement r.
intramedullary alignment r.
intramedullary Rush r.
Isola spinal implant system eye r.
Jackson r.
Jacobs distraction r.
Jacobs locking hook spinal r.
Kaneda r.
Knodt distraction r.
Kostuik r.
Küntscher r.
laser r.
Lincoff sponge r.
Luque r.
Maddox r.
McLaughlin laser vaginal
    measuring r.
McLaughlin quartz r.
measuring r.
Meckel r.
medullary r.
Mira silicone r.
modified Harrington r.
Moe modified Harrington r.
Moe subcutaneous r.
Moore measuring r.
Moss r.
Mouradian humeral r.
Olerud PSF r.
orthopedic r.
pediatric Cotrel-Dubousset r.
Perspex r.
Polarus humeral r.
precontoured unit r.
quartz r.
radiotranslucent r.
retracting r.
Richards locking r.
Richardson r.
rigid holding r.
Rogozinski r.
round-ended distraction r.
round extension r.
Rush r.
Russell-Taylor delta r.
Schneider r.
scleral sponge r.
screw alignment r.
silicone flexor r.
SinuScope rigid r.
slotted intramedullary r.
spinal r.
square-ended distraction r.
Stader connecting r.
Stenzel fracture r.
sterile transverse r.
R. TAG suture anchor system
telescoping r.
r. template
thermoluminescent dosimeter r.
threaded r.
unit spinal r.

rod *(continued)*
    vaginal laser measuring r.
    Veirs canaliculus r.
    Williams r.
    Wiltse system spinal r.
    Wissinger r.
    Zickel II subtrochanteric r.
    Zickel supracondylar r.
    Zielke r.
Rodenstock
    R. panfundoscope
    R. panfundus lens
    R. scanning laser ophthalmoscope
    R. slit lamp
    R. system
rod-hook construct
Rodin orbital implant
rod-lens system
Rodriguez-Alvarez catheter
Rodriguez catheter
Roe aortic tourniquet clamp
Roeder
    R. forceps
    R. manipulative aptitude test device
    R. towel clamp
Roeltsch forceps
Roentgen
    R. knife
    R. knife stereotaxic radiosurgical device
    R. meter
roentgenographic opaque marker
Rogan teleradiology system
Roger
    R. Anderson apparatus
    R. Anderson external skeletal fixation device
    R. Anderson fixation bar
    R. Anderson pin
    R. Anderson pin fixation appliance
    R. Anderson well-leg splint
    R. septal elevator
    R. septal knife
    R. submucous dissector
    R. system
    R. vascular-toothed hysterectomy forceps
    R. wire-cutting scissors
Rogers
    R. mammotome
    R. needle holder
    R. sphygmomanometer
    R. wire cutter
Rogozinski
    R. hook
    R. rod
    R. screw system
    R. spinal fixation system
    R. spinal rod system
Rohadur gait plate
Rohadur-Polydor orthotic
Rohadur-Schaefer orthotic
Rohadur-Whitman orthotic

Rohm and Haas PMMA intraocular lens
Roho
    R. bed
    R. Dry Flotation wheelchair pad
    R. heel pad
    R. heel protector
    R. high-profile cushion
    R. mattress
    R. Pack-It cushion
    R. pediatric seating system
    R. solid seat insert
Rohrschneider
    R. cannula
    R. probe
Roland dilator
rolandometer
Rolf
    R. jeweler's forceps
    R. lacrimal probe
    R. lance
    R. lance needle
    R. muscle hook
    R. punctum dilator
    R. utility forceps
Rolf-Jackson cannula
roll
    ACCO cotton r.
    Akton positioning r.
    Celluron dental r.
    cervical r.
    r. control bolster
    Dutchman's r.
    Fluftex gauze r.
    intrascapular r.
    Kerlix bandage r.
    Kling fluff r.
    Krinkle gauze r.
    Lakeside cotton r.
    lumbar r.
    McKenzie cervical r.
    McKenzie lumbar r.
    McKenzie night r.
    Medline r.
    3M Reston self-adhering foam pad & r.
    narrow gauze r.
    neck r.
    octagon r.
    silver mylar r.
    Skillbuilder half r.
    Stretch gauze r.
    Tensor elastic bandage r.
    Tumble Forms r.
    Veratex cotton r.
Roll-A-Bout mobility device
Rollator Nova walker
rolled Instat stent
roller
    r. bandage
    Devonshire r.
    r. dressing
    r. electrode
    r. forceps
    r. head perfusion pump

r. knife
r. pump
Spence cranioplastic r.
Toledo r.
tubing hand r.
RollerBack self-massage device
rollerball
roller-bar electrode
roller-barrel electrode
Rollerbottom Xtra Depth shoe
Roller pump suction tube
Rollet
R. anterior chamber irrigator
R. chisel
R. eye retractor
R. I&A unit
R. lacrimal probe
R. lacrimal sac retractor
R. lake retractor
R. refractor
R. rugine
R. skin retractor
R. strabismus hook
Rollocane
Rolloscope II
Rolnel catheter
Rolodermatome dermatome
Rolon spatula
Rolyan
R. arm elevator
R. Firm D-Ring wrist support
R. foot support
R. Gel Shell splint
R. Reach-N-Range pulley system
R. tibial fracture brace
Rolz massage tool
Roman laryngostat
Romano
R. curved surgical drill
R. surgical curved drilling system
romanoscope
Romhilt-Estes point scoring system
ROM knee brace
Rommel
R. cautery
R. electrocautery
Rommel-Hildreth
R.-H. cautery
R.-H. electrocautery
Rondic sponge dressing
Rondo inhaler
rongeur
Adson bone r.
Adson cranial r.
Andrews-Hartmann r.
Bacon cranial bone r.
Baer bone r.
Bailey aortic valve r.
Bane bone r.
Bane-Hartmann bone r.
Bane mastoid r.
Belz lacrimal sac r.
Beyer bone r.
Beyer endaural r.
Beyer laminectomy r.

Beyer-Lempert r.
Beyer-Stille bone r.
biting r.
Blakesley laminectomy r.
Blumenthal bone r.
Bogle r.
Böhler r.
Boies-Lombard mastoid r.
bone-biting r.
bone-cutting r.
bone punch r.
Bruening-Citelli r.
Bucy laminectomy r.
Cairns r.
Callahan lacrimal r.
Campbell laminectomy r.
Campbell nerve r.
Carroll r.
Caspar r.
cervical r.
Cherry-Kerrison laminectomy r.
Cicherelli bone r.
Citelli sphenoid r.
Cleveland bone r.
Cloward-English r.
Cloward-Harper laminectomy r.
Cloward intervertebral disk r.
Cloward laminectomy r.
Cloward pituitary r.
Codman cervical r.
Codman-Kerrison laminectomy r.
Codman laminectomy r.
Codman-Leksell laminectomy r.
Codman-Schlesinger cervical
    laminectomy r.
Cohen r.
Colclough laminectomy r.
Colclough-Love-Kerrison
    laminectomy r.
Converse-Lange r.
Converse nasal root r.
Corbett bone r.
Costen-Kerrison r.
Cottle-Jansen r.
cranial bone r.
Cushing bone r.
Cushing intervertebral disk r.
Cushing laminectomy r.
Cushing pituitary r.
Dahlgren r.
Dale first rib r.
Dale thoracic r.
Dawson-Yuhl-Kerrison r.
Dawson-Yuhl-Leksell r.
Dean bone r.
Decker microsurgical r.
Defourmental bone r.
Defourmental nasal r.
delicate intervertebral disk r.
Dench r.
dental r.
DePuy pituitary r.
DeVilbiss cranial r.
disk r.
double-action r.

rongeur *(continued)*
down-cutting r.
duckbill r.
Duggan r.
Echlin duckbill r.
Echlin laminectomy r.
end-biting blunt-nosed r.
Falconer r.
Ferris Smith disk r.
Ferris Smith-Gruenwald r.
Ferris Smith intervertebral disk r.
Ferris Smith-Kerrison disk r.
Ferris Smith-Kerrison laminectomy r.
Ferris Smith pituitary r.
Ferris Smith-Spurling disk r.
Ferris Smith-Takahashi r.
flat-bottomed Kerrison r.
FlexTip intervertebral r.
r. forceps
Friedman bone r.
Frykholm bone r.
Fukushima r.
Fulton laminectomy r.
Gam-Mer r.
Glover r.
Goldman-Kazanjian r.
gooseneck r.
Gruenwald-Love intervertebral
  disk r.
Gruenwald pituitary r.
Guleke bone r.
Hajek antral r.
Hajek-Claus r.
Hajek downbiting r.
Hajek-Koffler laminectomy r.
Hajek-Koffler sphenoidal r.
Hajek upbiting r.
Hakansson bone r.
Hakansson-Olivecrona r.
Hardy r.
Hartmann bone r.
Hartmann ear r.
Hartmann-Herzfeld ear r.
Hartmann mastoid r.
Hein r.
Henny laminectomy r.
Hoen intervertebral disk r.
Hoen laminectomy r.
Hoen pituitary r.
Hoffmann ear r.
Horsley cranial bone r.
Houghton r.
Husk mastoid r.
intervertebral disk r.
Ivy mastoid r.
Jackson intervertebral disk r.
Jansen bayonet r.
Jansen bone r.
Jansen-Cottle r.
Jansen ear r.
Jansen-Middleton r.
Jansen-Zaufel r.
Jarit-Kerrison r.
Jarit-Ruskin r.

jaw r.
Juers-Lempert endaural r.
Kazanjian-Goldman r.
Kerrison cervical r.
Kerrison-Costen r.
Kerrison-Ferris Smith r.
Kerrison lumbar r.
Kerrison mastoid r.
Kerrison-Morgenstein r.
Kerrison-Schwartz r.
Kerrison-Spurling r.
Killearn r.
Kleinert-Kutz bone r.
Kleinert-Kutz synovectomy r.
Koffler-Hajek laminectomy r.
lacrimal sac r.
laminectomy r.
Lange-Converse nasal root r.
Lebsche r.
Leksell bone r.
Leksell cardiovascular r.
Leksell laminectomy r.
Leksell-Stille thoracic r.
Lempert bone r.
Lempert endaural r.
Lempert-Juers r.
Lillie r.
Liston-Littauer r.
Liston-Luer-Whiting r.
Littauer r.
Littauer-West r.
Lombard r.
Lombard-Beyer r.
Lombard-Boies mastoid r.
Love-Gruenwald cranial r.
Love-Gruenwald intervertebral
  disk r.
Love-Gruenwald laminectomy r.
Love-Gruenwald pituitary r.
Love-Kerrison r.
Love pituitary r.
Lowman r.
Luer bone r.
Luer-Friedman bone r.
Luer-Hartmann r.
Luer-Liston-Wheeling r.
Luer-Stille r.
Luer thoracic r.
Luer-Whiting r.
Markwalder bone r.
Markwalder rib r.
Marquardt bone r.
mastoid r.
Mead bone r.
Mead dental r.
micropituitary r.
Middleton r.
Mollison mastoid r.
Montenovesi cranial r.
Morgenstein-Kerrison r.
narrow-bite bone r.
needle-nose r.
Nichols infundibulectomy r.
Nicola pituitary r.
Noyes r.

O'Brien r.
Oldberg intervertebral disk r.
Oldberg laminectomy r.
Oldberg pituitary r.
Olivecrona endaural r.
orthopedic r.
peapod intervertebral disk r.
Peiper-Beyer bone r.
Pennybacker r.
Pierce r.
Pilling-Ruskin r.
pituitary r.
Poppen intervertebral disk r.
Poppen laminectomy r.
Poppen pituitary r.
Prince r.
punch r.
Quervain r.
Raaf-Oldberg r.
Raney laminectomy r.
rat-tooth r.
Reiner r.
Rica bone r.
Rica cranial r.
Rica laminectomy r.
Rica mastoid r.
Rica spinal r.
Ronjair air-powered r.
Röttgen-Ruskin bone r.
round-nosed r.
Rowland nasal r.
Ruskin bone r.
Ruskin duckbill r.
Ruskin-Jay r.
Ruskin mastoid r.
Ruskin multiple-action r.
Ruskin-Storz r.
Sauerbruch r.
Sauerbruch-Coryllos rib r.
Sauerbruch-Lebsche r.
Scaglietti r.
Schlesinger cervical r.
Schlesinger intervertebral disk r.
Schlesinger laminectomy r.
Schwartz-Kerrison r.
Selverstone intervertebral disk r.
Selverstone laminectomy r.
Semb r.
Semb-Sauerbruch r.
Shearer bone r.
side-cutting r.
single-action r.
SMIC bone r.
SMIC cranial r.
SMIC laminectomy r.
SMIC mastoid r.
Smith-Petersen laminectomy r.
Smolik curved r.
Smolinski endaural r.
Spence intervertebral disk r.
Spurling intervertebral disk r.
Spurling-Kerrison r.
Spurling laminectomy r.
Spurling-Love-Gruenwald-Cushing r.
Spurling pituitary r.

Stellbrink synovectomy r.
Stille-Beyer r.
Stille bone r.
Stille-Horsley r.
Stille-Leksell r.
Stille-Liston r.
Stille-Luer angular duckbill r.
Stille-Luer bone r.
Stille-Luer-Echlin r.
Stille-Ruskin r.
Stille-Zaufal-Jansen r.
St. Luke's double-action r.
Stookey cranial r.
Storz duckbill r.
Struempel r.
Strully-Kerrison r.
Super Cut laminectomy r.
synovectomy r.
Takahashi r.
taper-jaw r.
Tiedmann r.
Tobey ear r.
Universal Kerrison r.
Urschel r.
Urschel-Leksell r.
von Seemen r.
Voris intervertebral disk r.
Wagner r.
Walton r.
Walton-Ruskin r.
Watson-Williams intervertebral
  disk r.
Weil-Blakesley r.
Weil pituitary r.
Weingartner r.
Whitcomb-Kerrison r.
Whiting mastoid r.
Wilde intervertebral disk r.
Young cystoscopic r.
Zaufal bone r.
Zaufel-Jansen bone r.

Ronis
  R. adenoidal punch
  R. cutting forceps
  R. tonsillar punch
Ronjair air-powered rongeur
**roof-reinforcement ring hip arthroplasty
  component**
roof wedge
Rooke perioperative boot
room humidifier
Roos
  R. brachial plexus root retractor
  R. first rib shears
Roosen clamp
Roosevelt
  R. gastroenterostomy clamp
  R. gastrointestinal clamp
root
  r. canal broach
  r. canal drill
  r. canal file
  r. canal spreader
  r. high-pull facebow
  r. needle

R

root *(continued)*
    r. pliers
    r. rubber dam clamp
    R. ZX apex locator
    R. ZX ultrasonic unit
root-form
    r.-f. dental implant
    r.-f. device
rope
    Bard AlgiDERM r.
    Kaltostat r.
Roper alpha-chymotrypsin cannula
Roper-Hall
    R.-H. localizer
    R.-H. locator
Roper-Rumel tourniquet
Rosa-Berens orbital implant
rosary bougie
Rosato fascial splitter
Rosch catheter
Roschke dropper sponge
Rosch-Thurmond fallopian tube catheterization set
Rose
    R. bed dressing
    R. disimpaction forceps
    R. double-ended retractor
    R. L-type nose bridge prosthesis
    R. tracheal retractor
Rosebud dissector
rosehead bur
Rosen
    R. angular elevator
    R. bayonet separator
    R. bur
    R. cartilage knife
    R. dissector
    R. ear incision knife
    R. ear probe
    R. endaural probe
    R. fenestrator
    R. fenestrometer
    R. incontinence device
    R. inflatable urinary incontinence prosthesis
    R. J-guide guidewire
    R. knife curette
    R. middle ear instrument
    R. needle
    R. nucleus paddle
    R. phaco splitter
    R. pick
    R. splint
    R. suction
    R. suction tube
Rosenbaum
    R. iris retractor
    R. pocket vision screener
Rosenbaum-Drews
    R.-D. iris retractor
    R.-D. plastic retractor
Rosenberg
    R. dissecting cannula
    R. dissector tip

    R. full-radius blade synovial retractor
    R. gynecomastia dissection instrument
    R. meniscal repair kit
Rosenberg-Sampson retractor
Rosenblatt scissors
Rosenblum rotating adapter
Rosenfeld hip prosthesis
Rosenmüller curette
Rosenthal
    R. aspiration needle
    R. urethral speculum
Rosenthal-French nebulization dosimeter
Roser
    R. mouthgag
    R. needle
Roser-Koenig mouthgag
rosette
    r. blade
    R. strain gauge
Rosner tonometer
Ross
    R. aortic valve retractor
    R. catheter
    R. needle
    R. pulmonary porcine valve
Rosser
    R. crypt hook
    R. signature series
Rossmax automatic wristwatch blood pressure monitor
Rotablator
    R. atherectomy device
    Heart Technology R.
    R. rotating bur
    R. system
    R. wire
Rotacamera
Rotacs
    R. guidewire
    R. motorized catheter
    R. rotational atherectomy device
    R. system
Rotaflex exerciser
Rotafloppy wire
Rotaglide total knee system
Rotahaler
Rotalok
    R. acetabular cup
    R. skin retractor
    R. wrist strap
rotary
    r. basket
    r. bur
    r. cutting instrument
    r. dissector
    r. hub saw
    r. scissors with cigar handle
    r. scissors with loop handle
rotatable
    r. coupling head
    r. polypectomy snare
    r. transsphenoidal enucleator

r. transsphenoidal horizontal ring curette
r. transsphenoidal knife handle
r. transsphenoidal right-angle hook
r. transsphenoidal round dissector
r. transsphenoidal spatula dissector
r. transsphenoidal vertical ring curette

rotating
r. adapter
r. air impactor
r. anode tube
r. arm impactor
r. brush
r. endo-scissors
r. forceps
r. gamma camera
r. hemostatic valve
r. laryngoscope
r. mechanism
r. morcellator
r. speculum anoscope
r. transilluminator
r. turner

rotating-hinge knee prosthesis
rotating-type cutter
rotational
r. ablation laser
r. atherectomy device
r. dynamic air therapy bed

rotation-stop washer
rotator
Bechert-Hoffer nucleus r.
Bechert nucleus r.
Hosmer above-knee r.
Howmedica monotube external r.
Jaffe-Bechert nucleus r.
Jarit r.
nucleus r.
Osher globe r.
Tennant nuclear ball r.

rotatory-variable-differential transducer
RotaWire
Rotex II biopsy needle
Roth
R. arch form
R. dental cement
R. endoscopy retrieval net
R. Grip-Tip suture guide
R. polyp retrieval net

Rothene catheter
Rothman
R.-Gilbard corneal punch
R. Institute femoral prosthesis
R. Institute porous femoral component

Rothon retractor
Roticulator
Cabot Optima laparoscopic R.
R. stapler

Roto
R. Kinetic bed
R. Rest delta kinetic therapy treatment table

RotoClix

rotoextractor
Douvas r.
roto-osteotome
rotor
Beckman J5.0 elutriation r.
Beckman JE-10X elutriation r.
Kontron TFT 45.6 r.
Ti r.
Roto-Rest bed
Rotorod sampler
rotoslide
Rotosnare device
rotosteotome rotary handpiece
Röttgen-Ruskin bone rongeur
Roubaix forceps
Roubin-Gianturco flexible coil stent
Roughton-Scholander
R.-S. apparatus
R.-S. syringe
rougine
round
r. body needle
r. chuck-end Kirschner wire
r. cutting bur
r. diamond bur
r. dissector
r. extension rod
r. Gigli saw
r. hole plate
r. optical zone marker
r. punch forceps
r. ruby knife
r. speculum
r. tapper
round-end cutter
round-ended distraction rod
round-handled forceps
round-loop electrode
round-nosed rongeur
round-tip
r.-t. catheter
r.-t. microscissors
round-tipped periosteal elevator
round-wire electrode
Rousek extender
Roush tonometer
Roussel-Fankhauser contact lens
router
power r.
trochanteric r.
Vortex r.
Roux
R. double-ended retractor
R. spatula
Roveda
R. lid everter
rove magnetic catheter
Rovenstine catheter-introducing forceps
Rowden uterine manipulator injector (RUMI)
Rowe
R. blanket
R. boathook retractor
R. bone-drilling forceps
R. bone elevator

R

Rowe *(continued)*
   R. disimpaction forceps
   R. glenoidal punch
   R. glenoidal reamer
   R. glenoid-reaming forceps
   R. humeral head retractor
   R. maxillary forceps
   R. modified-Harrison forceps
   R. orbital floor retractor
   R. scapular neck retractor
Rowe-Harrison bone-holding forceps
Rowe-Killey forceps
Rowen
   R. spatula
   R. spinal fusion gouge
Rowland
   R. double-action forceps
   R. hump forceps
   R. keratome
   R. nasal rongeur
   R. osteotome
   R. pouch
Rowland-Hughes osteotomy spline
Rowsey fixation cannula
Royal
   R. crown
   R. disposable skin stapler
   R. Flush angiographic flush catheter
   R. Hospital dilator
   R. spoon
Royale III denture resin
Royalite body jacket
Royalt-Street bougie
Roy-Camille plate
Royce
   R. bayonet ear knife
   R. forceps
   R. tympanum perforator
Roylan
   R. ergonomic hand exerciser
   R. Gel Shell spica splint
Royl-Derm
   R.-D. protectant powder
   R.-D. wound hydrogel nonadherent
      dressing
R-Port implantable vascular access
   system
RS4 pacemaker
RSDCP plate
R-synchronous VVT pacemaker
RT Advantage ultrasound
R-T nail
RT/SC 2000 frameless air support
   therapy
RTV total artificial heart
rubber
   r. acorn tip
   r. airway
   r. band ligator
   r. bite liner
   r. catheter
   r. drain
   r. finger cot
   r. Scan spray dressing

   r. shod clamp
   r. spa bowl
   r. spacer
   r. sponge
   r. suture
   r. walking heel
rubber-dam
   r.-d. clamp
   r.-d. drain
rubber-reinforced bandage
rubber-shod
   r.-s. catheter
   r.-s. forceps
Rubbs aortic dilator
Rubens pillow
Rubin
   R. blade
   R. bone planer
   R. bronchial clamp
   R. cartilage planer
   R. fallopian tube cannula
   R. gouge
   R. nasal chisel
   R. nasofrontal osteotome
   R. needle
   R. oblique rasp
   R. septal morcellizer
Rubin-Arnold needle
Rubin-Holth sclerectomy punch
Rubin-Lewis periosteal elevator
Rubinstein
   R. cryoextractor
   R. cryophake
   R. cryoprobe
   R. probe
Rubin-Wright forceps guard
Rubio
   R. needle holder
   R. scissors
   R. wire-holding clamp
Rubovits clamp
ruby
   r. diamond knife
   r. knife scalpel
   r. laser
Rudd
   R. Clinic hemorrhoidal forceps
   R. ligator
Rudderman "Frelevator" fragment
   elevator
Ruddock laparoscope
Ruddy
   R. dissector
   R. stapes calipers
   R. stapes prosthesis
Rudolf-Buck suturing device
Rudolph
   R. breathing system
   R. calibrated super syringe
   R. linear pneumotachometer
   R. mask
   R. one-way respiratory valve
   R. trowel retractor
Ruedemann
   R. eye implant

R. lacrimal dilator
R. tonometer
Ruedemann-Todd tendon tucker
Ruel forceps
Ruese bone graft
Rugby deep-surgery forceps
Rugelski arterial forceps
Ruggles
    R. microcurette
    R. surgical instruments
rugine
    Farabeuf r.
    Rollet r.
Ruiz
    R. adjustable marker
    R. fundal contact lens
    R. fundal laser lens
    R. microkeratome
    R. plano fundal lens
    R. plano fundal lens implant
Ruiz-Cohen round expander
Ruiz-Shepard marker
rulangemeter
ruler
    Berndt hip r.
    Bio-Pen biometric r.
    bronchoscopic r.
    r. calipers
    centimeter subtraction r.
    Charnow notched r.
    Helveston scleral marking r.
    Hyde astigmatism r.
    Hyde-Osher keratometric r.
    Joseph measuring r.
    Krinsky-Prince accommodation r.
    metal r.
    millimeter r.
    Pischel scleral r.
    Plexiglas radiographic r.
    Richard-Allan surgical r.
    Scott No. 2 curved r.
    stainless steel flexible r.
    steel r.
    Tabb r.
    Thornton corneal press-on r.
    Thornton double corneal r.
    ulnar r.
    V. Mueller r.
    Walker scleral r.
    Webster r.
    Weck astigmatism r.
Rultract internal mammary artery
    retractor
Rumel
    R. aluminum bridge splint
    R. cardiovascular tourniquet
    R. catheter
    R. dissecting forceps
    R. lobectomy forceps
    R. myocardial clamp
    R. ratchet tourniquet
    R. ratchet tourniquet eyed stylet
    R. retractor
    R. rubber clamp
    R. thoracic clamp

R. thoracic forceps
R. tourniquet-eyed obturator
Rumel-Belmont tourniquet
Rumex titanium instruments
RUMI
    Rowden uterine manipulator injector
    RUMI uterine manipulator
Rumi
    R. uterine manipulation system
Rumison side port fixation occluder
running nylon penetrating keratoplasty
    suture
ruptured disk curette
Rusch
    R. bougie
    R. bronchial catheter
    R. cleaning brush
    R. coudé catheter
    R. endotracheal tube cuff
    R. esophageal stethoscope
    R. external catheter
    R. filiform
    R. follower
    R. head strap
    R. laryngectomy tube
    R. laryngoscope
    R. laryngoscope blade
    R. laryngoscope handle
    R. laryngoscope lamp
    R. leg bag
    R. mucous trap
    R. perineal drape
    R. red rubber rectal tube
    R. stent
Ruschelit
    R. catheter
    R. polyvinyl chloride endotracheal
    tube
    R. urethral bougie
Rusch-Foley catheter
Rush
    R. awl reamer
    R. bone clamp
    R. driver
    R. driver-bender-extractor
    R. extractor
    R. intramedullary fixation pin
    R. intramedullary nail
    R. mallet
    R. pin reamer awl
    R. rod
Rushkin balloon
Ruskin
    R. antral trocar
    R. antral trocar needle
    R. bone-cutting forceps
    R. bone rongeur
    R. duckbill rongeur
    R. mastoid rongeur
    R. multiple-action rongeur
    R. rongeur forceps
    R. sphenopalatine ganglion needle
Ruskin-Jay rongeur
Ruskin-Liston bone-cutting forceps
Ruskin-Rowland bone-cutting forceps

R

Ruskin-Storz rongeur
Russ
    R. tumor forceps
    R. vascular forceps
Russell
    R. forceps
    R. frame
    R. gastrostomy kit
    R. gastrostomy tray
    R. hydrostatic dilator
    R. hysterectomy forceps
    R. peel-away sheath dilator
    R. percutaneous endoscopic
    gastrostomy
    R. skeletal traction
    R. splint
    R. suction tube
    R. traction device
Russell-Beck extension tractor
Russell-Davis forceps
Russell-Taylor
    R.-T. delta rod
    R.-T. delta tibial nail
    R.-T. femoral interlocking nail
    system
    R.-T. interlocking medullary nail
    R.-T. interlocking nail
    instrumentation
    R.-T. screw
Russian
    R. four-pronged fixation hook
    R. Péan forceps
    R. thumb forceps
    R. tissue forceps
Rust amputation saw
Ruth-Hedwig
    R.-H. pneumothorax apparatus
    R.-H. splitter
Rutkow sutureless plug and patch
Rutner
    R. biopsy needle

    R. nephrostomy balloon catheter
    R. stone basket
    R. stone extractor
    R. wedge catheter
Rutzen ileostomy bag
Ruuska meniscotome
RVAD
    right ventricular assist device
    RVAD centrifugal right ventricular
    assist device
RWuCath
    IntraEAR Round Window u
    Cath R.
RX
    RX Herculink 14 premounted stent
    system
    RX perfusion catheter
    RX stent delivery system
    RX Streak balloon catheter
RX-014 balloon catheter
Rx5000 cardiac pacing system
Rychener-Weve electrode
Rycroft
    R. cannula
    R. lamp
    R. needle
    R. tying forceps
Rydell nail
Rydel-Seiffert tuning fork
Ryder
    R. needle holder
    R. scissors
Ryecroft retractor
Ryerson
    R. bone retractor
    R. bone skid
    R. tenotome
    R. tenotome knife
Ryle duodenal tube
RZ mandibular matrix system

S

S root canal file
S stylet
Saalfeld comedo extractor
Sabbatsberg septum elevator
Sabel cast walker
saber-back scissors
Saber CBF-ICP trauma sensor
Sabina lift
sable
    S. balloon catheter
    s. brush
Sableflex anterior chamber intraocular lens
Sabra OMS 45 dental handpiece
Sabreloc
    S. spatula needle
    S. suture
sac (*See also* sack)
    aortic s.
    Lap S.
    Pleatman s.
SACH
    SACH foot
    SACH foot adapter
    SACH orthopaedic appliance
    SACH prosthesis
Sachs
    S. angled vein retractor
    S. brain-exploring cannula
    S. cervical punch
    S. dural hook
    S. dural separator
    S. needle
    S. nerve separator
    S. skull bur
    S. spatula
    S. suction tube
    S. tissue forceps
    S. urethrotome
Sachs-Cushing retractor
Sachs-Freer dissector
sack
    entrapment s.
    LapSac collection s.
    nylon surgical s.
Sacks
    S. biliary drain
    S. QuickStick catheter
    S. Single-Step catheter
Sacks-Vine
    S.-V. gastrostomy kit
    S.-V. PEG tube
sacral
    s. alar screw
    S. DISH pressure relief back cushion
    s. pedicle screw
    s. segmental nerve stimulation implantable neural prosthesis
    s. spine modular instrumentation

    s. spine Universal instrumentation
    s. support
sacroiliac cinch belt
saddle
    basal block cervical s.
    cervical s.
    Cloward surgical s.
    s. coil
    s. locator
    s. prosthesis
saddlebag
    Seidel s.
Sadler
    S. bone hook
    S. cartilage scissors
Sadowsky hook wire
SAE cast
Saeed Six-Shooter multi-band ligator
Saenger
    S. ovum forceps
    S. placental forceps
    S. suture
Safar-S airway
Safar ventilation bronchoscope
Safco
    S. alloy
    S. diamond instrument
    S. polycarbonate crown
Safe
    S. & Dry diaper
    S. & Dry pant
    S. & Dry undergarment
    S. & Dry underpad
    S. Response manual resuscitator
    S. spine thoracic-lumbar-sacral support
Safe-Cuff blood pressure cuff
Safe-Dwel Plus catheter
Safeset blood sampling system
Safestretch incontinence system
SafeTap tapered spinal needle
Safe-T-Coat heparin-coated thermodilution catheter
SafeTrak
    S. epidural catheter adapter
    S. ESP system
Safe-T-Tube
    Montgomery S.-T.-T.
    Montgomery-Lofgren tapered S.-T.-T.
Safe-T-Wheel pinwheel
safety
    S. AV fistula needle
    s. belt
    S. Clear Plus endotracheal tube
    s. glasses
    s. handle
    s. J-wire
    s. pessary
    s. pin
    s. pin closer
    s. pin splint
    s. plate

S

safety-bolt suture
Safe-Wrap gauze
Saf-Gel hydrogel dressing
SAFHS ultrasound device
Safian
    S. design prosthesis
    S. nasal splint
    S. rhinoplasty prosthesis
Safil synthetic absorbable surgical suture
Safir pin
Safsite
    S. IV therapy system
    S. valve
Saf-T
    S.-T. E-Z set
    S.-T. J guidewire
Saf-T-Coil intrauterine device
Saf-T-Fit amalgamator capsule
Saf-T-Flo
    S.-T.-F. T-tube connector
Saf-T-Intima intravenous catheter safety
  system
SafTouch catheter
SAF-T shield
Saf-T-Sound uterine sound
Sage
    S. driver-extractor
    S. Instruments syringe pump
    S. pin
    S. tonsillar snare
    S. wire
sagittal oscillating saw
Sahara
    S. clinical bone sonometer
    S. portable bone densitometer
    S. super absorbent reusable
    underpad
Sahli needle
Saint
    S. George knee prosthesis
    S. Jude prosthesis
    S. Mark dilator
Sajou laryngeal forceps
Sakler erysiphake
Salah sternal puncture needle
Salem
    S. pump
    S. sump action nasogastric tube
    S. sump drain
Salenius meniscal knife
SalEst preterm labor test system
Salibi carotid artery clamp
saline dressing
saline-filled
    s.-f. anatomical breast implant
    s.-f. expander
    s.-f. round breast implant
saline-saturated wool dressing
Saling amnioscope
Salinger reduction instrument
salivary bypass tube
Salman FES stent
Salmon-Rickham ventriculostomy
  reservoir

salpingeal
    s. curette
    s. probe
salpingograph
    Schultze s.
Salvage catheter
Salvati proctoscope
Salvatore-Maloney tracheotome
Salvatore umbilical cord ligator
Salzburg
    S. biconcave washer
    S. screw
Salz nucleus splitter
SAM
    SAM facial implant
    SAM facial implant material
    SAM module
    SAM system
Sam
    S. Roberts bronchial biopsy forceps
    S. Roberts esophagoscope
Samadhi cushion
Samb retractor
Samco tube
Sammons biplane goniometer
SampleMaster biopsy needle
sampler
    chorionic villus s.
    Cordguard umbilical cord s.
    Cytobrush Plus endocervical cell s.
    Endocell endometrial cell s.
    Endopap endometrial s.
    inertial suction s.
    Isaacs endometrial cell s.
    Johnson swab s.
    Mucat cervical s.
    Rotorod s.
    Sartorious air s.
    SelectCells Mini endometrial s.
    Wallach Endocell endometrial
    cell s.
Sampson
    S. fluted nail
    S. prosthesis
Samson-Davis infant suction tube
Samuels
    S. hemoclip-applying forceps
    S. valvulotome
    S. vein stripper
Samuels-Weck Hemoclip clip
Samway tourniquet
Sana-Lok syringe
Sanborn metabolator
Sanchez-Bulnes lacrimal sac self-retaining
  retractor
Sanchez-Perez automatic film cassette
  changer
Sandal
    Exercise S.
Sandalthotics postural support orthotic
sandbag
    neonatal s.
    pediatric s.
Sanders
    S. intubation laryngoscope

S. jet ventilation device respirator
S. oscillating bed
S. valve
S. vasectomy forceps
S. ventilation adapter
S. Venturi injector system
Sanders-Brown needle
Sanders-Brown-Shaw aneurysm needle
Sanders-Castroviejo suturing forceps
Sand-Eze EGD pillow
Sandhill
S. esophageal motility system
S. probe
Sandhill-800 TDS chart recorder
Sandman system
Sandow apparatus
Sandoz
S. balloon replacement tube
S. Caluso PEG
S. Caluso PEG gastrostomy tube
S. feeding/suction tube
S. nasogastric feeding tube
S. suction/feeding tube
S. suction tube
sandpaper dermabrader
Sandt
S. suture forceps
S. utility forceps
sandwich
Marlex methyl methacrylate s.
sandwich-type splint
Sanford ligator
Sani-Cloth
S.-C. HB disposable wipe
S.-C. Plus germicidal disposable
wipe
Sani-Garm waterproof pant
Sani-Grinder
Sani-Spec vaginal speculum
Sani Vac
Sano clip applier
Santa Casa wrench
Santulli clamp
Santy ring-end forceps
saphenous vein cannula
SaphFinder surgical balloon dissector
SaphLITE saphenous vein system
SAPHtrak balloon dissector
sapphire
s. crystal infrared photocoagulator
s. knife
s. lens
S. premium closed wound drainage
system
S. table
S. View arthroscope
Sapporo shunt tube
Saqalain dressing forceps
Saratoga
S. cycle
S. sump catheter
Sargis uterine tenaculum
Sargon implant

Sarmiento
S. brace
S. cast
Sarnoff aortic clamp
Sarns
S. aortic arch cannula
S. electric saw
S. intracardiac suction tube
S. 7000 MDX pump
S. membrane oxygenator
S. Siok II blood pump
S. soft-flow aortic cannula
S. temperature probe
S. two-stage cannula
S. venous drainage cannula
S. ventricular assist device
S. wire-reinforced catheter
Sarot
S. arterial clamp
S. arterial forceps
S. bronchus clamp
S. intrathoracic forceps
S. knife
S. needle
S. needle holder
S. pleurectomy forceps
S. thoracoscope
Sarot-Vital needle holder
Sarstedt system
Sartorious air sampler
Sartorius breast pump
SAS
SAS II brace
SAS shoe
Saso Variable Speed Massager
Sat-A-Lite contoured wedge seat cushion
Satalite cushion by Bodyline
Satellight needle holder forceps
Satellite
S. ear endoscope
S. Plus pulse oximeter
S. spirometer
Saticon vacuum chamber pickup tube
SatinCrescent implant knife
Satin Plus gloves
SatinShortCut implant knife
Satinsky
S. anastomosis clamp
S. aortic clamp
S. forceps
S. pediatric clamp
S. vascular clamp
S. vena cava clamp
S. vena caval scissors
SatinSlit
S. implant knife
S. keratome
Satlite pulse oximeter with earclip
Sato
S. cataract needle
S. corneal knife
S. lid retractor
S. speculum
Satterlee
S. advancement forceps

Satterlee *(continued)*
  S. amputating saw
  S. aseptic saw
  S. bone saw
  S. bone saw blade
  S. muscle forceps
saturated calomel electrode
SaturEyes contact lens
Saturn Splint
Satvioni cryptoscope
Sauer
  S. corneal debrider
  S. eye speculum
  S. hemostatic tonsillectome
  S. infant eye speculum
  S. outer ring forceps
  S. suture forceps
  S. suturing forceps
  S. tonometer
Sauerbruch
  S. implant
  S. pickup forceps
  S. prosthesis
  S. retractor
  S. rib elevator
  S. rib forceps
  S. rib guillotine
  S. rib shears
  S. rongeur
Sauerbruch-Britsch rib shears
Sauerbruch-Coryllos
  S.-C. rib rongeur
  S.-C. rib shears
Sauerbruch-Frey
  S.-F. raspatory
  S.-F. rib elevator
  S.-F. rib shears
Sauerbruch-Lebsche
  S.-L. rib shears
  S.-L. rongeur
Sauerbruch-Lillienthal rib spreader
Sauerbruch-Zukschwerdt rib retractor
Sauer-Sluder tonsillectome
Sauer-Storz
  S.-S. tonometer
  S.-S. tonsillectome
Sauflon PW hydrophilic contact lens
sauna
Saunders
  S. cataract needle
  S. cervical HomeTrac traction
  S. eye speculum
  S. mobilization wedge
Saunders-Paparella
  S.-P. marker
  S.-P. needle
  S.-P. pick
  S.-P. stapes hook
  S.-P. window rasp
Saurex spreader
Sauvage
  S. Bionit graft
  S. Dacron graft
  S. fabric graft prosthesis

  S. filamentous prosthesis
  S. filamentous velour graft
Savage intestinal decompressor
Savariaud-Reverdin needle
Savary
  S. bronchoscope
  S. esophageal dilator
  S. tapered thermoplastic dilator
Savary-Gilliard
  S.-G. esophageal dilator
  S.-G. metal olive
  S.-G. over-the-wire dilator
  S.-G. Silastic flexible bougie
  S.-G. tip
  S.-G. wire guide
  S.-G. wire-guided bougie
Savastano Hemi-Knee prosthesis
Save-A-Tooth tooth preserving system
Saver
  Haemonetics Cell S.
Saverburger irrigation/aspiration tip
Savlon splint
saw
  Accutome low-speed diamond s.
  Adams s.
  Adson Gigli s.
  air s.
  air-driven s.
  Albee bone s.
  amputation s.
  aseptic s.
  Bailey wire s.
  Becker-Joseph s.
  Bergman plaster s.
  Bier amputation s.
  Bishop oscillatory bone s.
  Bodenham s.
  bone s.
  Bosworth s.
  Bosworth-Joseph nasal s.
  Brown s.
  Brown-Joseph s.
  Butcher s.
  chain s.
  Charnley s.
  Charriere amputation s.
  Charriere aseptic metacarpal s.
  Charriere bone s.
  Clerf laryngeal s.
  Codman sternal s.
  Converse nasal s.
  Cottle-Joseph s.
  Cottle Universal nasal s.
  Crego-Gigli s.
  crown s.
  crurotomy s.
  Delrin-handle bone s.
  DeMartel conductor s.
  DeMartel T-wire s.
  diamond s.
  diamond wafering s.
  electric laryngofissure s.
  Engel plaster s.
  Farabeuf s.
  Farrior-Joseph bayonet s.

finger ring s.
Gigli solid-handle s.
Gigli-Strully s.
Gigli wire s.
gold s.
Goldman s.
Gottschalk transverse s.
Guilford-Wright bur s.
Guilford-Wullstein bur s.
Hall sagittal s.
Hall Versipower oscillating s.
Hall Versipower reciprocating s.
s. handle
helical tube s.
Hetherington circular s.
Hey skull s.
Hill-Bosworth s.
Hough crurotomy s.
Hough-Wullstein bur s.
Hub s.
humeral s.
Isomet low speed s.
Isomet Plus precision s.
Joseph bayonet s.
Joseph-Farrior s.
Joseph-Maltz angular nasal s.
Joseph nasal s.
Joseph-Stille s.
Joseph-Verner s.
Lamont nasal s.
Langenbeck metacarpal
  amputation s.
laryngeal s.
Lebsche wire s.
Lell laryngofissure s.
Luck-Bishop s.
Luck bone s.
Luxation patellar s.
Macewen s.
Magnuson circular twin s.
Magnuson double counter-rotating s.
Magnuson single circular s.
Maltz bayonet s.
McCabe crurotomy s.
metacarpal s.
Micro-Aire oscillating bone s.
microreciprocating s.
microsagittal s.
Miltex bone s.
Mueller s.
Myerson laryngectomy s.
nasal s.
Ogura nasal s.
Olivecrona-Gigli wire s.
Olivecrona wire s.
Orthair oscillating s.
Osada s.
oscillating s.
patella bone s.
Percy amputating s.
plaster s.
reciprocating s.
Rica wire s.
ring-cutting s.
rotary hub s.

round Gigli s.
Rust amputation s.
sagittal oscillating s.
Sarns electric s.
Satterlee amputating s.
Satterlee aseptic s.
Satterlee bone s.
Schwartz antral trocar s.
Seltzer s.
Shrady s.
single-sided bone s.
Skil s.
Sklar bone s.
Slaughter nasal s.
spinal s.
Stedman s.
sternal s.
sternum s.
Stille-Gigli wire s.
Stiwer finger-ring s.
Stryker autopsy s.
surgical s.
Tuke bone s.
Tyler-Gigli s.
Tyler spiral Gigli s.
Universal nasal s.
V. Mueller amputating s.
V. Mueller-Gigli s.
Wigmore plaster s.
wire s.
Woakes nasal s.
Xomed micro-oscillating s.
Zimmer s.
sawblade
  Stablecut s.
sawdust bed
Sawtell
  S. arterial forceps
  S. gallbladder forceps
  S. hemostat
  S. laryngeal applicator
  S. tonsillar forceps
Sawtell-Davis
  S.-D. forceps
  S.-D. hemostat
saw-toothed curette
Sawyer
  S. rectal retractor
  S. rectal speculum
Sayre
  S. bandage
  S. double-end periosteal elevator
  S. dressing
  S. head snare
  S. jacket
  S. periosteal raspatory
  S. retractor
  S. sling
  S. splint
  S. suspension apparatus
  S. suspension traction
Sbarbaro tibial prosthesis
SBE cast
SBQC cane
SC-1 needle

S

Scabbard needle
SCA-EX
    S.-E. ShortCutter catheter
    S.-E. ShortCutter catheter blade
scaffold, scaffolding
    biodegradable polymer s.
    collagen s.
    three-dimensional biocompatible s.
Scaglietti rongeur
scalar leads
scale
    balance beam s.
    bedside s.
    Braden s.
    Digitron dialysis chair s.
    Epworth Sleepiness S.
    Esterman s.
    Gosnell s.
    Health O Meter S.
    Job Attitude S.
    Kenna knee s.
    Miller s.
    Scotty the Scale stand-on s.
    Symptom Rating S.
scaler
    Amdent ultrasonic s.
    Brahler ultrasonic dental s.
    Buffalo ultrasonic s.
    Cavitron SPS ultrasonic s.
    Columbia s.
    Densco ultrasonic s.
    dental s.
    Ellman rotary s.
    loop s.
    Nordent s.
    Sonatron ultrasonic s.
    Steele s.
    Tamsco periodontic s.
    Titan s.
    ultrasonic s.
    Vivant ultrasonic s.
scalp
    s. clip-applying forceps
    s. electrode
    s. hemostasis clip
    s. self-retaining retractor
    s. vein needle
scalpel
    ASR s.
    Bard-Parker s.
    Bergman s.
    blade s.
    bone s.
    Bowen double-bladed s.
    B.U.S. Endotron-Lipectron
      ultrasonic s.
    carbon dioxide (CO_2) laser s.
    Cavitron s.
    Contact Laser s.
    Dieffenbach s.
    disposable s.
    Downing cartilage s.
    s. electrode
    Electrodes s.
    electrosurgical s.

    Endo-Assist retractable s.
    Endotron-Lipectron ultrasonic s.
    Epitome s.
    feather s.
    Green pendulum s.
    s. guard
    Guyton-Lundsgaard s.
    Hamer s.
    s. handle
    Harmonic s.
    Jackson tracheal s.
    John Green pendulum s.
    laser s.
    LaserSonics Nd:YAG LaserBlade s.
    lid s.
    Lipectron ultrasonic s.
    long s.
    Microcap s.
    Myocure blade s.
    Otocap myringotomy s.
    pendulum s.
    Personna Plus disposable Teflon s.
    plasma s.
    Pre-Cision miniature and
      microminiature s.
    razor s.
    ruby knife s.
    sculpturing s.
    Shaw I, II s.
    tracheal s.
    ultrasonically activated s.
    ultrasonic harmonic s.
    water s.
ScalpelTec
    S. keratome slit blade
    S. wound-enlargement blade
scalpene needle
scan
    bladder s.
    brain Neurolite SPECT s.
    computed tomography s. (CT scan)
    CT s.
      computed tomography scan
    DEXA s.
    fluorodopa positron emission
      tomographic s.
    gadolinium s.
    magnetic resonance imaging s.
    MRI s.
    Neurolite SPECT s.
    Opthascan Mini-A s.
    S. Pattern generator
    portal-phased spiral CT s.
    postgadolinium s.
    proton-density axial MR s.
    SPECT s.
    S. spray dressing
    T2-weighted s.
Scanditronix PET scanner
Scand pin
scanhead
    Entos vascular and abdominal
      intraoperative s.
Scanlan
    S. aneurysm clip

S. bipolar coagulator
S. laparoscopic forceps
S. ligator
S. ligature guide
S. microforceps
S. microneedle holder
S. micronerve hook
S. microrasp
S. microscissors
S. microvessel hook
S. pediatric retractor
S. plaster shears
S. rib shears
S. scissors
S. vascular tunneler
S. vessel dilator
Scanlan-Crafoord contractor
ScanLite scanner
Scanmaster
S. D x-ray film digitizer
S. DX system
S. DX x-ray film digitizer
S. DX x-ray film digitizer scanner
scanned-slot detector system
scanner
AccuScan CO_2 laser s.
Acoma s.
Acuson 128EP s.
Acuson ultrasound s.
Advanced NMR Systems s.
Agfa Medical s.
All-Tronics s.
Aloka SSD-720 real-time s.
Aloka ultrasound linear s.
Aloka ultrasound sector s.
American Shared-CuraCare s.
Analogic Anatom 2000 mobile
  CT s.
Aquilion CT s.
Artoscan MRI s.
A-scan s.
ATL duplex s.
ATL Mark 600 real-time sector s.
ATL Neurosector real-time s.
Aurora MR breast imaging
  system s.
Bergmann Optical laser s.
Biosound wide-angle monoplane
  ultrasound s.
Biospec MR imaging system s.
BladderManager portable
  ultrasound s.
BladderScan BVI2500 s.
Bruel & Kjaer ultrasound s.
Bruker s.
Canon s.
CardioData MK-3 Holter s.
Cemax/Icon s.
Cencit facial s.
Cencit surface s.
charge-coupled device s.
cine CT s.
conventional static s.
Corometrics Doppler s.
CTI 933/4 ECAT s.

CTI positron emission tomography
  (PET) s.
CT Max 640 s.
Delarnette s.
Del Mar Avionics s.
Diasonics Cardiovue SectOR s.
digital slide s.
Dine digital s.
Dornier s.
3D surface digitizer s.
DuPont s.
Dynamic Spacial Reconstructor s.
Eastman Kodak s.
electrical sector s.
electron beam CT s.
Elscint Excel 905 s.
Elscint MR s.
Elscint Twin CT s.
EMED s.
EMI CT s.
EUB-405 ultrasound s.
Evolution XP s.
Fonar Quad MRI s.
Fonar Stand-Up MRI s.
Galen Scan s.
Gammex RMI s.
GE Advance PET s.
GE CT Advantage s.
GE CT Max s.
GE CT Pace s.
GE Genesis CT s.
GE GN 500-MHz s.
GE 9800 high-resolution CT s.
GE HiSpeed Advantage helical
  CT s.
GE MR Max s.
GE MR Signa s.
GE MR Vectra s.
GE Omega 500-MHz s.
GE single-axis SR-230
  echoplanar s.
GE Spiral CT s.
GF-UM3 s.
Gyroscan S15 s.
Heidelberg laser tomographic s.
helical CT s.
Hewlett-Packard s.
high-field open MRI s.
high-resolution real-time s.
Hilight Advantage System CT s.
Hispeed CT s.
Hitachi CT, MR s.
Hitachi Open MRI System s.
Hologic 2000 s.
Hologic QDR 1000W dual-energy
  x-ray absorptiometry s.
Howtek Scanmaster DX s.
Imatron C-100 Ultrafast CT s.
Imatron Fastrac C-100 cine x-ray
  CT s.
Indomitable s.
infrared liver s.
Innervision MR s.
InstaScan s.
Integris 3000 s.

S

scanner *(continued)*
intensified radiographic imaging
  system s.
Interad whole body CT s.
Irex Exemplar ultrasound s.
IRIS s.
Konica s.
Kretz Combison 330 ultrasound s.
large-bore imaging system s.
s. laser ophthalmoscope
linear convex array s.
Lintro-Scan s.
Lumiscan s.
Lunar DPX total-body s.
LymphoScan nuclear imaging
  system s.
3M s.
Magna-SL s.
Magnes 2500 whole-blood s.
Magnetom s.
Magnex MR s.
Mallinckrodt s.
Max Plus MR s.
MedImage s.
Medison s.
Medspec MR imaging system s.
MedX s.
midget MRI s.
MKII automated s.
modified electron-beam CT s.
multiple jointed digitizer s.
multisensory structured light range
  digitizer s.
neurSector s.
Nishimoto Sangyo s.
Norland pQCT XCT2000 s.
OctreoScan s.
Ohio Nuclear Delta s.
Olympus endoscopic ultrasound s.
OmniMedia XRS s.
Opthascan Mini-A s.
Oxford 2-T large-bore imaging
  system s.
Pace Plus System s.
Park Medical Systems s.
Perception s.
PETite s.
Pfizer s.
Philips Gyroscan ACS s.
Philips Gyroscan NT-series s.
Philips Gyroscan S5 s.
Philips Gyroscan T5 s.
Philips small-bore system s.
Philips spiral CT s.
Philips Tomoscan SR 6000 CT s.
Picker CS, CT, MR s.
Picker PQ helical CT s.
Picker PQ spiral CT s.
Picker Synerview 600 s.
Picker Vista HPQ MRI s.
Picker Vista MagnaScanner s.
Polhemus 3 digitizer s.
Posicam HZ PET s.
ProSpeed CT s.

Quick CT9800 s.
real-time B s.
RIGHT 3200 Advantage
  ultrasound s.
Scanditronix PET s.
ScanLite s.
Scanmaster DX x-ray film
  digitizer s.
scintillation s.
scintiscanner s.
sector s.
Shimadzu CT, MR s.
Siemens DRH CT s.
Siemens ECAT 951/31R PET s.
Siemens Magnetom GBS II s.
Siemens Magnetom Vision s.
Siemens One Tesla s.
Siemens Somatom DR2, DR3
  whole-body s.
Siemens Sonoline Elegra
  ultrasound s.
SieScape ultrasound s.
Signa Horizon s.
SilkTouch CO_2 laser s.
single-field hyperthermia combined
  with radiation therapy and
  ultrasound s.
Sinvision ultrasound s.
Skinscan s.
SmartPrep s.
Softscan laser s.
Somatom DR CT s.
Somatom Plus S whole-body s.
Sonoline Siemens ultrasound s.
Sonos s.
spiral CT s.
spiral XCT s.
SwiftLase s.
Swissray s.
Technicare Delta 2020 s.
Tecmag Libra-S16 system s.
thermographic s.
Tomomatic brain s.
Toshiba brain s.
Toshiba helical CT s.
Toshiba MR s.
Toshiba 900S helical CT s.
Toshiba Xpress SX helical CT s.
Toshiba Xvision s.
Trionix s.
Twin Flash s.
ultrafast CT s.
Ultra-Image A-scan s.
Ultramark s.
Varian CT s.
Vidar s.
Vision MRI s.
Vision Ten V-scan s.
Vista American Health Tesla
  MRI s.
whole-body digital s.
Xpress/SW helical CT s.
Xpress/SX helical CT s.
scanning
  s. beam digital system

s. excimer laser
s. fluorometer
s. laser acoustic microscope
s. laser ophthalmoscope
s. laser polarimeter
s. prism
s. Radiometer
s. slit confocal microscope
s. transmission electron microscope
s. tunneling microscope
Scanpor
S. acrylate adhesive
S. surgical tape
Scanzoni forceps
Scaphoid-Microstaple system
scaphoid screw guide
scapular retractor
Scarborough prosthesis
scarf bandage
Scar Fx lightweight silicone sheeting
scarifier
Berkeley s.
Desmarres s.
Graefe s.
s. knife
Kuhnt corneal s.
scarifying curette
scarlet red gauze dressing
scattering
s. foil
s. foil compensator
s. system
scavenging tube
SCD
S. MaleFactor Pak
S. stockings
SCDT heart valve prosthesis
Sceratti goniometer
Schaaf foreign body forceps
Schachar
S. blepharostat
S. lens
Schachne-Desmarres lid everter
Schacht colostomy appliance
Schaedel
S. clip
S. cross-action towel clamp
Schaefer
S. ethmoid curette
S. fixation forceps
S. mastoid curette
S. sponge holder
Schaldach electrode pacemaker
Schall laryngectomy tube
Schaltenbrand-Wahren stereotactic atlas
Schamberg comedo extractor
Schanz
S. cannula
S. cautery
S. collar
S. collar brace
S. electrocautery
S. knife
S. needle
S. pin

S. Scheie blade
S. trephine
Schanzioni craniotomy forceps
Scharff
S. bipolar forceps
S. lens
Schatzki ring
Schatz-Palmaz tubular mesh stent
Schatz utility forceps
Schecter-Bryant aortic vent needle
Schede bone curette
Scheer
S. crimper forceps
S. elevator knife
S. hook
S. knife elevator
S. middle ear instrument
S. needle
S. oval window rasp
S. pick
S. Tef-wire prosthesis
Scheer-Wullstein cutting bur
Scheicher laminectomy punch
Scheie
S. anterior chamber cannula
S. blade
S. cataract-aspirating cannula
S. cataract-aspirating needle
S. electrocautery
S. goniopuncture knife
S. goniotomy knife
S. ophthalmic cautery
S. trephine
Scheie-Graefe fixation forceps
Scheie-Westcott corneal section scissors
Scheimpflug camera
Scheinmann
S. biting punch
S. biting tip
S. esophagoscopy forceps
S. laryngeal forceps
Schein syringe
Schepens
S. binocular indirect camera
S. boat silicone
S. eye cautery
S. forceps
S. grooved rubber silicone
S. hollow hemisphere implant
S. ophthalmoscope
S. orbital retractor
S. pad silicone
S. refractor
S. retinal detachment unit
S. scleral depressor
S. spoon
S. surface electrode
S. tantalum clip
Schepens-Pomerantzeff ophthalmoscope
Scherback-Porges vaginal speculum set
Scheuerlen raspatory
Schick
S. back support
S. forceps
Schilder plugger

S

709

Schillinger suture support
Schimelbusch inhaler
Schindler
   S. gastroscope
   S. optical esophagoscope
   S. peritoneal forceps
   S. retractor
Schink
   S. dermatome
   S. metatarsal retractor
Schiötz tonometer
Schirmer tear test strip
Schlein
   S. clamp
   S. shoulder holder
   S. shoulder positioner
   S. total elbow prosthesis
   S. trisurface ankle prosthesis
Schlesinger
   S. cervical punch
   S. cervical punch forceps
   S. cervical rongeur
   S. clamp
   S. Gigli-saw guide
   S. instrument
   S. intervertebral disk forceps
   S. intervertebral disk rongeur
   S. laminectomy rongeur
   S. meniscus-grasping forceps
   S. rongeur forceps
Schmeden tonsillar punch
Schmidt optics system
Schmid vascular spatula
Schmieden
   S. needle
   S. probe
Schmieden-Dick needle
Schmieden-Taylor
   S.-T. dissector
   S.-T. dural scissors
Schmiedt tube
Schmitt fan
Schmuth modification activator
Schnaudigel sclerotomy punch
Schneider
   S. catheter
   S. driver-extractor
   S. extractor
   S. intramedullary nail
   S. Magic Wallstent
   S. nail driver
   S. nail shaft reamer
   S. pelvimeter
   S. PTCA instruments
   S. raspatory
   S. rod
   S. self-broaching pin
   S. stent
   S. Wallstent biliary endoprosthesis
Schneider-Meier magnum system
Schneider-Sauerbruch raspatory
Schneider-Shiley
   S.-S. balloon
   S.-S. dilatation catheter

Schnidt
   S. clamp
   S. gall duct forceps
   S. hemostat
   S. thoracic forceps
   S. tonsillar forceps
Schnidt-Rumpler forceps
Schnitker scalp retractor
Schnitman skin hook
Schocket
   S. scleral depressor
   S. tube implant
Schoemaker
   S. intestinal clamp
   S. scissors
Schoemaker-Loth scissors
Schoenberg
   S. intestinal forceps
   S. uterine forceps
Schoenborn retractor
Schoenrock laser instrument set
Scholander apparatus
Scholar II vital sign monitor
Scholl
   S. meniscal knife
   S. pad
Scholten
   S. endomyocardial biopsy forceps
   S. endomyocardial bioptome
   S. sternal retractor
Schonander film changer
Schoonmaker
   S. femoral catheter
   S. multipurpose catheter
Schroeder
   S. episiotomy scissors
   S. interlocking uterine sound
   S. operating scissors
   S. tenaculum loop
   S. tissue forceps
   S. uterine curette
   S. uterine scoop
   S. uterine tenaculum
   S. uterine vulsellum forceps
   S. vulsellum
Schroeder-Braun uterine forceps
Schroeder-Van Doren tenaculum forceps
Schrotter catheter
Schubert
   S. cervical biopsy forceps
   S. uterine biopsy forceps
   S. uterine biopsy punch
Schuco
   S. 2000 nebulizer
Schuknecht
   S. chisel
   S. cutter
   S. elevator
   S. foreign body remover
   S. Gelfoam wire prosthesis
   S. gouge
   S. middle ear instrument
   S. needle
   S. pick

S. postauricular self-retaining
retractor
S. roller knife
S. sickle knife
S. spatula
S. stapes hook
S. suction tip
S. suction tube
S. Teflon wire piston prosthesis
S. Tef-Wire prosthesis
S. temporal trephine
S. whirlybird excavator
S. wire crimper
S. wire-cutting scissors
Schuknecht-Paparella wire-bending die
Schuknecht-Wullstein retractor
Schulec silver clip
Schuler aspiration/irrigation tube
Schuletz
S. antral curette
S. pacemaker
Schuletz-Simmons ethmoidal curette
Schultz
S. anterior capsule nibbler
S. iris retractor
Schultz-Crock binocular ophthalmoscope
Schultze
S. embryotomy knife
S. salpingograph
Schumacher
S. aortic clamp
S. biopsy forceps
S. sternal shears
S. umbilical cord scissors
Schumann giant eye magnet
Schumann-Schreus dermabrader
Schurring ossicle cup prosthesis
Schutte shovel-nose basket
Schutt needle
Schutz
S. clamp
S. clip
S. forceps
Schwarten
S. balloon dilatation catheter
S. LP balloon catheter
S. LP guidewire
S. Microglide LP balloon
Schwartz
S. antral trocar saw
S. arterial aneurysm clamp
S. bulldog clamp
S. cervical tenaculum hook
S. clip
S. clip applier
S. clip-applying forceps
S. cordotomy knife
S. endocervical curette
S. intracranial clamp
S. laminectomy self-retaining
retractor
S. multipurpose forceps
S. obstetrical forceps
S. plate
S. temporary clamp-applying forceps

S. trocar
S. vascular clamp
**Schwartz-Blajwas-Marcinko irrigation
system**
Schwartze chisel
Schwartz-Kerrison rongeur
Schwarz
S. arrow-forming pliers
S. bow-type activator
S. finger extension bow
S. traction bow
Schwasser
S. brain clip
S. microclip clip
Schwed Flexicut file
Schweigger
S. capsule forceps
S. extracapsular forceps
S. hand perimeter
Schweitzer
S. pin
S. spring plate
Schweizer
S. cervix-holding forceps
S. speculum
S. uterine forceps
Schwinn Air-Dyne bicycle
Scialom dental implant material
Science-Med balloon catheter
Scientec calorimeter
Scientronics magnet
Sci-Med
S.-M. angioplasty catheter
S.-M. Express Monorail balloon
S.-M. extracorporeal silicone rubber
reservoir
S.-M. guiding catheter
S.-M. Life Systems, Inc. membrane
artificial lung
S.-M. SSC "Skinny" catheter
Scimed-Choice floppy wire
Scimed rTRA-GC guiding catheter
scimitar blade
**Scinticore multicrystal scintillation
camera**
scintigraphic balloon
scintillation
s. counter
s. scanner
γ-scintillation camera
scintillator
aqueous s.
benzene s.
cyclohexane s.
organic liquid s.
scintimammography prone breast cushion
scintiscanner scanner
Scintiview nuclear computer system
Scintron IV nuclear computer system
scissors (*See also* shears)
abdominal s.
Ada s.
Adson ganglion s.
Aebli corneal s.
Aebli-Manson s.

scissors *(continued)*
Aebli tenotomy s.
alligator MacCarty s.
American umbilical s.
Anderson converse iris s.
angled s.
angular s.
Anis corneal s.
anterior chamber synechia s.
arteriotomy s.
Arthro Force hook s.
Aslan endoscopic s.
Aston facelift s.
Atkinson corneal s.
Atkinson-Walker s.
Aufricht s.
Azar corneal s.
baby Metzenbaum s.
Bahama suture s.
Bakst cardiac s.
ball tipped s.
Baltimore nasal s.
bandage s.
Bantam wire-cutting s.
Barkan s.
Barnes vessel s.
Barraquer corneal section s.
Barraquer-DeWecker iris s.
Barraquer iris s.
Barraquer-Karakashian s.
Barraquer vitreous strand s.
Barsky nasal s.
Baruch circumcision s.
bayonet s.
beaded-tip s.
Beall circumflex artery s.
Becker corneal section spatulated s.
Becker septal s.
Becker spatulated corneal section s.
Beckman nasal s.
Beebe wire-cutting s.
Bellucci alligator s.
Berens corneal transplant s.
Berens iridocapsulotomy s.
Bergman plaster s.
Berkeley Bioengineering
  mechanized s.
bipolar cautery s.
Birks Mark II trabeculectomy s.
Blanco s.
Blum arterial s.
Boettcher tonsillar s.
Bonn iris s.
Bowman iris s.
Bowman strabismus s.
Boyd dissecting s.
Boyd-Stille tonsillar s.
Boyd tonsillar s.
Bozeman s.
brain s.
Braun episiotomy s.
Braun-Stadler episiotomy s.
Brooks gallbladder s.
Brophy s.

Brown dissecting s.
Buerger-McCarthy s.
Buie rectal s.
bulldog s.
Bunge s.
Burnham bandage s.
Busch umbilical cord s.
calcified tissue s.
canalicular s.
cannular s.
Caplan angular s.
Caplan dorsal s.
Caplan nasal s.
capsulotomy s.
Carb-Edge s.
cardiovascular s.
cartilage s.
Castanares facelift s.
Castroviejo anterior synechia s.
Castroviejo corneal section s.
Castroviejo corneal transplant s.
Castroviejo iridocapsulotomy s.
Castroviejo iris s.
Castroviejo keratoplasty s.
Castroviejo-McPherson
  keratectomy s.
Castroviejo microcorneal s.
Castroviejo synechia s.
Castroviejo tenotomy s.
Castroviejo-Troutman s.
Castroviejo-Vannas capsulotomy s.
cataract s.
Caylor s.
Chadwick s.
Charnley cup-trimming s.
Cherry S-shape s.
Chevalier Jackson s.
Church pediatric s.
Cinelli-Fomon s.
circumflex artery s.
Classon pediatric s.
Clayman-Troutman corneal s.
Clayman-Vannas s.
Clayman-Westcott s.
clip-removing s.
Codman s.
Cohan-Vannas iris s.
Cohan-Westcott s.
Cohney s.
cold s.
collar s.
conjunctival s.
Converse nasal tip s.
Converse-Wilmer conjunctival s.
Cooley arteriotomy s.
Cooley cardiovascular s.
Cooley neonatal s.
Cooley probe-point s.
Cooley reverse-cut s.
corneal section-enlarging s.
corneal section spatulated s.
corneal spatulated s.
corneal transplant s.
corneoscleral s.
coronary artery s.

Costa wire suture s.
Cottle angular s.
Cottle bulldog s.
Cottle dorsal s.
Cottle dressing s.
Cottle heavy septal s.
Cottle nasal s.
Cottle spring s.
Crafoord lobectomy s.
Crafoord lung s.
Crafoord thoracic s.
Craig s.
craniotomy s.
crown s.
curved iris s.
curved-on-flat s.
curved operating s.
curved tenotomy s.
curved turbinate s.
curved turbinectomy s.
cuticle s.
Dahlgren iris s.
Dandy neurosurgical s.
Dandy trigeminal s.
Davis rhytidectomy s.
Dean dissecting s.
Dean tonsillar s.
Dean-Trussler s.
Deaver operating s.
DeBakey endarterectomy s.
DeBakey-Metzenbaum s.
DeBakey-Potts s.
DeBakey stitch s.
DeBakey valve s.
DeBakey vascular s.
Decker microsurgical s.
delicate operating s.
DeMartel neurosurgical s.
DeMartel vascular s.
Derf s.
DeWecker iridectomy s.
DeWecker iris s.
DeWecker-Pritikin iris s.
diamond-edge s.
diathermy s.
Diethrich circumflex artery s.
Diethrich coronary artery s.
Diethrich-Hegemann s.
Diethrich valve s.
dissecting s.
dissection s.
Dixon collar s.
dorsal angled s.
Douglas nasal s.
Doyen abdominal s.
Doyen dissecting s.
Doyen-Ferguson s.
dressing s.
Dubois decapitation s.
Duffield cardiovascular s.
Dumont thoracic s.
dural s.
Durotip s.
ear s.
East-Grinstead s.

Edelstein s.
Eiselsberg ligature s.
Electroscope disposable s.
electrosurgical curved s.
Emmet uterine s.
endarterectomy s.
endoscopic s.
enterotomy s.
enucleation s.
episiotomy s.
E-series s.
Esmarch bandage s.
esophageal s.
Essrig dissecting s.
Evershears bipolar curved s.
Evershears bipolar laparoscopic s.
eye stitch s.
eye suture s.
facelift s.
facial plastic surgery s.
Favaloro coronary s.
Federspiel s.
Ferguson abdominal s.
Ferguson-Metzenbaum s.
Fine suture s.
Finochietto thoracic s.
Fisch microcrurotomy s.
Fiskars s.
fistula s.
F. L. Fischer microsurgical
  neurectomy bayonet s.
Fomon angular s.
Fomon facelift s.
Fomon lower lateral s.
Fomon saber-back s.
Fomon upper lateral s.
s. forceps
Foster s.
Frahur s.
Frazier dural s.
Freeman rhytidectomy s.
Freeman-Schepens s.
Frost s.
Fulton pediatric s.
gallbladder s.
ganglion s.
gauze s.
Gellquist s.
Gene s.
general utility s.
Giardet corneal transplant s.
Giertz-Stille s.
Gill s.
Gill-Hess s.
Gillies suture s.
Gill-Welsh s.
Gill-Welsh-Vannas capsulotomy s.
Girard corneoscleral s.
Glasscock s.
Glassman thin-point s.
goiter s.
Goldman-Fox gum s.
Goldman septal s.
Good-Reiner s.
Good tonsillar s.

S

scissors *(continued)*
    Gorney facelift s.
    Gorney rhytidectomy s.
    Gradle stitch s.
    Graham pediatric s.
    Grieshaber vertical cutting s.
    Grieshaber vitreous s.
    Guggenheim s.
    Guggenheim-Schuknecht s.
    Guilford s.
    Guilford-Schuknecht wire-cutting s.
    Guilford-Wright s.
    guillotine s.
    Guist enucleation s.
    Guyton s.
    Haenig irrigating s.
    Haglund plaster s.
    Haimovici arteriotomy s.
    Halsey nail s.
    Halsted strabismus s.
    harmonic s.
    Harrington deep surgical s.
    Harrington-Mayo s.
    Harrison suture-removing s.
    Harvey wire-cutting s.
    Haynes s.
    Heath clip-removing s.
    Heath suture s.
    Heath suture-cutting s.
    Heath wire-cutting s.
    heavy septal s.
    Hegemann s.
    Heyman nasal s.
    Heyman-Paparella angular s.
    Hipp & Sohn dental s.
    Hoen laminectomy s.
    Holinger curved s.
    Holmes s.
    hook rotary s.
    Hooper pediatric s.
    Hoskins-Castroviejo corneal s.
    Hoskins-Westcott tenotomy s.
    Hough s.
    House alligator s.
    House-Bellucci alligator s.
    House-Bellucci-Shambaugh
      alligator s.
    Huey s.
    Huger diamond-back nasal s.
    Hunt chalazion s.
    IMA s.
    insulated curved s.
    insulated straight s.
    iridectomy s.
    iridocapsulotomy s.
    iridotomy s.
    iris s.
    Irvine corneal s.
    Irvine probe-pointed s.
    Jabaley s.
    Jabaley-Stille s.
    Jackson esophageal s.
    Jackson laryngeal s.
    Jackson turbinate s.

    Jacobson bayonet-shaped s.
    Jacobson spring-handled s.
    Jako microlaryngeal s.
    Jameson facelift s.
    Jameson-Metzenbaum s.
    Jameson-Werber s.
    Jannetta bayonet s.
    Jannetta bayonet-shaped s.
    Jannetta-Kurze dissecting s.
    Jansen-Middleton s.
    Jarit dissecting s.
    Jarit endarterectomy s.
    Jarit flat-tip s.
    Jarit lower lateral s.
    Jarit microstitch s.
    Jarit microsurgery s.
    Jarit peripheral vascular s.
    Jarit stitch s.
    Jesco s.
    Jones dissecting s.
    Jones IMA s.
    Jorgenson dissecting s.
    Jorgenson gallbladder s.
    Jorgenson thoracic s.
    Joseph-Maltz s.
    Joseph nasal s.
    Joseph serrated s.
    Kahn s.
    Karakashian-Barraquer s.
    Karmody venous s.
    Katzeff cartilage s.
    Katzin corneal transplant s.
    Katzin-Troutman s.
    Kaye blepharoplasty s.
    Kaye facelift s.
    Kaye fine-dissecting s.
    Kazanjian s.
    Keeler intravitreal s.
    Kelly fistular s.
    Kelly uterine s.
    keratectomy s.
    keratoplasty s.
    Kirby s.
    Kitner dissecting s.
    Kleinsasser microlaryngeal s.
    Klinkenbergh-Loth s.
    Knapp iris s.
    Knapp strabismus s.
    Knight nasal s.
    Knowles bandage s.
    Koenig nail-splitting s.
    Koenig-Stille s.
    Koros EndoMax s.
    Kramp s.
    Kreiger-Spitznas vibrating s.
    Kreuscher semilunar cartilage s.
    Kurze dissecting s.
    Lagrange eye s.
    Lagrange sclerectomy s.
    Lahey Carb-Edge s.
    Lahey delicate s.
    Lahey dissecting s.
    Lahey operating s.
    Lahey thyroid s.
    Lakeside nasal s.

Lambert-Heiman s.
Landolt enucleation s.
laparoscopic s.
laryngeal s.
Laschal suture s.
laser tubal s.
Lawrie modified circumflex s.
Lawton corneal s.
Leather-Karmody in-situ valve s.
left-handed cornea s.
Lexer dissecting s.
Lexer-Durotip dissecting s.
ligature s.
Lillie tonsillar s.
Lincoln-Metzenbaum s.
Lincoln pediatric s.
Lindley s.
Lipshultz epididymovasostomy
   microdissection s.
Lister bandage s.
Liston plaster-of-Paris s.
Littauer dissecting s.
Littauer stitch s.
Littauer suture s.
Littler dissecting s.
Littler suture-carrying s.
Litwak mitral valve s.
Litwin s.
Lloyd-Davies rectal s.
lobectomy s.
loop s.
Lorenz PC/TC s.
lung dissecting s.
Lynch s.
MacKenty s.
Maclay tonsillar s.
Maki s.
Malis neurosurgical s.
Mancusi-Ungaro s.
Manson-Aebli corneal section s.
Marbach episiotomy s.
marking s.
Martin ballpoint s.
Martin cartilage s.
Martin throat s.
Mattis corneal s.
Mattox-Potts s.
Maunoir iris s.
Max Fine s.
Mayo curved s.
Mayo-Harrington s.
Mayo-Harrington dissecting s.
Mayo-Lexer s.
Mayo long dissecting s.
Mayo-New s.
Mayo-Noble dissecting s.
Mayo operating s.
Mayo-Potts dissecting s.
Mayo round blade s.
Mayo-Sims dissecting s.
Mayo-Stille operating s.
Mayo straight s.
Mayo uterine s.
McAllister s.
McClure iris s.

McGuire corneal s.
McIndoe s.
McLean capsulotomy s.
McPherson-Castroviejo corneal
   section s.
McPherson-Castroviejo
   microcorneal s.
McPherson corneal section s.
McPherson microconjunctival s.
McPherson microtenotomy s.
McPherson-Vannas iris s.
McPherson-Vannas microiris s.
McPherson-Westcott conjunctival s.
McPherson-Westcott stitch s.
McReynolds pterygium s.
meatotomy s.
mechanized s.
meniscal hook s.
meniscectomy s.
Metzenbaum delicate s.
Metzenbaum dissecting s.
Metzenbaum-Lipsett s.
Metzenbaum long s.
Metzenbaum operating s.
micro s.
microconjunctival s.
microcorneal s.
microiris s.
microlaryngeal s.
micromosquito curved s.
micromosquito straight s.
micropituitary s.
microscopic s.
microsurgical s.
Microtek s.
microtenotomy s.
microvascular s.
Microvit s.
Microwec s.
micro Westcott s.
Miller dissecting s.
Miller operating s.
Miller rectal s.
Millesi s.
Mills circumflex s.
Milteck s.
mini-keratoplasty stitch s.
mitral valve s.
Mixter operating s.
Moore-Troutman corneal s.
Morse backward-cutting aortic s.
MPC automated intravitreal s.
Munro brain s.
Murphy s.
Nadler superior radial s.
nail s.
s. nail drill
nail-nipper s.
nasal s.
Nelson lobectomy s.
Nelson lung-dissecting s.
Nelson-Metzenbaum s.
Nelson-Vital dissecting s.
neonatal s.
Neumann s.

S

scissors *(continued)*
neurosurgical s.
neurovascular s.
New suture s.
Noble s.
Northbent suture s.
Noyes iridectomy s.
Noyes iris s.
Noyes-Shambaugh s.
Nugent-Gradle stitch s.
Nu-Tip laparoscopic s.
O'Brien-Mayo s.
O'Brien stitch s.
O'Brien suture s.
Ochsner s.
Ochsner ball-tipped s.
Ochsner diamond-edged s.
Olivecrona angular s.
Olivecrona dural s.
Olivecrona guillotine s.
O'Neill cardiac surgical s.
Ong capsulotomy s.
Ormco band s.
orthopedic s.
Osher corneal s.
otologic s.
Panzer gallbladder s.
Paparella wire-cutting s.
Par s.
pattern umbilical s.
Péan s.
Peck-Joseph s.
pericardiotomy s.
Peyman vitreous s.
Phaneuf uterine artery s.
Pickett s.
plain rotary s.
s. plaster shears
plastic surgery s.
plastic utility s.
Poppen sympathectomy s.
Potts-DeMartel gall duct s.
Potts-Smith arterial s.
Potts-Smith dissecting s.
Potts-Smith reverse s.
Potts tenotomy s.
Potts vascular s.
Potts-Yasargil s.
PowerStar bipolar s.
Pratt rectal s.
Prince dissecting s.
Prince-Potts s.
Prince tonsillar s.
s. probe
probe point s.
pterygium s.
ptosis s.
pupillary membrane s.
Quimby gum s.
radial iridotomy s.
Ragnell undermining s.
Rappazzo foreign body s.
Rappazzo haptic s.
Real s.

Reeh stitch s.
Rees face lift s.
Reichling corneal s.
Reinhoff thoracic s.
Resano thoracic s.
Reul coronary artery s.
reverse s.
reverse-cutting s.
Reynolds dissecting s.
Reynolds-Jameson vessel s.
Rhoton bayonet s.
Rhoton microsurgical s.
rhytidectomy s.
Rica ear polypus s.
Richter s.
right-angle s.
right-handed corneal s.
Rizzuti keratoplasty s.
Rizzuti-McGuire corneal section s.
Roberts episiotomy s.
Rochester s.
Rochester-Ferguson s.
Rochester-Ochsner s.
Roger wire-cutting s.
Rosenblatt s.
rotary s. with cigar handle
rotary s. with loop handle
Rubio s.
Ryder s.
saber-back s.
Sadler cartilage s.
Satinsky vena caval s.
Scanlan s.
Scheie-Westcott corneal section s.
Schmieden-Taylor dural s.
Schoemaker s.
Schoemaker-Loth s.
Schroeder episiotomy s.
Schroeder operating s.
Schuknecht wire-cutting s.
Schumacher umbilical cord s.
Scott dissecting s.
Scott right-angle s.
Scoville s.
Sealy dissecting s.
Seiler turbinate s.
Semb dissecting s.
serrated iris s.
Serratex s.
Seutin s.
Shapshay-Healy laryngeal s.
Shea-Bellucci s.
Shea vein graft s.
Shepard-Westcott s.
Shield iridotomy s.
Shortbent suture s.
Shutt s.
sickle s.
Siebold uterine s.
Sims-Siebold uterine s.
Sims uterine s.
Sistron s.
Sistrunk dissecting s.
in situ valve s.
Slip-N-Snip s.

Smart enucleation s.
Smellie obstetrical s.
SMIC collar s.
SMIC ear polypus s.
Smith bandage s.
Smith suture wire s.
Snowden-Pencer Super-Cut s.
Southbent s.
Spencer eye suture s.
Spencer stitch s.
Spetzler s.
spring s.
spring-handled s.
Spring iris s.
Stalzner rectal s.
StaySharp face lift Super-Cut s.
Stevens eye s.
Stevenson alligator s.
Stevens stitch s.
Stevens tenotomy s.
Stille dissecting s.
Stille-Mayo dissecting s.
Stille Super Cut s.
stitch s.
Stiwer s.
Storz intraocular s.
Storz iris s.
Storz stitch s.
Storz-Westcott conjunctival s.
Storz wire-cutting s.
strabismus s.
straight tenotomy s.
Strully cardiovascular s.
Strully dissecting s.
Strully dural s.
Strully hook s.
Strully neurosurgical s.
Sullival gum s.
Super-Cut s.
superior radial tenotomy s.
surgical s.
Sutherland eye s.
Sutherland-Grieshaber s.
suture wire-cutting s.
Sweet delicate pituitary s.
Sweet esophageal s.
Take-apart s.
Tamsco wire-cutting s.
Taylor brain s.
Taylor dural s.
tenotomy s.
thin-shaft nasal s.
Thomas s.
Thomson-Walker s.
thoracic s.
Thorek-Feldman gallbladder s.
Thorek gallbladder s.
Thorek thoracic s.
Thorpe-Castroviejo cataract s.
Thorpe pupillary membrane s.
Thorpe-Westcott cataract s.
Tindall s.
tissue s.
Toennis-Adson dural s.
Toennis dissecting s.

tonsillar s.
Torchia conjunctival s.
Torchia microcorneal s.
Torchia-Vannas micro-iris s.
trigeminal s.
Troutman-Castroviejo corneal
  section s.
Troutman conjunctival s.
Troutman-Katzin corneal
  transplant s.
Troutman microsurgical s.
Troutman suture s.
Trusler-Dean s.
tubal s.
turbinate s.
turbinectomy s.
Turner-Warwick diathermy s.
Twisk s.
umbilical s.
Universal wire s.
upper lateral s.
U. S. Army gauze s.
U. S. Army umbilical s.
uterine s.
utility bandage s.
valve leaflet excision s.
Vannas capsulotomy s.
Vannas corneal s.
Vannas iridocapsulotomy s.
vascular s.
Verhoeff dissecting s.
Verner-Joseph s.
Vernon wire-cutting s.
Vezien abdominal s.
vibrating s.
Vital-Cooley operating s.
Vital-Cooley wire-cutting s.
Vital-Cottle dorsal angled s.
Vital-Fomon angular s.
Vital-Knapp iris s.
Vital-Knapp strabismus s.
Vital-Mayo dissecting s.
Vital-Metzenbaum s.
Vital-Metzenbaum dissecting s.
Vital-Nelson dissecting s.
Vital operating s.
Vital wire-cutting s.
vitreous strand s.
V. Mueller curved operating s.
V. Mueller laser tubal s.
V. Mueller operating s.
V. Mueller-Vital laser Mayo
  dissecting s.
Wadsworth s.
Walker-Apple s.
Walker-Atkinson s.
Walker corneal s.
Walton s.
Weber tissue s.
Weck iris s.
Weck-Spencer suture s.
Weck suture s.
Weck suture-removal s.
Weck wire-cutting s.
Weller cartilage s.

S

scissors *(continued)*
  Werb s.
  Wertheim deep surgery s.
  Westcott conjunctival s.
  Westcott double-end s.
  Westcott micro s.
  Westcott-Scheie s.
  Westcott spring-action s.
  Westcott stitch s.
  Westcott tenotomy s.
  Westcott utility s.
  Wester meniscectomy s.
  White s.
  Wiechel s.
  Wiechel-Stille bile duct s.
  Wiet otologic s.
  Wilde-Blakesley s.
  Willauer s.
  Williamson-Noble s.
  Wilmer conjunctival s.
  Wilmer-Converse conjunctival s.
  Wilmer iris s.
  Wilson intraocular s.
  Wincor enucleation s.
  wire s.
  wire-cutting suture s.
  Wong-Staal s.
  Wullstein ear s.
  Wutzler s.
  Yankauer s.
  Yasargil bayonet s.
  Yasargil microvascular bayonet s.
  Zoellner s.
  Z-Scissors hysterectomy s.
  Zylik-Michaels s.
scleral
  s. blade
  s. buckle eye implant
  s. buckler implant
  s. buckling catheter
  s. depressor
  s. expander ring
  s. hook
  s. marker
  s. pick
  s. plug
  s. punch
  s. resection knife
  s. shell
  s. shield
  s. shortening clip
  s. spatula needle
  s. sponge rod
  s. twist fixation hook
  s. twist-grip forceps
  s. wound retractor
sclerectomy
  s. punch
  s. punch forceps
ScleroLASER
ScleroPLUS LongPulse dye laser
sclerostomy needle
sclerotherapy needle

sclerotome
  Alvis-Lancaster s.
  Atkinson s.
  s. blade
  Castroviejo s.
  Curdy s.
  Guyton-Lundsgaard s.
  Lancaster s.
  Lundsgaard s.
  Lundsgaard-Burch s.
  s. pain chart
  Walker-Lee s.
sclerotomy punch
Scobee-Allis forceps
Scobee oblique muscle hook
SCOI brace
scoliometer
scoliosis brace
ScoliTron instrument
scoop
  Abbott s.
  abdominal s.
  abortion s.
  Arlt fenestrated lens s.
  Asch uterine secretion s.
  Beck abdominal s.
  Beck gastrostomy s.
  Berens common duct s.
  Berens lens s.
  Bruus s.
  S. 1, 2 catheter
  common duct stone s.
  Councill stone s.
  cystic duct s.
  Daviel lens s.
  Desjardins gall duct s.
  Desjardins gallstone s.
  s. dish
  duct s.
  Elschnig lens s.
  enucleation s.
  Ferguson gallstone s.
  Ferris common duct s.
  French s.
  gallbladder s.
  gall duct s.
  gallstone s.
  Goudet uterine s.
  Green lens s.
  Hess lens s.
  Hibbs s.
  Klebanoff gallstone s.
  Knapp lens s.
  Lang eye s.
  lens enucleation s.
  Lewis lens s.
  Luer s.
  Luer-Koerte gallstone s.
  Mayo common duct s.
  Mayo cystic duct s.
  Mayo gallbladder s.
  Mayo gall duct s.
  Mayo gallstone s.
  Mayo-Robson gallstone s.
  microbayonet s.

Moore gall duct s.
Moore gallstone s.
Moynihan gallstone s.
Mules s.
Pagenstecher lens s.
Schroeder uterine s.
Simon uterine s.
Snellen lens s.
Syrrat s.
S. transtracheal catheter
uterine s.
Volkmann s.
Wallich abortion s.
Wallich placental s.
Weber lens s.
Wells enucleation s.
Wilder lens s.
Yasargil s.
Zarski gallstone s.

Scoot-Gard mat
scope
baby s.
Doppler s.
Electro-Acuscope s.
endocervicometer s.
ENT s.
fixed-focus s.
Gamboscope s.
GO s.
KeraCorneoScope s.
keratoiridoscope s.
KeyMed fiberoptic s.
Lixiscope s.
MaculoScope s.
Olympus ENF-P2 s.
Olympus fiberoptic s.
Olympus OSF s.
Oral Video S.
SinuScope s.
Smart S.
variable-focus s.
Welch Allyn pocket s.
Scopemaster contact hysteroscope
ScopeTrac support device
Scopette device
Scorpio total knee system
Scotch boot
Scotchcast
S. 2 casting tape
S. length splinting system
scotometer
Bjerrum s.
scotoscope
Scott
S. AMS inflatable penile prosthesis
S. attic cannula
S. chronic wound care system
S. dissecting scissors
S. ear speculum
S. humeral splint
S. lens-insertion forceps
S. nasal suction tube
S. No. 2 curved ruler
S. right-angle scissors

S. rotating resectoscope
S. rubber ventricular cannula
Scott-Craig orthosis
Scott-Harden tube
Scottish
S. Rite brace
S. Rite hip orthosis
S. Rite splint
Scott-McCracken periosteal elevator
Scott-RCE osteotomy guide
Scotty
S. the Scale stand-on scale
S. stainless ankle joint
Scoville
S. blunt hook
S. brain forceps
S. Britetrac retractor
S. cervical disk self-retaining
retractor
S. clip
S. clip applier
S. clip-applying forceps
S. curved nerve hook
S. dural hook
S. flat brain spatula
S. hemilaminectomy self-retaining
retractor
S. laminectomy retractor
S. nerve root retractor
S. psoas muscle retractor
S. retractor blade
S. retractor hook
S. ruptured disk curette
S. scissors
S. self-retaining retractor
S. skull trephine
S. ventricular needle
Scoville-Drew clip applier
Scoville-Greenwood bayonet neurosurgical
bipolar forceps
Scoville-Haverfield laminectomy retractor
Scoville-Hurteau forceps
Scoville-Lewis
S.-L. aneurysm clip
S.-L. clamp
Scoville-Richter self-retaining retractor
SCRAM face mask
scraper
amalgam s.
capsular s.
Charnley acetabular s.
drum s.
epithelial s.
Hough drum s.
Knolle capsular s.
Kratz capsular s.
Lewicky capsular s.
Simcoe capsular s.
Tano membrane s.
scraping brush
scratcher
Jensen capsular s.
Knolle capsular s.
Kratz capsular s.
Kratz-Jensen capsular s.

S

screen
Bernell tangent s.
Bjerrum s.
ether s.
Fast Lanex rare earth s.
Grey-Hess s.
guilt s.
Hess diplopia s.
Hess-Lee s.
homogeneous s.
intensifying s.
Lancaster red-green s.
Lanex medium s.
split s.
tangent s.
screener
Algo newborn hearing s.
AutoPap 300 QC automatic Pap s.
Rosenbaum pocket vision s.
Smart Screener infant hearing s.
screw
Absolute absorbable s.
Acutrak s.
alar s.
s. alignment bar
s. alignment rod
Alta cancellous s.
Alta cortical s.
Alta cross-locking s.
Alta lag s.
Alta supracondylar s.
Alta transverse s.
amputation s.
anchor s.
Arthrex sheathed interference s.
Asnis guided s.
Asnis 2 guided s.
Asnis III cannulated s.
Aten olecranon s.
Barouk cannulated bone s.
Basile hip s.
bicortical superior border s.
bioabsorbable interference s.
Biofix absorbable s.
biointerference s.
Biologically Quiet interference s.
Biologically Quiet reconstruction s.
Bionix self-reinforced PLLA
  smart s.
BioSorb endoscopic browlift s.
bone s.
Bone Mulch s.
Bosworth coracoclavicular s.
brow lift suspension s.
Buttress thread s.
Calcitek retaining s.
Camino subdural s.
cancellous bone s.
cannulated cancellous lag s.
Carol Gerard s.
carpal scaphoid s.
Carrel-Girard s.
Caspar cervical s.
Clearfix meniscal s.
Cohort bone s.

Collison s.
compression hip s. (CHS)
s. compressor
Concise compression hip s.
cortex s.
cortical s.
Cotrel pedicle s.
cover s.
craniomaxillofacial s.
Crites laryngeal cotton s.
crown drill s.
cruciate head bone s.
cruciform head bone s.
Cubbins s.
Demuth hip s.
dental implant cover s.
Dentatus s.
s. depth calibrator
s. depth gauge
DePuy interference s.
Deyerle s.
distal locking s.
distraction s.
Doyen myoma s.
Doyen tumor s.
Duo-Drive cortical s.
Dwyer spinal s.
dynamic condylar s.
dynamic hip s.
Edwards sacral s.
Eggers s.
encased s.
endocardial s.
EndoFix absorbable interference s.
expansion s.
Fabian s.
Fixateur Interne s.
fixation s.
foreign body s.
four-tap s.
Geckeler s.
Gentle Threads interference s.
Glasser fixation s.
glenoid fixation s.
s. grip
Guardsman femoral interference s.
Hahn s.
Hall-Morris biphase s.
Hall spinal s.
healing s.
Heck s.
Herbert bone s.
Herbert scaphoid s.
Herbert-Whipple bone s.
Howmedica Universal
  compression s.
iliac s.
iliosacral s.
Ilizarov s.
ImplaMed gold s.
Implant Innovations titanium s.
Implant Support Systems titanium
Instrument Makar biodegradable
  interference s.
Integrity acetabular cup s.

interference s.
interfragmentary lag s.
intracranial pressure monitor s.
Isola spinal implant system iliac s.
Isola vertebral s.
Jeter lag s.
Jeter position s.
Jewett pickup s.
Johannson lag s.
Johannson-Stille lag s.
KLS Centre-Drive s.
KLS-Martin Centre-Drive s.
Kostuik s.
Kristiansen eyelet lag s.
Kurosaka interference-fit s.
lag s.
Lane bone s.
lateral s.
Leibinger Micro Plus s.
Leibinger Mini Würzburg s.
Leibinger Würzburg s.
Leinbach olecranon s.
Leone expansion s.
Lewis tonsillar s.
Lindorf lag s.
Lindorf position s.
Linvatec absorbable s.
Linvatec bioabsorbable
  interference s.
locking s.
Lorenz s.
Luhr implant s.
Luhr Vitallium s.
lumbar pedicle s.
Lundholm s.
Luque II s.
mandibular angle fracture intraoral
  open reduction s.
Marion s.
maxillofacial bone s.
McLaughlin carpal scaphoid s.
medial bicortical s.
medial unicortical s.
metallic s.
Micro Plus s.
Mille Pattes s.
mini lag s.
mini Würzburg s.
monocortical s.
Morris biphase s.
multiaxial s.
myoma s.
navicular s.
Neufeld s.
Nobelpharma gold prosthetic
  retaining s.
No-Lok compression s.
s. occlusive clamp
Olerud PSF s.
Omega compression hip s.
oral s.
Orion plate and s.
Orthex cannulated titanium bone s.
Orthofix s.
orthopedic s.

Osteomed s.
Palex expansion s.
pedicle s.
PerFixation s.
Periotest Implant Innovations
  gold s.
Phantom interference s.
Phillips recessed-head s.
Pilot point s.
polyaxial cervical s.
polylactide absorbable s.
pretapped Synthes lag s.
Pro/Pel cannulated interference s.
pull s.
Quiet interference s.
Reddick-Saye s.
resorbable plate and s.
ReUnite orthopedic s.
reverse-threaded s.
Revo retrievable cancellous s.
Richards classic compression hip s.
Richmond subarachnoid s.
rigid pedicle s.
Rockwood shoulder s.
Russell-Taylor s.
sacral alar s.
sacral pedicle s.
Salzburg s.
Scuderi s.
self-tapping bone s.
self-tapping Leibinger lag s.
set s.
Sharpey s.
Sherman bone s.
silk s.
Simmons double-hole spinal s.
Simmons-Martin s.
SmartScrew s.
Smith & Nephew s.
Spiessel lag s.
Spiessel position s.
stainless steel s.
Steinhauser lag s.
Steinhauser position s.
step s.
Stryker lag s.
subarachnoid s.
superior thoracic pedicle s.
superlag s.
syndesmotic s.
Synthes s.
Synthes compression hip s.
s. tap
Texas Scottish Rite Hospital
  pedicle s.
Thatcher s.
thoracolumbar pedicle s.
ThreadLoc driver mount s.
ThreadLoc retaining s.
Ti alloy s.
TiMesh s.
titanium s.
tonsillar s.
Townley bone graft s.
Townsend-Gilfillan s.

S

screw *(continued)*
TPS-coated s.
traction tongs s.
transarticular s.
transfixion s.
transpedicular s.
triangulated pedicle s.
tulip pedicle s.
tumor s.
Venable s.
Vilex cannulated s.
Virgin hip s.
Vitallium s.
Weise jack s.
Wood s.
Woodruff s.
Yuan s.
Zielke s.
Zimmer s.
screwdriver
Allen-headed s.
automatic s.
Becker s.
Bosworth s.
Children's Hospital s.
Collison s.
cross-slot s.
cruciform s.
Cubbins s.
DePuy s.
Dorsey s.
Hall s.
heavy cross-slot s.
hexhead s.
s. instrument
Johnson s.
Ken s.
KLS Centre-Drive s.
Lane s.
light cross-slot s.
Lok-it s.
Lok-screw double-slot s.
Massie s.
Master s.
Moore-Blount s.
Phillips s.
plain s.
Richards Phillips s.
Richter s.
right-angle s.
Shallcross s.
Sherman s.
Sherman-Pierce s.
single cross-slot s.
skull plate s.
Stab-and-Grab s.
straight hex s.
Stryker s.
Trinkle s.
Universal s.
Universal hex s.
V. Mueller s.
White s.
Williams s.

Woodruff s.
Zimmer s.
screw-holding forceps
screw-in
s.-i. epicardial electrode
s.-i. lead
s.-i. lead pacemaker
s.-i. sutureless myocardial electrode
screw-on lead
screw-tipped intraosseous needle
screw-to-screw compression construct
screw-type implant
Screw-Vent
S.-V. implant
S.-V. implant system
Scribner shunt
Script Stat, Inc. dispensing system
scrotal
s. dressing
s. truss
scrub
s. brush
s. file
scrubber
capsular s.
posterior capsule s.
Simcoe anterior chamber capsule s.
Simcoe posterior capsule s.
Scudder
S. intestinal clamp
S. intestinal forceps
S. skid
S. stomach clamp
Scuderi
S. bipolar coagulating forceps
S. prosthesis
S. screw
Scuderi-Callahan flange
Scully Hip S'port functional hip suppor
sculp knife
Sculptor
S. annuloplasty ring
S. flexible annuloplasty ring
sculpturing scalpel
scultetus
s. bandage
s. binder band
s. binder dressing
Scurasil device prosthesis
Scutan temporary splint material
SD-1 stone disintegrator
S.D.port
S-D-Sorb
S.-D.-S. E-Z TAC implant
S.-D.-S. E-Z Tac system
S.-D.-S. suture anchor system
SDsorb meniscal stapler
SDU-400 EchoView ultrasound machine
SE-100 smoke aspiration tip
Sea-Band acupressure wristband
Seabands
seal
a-fiX cannula s.
Asherman chest s.

Bennett s.
iLEX stomal s.
SealEasy resuscitation mask
sealing window plug
Seal-Tight cast protector
Seal-Tite adhesive gasket
Sealy dissecting scissors
SeamGuard staple line material
seamless
s. graft
s. prosthesis
seam-sealer gun
searcher
Allport-Babcock mastoid s.
Allport mastoid s.
mastoid s.
Proctor-Bruce mastoid s.
Shea s.
Shuletz s.
Searcy
S. anchor/fixation
S. capsular forceps
S. chalazion trephine
S. fixation
S. fixation anchor
S. fixation hook
S. oval cup erysiphake
S. tonsillectome
Searle volume ventilator
Sears Wee Alert
SeaSorb alginate wound dressing
seat
Backjoy s.
Carrie car s.
Dream Ride car s.
Heffington lumbar s.
Ingram bicycle s.
Maddacare child bath s.
orthopedic positioning s.
Posey drop s.
Renolux convertible car s.
Snug s.
Special S.
Spelcast car s.
Tall-ette toilet s.
Tubsider Kneeling S.
Seated
S. Cable Row exerciser
S. Hamstring Curl exercise chair
Seattle
S. Foot prosthesis
S. orthosis
S. splint
Sebbin
S. ultrasound-assisted lipoplasty
machine
S. ultrasound device
Sebileau periosteal elevator
Sebra arm tourniquet
Sechrist
S. infant ventilator
S. Model 2500E, 3200E, 7200
hyperbaric chamber
S. monoplace hyperbaric chamber
S. neonatal ventilator

second
s. generation lithotriptor
s. skin pad
Secor system
Secto
S. dissector
S. tonsillar sponge
sector scanner
Secu clip
Securat suction tube
SeCure
S. therapeutic mattress
Secure
S. closed pressure monitoring and
blood sampling system
S. Yet Gentle surgical dressing
system
SecureEasy endotracheal harness
SecureStrand
S. cable
S. cervical fusion system
Secur-Its silicon cushion mat
Security+ self-sealing Urisheath external
catheter
Sedan
S. cannula
S. goniometer
Sedan-Nashold needle
Seddon nerve graft
Sédillot
S. periosteal elevator
S. raspatory
Seeburger implant
Seecor pacemaker
seed implant
seeker
ball-tipped s.
S. guidewire
Kuhn-Bolger s.
ostium s.
Seeman-Seiffert mouthgag
Seep-Pruf ileostomy appliance
SeeQuence disposable contact lens
Seer cardiac monitor
segmental
s. compression construct
s. spinal correction system
s. spinal instrumentation
segmented ring tripolar lead
Segond
S. abdominal retractor
S. hysterectomy forceps
S. myomatome
S. tumor forceps
S. vaginal spatula
Segond-Landau hysterectomy forceps
Séguin formboard
Segura
S. CBD basket
S. stone basket
Segura-Dretler stone basket
Sehrt
S. clamp
S. compressor
Seibel nucleus chopper

S

Seidel
- S. bone-holding clamp
- S. catheter
- S. humeral locking nail
- S. intramedullary fixation
- S. plug
- S. saddlebag

Seiffert
- S. esophagoscopy forceps
- S. grasping punch
- S. laryngeal forceps
- S. tonsillectome

Seiff frontalis suspension set

Seiler
- S. MC-M900 surgical microscope
- S. tonsillar knife
- S. turbinate scissors

Seirin acupuncture needle

Seitzinger tripolar cutting forceps

seizing forceps

Sekomic SS-100F recorder

Selby II hook

Seldin
- S. dental retractor
- S. elevator

Seldinger
- S. apparatus
- S. arterial needle
- S. cardiac catheter
- S. gastrostomy needle
- S. retrograde wire

Selecon coronary angiography catheter

Select
- S. ankle prosthesis
- S. GT blood glucose system
- S. joint orthosis
- S. shoulder prosthesis

SelectCells Mini endometrial sampler

selective
- s. imaging and graphics for stereotactic surgery
- s. tubal occlusion procedure system

Selective-HI catheter

Selectives
- Theraform S.

selector
- Leksell s.
- sleeve s.
- S. ultrasonic aspirator

Selectron system

Seletz
- S. catheter
- S. foramen-plugging forceps
- S. Universal Kerrison punch
- S. ventricular cannula

Seletz-Gelpi self-retaining retractor

self-adhering
- s.-a. lid retractor
- s.-a. varus/valgus wedge

self-aligning knee

self-articulating femoral prosthesis

self-aspirating cut-biopsy needle

Selfast dental cement

self-broaching pin

Self-Cath
- S.-C. closed catheterization system
- S.-C. coudé tipped catheter
- S.-C. coude tipped catheter with guide stripe
- S.-C. soft catheter
- S.-C. straight tipped female catheter
- S.-C. straight tipped pediatric catheter
- S.-C. straight tipped soft catheter

self-catheter
- Mentor female s.-c.

self-centering
- s.-c. micromanipulator
- s.-c. Universal hip prosthesis

self-contained
- s.-c. underwater breathing apparatus

self-examination
- BD Sensability breast s.-e.

self-expandable
- s.-e. metallic stent
- s.-e. stainless steel braided endoprosthesis

self-expanding
- s.-e. coil stent
- s.-e. metallic endoprosthesis
- s.-e. metallic stent
- s.-e. stainless steel stent
- s.-e. tulip sheath
- s.-e. Wallstent endoprosthesis

self-guiding catheter

self-inflating
- s.-i. bulb
- s.-i. tissue expander

self-opening
- s.-o. forceps
- s.-o. rigid snare

self-propelling wheelchair

self-retaining
- s.-r. abdominal retractor
- s.-r. bone forceps
- s.-r. brain retractor
- s.-r. brain retractor frame
- s.-r. catheter
- s.-r. chamber maintainer
- s.-r. coil stent
- s.-r. infusion cannula
- s.-r. irrigating cannula
- s.-r. laryngoscope
- s.-r. retractor blade
- s.-r. ring retractor
- s.-r. skin retractor
- s.-r. spring retractor

self-sealing cannula

Self Snag strap

self-stabilizing vitrectomy lens

self-stopping drill point

self-tapering pin

self-tapping
- s.-t. bone screw
- s.-t. Leibinger lag screw
- s.-t. screw-type implant

Selker ventriculostomy reservoir

sellar punch

Sellheim
   S. elevating spoon
   S. obstetrical lever
   S. uterine catheter
Sellor
   S. clamp
   S. mitral valve knife
   S. rib contractor
   S. rib retractor
   S. valvulotome
Sellotape tie-over dressing
Selman
   S. clamp
   S. clip
   S. nonslip tissue forceps
   S. peripheral blood vessel forceps
   S. tissue forceps
   S. vessel forceps
Selofix dressing
Selopor dressing
Seloris balloon
Selrodo
   S. bulb
   S. nebulizer
Selsi sport telescope
Seltzer saw
Selverstone
   S. carotid artery clamp
   S. cordotomy hook
   S. embolus forceps
   S. intervertebral disk forceps
   S. intervertebral disk rongeur
   S. laminectomy rongeur
   S. rongeur forceps
Semb
   S. bone-cutting forceps
   S. bone forceps
   S. bone-holding clamp
   S. bone-holding forceps
   S. bronchus clamp
   S. dissecting forceps
   S. dissecting scissors
   S. ligature-carrying forceps
   S. ligature forceps
   S. lung retractor
   S. rib forceps
   S. rib raspatory
   S. rongeur
   S. rongeur forceps
   S. self-retaining retractor
   S. shears
   S. vaginal speculum
Semb-Ghazi dissecting forceps
Semb-Sauerbruch rongeur
semi-adjustable articulator
semicircular gouge
semicompressive dressing
semiflat tip electrode
semiflexible
   s. endoscope
   s. intraocular lens
semilunar cartilage knife
semilunar-tip blade
semiocclusive moisture-retentive dressing
semipermeable membrane dressing

semipressure dressing
semirigid
   s. catheter
   s. endoscope
   s. fiberglass cast
   s. intraocular lens
   s. polypropylene ankle-foot orthosis
semishell eye implant
semitubular blade plate
Semken
   S. bipolar forceps
   S. dressing forceps
   S. infant forceps
   S. microbipolar neurosurgical forceps
   S. thumb forceps
   S. tissue forceps
Semm
   S. CO_2 pneumatometer
   S. morcellator
   S. Pelvi-Pneu insufflator
   S. pneumoperitoneum apparatus
   S. uterine vacuum cannula
   S. uterine vacuum catheter
Semmes
   S. curette
   S. dural forceps
Semmes-Weinstein
   S.-W. monofilament instrument
   S.-W. nylon monofilament
   S.-W. pressure aesthesiometer filament
   S.-W. pressure anesthesiometer
Seneliners
Senepads
   S. underpad
Sengstaken
   S. balloon
   S. nasogastric tube
Sengstaken-Blakemore
   S.-B. esophageal balloon
   S.-B. esophagogastric tamponade tube
Senn
   S. bone plate
   S. double-ended retractor
   S. mastoid retractor
   S. self-retaining retractor
Senn-Dingman double-ended retractor
Senn-Green retractor
Sennheiser electric condenser ME 40-3 microphone
Senning
   S. cardiovascular forceps
   S. featherweight bulldog clamp
   S. intraatrial baffle
Senning-Stille clamp
Senn-Kanavel double-ended retractor
Senn-Miller retractor
Senoran aspirator
Sensability Breast Self-Examination Aid
Sens-A-Ray digital dental imaging system
Sensatec
   S. endoscope

Sensation
 S. intra-aortic balloon catheter
 S. Short Throw snare
Sens dissector
Sense-of-Feel prosthesis
SensiCath
 S. blood gas measurement system
 S. optical sensor
Sensimatic electrosurgical unit
sensing
 s. catheter
 s. coil
Sensitometer
 Poppen Ridge S.
Sensi-Touch anesthesia delivery system
Sensiv endotracheal tube
Senso
 S. completely-in-the-canal digital
  hearing aid
 S. listening device
Sensolog II, III pacemaker
Sensonic plaque removal instrument
sensor
 Albin-Bunegin pressure s.
 anal EMG PerryMeter s.
 anterior aspect esophageal s.
 BIS S.
 capacitive s.
 Capnostat CO_2 s.
 CardioSearch s.
 ClipTip reusable s.
 Cross Top replacement oxygen s.
 DC SQUID s.
 DermaTemp infrared
  thermographic s.
 Diasensor 1000 s.
 differential temperature s.
 disposable Doppler-constant
  thermocouple s.
 electromyogram s.
 ENDEX apex s.
 fiberoptic PCO_2 s.
 finger clip s.
 FlexiSensor s.
 Infinity s.
 S. Kelvin pacemaker
 Ladd intracranial pressure s.
 manometric s.
 MEG s.
 MicroMirror gold s.
 multiparameter s.
 MyoScan s.
 Nellcor FS-series oximeter s.
 Novametrix combination O_2/CO_2 s.
 oximetry s.
 Oxisensor II adult adhesive s.
 OxyTip s.
 s. pad
 Paratrend 7+ s.
 Paratrend 7 fiberoptic PCO_2 s.
 Perry s.
 PerryAnal/PerryVaginal EMG s.
 PerryMeter anal EMG s.
 Pulsar Max s.
 Richmond subarachnoid screw s.

 Saber CBF-ICP trauma s.
 SensiCath optical s.
 Servo Pro force s.
 Shell s.
 SpiroSense flow s.
 telemetric intracranial pressure s.
 three-dimensional magnetic s.
 ultrasonic tactile s.
sensor-based single-chamber pacemaker
SensorMedics pressure transducer
sensory stimulation kit
SensoScan mammography system
Sentalloy digital calipers
SentiLite neurological monitor
Sentinel-4 neurological monitor
Sentron
 S. pigtail angiographic
  micromanometer catheter
 S. pigtail microtip-manometer
  catheter
Senturia
 S. forceps
 S. pharyngeal speculum
 S. retractor
Senturia-Alden specimen collector
separating strip
separator
 Allen stereo s.
 Amicus blood collection s.
 Asahi Plasmaflo plasma s.
 bayonet s.
 Benson baby pyloric s.
 blood cell s.
 Cobe blood cell s.
 Davis nerve s.
 Dorsey dural s.
 dural s.
 Elast-O-Chain s.
 Fenwal CS3000 Plus cell s.
 Ferrier s.
 finger s.
 Frazier dural s.
 Grant dural s.
 Harris s.
 head spoon s.
 Hoen dural s.
 Horsley dural s.
 House ear s.
 Hunter s.
 iliac graft s.
 Kirby curved zonular s.
 Kirby cylindrical zonular s.
 Kirby double-ball s.
 Kirby flat zonular s.
 Lig-A-Ring s.
 Luys s.
 mechanical s.
 noninterfering s.
 Remy s.
 Rosen bayonet s.
 Sachs dural s.
 Sachs nerve s.
 Sep-A-Ring s.
 Silverstein nerve s.
 stem spoon s.

synovial s.
True s.
s. tube
Woodson dural s.
zonule s.
Sep-A-Ring separator
Sephadex bead
Seprafilm bioresorbable membrane
Sepramesh biosurgical composite
S-E prosthesis
septal
s. bone forceps
s. chisel
s. clamp
s. compression forceps
s. dissector
s. elevator
s. knife
s. needle
s. ridge forceps
s. straightener
Septer closed wound drainage system
Septi-Chek culture system
Septisol soap dressing
Septobal bead
Septoject needle
Septopack periodontal dressing
Septopal implant
Septosil impression material
septostomy balloon catheter
septum-cutting forceps
septum-straightening forceps
Sep-T-Vac suction cannister
Sequel compression system
sequencer
ALF DNA S. II
automated laser-fluorescence s.
automatic gas s.
sequencing bead patterns set
sequential
s. circulator
s. compression device
s. compression stockings
s. extremity pump
s. multiple analyzer
S. Multiple Analyzer Computer (SMAC)
s. pressure
s. video converter
Sequestra 1000 blood processing system
sequestrum forceps
Sequicor
S. II, III pacemaker
Sequoia
S. Acuson system
S. echocardiography system
S. ultrasound system
Seraflo
S. AV fistular needle
S. blood line
S. transducer protector
Seraphim clip
Seraton dialysis control system
Serature spur clip

Serdarevic
S. Circle of Light
S. speculum
S. suture adjuster
Serena
S. Mx apnea recorder/analyzer
S. Mx hand-held apnea detection device
series
HESSCO 300, 500 s.
Leksell gamma knife target s.
Mist 14-gauge Eubanks instrument s.
Option Orthotic S.
RingLoc acetabular s.
Rosser signature s.
Sevrain cranial clamp 200 s.
St. Jude medical heart valve hemodynamic plus s.
Vmax s.
Series-II humeral head
Serola sacroiliac belt
Seroma-Cath
S.-C. drainage tube
S.-C. feeding tube
S.-C. wound drainage catheter
S.-C. wound drainage system
Serono SR1 FSH analyzer
serpentine bone plate
serrated
s. amalgam plugger
s. blade
s. catheter
s. conjunctival forceps
s. curette
s. fine-cutting knife
s. iris scissors
s. retractor
s. suture
s. T-spatula
Serratex scissors
serrefine
Blair s.
Brunswick s.
s. clamp
Dieffenbach s.
s. forceps
Hess s.
s. implant
Lemoine s.
Mack s.
s. retractor
SERTEC International, Inc.
Serter
C-wire S.
serum pregnancy assay cartridge
Servo
S. Pro force sensor
S. pump
S. ventilator
servo-mechanism sphincter
Servox
S. amplifier
S. device

Servox *(continued)*
  S. electronic speech aid
  S. Inton speech aid
sesamoidectomy dissector
set
  Ackrad Tampa catheter s.
  Acland-Banis arteriotomy s.
  ACS percutaneous introducer s.
  Alken s.
  Amicon arteriovenous blood
    tubing s.
  Arnold-Bruening intracordal
    injection s.
  Bankart shoulder repair s.
  Bantam irrigation s.
  Bio-Medicus percutaneous cannula s.
  Biostil blood transfusion s.
  Bloomberg trabeculotome s.
  Borst side-arm introducer s.
  Bremer halo crown traction s.
  Brodmerkel colon decompression s.
  Brown-Mueller T-fastener s.
  Bruening-Arnold intracordal
    injection s.
  Bruening intracordal injection s.
  Bruening otoscope s.
  Catalano intubation s.
  Ciaglia Blue Rhino percutaneous
    tracheostomy introducer s.
  Ciaglia percutaneous tracheostomy
    introducer s.
  Cliniset infusion s.
  Cloward cervical retractor s.
  coaxial micropuncture introducer s.
  Codman external drainage
    ventricular s.
  Colapinto transjugular biopsy s.
  Collis Universal laminectomy s.
  Coloplast economy irrigation s.
  Coloplast hospital irrigation s.
  Coloplast two-piece sterile post-
    op s.
  Cone-Bucy suction cannula s.
  Cook drainage pouch s.
  Cope gastrointestinal suture
    anchor s.
  Corpak enteral Y extension s.
  Cotton-Huibregtse biliary stent s.
  Cotton-Leung biliary stent s.
  Craig vertebral body biopsy
    instrument s.
  Crampton-Tsang percutaneous
    endoscopic biliary stent s.
  Crawford lacrimal s.
  Criticare HN-Isocal tube feeding s.
  Dansac colostomy irrigation s.
  DePuy small-joint arthroscopy
    instrument s.
  Desilets-Hoffman introducer s.
  Diethrich coronary artery s.
  DORC subretinal instrument s.
  DSP Micro Diamond-Point
    microsurgery s.
  Dujovny microsuction dissection s.

  Dynacor vaginal irrigator s.
  Echosight Jansen-Anderson
    intrauterine catheter s.
  Echosight Patton coaxial catheter s.
  Echotip Baker amniocentesis s.
  Echotip Dominion needle s.
  Echotip Kato-Asch needle s.
  Eiken-Kizai hemodialysis blood
    tubing s.
  Eliminator nasal biliary catheter s.
  Embryon GIFT transfer catheter s.
  Endo-Suction sinus microstat s.
  Entrex small-joint arthroscopy
    instrument s.
  Freiburg biopsy s.
  Garcia endometrial biopsy s.
  Grandon cortex extractor s.
  Greenberg retractor s.
  Guardian one-piece ostomy system:
    sterile drainage O.R. s.
  Guardian two-piece ostomy system:
    sterile drainage loop s.
  Guibor canaliculus intubation s.
  Harvard microbore intravenous
    extension s.
  Henning instrument s.
  Heyer-Schulte Small-Carrion
    sizing s.
  Hobbs stent s.
  Huibregtse biliary stent s.
  Hulbert endo-electrode s.
  Impex/Lerner foldable lens
    removing s.
  Inpersol peritoneal dialysis s.
  Jackson lacrimal intubation s.
  Jackson magnification ruler s.
  Jaffe laser blepharoplasty and facial
    resurfacing s.
  Janacek reimplantation s.
  Jeffrey introducer s.
  Kawasumi infusion s.
  KeyMed advanced oesophageal
    dilator s.
  Kish urethral illuminated catheter s.
  Klippel retractor s.
  Küntscher nail s.
  Leung endoscopic nasal biliary
    drainage s.
  Level One normothermic IV
    fluid s.
  LifePort infusion s.
  Liguory endoscopic nasal biliary
    drainage s.
  Loversan infusion s.
  Maciol suture needle s.
  Malis irrigation tubing s.
  Marcon colon decompression s.
  Mardis-Dangler ureteral stent s.
  McIntyre guarded irrigating
    cystitome s.
  McIntyre infusion s.
  MegaFlo infusion s.
  Mentanium vitreoretinal
    instrument s.
  Messerklinger sinus endoscopy s.

Mills coronary endarterectomy s.
Mi-Mark endocervical curette s.
Molina mandibular distractor s.
Moore nail s.
Mullan percutaneous trigeminal
ganglion microcompression s.
Mullan trigeminal ganglion
microcompression s.
Myelo-Nate s.
Nagaraja endoscopic nasal biliary
drainage s.
Neff percutaneous access s.
Neo-Sert umbilical vessel catheter
insertion s.
NephroMax catheter s.
New Orleans endarterectomy
stripper s.
Novack special extraction s.
Palex colostomy irrigation starter s.
Parker-Glassman intestinal clamp s.
parquetry s.
Peel-Away introducer s.
Pettigrove laser-assisted intrastromal
keratomileusis s.
Pettigrove LASIK s.
Porter-Kolpe biliary biopsy s.
Price Donor Cornea Punch s.
prothelen s.
Ramel s.
Re-Entry Malecot catheter s.
Rica esophagoscopy s.
Rica skull perforator s.
Rosch-Thurmond fallopian tube
catheterization s.
Saf-T E-Z s.
Scherback-Porges vaginal
speculum s.
Schoenrock laser instrument s.
s. screw
Seiff frontalis suspension s.
sequencing bead patterns s.
Simcoe lens-positioning s.
Sippy esophageal dilating s.
Sobel-Kaplitt-Sawyer gas
endarterectomy s.
Soehendra lithotripsy s.
Soluset IV s.
Steinert laser-assisted intrastromal
keratomileusis s.
Stille bone drill s.
Stille-pattern trephine and bone
drill s.
Storz ear knife s.
Surewing winged infusion s.
Sur-Fit night drainage container s.
Surflo winged infusion s.
Surgimedics TMP multiperfusion s.
Szabo-Berci endoscopic needle
driver s.
Tebbets rhinoplasty s.
Tender subcutaneous infusion s.
Thomas subretinal instrument s. II
Toomey surgical steel instrument s.
Turkel bone biopsy trephine s.
U-Mid-O_2 Jet s.

Universal laminectomy s.
Veirs dacryocystorhinostomy s.
Vennes pancreatic dilation s.
VISI-FLOW irrigation starter s.
VPI-Jacobellis microhematuria
catheter s.
Wiegerinck culdocentesis puncture s.
Wilson-Cook Carey capsule s.
Wilson-Cook low-profile esophageal
prosthesis s.
Wissinger s.
Wylie endarterectomy s.
Zimmon endoscopic biliary stent s.
Zimmon endoscopic pancreatic
stent s.
Zimmon esophagogastric balloon
tamponade s.
Setacure denture repair acrylic
Setma hydrotherapy system
seton
    S. drain
    S. hip brace
    Molteno s.
    s. needle
    s. suture
Set-Op myringotomy kit
Setopress
    S. dressing
    S. high-compression bandage
setter
    Eby band s.
    Klauber band s.
    Ormco band s.
    orthodontic band s.
SET three-lumen thrombectomy catheter
Seutin
    S. bandage
    S. plaster shears
    S. scissors
seven-hole plate
seven-pin staple
Seven-Star acupuncture needle
severance transurethral bag
Severin
    S. implant
    S. multiple closed-loop intraocular
    lens
Severinghaus electrode
Sevrain cranial clamp 200 series
Sewall
    S. antral cannula
    S. antral trocar
    S. brain clip-applying forceps
    S. ethmoidal chisel
    S. ethmoidal elevator
    S. mucoperiosteal elevator
    S. orbital retractor
    S. raspatory
sewing ring
sewn-in waterproof drape
sew-on electrode
sex reassignment surgery
Sexton ear knife
Seyand vulsellum

S

Seyfert
  S. forceps
  S. vaginal speculum
SF-9 baculovirus-insect cell system
SFB-I right-angled bronchoscope
Sgarlato hammertoe implant
S-G catheter
SGIA
  SGIA 50 disposable stapler
  SGIA stapling device
Shaaf
  S. eye forceps
  S. foreign body forceps
Shack-Hartmann aberrometer
shadow
  S. balloon
  S. over-the-wire balloon catheter
shadow-free laryngoscope
Shadow-Line ACF spine retractor system
shadow shield
Shadow-Stripe catheter
Shaeffer rigid orthosis
Shaffer modification of Barkan knife
Shaffner orthopaedic inserter
shaft
  Adante Monorail catheter s.
  Cloward drill s.
  cup pusher s.
  Marlow Primus s.
  s. prosthesis
  s. reamer
Shah
  S. aural dressing
  S. grommet
  S. myringotomy tube
  S. nasal splint
  S. permanent ventilation tube
Shahan thermopore
Shahinian lacrimal cannula
Shah-Shah intraocular lens
Shaldach pacemaker
Shaldon catheter
Shallcross
  S. cystic duct forceps
  S. gallbladder forceps
  S. hemostat
  S. nasal forceps
  S. screwdriver
Shallcross-Dean gall duct forceps
Shambaugh
  S. adenoidal curette
  S. endaural hook
  S. endaural self-retaining retractor
  S. fistula hook
  S. irrigator
  S. knife
  S. microscopic hook
  S. narrow elevator
  S. palpating needle
  S. reverse adenotome
Shambaugh-Derlacki
  S.-D. chisel
  S.-D. duckbill elevator
  S.-D. microhook
Shambaugh-Lempert knife

Shampaine
  S. headholder
  S. orthopaedic table
Shandon
  S. Candenza immunostainer
  S. cytospin chamber
shank
  Crowley s.
  S. electrode
  grater-type reamer with Zimmer-Hudson s.
  Hudson s.
  taper with Zimmer s.
  Zimmer-Hudson s.
Shannon bur
Shantz
  S. dressing
  S. pin
Shape
  S. Maker system
shape memory alloy stent
shaper
  automated corneal s. (ACS)
  Chiron automated corneal s.
  interspace s.
  ProFile orifice s.
Shapleigh
  S. ear wax curette
Shapshay-Healy
  S.-H. laryngeal alligator forceps
  S.-H. laryngeal scissors
  S.-H. operating laryngoscope
  S.-H. phonatory laryngoscope
Shapshay laser bronchoscope
Sharbaro driver
shark
  s. fin papillotome
  s. fin sphincterotome
  S. forceps
shark-mouth cannula
shark-tooth forceps
Sharman curette
sharp
  s. dermal curette
  s. hook
  s. knife
  s. loop curette
  S. point-tip cystitome
  s. trocar
Sharpey screw
Sharplan
  S. argon laser
  S. CO_2 laser
  S. Erbium SilkLaser
  S. FeatherTouch SilkLaser
  S. Laser 710 Acuspot
  S. Medilas Nd:YAG surgical laser
  S. sight system
  S. SilkTouch flashscan surgical laser
  S. Ultra ultrasonic aspirator
SharpLase Nd:YAG laser
Sharplav laparoscope
Sharpley hook

Sharpoint
- S. cutting instrument
- S. knife
- S. microsuture
- S. ophthalmic microsurgical suture
- S. spoon blade
- S. Ultra-Guide ophthalmic needle
- V-lance S.
- S. V-lance blade

sharp-pointed forceps
sharp-pronged retractor
Sharptome
- S. crescent blade
- S. microblade

Shar-Tek foot positioning grid
Sharvelle side port splitter
Shasta alloy
shattering needle
shaver
- Aggressor meniscal s.
- s. catheter
- Concept s.
- DORC vitreous s.
- dragon s.
- Gator s.
- Grierson meniscal s.
- Kuda s.
- Microsect s.
- motorized meniscal s.
- Rhinotec s.
- Richardson s.
- Stryker s.
- sucker s.
- Xomed skimmer s.

Shaw
- S. carotid artery clot stripper
- S. catheter
- S. I, II scalpel

Shea
- S. bur
- S. curette
- S. ear drill
- S. elevator
- S. fenestration hook
- S. fistular hook
- S. headrest
- S. incision knife
- S. irrigator
- S. microdrill
- S. middle ear instrument
- S. oblique hook
- S. pick
- S. polyethylene prosthesis
- S. searcher
- S. speculum
- S. speculum holder
- S. stapes hook
- S. Teflon piston prosthesis
- S. vein graft scissors

Shea-Anthony
- S.-A. bag
- S.-A. balloon

Shea-Bellucci scissors
Shealy facet rhizotomy electrode

Shearer
- S. bone rongeur
- S. chicken-bill forceps
- S. lip retractor

ShearGuard low-friction interface
Shearing
- S. J-Loop intraocular lens
- S. posterior chamber implant material
- S. posterior chamber intraocular lens
- S. posterior chamber intraocular lens implant
- S. S-style anterior chamber intraocular lens
- S. suction kit

shears (*See also* scissors)
- ADC Medicut s.
- Bacon s.
- Baer rib s.
- bandage plaster s.
- Bethune-Coryllos rib s.
- Bethune rib s.
- Bortone s.
- Braun-Stadler sternal s.
- Brunner rib s.
- Brun plaster s.
- Clayton laminectomy s.
- Collin rib s.
- Cooley first-rib s.
- Cooley-Pontius sternal s.
- Cooley rib s.
- Coryllos-Bethune rib s.
- Coryllos-Moure rib s.
- Coryllos rib s.
- Coryllos-Shoemaker rib s.
- Duval-Coryllos rib s.
- Eccentric locked rib s.
- Endo S.
- Esmarch plaster s.
- Felt s.
- first rib s.
- Frey-Sauerbruch rib s.
- Giertz rib s.
- Giertz-Shoemaker rib s.
- Giertz-Stille rib s.
- Gluck rib s.
- Hercules plaster s.
- Horgan-Coryllos-Moure rib s.
- Horgan-Wells rib s.
- infant rib s.
- Jackson esophageal s.
- Jackson-Moore s.
- Jarit plaster s.
- Jarit utility s.
- LaparoSonic coagulating s.
- Lebsche sternal s.
- Lefferts rib s.
- Liston s.
- Liston-Key-Horsley rib s.
- Liston-Ruskin s.
- Moure-Coryllos rib s.
- Nelson-Bethune s.
- Pilling laryngofissure s.
- plain rib s.

S

shears *(continued)*
plaster s.
pleural biopsy needle s.
Potts infant rib s.
rib s.
Roos first rib s.
Sauerbruch-Britsch rib s.
Sauerbruch-Coryllos rib s.
Sauerbruch-Frey rib s.
Sauerbruch-Lebsche rib s.
Sauerbruch rib s.
Scanlan plaster s.
Scanlan rib s.
Schumacher sternal s.
scissors plaster s.
Semb s.
Seutin plaster s.
Shoemaker rib s.
Shuletz rib s.
sternal s.
Stille-Aesculap plaster s.
Stille-Ericksson rib s.
Stille-Giertz s.
Stille-Horsley s.
Stille plaster s.
Stille-Stiwer plaster s.
Thompson rib s.
Thomsen rib s.
Tudor-Edwards rib s.
UltraCision harmonic laparoscopic
cutting s.
utility s.
Walton rib s.
Weck s.

sheath
Amplatz s.
angioplasty s.
Appel-Bercie s.
Arrow s.
ArrowFlex s.
Bakelite cystoscopy s.
Banana peel s.
beaked s.
blue Cook s.
catheter s.
check-valve s.
Colapinto s.
concave s.
convex s.
Cordis Bioptone s.
Desilets-Hoffman s.
s. and dilator system
double-channel operating s.
Electroshield reusable s.
ERA resectoscope s.
femoral introducer s.
fiberoptic s.
French s.
Futura resectoscope s.
Hemaflex s.
hysteroscope s.
incandescent s.
Insul-Sheath vaginal speculum s.
introducer s.

Introducer II s.
irrigating s.
IVT percutaneous catheter
introducer s.
Klein transseptal introducer s.
Mapper hemostasis EP mapping s.
Medi-Tech s.
MicroSpan s.
Mullins transseptal catheterization
s. and obturator
O'Connor s.
Passager introducing s.
peel-away s.
percutaneous brachial s.
Pfister-Schwartz s.
Pinnacle introducer s.
PRO/Covers ultrasound probe s.
ProSys Samec D, self-adhering,
nonlatex male external catheter,
short s.
ProSys Samec NL, self-adhering,
nonlatex male external catheter,
normal length s.
quill s.
resectoscope s.
retroflexed cystoscopy s.
self-expanding tulip s.
short monorail polyethylene
imaging s.
Silipos Distal Dip prosthetic s.
single-channel operating s.
Spectranetics laser s.
Storz s.
Super Arrow-Flex catheterization s.
tear-away introducer s.
Teflon s.
Terumo Radiofocus s.
tulip s.
UMI Cath-Seal s.
Universal s.
ureterorenoscope procedure s.
vascular s.
Warne penile s.
water-filled balloon s.
s. with side-arm adapter
sheathed flexible sigmoidoscope
Sheathes ultrasound probe cover
Shea-type parasol myringotomy tube
Sheehan
S. gouge
S. knee prosthesis
S. nasal chisel
S. osteotome
S. retractor
Sheehan-Gillies needle holder
Sheehy
S. canal knife
S. collar button
S. collar-button ventilating tube
S. fascial press
S. incus replacement prosthesis
S. myringotomy knife
S. ossicle-holding clamp
S. ossicle-holding forceps
S. Pate Collector

S. round knife
S. Tytan ventilation tube
Sheehy-House
S.-H. chisel
S.-H. curette
S.-H. knife
Sheehy-Urban sliding lens adapter
Sheen tip graft
sheepskin
s. boot
s. dressing
Sheer
S. Plus pouch
S. probe
S. wire crimper
sheet
Abanda drape s.
AcryDerm hydrogel s.
Barrier lower extremity s.
Biobrane s.
casting wax s.
craniomaxillofacial s.
Dacron-impregnated Silastic s.
Derma-Gel hydrogel s.
Elasto-Gel hydrogel s.
FlexDerm hydrogel s.
foil s.
Grafton flexible s.
HK s.
s. holder
hydrogel s.
impervious s.
Ioban 2 iodophor cesarean s.
iodoform-impregnated plastic s.
KINS draw s.
Korex cork s.
mandibular s.
Moran-Karaya s.
Ortholen s.
polydioxanone s.
PPT s.
Prolene mesh s.
ReJuveness scar silicone s.
Silastic s.
Silk Skin s.
sterile s.
Subortholen s.
Supramid s.
Teflon s.
Tegagel hydrogel s.
Teknamed drape s.
sheeting
Carboplast II s.
DermaSof gel s.
Epi-Derm silicone gel s.
gel s.
Kelocote s.
micromesh s.
New Beginnings GelShapes silicone gel s.
New Beginnings topical gel s.
NovaGel silicone gel s.
ReJuveness pure silicone s.
Scar Fx lightweight silicone s.

silicone gel s.
Silon silicone elastomer s.
Sheets
S. closed-loop posterior chamber intraocular lens
S. intraocular glide
S. iris hook
S. irrigating vectis
S. irrigating vectis cannula
S. lens cutter
S. lens forceps
S. lens glide
S. lens spatula
Sheets-Hirsch spatula
Sheets-McPherson
S.-M. angled forceps
S.-M. tying forceps
sheet-wadding dressing
Sheffield
S. gamma unit
S. splint
Sheinmann laryngeal forceps
Sheldon
S. catheter
S. clamp
S. hemilaminectomy self-retaining retractor
S. spreader
Sheldon-Gosset self-retaining retractor
Sheldon-Pudenz dissector
Sheldon-Spatz vertebral arteriogram needle
Sheldon-Swann needle
shelf reamer
shelf-type implant
Shelhigh No React VascuPatch
shell
chest s.
elastomer s.
s. eye implant
fibrous s.
Harris protrusio s.
s. impactor
implant elastomer s.
s. implant material
Integrity s.
KM-series s.
protrusio s.
Restoration Secur-Fit X'tra acetabular s.
scleral s.
S. sensor
Terino malar s.
shellac-covered catheter
Shenstone tourniquet
Shepard
S. bipolar forceps
S. calipers block
S. curved intraocular lens forceps
S. drain tube
S. flexible anterior chamber intraocular lens
S. grommet
S. grommet ventilation tube
S. incision depth gauge

S

Shepard (*continued*)
- S. incision irrigating cannula
- S. intraocular lens implant
- S. lens forceps
- S. optical center marker
- S. radial keratotomy irrigating cannula
- S. reversed iris hook
- S. tying forceps
- S. Universal intraocular lens

Shepard-Kramer calipers block
Shepard-Reinstein intraocular lens forceps
Shepard-Westcott scissors
shepherd's hook catheter
Shepherd Tomahawk chopper
Sheridan endotracheal tube cuff
Sherlock bone screw suture/anchor system
Sherman
- S. bone plate
- S. bone screw
- S. knife
- S. remote podiatric vacuum system
- S. screwdriver
- S. suction tube

Sherman-Pierce screwdriver
Sherman-Stille drill
Sherpa guiding catheter
Sherwin self-retaining retractor
Sherwood
- S. intrascopic suction/irrigation system
- S. retractor

ShiatsuBACK support
shield
- aluminum eye s.
- American Medical Electronics PinSite s.
- Atkins-Tucker surgical s.
- Barraquer eye s.
- bili mask eye s.
- binocular s.
- bronchoscopic face s.
- Buller eye s.
- bunion s.
- Carapace face s.
- Cartella eye s.
- circumcisional s.
- collagen s.
- ComPly panty s.
- contact s.
- corneal light s.
- Cox II ocular laser s.
- Dacron s.
- Dalkon s.
- dental s.
- designs for vision side s.
- Durette dental s.
- Durette external laser s.
- Electroshield cylindrical conductive s.
- Expo Bubble eye s.
- eye s.

- face s.
- Face-It protective s.
- Faraday s.
- Fox aluminum eye s.
- Fuller perianal s.
- Garter s.
- gastric s.
- Goffman blue eye garter s.
- gonad s.
- Gottesman splash s.
- Grafco eye s.
- Green eye s.
- Guibor s.
- Hessburg corneal s.
- Hessburg eye s.
- high-humidity tracheostomy s.
- S. iridotomy scissors
- Jardon eye s.
- Jet s.
- Lea s.
- lead eye s.
- metal Fox s.
- metal scleral s.
- Mueller eye s.
- Nolan system collimator mounted contact s.
- Paton eye s.
- plastic eye s.
- pressure s.
- probe s.
- Pro-Ophtha type-K, -S s.
- Proshield collagen corneal s.
- Pro-Tex face s.
- ring cataract mask s.
- ring cataract mask eye s.
- SAF-T s.
- scleral s.
- shadow s.
- Simmons eye s.
- SlimStem metal scleral s.
- Sof-Gel palm s.
- Soft Shield collagen corneal s.
- Sportelli system collimator mounted contact s.
- Storz Easy s.
- Surety s.
- Surgical Patient Arm s.
- Trelles metal scleral s.
- tungsten eye s.
- Universal eye s.
- Visitec corneal s.
- Weck eye s.

shielded open-end cone
shielding block
Shields forceps
Shier knee prosthesis
Shiffrin bone wire tightener
shifting pacemaker
Shikani middle meatal antrostomy stent
Shiley
- S. cardioplegia system
- S. cardiotomy reservoir
- S. catheter distention system
- S. convexoconcave heart valve
- S. cuffless fenestrated tube

S. cuffless tracheostomy tube
S. decannulation plug
S. disposable cannula low pressure cuffed tracheostomy tube
S. distention kit
S. extra-length single cannula tracheostomy tube
S. fenestrated low pressure cuffed tracheostomy tube
S. French sump tube
S. guiding catheter
S. Infusaid pump
S. irrigation catheter
S. laryngectomy tube
S. low-pressure cuffed tracheostomy tube
S. low-pressure cuffed tracheostomy tube with pressure relief valve
S. monostrut heart valve
S. MultiPro catheter
S. neonatal tracheostomy tube
S. oxygenator
S. pediatric tracheostomy tube
S. Phonate speaking valve
S. pressure-relief adapter
S. saphenous vein irrigation and pressurization device
S. single cannula cuffed tracheostomy tube
S. soft-tip guiding catheter
S. Tetraflex vascular graft
Shiley-Ionescu catheter
shim
    s. coil
    s. magnet
Shimadzu
    S. cardiac ultrasound
    S. CT, MR scanner
    S. DAR-2400 coronary arteriographic analyzer
    S. IIQ ultrasound
    S. SDU-400 ultrasound
    S. ultrasound system
Shimatzu RF-5301 PC spectrometer
shimmed magnet
Shimstock occlusion foil
SHIP
    SHIP hammertoe implant
SHIP-Shaw rod hammertoe implant
Shirakable nasal implant
Shirlee spline
Shirley sump wound drain
Shirodkar
    S. aneurysm needle
    S. cervical needle
    S. probe
    S. suture
SHJR4, SHJR4s catheter
Shoch
    S. foreign body pickups
    S. suture
shock
    s. block
    s. suit
    s. wave lithotriptor

shocker
    Take-Me-Along Personal Shocker pocket s.
Shockmaster heel cushion
shoe
    Ambulator H1200 healing s.
    Balmoral s.
    beach bum rocker-bottom cast sandal s.
    Blucher low-quarter s.
    cast s.
    COMED postoperative s.
    Darby surgical s.
    Darco MedSurg s.
    Darco Wedge s.
    decubitus boot s.
    diabetic pressure relief s.
    extra-depth s.
    Gard-all boot s.
    healing s.
    Hi-Top s.
    H-series healing s.
    in-depth s.
    ipos heel relief s.
    Kunzli orthopaedic sports s.
    s. lift
    low quarter Blucher s.
    Mala-paedic s.
    Markell Mobility S.'s
    Markell open-toe s.
    Markell tarso medius straight s.
    Markell tarso pronator outflare s.
    OrthoWedge healing s.
    Pedors orthopaedic s.
    Plastizote s.
    postoperative s.
    Power Anthro s.
    pressure relief s.
    Reece orthopaedic s.
    Reece PO s.
    rocker-bottom cast boot s.
    Rollerbottom Xtra Depth s.
    SAS s.
    Shoethotic s.
    Softie s.
    s. stretcher
    Thera-Medic s.
    Tru-Fit custom molded s.
    Tru-Mold s.
    Vibram rockerbottom s.
    WACH s.
    wedge adjustable cushioned heel s.
shoehorn speculum
Shoemaker
    S. intraocular lens forceps
    S. rib shears
Shoethotic shoe
Shofu
    S. dental cement
    S. porcelain stain kit
shooter
    S. Saeed multiband irrigator
    Wilson-Cook Saaed six s.
short
    s. above-elbow cast

S

short *(continued)*
s. arm cylinder cast
s. arm navicular cast
s. arm plaster splint
s. arm posterior molded splint
s. below-elbow cast
S. bridge
s. C-loop intraocular lens
s. coarse bur
s. fine bur
s. Heaney retractor
s. leg caliper brace
s. leg cylinder cast
s. leg nonwalking cast
s. leg nonweightbearing cast
s. leg plaster cast
s. leg splint
s. leg walker
s. leg walking cast
s. monorail polyethylene imaging sheath
s. needle
s. occluder
S. Speedy balloon
s. tooth forceps
short-arm Grollman catheter
Shortbent suture scissors
short-bore magnet
ShortCut A-OK small-incision knife
ShortCutter catheter
shorthand vertical mattress stitch
short-stretch bandage
short-term
flow-assisted s.-t. (FAST)
short-tip hemostatic bag
shot compressor
shotted suture
shoulder
s. abduction immobilizer
s. abduction pillow
s. abduction positioner
s. blade
s. controller
s. cuff
S. Ease abduction support
s. ladder
s. orthosis
s. prosthesis
s. pulley
s. ROM arc
s. saddle sling
s. subluxation inhibitor brace
s. surface coil
s. wheel
shoulder-elbow-wrist-hand orthosis
shoulderRAP wrap
shower
chair s.
Hydrokinetic Vichy s.
ShowerSafe
S. protector material
S. waterproof cast and bandage cover

S. waterproof cast and bandage protector
Show'rbag cast and dressing cover
SH popoff suture
Shrader fitting
Shrady saw
Shriners
S. Hospital interlocking retractor
S. Hospital pin
shrinker
Juzo s.
Shuco-Myst nebulizer
Shug male contraceptive device
Shulec adenotome
Shuletz
S. pusher
S. raspatory
S. rib shears
S. searcher
S. spring
Shuletz-Damian raspatory
Shuletz-Paul rib retractor
Shulitz catheter
shunt
Accura hydrocephalus s.
Ames ventriculoperitoneal s.
Anastaflo intravascular s.
angiographic portacaval s.
aortopulmonary s.
aqueous tube s.
Austin endolymph dispersement s.
Baerveldt s.
balloon s.
bidirectional s.
Blalock s.
Blalock-Taussig s.
Brenner carotid bypass s.
Brescia-Cimino s.
Brisman-Nova carotid endarterectomy s.
Buselmeier s.
capillary bed s.
cardiovascular s.
cavernospongiosum s.
cerebrospinal fluid s.
Cimino arteriovenous s.
Cimino dialysis s.
Cobe AV s.
Codman Accu-Flow s.
Cordis-Hakim s.
coronary anastomotic s.
CSF T-tube s.
CUI s.
Denver ascites s.
Denver hydrocephalus s.
Denver peritoneovenous s.
Denver pleuroperitoneal s.
Denver valve s.
dialysis s.
Drapanas mesocaval s.
Edwards-Barbaro T-shaped syringeal s.
endolymphatic-subarachnoid s.
extracardiac right-to-left s.
extrahepatic s.

s. filter
Flo-Thru intraluminal s.
Gibson inner ear s.
Glenn s.
Gore-Tex s.
Gott s.
Hakim s.
Hallin carotid endarterectomy s.
Hashmat s.
Hashmat-Waterhouse s.
hepatofugal porto-systemic venous s.
Heyer-Schulte hydrocephalus s.
Heyer-Schulte-Spetzler lumbar
  peritoneal s.
H-H neonatal s.
Holter s.
House endolymphatic s.
House and Pulec otic-periotic s.
indwelling nonvascular s.
intracardial s.
Javid carotid s.
Kasai peritoneal venous s.
s. kit
LaRivetti-Levinson intraluminal s.
left-to-right s.
LeVeen ascites s.
LeVeen dialysis s.
LeVeen peritoneal s.
LeVeen peritoneovenous s.
loop s.
mesocaval H-graft s.
Mischler s.
Mischler-Pudenz s.
Ommaya s.
one-piece s. with reservoir
parietal s.
PC s.
pentose phosphate s.
percutaneous thecoperitoneal s.
peritoneojugular s.
peritoneovenous s.
portacaval s.
portosystemic s.
Potts s.
Pruitt-Inahara carotid s.
Pruitt-Inahara vascular s.
Pruitt vascular s.
PTFE s.
Pudenz-Schulte thecoperitoneal s.
Pudenz valve-flushing s.
Quinton-Scribner s.
radiologic portacaval s.
Raimondi low-pressure s.
Ramirez s.
Reynold-Southwick H-graft
  portacaval s.
Rickham reservoir s.
Scribner s.
side-to-side portacaval s.
Silastic Ames s.
Silastic ventriculoperitoneal s.
Simeone-Erlik side-to-end
  portorenal s.
Spetzler lumbar-peritoneal s.
splenorenal bypass s.

subduroperitoneal s.
Sundt carotid endarterectomy s.
syrinx s.
TDMAC heparin s.
thecoperitoneal Pudenz-Schulte s.
Thomas femoral s.
tracheoesophageal s.
tracheopharyngeal s.
transhepatic portacaval s.
transjugular intrahepatic portal
  systemic s.
T-shaped Edwards-Barbaro
  syringeal s.
s. tubing
Uni-Shunt hydrocephalus s.
Uresil Vascu-Flo carotid s.
USCI s.
Vascushunt carotid balloon s.
ventriculoperitoneal s.
vesicoamniotic s.
Vitagraft arteriovenous s.
VS s.
White glaucoma pump s.
Winter s.
Shuppe biting forceps
Shur-Band self-closure elastic bandage
Shurly tracheal retractor
Shur resin
Shur-Strip wound closure tape
Shuster
  S. suture forceps
  S. tonsillar forceps
shutoff clamp
Shutt
  S. Aggressor forceps
  S. alligator forceps
  S. basket forceps
  S. B-scoop forceps
  S. grasping forceps
  S. Mantis retrograde forceps
  S. microscissors
  S. Mini-Aggressor forceps
  S. minibasket
  S. retrograde forceps
  S. scissors
  S. shovel-nosed forceps
  S. suction forceps
  S. suture punch system
shuttle
  S. cardiomuscular conditioner
  Caspari s.
Shuttle-Relay suture passer
sialography needle
Siamese twin bracket
Sichel
  S. iris knife
  S. movable orbital implant
Sichi implant
sickle
  s. blade
  s. knife
  s. scissors
sickle-shaped Beaver blade
**SICOR cardiac catheterization recording
  system**

side
 s. blade
 S. Branch Occlusion system
 s. mouthgag
 s. plate
side-arm
 s.-a. adapter
 s.-a. nebulizer
side-biting
 s.-b. clamp
 s.-b. ostrum punch
 s.-b. spatula
 s.-b. Stammberger punch forceps
side-curved forceps
side-cut pin cutter
side-cutting
 s.-c. basket forceps
 s.-c. blade
 s.-c. cannula
 s.-c. irrigating cystitome
 s.-c. rasp
 s.-c. rongeur
 s.-c. spatula
 s.-c. spatulated needle
 s.-c. Swanson bur
SideFire laser
side-flattened needle
side-grasping forceps
side-hole
 s.-h. cannulated probe
 s.-h. Judkins right, 4-cm curved,
 short catheter
 s.-h. pigtail catheter
Sidekick foot support
side-lip forceps
side-opening laminar hook
side-port
 s.-p. cannula
 s.-p. flat-bottomed Ommaya reservoir
SidePort AutoControl airway connector
Sideris adjustable buttoned device
sidestream spirometer
side-to-side portacaval shunt
side-viewing
 s.-v. duodenoscope
 s.-v. endoscope
 s.-v. fiberscope
sidewall
 s. holed needle
 s. infusion cannula
sidewinder
 s. aortic clamp
 s. percutaneous intra-aortic balloon
 catheter
Sidney Stephenson corneal trephine
Siebold uterine scissors
Siegel
 S. pneumatic otoscope
 S. stent
Siegel-Cohen dilating catheter
Sieger insufflator
Siegle
 S. ear speculum
 S. otoscope
Siegler biopsy forceps

Siegler-Hellman clamp
Sielaff gastroscope
Siemens
 S. BICOR cardioscope
 S. couch
 S. DRH CT scanner
 S. ECAT 951/31R PET scanner
 S. Endo-P endorectal transducer
 S. HICOR cardioscope
 S. Hicor II
 S. linear probe
 S. Lithostar Plus
 S. Lithostar Plus System C
 lithotriptor
 S. Magnetom GBS II scanner
 S. Magnetom Vision scanner
 S. Mevatron 74 linear accelerator
 S. MRI unit
 S. One Tesla scanner
 S. open-heart table
 S. Orbiter gamma camera
 S. PTCA open-heart suture
 S. Quantum 2000 Color Doppler
 S. Satellite CT evaluation console
 S. Servo ventilator
 S. Siecure implantable cardioverter-
 defibrillator
 S. SI 400 ultrasound
 S. somatoma plus DCT system
 S. Somatom DR2, DR3 whole-body
 scanner
 S. Somatom DRH CT analyzer
 S. Somatom DRH CT analyzer unit
 S. Somatom Plus
 S. Sonoline Elegra ultrasound
 S. Sonoline Elegra ultrasound
 scanner
 S. Sonoline Prima ultrasound
 S. Sonoline SI-400 ultrasound
 system
 S. Sonoline SL-2 echocardiograph
 S. Sonoline ultrasonography
 S. vaginal probe
 S. Vision MRI
Siemens-Albis bicycle ergometer
Siemens-Elema
 S.-E. AG bicycle ergometer
 S.-E. multiprogrammable pacemaker
 S.-E. Servo 900C ventilator
Siemens-Pacesetter pacemaker
Siepser intraocular lens
Sierra alloy
Sierra-Sheldon tracheotome
SieScape
 S. ultrasound
 S. ultrasound scanner
sieve
 s. graft
 Mobin-Uddin s.
 molecular s.
Sievert unit
SIF10 Olympus enteroscope
Sifoam padding
Sigma
 S. II Dualplace

S. II hyperbaric system
S. 6000+ infusion pump
S. TMB assay kit
sigmoid
  s. anastomosis clamp
  s. notch retractor
sigmoidofiberscope
  Pentax s.
sigmoidoscope
  ACMI flexible s.
  adult s.
  Boehm s.
  Buie s.
  disposable sheathed flexible s.
  Eder s.
  ESI s.
  fiberoptic s.
  flexible s.
  Frankfeldt s.
  Fujinon ES-200ER s.
  Fujinon flexible s.
  Fujinon FS-100ER s.
  Gorsch s.
  Heinkel s.
  Hopkins s.
  Kelly s.
  KleenSpec fiberoptic disposable s.
  Lieberman s.
  s. light carrier
  Lloyd-Davies s.
  Montague s.
  Olympus CF-L-series flexible s.
  Olympus CF-OSF-series flexible s.
  Olympus CF-series flexible s.
  Olympus fiberoptic s.
  Pentax flexible s.
  Pentax FS-series fiberoptic s.
  Reichert fiberoptic s.
  Reichert flexible s.
  s. replacement lamp
  rigid s.
  sheathed flexible s.
  Solow s.
  Strauss s.
  Turrell s.
  Tuttle s.
  Vernon David s.
  Visiline disposable s.
  VSI 2000 s.
  Welch Allyn disposable s.
  Welch Allyn fiberoptic s.
  Welch Allyn flexible s.
  Welch Allyn KleenSpec fiberoptic
    disposable s.
  Yeoman s.
Signa
  S. Advantage system
  S. GEMS MR imaging system
  S. Horizon scanner
  S. imager
  S. Pad
  S. 1.5 Tesla unit
SignaDress hydrocolloid dressing
signal-averaged electrocardiograph
Signal system

Signature Edition infusion system
Signet
  S. disposable skin stapler
  S. Optical lens
Signorini tourniquet
Sigvaris
  S. compression stockings
  S. medical stockings
Siker mirror laryngoscope
silanated slide
Silastic
  S. Ames shunt
  S. ball
  S. ball spacer prosthesis
  S. band
  S. bead embolization
  S. Brand sterile Foley catheter
  S. bur hole cover
  S. catheter
  S. chin implant
  S. chin prosthesis
  S. collar-reinforced stoma
  S. corneal eye implant
  S. coronary artery cannula
  S. Cronin implant
  S. cup extractor
  S. elastomer infusion catheter
  S. eustachian tube
  S. eye implant
  S. fimbrial prosthesis
  S. finger implant
  S. foam dressing
  S. gel dressing
  S. graft
  S. grommet
  S. ileal reservoir catheter
  S. indwelling ureteral stent
  S. intestinal tube
  S. mammary prosthesis
  S. medical adhesive
  S. midfacial malar implant
  S. mold
  S. mushroom catheter
  S. obstetrical vacuum cup
  S. otoplasty prosthesis
  S. penile implant
  S. penile prosthesis
  S. plate
  S. rhinoplasty implant
  S. ring
  S. scleral buckle implant
  S. scleral buckler eye implant
  S. sheet
  S. sheeting keel prosthesis
  S. silicone rubber implant
  S. sling
  S. sphere
  S. sponge
  S. spring-loaded silo
  S. standard elastometer prosthesis
  S. strain gauge
  S. strap
  S. subdermal implant
  S. sucker suction tube
  S. suture button

S

Silastic *(continued)*
  S. testicular implant
  S. testicular prosthesis
  S. thoracic drain
  S. thyroid drain
  S. toe implant
  S. tracheostomy tube
  S. T-tube
  S. tubing
  S. ventriculoperitoneal shunt
  S. wick
Silber
  S. microneedle holder
  S. microvascular clamp
  S. vasovasostomy clamp
Silberg E.U.A. system
Silcath subclavian catheter
Silc extractor
Silcock dissection forceps
Silent
  S. Nite alarm
  S. Speaker communication system
Silesian bandage
Silflex intramedullary prosthesis
Silhouette
  S. endoscopic laser
  S. spinal system
  S. therapeutic massage system
  S. therapeutic mattress
  S. therapeutic surface
silica contact lens
silicate cement
silicon
  S. Graphics Indigo 2 computer
  S. Graphics Reality Engine system
silicon-controlled
  s.-c. rectifier
  s.-c. switch
silicone
  s. adhesive
  s. ball heart valve
  Biocell textured s.
  s. block
  s. buckling implant
  s. button
  s. button eye implant
  s. cannula
  s. conformer
  s. diode dosimeter
  s. disk heart valve
  s. doughnut prosthesis
  s. dressing
  s. elastomer
  s. elastomer band
  s. elastomer infusion catheter
  s. elastomer lens
  s. elastomer prosthesis
  s. elastomer ring
  s. elastomer rubber ball implant
  s. epistaxis catheter
  s. eye sphere
  s. flexor rod
  s. gel prosthesis
  s. gel sheeting

  s. hubless flat drain
  s. insole
  s. introducer
  s. meshed motility implant
  s. microimplant
  s. mold
  s. MP implant
  s. nasal strut implant
  s. pad eye implant
  s. Robinson catheter
  s. rod implant
  s. rod and sleeve forceps
  s. round drain
  s. rubber Dacron-cuffed catheter
  Schepens boat s.
  Schepens grooved rubber s.
  Schepens pad s.
  s. sizer
  s. sleeve eye implant
  s. sponge
  s. sponge forceps
  s. sponge implant
  s. strip
  s. strip eye implant
  s. sump drain
  s. textured mammary implant
  s. thoracic drain
  s. tire
  s. tire eye implant
  tire-grooved s.
  s. trapezium prosthesis
  s. T-tube
  s. tube
silicone-coated, metallic self-expanding stent
silicone-filled
  s.-f. anatomical breast implant
  s.-f. mammary implant
  s.-f. round breast implant
silicone-gel breast implant
silicone-lubricated endotracheal tube
silicone-spiked mat
silicone-treated surgical silk suture
Silicore catheter
Sili-Gel impression material
Silikon 1000 retinal tamponade
Silima breast prosthesis
Silipos
  S. digital pad
  S. Distal Dip
  S. Distal Dip prosthetic sheath
  S. mesh cap
  S. mesh tubing
  S. silicone wonder cup
  S. suspension sleeve
Silitek
  S. catheter
  S. ureteral stent
  S. Uropass stent
silk
  s. braided suture
  S. guide wire
  s. guidewire
  s. Mersilene suture
  s. nonabsorbable suture

Owens s.
s. pop-off suture
s. screw
S. Skin sheet
s. stay suture
s. traction suture
silk-and-wax catheter
SilkLaser
EpiTouch Ruby S.
FeatherTouch S.
Sharplan Erbium S.
Sharplan FeatherTouch S.
Sil-K OB barrier
SilkTouch
S. CO_2 laser scanner
S. laser
silkworm gut suture
Silky Polydek suture
Sil-Med
S.-M. catheter
S.-M. instrument paws
silo
Prolene mesh s.
removal mesh s.
Silastic spring-loaded s.
SI-LOC sacroiliac belt
SiloLiner
Silon
S. silicone thermoplastic splinting
material
S. tent
S. wound dressing
Silon silicone elastomer sheeting
Silopad
S. body sleeve
S. toe sleeve
Silosheath
S. gel liner
S. sock
Siloskin dressing
Silovi saphenous vein graft
Siloxane
S. graft
S. implant
S. prosthesis
Silsoft extended wear contact lens
Siltex
S. Becker 50 breast prosthesis
S. mammary implant
Silva-Packer
silver
s. bead electrode
S. cannula
s. catheter
S. chisel
s. clip
S. endaural forceps
S. knife
s. mylar roll
S. nasal osteotome
s. needle
s. probe
s. suture
silver-coated stent
silvered contact lens

silverized catgut suture
Silverman biopsy needle
Silverman-Boeker
S.-B. cannula
S.-B. needle
Silverstein
S. arachnoid dissector
S. auditory canal dissector
S. dressing
S. dural elevator
S. facial nerve monitor
S. lateral venous sinus retractor
S. micromirror
S. nerve separator
S. permanent aeration tube
S. round knife
S. sickle knife
S. stimulator probe
Simal cervical stabilization system
Simcoe
S. anterior chamber capsule
scrubber
S. anterior chamber receiving needle
S. anterior chamber retaining wire
S. cannula tip
S. capsular scraper
S. C-loop intraocular lens
S. connecting tubing
S. corneal marker
S. cortex cannula
S. cortex extractor
S. double-barreled cannula
S. double-end lens loop
S. eye speculum
S. I&A system
S. II PC aspirating needle
S. II PC double cannula
S. II PC nucleus delivery loupe
S. II posterior chamber nucleus
delivery loop
S. implantation forceps
S. interchangeable tip
S. intraocular lens implant
S. irrigating-positioning needle
S. lens-inserting forceps
S. lens-positioning set
S. microhook
S. notched irrigating spatula
S. nucleus delivery cannula
S. nucleus erysiphake
S. nucleus forceps
S. nucleus lens loop
S. nucleus spatula
S. posterior capsule scrubber
S. posterior chamber forceps
S. reverse-aperture cannula
S. reverse I&A cannula
S. superior rectus forceps
S. suture needle
S. wire speculum
Simcoe-AMO eye implant
Simcoe-Barraquer eye speculum
Simeone-Erlik side-to-end portorenal
shunt

S

Simmonds
- S. cricothyrotomy needle
- S. vaginal speculum

Simmons
- S. 1, 2, 3 catheter
- S. chisel
- S. double-hole spinal screw
- S. eye shield
- S. II, III catheter
- S. plating system
- S. sidewinder catheter

Simmons-Kimbrough glaucoma spatula
Simmons-Martin screw
Simon
- S. bone curette
- S. cup uterine curette
- S. dermatome
- S. expansion arch
- S. fistula hook
- S. fistula knife
- S. nitinol inferior vena cava (IVC) filter
- S. spinal curette
- S. uterine scoop
- S. vaginal retractor

Simonart
- S. band
- S. bar

Simons
- S. cleft palate knife
- S. stone-removing forceps

Simpa denture reliner
Simplastic catheter
Simplex cement adhesive
Simplex-P bone cement
Simplicity adult disposable contoured undergarment liner system
Simplus
- S. PE/t dilatation catheter

Simply Wet table
Simpson
- S. antral curette
- S. atherectomy catheter
- S. coronary AtheroCath
- S. coronary AtheroCath catheter
- S. directional coronary atherectomy device
- S. endoscope
- S. epistaxis balloon
- S. lacrimal dilator
- S. obstetrical forceps
- S. peripheral AtheroCath
- S. PET balloon atherectomy device
- S. sterling lacrimal probe
- S. suction catheter
- S. sugar-tong splint
- S. Ultra Lo-Profile II balloon catheter
- S. uterine dilator
- S. uterine sound

Simpson-Braun obstetrical forceps
Simpson-Luikart obstetrical forceps
Simpson-Robert
- S.-R. ACS dilatation catheter
- S.-R. vascular dilation system

Simpulse
- S. irrigation system
- S. lavage system
- S. pulsing lavage

Simrock speculum
Sims
- S. abdominal needle
- S. anoscope
- S. cannula
- S. double-ended retractor
- S. double-ended vaginal speculum
- S. irrigating uterine curette
- S. knife
- S. Per-fit percutaneous tracheostomy kit
- S. proctoscope
- S. rectal retractor
- S. rectal speculum
- S. sponge holder
- S. suction tip
- S. suture
- S. uterine depressor
- S. uterine dilator
- S. uterine probe
- S. uterine scissors
- S. uterine sound
- S. vaginal decompressor
- S. vaginal plug
- S. vaginal retractor
- S. vaginal speculum

Sims-Kelly vaginal retractor
Sims-Maier
- S.-M. clamp
- S.-M. sponge and dressing forceps

Sims-Siebold uterine scissors
simulator
- AcQsim CT s.
- Boston Dynamics surgical s.
- BTE Work S.
- Ergos work s.
- flexible bronchoscopy s.
- Lido WorkSET work s.
- Maxwell 3D field s.
- MR s.
- Nucletron s.
- radiation s.
- spinal physiotherapy s.
- virtual reality s.
- Ximatron s.

simultaneous thermal diffusion blood flow and pressure probe
Sinai system
Sinclair spatula
Sine-U-View nasal endoscope
Sinexon dilator
Singer
- S. needle
- S. portable pneumothorax apparatus

Singer-Blom
- S.-B. ossicular prosthesis
- S.-B. tube
- S.-B. valve

Singh speech system voice rehabilitation prosthesis

single
  s. cross-slot screwdriver
  s. hook
  s. occluder
  s. patient system
  s. pigtail stent
  s. port
  s. safe-sided chisel
  s. width bracket
single-action
  s.-a. pumping system
  s.-a. rongeur
single-armed suture
single-axis
  s.-a. ankle prosthesis
  s.-a. friction knee
  s.-a. locking knee
  s.-a. Syme DYCOR foot
single-base cane
single-beveled cutting instrument
single-blade retractor
single-chamber pacemaker
single-channel
  s.-c. analyzer
  s.-c. cochlear implant
  s.-c. electromyograph oscilloscope
  s.-c. fiberoptic bronchoscope
  s.-c. nonfade oscilloscope
  s.-c. operating sheath
  s.-c. in vivo light dosimeter
  s.-c. wire-guided sphincterotome
single-crystal gamma camera
Single-Day Baxter infuser
single-energy x-ray absorptiometer
single-fiber EMG electrode
single-field hyperthermia combined with radiation therapy and ultrasound scanner
single-head rotating gamma camera
single-hook retractor
single-incision system
single-J urinary diversion stent
single-loop tourniquet
single-lumen
  s.-l. balloon stone extractor catheter
  s.-l. cannula
  s.-l. infusion catheter
single-mirror goniolens
single-needle device
single-pass
  s.-p. lead
  s.-p. pacemaker
single-photon
  s.-p. densitometer
  s.-p. electrospinal orthosis
single-plane instrument
single-prong broad acetabular retractor
single-reference-point instrument
single-rod construct
single-running suture
single-sided bone saw
single-stage
  s.-s. catheter
  s.-s. screw implant
single-stemmed silicone hemiprosthesis

SingleStitch PhacoFlex lens
Singleton empyema trocar
single-tooth
  s.-t. forceps
  s.-t. subperiosteal implant
  s.-t. tenaculum
single-use
  s.-u. dermatome
  s.-u. electrode
single-wire electrode
Singley
  S. intestinal clamp
  S. intestinal forceps
  S. tissue forceps
Singley-Tuttle
  S.-T. dressing forceps
  S.-T. intestinal forceps
  S.-T. tissue forceps
Singular oval polypectomy snare
Siniscal eyelid clamp
Siniscal-Smith lid everter
sinoscopy
  s. cannula
  s. trocar
Sinskey
  S. intraocular lens forceps
  S. iris hook
  S. J-loop intraocular lens
  S. lens implant
  S. lens-manipulating hook
  S. lens manipulator
  S. microlens hook
  S. microtying forceps
  S. needle holder
  S. nucleus spatula
  S. pick
Sinskey-McPherson forceps
Sinskey-Wilson
  S.-W. foreign body forceps
sintered titanium mesh
Sinterlock
  S. implant
  S. implant metal prosthesis
sinus
  s. antral cannula
  s. balloon
  s. biopsy forceps
  s. bur
  s. chisel
  s. curette
  s. dilator
  s. irrigating cannula
  s. irrigator
  s. lift osteotome
  s. node pacemaker
  s. probe
  s. trephine
  s. tympani excavator
SinuScope
  S. rigid rod
  S. rigid rod lens optics
  S. scope
  S. system
SinuSeal nasal packing
SinuSpacer turbinate stent

S

Sinvision ultrasound scanner
siphon
    Duguet s.
    Moniz carotid s.
    Nichols nasal s.
    s. suction tube
Sippy
    S. esophageal dilating set
    S. esophageal dilator
    S. esophageal dilator piano-wire
    staff
    S. esophageal dilator pusher wire
Sirecust 404N neonatal monitoring
    system
Siremobil
    S. C-arm
    S. C-arm unit
Sirognathograph
SISCO spectrometer
Sisler lacrimal trephine
Sisson
    S. forceps
    S. fracture-reducing elevator
    S. spring hook
    S. spring retractor
Sisson-Cottle speculum
Sisson-Love retractor
Sisson-Vienna speculum
Sister
    S. Helen Mustard ENT table
sister-hook forceps
Sistron scissors
Sistrunk
    S. band retractor
    S. dissecting scissors
    S. double-ended retractor
SITE
    SITE argon laser
    SITE guillotine cutting tip
    SITE I&A instrument
    SITE I&A needle
    SITE I&A unit
    SITE macrobore plus needle
    SITE phaco I&A needle
    SITE Phaco II handpiece
    SITE TXR diaphragmatic
    microsurgical system
    SITE TXR 2200 microsurgical unit
    SITE TXR peristaltic microsurgical
    system
    SITE TXR phacoemulsification
    system
SiteGuard transparent dressing
SITElite
SITEprobe
SiteSelect percutaneous incisional breast
    biopsy system
SITEtrac
    S. spinal surgery system
sit/stand chair
Sit-Straight wheelchair cushion
sitz bath
Sitzmarks radiopaque marker
Sivash hip prosthesis
six-degrees-of-freedom electrogoniometer

six-eye catheter
six-hole mandibular plate
six-point knee brace
six-prong rake retractor
six-wire spiral-tip Segura basket
sizer
    Björk-Shiley heart valve s.
    Brannock device shoe s.
    Meadox graft s.
    silicone s.
    voice prosthesis s.
sizing
    s. balloon
    s. ring
SJM
    S. Sequin annuloplasty ring
    S. Tailor annuloplasty ring
    S. X-Cell cardiac bioprosthesis
SkareKare silicon gel-filled cushion
Skatron apparatus
Skeele
    S. chalazion curette
    S. corneal curette
    S. eye curette
Skeeter otologic drill
skeletal pin
Skeleton fine forceps
Skene
    S. catheter
    S. tenaculum forceps
    S. uterine forceps
    S. uterine spoon
    S. uterine tenaculum
    S. vulsellum
    S. vulsellum forceps
skiameter
skiascope
skiascopy bar
skid
    acetabular s.
    Austin Moore-Murphy bone s.
    bone s.
    s. curette
    Davis bone s.
    hip s.
    MacAusland hip s.
    Meyerding bone s.
    Meyerding hip s.
    Meyerding shoulder s.
    Murphy bone s.
    Murphy-Lane bone s.
    Ryerson bone s.
    Scudder s.
    Yund acetabular s.
SKI knee prosthesis
Skil-Care
    S.-C. cushion grip
    S.-C. reclining wheelchair
Skil-CARE
    S.-C. Alarm cushion
Skillbuilder half roll
Skillern
    S. phimosis forceps
    S. punch
    S. sinus curette

S. sphenoidal probe
S. sphenoid cannula
Skillman
S. arterial forceps
S. mosquito forceps
S. prepuce forceps
Skil saw
Skimmer
S. blade
S. laryngeal blade tip
skin
s. clip
Composite Cultured S.
s. elevator
Epigard synthetic s.
s. flap retractor
s. forceps
s. graft expander mesh
s. graft mesher
s. grinder
s. gun
s. hook
s. hook retractor
Integra artificial s.
s. marker
s. marking pen
s. punch
s. self-retaining retractor
S. Skribe marker
S. Skribe pen
s. splint
s. staple
Skin-Bond skin cement
ski needle
skinfold calipers
SkinLaser system
Skinlight
S. erbium yttrium-aluminum-garnet
laser
S. Er:YAG laser
Skinny
S. balloon catheter
S. Chiba needle
S. dilatation catheter
S. over-the-wire balloon catheter
Skin-Prep protective dressing
Skinscan scanner
Skinsense glove
SkinSleeves
Posey S.
SkinTech medical tattooing device
SkinTegrity
S. hydrogel
S. hydrogel dressing
SkinTemp biosynthetic collagen dressing
Skirrow agar plate
skiving knife
Sklar
S. anoscope
S. bone drill
S. bone saw
S. brush
S. evacuator
S. ligature needle
S. medical breast stamp

S. pin cutter
S. tonometer
S. wire tightener
Sklar-Junior Tompkins aspirator
Sklar-Schitz jewel tonometer
SklarScribe skin marker
Skoog nasal chisel
skull
s. bur
s. clamp
s. elevator
s. plate
s. plate screwdriver
s. punch
s. raspatory
s. traction drill
s. traction tongs
s. trephine
Sky-Boot stirrup system
SKY epidural pain control system
Skylark
S. surface electrode
S. TENS unit
Skylight
S. gantry-free nuclear medicine
gamma camera
S. system
Skytron
S. air-fluidized bed
S. surgical table
Slade cannula
Slalom balloon
Slam'r wheelchair
Slant
S. haptic
S. haptic intraocular lens
slant hole collimator
slaphammer
BIAS s.
Slatis frame
slatted plinth table
**Slattery-McGrouther dynamic flexion
splint**
Slaughter nasal saw
Sled implant
Sleds
Penco Walker S.
Sleek catheter
sleep
s. apnea monitor
S. Right nasal strips
Sleepscan polysomnograph
sleeve
s. adapter
s. bag
Bard irrigation s.
biocompression pneumatic s.
Charles anterior segment s.
Charles infusion s.
Charles vitrector with s.
Coloplast transparent irrigation s.
Cunningham-Cotton s.
delivery assistance s.
Dexterity Pneumo S.
drug infusion s.

sleeve *(continued)*
  Dunlop s.
  Easy S.
  Edwards-Levine s.
  elbow s.
  Electro-Mesh s.
  epX suspension s.
  gel suspension s.
  heel s.
  Iceflex Endurance suction
    suspension s.
  ICEROSS s.
  implant s.
  s. implant
  Jobst s.
  Ken Drive s.
  Knit-Rite suspension s.
  laparoscopic s.
  LocalMed catheter infusion s.
  malleolar gel s.
  Mentor Foley catheter with
    comfort s.
  MICA 3x s.
  neoprene elbow s.
  PMMA centering s.
  pneumo s.
  Preclude IMA s.
  release s.
  retinal probe s.
  s. selector
  Silipos suspension s.
  Silopad body s.
  Silopad toe s.
  Steri-Sleeve s.
  Stevens-Charles s.
  Super Grip s.
  Supramid eye muscle s.
  SupraSLEEVES nylon s.
  Sur-Fit colostomy irrigation s.
  Surgiport trocar and s.
  tri-point K-wire s.
  Ultra Duet Colostomy irrigating s.
  Watzke silicone s.
sleeved nut
sleeve/multiple sidehole manometric
  assemble
sleeve-spreading forceps
Sleuth
  CO S.
  ETO S.
  HBT S.
Slick stylette endotracheal tube guide
slide
  Cyto-Rich cervical cytology s.
  Fisher-plus s.
  gelatin-subbed s.
  s. hammer
  Hemoccult Sensa s.
  Polaroid vectograph s.
  poly-L-lysine-coated glass s.
  silanated s.
  Tanner s.
  Testsimplets prestained s.
Slide-On EndoSheath

Slider
  S. balloon
  S. catheter
Slidewire extension guide
sliding
  s. AFO
  s. barrel hook
  s. capsular forceps
  s. hammer
  s. laryngoscope
  s. lock
sliding-rail catheter
slightly-curved ear pick
Slik-Pak non-stick nasal pack
Slim
  S. Fit flex clamp
  S. Option shoe orthosis
  S. and Trim brief
slimcut blade
Slimfit lens
SlimLine
  S. cast boot
  S. disposable brief
  S. fitted liner
  S. peach sheet care pad
Slimline
  S. clip
Slimrest
  Core S.
SlimStem metal scleral shield
Slimthetics orthotic
sling
  Aldridge rectus fascia s.
  Ampoxen s.
  Arjo Loop S.
  arm elevator s.
  Barton s.
  Böhler-Braun leg s.
  cardiac s.
  clip-reinforced cotton s.
  Colles s.
  cradle arm s.
  CVA S.
  DLP cardiac s.
  s. dressing
  envelope arm s.
  finger s.
  Fits-All s.
  s. frame
  hanging cast s.
  Harris Hemi Arm s.
  Harris splint s.
  head s.
  Hemi s.
  Kodel s.
  leg s.
  Mersilene mesh s.
  Murphy s.
  Nada-Chair Back-Up portable
    back s.
  Perthes s.
  platysma inerlocking suture s.
  Posey s.
  pouch-type s.
  pressure s.

pulmonary artery s.
Rauchfuss s.
resting foot s.
Sayre s.
shoulder saddle s.
Silastic s.
slinger-style envelope s.
sling and swathe s.
static s.
Stratasis urethral s.
suburethral s.
Suspend pubovaginal s.
s. and swathe (S&S)
temporalis s.
Thomas Kodel s.
triangular arm s.
UltraSling glenohumeral joint s.
Uni-Versatil s.
Velpeau s.
Weil pelvic s.
Westfield-style envelope s.
sling-and-swathe bandage
slinger-style envelope sling
Slinky
S. balloon
S. balloon catheter
S. PTCA catheter
Slip-Coat tip
slip-joint pliers
Slip-N-Snip scissors
slipper-tipped guidewire
Slippery Slider transport board
slip-ring camera
Slip-Sheen catheter
slit
s. blade
s. blade knife
s. illuminator
s. lamp
slit-lamp, slitlamp (*See also* lamp)
s.-l. cup
s.-l. fluorophotometer
Gullstrand s.-l.
s.-l. microscope
SLM-8000 fluorescence spectrophotometer
Sloan
S. goiter flap dissector
S. goiter self-retaining retractor
Slocum meniscal clamp
Slocum-Smith-Petersen nail
Slo-Mo ball
slot
S. distraction device
s. table
slotted
s. anoscope
s. bone plate
s. instrument
s. intramedullary rod
s. laryngoscope
s. mallet
s. nail
s. needle
s. nerve clamp
s. tendon stripper

s. tube articulated stent
s. whisker
s. wrench
slotting bur
slotting-bur osteotome
slow palatal expander
SL-Plus stem
SLS Chromos long pulse ruby laser system
SLT
S. CL MD/Dual Contact laser
S. Contact ArthroProbe
S. Contact MTRL laser
S. FiberTact/Contact laser fiber
Sluder
S. adenotome
S. cautery electrode
S. headband
S. knife
S. needle
S. palate retractor
S. sphenoidal hook
S. sphenoidal speculum
S. tonometer
S. tonsillar guillotine
S. tonsillar tonsillectome
Sluder-Ballenger
S.-B. tonsillar punch forceps
S.-B. tonsillectome
Sluder-Demarest
S.-D. tonometer
S.-D. tonsillectome
Sluder-Ferguson mouthgag
Sluder-Jansen mouthgag
Sluder-Mehta electrode
Sluder-Sauer
S.-S. tonsillar guillotine
S.-S. tonsillectome
Sluijter-Mehta SMK-C10 cannula
SMAC
Sequential Multiple Analyzer Computer
small
s. aperture Steri-Drape drape
s. cup biopsy forceps
s. nail spicule bur
S. rake retractor
S. tissue retractor
s. volume nebulizer
small-based quad cane
small-bore
s.-b. cannula
s.-b. needle
small-caliber needle
Small-Carrion
S.-C. penile implant material
S.-C. penile prosthesis
S.-C. Silastic rod for penile implant
small-diameter endosonographic instrument
SmallHand polpypectomy snare
small-loop electrode
SmallPort needle
SMART
SMART Balance Master

S.M.A.R.T.
    S. bile duct stent
    S. biliary stent
Smart
    S. chalazion forceps
    S. enucleation scissors
    S. nonslipping chalazion forceps
    S. position-sensing catheter
    S. Scope
    S. Screener infant hearing screener
    S. Splint
    S. System irrigation/suction system
    S. Trigger
    S. Trigger Bear 1000 ventilator
SmartAnchor-D suture anchor
SmartAnchor-L suture anchor
SmartBrace brace
Smartdop Doppler
SmartDose infusion system
SmartKard digital Holter system
SmartKnit seamless sock
SmartMist asthma management system
SmartNeedle needle
SmartPins fastener
SmartPrep scanner
SmarTracking
SmartScrew
    S. bioabsorbable implant
    S. screw
SmartSite needleless system
SmartSpot high-resolution digital imaging system
SmartTack tack
SmartWrap elbow brace
Smedberg
    S. brace
    S. dilator
    S. hand drill
    S. twist drill
Smeden tonsillar punch
Smedley dynamometer
SMEI
    SMEI ultrasound-assisted lipoplasty machine
Smellie
    S. obstetrical forceps
    S. obstetrical hook
    S. obstetrical perforator
    S. obstetrical scissors
Smeloff-Cutter
    S.-C. ball-cage prosthetic valve
    S.-C. ball-valve prosthesis
Smeloff heart valve
SMIC
    SMIC abdominal spatula
    SMIC anterior commisure laryngoscope
    SMIC auricular tourniquet
    SMIC bone chisel
    SMIC bone file
    SMIC bone hammer
    SMIC bone rongeur
    SMIC brain spatula
    SMIC burnisher
    SMIC carver

SMIC cerumen hook
SMIC cheek retractor
SMIC collar scissors
SMIC cranial rongeur
SMIC dermatome
SMIC ear curette
SMIC ear polypus scissors
SMIC ear speculum
SMIC eustachian catheter
SMIC excavator
SMIC explorer
SMIC intestinal clamp
SMIC laminectomy rongeur
SMIC malleus head nipper
SMIC mastoid chisel
SMIC mastoid curette
SMIC mastoid gouge
SMIC mastoid rongeur
SMIC mastoid suction tube
SMIC mouth mirror
SMIC myringotome
SMIC nasal septal speculum
SMIC nylon thread
SMIC periodontal abscess probe
SMIC periodontal file
SMIC periosteal elevator
SMIC pituitary curette
SMIC pliers
SMIC pneumatic otoscope
SMIC powder blower
SMIC root canal plugger
SMIC sternal chisel
SMIC sternal drill
SMIC sternal knife
SMIC surgical catgut
SMIC surgical mallet
SMIC suture needle
SMIC tonsillar guillotine
SMIC tuning fork
Smiley-Williams arteriography needle
SmiLine abutment system
Smillie
    S. cartilage chisel
    S. knee joint retractor
    S. meniscal cartilage knife
    S. meniscectomy chisel
    S. meniscotome
    S. nail
    S. nail punch
    S. pin
Smirmaul
    S. eyelid speculum
    S. nucleus extractor
Smith
    S. anal retractor
    S. anal speculum
    S. aneurysm clip
    S. anoscope
    S. bandage scissors
    S. bone clamp
    S. cartilage knife
    S. cataract knife
    S. cordotomy clamp
    S. cordotomy knife
    S. drill

S. endoscopic electrode
S. expressor hook
S. eye speculum
S. grasping forceps
S. intraocular capsular amputator
S. intraocular implant lens
S. lens expressor
S. lid expressor
S. lid-retracting hook
S. lion-jaw forceps
S. marginal clamp
S. & Nephew ENT nasopharyngoscope
S. & Nephew medium barbed staple
S. & Nephew reflection acetabular cup implant component
S. & Nephew Richards bipolar forceps
S. & Nephew screw
S. & Nephew small barbed staple
S. nerve root suction retractor
S. obstetrical forceps
S. orbital floor implant
S. perforator
S. posterior cartilage stripper
S. rectal self-retaining retractor
S. retroversion pessary
S. STA-peg
S. suture wire scissors
S. tonsillar dissector
S. total ankle prosthesis
S. tube
S. vaginal self-retaining retractor
Smith-Buie
S.-B. anal retractor
S.-B. rectal speculum
S.-B. self-retaining rectal retractor
Smith-Fisher
S.-F. cataract knife
S.-F. cataract spatula
S.-F. iris replacer
S.-F. iris spatula
Smith-Green
S.-G. cataract knife
S.-G. double-ended spatula
Smith-Hodge pessary
Smith-Leiske
S.-L. cross-action intraocular lens forceps
S.-L. lens manipulator
Smith-Miller-Patch cryosurgical instrument
Smith-Petersen
S.-P. bone gouge
S.-P. bone plate
S.-P. cannulated nail
S.-P. capsular retractor
S.-P. chisel
S.-P. cup
S.-P. curette
S.-P. curved gouge
S.-P. curved osteotome
S.-P. elevator
S.-P. extractor

S.-P. femoral neck nail
S.-P. forceps
S.-P. fracture pin
S.-P. hammer
S.-P. hip cup prosthesis
S.-P. hip reamer
S.-P. impactor
S.-P. intertrochanteric plate
S.-P. laminectomy rongeur
S.-P. mallet
S.-P. spatula
S.-P. straight osteotome
S.-P. transarticular nail
S.-P. tucker
Smith-Richards instrumentation
Smithuysen sphenoidal punch
Smithwick
S. anastomotic clamp
S. buttonhook
S. buttonhook button
S. clip-applying forceps
S. ganglion hook
S. nerve dissector
S. nerve hook
S. retractor
S. silver clip
S. sympathectomy hook
Smithwick-Hartmann forceps
SMo
SMo Moore pin
SMo plate
SMo prosthesis
smoke
s. Controller device
s. Control Porta-Pack aversive stimulator
s. evacuator
s. evacuator suction tube
s. removal tube
Smokeeter tube
SmokEvac
S. electrosurgical probe
S. smoke evacuator
S. trumpet valve
Smolik curved rongeur
Smolinski endaural rongeur
smooth
s. cannula
s. dressing forceps
s. endoprosthesis
s. pin
s. staple implant
s. tissue forceps
s. transfixion wire
Smoothie Junior bur
smooth-tipped jeweler's forceps
smooth-tooth forceps
Smuckler tucker
SMZ zoom stereo microscope
snail-headed catheter retriever
SNAP
SNAP sleep recorder
Snap
S. fixation pin
S. Lock wire/pin extractor

S

Snap-Gauge gauge
snap-lock brace
snap-on inserter plate
Snap-pak
    Mitek GII S.-p.
snare
    AcuSnare s.
    Alfred s.
    Amplatz retinal s.
    automatic ratchet s.
    Banner enucleation s.
    barbed s.
    Beck-Schenck tonsillar s.
    Beck-Storz tonsillar s.
    BiSNARE bipolar polypectomy s.
    Boettcher-Farlow s.
    Bosworth nasal s.
    Brown tonsillar s.
    Bruening ear s.
    Bruening nasal s.
    Bruening tonsillar s.
    Buerger s.
    Captiflex polypectomy s.
    Captivator polypectomy s.
    Castroviejo enucleation s.
    s. catheter
    cautery s.
    coaxial s.
    Colles s.
    Cox polypectomy s.
    Crapeau nasal s.
    crescent s.
    diathermal s.
    diathermic s.
    Douglas nasal s.
    Douglas tonsillar s.
    ear polyp s.
    Electrosurgery s.
    enucleation wire s.
    s. enucleator
    EUE tonsillar s.
    Eves-Neivert tonsillar s.
    Eves tonsillar s.
    Farlow-Boettcher s.
    Farlow tonsillar s.
    fascial s.
    Foerster enucleation s.
    Förster enucleation s.
    Frankfeldt diathermy s.
    Frankfeldt rectal s.
    Freidenwald-Guyton s.
    frontalis s.
    Glegg nasal polyp s.
    Glisson s.
    Goebel-Stoeckel s.
    gooseneck s.
    hand cock-up s.
    Harris s.
    hexagon s.
    Hobbs polypectomy s.
    Hoyer s.
    Jarvis s.
    Krause ear polyp s.
    Krause laryngeal s.
    Krause nasal polyp s.

    laryngeal s.
    lasso s.
    levator s.
    Lewis tonsillar s.
    Marlex mesh s.
    Martin s.
    Mason-Allen s.
    Meek s.
    Microvena Amplatz Goose Neck s
    Milwaukee s.
    Myles tonsillectome s.
    Nakao s. I, II
    nasal s.
    Neivert-Eves tonsillar s.
    Nesbit tonsillar s.
    Newhart-Casselberry s.
    Norwood rectal s.
    Olympus SD-5L semicircular s.
    open electrocautery s.
    oval s.
    pelvic s.
    pericardial s.
    polypectomy s.
    Posey s.
    Profile pediatric polypectomy s.
    ptosis s.
    pulmonary arterial s.
    Pynchon ear s.
    Quire mechanical finger s.
    Rainbow envelope arm s.
    Rauchfuss s.
    rectal cautery s.
    Reiner-Beck tonsillar s.
    Robert nasal s.
    rotatable polypectomy s.
    Sage tonsillar s.
    Sayre head s.
    self-opening rigid s.
    Sensation Short Throw s.
    Singular oval polypectomy s.
    SmallHand polpypectomy s.
    standard endoscopy polypectomy s.
    Stewart lenticular nuclear s.
    Stiegler unipolar nasal s.
    Storz-Beck tonsillar s.
    Stutsman nasal s.
    Supramid s.
    surgical s.
    Teare s.
    tonsillar s.
    Tydings automatic ratchet s.
    Tydings tonsillar s.
    UroSnare cystoscopic tumor s.
    Veeder tip s.
    Velpeau s.
    Wappler polypectomy s.
    Weil pelvic s.
    Weston rectal s.
    Wilde-Bruening ear s.
    Wilde-Bruening nasal s.
    Wilde ear polyp s.
    Wilde nasal s.
    Wilson-Cook polypectomy s.
    s. wire
    wire s.

Wright nasal s.
Wright tonsillar s.
Zimmer s.
Snellen
S. chart
S. conventional reform eye implant
S. entropion forceps
S. lens loop
S. lens scoop
S. reform eye
S. soft contact lens
S. suture
S. vectis
Snitman endaural self-retaining retractor
Snornomor device
Snowden-Pencer
S.-P. insufflator
S.-P. internal heater
S.-P. laparoscopic cholecystectomy instrument
S.-P. Super-Cut scissors
Snowflake laparotomy sponge
snow plow rasp
Snug
S. denture cushion
S. seat
Snugfit eye patch
Snuggle Warm convective warming system
Snugs
S. dressing
S. tapeless wound care system
Snyder
S. breast prosthesis
S. corneal spring forceps
S. deep-surgery forceps
S. Hemovac evacuator
S. Hemovac silicone sump drain
S. Hemovac suction tube
S. suction device
S. Surgivac drainage
S. Surgivac suction tube
S. Urevac suction tube
S. Urevac trocar
Sobel-Kaplitt-Sawyer gas endarterectomy set
Soccer Sporthotic
sock
s. aid
Bio-Wick s.
Carolon AFO s.
Comfort Ag prosthetic s.
Dero hole-in-one prosthetic s.
diabetic s.
edema s.
electrode s.
gel stump s.
molding s.
polytetrafluoroethylene s.
Regal Acrylic/Stretch prosthetic s.
Silosheath s.
SmartKnit seamless s.
Soft Walk gel s.
STS molding s.

socket
APOPPS, transtibial prosthetic s.
concave loading s.
flexible s.
Flo-Tech prosthetic s.
hard s.
Iceross silicone s.
ICEX s.
ischial containment s.
ischial-gluteal weightbearing s.
metal-backed s.
polyethylene s.
prosthetic s.
Pump-It-Up pneumatic s.
standard s.
SuperClearPro suction s.
supracondylar s.
suspension-type s.
s. wrench
Socon spinal system
Sodas spheroidal oral drug absorption system
Soderstrom-Corson electrode
sodium
s. alginate wool mold
s. chloride-impregnated gauze
s. detector
S. hyaluronate-based bioresorbable membrane
s. hyaluronate viscoelastic
Soehendra
S. BII papillotome/sphincterotome
S. catheter dilator
S. catheter system
S. dilating catheter
S. endoscopic biliary stent system
S. lithotripsy set
S. Precut papillotome/sphincterotome
S. stent extractor
S. stent retrieval device
S. stent retriever
S. Universal catheter
Sofamor
S. spinal instrument
S. spinal instrumentation device
Sof-Band bulky bandage
Sof-Care
S.-C. chair cushion
S.-C. Plus cushion
Sof.Care mattress
Sofflex mattress
Sof-Foam dressing
Sof-Form conforming gauze
Sof Gel HeelCup orthosis
Sof-Gel palm shield
Sofield
S. retractor
S. retractor blade
S. retractor clip
Sof-Kling conforming bandage
Soflens contact lens
SoFlex lens
Sof-Matt pressure reducing mattress
Sofnit
S. Birdseye reusable underpad

S

751

Sofnit *(continued)*
   S. 300 fitted brief
   S. 300 reusable underpad
Sofomor-Danek component
SofPulse electrotherapy device
Sof-Rol
   S.-R. cast pad
   S.-R. dressing
SofSeat pressure relief pad
Sofsilk
   S. coated and braided suture
   S. nonabsorbable silk suture
SofSorb absorptive dressing
SofStep wheelchair footplate cover
SOF-T
   S.-T. guidewire
   S.-T. guiding catheter
soft
   s. ankle, cushioned heel
   s. ankle, cushioned heel orthopaedic appliance
   s. cataract aspirator
   s. contact lens
   S. Guard XL fecal incontinence bag
   s. intraocular lens
   s. palate retractor
   s. rubber curette
   s. rubber drain
   s. scrub brush
   S. & Secure 1-piece spouted pouch system
   S. & Secure 2-piece spouted pouch system
   S. Shield collagen corneal shield
   S. & Silent diaper pant
   S. & Silent vinyl pull-on brief
   S. & Silent vinyl snap-on brief
   s. silicone sphere implant
   s. silicone sponge
   S. Super Sport orthotic
   S. Support Preforms orthotic
   S. Thoracoport
   s. tissue blade retractor
   s. tissue shaving cannula
   S. Torque uterine catheter
   S. Touch cup
   S. Touch hand exerciser
   S. Touch lancet device
   S. Walk gel sock
   s. wire loop
   s. x-ray film
Soft-Cell permanent dual-lumen catheter
SoftCloth absorptive dressing
Softech endotracheal tube
Softepil tweezer epilation device
Softexe non-adherent sub-bandage padding
Softeze
   S. self-adhering foam pad
   S. water pillow
Soft-EZ reusable electrode
Softflo fiber optic probe

SoftForm
   S. facial implant
   S. tube
Softgut surgical chromic catgut suture
Softie shoe
Softip
   S. arteriography catheter
   S. diagnostic catheter
SofTip monofilament
Softjaw
   S. clamp
   S. insert
SoftLight
   S. laser
   S. laser hair removal system
soft-lined denture
Softopac intraoral film
Softouch
   S. Cobra 1, 2 catheter
   S. Cold/Hot Pack
   S. Headhunter 1 catheter
   S. Multipurpose B2 catheter
   S. Simmons 1, 2 catheter
   S. spinal angiography catheter
   S. UHF cardiac pigtail catheter
SofTouch vacuum erection device
Softpatch
Softplate
Softrace gel electrode
Softrac-PTA catheter
Softscan laser scanner
SoftSITE high add aspheric multifocal contact lens
Softsplint foot splint
soft-tipped
   s.-t. cannula
   s.-t. extrusion handpiece
soft-tissue Super Sport orthotic
Soft-Touch A-Probe
Soft-Vu
   S.-V. angiographic catheter
   S.-V. Omni flush catheter
Soft-Wand
   S.-W. atraumatic tissue manipulator balloon
Sof-Wick
   S.-W. drain
   S.-W. drain sponge
   S.-W. dressing
   S.-W. lap pad
Sofwire cable system
SOF'WIRE spinal fixation
Sohes pacemaker
Soileau Tytan ventilation tube
Sokolec elevator
Sokolow electrocardiographic index
Sokolowski antral punch
Sola
   S. Optical USA Spectralite high-index lens
   S. VIP lens
SolAiris III oxygen concentrator
Solar
   S. Beam medical examination light
   S. pacemaker

SolarEar hearing aid
Solcotrans
  S. autotransfusion system
  S. autotransfusion unit
  S. closed vacuum-drainage system
  S. drainage/reinfusion system
  S. orthopaedic drainage-refusion
    system
  S. Plus drainage-reinfusion system
Solcovac closed wound drainage system
solder
  PF Universal s.
  tissue s.
soldering tweezers
sole
  D-Soles foot s.
  S. Primeur 33D analyzer
solenoid surface coil
SOLEutions
  S. custom orthosis
  S. custom orthotic device
  S. orthotic
  S. Prefab orthotic device
Solfy ZX ultrasonic unit
solid
  s. buckling implant material
  s. copper head mallet
  S. Creation System
  s. hex bolt
  s. silicone buttock implant
  s. silicone exoplant implant material
  s. silicone orbital prosthesis
  s. silicone with Supramid mesh
    implant
solid-ankle,
  s.-a. cushioned-heel
  s.-a. cushioned-heel foot prosthesis
solid-phase
  s.-p. extraction chromatograph
  s.-p. extraction tube
solid-rod rigid telescope
solid-state
  s.-s. coagulator
  s.-s. esophageal manometry catheter
  s.-s. instrument
  s.-s. nuclear track detector
solid-tip catheter
Solis pacemaker
Solitaire needle
Solitens
  S. TENS unit
  S. transcutaneous electrical nerve
    stimulation unit
Soll suture and incision marker
Solo
  S. catheter
  S. catheter with Pro/Pel coating
SoloPass
  S. catheter
  S. Percuflex biliary stent
Solos
  S. disposable cannula
  S. disposable trocar
  S. endoscopy diagnostic laparoscope
SoloSite hydrogel dressing

SOLO-Surg Colo-Rectal self-retaining
  retractor system
Solo-Tach resin
Solow sigmoidoscope
Soluset
  intravenous S.
  S. IV set
Solus pacemaker
Solvang graft
Soma
  S. Gonio system
  S. pulley system
  S. sacroiliac stabilization belt
Somanetics INVOS 3100 cerebral
  oximeter
SomaSensor
  S. device
  S. pad
Somatics
  S. monitoring electrode
  S. mouth guard
Somatom
  S. DR CT scanner
  S. Plus S whole-body scanner
Somers
  S. uterine clamp
  S. uterine forceps
Somerset bur
Somer uterine elevator
SOMI
  SOMI brace
  SOMI Jr. brace
  SOMI orthosis
Sommers compression dressing
SomnoStar apnea testing device
Sonablate transrectal probe
Sonatron ultrasonic scaler
Sonde enteroscope
Sones
  S. Cardio-Marker catheter
  S. coronary catheter
  S. guidewire
  S. hemostatic bag
  S. Hi-Flow catheter
  S. Positrol catheter
  S. vent catheter
  S. woven Dacron catheter
Songer
  S. cable
  S. cable system
  S. tonsillar forceps
Song stent
sonic
  s. accelerated fracture healing
    system
  S. Air 1500 device
  S. Boom alarm clock
  s. curette
  S. Hedgehog
Sonicaid
  S. Axis monitor
  S. system 8000 fetal monitor
  S. Vasoflow Doppler system
Sonicare Plus

S

Sonicath
  S. endoluminal ultrasound catheter
  S. imaging catheter
  S. intravascular ultrasound catheter
Sonicator portable ultrasound
Sonifer sonicating system
Sonnenberg sump drain
Sonnenschein nasal speculum
Sonoblate ablation device
Sonocath ultrasound probe
Sonoclot
  S. coagulation analyzer
Sonocut ultrasonic aspirator
Sonogage
  S. System Corneo-Gage 20 MHz center frequency transducer
  S. ultrasound pachymeter
Sono-Gram fetal ultrasound image card
sonography
  Toshiba SSA-340A Doppler s.
SonoHeart hand-held, all digital echocardiography system
Sonoline
  S. Elegra ultrasound system
  S. Prima ultrasound
  S. Siemens ultrasound scanner
  S. Sierra ultrasound imaging system
  S. SI-200/250 ultrasound imaging system
Sonolith 3000 lithotriptor
Sonomed A/B-Scan system
sonometer
  Sahara clinical bone s.
  SoundScan 2000 bone s.
  SoundScan Compact bone s.
Sonometric Ocuscan
Sonop
  S. handpiece
  S. ultrasonic aspirator
Sonoprobe
  SP-501 S.
Sonopsy
  S. biopsy imaging system
  S. ultrasound-guided breast biopsy system
Sonoran dehumidifier
Sonos
  S. 5500 cardiovascular ultrasound
  S. imaging system
  S. scanner
  S. ultrasonographic transducer
  S. ultrasound imager
Sono-stat
  S.-s. Plus EMG machine
Sono-Stat Plus sound device
Sonotrode lithotriptor
SonoVu US aspiration needle
Sontec pliers
Sony
  S. CCD/RGB DXC-151 color video camera
  S. Promavica still capture device
  S. video recorder

Soonawalla
  S. uterine elevator
  S. vasectomy forceps
Sopha Medical gamma camera
Sopher ovum forceps
Sophie mammagraphy unit
Sophy
  S. high-resolution collimator
  S. mini programmable pressure valve
Soprano
  S. cryoablation system
  S. cryotherapy unit
SorbaView composite wound dressing
Sorbex
  S. Thin hydrocolloid dressing
Sorbiclear dialyzer
Sorbie-Questor total elbow system
Sorb-It II dressing
Sorbothane orthotic device
Sorbsan
  S. alginate dressing
  S. gel block topical wound dressi
Sorbuthane II heel cup
Sorensen
  S. aspirator
  S. reusable cannister
Sorenson thermodilution catheter
Soresi cannula
Sorin
  S. mitral valve prosthesis
  S. pacemaker
  S. prosthetic valve
Sorrells
  S. hip arthroplasty retractor system
  S. Mark II hip arthroplasty retrac system
sorter
  FACSVantage cell s.
  fluorescence-activated cell s.
  magnetically activated cell s.
Soto USCI balloon
Soules intrauterine insemination cathete
sound
  Allport mastoid s.
  Bellocq s.
  Béniqué s.
  bladder s.
  bronchocele s.
  Campbell-French s.
  Campbell miniature urethral s.
  Davis interlocking s.
  Dittel urethral s.
  Dittel uterine s.
  Ellik s.
  female s.
  flexible s.
  Fowler urethral s.
  French steel s.
  Gouley tunneled urethral s.
  Greenwald s.
  Guyon-Benique urethral s.
  Guyon dilating s.
  Guyon urethral s.
  Hishida pine-needle s.

Hunt metal s.
interlocking s.
Jewett urethral s.
Jewett uterine s.
Klebanoff common duct s.
Kocher bronchocele s.
Korotkoff s.
lacrimal s.
LeFort urethral s.
LeFort uterine s.
s. level meter
Mark-7 intrauterine s.
Martin uterine s.
McCrea infant s.
meatal s.
Mercier s.
miniature s.
Otis urethral s.
Pharmaseal disposable uterine s.
Pratt urethral s.
radiolucent s.
Rica uterine s.
rigid s.
Rissler vein s.
Ritter s.
Saf-T-Sound uterine s.
Schroeder interlocking uterine s.
Simpson uterine s.
Sims uterine s.
urethral s.
uterine s.
Van Buren canvas roll s.
Van Buren dilating s.
Van Buren urethral s.
Walther urethral s.
Winternitz s.
Woodward s.
soundbridge
Symphonix Vibrant s.
Vibrant D, P s.
sounder
mini-echo s.
pedicle s.
SoundScan
S. 2000 bone sonometer
S. Compact bone sonometer
source
Arclite light s.
cesium s.
dummy s.
DyoBrite Xenon light s.
ESI fiberoptic light s.
fiberoptic light s.
halogen light s.
Heyman-Simon s.
Maxenon 300 watt xenon light s.
Maxillume 250 watt quartz halogen
light s.
Medicam light s.
Minimax 200 watt light s.
MX2-300 xenon quality light s.
Olympus CLV-U 20 endoscopic
halogen light s.
Teclite fiberoptic light s.

xenon light s.
Zeiss Super Lux 40 light s.
Sourdille forceps
Souter Strathclyde total elbow system
Southbent scissors
**Southern Eye Bank corneal cutting
block**
Southey
S. anasarca trocar
S. cannula
S. capillary drainage tube
Southey-Leech trocar
Southwick
S. clamp
S. screw extractor
Southworth rasp
Souttar
S. cautery
S. esophageal conductor
S. tube
Sovak reamer
Sovally suprapubic suction cup drain
Sovereign
S. bifocal lens
S. Shield system
Soviet mechanical bronchial stapler
Sox
Champion Power S.
SP-10 spirometer
SP-501 Sonoprobe
SP6 camera
Spa
S. Bed
S. Champion PowerSox for Men
gradient pressure therapy hosiery
S. Ready-To-Wear gradient pressure
therapy hosiery
S. SoftBasics gradient pressure
therapy hosiery
S. UltraSilk Sheers gradient
pressure therapy hosiery
space-age wire
Spacekeeper retractor
SpaceLabs
S. Event Master
S. Holter monitor
S. pulse oximeter
space-maintaining barrier
Spacemaker
S. hernia balloon dissector
S. II balloon
Space-OR retractor
spacer
Barouk s.
Barouk button s.
Bio-Moore II provisional neck s.
button s.
ceramic vertebral s.
dummy s.
Ellipse compact s.
eyelid s.
GAIT s.
s. inserter
Kinemax s.
methyl methacrylate s.

S

spacer *(continued)*
    Plexiglas s.
    proximal cement s.
    rubber s.
    suture s.
space retainer
SpaceSEAL balloon tip cannula
Spadafora MemoryLens dialer
spade-shaped valvotome
spaghetti drain
Spaide depressor
Spaleck forceps
Spandage
    S. bandage
    S. elastic
Spand-Gel
Span+Guard
Spanish
    S. blue virgin silk suture
spanner
    Codman s.
    s. gauge
    s. wrench
spanning external fixator
spark-gap
    s.-g. instrument
    s.-g. shock wave generator
Spark handheld dynamometer
Sparks
    S. atrioseptal punch
    S. mandrel prosthesis
Sparta
    S. microforceps
    S. micro-iris forceps
SPART analyzer
Spartan jaw wire cutter
SpaTouch PhotoEpilation system
spatula
    Allison lung s.
    angled iris s.
    angulated iris s.
    Ayers s.
    Aylesbury cervical s.
    Ayre cervical s.
    Bakelite s.
    Banaji s.
    Bangerter angled iris s.
    Barraquer cyclodialysis s.
    Barraquer iris s.
    Barraquer irrigator s.
    Bechert s.
    Berens s.
    Birks Mark II micro push/pull s.
    brain s.
    s. cannula
    s. cannula tip
    capsule fragment s.
    Castroviejo cyclodialysis s.
    Castroviejo double-end s.
    Castroviejo synechia s.
    Cave scaphoid s.
    cement s.
    Children's Hospital brain s.
    Clayman s.

    Cleasby iris s.
    corneal fascia lata s.
    corneal graft s.
    coronary endarterectomy s.
    Crile s.
    Culler iris s.
    curved-tipped s.
    Cushing S-shaped brain s.
    cyclodialysis s.
    Cytobrush s.
    Davis brain s.
    D'Errico brain s.
    DeWecker iris s.
    s. dissector
    Dixey s.
    Dorsey s.
    double s.
    double-vector brain s.
    Doyen s.
    Drews-Sato capsular fragment s.
    Drews-Sato suture-pickup s.
    duck-billed anodized s.
    electrosurgical s.
    s. electrosurgical probe
    Elschnig cyclodialysis s.
    endarterectomy s.
    Fisher-Smith s.
    fishtail s.
    flat s.
    s. forceps
    Freer nasal s.
    French hook s.
    French lacrimal s.
    French-pattern s.
    Fukusaku s.
    Fukushima malleable brain s.
    Galin lens s.
    Garron s.
    Gill-Welsh s.
    Girard synechia s.
    Green double s.
    Green lens s.
    Green replacer s.
    Gross brain s.
    Guimaraes ophthalmic flap s.
    Haberer s.
    Halle vascular s.
    Heifitz s.
    Hersh LASIK retreatment s.
    Hertzog lens s.
    Hirschman iris s.
    Hirschman lens s.
    s. hook
    hook s.
    Hough s.
    Interstate s.
    iridodialysis s.
    iris s.
    irrigating notched s.
    Jacobson endarterectomy s.
    Jaffe intraocular s.
    Jaffe lens s.
    Johnson s.
    Kader intestinal s.
    Kallmorgen vaginal s.

Katena iris s.
Kellman-Elschnig s.
Kennerdell s.
Killian laryngeal s.
Kimura platinum s.
Kirby angulated iris s.
Knapp cyclodialysis s.
Knapp iris s.
Knolle lens cortex s.
Knolle lens nucleus s.
Kocher bladder s.
Korte abdominal s.
Krause-Davis s.
Kummel intestinal s.
Kwitko lens s.
Laird s.
Legueu s.
lens s.
Leriche s.
Lewicky IOL s.
Lieppman s.
Lindner cyclodialysis s.
lingual s.
Lynch s.
MacRae flap flipper/retreatment s.
Maddox LASIK s.
malleable s.
Manhattan Eye & Ear s.
Masket phaco s.
Maumenee-Barraquer vitreous
 sweep s.
Maumenee vitreous sweep s.
Mayfield malleable brain s.
McIntyre irrigating s.
McPherson iris s.
McReynolds eye s.
Medscand cervical s.
Meller cyclodialysis s.
microvitreoretinal s.
Mikulicz s.
Milex s.
Millin bladder s.
Mills coronary endarterectomy s.
Morgenstein s.
needle s.
nerve separator s.
nucleus s.
O'Brien s.
Obstbaum lens s.
Obstbaum synechia s.
Olivecrona brain s.
Olk retinal s.
Olk vitreoretinal s.
Pallin lens s.
Paton double s.
Paton single s.
Paton transplant s.
Peyton brain s.
phacodialysis s.
plaster s.
platinum probe s.
probe s.
Pucci-Seed s.
Raaf flexible lighted s.
Rainin lens s.

Ray brain s.
rectangular brain s.
Reverdin abdominal s.
Rica brain s.
Rizzuti graft carrier s.
Rolon s.
Roux s.
Rowen s.
Sachs s.
Schmid vascular s.
Schuknecht s.
Scoville flat brain s.
Segond vaginal s.
serrated T-s.
Sheets-Hirsch s.
Sheets lens s.
side-biting s.
side-cutting s.
Simcoe notched irrigating s.
Simcoe nucleus s.
Simmons-Kimbrough glaucoma s.
Sinclair s.
Sinskey nucleus s.
SMIC abdominal s.
SMIC brain s.
Smith-Fisher cataract s.
Smith-Fisher iris s.
Smith-Green double-ended s.
Smith-Petersen s.
s. split needle
s. spoon
spoon s.
S-shaped brain s.
stainless s.
Sterling iris s.
Suker cyclodialysis s.
surgical s.
suture pickup s.
synechia s.
"T" s.
Tan s.
tapered brain s.
Tauber vaginal s.
Tennant s.
Thomas s.
Thornton malleable s.
Tooke s.
Troutman-Barraquer iris s.
Troutman lens s.
Tuffier abdominal s.
University of Kansas s.
vaginal s.
vitreous sweep s.
wax-removing s.
Weary brain s.
Wheeler cyclodialysis s.
Wheeler iris s.
Woodson s.
Wullstein transplant s.
Wurmuth s.
Wylie s.

spatulated
 s. half-circle needle
speaking tube

S

spear
s. blade
eye s.
LASIK s.
Merocel surgical s.
PVA s.
Speare dural hook
spear-ended chrome probe
spear-pointed nickelene probe
Spears USCI laser balloon
special
s. Colles splint
S. Seat
specialized tissue-aspirating resectoscope
specimen forceps
Speck-Ange cutter
Speck introducer
SPECT
SPECT ADAC/Cirrus single-headed
camera
SPECT ADAC/Vertex dual-headed
camera
SPECT high-resolution brain system
SPECT scan
spectacles
bronchoscopic s.
compound s.
decentered s.
Franklin s.
Fresnel nystagmus s.
Hallauer s.
industrial s.
Masselon s.
mica s.
periscopic s.
prismatic s.
tinted s.
wire frame s.
Spect-Align laser system
Spectra
S. 400 extended surveillance and
alert system
S. pad
S. quilted underpad
Spectra-Cath
S.-C. STP catheter
Spectra-Diasonics ultrasound
Spectraflex pacemaker
spectral Doppler
Spectralite Transitions lens
Spectramed transducer
Spectranetics
S. laser
S. laser sheath
S. P23 Statham transducer
Spectra-Physics
S.-P. argon laser
S.-P. microsurgical laser
Spectraprobe-Max probe
**Spectraprobe-PLS laser angioplasty
catheter**
SpectraScience optical biopsy system
Spectra-System
S.-S. abutment
S.-S. implant

Spectrax
S. bipolar pacemaker
S. programmable Medtronic
pacemaker
S. SX, SX-HT, SXT, VL, VM,
pacemaker
S. SXT pulse generator
spectrocolorimeter
spectrometer
Bruker AMX 300 NMR s.
Centronic 200 MGA respiratory
mass s.
Compton suppression s.
EDXRF s.
gamma-ray s.
gas isotope ratio mass s.
GE GN300 7.5-T/89-mm bore
multinuclear s.
GE NMR s.
hard x-ray imaging s.
IBM NMR s.
liquid scintillation s.
mass s.
Mossbauer s.
Nicolet NMR s.
NMR s.
PROBE-SV s.
Shimatzu RF-5301 PC s.
SISCO s.
Varian Associates 11.7-T, 51-mm
bore s.
Varian NMR s.
x-ray s.
Spectron
S. EF total hip system
S. prosthesis
Spectronic 20 spectrophotometer
spectrophotometer
atomic absorbance s.
Beckman UV s.
digital imaging s. (DISEASE)
F-series fluorescence s.
Genetics Systems microplate
reader s.
Hitachi F-series fluorescence s.
Hitachi U-series s.
liquid scintillation s.
mass s.
Model IL 750, AA s.
Perkin-Elmer model 5000 atomic
absorption s.
reflectance s.
SLM-8000 fluorescence s.
Spectronic 20 s.
U-1100 UV-Vis s.
Varian Assoc. Cary 118C s.
spectroscope
Auger electron s. (AES)
near-infrared s.
Ohmeda Rascal II Raman s.
two-wavelength near-infrared s.
spectroscopy
Fourier transform infrared s.
gas chromatography/mass s.
H-1 MR s.

laser-Doppler s.
magnetic resonance s.
Model 3-60 mass s.
MR proton s.
nuclear magnetic resonance s.
point resolved s.
proton MR s.
in vivo H' magnetic resonance s.
spectroscopy-directed laser
spectrum
    DermaGard s.
    S. Designs facial implant
    S. DG-P pediatric cradle
    S. K1 laser
    S. lens analysis system
    S. ruby laser
    S. stethoscope
    S. tissue repair system
SPECTurn chair
specula (*pl. of* speculum)
specula
    Prima Series s.
specular
    s. attachment
    S. reflex slit lamp
Speculite
speculoscopy
    Pap Plus s.
speculum, pl. **specula**
    adolescent vaginal s.
    Adson s.
    Agrikola eye s.
    Alfonso eyelid s.
    Allen-Heffernan nasal s.
    Allingham rectal s.
    Amko vaginal s.
    anal s.
    s. anoscope
    Arruga eye s.
    Arruga globe s.
    Artisan wide-angle vaginal s.
    Aufricht septal s.
    aural s.
    Auvard Britetrac s.
    Auvard-Remine vaginal s.
    Auvard weighted vaginal s.
    Azar lid s.
    Bárány s.
    Barr anal s.
    Barraquer-Colibri eye s.
    Barraquer-Douvas eye s.
    Barraquer eye s.
    Barraquer-Floyd s.
    Barraquer solid s.
    Barraquer wire s.
    Barr rectal s.
    Barr-Shuford s.
    basket-style scleral supporter s.
    Beard eye s.
    Becker-Park s.
    Beckman-Colver nasal s.
    Beckman nasal s.
    Bedrossian eye s.
    Bercovici wire lid s.
    Berens eye s.

Berlind-Auvard vaginal s.
Bionix nasal s.
bivalved anal s.
blackened s.
Bodenheimer rectal s.
Bosworth nasal wire s.
Boucheron ear s.
Bovin-Stille vaginal s.
Bovin vaginal s.
Bowman eye s.
Bozeman s.
Braun s.
Breisky-Navratil vaginal s.
Breisky-Stille s.
Breisky vaginal s.
Brewer vaginal s.
Brinkerhoff rectal s.
Britetrac s.
Bronson s.
Bronson-Park s.
Bronson-Turtz s.
Brown ear s.
Bruening s.
Bruner vaginal s.
Buie-Smith rectal s.
Burnett Sani-Spec disposable s.
Callahan modification s.
Carpel s.
Carter septal s.
Caspar s.
Castallo eye s.
Castroviejo eye s.
Chelsea-Eaton anal s.
Chevalier Jackson laryngeal s.
Clark eye s.
Coakley nasal s.
Collin vaginal s.
Converse nasal s.
Conway lid s.
Cook eye s.
Cook rectal s.
Cottle nasal s.
Cottle septal s.
Critchett eye s.
Culler iris s.
Cusco vaginal s.
Cushing-Landolt transsphenoidal s.
Czerny rectal s.
David rectal s.
DeLee s.
DeRoaldes s.
Desmarres eye s.
Desmarres lid s.
DeVilbiss-Stacy s.
DeVilbiss vaginal s.
Disposo-Spec disposable s.
Docherty cheek s.
Douglas mucosal s.
Douvas-Barraquer s.
Downes nasal s.
Doyen vaginal s.
duckbill s.
Dudley-Smith rectal s.
Duplay-Lynch nasal s.
Duplay nasal s.

S

speculum *(continued)*
Dynacor vaginal s.
ear s.
Eaton nasal s.
Eisenhammer s.
endaural s.
ENT s.
Erhardt ear s.
Erosa-Spec vaginal s.
eye s.
Fansler rectal s.
Fanta s.
Farkas urethral s.
Farrior ear s.
Farrior oval s.
Fergusson tubular vaginal s.
fiberoptic vaginal s.
fine-wire s.
Flannery ear s.
flat-bladed nasal s.
Flint glass s.
Floyd-Barraquer wire s.
Forbes esophageal s.
s. forceps
Foster-Ballenger nasal s.
four-prong finger s.
Fox eye s.
Fränkel s.
Gaffee s.
Garrigue weighted vaginal s.
Gerzog nasal s.
Gilbert-Graves s.
Gleason s.
Goldbacher anoscope s.
Goldstein septal s.
Goligher s.
Graefe eye s.
Graves bivalve s.
Graves Britetrac vaginal s.
Graves Coldlite s.
Graves open-side vaginal s.
Gruber ear s.
Guild-Pratt rectal s.
Guilford-Wright bivalve s.
Guist s.
Guist-Black eye s.
Guist-Bloch s.
Gutter s.
Guttmann vaginal s.
Guyton-Maumenee s.
Guyton-Park eye s.
Gyn-A-Lite vaginal s.
Haglund-Stille vaginal s.
Haglund vaginal s.
Halle infant nasal s.
Halle-Tieck nasal s.
Hardy bivalve s.
Hardy-Duddy s.
Hardy nasal bivalve s.
Hartmann dewaxer s.
Hartmann ear s.
Hartmann nasal s.
Hayes vaginal s.
Heffernan nasal s.

Helmholtz s.
Helmont s.
Henrotin weighted vaginal s.
Hertel nephrostomy s.
Higbee vaginal s.
Hinkle-James rectal s.
Hirschman anoscope rectal s.
s. holder
Holinger infant esophageal s.
Hood-Graves vaginal s.
Hough-Boucheron ear s.
House stapes s.
Huffman-Graves adolescent
  vaginal s.
Huffman-Graves vaginal s.
Huffman infant vaginal s.
Iliff-Park s.
illuminated s.
s. illuminator transilluminator
Ingals nasal s.
Ives rectal s.
Jackson vaginal s.
Jaffe eyelid s.
Jarit-Graves vaginal s.
Jarit-Pederson vaginal s.
Jonas-Graves vaginal s.
Kahn-Graves vaginal s.
Kaiser s.
Kalinowski ear s.
Kalinowski-Verner ear s.
Katena s.
Keeler-Pierse eye s.
Keizer-Lancaster eye s.
Kelly rectal s.
Killian-Halle nasal s.
Killian nasal s.
Killian rectal s.
Killian septal s.
Klaff septal s.
KleenSpec disposable vaginal s.
Knapp-Culler s.
Knapp eye s.
Knolle lens s.
Kogan endocervical s.
Kogan urethra s.
Kramer ear s.
Kratz aspirating s.
Kratz-Barraquer wire lid s.
Kristeller vaginal s.
Kyle nasal s.
Lancaster eye s.
Lancaster lid s.
Lancaster-O'Connor s.
Landau s.
Lang eye s.
Lawford s.
LeFort s.
Lempert-Beckman-Colver endaural s.
Lempert-Colver endaural s.
Lester-Burch eye s.
lid s.
LidFix s.
Lieberman aspirating s.
Lieberman K-Wire s.
lighted s.

Lillie nasal s.
Lindstrom-Chu aspirating s.
Lister-Burch eye s.
Lofberg vaginal s.
Lucae ear s.
Luer eye s.
Machat adjustable aspirating wire s.
Macon Hospital s.
Mahoney intranasal antral s.
Manche LASIK s.
Martin rectal s.
Martin vaginal s.
Mason-Auvard weighted vaginal s.
Mathews rectal s.
Matzenauer vaginal s.
Maumenee-Park eye s.
Mayer s.
McBratney aspirating s.
McHugh oval s.
McKee s.
McKinney eye s.
McLaughlin s.
McPherson eye s.
Mellinger-Axenfeld eye s.
Mellinger eye s.
Mellinger fenestrated blades s.
Merz-Vienna nasal s.
Metcher eye s.
Miller vaginal s.
Milligan s.
Montgomery-Bernstine s.
Montgomery vaginal s.
Moria one-piece s.
Mosher nasal s.
Mosher urethral s.
Moynihan s.
Mueller eye s.
Muir rectal s.
Murdock eye s.
Murdock-Wiener eye s.
Murdoon eye s.
Myles nasal s.
Myles-Ray s.
nasal bivalve s.
Nasa-Spec nasal s.
nasopharyngeal s.
National ear s.
National Graves vaginal s.
Nott-Gutmann vaginal s.
Nott vaginal s.
Noyes s.
Omni-Park s.
one-hand s.
open-side vaginal s.
O'Sullivan-O'Connor vaginal s.
oval s.
Pannu-Kratz-Barraquer s.
Park eye s.
Park-Guyton-Callahan eye s.
Park-Guyton eye s.
Park-Guyton-Maumenee s.
Park-Maumenee s.
Parks anal s.
Patton septal s.
Pearce eye s.

Pederson vaginal s.
pediatric s.
pediatric lid s.
Pennington rectal s.
Picot vaginal s.
Pierse eye s.
Pilling-Hartmann s.
plain wire s.
Politzer ear s.
post-urethroplasty review s.
Pratt bivalve s.
Pratt rectal s.
Preefer eye s.
Prima Series LEEP s.
Prospec disposable s.
Proud infant turbinate s.
Pynchon nasal s.
Rappazzo s.
Ray nasal s.
rectal s.
Reipen s.
Relat vaginal s.
reversible lid s.
Rica ear s.
Rica nasal septal s.
Rica vaginal s.
Richard Gruber s.
Richnau-Holmgren ear s.
Roberts esophageal s.
Roberts oval s.
Rosenthal urethral s.
round s.
Sani-Spec vaginal s.
Sato s.
Sauer eye s.
Sauer infant eye s.
Saunders eye s.
Sawyer rectal s.
Schweizer s.
Scott ear s.
Semb vaginal s.
Senturia pharyngeal s.
Serdarevic s.
Seyfert vaginal s.
Shea s.
shoehorn s.
Siegle ear s.
Simcoe-Barraquer eye s.
Simcoe eye s.
Simcoe wire s.
Simmonds vaginal s.
Simrock s.
Sims double-ended vaginal s.
Sims rectal s.
Sims vaginal s.
Sisson-Cottle s.
Sisson-Vienna s.
Sluder sphenoidal s.
SMIC ear s.
SMIC nasal septal s.
Smirmaul eyelid s.
Smith anal s.
Smith-Buie rectal s.
Smith eye s.
Sonnenschein nasal s.

S

speculum *(continued)*
  stapes s.
  Stearnes s.
  Steiner-Auvard s.
  Stop eye s.
  Storz nasal s.
  Storz septal s.
  Storz-Vienna nasal s.
  Sutherland-Grieshaber s.
  Sweeney posterior vaginal s.
  Swiss-pattern s.
  Swolin self-retaining vaginal s.
  Tauber s.
  Taylor vaginal s.
  Terson s.
  Thornton open-wire lid s.
  Thudichum nasal s.
  Tieck-Halle infant nasal s.
  Tieck nasal s.
  Torchia eye s.
  Toynbee ear s.
  transsphenoidal s.
  Trelat vaginal s.
  Troeltsch ear s.
  Turner-Warwick post-urethroplasty
    review s.
  Ullrich vaginal s.
  Universal s.
  vaginal s.
  Vaginard metal s.
  Vauban s.
  Verner s.
  Verner-Kalinowski s.
  Vernon-David rectal s.
  Vienna Britetrac nasal s.
  Voltolini nasal s.
  Vu-Max vaginal s.
  Watson s.
  Weeks eye s.
  weighted vaginal s.
  Weiner s.
  Weisman-Graves open-sided
    vaginal s.
  Weiss s.
  Weissbarth vaginal s.
  Welch Allyn illuminated s.
  Welch Allyn KleenSpec vaginal s.
  Wellington Hospital vaginal s.
  Wiener eye s.
  Williams eye s.
  Wilson-Kirbe s.
  wire bivalve vaginal s.
  wire lid s.
  Worcester City Hospital s.
  Yankauer nasopharyngeal s.
  Ziegler eye s.
  Zower s.
  Zylik-Michaels s.
Speed
  S. brace
  S. hand splint
  S. Lok soft stent
  S. osteotomy graft
  S. radius cap prosthesis

Speedband
  S. ligature
  S. multiple band ligator
Speed-E-Rim denture bite block
Speedi-Pak sinus pack
SpeedReducer instrument
Speed-Sprague knife
Speedy-1 Auto refractometer
Speedy balloon catheter
Speer
  S. periosteotome
  S. suture hook
Spelcast car seat
Spembly cryoprobe
Spence
  S. cranioplastic roller
  S. intervertebral disk rongeur
  S. rongeur forceps
Spence-Adson forceps
Spencer
  S. biopsy forceps
  S. cannula
  S. chalazion forceps
  S. eye suture scissors
  S. incontinence device
  S. labyrinth exploration probe
  S. oval punch
  S. oval tip
  S. plication forceps
  S. probe depth electrode
  S. stitch scissors
  S. trachelotome
  S. triangular adenoid punch
  S. triangular tip
  S. Universal adenoid punch tip
Spencer-Wells
  S.-W. arterial forceps
  S.-W. chalazion forceps
Spenco
  S. arch support
  S. boot
  S. external breast form
  S. insole
  S. orthotic device
  S. top cover
Sperma-Tex preshaped mesh
Sperm Select sperm recovery system
Spero meibomian forceps
Spetzler
  S. clip applier
  S. dissector
  S. forceps
  S. lumbar-peritoneal shunt
  S. MacroVac surgical suction device
  S. MicroVac suction tube
  S. needle holder
  S. scissors
  S. subarachnoid catheter
  S. titanium aneurysm clip
SpF spinal fusion stimulator
SpF-XL stimulator
sphenoidal
  s. bone punch
  s. bur
  s. cannula

s. probe
s. punch forceps
sphenopalatine ganglion needle
sphere
 AccuPoint targeting s.
 American Heyer-Schulte s.
 Carter s.
 Doherty s.
 s. introducer
 Mules vitreous s.
 porous hydroxyapatite s.
 Pyrex eye s.
 resin s.
 Silastic s.
 silicone eye s.
spherical
 s. bur
 s. eye implant
spherocentric knee prosthesis
spherocylinder
spherocylindrical lens
Sphero Flex implant
sphincter
 AMD artificial urinary s.
 American Medical Systems
  urethral s.
 AMS 800 artificial urethral s.
 artificial s.
 AS-800 artificial s.
 s. dilator
 double-cuff urinary s.
 Hydroflex s.
 servo-mechanism s.
sphincteroscope
 Kelly s.
sphincterotome
 Bitome bipolar s.
 Cotton s.
 Cremer-Ikeda s.
 Doubilet s.
 double-channel s.
 ERCP s.
 Fluorotome double-lumen s.
 Frimberger-Karpiel 12 O'Clock s.
 Howell rotatable BII s.
 Huibregtse-Katon s.
 Koch-Julian s.
 long-nosed s.
 needle-tipped s.
 open s.
 shark fin s.
 single-channel wire-guided s.
 Ultratome double-lumen s.
 Ultratome XL triple-lumen s.
 Wilson-Cook double-channel s.
 Wilson-Cook wire-guided s.
 wire-guided s.
 Zimmon s.
sphincterotomy basket
sphygmomanometer
 s. cuff
 Erlanger s.
 Faught s.
 Hader aneroid s.
 Hawksley random zero mercury s.

Janeway s.
Mosso s.
Physio-Control Lifestat s.
random-zero s.
Riva Rocci s.
Rogers s.
sphygmometer
 Honan s.
sphygmoscope
 Bishop s.
SPI-Argent II peritoneal dialysis catheter
spica
 s. bandage
 s. cast
 s. dressing
 s. splint
 s. table
spicule forceps
Spiegel-Wycis
 S.-W. human apparatus
 S.-W. stereoencephalotome
Spielberg
 S. dilator
 S. sinus cannula
Spies ethmoidal punch
Spiesman fistular probe
Spiessel
 S. internal screw fixation
 S. lag screw
 S. position screw
Spigelman baseball finger splint
spike
 cemental s.
 Gissane s.
 Monoscopy locking trocar with
  Woodford s.
 s. retractor
 Spitzy s.
 s. staple
spiked washer
spinal
 s. arthroscope
 s. catheter
 s. cord retractor
 s. cord stimulator
 s. fusion chisel
 s. fusion curette
 s. fusion gouge
 s. needle
 s. physiotherapy simulator
 s. retractor blade
 s. rod
 s. rod cross-bracing
 s. saw
 s. slip wrench
 S. Technology bivalve TLSO brace
 s. turning frame
SpinaLase
 S. neodymium:yytrium-aluminum-
  garnet (Nd:YAG) surgical laser
  system
SpinaLogic 1000 bone growth stimulator
SpinalPak fusion stimulator
spinal-perforating forceps
SpineCATH intradiscal catheter

S

SpineLink system
Spinelli biopsy needle
Spine Power pelvic stabilizer belt
SpineScope
   Clarus S.
SpineStat side-directed diskectomy probe
Spinhaler
   S. inhaler
   S. Turbo-Inhaler
spinning
   s. disk nebulizer
   s. probe
Spinoscope noninasive imaging system
spinous
   s. process spreader
   s. process wire
spiral
   s. coil stent
   s. CT
   s. CT scanner
   s. drill
   s. electrode
   s. endosteal implant
   s. filler
   s. fluted tungsten carbide bur
   s. forceps
   S. Mark V portable ultrasonic drug
     inhaler
   s. probe
   s. reverse bandage
   s. stone dislodger
   s. trochanteric reamer
   s. vein stripper
   s. XCT scanner
SpiralGold oxygenator
spiral-tipped
   s.-t. bougie
   s.-t. catheter
spiral-wound endotracheal tube
SpiraStent stent
Spirea adjustable foldable wheelchair
Spirec drill
Spirette
   CCD S.
SpiroFlo bioabsorbable prostate stent
Spir-O-Flow peak flow monitor
Spirolyte 201 bedside spirometer
spirometer
   Barnes s.
   bedside s.
   Benedict-Roth s.
   Bennett monitoring s.
   Buhl s.
   Calculair s.
   Capnomac Ultima sidestream s.
   Cardiovit s.
   Coach incentive s.
   Collins Dry s.
   Collins Survey s.
   Collis s.
   Datex Ultima s.
   Douglas bag s.
   Eagle II survey s.
   Flash portable s.
   flow-sensing s.

   incentive s.
   Inspirx incentive s.
   KoKo s.
   Krogh apparatus s.
   low-resistance rolling seal s.
   Microloop s.
   Micro Plus s.
   Respirex incentive s.
   Satellite s.
   sidestream s.
   SP-10 s.
   Spirolyte 201 bedside s.
   Spirovit SP-1 portable s.
   Timeter pocket s.
   Tissot s.
   Tri-flow incentive s.
   Venturi s.
   Vitalograph s.
   Volurex incentive s.
   water-sealed s.
spirometry
SpiroSense
   S. flow sensor
   S. system
Spirovit
   S. SP-1 portable spirometer
Spitz-Holter
   S.-H. flushing device
   S.-H. valve
   S.-H. valve implant material
Spitzy
   S. button
   S. spike
Spivack valve
Spivey iris retractor
Spizziri cannula knife
Spizziri-Simcoe cannula
splanchnic retractor
Splashield
   Zerowet S.
splaytooth forceps
splenorenal bypass shunt
splice
   breakaway s.
spline
   Bosworth osteotomy s.
   Calcitek s.
   S. dental implant system
   Keys-Briston type s.
   Rowland-Hughes osteotomy s.
   Shirlee s.
   S. Twist microtextured titanium
     implant
splint
   abduction finger s.
   acrylic cap s.
   acrylic wafer TMJ s.
   Adam and Eve rib belt s.
   Adjusta-Wrist s.
   aeroplane s.
   Agnew s.
   Ainslie acrylic s.
   air s.
   AirFlex carpal tunnel s.
   airfoam s.

airplane s.
AliMed diabetic night s.
Alumafoam nasal s.
aluminum fence s.
aluminum finger cot s.
anchor s.
Anderson s.
angle s.
ankle-foot orthotic s.
Aquaplast s.
Asch nasal s.
Ashhurst leg s.
A-splint dental s.
Atkins nasal s.
Balkan femoral s.
ball-peen s.
banana finger extension s.
banjo s.
baseball finger s.
Basswood s.
Bavarian s.
Baylor adjustable cross s.
Baylor metatarsal s.
Bend-A-Boot foot s.
Bilson fixable-removable cross arch
  bar s.
birdcage s.
Blount s.
board s.
Body prop positioning s.
Böhler-Braun s.
Böhler wire s.
Bond arm s.
boutonniere s.
Bowlby arm s.
bracketed s.
Brady balanced suspension s.
Brant aluminum s.
bridge s.
Bridgemaster nasal s.
Brooke Army Hospital s.
Browne s.
Brown nasal s.
Buck extension s.
Buck traction s.
Budin hammertoe s.
Budin toe s.
Bunnell active hand s.
Bunnell finger extension s.
Bunnell gutter s.
Bunnell knuckle-bender s.
Bunnell outrigger s.
Bunnell reverse knuckle bender s.
Bunnell safety-pin s.
Bunny Boot foot s.
Burget nasal s.
Cabot leg s.
calibrated clubfoot s.
Camo disposable dental s.
Campbell airplane s.
Campbell traction s.
Cannon Bio-Flek nasal s.
cap s.
Capener coil s.
Capener finger s.

Carpal Lock cock-up wrist s.
Carter intranasal s.
cartilage elastic pullover kneecap s.
cast lingual s.
Cawood nasal s.
Chandler felt collar s.
Chatfield-Girdlestone s.
clubfoot s.
coaptation s.
cock-up arm s.
Colles s.
Comfy elbow s.
composite spring elastic s.
compression sleeve shin s.
compressive plastic s.
Comprifix ankle s.
Cone s.
Converse s.
copper band-acrylic s.
Cordon Colles fracture s.
Cosmolon closure for s.
counterrotational s.
Craig abduction s.
Cramer wire s.
crib s.
CTS Gripfit s.
Culley ulna s.
Curry walking s.
Darco toe alignment s.
Davis metacarpal s.
Delbet s.
Denis Browne clubfoot s.
Denis Browne hip s.
Denis Browne talipes hobble s.
Denver nasal s.
DePuy aeroplane s.
DePuy any-angle s.
DePuy coaptation s.
DePuy open-thimble s.
DePuy-Pott s.
DePuy rocking leg s.
DePuy rolled Colles s.
DeRoyal/LMB finger s.
digit s.
Digit Aid s.
DonJoy knee s.
dorsal wrist s. with outrigger
Dorsiwedge night s.
double-occlusal s.
Doyle bi-valved airway s.
Doyle Combo nasal airway s.
Doyle intranasal airway s.
Doyle Shark nasal s.
drop-foot s.
Dupuytren s.
dynamic s.
Early Fit night s.
Easton cock-up s.
Easy Access foot s.
Eggers contact s.
elastic plastic s.
elbow extension s.
elbow flexion s.
EnduraSplint s.
Engelmann thigh s.

S

splint *(continued)*
Engen palmar wrist s.
Epitrain elbow s.
Erich maxillary s.
Erich nasal s.
Extend-It finger s.
Ezeform s.
Fasplint s.
fence s.
Ferciot tip-toe s.
Fillauer night s.
finger cot s.
finger extension clockspring s.
finger flexion s.
Finger-Hugger s.
folded aluminum ear s.
fold-over finger s.
foot drop night s.
Formatray mandibular s.
Forrester head s.
four-prong finger s.
Fox clavicular s.
FracSure s.
Fractomed s.
fracture s.
Framer s.
Freedom Neutral Position S.
Freedom Omni Progressive S.
Freedom Progressive Resting S.
Freedom Sportsfit S.
Freedom Ultimate Grip S.
Freidman s.
Frejka pillow s.
Friedman s.
frog s.
frog-leg s.
Froimson s.
Fruehevald s.
full-hand s.
full-occlusal s.
functional resting position s.
Funsten supination s.
Futuro s.
gait lock s.
Gallows s.
Galveston s.
Ganley s.
Gibson s.
Gilmer dental s.
Gilmer tooth s.
Gooch s.
Goode Magne-Splint magnetic
  nasal s.
Gordon s.
Granberry s.
Gunning jaw s.
Hammond orthodontic s.
hand cock-up s.
Hare compact traction s.
Hart extension finger s.
Haynes-Griffin mandibular s.
Heel Free s.
Hexcelite sheet s.
hinged Thomas s.

HIPciser abduction s.
Hirschtick utility shoulder s.
Hodgen hip s.
Hodgen leg s.
HV NightSplint s.
HV SoftSplint s.
Ilfeld s.
indexed s.
infant abduction s.
inflatable elbow s.
Innoboot night s.
interdental s.
intermediate s.
intranasal bivalve s.
Isoprene plastic s.
Jacoby heel s.
Jelenko s.
Jet-Air s.
Joint-Jack finger s.
Jonell countertraction finger s.
Jonell thumb s.
Jones arm s.
Jones forearm s.
Jones metacarpal s.
Jones nasal s.
Jones traction s.
Joseph nasal s.
Joseph septal s.
Kanavel cock-up s.
Kazanjian nasal s.
Keller-Blake leg s.
Kenny-Howard s.
Kerr abduction s.
Keystone s.
kidney internal s.
Kingsley s.
Kirschner wire s.
Kleinert s.
Klenzak double-upright s.
knee brace s.
knee immobilizer s.
knuckle-bender s.
Lambrinudi s.
leaf s.
Levis arm s.
Lewin baseball finger s.
Lewin-Stern finger s.
Lewin-Stern thumb s.
Liberty One s.
s. liner
Link stack split s.
Link toe s.
Liston s.
live s.
long arm s.
long leg s.
long leg posterior molded s.
Love nasal s.
Lynch septal s.
Lytle metacarpal s.
MacKay nasal s.
magnet s.
Magnuson abduction humeral s.
malleable metal finger s.
Malmö hip s.

Mason s.
Mason-Allen hand s.
Mayer nasal s.
McGee s.
McIntire s.
McLeod padded clavicular s.
memory s.
metal s.
Middledorpf s.
MindSet toe s.
modified Oppenheimer s.
Mohr finger s.
Morris s.
M.S. s.
Murphy s.
Murray-Jones arm s.
Murray-Thomas arm s.
nasal s.
Neiman nasal s.
Neubeiser adjustable forearm s.
neutral position s.
New Mind Set toe s.
N'ice Stretch night s.
nose guard s.
OCL volar s.
O'Donoghue knee s.
O'Donoghue stirrup s.
O'Malley jaw fracture s.
Oppenheimer knuckle-bender s.
Oppenheimer spring wire s.
Oppenheim spring wire s.
opponens s.
Orfit s.
Ortho-last s.
Orthomedics Stretch and Heel s.
Ortho-Mold s.
orthopedic strap clavicle s.
Orthoplast isoprene s.
outrigger s.
oyster s.
padded aluminum s.
padded board s.
padded plywood s.
s. padding
palmar s.
Pavlik harness s.
Peabody s.
PF night s.
Phelps s.
Phemister s.
Phoenix outrigger s.
Pil-O-Splint wrist s.
plantar fasciitis night s.
Plastalume bulb-ended s.
Plastalume straight s.
plaster s.
plaster-of-Paris s.
Polyform s.
Polymed s.
polymethyl methacrylate ear s.
polyvinyl alcohol s.
Ponseti s.
Poroplastic s.
Porzett s.
Potts s.

Pro-glide s.
Protecto s.
Pucci s.
Puth abduction s.
Putti s.
QualCraft s.
QuickCast s.
Quik s.
radiolucent s.
Rancho Los Amigos s.
Rauchfuss sling s.
Redi-Around finger s.
replant s.
reverse Kingsley s.
reverse knuckle-bender s.
Robert Jones s.
Roger Anderson well-leg s.
Rolyan Gel Shell s.
Rosen s.
Roylan Gel Shell spica s.
Rumel aluminum bridge s.
Russell s.
safety pin s.
Safian nasal s.
sandwich-type s.
Saturn S.
Savlon s.
Sayre s.
Scott humeral s.
Scottish Rite s.
Seattle s.
Shah nasal s.
Sheffield s.
short arm plaster s.
short arm posterior molded s.
short leg s.
Simpson sugar-tong s.
skin s.
Slattery-McGrouther dynamic flexion s.
Smart S.
Softsplint foot s.
special Colles s.
Speed hand s.
spica s.
Spigelman baseball finger s.
spreading hand s.
spring cock-up s.
spring wire safety pin s.
Stack s.
Stader s.
Stax fingertip s.
Stock finger s.
Strampelli eye s.
strap clavicle s.
Stretch and Heel s.
Stromeyer s.
Stuart Gordon hand s.
Stulberg HIPciser abduction s.
sugar-tong s.
Supramead nose s.
swan-neck s.
Swanson dynamic toe s.
Swanson hand s.
synergistic wrist motion s.

S

splint *(continued)*
    Synergy s.
    talipes hobble s.
    Taylor s.
    Teare arm s.
    tennis elbow s.
    T-finger s.
    therapeutic s.
    thermoplastic s.
    Thomas full-ring s.
    Thomas hinged s.
    Thomas knee s.
    Thomas leg s.
    Thomas posterior s.
    Thomas suspension s.
    Thomas s. with Pearson attachment
    Thompson modification of Denis
      Browne s.
    ThumZ'Up functional thumb s.
    Ticonium s.
    Titus forearm s.
    Titus wrist s.
    Toad finger s.
    Tobruk s.
    Toronto s.
    torsion bar s.
    turnbuckle elbow s.
    turnbuckle functional position s.
    Ultraflex ankle dorsiflexion
      dynamic s.
    Universal support s.
    Urias pressure s.
    U-splint s.
    Valentine s.
    Van Rosen s.
    Velcro extenders s.
    Volkmann s.
    von Rosen s.
    Wertheim s.
    Winter s.
    wire s.
    Xomed Doyle nasal airway s.
    Xomed Silastic s.
    Yucca wood s.
    Zimfoam s.
    Zimmer airplane s.
    Zimmer clavicular cross s.
    Zim-Trac traction s.
    Zim-Zip rib belt s.
    Zollinger s.
    Zucker s.
splinter forceps
Splintline acrylic
Splintrex
    S. instrument
SplintsRite stabilization device
split
    s. drape
    s. overtube
    s. Russell skeletal traction
    s. screen
split-finger hook

split-sheath
    s.-s. catheter
    s.-s. introducer
splitter
    beam s.
    Brierley nucleus s.
    Goldberg side port s.
    Koch-Salz nucleus s.
    Kraff nucleus s.
    Rosato fascial s.
    Rosen phaco s.
    Ruth-Hedwig s.
    Salz nucleus s.
    Sharvelle side port s.
    Tooke angled s.
    Troutman corneal s.
    Zeiss small beam s.
split-thickness implant
splitting
    s. chisel
    s. forceps
Spli-Tube
S-P needle holder
SpO$_2$-5001 oximeter
Spondex sponge ball
spondylitic bar
spondylophyte
    s. annular dissector perforator
    s. impactor
sponge
    Accu-Sorb gauze s.
    Actifoam collagen s.
    Actifoam hemostat s.
    Alcon s.
    Bernay s.
    Bicol collagen s.
    Bohm dropper s.
    Boston gauze s.
    bronchoscopic s.
    buffing s.
    Bulkee super fluff s.
    s. carrier
    cellulose surgical s.
    cherry s.
    s. clamp
    Codman Bicol s.
    collagen s.
    Collostat s.
    cotton ball s.
    Curity cover s.
    Curity disposable laparotomy s.
    Curity gauze s.
    Custodis s.
    cylindrical s.
    DeRoyal laparotomy s.
    s. dissector
    s. ear curette
    EndoZime s.
    Excilon drain s.
    Excilon dressing s.
    Excilon IV s.
    Expandacell s.
    Fluftex gauze rolls and s.
    s. forceps
    Fuller silicone s.

Gardlok neurosurgical s.
gauze dissector s.
gauze rosebud s.
gelatin s.
s. graft
Graham Clark silicone s.
grooved silicone s.
Helistat absorbable collagen
  hemostatic s.
Heros chiropody s.
Hibbs s.
implant s.
s. implant
Incert s.
Incert bioabsorbable implantable s.
InstruWipes surgical s.
Ivalon s.
Ivalon embolic s.
Johnson gauze s.
Johnson & Johnson gauze s.
K dissector s.
Kenwood laparotomy s.
Kerlix laparotomy s.
Kerlix packing s.
Kerlix super s.
King fluff rolls & s.
Kling s.
Krukenberg s.
K-Sponge hydrocellulose s.
laminectomy wedge s.
laparotomy s.
Lapwall laparotomy s.
Lincoff lens s.
lint-free s.
LISCO s.
Masciuli silicone s.
Mediskin hemostatic s.
Medline gauze s.
Merocel s.
Microsponge Teardrop s.
Mikulicz s.
Miragel s.
Mirasorb s.
nasal tampon s.
Naso-Tamp nasal packing s.
neurological s.
nonwoven s.
Nu-Brede packing and
  debridement s.
Nu Gauze s.
ophthalmic s.
Optipore scrub s.
Optipore wound-cleaning s.
Packer tunnel silicone s.
peanut s.
Pedic s.
pledget s.
polyvinyl alcohol s.
Porolon s.
Pro-Ophtha absorbent stick s.
Protectaid contraceptive s.
radial s.
Ray-Tec x-ray detectable surgical s.
Reston s.
s. ring

Roschke dropper s.
rubber s.
Secto tonsillar s.
Silastic s.
silicone s.
s. silicone implant material
Snowflake laparotomy s.
soft silicone s.
Sof-Wick drain s.
s. stick
strip and point s.
Taka microneurosurgical s.
tonsillar s.
Topper dressing s.
tracheotomy s.
two-by-two strung s.
Vaiser s.
Venture s.
Versalon all purpose s.
Visi-Spear eye s.
Vistec x-ray detectable s.
vitrectomy s.
Weck s.
Weck-cel surgical spear s.
Wextran s.
x-ray detectable laparotomy s.

sponge-holding forceps
spongiosa bone graft
spoon
  s. anastomosis clamp
  Ballance mastoid s.
  Bunge evisceration s.
  Bunge exenteration s.
  Castroviejo lens s.
  cataract s.
  Coyne s.
  Culler lens s.
  s. curette
  Cushing pituitary s.
  Cushing spatula s.
  Cutler lens s.
  Daviel cataract s.
  Daviel lens s.
  ear s.
  Elschnig cataract s.
  Elschnig eye s.
  Elschnig lens s.
  enucleation s.
  evisceration s.
  exenteration s.
  Falk appendectomy s.
  Fisher eye s.
  s. forceps
  gallbladder s.
  Graefe cataract s.
  graft carrier s.
  Gross ear s.
  Hardy pituitary s.
  Hatt s.
  Hess lens s.
  Hiebert esophageal suture s.
  Hoke s.
  Hoke-Roberts s.
  Kalt eye s.
  Kirby intracapsular lens s.

S

spoon *(continued)*
    Knapp cataract s.
    Knapp lens s.
    Kocher brain s.
    laser-assisted intrastromal
      keratomileusis aspiration s.
    LASIK aspiration s.
    lens s.
    Lindner cyclodialysis s.
    MacNamara cataract s.
    maroon s.
    meniscal s.
    Moore gallbladder s.
    s. needle
    needle s.
    obstetrical s.
    Olivecrona brain s.
    pituitary s.
    plain ear s.
    Ray brain s.
    s. retractor
    Rizzuti graft carrier s.
    Royal s.
    Schepens s.
    Sellheim elevating s.
    Skene uterine s.
    spatula s.
    s. spatula
    spoon and spatula s.
    Turner-Warwick malleable s.
    Volkmann s.
    Wells enucleation s.
    Wills s. with spatula
    Woodson obstetrical s.
spoon-shaped forceps
S'port
    S. Max back support
    Posture S.
Sport
    S. Cord
    S. Preforms orthotic
Sportape tape
Sportelli system collimator mounted
   contact shield
Sporthotic
    Soccer S.
Sportorno cementless hip arthroplasty
   system
Sports-Caster I, II knee brace
SportsFit thumb orthosis
Sports Plus II back belt
sportstape
Sport-Stirrup orthosis
SporTX
    S. pulsed direct current stimulator
    S. stimulation device
spot
    s. face reamer
    s. retinoscope
SpotCheck+ handheld pulse oximeter
spot-compression paddle
spotlight
    examining s.
    KDC-Healthdyne nonfluorescent s.

Sprague ear curette
Spratt
    S. bone curette
    S. ear curette
    S. mastoid curette
    S. nasofrontal rasp
spray
    s. bandage
    S. Band dressing
SprayGel Adhesion Barrier system
spreader
    Assistant Free calibrated femoral-
      tibial s.
    Assistant Free calibrated femoral
      tibial s.
    Athens suture s.
    baby Inge bone s.
    baby Inge laminar s.
    Bailey rib s.
    s. bar
    Beeson cast s.
    Benson pylorus s.
    Blanco valve s.
    Blount bone s.
    Blount laminar s.
    Bobechko s.
    Bores incision s.
    Burford-Finochietto infant rib s.
    Burford-Finochietto rib s.
    Burford rib s.
    Caspar disk space s.
    Caspar vertebral body s.
    cast s.
    Cloward s.
    Cloward vertebral s.
    conjunctival s.
    Costenbader incision s.
    Cox metatarsal s.
    Davis modified Finochietto rib s.
    Davis rib s.
    DeBakey infant and child rib s.
    Doyen rib s.
    Endotec s.
    Favaloro-Morse rib s.
    Finochietto-Burford rib s.
    Finochietto rib s.
    Finochietto-Stille rib s.
    Gerbode modified Burford rib s.
    Gerbode rib s.
    Gill incision s.
    s. graft
    Gross ductus s.
    Haglund s.
    Haglund-Stille plaster s.
    Haight-Finochietto rib s.
    Haight pediatric rib s.
    Harken rib s.
    Harrington s.
    Henning cast s.
    Henning plaster s.
    Hertzler rib s.
    incision s.
    Inge laminar s.
    intervertebral s.
    Jarit three-prong cast s.

jaw s.
Kimpton vein s.
Kirschner wire s.
Kwitko conjunctival s.
lamina s.
Landolt s.
Lefferts rib s.
Leksell sternal s.
Lemmon sternal s.
Lilienthal rib s.
Lilienthal-Sauerbruch rib s.
McGuire rib s.
Medicon rib s.
Millin-Bacon bladder neck s.
Millin bladder neck s.
Miltex rib s.
Mity s.
Morris mitral valve s.
Morse sternal s.
M-Pact cast s.
Nelson rib s.
Nissen rib s.
Overholt-Finochietto rib s.
Overholt rib s.
Park rectal s.
plaster s.
Quervain rib s.
Rehbein rib s.
Reinhoff-Finochietto rib s.
Reinhoff rib s.
rib s.
Ridlon s.
root canal s.
Sauerbruch-Lillienthal rib s.
Saurex s.
Sheldon s.
spinous process s.
sternal s.
Stille plaster s.
Stille-Quervain s.
Struck s.
Suarez s.
Sweet-Burford rib s.
Sweet rib s.
Tessier s.
Texas Scottish Rite Hospital
  eyebolt s.
Theis infant rib s.
Tudor-Edwards rib s.
Tuffier rib s.
Turek spinous process s.
Turner-Warwick bladder neck s.
USA plaster s.
Ventura s.
Weinberg rib s.
Wilder band s.
Wilson rib s.
Wiltberger spinous process s.
Wölfe-Böhler plaster cast s.

spreading
  s. forceps
  s. hand splint
spring
  S. catheter
  S. catheter with Pro/Pel coating

s. clip
s. cock-up splint
coiled s.
compression s.
Gruca s.
Gruca-Weiss s.
s. hook
INSTRA-mate instrument-holding s.
internal fixation s.
S. iris scissors
Kesling tooth-spacing s.
s. loaded biopsy instrument
s. mechanism
Mershon s.
s. needle holder
s. pin
s. plate
s. retractor
s. scissors
Shuletz s.
Strach s.
Weiss s.
s. wire loop
s. wire safety pin splint
spring-assisted syringe
spring-eye needle
spring-handled
  s.-h. forceps
  s.-h. needle holder
  s.-h. scissors
spring-hook wire needle
Springlite
  S. Advantage DP
  S. G foot component
  S. II foot component
  S. lower limb prosthesis
  S. low-profile Symes II
  S. polyolefin BK cover
  S. polyurethane AK, BK conical
    cover
  S. super low-profile Symes II
  S. toe filler
spring-loaded
  s.-l. biopsy gun
  s.-l. nail
  s.-l. self-retaining retractor
  s.-l. vascular stent
spring-mounted electromagnet
spring-wire retractor
Sprint
  S. catheter
  S. Climber
  S. cross trainer
Spri Xercise board
Sprotte
  S. epidural needle
  S. spinal needle
SPR.Plus II mattress
sprue pin
SPTL-1b vascular lesion layer
SPTL vascular lesion laser
S.P. 100 transcutaneous electrical neural
  stimulator
SPTU Soviet stapler

S

spud
Alvis foreign body s.
Bahn s.
Bennett foreign body s.
Bishop-Harman s.
Corbett foreign body s.
corneal s.
curved needle s.
Davis foreign body s.
s. dissector
Dix eye s.
Dix foreign body s.
Ellis foreign body s.
Fisher s.
flat needle s.
foreign body s.
Francis knife s.
Goldstein golf club s.
golf-club s.
s. gouge
gouge s.
Gross ear s.
Hosford foreign body s.
knife s.
LaForce golf-club knife s.
Levine curetting s.
Levine foreign body s.
needle s.
s. needle
Nicati foreign body s.
O'Brien foreign body s.
Plange s.
s. tool
Walter corneal s.
Walton round gauge s.
Whittle s.
spur-crushing clamp
Spurling
S. intervertebral disk forceps
S. intervertebral disk rongeur
S. laminectomy rongeur
S. periosteal elevator
S. pituitary rongeur
S. retractor
S. rongeur forceps
S. tissue forceps
Spurling-Kerrison
S.-K. laminectomy punch
S.-K. rongeur
S.-K. rongeur forceps
Spurling-Love-Gruenwald-Cushing rongeur
Sputnik Russian razor blade
Spyrogel hydrogel wound dressing
spyrolace shoe lace
SQS-20 subcuticular skin stapler
square
S. Module Seating System
s. prism
s. specimen forceps
s. wire
square-ended
s.-e. distraction rod
s.-e. hook
square-end pliers
square-hole broach

squares of dressing
square-shaped occluder
square-tipped arterial dissector
squeeze
s. ball
s. exerciser
squeeze-handle forceps
Squeeze-Mark surgical marker
squeezer
lemon s.
Squibb
S. catheter
S. system
S. urostomy pouch
squint hook
Squire catheter
Squirt wound irrigation system
^{89}Sr bracelet
SRI automated immunoassay analyzer
SR-Isosit dental restorative material
SR-Ivocap denture material
SR-Ivolen impression material
SR-Ivoseal impression material
SR-IV Programmed Subjective refracto
^{90}Sr-loaded eye applicator
S-ROM
S-ROM acetabular cup
S-ROM femoral stem prosthesis
S-ROM hip prosthesis
S-ROM hip replacement system
S-ROM modular total knee system
S-ROM Poly-Dial insert
S-ROM proximally modular total hip system
SRR-5 digital-analogue converter
SS
SS bobbin drain tube
SS bobbin myringotomy tube
SS suture
S&S
sling and swathe
Ssabanejeu-Frank gastrostomy
S-shaped
S.-s. brain retractor
S.-s. brain spatula
S.-s. peripheral vascular clamp
S.-s. retractor
S-Soles insole
S. S. White
S. S. White clamp
S. S. White J-Notch surgical handpiece bur
S. S. White 100 K surgical handpiece bur
St.
St. Bartholomew barium catheter
St. Clair forceps
St. Clair-Thompson adenoidal cure
St. Clair-Thompson adenoidal forceps
St. Clair-Thompson adenotome
St. Clair-Thompson peritonsillar abscess forceps
St. George total elbow prosthesis
St. Jude annuloplasty ring

St. Jude bileaflet prosthetic valve
St. Jude cardiac device
St. Jude composite valve graft
St. Jude Medical bileaflet tilting-disk aortic valve
St. Jude Medical BioImplant valve
St. Jude medical heart valve hemodynamic plus series
St. Jude Medical Port-Access
St. Jude Medical prosthesis
St. Jude mitral valve prosthesis
St. Luke's double-action rongeur
St. Luke's retractor
St. Mark clamp
St. Mark pudendal electrode
St. Mark's Hospital retractor
St. Mark's lipped retractor
St. Mark's pelvis retractor
St. Martin eye forceps
St. Martin-Franceschetti cataract hook
St. Martin suturing forceps
St. Vincent tube clamp
St. Vincent tube-occluding forceps

ST3 stethoscope
Staar
S. foldable intraocular lens
S. glaucoma wick
S. implantable contact lens
S. low-diopter IOL
S. Toric IOL
S. Toric IOL lens for astigmatism
S. Toric lens

stab
s. electrode
s. needle

Stab-and-Grab screwdriver
Stabident system
Stability total hip system
stabilization plate
stabilizer
Claussen fragment s.
Cohn cardiac s.
Dynamic foot s.
foot s.
Freedom Thumb S.
Goldstein Grasp atraumatic cervical s.
Heel Hugger therapeutic heel s.
Insall-Burstein posterior s.
kneecap s.
KT1000 foot s.
Kwik Board IV and arterial line s.
Medline lateral s.
Palumbo ankle s.
Stamler corneal transplant s.
subpectoral s.

stabilizing
s. bar
s. guide pin

stabilocondylar knee prosthesis
Stabilor alloy
stab-in epicardial electrode
stable access cannula
Stablecut sawblade

Stableflex lens
Stableloc
S. Colles fracture external fixator
S. external wrist fixation system
S. II external fixator system

Stable-Lok nut
stab-wound drain
Stack
S. autoperfusion balloon
S. perfusion coronary dilatation catheter
S. retractor
S. splint

Stacke
S. gouge
S. probe

stacking cone
Stader
S. connecting rod
S. extraoral apparatus
S. pin
S. pin guide
S. splint
S. wrench

Stadie-Riggs microtome
stadiometer
Harpenden s.
Heightronic s.
Hita-Rite s.
Photonic s.

staff
fiberglass s.
piano-wire s.
Sippy esophageal dilator piano-wire s.
Turner-Warwick urethral s.
urethral s.

Sta-Fix tape
Stage
S. IV crib overlay
S. IV mattress replacement

Stage-1 single-stage dental implant system
Stagnara gouge
Stahl
S. calipers block
S. calipers plate
S. lens gauge
S. nucleus expressor
S. ophthalmic calipers

stainless
s. spatula
s. steel AO plate
s. steel balloon expandable stent
s. steel blade
s. steel clamp
s. steel crown
s. steel cup
s. steel flexible ruler
s. steel guidewire
s. steel implant
s. steel mesh
s. steel mesh stent
s. steel screw

S

stainless *(continued)*
  s. steel wire
  s. steel wire suture
StairClimber assist device
StairMaster exercise system
Stalite root canal post
Stallard
  S. blunt dissector
  S. head clamp
  S. scleral hook
  S. stricturotome
Stallard-Liegard suture
stall bar
Stallerpointe needle
Stalzner rectal scissors
Stamey
  S. dorsal vein apical retractor
  S. Malecot catheter
  S. needle
  S. open-tip ureteral catheter
Stamler
  S. corneal transplant stabilizer
  S. side-port fixation hook
Stamm
  S. bone-cutting forceps
  S. gastrostomy tube
Stammberger
  S. antral punch
  S. side-biting punch forceps
stamp
  Sklar medical breast s.
StanceGuard internal support
stand
  Brown-Roberts-Wells floor s.
  Cherf cast s.
  Contraves s.
  Grand Stand support s.
  IMP turnstile casting s.
  Keeler lightsource s.
  KINEX anatomic specimen s.
  Mayo s.
  turnstile casting s.
  Wilson-Mayo s.
standard
  s. above-elbow cast
  s. arterial forceps
  S. Care sterile urethral catheter
  s. colonoscope
  s. duodenoscope
  s. endoscopy polypectomy snare
  s. ERCP catheter
  S. E-Z-On Vest
  s. full-lumen esophagoscope
  s. head halter
  s. hook electrosurgical probe
  s. Jackson laryngoscope
  s. Lehman catheter
  s. needle
  s. pattern mallet
  s. socket
  s. wire gauge
standby pacemaker
standing frame orthosis

Stanford
  S. bioptome
  S. end-hole pigtail catheter
  S. and Wheatstone stereoscope
Stanford-Caves bioptome
Stangel
  S. fallopian tube cannula
  S. fallopian tube miniclip
  S. modified Barraquer microsurgical
    needle holder
Stange laryngoscope
Stanicor
  S. Gamma pacemaker
  S. Lambda demand pacemaker
Stankiewicz iris clip intraocular lens
Stanmore
  S. shoulder arthroplasty
  S. shoulder prosthesis
  S. total knee
Stanton cautery clamp
Stanzel needle holder
Staodyne EMS+2 neurostimulator
Staodyn Insight point locator
stapedectomy
  s. footplate pick
  s. forceps
  s. knife
  s. prosthesis
STA-peg
  Smith S.-p.
STA-Pen writer pen
stapes
  s. chisel
  s. curette
  s. dilator
  s. elevator
  s. excavator
  s. forceps
  s. hoe
  s. hook
  s. needle
  s. pick
  s. speculum
Staph-Chek pad
staphylorrhaphy
  s. elevator
  s. needle
staple
  barbed Richards s.
  bioabsorbable s.
  Blount epiphyseal s.
  Blount fracture s.
  s. bone plate
  Bostick s.
  DePalma s.
  duToit shoulder s.
  Ellison fixation s.
  Fastlok implantable s.
  five-pin s.
  s. forceps
  GIA s.
  Hernandez-Ros bone s.
  Krackow HTO blade s.
  Lactomer absorbable subcuticular
    skin s.

meniscal s.
metallic s.
Nakayama s.
orthopedic s.
Polysorb absorbable s.
Richards fixation s.
seven-pin s.
skin s.
Smith & Nephew medium
  barbed s.
Smith & Nephew small barbed s.
spike s.
stone s.
TA metallic s.
TA Premium-series s.
titanium mandibular s.
Wiberg fracture s.
Zimaloy epiphyseal s.

stapler
American vascular s.
Appose skin s.
arcuate skin s.
Auto Suture Multifire Endo GIA
  30 s.
Auto Suture Premium CEEA s.
Auto Suture surgical s.
barbed s.
CDH s.
CEEA s.
circular intraluminal s.
circular mechanical s.
Concorde disposable skin s.
copolymer s.
Coventry s.
Cricket disposable skin s.
curved intraluminal s.
Day s.
disposable intraluminal s.
Downing s.
duToit s.
Dwyer spinal mechanical s.
EEA Auto Suture s.
end-end s.
Endo Babcock s.
Endo GIA s.
Endo Hernia s.
Endopath EMS hernia s.
Endopath endoscopic articulating s.
Endopath ES endoscopic s.
Endopath Stealth s.
Ethicon Endosurgery circular s.
gastroplasty s.
Graftac-S skin s.
Hall double-hole spinal s.
hernia s.
ILA s.
Imagyn surgical s.
Inokucki vascular s.
intraluminal s.
Lactomer copolymer absorbable s.
ligating and dividing s.
linear s.
Multifire GIA-series s.
Multifire TA-series s.
Nakayama microvascular s.

Ni-Ti Shape Memory alloy
  compression s.
One-Time disposable skin s.
Oswestry-O'Brien spinal s.
PC EEA s.
PI disposable s.
PKS-25 apparatus s.
Polysorb 55 s.
Precise disposable skin s.
Premium CEEA circular s.
Premium Plus CEEA disposable s.
Premium Poly CS-57 s.
Proximate disposable skin s.
Proximate flexible linear s.
Proximate-ILS curved intraluminal s.
PSS Powered disposable skin s.
Reflex skin s.
Roticulator s.
Royal disposable skin s.
SDsorb meniscal s.
SGIA 50 disposable s.
Signet disposable skin s.
Soviet mechanical bronchial s.
SPTU Soviet s.
SQS-20 subcuticular skin s.
STI-1 needle-shaped tissue s.
Surgeons Choice surgical s.
Surgiport s.
TA 55 s.
thoracoabdominal (TA) 55 s.
TL-90 s.
UG-70 s.
United States Surgical circular s.
UPO-16 s.
Versatack s.
Vista disposable skin s.
Vital skin s.
Vogelfanger-Beattie s.
Vogelfanger blood vessel s.
Wiberg fracture s.
Yamagishi s.

Staples osteotomy nail
stapling device
Star
  S. Optica hearing aid
  S. S2 SmoothScan excimer laser
    system
  S. ventilator
  S. X carbon dioxide laser
Starcam camera
starch bandage
starch-based copolymer dressing
Starck dilator
Stargate falloposcopy catheter
Starkey
  S. hearing aid
  S. stethoscope
Stark vulsellum forceps
Starlinger uterine dilator
Starlite
  S. endodontic implant starter kit
  S. Omni-AT bur
  S. point
STAR-LOCK Press-Fit cylinder implant
StarMed video otoscope

Starr
S. ball heart prosthesis
S. ball heart valve
S. fixation forceps
S. Surgical polyimide loop
   intraocular lens
Starr-Edwards
S.-E. aortic valve prosthesis
S.-E. ball-cage valve
S.-E. ball valve prosthesis
S.-E. cloth-covered metallic ball
   heart valve
S.-E. heart valve
S.-E. hermetically-sealed pacemaker
S.-E. mitral prosthesis
S.-E. pacemaker
S.-E. prosthetic aortic valve
S.-E. prosthetic mitral valve
S.-E. Silastic valve
S.-E. silicone rubber ball valve
Starrett pin vise
STARRT falloposcopy system
Startanius blade implant
starter
s. awl
s. broach
Ritchey nail s.
Ritchie nail s.
Star/Vent one-stage dental screw implant
Stat
S. aspirator
S. 2 Pumpette
S. 2 Pumpette disposable IV pump
S. Scrub handwasher machine
Statak
S. anchor system
S. soft tissue attachment device
S. suture anchor
Statham
S. cautery
S. electromagnetic flow meter
S. external transducer
S. flowmeter
static
s. air mattress
s. gray scale ultrasound equipment
s. sling
s. topical occlusive hemostatic
   pressure device
stationary
s. angle guide
s. ankle flexible endoskeleton
Sta-tite
S.-t. 2ply elastic roll gauze
Sta-Tite gauze dressing
StatLock-Foley catheter
Stat-padz defibrillator patch
Stat-Temp
S.-T. II liquid crystal temperature
   monitor
S.-T. II temperature device
Stat-Trace electrode
Status-X machine

Staude
S. tenaculum forceps
S. uterine tenaculum
Staude-Jackson
S.-J. tenaculum forceps
S.-J. uterine tenaculum
Staude-Moore
S.-M. uterine tenaculum
S.-M. uterine tenaculum forceps
Stavis fixation forceps
Stax
S. fingertip splint
Stayce adjustable clamp
Stay-Erec system
Stayoden 9000F TENS unit
Stay-Rite clamp
StaySharp face lift Super-Cut scissors
stay suture retractor
STC 900-series travel chair
STD+ titanium total hip prosthesis
Stealth
S. angioplasty balloon catheter
S. catheter balloon
S. DBO diamond blade
S. DBO free-hand diamond knife
S. frame
StealthStation
S. image-guided system
S. image-interactive system
S. treatment guidance platform
steam
s. box
s. tent
steam-shaping mandrel
Stearnes speculum
Stecher
S. arachnoid knife
S. microruler
Stedman
S. awl
S. continuous suction tube
S. saw
S. suction pump aspirator
steel
s. embolization coil
s. mesh suture
s. ruler
Steele
S. articulator
S. bronchial dilator
S. fiberoptic system
S. filling instrument
S. periosteal elevator
S. scaler
steel-slotted plastic bracket
steel-winged butterfly needle
Steeper powered Gripper
steerable
s. angioplastic guidewire
s. decapolar electrode catheter
s. guidewire catheter
s. guide wire system
steering catheter
Steerocath catheter
Steers replicator

Steffee
  S. pedicle plate
  S. pedicle screw-plate system
  S. screw plate
  S. spinal instrumentation
  S. variable spine plating system
Steffensmeier board
Steigmann-Goff endoscopic ligature
  overtube
Steinbach mallet
Steiner
  S. bracket
  S. electromechanical morcellator
Steiner-Auvard
  S.-A. speculum
  S.-A. vaginal retractor
Steinert
  S. double-ended claw chopper
  S. laser-assisted intrastromal
    keratomileusis set
Steinert-Deacon incision gauge
Steinhauser
  S. bone clamp
  S. electromucotome
  S. internal screw fixation
  S. lag screw
  S. orotome
  S. plate
  S. position screw
Steinhauser-Castroviejo electromucotome
Steinmann
  S. calibrated pin
  S. extension bow
  S. extension nail
  S. fixation pin
  S. holder
  S. intestinal forceps
  S. pin chuck
  S. tendon forceps
  S. traction
  S. traction tractor
Stein membrane perforator
Steis bone marrow transplant needle
Stela electrode lead
Steldent alloy
Stellbrink
  S. fixation device
  S. synovectomy rongeur
Stellite
  S. ball-cage heart valve
  S. ring material
  S. ring material of prosthetic valve
stem
  APF Moore-type femoral s.
  APR I femoral s.
  autologous s.
  Bio-Groove s.
  Biomet hip s.
  calcar replacement s.
  s. cell concentrator
  Cementless Sportorno hip
    arthroplasty s.
  collarless s.
  contoured femoral s. (CFS)
  Corail HA-coated s.

Deon s.
Extend s.
s. extractor
femoral s.
fenestrated Moore-type femoral s.
F2L Multineck femoral s.
Howmedica hip fracture s.
hydroxyapatite-coated s.
Iowa s.
Kirschner II-C shoulder system s.
KMP fenestrated femoral s.
Linear hip s.
Link microporous hip s.
MAPF (textured surface) femoral s.
modular calcar replacement s.
Moore hip endoprosthesis system s.
Morse taper s.
Natural-Hip titanium hip s.
nonfenestrated Moore-type femoral s.
Omnifit HA hip s.
Osteonics Omnifit-HA hip s.
PCA total hip s.
Perfecta femoral s.
s. pessary
Precident s.
Precision Osteolock s.
Press-Fit s.
Profix metaphyseal tibial s.
quadrature surface coil system s.
Ranawat-Burstein porous s.
rectal snare insulated s.
ReVision hip s.
RIGS system s.
SL-Plus s.
s. spoon separator
Strata hip system s.
Taperloc femoral s.
TC femoral s.
VS femoral s.
stemmed tibial prosthesis
Stemp clamp
stencil
  Etch-Master electronic s.
stenopaic goggles
Stenosimeter
stenosis clamp
Stenstrom
  S. nerve holder
  S. rasp
  S. raspatory
stent
  absorbable s.
  ACS Multi-Link Duet coronary s.
  ACS Multi-Link Tristar coronary s.
  ACS RX multilink s.
  activated balloon expandable
    intravascular s.
  ACT-one coronary s.
  adherent s.
  adjustable vaginal s.
  American Heyer-Schulte s.
  Amsterdam biliary s.
  AMS urethral s.
  Anastaflo s.
  AngioStent s.

S

stent *(continued)*
antegrade internal s.
antegrade ureteral s.
antibiotic-coated s.
Atkinson tube s.
AVE GFX coronary s.
AVE Micro s.
bailout s.
balloon-expandable flexible coil s.
balloon-expandable intravascular s.
balloon-expandable metallic s.
Bard coil s.
Bardex s.
Bard soft double-pigtail s.
Bard XT coronary s.
Beamer s.
beStent balloon-expandable s.
beStent 2 coronary s.
biliary s.
bioabsorbable double-spiral s.
biodegradable s.
BioDivYsio s.
Black Beauty ureteral s.
Braun s.
Bx Velocity coronary artery s.
Carcon s.
CardioCoil coronary s.
CardioCoil self-expanding
coronary s.
Carey-Coons soft s.
carotid s.
CarotidCoil s.
Carpentier s.
Carson internal/external
endopyelotomy s.
cell-seeded s.
C-Flex Amsterdam s.
C-Flex ureteral s.
coil vascular s.
composite polymer s.
Conley tracheal s.
conventional s.
Cook FlexStent s.
Cook intracoronary s.
Cook ureteral s.
Cook Urosoft s.
Cordis Crossflex s.
Cordis radiopaque tantalum s.
Corvita s.
Cotton-Huibregtse double pigtail s.
Cotton-Leung biliary s.
covered Gianturco s.
Cragg s.
CrossFlex coil s.
CrossFlex LC coronary artery s.
Crown s.
s. cutter
Cysto Flex s.
Dacron s.
Dacron-covered s.
Dart coronary s.
Devon-Pura s.
diversion s.
Dobbhoff biliary s.

double-J dangle s.
double-J indwelling catheter s.
double-J silicone internal ureteral
catheter s.
double-J ureteral s.
double-pigtail s.
Doyle II silicone s.
s. dressing
drug-coated s.
Duet coronary s.
Dumon silicone s.
Dumon tracheobronchial s.
Dynamic Y s.
Elastalloy esophageal s.
Elastalloy Ultraflex Strecker
nitinol s.
Eliminator biliary s.
Eliminator pancreatic s.
eluting s.
endobiliary s.
EndoCoil biliary s.
EndoCoil esophageal s.
endoesophageal s.
endoluminal s.
endovascular s.
Entract s.
EsophaCoil biliary s.
EsophaCoil self-expanding
esophageal s.
esophageal Strecker s.
Esophageal Z-Stent s.
expandable esophageal s.
expandable intrahepatic portacaval
shunt s.
expandable metallic s.
expulsion s.
Fader Tip ureteral s.
fibrin film s.
flat wire coil s.
Flex s.
Flexima biliary s.
FlexStent s.
foam rubber vaginal s.
FocalSeal-R neurosurgical s.
Freedom s.
free-standing s.
Freitag s.
French s.
s. funnel
gauze s.
Geenan pancreatic s.
gelatin-covered mesh s.
gfx coronary s.
Gianturco expandable metallic
biliary s.
Gianturco expanding metallic s.
Gianturco metal urethral s.
Gianturco-Rosch self-expandable
biliary Z s.
Gianturco-Roubin flexible coil s.
Gianturco-Roubin FlexStent
coronary s.
Gianturco zigzag s.
Gibbon indwelling ureteral s.
Global Therapeutics Freedom s.

Global Therapeutics V-Flex s.
Guidant s.
hand-crimped s.
hand-mounted s.
heat-expandable s.
helical coil s.
helical-ridged ureteral s.
Hepamed-coated Wiktor s.
heparin-coated Palmaz-Schatz s.
Hood stoma s.
Hood-Westaby T-Y s.
Huibregtse biliary s.
Hydromer coated polyurethane s.
HydroPlus s.
iliac artery s.
indwelling ureteral s.
InStent CarotidCoil s.
interdigitating coil s.
intracoronary s.
intraoral s.
Intra-Prostatic s.
intravascular s.
s. introducer
INX s.
iridium-192 s.
J-s.
s. jail
Jasin Frontal Ostent s.
JJIS s.
J-Maxx s.
Johnson & Johnson biliary s.
Johnson & Johnson coronary s.
Jomed s.
JoStent coronary s.
Kaminsky s.
keel s.
kidney internal s.
kissing s.
lacrimal s.
laryngeal s.
lighted s.
Lubri-Flex ureteral s.
Lubri-Flex urologic s.
luminal s.
Magic-Wall s.
magnetic internal ureteral s.
main pancreatic duct s.
Mardis soft s.
Medinol NIRside slotted s.
Medivent self-expanding coronary s.
Medivent vascular s.
Medtronic AVE S660 coronary s.
Medtronic Bestent s.
Medtronic interventional vascular s.
MegaLink biliary s.
Memotherm colorectal s.
Memotherm Flexx biliary s.
Mentor biliary s.
Merogel s.
mesh s.
metal-augmented polymer s.
metal-coated s.
metallic s.
Metal Z s.
methyl methacrylate ear s.

Micro S. II
Microvasive s.
Montgomery laryngeal s.
MPD s.
multicellular s.
Multi-Flex s.
Multilink s.
Navius s.
Neville s.
NexStent carotid s.
NIR ON Ranger balloon
  expandable s.
NIROYAL Advance balloon
  expandable s.
NIR Primo balloon expandable s.
NIRstent s.
NIR with SOX over-the-wire
  coronary s.
nitinol mesh s.
nitinol self-expanding coil s.
nitinol subglottic stenosis s.
nitinol thermal memory s.
Novastent s.
OmniStent s.
Orlowski s.
Ossoff-Sisson surgical s.
osteomeatal s.
Palmaz arterial s.
Palmaz balloon-expandable iliac s.
Palmaz biliary s.
Palmaz Corinthian transhepatic
  biliary s.
Palmaz-Schatz balloon-expandable s.
Palmaz-Schatz biliary s.
Palmaz-Schatz coronary s.
Palmaz-Schatz Crown balloon-
  expandable s.
Palmaz vascular s.
pancreatic duct s.
Paragon Champion s.
Paragon coronary s.
Paragon nitinol s.
Passager s.
patent s.
Percuflex Amsterdam s.
Percuflex biliary s.
Percuflex endopyelotomy s.
Percuflex flexible biliary s.
Percuflex Plus ureteral s.
percutaneous ureteral s.
Perflex stainless steel stent and
  delivery system bilary s.
piano-style guidewire s.
pigtail biliary s.
plastic s.
polyethylene s.
polymer-coated, drug-eluting s.
polymeric endoluminal paving s.
polytetraflouroethylene-covered s.
polyurethane s.
porous metallic s.
PowerGrip s.
premounted s.
ProstaCoil self-expanding s.
Prostakath urethral s.

S

stent *(continued)*
prostatic s.
PTFE-covered Palmaz s.
Pura-Vario s.
radioactive s.
radioisotope s.
radiopaque nitinol s.
radiopaque tantalum s.
Radius self-expanding s.
Reliance urinary control s.
renovascular s.
Retromax endopyelotomy s.
ring biliary s.
rolled Instat s.
Roubin-Gianturco flexible coil s.
Rusch s.
Salman FES s.
Schatz-Palmaz tubular mesh s.
Schneider s.
self-expandable metallic s.
self-expanding coil s.
self-expanding metallic s.
self-expanding stainless steel s.
self-retaining coil s.
shape memory alloy s.
Shikani middle meatal antrostomy s.
Siegel s.
Silastic indwelling ureteral s.
silicone-coated, metallic self-
  expanding s.
Silitek ureteral s.
Silitek Uropass s.
silver-coated s.
single-J urinary diversion s.
single pigtail s.
SinuSpacer turbinate s.
slotted tube articulated s.
S.M.A.R.T. bile duct s.
S.M.A.R.T. biliary s.
SoloPass Percuflex biliary s.
Song s.
Speed Lok soft s.
spiral coil s.
SpiraStent s.
SpiroFlo bioabsorbable prostate s.
spring-loaded vascular s.
stainless steel balloon expandable s.
stainless steel mesh s.
straight s.
Strecker balloon-expandable s.
Strecker coronary s.
Strecker esophageal s.
Strecker tantalum s.
s. strut
Supramid occluding s.
Surgitek Double-J II closed-tip
  ureteral s.
Surgitek Quadra-Coil ureteral s.
Surgitek Tractfinder ureteral s.
Surgitek Uropass s.
Symphony s.
synthetic s.
tandem s.
Tannenbaum s.

tantalum balloon-expandable s.
tantalum-wire s.
Tenax coronary s.
Tensum coronary s.
thermal memory s.
thermoexpandable s.
thermoplastic s.
Titan s.
titanium urethral s.
Tower s.
transhepatic biliary s.
transpapillary cystopancreatic s.
Trimble suture s.
T-tube s.
tubular slotted s.
T-Y s.
Ultraflex Microvasive s.
Ultraflex nitinol expandable
  esophageal s.
Ultraflex self-expanding s.
uncoated mesh s.
Universal s.
ureteral s.
UroCoil self-expanding s.
Uro-Guide s.
Urolume urethral s.
Urosoft s.
Urospiral urethral s.
U-tube s.
vaginal s.
Vantec urinary s.
VascuCoil peripheral vascular s.
vein-coated s.
vein graft stenting s.
Velocity s.
s. and vent system
Vistaflex balloon expandable,
  platinum alloy biliary s.
Wallstent spring-loaded s.
whistle s.
Wiktor balloon-expandable
  coronary s.
Wiktor GX coronary s.
Wilson-Cook French s.
wire-mesh self-expandable s.
Z s.
zigzag s.
Zimmon biliary s.

stented
s. bioprosthetic valve
s. homografts heart valve

stenting catheter

stentless
s. porcine aortic valve
s. porcine aortic valve prosthesis

stent-mounted
s.-m. allograft valve
s.-m. heterograft valve

Stenzel
S. fracture rod
S. rod prosthesis

step
S. device
s. drill
S. laparoscopic entry system

S. laparoscopic trocar
s. screw
step-down
s.-d. cannula
s.-d. drill
s.-d. transformer
Stephen-Slater valve
Stephenson needle holder
Stephens soft IOL-inserting forceps
Stepita meatal clamp
Step-Knife diamond blade knife
stepped-down cautery
stepper
NuStep total body recumbent s.
Stepty P hemostasis bandage
step-up transformer
Stereo
stereo
s. campimeter
stereoencephalotome
Spiegel-Wycis s.
StereoGuide
S. breast biopsy equipment
S. collimator
LORAD S.
S. needle
S. stereotactic breast biopsy system
stereolithography cage
stereomicroscope
Zeiss OPMI-6 surgical s.
stereoscope
Krumeich s.
Stanford and Wheatstone s.
stereoscopic microscope
stereotactic (*See also* stereotaxic)
s. atlas
s. breast biopsy needle
s. head frame
s. instrumentation
s. localization frame
s. retractor
stereotactic-assisted radiation therapy kit
stereotaxic (*See also* stereotactic)
s. device
s. instrument
s. laser
Stereotaxis magnetic surgery system
Steri-Band bandage
SteriCam Endoscopic camera
Stericare
S. copolymer absorbent dressing
S. glycerin hydrogel
S. hydrogel gauze dressing
Steri-Cath catheter
Steri-Clamp
IMP S.-C.
Innovative Medical Products S.-C.
Steri-Cuff
S.-C. disposable tourniquet cuff
S.-C. Plus
Steri-Dent dry heat sterilizer
Steri-Drape drape
Steriflex-Braun bacterial filter
Steriking sterilization system

sterile
s. adhesive bubble dressing
s. compression dressing
s. drape
s. dry dressing
s. electrodermatome blade
s. field barrier
s. forceps holder
s. isolation bag
s. sheet
s. stockinette
s. transverse rod
sterilizer
Anprolene s.
autoclave s.
Bard s.
s. box
Dry-Therm s.
Esquire dental s.
glass bead s.
Harvey vapor s.
hot salt s.
Steri-Dent dry heat s.
Stermatic s.
Wallach Bio-Tool s.
sterilizing
s. basket
s. forceps
Steri-Oss
S.-O. dental implant device
S.-O. endosteal dental implant
S.-O. implant system
Steri-Pad gauze pad
Steri-Probe explorer
Steris automatic reprocessor
Steriseal disposable cannula
Steri-Sleeve sleeve
Steri-Strips bandage
Steri-Strip skin closure
Steritapes closure
Steritek ICP mini monitor
Steri-Vac drain
Sterling iris spatula
Sterling-Spring orthodontic wire
Sterling-Sylva irrigator
Stermatic sterilizer
Sterna-Band self-locking suture
sternal
s. approximator
s. clip
s. knife
s. needle holder
s. notch stethoscope
s. perforating awl
s. punch forceps
s. puncture needle
s. retractor
s. retractor blade
s. saw
s. shears
s. spreader
s. wire suture
Stern-Castroviejo
S.-C. locking forceps
S.-C. suturing forceps

S

Stern dental attachment
Stern-McCarthry panendoscope
Stern-McCarthy
    S.-M. electrode
    S.-M. electrotome
    S.-M. electrotome resectoscope
sternooccipital-mandibular immobilization
    orthosis
sterno-occipital-mandibular immobilizer
    brace (SOMI brace)
sternooccipitomanubrial immobilizer
sternotome
sternotomy retractor
sternum-perforating awl
sternum saw
SteroGuide
    Lorad S.
steroid eluting electrode
Ster-O$_2$-Mist ultrasonic cup
Sterrad sterilization system
Stertzer brachial guiding catheter
Stertzer-Myler extension wire
StethoDop
    Imex S.
stethoscope
    Acoustascope esophageal s.
    Allen fetal s.
    Andries s.
    Argyle esophageal s.
    Boston s.
    Cammann s.
    Cardiocare s.
    Cardiology II s.
    Classic II s.
    DeLee fetal s.
    DeLee-Hillis fetal s.
    Doppler fetal s.
    Doppler ultrasound s.
    Doptone fetal s.
    electronic s.
    electronic-amplified s.
    E-Scope electronic s.
    esophageal s.
    fetal s.
    First Beat ultrasound s.
    Harvey Elite s.
    Hillis fetal s.
    Labtron s.
    Leff s.
    Littmann Master Classic II s.
    MedaSonics ultrasound BF4A,
      BF5A s.
    oral esophageal s.
    pacing esophageal s.
    Pinard fetal s.
    Pocket-Dop fetal s.
    precordial s.
    Rappaport-Sprague s.
    Rusch esophageal s.
    Spectrum s.
    ST3 s.
    Starkey s.
    sternal notch s.
    Tapscope esophageal pacing s.
    ultrasound s.

Stetten
    S. intestinal clamp
    S. spur crusher
Stevens
    S. eye scissors
    S. fixation forceps
    S. iris forceps
    S. lacrimal retractor
    S. muscle hook
    S. muscle hook retractor
    S. needle holder
    S. stitch scissors
    S. tenotomy hook
    S. tenotomy scissors
Stevens-Charles sleeve
Stevenson
    S. alligator forceps
    S. alligator scissors
    S. capsular punch
    S. clamp
    S. cupped-jaw forceps
    S. grasping forceps
    S. lacrimal sac retractor
    S. microsurgical forceps
    S. needle holder
    S. refractor
Stevenson-LaForce adenotome
Stevens-Street elbow prosthesis
Stewart
    S. cartilage knife
    S. cruciate ligament guide
    S. crypt hook
    S. lenticular nuclear snare
    S. rectal hook
STI-1 needle-shaped tissue stapler
Stichs wound clip
stick
    bite s.
    dextrose s.
    Disstik dissection s.
    dressing s.
    FMS Intracell s.
    Grafco seizure s.
    Intracell Sprinter s.
    lollipop s.
    percutaneous s.
    Pro-Ophtha s.
    sponge s.
    switching s.
"stick-and-carrot" appliance
stick-on electrode
Stiegler unipolar nasal snare
Stieglitz splinter forceps
Stiegmann-Goff Clearvue endoscopic
    ligator
Stierlen lens loop
Stifcore transbronchial aspiration needle
stiffening wire
Stik-Temp thermometer
stiletto
    Berkeley Bioengineering s.
    Blair s.
    s. knife
    s. ureteroscope

Stilith implantable cardiac pulse generator
Stille
  S. bone biter
  S. bone chisel
  S. bone drill
  S. bone drill set
  S. bone gouge
  S. bone rongeur
  S. brace
  S. bur
  S. cast cutter
  S. cheek retractor
  S. coarctation hook
  S. conchotome
  S. cranial drill
  S. dissecting scissors
  S. flat pliers
  S. gallstone forceps
  S. Gigli-saw guide
  S. hand drill
  S. heart retractor
  S. insufflator
  S. kidney clamp
  S. kidney forceps
  S. laryngeal applicator
  S. mallet
  S. osteotome
  S. periosteal elevator
  S. plaster shears
  S. plaster spreader
  S. rongeur forceps
  S. Super Cut scissors
  S. tissue forceps
  S. trephine
  S. uterine dilator
  S. vessel clamp
  S. wrench
Stille-Adson forceps
Stille-Aesculap plaster shears
Stille-Babcock forceps
Stille-Bailey-Senning rib contractor
Stille-Barraya
  S.-B. intestinal forceps
  S.-B. vascular forceps
Stille-Beyer rongeur
Stille-Björk forceps
Stille-Broback knee retractor
Stille-Crafoord
  S.-C. forceps
  S.-C. raspatory
Stille-Crawford coarctation clamp
Stille-Crile forceps
Stille-Doyen raspatory
Stille-Edwards raspatory
Stille-Ericksson rib shears
Stille-French cardiovascular needle holder
Stille-Giertz shears
Stille-Gigli wire saw
Stille-Halsted forceps
Stille-Horsley
  S.-H. bone-cutting forceps
  S.-H. rib forceps
  S.-H. rongeur
  S.-H. shears

Stille-Langenbeck elevator
Stille-Leksell rongeur
Stille-Liston
  S.-L. bone forceps
  S.-L. rib-cutting forceps
  S.-L. rongeur
Stille-Luer
  S.-L. angular duckbill rongeur
  S.-L. bone rongeur
  S.-L. rongeur forceps
Stille-Luer-Echlin rongeur
Stille-Mayo dissecting scissors
Stille-Mayo-Hegar needle
Stillenberg raspatory
Stille-pattern trephine and bone drill set
Stille-Quervain spreader
Stille-Ruskin rongeur
Stille-Russian forceps
Stille-Seldinger needle
Stille-Sherman bone drill
Stille-Stiwer
  S.-S. gouge
  S.-S. osteotome
  S.-S. plaster shears
Stille-Waugh forceps
Stille-Zaufal-Jansen rongeur
Stimitrode electrode
Stimoceiver implant material
Stim Plus hand-held microcurrent stimulator
Stimprene
  S. electrotherapy brace
  S. wrap
Stimson
  S. dressing
  S. pedicle clamp
stimulating
  s. catheter
  s. electrode
stimulator
  Acuscope microcurrent s.
  ACUTENS transcutaneous nerve s.
  Anustim electronic neuromuscular s.
  Arzco model 7 cardiac s.
  Axostim nerve s.
  Baltimore Therapeutic Equipment work s.
  Bard Neurostim peripheral nerve s.
  Bionicare s.
  Bipulse s.
  Bloom programmable s.
  Butler s.
  CAM s.
  Concept nerve s.
  constant current s.
  Digitimer pattern reversal s.
  direct-current bone growth s.
  direct electrical nerve s.
  Dormed cranial electrotherapy s.
  dorsal column s.
  EBI SPF-2 implantable bone s.
  electrical brain s.
  electric nerve s.
  Electro-Acuscope s.
  electronic muscle s.

S

stimulator *(continued)*
EMG s.
EMHI galvanic electrode s.
EMS 2000 neuromuscular s.
Endo Multi-Mode s.
external functional neuromuscular s.
facial nerve s.
fastSTART EMS neuromuscular s.
fastSTART HVPC pulsed s.
Freedom Micro Pro s.
galvanic electrode s.
Ganzfeld s.
Gatron nerve s.
G5 Porta-Plus muscle s.
Grass Model S9 s.
Grass S88 muscle s.
Hilger facial nerve s.
implantable neural s.
Innova pelvic floor s.
InSync cardiac s.
Intelect Legend s.
Intelect 600MP microcurrent s.
interferential s.
JACE-STIM electrical s.
magnetic s.
Magstim 200 s.
Master-Stim interferential s.
Maxima II transcutaneous electrical
 nerve s.
Medi-Stim s.
metabolic heat load s.
microamperage electrical nerve s.
Micro-Z neuromuscular s.
Myogyn II s.
Myopulse muscle s.
Myosynchron muscle s.
Myotest train-of-four nerve s.
nerve s.
neuromuscular electrical s. (NMES)
neuromuscular III s.
Neuro Stim 2000 Mk$_1$ s.
Nicolet SM-300 s.
Nuwave transcutaneous electrical
 nerve s.
oculogyric s.
Optokinetic s.
Ortho Dx electromedical s.
Orthofix Cervical-Stim s.
Orthofuse implantable growth s.
OrthoGen bone growth s.
OrthoLogic bone growth s.
OrthoPak II bone growth s.
OsteoGen implantable s.
OsteoStim implantable bone
 grown s.
percutaneous epidural nerve s.
photic-evoked response s.
Physio-Stim Lite bone growth s.
piezoelectrical s.
Prizm Electro-Mesh Z-Stim-II s.
Pulsatron II hand-held nerve s.
pulsed galvanic s.
Reese s.

Smoke Control Porta-Pack
 aversive s.
SpF spinal fusion s.
SpF-XL s.
spinal cord s.
SpinaLogic 1000 bone growth s.
SpinalPak fusion s.
SporTX pulsed direct current s.
S.P. 100 transcutaneous electrical
 neural s.
Stim Plus hand-held microcurrent
Stimuplex-S nerve s.
Super Stimm MF s.
surgical nerve s.
Synchrosonic s.
SysStim muscle s.
Theramini 1, 2 electrotherapy s.
Theratouch 4.7 s.
ThermaStim muscule s.
Toennis ES stand-alone constant-
 current electrical s.
transcutaneous cranial electrical s.
transcutaneous electrical nerve s.
transcutaneous electrical
 neuromuscular s. (TENS)
transcutaneous neuromuscular
 electrical s.
transelectrical nerve s.
transmural electrical s.
Ultratone electrical transcutaneous
 neuromuscular s.
URYS 800 nerve s.
Vari-Stim III hand-held nerve s.
Waters muscle s.
Whistle-Stop wireless aversive s.
Stimulite
 S. honeycomb mattress overlay
 S. honeycomb seating pad
Stimuplex block needle
Stimuplex-S nerve stimulator
sting mat
stirrup, pl. **stirrups**
 Allen laparoscopic stirrups
 ankle air s.
 s. brace
 candy-cane stirrups
 Comfort Cast s.
 Finochietto s.
 Infinity stirrups
 Lloyd-Davies stirrups
 Navratil stirrups
 Swivel-Strap ankle s.
stirrup-loop curette
stitch
 Endo S.
 Frost s.
 Kessler s.
 Mersilene Kessler s.
 Prolene s.
 s. scissors
 shorthand vertical mattress s.
 tracheal safety s.
stitch-removing knife
Stitt catheter

Stiwer
S. biopsy forceps
S. bone-holding forceps
S. curette
S. dressing forceps
S. finger-ring saw
S. furuncle knife
S. grooved director
S. hand drill
S. laryngeal mirror
S. retractor
S. scalpel handle
S. scissors
S. sponge forceps
S. tendon dissector
S. tissue forceps
S. towel clamp
S. trocar
S&T Lalonde hook forceps
Stock
S. eye trephine
S. finger splint
Stocker
S. cyclodiathermy puncture needle
Stockert cardiac pacing electrode
Stockfisch appliance
stockinette
s. amputation bandage
Bias s.
s. dressing
impervious s.
orthopedic s.
sterile s.
Velpeau s.
stocking, pl. **stockings**
adjustable thigh antiembolism stockings (ATS)
antiembolic stockings (AES)
antiembolism stockings
A-T antiembolism stockings
Atkins-Tucker antiembolism stockings
Bellavar medical support stockings
Camp-Sigvaris stockings
Carolon life support antiembolism stockings
Circ-Aid elastic stockings
compression stockings
Compriform support stockings
Comtesse medical support stockings
drop-foot redression stockings
elastic stockings
Florex medical compression stockings
graduated compression stockings
Jobst-Stride support stockings
Jobst-Stridette support stockings
Jobst VPGS stockings
Juzo stockings
Juzo-Hostess two-way stretch compression stockings
Kendall compression stockings
Linton elastic stockings
Medi Plus compression stockings
Medi-Strumpf stockings
Medi vascular stockings
Orthawear antiembolism stockings
Planostretch stockings
pneumatic antiembolic stockings
pneumatic compression stockings
SCD stockings
sequential compression stockings
Sigvaris compression stockings
Sigvaris medical stockings
Stride support stockings
TED antiembolism stockings
thigh-high antiembolic stockings
thromboembolic disease stockings
True Form support stockings
Twee alternating cut-off compressor stockings
Vairox high-compression vascular stockings
Venofit medical compression stockings
Venoflex medical compression stockings
venous pressure gradient support stockings
Zimmer antiembolism stockings
Zipzoc stockings
Stockman
S. meatal clamp
S. penile clamp
Stoesser stripper
Stokes lens
Stolte
S. capsulorhexis forceps
S. tonsillar dissector
Stolte-Stille elevator
Stoltz laparoscope
stoma
Bard regular one-piece s.
s. button
s. cap microporous adhesive
s. cone
s. irrigator drain
Silastic collar-reinforced s.
stoma-centering guide
stomach
s. brush
s. clamp
s. tube
Stomahesive
S. powder
S. sterile wafer
stomal bag
stoma-measuring device
Stomate
S. decompression tube
S. extension tube
S. low-profile gastrostomy kit
stone
s. basket
s. basket screw mounted handle
S. clamp-applying forceps
s. clamp-locking device
s. dislodger
S. eye implant
S. intestinal clamp

stone *(continued)*
S. intestinal forceps
S. lens nucleus prolapser
pumice s.
s. recognition system
s. retriever
s. staple
S. stomach clamp
S. tissue forceps
stone-crushing forceps
stone-extraction forceps
stone-grasping forceps
Stone-Holcombe
S.-H. anastomosis clamp
S.-H. intestinal clamp
stone-holding basket
Stoneman forceps
stone-retrieval
s.-r. balloon
s.-r. basket
StoneRisk diagnostic monitoring kit
stone-tissue
s.-t. detection system
s.-t. recognition system
Stonetome stone removal device
Stony splenorenal shunt clamp
Stookey
S. cranial rongeur
S. retractor
stool
s. collector
foot s.
Fuchs surgical s.
nested step s.
STOO Series Ten Thousand ocutome
stop
Bowman needle s.
Castroviejo corneal scissors with
inside s.
s. cock
s. collar telescope
Devonshire-Mack s.
Elite posterior adjustable s.
Endo s.
S. eye speculum
footdrop s.
Krueger instrument s.
s. needle
stopcock
Accel s.
Burron Discofix s.
Discofix s.
Luer-Lok s.
Manometer s.
Morse s.
Stopko irrigator
Stop-Leak
S.-L. gel flotation cushion
S.-L. gel flotation mattress
Storer thoracoabdominal retractor
Storey
S. clamp
S. gall duct forceps
S. thoracic forceps

Storey-Hillar dissecting forceps
Stormby brush
Storm Von Leeuwen chamber
Story orbital elevator
Storz
S. adjustable headrest
S. anterior commissure laryngoscop
S. applicator
S. arthroscope
S. aspiration biopsy needle
S. band
S. biopsy forceps
S. bronchial catheter
S. bronchoscopic forceps
S. bronchoscopic telescope
S. calipers
S. camera
S. capsular forceps
S. Capsulor blue intraocular lens
S. cataract knife
S. catheter adapter
S. ceiling-mounted microscope
system
S. chalazion trephine
S. cholangiograsper
S. choledochoscope-nephroscope
S. ciliary forceps
S. cleaning brush
S. continuous-flow rectoscope
S. corneal bur
S. corneal forceps
S. corneal trephine
S. corneoscleral punch
S. cotton carrier
S. curved forceps
S. cystoscope
S. cystoscopic electrode
S. cystoscopic forceps
S. diagnostic laparoscope
S. DiaPhine trephine
S. direct-view resectoscope
S. disposable blade
S. disposable cannula
S. disposable fiberoptic light pipe
S. disposable trocar
S. duckbill rongeur
S. ear knife handle
S. ear knife set
S. ear, nose and throat camera
system
S. Easy shield
S. esophagoscopic forceps
S. face shield headband
S. flexible injection needle
S. folding-handle ear knife
S. grasping biopsy forceps
S. hair transplant trephine
S. handpiece
S. head holder
S. hysteroscope
S. infant bronchoscope
S. infection ventilation laryngoscop
S. inserter

S. intranasal antral punch
S. intraocular scissors
S. iris hook
S. iris scissors
S. keratome
S. keratometer
S. kidney stone forceps
S. Laparocam
S. Laparoflator insufflator
S. laser
S. laser resectoscope
S. magnet
S. meatal clamp
S. microcalipers
S. microscope
S. MicroSeal
S. microserrefine
S. microsurgical bipolar coagulator
S. Microsystems drill bit
S. Microsystems plate cutter
S. Microsystems plate-holding forceps
S. Millennium microsurgical system
S. miniature forceps
S. miniplate
S. Monolith lithotriptor
S. nasal speculum
S. nasopharyngeal biopsy forceps
S. needle cannula
S. needle holder
S. nephroscope
S. operating esophagoscope
S. operating laparoscope
S. optical biopsy forceps
S. optical esophagoscope
S. panendoscope
S. pediatric esophagoscope
S. pigtail probe
S. plate
S. Premiere Microvit vitrector
S. radial incision marker
S. resectoscope curette
S. resectoscope electrode
S. retractor
S. rhinomanometer
S. scleral buckling balloon catheter
S. septal speculum
S. sheath
S. sheath-handle ear knife
S. Sine-U-View endoscope
S. sinus biopsy forceps
S. 27022 SK ureteroscope
S. stitch scissors
S. stone-crushing forceps
S. stone dislodger
S. stone-extraction forceps
S. suction tube
S. syringe
S. Teflon forceps guard
S. thoracoscope
S. tonometer
S. tracheoscope
S. twisted snare wire
S. twist hook
S. Universal lens loop
S. urethrotome

S. vent tube introducer
S. wire-cutting scissors
Storz-Atlas eye magnet
Storz-Beck tonsillar snare
Storz-Bell erysiphake
Storz-Bonn suturing forceps
Storz-Bowman lacrimal probe
Storz-Bruening
   S.-B. anastigmatic aural magnifier
   S.-B. diagnostic head
Storz-DeKock two-way bronchial catheter
Storz-Duredge
   S.-D. keratome
   S.-D. steel cataract knife
Storz-Hopkins
   S.-H. laryngoscope
   S.-H. system
   S.-H. telescope
Storz-Iglesias resectoscope
Storz-Kirkheim urethrotome
Storz-LaForce adenotome
Storz-LaForce-Stevenson adenotome
Storz-Moltz tonsillectome
Storz-Riecker laryngoscope
Storz-Schitz tonometer
Storz-Shapshay tracheoscope
Storz-Utrata forceps
Storz-Vienna nasal speculum
Storz-Walker retinal detachment unit
Storz-Westcott conjunctival scissors
Stott Reformers
Stough punch
stout-neck curette
strabismus
   s. forceps
   s. hook
   s. needle
   s. scissors
Strach spring
straight
   s. ahead bronchoscopic telescope
   s. aneurysm clip
   s. bipolar pencil
   s. bistoury
   s. blade
   s. burnisher
   s. catheter guide
   s. chest tube
   s. coagulating forceps
   s. connector
   s. fissure bur
   s. flush percutaneous catheter
   s. guidewire
   s. hex screwdriver
   s. inclined plane elevator
   s. knot-tying forceps
   s. lacrimal cannula
   s. laryngeal mirror
   s. line bayonet forceps
   s. magnifying mirror
   s. Maryland forceps
   s. microbipolar forceps
   s. micromonopolar forceps
   s. microscissors

S

straight *(continued)*
   s. monopolar electrosurgical dissector
   s. mosquito clamp
   s. mosquito hemostat
   s. nerve hook
   s. osteotome
   s. periosteal elevator
   s. rasp
   s. reamer
   s. retinal probe
   s. retractor
   s. ring curette
   s. shank bur
   s. single tenaculum forceps
   s. stent
   s. suturing needle
   s. tenaculum
   s. tenotomy scissors
   s. tube stylet
   s. tying forceps
   s. tympanoplasty knife
   s. walker brace
straight-blade
   s.-b. electrode
   s.-b. laryngoscope
straight-end cup forceps
straightener
   Asch septal s.
   Cottle-Walsham septal s.
   septal s.
   Walsham septal s.
straightening cannula
Straight-In surgical system
straight-needle electrode
straight-point
   s.-p. electrode
   s.-p. needle
straight-tip
   s.-t. bipolar forceps
   s.-t. electrode
   s.-t. jeweler's bipolar forceps
straight-wire electrode
strain
   s. gauge
   s. gauge transducer
Straith
   S. chin implant
   S. nasal implant
   S. nasal splint kit
   S. profilometer
Strampelli
   S. eye splint
   S. implant
   S. lens
Strandell retractor
Strandell-Stille
   S.-S. retractor
   S.-S. tendon hook
strands
   AcryDerm S.
   FlexiGel s.
strap
   API Universal foam chin s.

Band-It tennis elbow s.
Bard catheter s.
Bard wide leg bag s.
Beta Pile II, III splint s.
buddy s.
Butterfly cushion with s.
catheter leg s.
chest s.
Cho-Pat Achilles tendon s.
Cho-Pat elbow s.
Cho-Pat knee s.
Circumpress chin s.
s. clavicle splint
comfort leg bag s.
control adjustment s.
Conveen leg bag s.
deluxe leg bag s.
Dermicel Montgomery s.
distal over-shoulder s.
D-ring s.
Eclipse Gel elbow s.
elastic back s.
extremity mobilization s.
fabric leg bag s.
figure-of-eight clavicle s.
Fitz-all fabric leg s.
Flushmesh s.
forearm flexion control s.
front support s.
latex rubber tourniquet s.
Lema s.
S. Lok ankle brace
Meek-style clavicular s.
Montgomery s.
neoprene wrist s.
Nylatex s.
s. on undergarment
over-shoulder s.
PIP/DIP s.
ProSys leg bag comfort s.
proximal over-shoulder s.
QualCraft s.
Rotalok wrist s.
Rusch head s.
Self Snag s.
Silastic s.
stretch-out s.
tourniquet s.
Strap-Pad
   Daw S.-P.
strapping
   loop & hook s.
   LowDye s.
Strasbourg-Fairfax in vitro fertilization needle
Strassburger tissue forceps
Strassmann uterine forceps
Strata
   S. hip system
   S. hip system stem
   ProForm S.
Stratagene SCS-96 thermocycler cycle
Stratasis urethral sling
StrataSorb composite wound dressing
Stratasys FDM Med Modeler system

Stratis II MRI system
Stratos orthotic
Stratte
  S. forceps
  S. kidney clamp
  S. needle holder
Stratus
  S. impact reducing pylon
  S. instrument
Straus curved retrobulbar needle
Strauss
  S. cannula
  S. dental attachment
  S. meatal clamp
  S. penile clamp
  S. sigmoidoscope
Strauss-Valentine penile clamp
Strayer meniscal knife
Streak resectoscope
Streamline peripheral catheter
Strecker
  S. balloon-expandable stent
  S. coronary stent
  S. esophageal stent
  S. tantalum stent
Street pin
Streli forceps
Strelinger
  S. catheter-introducing forceps
  S. colon clamp
Strempel dermatome
strengthening exerciser
StressCath catheter
Stress echo bed
Stress-Ray varus-valgus device
Stretch
  S. balloon
  S. cardiac device
  S. gauze roll
  S. and Heel splint
  S. Net wound dressing
stretcher
  Brandy scalp s.
  Kuttner wound s.
  Lumex shower s.
  shoe s.
stretch-out strap
Stretzer bent-tip USCI catheter
striascope
Stribs strut
stricturotome
  Stallard s.
  Werb angled s.
Stride
  S. analyzer
  S. cardiac pacemaker
  S. support stockings
string drawing board
Stringer
  S. catheter-introducing forceps
  S. newborn throat forceps
  S. tracheal catheter
stringing peg
strip
  blood glucose reagent s.

boxing s.
Breathe Right nasal s.'s
Codman surgical s.
Color Bar Schirmer s.
Cover-Strip wound closure s.
demineralized flexible laminar
  bone s.
DisIntek reagent s.
Excel GE electrochemical glucose
  monitoring test s.
EyeClose Adhesive s.
flexible laminar bone s.
Flu-Glow s.
G-C polishing s.
GHM polishing s.
Gore-Tex s.
LC s.
leucocyte detection s.
Microflo test s.
Mosher s.
NEURAY neurosurgical s.
Nu-Hope skin barrier s.
Pacific Coast flexible laminar
  bone s.
packing s.
PD polishing s.
plastic s.
s. and point sponge
polishing s.
ProSys Urahesive system LA latex
  male external condom catheter
  with Urahesive s.
Schirmer tear test s.
separating s.
silicone s.
Sleep Right nasal s.'s
Suture S.
tear s.
Telfa s.
Thera-Band s.
UC s.
Urihesive moldable adhesive s.
Visidex II blood glucose testing s.
stripe
  Quad-Lumen drain with
  radiopaque s.
  Self-Cath coude tipped catheter with
  guide s.
stripper
  Babcock jointed vein s.
  Bartlett fascial s.
  Brand tendon s.
  Bunnell tendon s.
  Bunt tendon s.
  Cannon-type s.
  Carroll forearm tendon s.
  chest tube s.
  Clark vein s.
  Codman vein s.
  Cole polyethylene vein s.
  Crawford fascial s.
  Crile vagotomy s.
  DeBakey intraluminal s.
  Dorian rib s.
  Doyen rib s.

S

stripper *(continued)*
 Doyle vein s.
 Dunlop thrombus s.
 Emerson vein s.
 endonerve s.
 Endostat fiber s.
 external vein s.
 fascia lata s.
 Fischer tendon s.
 Friedman olive-tip vein s.
 Furlong tendon s.
 Grierson tendon s.
 Hall-Chevalier s.
 hydraulic vein s.
 IM tendon s.
 interchangeable vein s.
 Joplin tendon s.
 Keeley vein s.
 Kurtin vein s.
 LaVeen helical s.
 Lempka vein s.
 Levy-Okun s.
 Linton vein s.
 Martin endarterectomy s.
 Masson fascial s.
 Matson-Alexander rib s.
 Matson-Mead periosteum s.
 Matson rib s.
 Mayo external vein s.
 Mayo-Myers external vein s.
 Meyer olive-tipped vein s.
 Meyer spiral vein s.
 Nabatoff vein s.
 Nelson rib s.
 Nelson-Roberts s.
 New Orleans endarterectomy s.
 orthopedic surgical s.
 Phelan vein s.
 pigtail tendon s.
 Price-Thomas rib s.
 ramus s.
 reusable vein s.
 rib edge s.
 ring s.
 Roberts-Nelson rib s.
 Samuels vein s.
 Shaw carotid artery clot s.
 slotted tendon s.
 Smith posterior cartilage s.
 spiral vein s.
 Stoesser s.
 Stukey s.
 surgical s.
 tendon s.
 thrombus s.
 Trace hydraulic vein s.
 vagotomy s.
 vein s.
 Verner s.
 Webb interchangable vein s.
 Wilson vein s.
 Wurth vein s.
 Wylie endarterectomy s.

 Zollinger-Gilmore vein s.
 zonule s.
strips
 bovine pericardium s.
 CarraGauze packing s.
 DermAssist hydrogel packing s.
 Medline Packing s.
Stripseal catheter
Strobex Mark II electrosurgical unit
stroboscope
 Kay rhinolaryngeal s.
 rhinolarynx s.
Stromeyer splint
Stromgren ankle brace
Stronghands hand exerciser
strontium-90 ophthalmic beta ray
  applicator
Stroud-Baron ear suction tube
Strow corneal forceps
Strubel lid everter
Struck spreader
structured coil electromagnet
Struempel
 S. ear alligator forceps
 S. ear punch forceps
 S. rongeur
Struempel-Voss
 S.-V. ethmoidal forceps
 S.-V. nasal forceps
Strully
 S. cardiovascular scissors
 S. dissecting scissors
 S. dressing forceps
 S. dural scissors
 S. dural twist hook
 S. Gigli-saw handle
 S. hook scissors
 S. nerve root retractor
 S. neurosurgical scissors
 S. ruptured-disk curette
 S. tissue forceps
Strully-Kerrison rongeur
strut
 Adkins s.
 Anderson nasal s.
 s. bar
 s. bar hook
 s. calipers
 s. forceps
 George Washington s.
 s. graft
 Harrington s.
 House calipers s.
 Judet s.
 Magnuson s.
 s. measuring instrument
 miniplate s.
 Nalebuff-Goldman s.
 s. pick
 polyethylene s.
 Rehbein internal steel s.
 Robinson s.
 stent s.
 Stribs s.
 Teflon s.

TORP s.
tricuspid valve s.
valve outflow s.
wire-loop s.
strut-type pin
Struyken
    S. angular punch tip
    S. conchotome
    S. ear forceps
    S. nasal-cutting forceps
    S. nasal forceps
    S. punch
    S. turbinate forceps
Stryker
    S. arthrometer
    S. arthroscope
    S. autopsy saw
    S. blade
    S. bur
    S. cartilage knife
    S. cast cutter
    S. chip camera
    S. chondrotome
    S. CircOlectric bed
    S. CircOlectric fracture frame
    S. Constavac closed-wound suction
      apparatus
    S. CPM exerciser
    S. drain
    S. drill
    S. fracture table
    S. lag screw
    S. leg exerciser
    S. microdebrider
    S. microirrigator
    S. microshaver
    S. power instrumentation
    S. resector
    S. Rolo-dermatome
    S. screwdriver
    S. SE3 drive system
    S. shaver
    S. suction irrigator
    S. turning fracture frame
Stryker-School meniscal knife
STS
    STS lithotripsy system
    STS molding sock
STTOdx ophthalmic surgery system
Stuart
    S. articulator
    S. Gordon hand splint
Stubbs adenoidal curette
Stucker bile duct dilator
Stuckrad magnifying
    laryngopharyngoscope
Stuck self-retaining laminectomy
    retractor
Studer pouch
Stuhler-Heise fixator
Stukey stripper
Stulberg
    S. HIPciser abduction splint
    S. hip positioner
    S. Mark II leg positioner

Stumer perforating bur
Sturmdorf
    S. cervical needle
    S. cervical reamer
    S. pedicle needle
    S. suture
Stutsman nasal snare
STx Saunders lumbar disk device
Stycar graded ball
Styles forceps
stylet, stylette
    Bing s.
    bipolar irrigating s.
    Bruening forceps s.
    cardiovascular s.
    Cook locking s.
    Cooper endotracheal s.
    Frazier s.
    Frigitronics disposable
      cryosurgical s.
    illuminating s.
    Inrad HiLiter ultrasound-enhanced s.
    Jelco intravenous s.
    jet s.
    K s.
    L s.
    lighted s.
    locking s.
    Malis irrigating forceps s.
    malleable s.
    retractable s.
    Rumel ratchet tourniquet eyed s.
    S s.
    straight tube s.
    surgical s.
    The Hockey Stick articulating s.
    tourniquet-eyed ratchet s.
    Trachlight lighted intubating s.
    transmyocardial pacing s.
    transthoracic pacing s.
    Tubestat lighted s.
    Universal curved-tube s.
    Universal straight-tube s.
    ureteral s.
    wire s.
stylet-scope endoscope
styletted tracheobronchial catheter
stylus
    S. cardiovascular suture
    IM/EM tibial resection s.
    S. suture needle
    tibial s.
S-type dental implant
Styrofoam dressing
Suarez
    S. retractor
    S. spreader
Suarz continence ring
Sub-4
    S. Platinum Plus wire kit
    S. small-vessel balloon dilatation
      catheter
subannular mattress suture
subarachnoid screw

S

subclavian
    s. apheresis catheter
    s. cannula
    s. dialysis catheter
    s. hemodialysis catheter
    s. Tegaderm dressing
    s. vein access catheter
Subco needle
subconjunctival needle
subcostal trocar
subcutaneous
    s. augmentation material
    s. morphine pump
    s. patch electrode
    s. peritoneal administration device
    s. suture
    s. tunneling device
subcuticular suture
subdermal implant
subdural
    s. grid electrode
    s. strip electrode
subduroperitoneal shunt
subgaleal drain
subglottic forceps
subglottiscope
    Healy-Jako pediatric s.
sublaminar wire
submammary dissector
submicroinfusion catheter
submucosal implant
submucous
    s. chisel
    s. curette
    s. dissector
    s. retractor
suboccipital Ommaya reservoir
Subortholen sheet
subpectoral stabilizer
subperiosteal
    s. glass bead inserter
    s. implant
    s. tissue expander
Sub-Q-Set
    S.-Q.-S. subcutaneous continuous
    infusion device
Subramanian
    S. classic miniature aortic clamp
    S. sidewinder aortic clamp
subretinal fluid cannula
Subrini penile prosthesis
substitute
    Accu-Flo dural s.
    AlloMatrix injectable putty bone
    graft s.
    Biobrane/HF experimental skin s.
    Dermagraft skin s.
    Dermagraft-TC temporary skin s.
    dural s.
    HemAssist blood s.
    OrthoDyn bone s.
    OsteoSet bone graft s.
    TransCyte temporary skin s.
    U-channel stripping dural s.
sub-Tenon anesthesia cannula

suburethral sling
Sub-Vent implant system
sucker
    Churchill s.
    intercardiac s.
    intracardiac s.
    KAM Super S.
    malleable s.
    s. shaver
    s. tip
suction
    s. adapter
    s. apparatus
    s. aspirator
    Barton s.
    s. biopsy needle
    s. biter
    Bowen s.
    S. Buster catheter
    s. cannula
    s. catheter
    s. cautery
    s. cup
    s. cylinder
    s. device
    s. dissector
    s. drain
    ear forceps with s.
    s. elevator
    Ferguson s.
    s. forceps
    Frazier s.
    s. irrigator
    s. magnet
    Ortholav s.
    perilimbal s.
    Pleur-evac s.
    s. probe
    s. pump
    s. punch
    s. Regugauge regulator
    s. ring
    Rosen s.
    SureTran s.
    s. tip
    s. tip curette
    Tis-U-Trap endometrial s.
    s. tonsillar dissector
    s. tube
    s. tube clip
    s. tube obturator
    Vactro perilimbal s.
    Wangensteen s.
    Yankauer s.
suction-coagulation tube
suction-irrigator
    Brackmann s.-i.
    FlowGun s.-i.
    Jako s.-i.
    Kurze s.-i.
    Nezhat-Dorsey s.-i.
    PMT MacroVac s.-i.
    William-House s.-i.
Sudan needle
Sudarsky cryoprobe

Sudbury system
Suetens-Gybels-Vandermeulen
  angiographic localizer
Sugar aneurysm clip
Sugarbaker retrocolic clamp
sugar-tong
  s.-t. cast
  s.-t. splint
Suggs catheter
Sugita
  S. aneurysm clip
  S. catheter
  S. cross-legged clip
  S. fork
  S. head clamp
  S. head holder
  S. headholder
  S. jaws clip applier
  S. microsurgical table
  S. multipurpose head frame
  S. retractor
  S. side-curved bayonet clip
  S. temporary straight clip
Sugita-Ikakogyo clip
Suh ventilation tube
suit
  antishock s.
  body-exhaust s.
  Gladiator shock s.
  hot-water circulating s.
  Life S.
  MAST s.
  total-body compression s.
Suker
  S. cyclodialysis spatula
  S. iris forceps
  S. spatula knife
Sukhtian-Hughes fixation device
Sulcabrush
Sulfix-6 cement
Sullival gum scissors
Sullivan
  S. bubble cushion
  S. III nasal continuous positive air
    pressure device
  S. nasal variable positive airway
    pressure unit
  S. sinus rasp
  S. variable stiffness cable
  S. VPAP II
Sully shoulder stabilizer brace
SULP II balloon catheter
Sulze diamond-point needle
Sulzer prosthesis
Summar alloy
SummaSketch III digitizing board
Summit
  S. alloy
  S. excimer laser
  S. Krumeich-Barraquer
    Microkeratome
  S. LoDose collimator
  S. Omnimed excimer laser
  S. SVS Apex laser
  S. UV 200 Excimed laser

Sumner clamp
sump
  Argyle silicone Salem s.
  Cooley ventricular s.
  DLP pericardial s.
  s. drain
  Grice laparoscopic s.
  s. pump
  s. pump catheter
  s. tube
  ventricular s.
Sumpter clasp spring-lock
sunburst mechanism
Sunday staphylorrhaphy elevator
Sundt
  S. aneurysm clip-applier
  S. AVM clip system
  S. AVM microclip system
  S. booster clip
  S. carotid endarterectomy shunt
  S. cross-legged clip
  S. encircling clip
  S. straddling clip
  S. suction system
Sundt-Kees
  S.-K. aneurysm clip
  S.-K. booster clip
  S.-K. encircling patch clip
  S.-K. graft clip
  S.-K. Slimline clip
Sung reverse nucleus chopper
Sunrise LTK system
Sun SPARCstation system
SunVideo frame grabber
Super
  S. Arrow-Flex catheterization sheath
  S. Cut laminectomy rongeur
  S. Dopplex SDI vascular test unit
  S. Eidersoft bed pad
  S. Epitron high-frequency epilator
  S. Field NC slit lamp lens
  S. Grip sleeve
  S. "M" vacuum extractor cup
  S. Pak posterior nasal pack
  S. PEG tube
  S. Pinky ball
  S. Pinky device
  S. punctum plug
  S. Stimm MF stimulator
  S. Torque Plus catheter
Super-9
  S. guiding cardiac device
  S. guiding catheter
superabsorbent polymer
super-absorptive polymer dressing
Superblade
  Bishop-Harman S.
  S. No. 75 blade
  S. trapezoid
Super-Bright microsphere
Supercath intravenous catheter
SuperCat self-tapping implant
SuperClearPro suction socket

superconducting
  s. magnet
  s. quantum interference device
SuperCup acetabular cup prosthesis
Super-Cut
  S.-C. blade
  S.-C. diamond bur
  S.-C. scissors
Super-Dent orthodontic cement
SuperEBA cement
superficial implant
superfine fiberscope
Superflex elastic dressing
Superflow guiding catheter
Superform Contours orthotic
Superglue adhesive
superior
  s. border plate
  s. radial tenotomy scissors
  s. rectus forceps
  S. suction catheter
  s. thoracic pedicle screw
superlag screw
Super-Plus Trimshield pad
SuperQuad assistive device
Superscript preamplification system
Superselector Y-K guidewire
Superset exercise system
SuperSkin thin film dressing
Super-Soft denture reliner
Superstabilizer
  S. cemented stem extender
  S. press-fit stem extender
Super-Trac adhesive traction dressing
supervoltage generator
super wrap
supine C-Trax traction
Supolene suture
support
  Achillotrain active Achilles
    tendon s.
  Act joint s.
  Airprene hinged knee s.
  AliMed Freedom arthritis s.
  AliMed QualCraft wrist s.
  arch s.
  Back-Huggar lumbar s.
  BackThing lumbar s.
  BIOflex Magnet Back S.
  BioSkin s.
  Birkenstock Blue Footbed arch s.
  Birkenstock high-flange arch s.
  Body Gard neoprene s.
  Carabelt lower back s.
  cardiopulmonary s.
  Castech extremity s.
  chin s.
  ChinUpps cervicofacial s.
  cock-up wrist s.
  Comprifix active ankle s.
  Conve back s.
  Corfit System 7000 Series
    Lumbosacral S.
  Dale oxygen cannula s.
  Dale ventilator tubing s.

DayTimer carpal tunnel s.
DePuy s.
Desk-Rest arm s.
Dr. Gibaud thermal health s.
Dr. Kho's CMC S.
Epitrain active elbow s.
Epitrain elastic elbow s.
Ergo Cush back s.
Ergoflex Premiere back s.
Ezy Wrap lumbosacral s.
facial s.
Firm D-Ring wrist s.
flat brain spatula s.
FlexLite hinged knee s.
Flex-Rite lumbar s.
Foot Hugger foot s.
Freedom arthritis s.
Freedom Back S.
Freedom Elastic Long Wrist S.
Futuro wrist s.
Genutrain P3 active knee s.
geriatric chair trunk s.
Grotena abdominal s.
Hand-Aid arterial wrist s.
IMP-Capello arm s.
Kallassy ankle s.
Lo Bak spinal s.
Malleotrain ankle s.
McKenzie AirBack s.
MKG knee s.
Mold-In-Place back s.
Momma-Too Maternity S.
Monitor Master monitor s.
Morton toe s.
Mother-To-Be abdominal s.
Mother-To-Be Support Maternity
MouseMitt Keyboarders wrist s.
neck s.
neoprene ankle s.
neoprene back s.
Nightimer carpal tunnel s.
Norco ulnar deviation s.
obese s.
OBUS back s.
Olympia Vacpac s.
Orion lumbar s.
Ortho-Pal body s.
OSI Well Leg S.
Parham s.
PattStrap knee s.
percutaneous cardiopulmonary
  bypass s.
Plastizote arch s.
postoperative mammary s.
ProFlex wrist s.
QualCraft ankle s.
QualCraft short elastic wrist s.
Rolyan Firm D-Ring wrist s.
Rolyan foot s.
sacral s.
Safe spine thoracic-lumbar-sacral s
Schick back s.
Schillinger suture s.
Scully Hip S'port functional hip
ShiatsuBACK s.

Shoulder Ease abduction s.
Sidekick foot s.
Spenco arch s.
S'port Max back s.
StanceGuard internal s.
Surgi-Bra breast s.
Taylor clavicle s.
Tecnol ankle s.
Tecnol back s.
Tecnol elbow s.
Tecnol knee s.
Tecnol wrist s.
Thompson chin s.
Three-D worker's back s.
tibial fracture brace proximal s.
wedge-shaped s.
well-leg s.
Whitman arch s.
Wristaleve s.
SupraCAPS quarter-globe cap
supracondylar
  s. barrel/plate component
  s. knee-ankle orthosis
  s. nail
  s. plate
  s. socket
SupraFoley
  S. catheter
  S. suprapubic introducer
Supralen
  S. cradle orthotic
  S. Schaefer orthotic
supramalleolar orthosis
Supramead nose splint
Supramid
  S. bridle collagen suture
  S. Extra suture
  S. eye muscle sleeve
  S. graft
  S. implant
  S. lens
  S. lens implant suture
  S. occluding stent
  S. polyamide mesh
  S. prosthesis
  S. sheet
  S. snare
Supramid-Allen implant
suprapubic
  s. cannula
  s. catheter
  s. hemostatic bag
  s. self-retaining retractor
  s. suction drain
  s. trocar
suprarenal Greenfield filter
SupraSLEEVES nylon sleeve
Supratusion system
Supreme II blood glucose meter
Suraci
  S. elevator hook
  S. zygoma hook elevator
Surbaugh legholder

Surcan
  S. knee holder
  S. leg holder
Sur-Catch paired-wire basket
surcingle
  Von Lackum s.
Sure
  S. Seal Golden Drain catheter
  S. Sport pad
  S. Step brace
SureBite biopsy forceps
SureCare/Medical disposable underpad
SureCath port access catheter
Sure-Closure
  S.-C. closure
  S.-C. device
  S.-C. skin closure system
  S.-C. wound closure tape
Sure-Cut biopsy needle
Surefit intraocular lens
Sure-Flex III prosthetic foot
SureFlex nickel-titanium file
Sure-Gait folding walker
SureGrip
  S. breathing bag
  S. manual resuscitator
Surelite blood lancet
SurePress
  S. absorbent padding
  S. compression dressing
  S. compression wrap
  S. high-compression bandage
SureScan
  S. scanning handpiece
  S. system
Sureseal
  S. cellulose sponge bandage
  S. pressure bandage
Suresharp
  S. blood collecting needle
  S. dental needle
SureSite transparent adhesive film dressing
Sure-Snare tourniquet
SureStart imaging system
SureStep
  S. ankle support system
  S. glucose meter
  S. glucose monitor
Suretac bioabsorbable shoulder fixation device
SureTemp4 oral thermometer
SureTrans autotransfusion system
SureTran suction
Surety shield
Surevue contact lens
Surewing winged infusion set
surface
  Advance Dynamicaire sleep s.
  Advance Zoneaire sleep s.
  ALPHA ACTIVE pressure-relieving support s.
  s. coil
  DeCube therapeutic s.
  DermaGard II seating s.

S

surface *(continued)*
    DermaGard TRIAD seating s.
    s. electrode
    s. eye implant
    ISCH-DISH CFT pressure relieving seat s.
    NewLife therapeutic s.
    Silhouette therapeutic s.
surface-coil MRI
Surfasoft dressing
Sur-Fast needle
Sur-Fit
    S.-F. colostomy bag
    S.-F. colostomy irrigation sleeve
    S.-F. disposable Convex insert
    S.-F. flange cap
    S.-F. flexible and drainable pouch
    S.-F. irrigation adapter faceplate
    S.-F. irrigation sleeve tail closure
    S.-F. loop
    S.-F. Mini-Pouch
    S.-F. Natura pouch
    S.-F. night drainage container set
    S.-F. night drainage container tubing
    S.-F. urinary drainage bag
    S.-F. urostomy pouch
    S.-F. wafer and drainable pouch
Sur-Fit/ACTIVE LIFE tail closure
Surfit adhesive
Surflo
    S. IV catheter
    S. winged infusion set
Surgair bur
Surgairtome air drill
Surgaloy metallic suture
Surgamid polyamide suture material
SurgAssist
    S. leg positioner
    S. surgical leg holder
Surgenomic endoscope
Surgeons
    S. Choice stapling system
    S. Choice surgical stapler
surgery
    Bosker TMI s.
    collimated beam handpiece (CBH-1) for laser s.
    Elite Farley retractor for spinal s.
    fracture computer-aided s.
    hand-assisted laparoscopic s.
    InstaTrak System image-guided s.
    percutaneous vascular s.
    ProTrac system for knee s.
    selective imaging and graphics for stereotactic s.
    sex reassignment s.
Surg-E-Trol
    S.-E.-T. I/A/R system
    S.-E.-T. I/A system
SurgiBlade
    LaserSonics S.
Surgibone
    S. implant
Surgi-Bra breast support

Surgica K6 laser
surgical
    s. appliance
    s. appliance adhesive
    s. aspirator
    s. bur
    s. cannula
    s. chromic suture
    s. clip
    s. clip applier
    s. compression garment
    s. contractor
    s. curette
    s. cutter
    s. drain
    s. drape
    s. dressing
    s. electrode
    s. exhaust apparatus
    s. file
    s. general rasp
    s. gouge
    s. gut suture
    s. hammer
    s. handle
    s. hood
    s. instrument guide
    s. instrument post
    s. keratometer
    s. laser
    s. leg pedestal
    s. linen suture
    s. loupe
    s. mallet
    s. marking pen
    s. mask
    s. metallic mesh
    s. microscope
    s. nerve stimulator
    S. No Bounce mallet
    S. Nu-Knit absorbable hemostatic material
    s. otoscope
    S. Patient Arm shield
    s. pin driver
    s. power magnet
    s. retractor
    s. saw
    s. saw blade
    s. scissors
    s. silk suture
    S. Simplex P radiopaque adhesive
    S. Simplex P radiopaque bone cement
    s. skin graft expander
    s. snare
    s. spatula
    s. stapling gun
    s. steel gauze
    s. steel suture
    s. stripper
    s. stylet
    s. suction pump
    s. telescope

surgically implanted hemodialysis catheter
surgical-orthopaedic drill
Surgicel
    S. fibrillator absorbable hemostat
    S. gauze
    S. gauze dressing
    S. implant
    S. Nu-Knit
    S. Nu-Knit absorbable hemostat
    S. Nu-Knit absorbable hemostatic agent
    S. Nu-Knit dressing
Surgicenter 40 CO$_2$ laser
Surgiclip
    S. clip
    McDermott S.
    McFadden S.
Surgicraft
    S. Copeland fetal scalp electrode
    S. pacemaker electrode
    S. suture
    S. suture needle
Surgicutt incision device
Surgidac suture
Surgidev
    S. iris clip
    S. Leiske anterior chamber intraocular lens
    S. suture
Surgi-Fine reusable cannula tip
SurgiFish visceral retainer
Surgifix dressing
Surgiflex
    S. bandage
    S. dressing
    S. WAVE suction-irrigation device
    S. WAVE XP suction/irrigation probe
Surgi-Flo leg bag
Surgigut suture
Surgikit Velcro tourniquet
Surgikos disposable drape
Surgilar suture
Surgilase
    S. CO$_2$ laser
    S. ECS.1 smoke evacuator
    S. 150 high-powered CO$_2$ laser
    S. 55W laser
Surgilast tubular elastic dressing
Surgilav
    S. drain
    S. machine
Surgilene blue monofilament polypropylene suture
Surgiloid suture
Surgilon
    S. braided nylon suture
    S. monofilament polypropylene suture
Surg-I-Loop
Surgilope suture
SurgiMed
    S. clamp

    S. suture
    S. umbiliclamp
Surgimedics
    S. cholangiography catheter
    S. TMP air aspirator needle
    S. TMP multiperfusion set
Surgin
    S. hemorrhage occluder pin
    S. insufflation tubing
Surgineedle
    S. pneumoperitoneum needle
Surgi-Pad combined dressing
SurgiPeace analgesia pump
Surgi-PEG replacement gastrostomy feeding system
Surgiport
    S. disposable trocar
    S. stapler
    S. trocar and sleeve
Surgipro
    S. hernia mesh
    S. suture
Surgipulse XJ 150 CO$_2$ laser
SurgiScope
    Marco S.
Surgiscribe
Surgiset suture
Surgi-Site Incise drape
Surgi-Spec telescope
Surgistar
    S. corneal trephine
    S. ophthalmic blade
Surgitable hand surgery table
Surgitek
    S. button
    S. Double-J II closed-tip ureteral stent
    S. Double-J ureteral catheter
    S. Flexi-Flate II penile implant
    S. graduated cystoscope
    S. handpiece
    S. mammary implant
    S. mammary prosthesis
    S. OM-5 urodynamic system
    S. One Step percutaneous endoscopic gastrostomy
    S. penile prosthesis
    S. Quadra-Coil ureteral stent
    S. Tractfinder ureteral stent
    S. Uropass stent
Surgitite ligating loop
Surgitome bur
Surgitron
    S. portable radiosurgical unit
    S. ultrasound-assisted lipoplasty machine
    S. 3000 ultrasound device
Surgi-Tron thoracoscopic instrument
Surgitube
    S. dressing
    S. tubular gauze
Surgivac drain
Surgiview multi-use disposable laparoscope
Surgiwand suction/irrigation device

S

Surgiwip suture ligature
Surgtech gloves
Surpass guidewire
Surveyor monitor
Suspend
    S. pubovaginal sling
    S. Tutoplast processed fascia lata
suspended operating illuminator
suspension
    s. apparatus
    s. feeder
    s. laryngoscope
suspension-type socket
suspensor
    elastic s.
suspensory
    s. bandage
    s. dressing
Sussman four-mirror gonioscope
Sustagen nasogastric tube
Sustain
    S. dental implant system
    S. HA-coated screw implant
    S. hydroxyapatite biointegrated
        dental implant
Sustainer
    Akahoshi Nucleus S.
Sutcliffe laser shield and retracting
  instrument
Sutherland
    S. eye scissors
    S. lens
    S. rotatable microsurgery instrument
    S. vitreous forceps
Sutherland-Grieshaber
    S.-G. forceps
    S.-G. scissors
    S.-G. speculum
Sutter
    S. double-stem silicone implant
      prosthesis
    S. hinged great toe implant
    S. MCP finger joint prosthesis
Sutter-CPM knee device
Sutter-Smeloff heart valve prosthesis
Sutton biopsy needle
Sutupak suture
Suturamid suture
suture
    Acier stainless steel s.
    Acufex bioabsorbable Suretac s.
    Acutrol s.
    Alcon s.
    already-threaded s.
    aluminum-bronze wire s.
    American silk s.
    Ancap braided silk s.
    s. anchor
    angiocatheter with looped
      polypropylene s.
    arterial silk s.
    S. Assistant
    S. Assistant instrument
    atraumatic braided silk s.
    atraumatic chromic s.

Aureomycin s.
Auto S. (AS)
Barraquer silk s.
bastard s.
basting s.
BioSorb s.
Biosyn s.
black braided s.
black braided nylon s.
black braided silk s.
black twisted s.
Blalock s.
blanket s.
blue-black monofilament s.
blue twisted cotton s.
bolster s.
Bondek absorbable s.
bone wax s.
Bozeman s.
braided Ethibond s.
braided Mersilene s.
braided Nurolon s.
braided nylon s.
braided polyamide s.
braided polyester s.
braided silk s.
braided Vicryl s.
braided wire s.
Bralon s.
bridle s.
bronze wire s.
Brown-Sharp gauge s., B&S
  gauge s.
Bunnell wire pull-out s.
s. button
cable wire s.
capitonnage s.
Caprolactam s.
cardinal s.
Cardioflon s.
Cardionyl s.
cardiovascular Prolene s.
cardiovascular silk s.
Carrel s.
s. carrier
catgut s.
celluloid linen s.
cervical s.
Chinese fingertrap s.
Chinese twisted silk s.
chloramine catgut s.
chromated catgut s.
chromic blue dyed s.
chromic catgut s.
chromic collagen s.
chromic gut s.
chromicized catgut s.
circular s.
circumcisional s.
s. clip forceps
coated polyester s.
coated Vicryl Rapide s.
cocoon thread s.
collagen absorbable s.
compound s.

Connell s.
coronal s.
cotton Deknatel s.
cotton nonabsorbable s.
Cottony Dacron hollow s.
cranial s.
CT1 s.
Cushing Cushing s.
s. cushion
Custodis s.
s. cutter
Czerny s.
Czerny-Lembert s.
Dacron bolstered s.
Dacron traction s.
Dafilon s.
Dagrofil s.
Davis-Geck s.
Degnon s.
Deklene polypropylene s.
Deknatel silk s.
delayed s.
dermal s.
Dermalene polyethylene s.
Dermalon cuticular s.
Dexon absorbable synthetic
  polyglycolic acid s.
Dexon II s.
Dexon Plus s.
DG Softgut s.
Docktor s.
double-armed s.
double right-angle s.
double-running penetrating
  keratoplasty s.
Dulox s.
Dupuytren s.
Edinburgh s.
EEA Auto s.
elastic s.
Endo Knot s.
Endoloop s.
EPTFE vascular s.
Equisetene s.
Ethibond polybutilate-coated
  polyester s.
Ethibond polyester s.
Ethicon-Atraloc s.
Ethicon micropoint s.
Ethicon Sabreloc s.
Ethicon silk s.
Ethiflex retention s.
Ethilon nylon s.
Ethi-pack s.
everting mattress s.
expanded polytetrafluoroethylene
  (EPTFE) s.
extrachromic s.
figure-of-eight s.
filament s.
fine chromic s.
fine silk s.
fingertrap s.
Flaxedil s.
Flexitone s.

Flexon steel s.
formaldehyde catgut s.
Foster s.
Fothergill s.
Frater s.
Frost s.
Gaillard-Arlt s.
Gambee s.
gastrointestinal surgical gut s.
gastrointestinal surgical linen s.
gastrointestinal surgical silk s.
Gély s.
general closure s.
Gillies horizontal dermal s.
GI pop-off silk s.
glue-in s.
Gore-Tex s.
gossamer silk s.
Gould s.
green braided s.
green Mersilene s.
green monofilament polyglyconate s.
groove s.
s. guide
Gussenbauer s.
gut s.
guy s.
guy-steading s.
Guyton-Friedenwald s.
Halsted mattress s.
Heaney s.
heavy-gauge s.
heavy monofilament s.
heavy retention s.
heavy silk retention s.
heavy wire s.
helical s.
hemostatic s.
Herculon s.
s. holder
s. hole drill
Horsley s.
Hu-Friedy PermaSharp s.
IKI catgut s.
India rubber s.
interrupted pledgeted s.
intraluminal s.
Investa s.
iodine catgut s.
iodized surgical gut s.
iodochromic catgut s.
Ivalon s.
Jobert de Lamballe s.
Kal-Dermic s.
kangaroo tendon s.
Kessler-Kleinert s.
Kirschner s.
Krackow s.
Küstner s.
lacidem s.
lambdoidal s.
s. lancet
lancet s.
Lang s.
Lapra-Ty s.

S

suture *(continued)*
large-caliber nonabsorbable s.
lateral trap s.
lead s.
lead-shot tie s.
LeFort s.
Lembert s.
Ligapak s.
Linatrix s.
Lindner corneoscleral s.
linen s.
Linvatec meniscal BioStinger
  anchor s.
S. Lok device
Look s.
Lukens catgut s.
malar periosteum-SMAS flap
  fixation s.
Mannis s.
Marlex s.
Marshall V-s.
mattress s.
Maxam s.
Maxon absorbable s.
Mayo linen s.
McCannel s.
McLean s.
Measuroll s.
Medrafil wire s.
Meigs s.
Mersilene braided nonabsorbable s.
Mersilk s.
mesh s.
metal band s.
metallic s.
Micrins microsurgical s.
Micro-Glide corneal s.
MicroMite anchor s.
micropoint s.
middle palatine s.
Millipore s.
Miralene s.
Monocryl poliglecaprone s.
monofilament absorbable s.
monofilament clear s.
monofilament green s.
monofilament nylon s.
monofilament polypropylene s.
monofilament skin s.
monofilament steel s.
monofilament wire s.
Monosof s.
multifilament steel s.
multistrand s.
nasofrontal s.
natural s.
Needle-Less S.
neurosurgical s.
Nissen s.
nonabsorbable surgical s.
Nurolon s.
nylon 66 s.
nylon monofilament s.
nylon retention s.

oiled silk s.
opaque wire s.
Ophthalon s.
Oyloidin s.
Pagenstecher linen thread s.
Palfyn s.
Panacryl s.
Panalok absorbable s.
Pancoast s.
Paré s.
Parker-Kerr basting s.
s. passer
PDS II Endoloop s.
PDS Vicryl s.
Pearsall Chinese twisted s.
Pearsall silk s.
Perlon s.
Perma-Hand braided silk s.
PermaSharp PGA s.
s. pickup hook
pickup spatula s.
s. pickup spatula
pin s.
pink twisted cotton s.
plain catgut s.
plain collagen s.
plain gut s.
plastic s.
pledget s.
pledgeted Ethibond s.
pledgeted mattress s.
poliglecaprone 25 s.
polyamide s.
polybutester s.
Polydek s.
polydioxanone s. (PDS)
polyester fiber s.
polyethylene s.
polyfilament s.
polygalactic acid s.
polyglactin 910 s.
polyglecaprone 25 s.
polyglycolate s.
polyglycolic acid s.
polyglyconate s.
polypropylene button s.
Polysorb s.
pop-off s.
preplaced s.
presphenoethmoid s.
Prolene polypropylene s.
Pronova s.
Proxi-Strip s.
Pulvertaft s.
Purlon s.
PVB s.
pyoktanin catgut s.
pyroglycolic acid s.
Quickert s.
Ramsey County pyoktanin catgut
Rankin s.
Rapide wound s.
RB1 s.
reabsorbable s.
Reo Macrodex s.

ribbon gut s.
s. ring
rip-cord s.
rubber s.
running nylon penetrating
  keratoplasty s.
Sabreloc s.
Saenger s.
safety-bolt s.
Safil synthetic absorbable surgical s.
serrated s.
seton s.
Sharpoint ophthalmic
  microsurgical s.
Shirodkar s.
Shoch s.
shotted s.
SH popoff s.
Siemens PTCA open-heart s.
silicone-treated surgical silk s.
silk braided s.
silk Mersilene s.
silk nonabsorbable s.
silk pop-off s.
silk stay s.
silk traction s.
silkworm gut s.
Silky Polydek s.
silver s.
silverized catgut s.
Sims s.
single-armed s.
single-running s.
Snellen s.
Sofsilk coated and braided s.
Sofsilk nonabsorbable silk s.
Softgut surgical chromic catgut s.
s. spacer
Spanish blue virgin silk s.
SS s.
stainless steel wire s.
Stallard-Liegard s.
steel mesh s.
Sterna-Band self-locking s.
sternal wire s.
S. Strip
S. Strip Plus
Sturmdorf s.
Stylus cardiovascular s.
subannular mattress s.
subcutaneous s.
subcuticular s.
Supolene s.
Supramid bridle collagen s.
Supramid Extra s.
Supramid lens implant s.
Surgaloy metallic s.
surgical chromic s.
surgical gut s.
surgical linen s.
surgical silk s.
surgical steel s.
Surgicraft s.
Surgidac s.
Surgidev s.

Surgigut s.
Surgilar s.
Surgilene blue monofilament
  polypropylene s.
Surgiloid s.
Surgilon braided nylon s.
Surgilon monofilament
  polypropylene s.
Surgilope s.
SurgiMed s.
Surgipro s.
Surgiset s.
Sutupak s.
Suturamid s.
Sutureloop colposuspension s.
swaged s.
swaged-on s.
Swedgeon s.
Swiss blue virgin silk s.
synthetic absorbable s.
Synthofil s.
s. tag forceps
tantalum wire monofilament s.
Tapercut s.
Teflon-coated Dacron s.
Teflon-pledgeted s.
tension-requiring s.
tentalum wire tension s.
Tevdek pledgeted s.
Thermo-Flex s.
Thiersch s.
thread s.
through-and-through reabsorbable s.
through-the-wall mattress s.
Ti-Cron s.
tiger gut s.
Tinel s.
transfixion s.
transosseous s.
transscleral s.
twisted cotton s.
twisted dermal s.
twisted linen s.
twisted silk s.
twisted virgin silk s.
Tycron s.
tympanomastoid s.
Tyrrell-Gray s.
UltraFix MicroMite anchor s.
umbilical tape s.
unabsorbable s.
undyed s.
vascular silk s.
Verhoeff s.
S. VesiBand organizer
Vicryl pop-off s.
Vicryl Rapide s.
Vicryl SH s.
Vienna wire s.
virgin silk s.
Viro-Tec s.
white braided silk s.
white nylon s.
white twisted s.
wing s.

suture *(continued)*
   s. wire
   s. wire-cutting scissors
   wire Zytor s.
sutured plaque electrode
sutureless pacemaker electrode
Sutureloop
   S. colposuspension suture
SutureMate needle rest
SutureStrip Plus wound closure
suture-tying platform forceps
suturing
   s. forceps
   s. instrument
   s. needle
Sven
   S. Johansson driver
   S. Johansson extender
   S. Johansson femoral neck nail
swab
   calcium alginate s.
   Chamois s.
   Janet bladder s.
   KBM gauze s.
   Koenig tonsillar s.
   Merthiolate s.
   Phenol EZ s.
   Puritan s.
   Q-Tee cleaning s.
swaged
   s. needle
   s. suture
swaged-on
   s.-o. needle
   s.-o. suture
Swan
   S. aortic clamp
   S. corneoscleral punch
   S. discission knife
   S. eye needle holder
   S. knife-needle
   S. lancet
   S. needle
   S. spade-type needle knife
Swan-Brown arterial forceps
Swan-Ganz
   S.-G. balloon flotation catheter
   S.-G. bipolar pacing catheter
   S.-G. flow-directed catheter
   S.-G. guidewire TD catheter
   S.-G. Pacing TD catheter
   S.-G. pulmonary artery catheter
   S.-G. thermodilution catheter
   S.-G. tube
Swank high-flow arterial blood filter
swan-neck
   s.-n. clamp
   s.-n. gouge
   s.-n. Missouri catheter
   s.-n. pediatric Coil-Cath catheter
   s.-n. splint
Swann-Morton surgical blade
Swanson
   S. carpal lunate implant

   S. carpal scaphoid implant
   S. dynamic toe splint
   S. elevator
   S. finger joint implant
   S. finger joint prosthesis
   S. flexible hallux valgus prosthesis
   S. great toe implant
   S. great toe prosthesis
   S. Grip-X hand exerciser
   S. hand splint
   S. intramedullary broach
   S. mallet
   S. metacarpal prosthesis
   S. metacarpophalangeal implant
   S. metatarsal broach
   S. metatarsal prosthesis
   S. osteotome
   S. radial head implant
   S. radiocarpal implant
   S. reamer
   S. scaphoid awl
   S. Silastic elbow prosthesis
   S. Silastic implant
   S. small joint implant
   S. trapezium implant
   S. ulnar head implant
   S. wrist joint implant
   S. wrist prosthesis
swathe
   sling and s. (S&S)
Sweaper curette
Swede-O
   S.-O. ankle brace
   S.-O. Arch-lok
Swede-O-Universal
   S.-O.-U. brace
   S.-O.-U. orthosis
Swede-Vent TL self-tapping external implant
Swedgeon
   S. already-threaded needle
   S. suture
Swedish
   S. Helparm device
   S. knee cage
Swedish-pattern chisel
Sween-A-Peel wound dressing
Sweeney
   S. posterior vaginal retractor
   S. posterior vaginal speculum
sweep
   Barraquer s.
   The Cell S.
sweeper
   Cottle spicule s.
   periosteal spicule s.
   Tiko zonule s.
Sweet
   S. amputation retractor
   S. antral trocar
   S. clip-applying forceps
   S. delicate pituitary scissors
   S. dissecting forceps
   S. esophageal scissors
   S. eye magnet

S. ligature forceps
S. locator
S. original magnet
S. rib spreader
S. sternal punch
S. two-point discriminator
Sweet-Burford rib spreader
sweetheart retractor
Sweet-Tip bipolar lead
Swenko
S. bag
S. gastric-cooling apparatus
Swenson
S. cholangiography tube
S. papillotome
S. ring-jawed holding clamp
S. wire-guided
   papillotome/sphincterotome
Swets
S. goniotomy cannula
S. goniotomy knife
Swiderski nasal chisel
swift-cut phaco incision knife
SwiftLase scanner
SwimEx
S. hydrotherapy system
S. pool
swimmer's goggles
SwingAlong walker caddie
Swing DR1 DDDR pacemaker
Swinger car bed
Swiss
S. Balance orthotic
S. ball
S. blade
S. bladebreaker
S. blade holder
S. blue virgin silk suture
S. bulldog clamp
S. Kiss intrastent balloon inflation
   device
S. Lithoclast
S. Lithoclast pneumatic lithotripsy
   probe
S. MP joint implant
S. Precision cannula system
S. Therapy eye mask
Swissedent wax
Swiss-pattern speculum
Swissray scanner
switch
s. box
silicon-controlled s.
The Trigger s.
switching stick
Switzerland dilatation catheter
swivel
s. adapter
Erich s.
s. joint suture holder
s. knife
Universal s.
swivel-arm system

Swivel-Strap
S.-S. ankle brace
S.-S. ankle stirrup
Swolin self-retaining vaginal speculum
sword knife
Swyrls swim mold
Syark vulsellum forceps
Sydenham mouthgag
Syed
S. template
S. template implant
Syed-Neblett
S.-N. implant
S.-N. template
Syed-Puthawala-Hedger esophageal
   applicator
Sylva
S. anterior chamber irrigator
S. I&A unit
S. irrigating cannula
Sylver-Wax dental wax
Symbion
S. cardiac device
S. Jarvik-7 artificial heart
S. pneumatic assist device
S. total artificial heart
Symbion/CardioWest 100 mL total
   artificial heart
Symbios pacemaker
symblepharon ring
Syme
S. amputation prosthesis
S. Dycor prosthetic foot
S. foot prosthesis
symmetrical
s. sacral plate
s. thoracic vertebral plate
Symmetry endobipolar generator
Symmonds
S. hysterectomy retractor
S. needle
sympathectomy
s. hook
s. retractor
sympathetic raspatory
Symphonix Vibrant soundbridge
Symphony
S. patient monitoring system
S. stent
Symptom Rating Scale
Syms
S. traction
S. tractor
Synaptic 2000 pain management system
Synatomic total knee prosthesis
SynchroMed
S. drug administration device
S. implantable pump
S. infusion system
S. programmable pump
Synchron CX-series automated analyzer
synchronizer
CardioSync cardiac s.

S

synchronous
s. burst pacemaker
s. mode pacemaker
Synchrony I, II pacemaker
Synchrosonic stimulator
syndesmotic screw
synechia spatula
Synectics-Dantec Flo-Lab II uroflowmeter
Synectics 6000 digital pH meter
synergistic wrist motion splint
Synergist vacuum erection device
Synergy
S. frameless air support therapy
S. neurostimulation system
S. Plus
S. posterior titanium spinal system
S. Pulse frameless air support therapy
S. splint
S. ultrasound
Synergyst
S. DDD pacemaker
S. II pacemaker
Synevac vacuum curettage system
SynMesh mesh
Syn-optics camera
synoptoscope
Synovator arthroscopic blade
synovectomy
s. blade
s. rongeur
synovial
s. dissector
s. separator
synovium biopsy forceps
Synthaderm occlusive wound dressing
Synthes
S. AO reconstruction plate
S. Cervifix system
S. compression hip screw
S. dorsal distal radius plate
S. drill
S. facial curette
S. genioplate
S. guide pin
S. ligament washer
S. maxillofacial locking reconstruction plate
S. maxillofacial titanium plate
S. Microsystem drill bit
S. Microsystem plate cutter
S. mini-depth gauge
S. mini L-plate
S. Schuhli implant system
S. screw
S. stainless steel minifragment plate
S. titanium elastic nail
S. titanium minifragment plate
S. transbuccal trocar
S. Universal spinal system
synthetic
s. absorbable suture
s. hygroscopic cervical dilator
s. mesh

s. sapphire tip
s. stent
Synthetics dual-channel, solid-state Digitrapper
Synthofil suture
Syracuse anterior I-plate
Syrex syringe
Syrijet Mark II Needleless Injector
syringe
Accuguide s.
Alcock bladder s.
Alexander-Reiner ear s.
Anel s.
Arnold-Bruening s.
Arrow Raulerson introducer s.
Asepto bulb s.
aspirating s.
Autoblock safety s.
BD Luer s.
Boehm drop s.
Bruening pressure s.
bulb s.
bulbous-tip ear s.
Canyons irrigation s.
s. cap
Carti-Loid s.
Centrix s.
Cilacalcin double-chambered s.
Concord line draw s.
C-R resin s.
Cuchica s.
D s.
Davidson s.
DeVilbiss s.
Dynacor ear s.
Dynacor ulcer s.
ear s.
electric s.
ENSI s.
ExtraSafe s.
E-Z s.
Fink-Weinstein two-way s.
Fluorescite s.
FNA-21 s.
Fortuna s.
Fragmatome flute s.
Fuchs retinal detachment s.
Fuchs two-way eye s.
Gabriel s.
Gas lyte ABG s.
G-C s.
Gemini s.
glycerine s.
Goldstein anterior chamber s.
Goldstein lacrimal s.
Green-Armytage s.
Higginson irrigation s.
Ilopan disposable s.
impression material s.
Infuset GP s.
intraligamentary s.
IPAS s.
Irrigo s.
Irrivac s.
Isosal s.

laryngeal s.
LeVeen inflation s.
Lewy Teflon glycerine-mixture s.
Ligmajet s.
Luer s.
Luer-Lok B-D s.
Max-I-Probe endodontic irrigation s.
MPL aspirating s.
Multi-Fit Luer-Lok control
  tonsillar s.
Namic angiographic s.
Neisser s.
Nourse bladder s.
Osciflator balloon inflation s.
OutBound s.
Pallin spring-assisted s.
Parker-Heath anterior chamber s.
PDL intraligamentary s.
PermaRidge delivery s.
Pitkin s.
Politzer air s.
Pomeroy ear s.
Pritchard s.
Proetz s.
Pulsator anaerobic s.
s. pump
Raulerson introducer s.
Reiner-Alexander ear s.
Reiner ear s.
retinal detachment s.
Riches bladder s.
Rochester s.
Roughton-Scholander s.
Rudolph calibrated super s.
Sana-Lok s.
Schein s.
spring-assisted s.
Storz s.
Syrex s.
tapered-tip ear s.
Teflon glycerine-mixture s.
Terumo insulin s.
Tobald s.
tonsillar s.
Toomey s.
tuberculin s.
Tubex metal s.
two-way s.
Ultraject contrast media s.
Ultraject prefilled s.
VanishPoint s.
Visitec s.
Yale Luer-Lok s.
syringe-driven system
syringe-type infusion pump
syrinx shunt
Syrrat scoop
Sysmex
  S. HS-330 robotic hematology
    system
  S. NE-8000 CBC analyzer
  S. R-1000 reticulocyte counter
SysStim muscle stimulator
System-1
  Topographic Modeling S.

System-4
  GENTLE TOUCH Loop Ostomy S.
System-
system
  ABaer s.
  ABBI s.
  Abbott LifeCare PCA Plus II
    infusion s.
  Abbott Lifeshield needleless s.
  ABG cement-free hip s.
  Abiomed biventricular support s.
  ABL520 blood gas measurement s.
  Above-Knee Suction Enhancement s.
  Accents s.
  Access MV s.
  Accu-Chek Advantage non-wipe
    blood glucose monitoring s.
  Accu-Chek InstantPlus s.
  accuDEXA bone mineral density
    assessment s.
  AccuLength arthroplasty
    measuring s.
  AccuMeter cholesterol test s.
  Accurus vitrectomy s.
  AccuSway balance measurement s.
  Ace intramedullary femoral nail s.
  Acra-clip s.
  Acra-gun s.
  Acryl-X orthopaedic cement
    removal s.
  Action traction s.
  Activa tremor control s.
  ACTIVE LIFE FLUSHAWAY one-
    piece flushable closed-end
    pouch s.
  ACT MicroCoil delivery s.
  Acucair continuous airflow s.
  AcuFix anterior cervical plate s.
  Acuson 128XP ultrasound s.
  Acutrak bone fixation s.
  Acutrak bone replacement s.
  Acutrak fusion s.
  Adapteur power s.
  Add-On Bucky digital x-ray image
    acquisition s.
  Adjustaback wheelchair backrest s.
  Adolph Gasser camera s.
  Advanced Cardiovascular S. (ACS)
  Advanced Medical Systems fetal
    monitoring s.
  Advancit guidewire s.
  Advantim revision knee s.
  Advantx LC+ cardiovascular
    imaging s.
  AEGIS sonography management s.
  AERx diabetes management s.
  AERx pain management s.
  AERx pulmonary drug delivery s.
  Affirm VP microbial
    identification s.
  Affymetrix GeneChip s.
  AGC Biomet total knee s.
  Agee carpal tunnel release s.
  Agee WristJack fracture reduction s.
  Agfa CR s.

S

system *(continued)*
Agfa PACS s.
AI 5200 diagnostic ultrasound s.
AIM femoral nail s.
Air-Back spinal s.
AirFlo alternating pressure s.
Airis II MRI s.
Air-Limb edema control s.
AI 5200 S open color Doppler
    imaging s.
AITA modular trauma s.
AlaSTAT allergy immunoassay s.
Albert Grass Heritage digital
    EEG s.
Alcon Closure S. (ACS)
Alexa 1000 breast diagnostic s.
Alice 4 diagnostic sleep s.
All Access laser s.
Allen traction s.
Allen Universal stirrup s.
Alliance integrated inflation s.
Alliance rehabilitation s.
AlloMune s.
Allo-Pro hip s.
Aloka color Doppler s.
Aloka SD, SSD ultrasound s.
Alphatec mini lag-screw s.
Alphatec small fragment s.
Alta modular trauma s.
S. 2000 alternating pressure pump
    & pad overlay
ALTERNS therapeutic seating s.
ALT ultrasound s.
AMBI compression hip screw s.
AMK total knee s.
AMO Prestige advanced cataract
    extraction s.
AMO-Prestige phaco s.
Amplatz anchor s.
Amplatz TractMaster s.
Amset anterior locking plate s.
Anatomic hip s.
Anchor IIa osseointegrated titanium
    implant s.
Anchorlok s.
ANCOR imaging s.
Ancure s.
AngeCool RF catheter ablation s.
Anger gamma camera s.
AngioJet rheolytic thrombectomy s.
Angiomat 6000 contrast delivery s.
AngioRad radiation s.
Angio-Seal hemostasis s.
AngioVista angiographic s.
AnkleTough ankle rehabilitation s.
Anspach 65K instrument s.
anterior cervical plate fixation s.
    (ACFS)
AOA/CHICK ambulatory halo s.
AO/ASIF titanium craniofacial s.
AO mandibular s.
Aortic Connector s.
Apex irrigation s.
Apogee CX 200 echo s.

Apogee 800 ultrasound s.
Apollo DXA bone densitometry s
Apollo 95E tooth-whitening and
    curing s.
Apollo hip s.
APR total hip s.
Aqua-Cel heating pad s.
Aquanex hydrodynamic
    measurement s.
AquaSens FMS 1000 fluid
    monitoring s.
AquaSens FMS 1000 fluid
    monitoring s.
Aqua Spray debridement s.
Arcitumomab diagnostic imaging s
arc-quadrant stereotactic s.
Argyle-Turkel safety thoracentesis
Arndorfer infusion s.
Arndorfer pneumohydraulic capillar
    infusion s.
Arnett-TMP s.
arrhythmia mapping s.
Arrow UserGard injection cap s.
ArthroCare multielectrode s.
Arthro-Flo powered irrigation s.
Arthro-Lok s.
Arthroscan video s.
ArthroSew suturing s.
Artoscan MRI s.
Artus power s.
ASAP Stacker automated multi-
    sample biopsy s.
Ascent total knee s.
Aspen digital ultrasound s.
Aspen echocardiography s.
AspenVAC smoke evacuation s.
Aspire continuous imaging s.
Assure blood glucose monitoring
Aston cartilage reduction s.
Astro-Med Albert Grass Heritage
    digital EEG s.
Atakr s.
Athena high frequency
    mammography s.
Atlas 2.0 diagnostic ultrasound s.
AtLast blood glucose s.
ATL high definition imaging s.'s
A-Trac atraumatic clamping s.
Atridox drug delivery s.
Atrigel drug delivery s.
Atrium Blood Recovery S.
ATS 500/1500 tourniquet s.
AuRA cemented total hip s.
Aura laser s.
Aurora dedicated breast MRI s.
Aurora diode-based dental laser s.
Aurora MR breast imaging s.
AutoCyte Image Analysis s.
autoLog autotransfusion s.
automated angle-encoder s.
automated cellular imaging s.
Autoread centrifuge hematology s.
AutoSet portable s.
Auto Suture ABBI s.
Autovac LF autotransfusion s.

Avi lens s.
Aviva mammography s.
Axiom modular knee s.
AxyaWeld bone anchor s.
BABE OB ultrasound reporting s.
Babyflex heated ventilation s.
BacFix s.
Back Bull lumbar support s.
BacT/Alert automated blood
culture s.
BACTEC automated blood
culture s.
Badal stimulus s.
BAK/C interbody fusion s.
BAK interbody fusion s.
BAK-1 interbody fusion s.
BAK/T interbody fusion s.
Balance Master training and
assessment s.
Bard cardiopulmonary support
(CPS) s.
Bard percutaneous cardiopulmonary
support s.
Bard rotary atherectomy s.
Bard urinary sterile collection s.
Bard Urolase fiber laser s.
BariKare advanced power s.
BAT s.
Bateman UPF II bipolar knee s.
Baxter Interline IV s.
Baxter InterLink needle s.
Baylor autologous transfusion s.
BCELL-HDM - filtering s.
BDProbeTec ET s.
Beamer injection stent s.
Becker orthopaedic spinal s.
(BOSS)
Becker orthopaedic thermoformable
ankle s.
Becker-Rojas Sub-Sonic surgical s.
Becker vibrating cannula s.
Beckman ICS Nephelometer s.
bedside sterile drainage collection s.
Bennett contour mammography s.
Benzaquen-Chajchir
extraction/reinjection s.
Betaseron needle-free delivery s.
Better Than Another Pair of Hands
retractor s.
Bevalac s.
BIAcore s.
Biad SPECT imaging s.
BIAS total hip s.
bilateral variable screw placement s.
Bilibed phototherapy s.
BiliBlanket phototherapy s.
BiliCheck battery-powered s.
Biodex Unweighing s.
BioDimensional s.
Biodynamic molding s.
Bio-Esthetic abutment s.
Bio-Fit total hip s.
Bio Flote air flotation s.
Biogel Reveal puncture indication s.

Biojector 2000 needle-free injection
management s.
BioLab modular motility s.
BioLogic DT-HT s.
BioMedx portable air flotation s.
Biomet Ascent total knee s.
Biomet Finn salvage/oncology knee
reconstruction s.
Biomet Genus uniknee s.
Biomet Maxim revision knee s.
Biomet Maxim total knee s.
Biomet Ultra-Drive ultrasonic
revision s.
Bio-Modular total shoulder s.
Bionicare 1000 stimulator s.
Bio-Optics Bambi cell analysis s.
Bio-Optics Bambi image analysis s.
Bioplate screw fixation s.
Bioport collection and transport s.
bioptic amorphic lens s.
BioRad Model 5000 Titanium s.
bioresorbable drug delivery s.
Biosense NOGA catheter-based
endocardial mapping s.
Biosound AU (Advanced
Ultrasonography) s.
Biosound Phase 2 ultrasound s.
Biospec MR imaging s.
BioStinger fixation s.
biotelemetry s.
BIOWARE software for Biodex
isokinetic exercise s.
BioZ s.
biphasic s.
BI-RADS breast imaging and
reporting data s.
BIRO s.
Bitome bipolar s.
BKS refractive s.
Blade-Vent implant s.
Blajwas-Schwartz-Marcinko irrigation
drainage s.
BMP cabling and plating s.
Body Logic rehabilitation s.
Body Masters MD 510 hi-lo
pulley s.
Body Response s.
Boehringer Autovac
autotransfusion s.
Bolin wedge filter s.
Bonchek-Shiley vein distention s.
bone tack s.
Bosker TMI Reconstruction s.
Bosker transmandibular reconstructive
surgical s.
BosPac cardiopulmonary bypass s.
Boston elbow s.
Bottoms-Up posture s.
Bracco s.
BrachyVision brachytherapy
planning s.
Brackmann II EMG s.
BrainLAB VectorVision
neuronavigational s.
BrainSCAN computer planning s.

S

system *(continued)*
BrainSCAN Linac radiosurgery s.
Branemark implant s.
Bremer halo crown s.
Bridge hip s.
Bristol-Myers s.
BriteSmile laser tooth whitening s.
Broselow/Hinkle s.
Browlift Bone Bridge s.
Brown-Roberts-Wells stereotactic s.
Bruel & Kjaer 1846 ultrasound s.
Bruker Biospec s.
Bruker CSI MR s.
Bruker S 200 MR s.
BRW stereotactic s.
BTA S-2000 biofeedback s.
Budde halo retractor s.
Burette multiple patient delivery s.
Buzard Diamond Barraqueratome
  Microkeratome s.
BWM spine s.
CADD-Prizm pain control s.
CADD-TPN ambulatory infusion s.
Cadence tiered therapy
  defibrillator s.
Cafet s.
Calasept medicament delivery s.
Calcitek drill s.
Calcitek implant s.
caliceal s.
Camino intracranial pressure
  monitoring s.
Canal Finder s.
Candela videoimaging s.
Cannulated Plus screw s.
Can-Opt dual-lumen ERCP s.
Capasee diagnostic ultrasound s.
Capintec VEST s.
Capiox SX gas and heat exchange
  oxygenation s.
CAPIS bone plate s.
CAP/3SBII angiogram projection s.
capsule applier s.
Carbon Monotube long bone
  fracture external fixation s.
CardiData Prodigy s.
CardioCamera imaging s.
Cardio3DScope imaging s.
Cardiofreezer cryosurgical s.
CardioGenesis PMR s.
cardiopulmonary support s.
cardioscope U s.
Cardiovascular Angiography
  Analysis S. (CAAS)
Cardiovit AT-10 ECG/spirometry
  combination s.
cartesian reference coordinate s.
Cascade Up and About s.
CASE computerized exercise
  EKG s.
CASE Marquette 16 exercise s.
CASS whole-brain mapping s.
Castle Daystar surgical television s.
Catarex cataract removal s.

catheter-tip micromanometer s.
Cath-Finder catheter tracking s.
CathTrack catheter locator s.
CatsEye digital camera s.
Cavi-Endo ultrasonic s.
Cavitron I&A s.
Cavitron-Kelman I&A s.
CB Erbium/2.94 laser s.
CC Rider closed-chain
  rehabilitation s.
CDI 2000 blood gas monitoring s.
CDRPan digital x-ray s.
Ceegraph 128 EEG s.
Celay s.
Cell Analysis s.
CellFIT acquisition s.
Cell Recovery S.
Cell Saver Haemonetics
  autotransfusion s.
Cell Soft s.
Cemex s.
Cencit imaging s.
Cenflex central monitoring s.
Centauri Er:YAG laser s.
Centrax bipolar s.
CeraOne implant s.
CerviFix s.
CFC BioScanner s.
CGR biplane angiographic s.
ChamberLift 2000 patient lift s.
Champy miniplate rigid fixation s.
Charnley Howorth ExFlow s.
Chattanooga Balance s.
ChemoBloc vial venting s.
Chemo-Port perivena catheter s.
C-2 hip s.
Chirotech x-ray s.
Chocstruct chondral repair s.
Cholestech L-D-X office lab s.
Chromos imager s.
ChromoVision video s.
Cinch bladder neck suspension
  anchor s.
Cineloop image review ultrasound s.
CineView Plus Freeland s.
CircPlus bandage/wrap s.
Circulaire aerosol drug delivery s.
Circul'Air shoe s.
Circulator boot s.
CIS-2 s.
CKS knee s.
Clark hemoperfusion s.
Clave needleless s.
Clensicair incontinence
  management s.
Clinac 600SR stereotactic radiation
  treatment s.
Clinical HandMaster s.
Clini-Care low-air-loss s.
Clini.Float flotation therapy bed s.
closed-circuit television vision
  enhancement s.
CMI vacuum delivery s.
COBE Spectra apheresis s.
Coburn I&A s.

Codman anterior cervical plating (ACP) s.
Codman external drainage s.
Codman neurological headrest s.
Codman Ti-frame posterior fixation s.
COER-24 delivery s.
Cofield 2 total shoulder s.
Cohort anterior plate s.
Co₂ject s.
Coleman microinfiltration s.
Colin Electronics BP-508 tonometry s.
CollectFirst s.
Colopast Sween sealed dispensing s.
Coltene direct inlay s.
Combi Multi-Traction s.
Comfort Care bed s.
Comfort Cast casting s.
Command hip instrumentation s.
Companion 314, 318 nasal CPAP s.
Compass arc-quadrant stereotactic s.
Compass CT stereotaxic adaptation s.
Compass frame-based stereotactic s.
Complement C31 desArg Biotrack RIA s.
Compton suppression s.
Computed Anatomy Corneal Modeling S.
computer-aided sleep s.
computer-assisted neurosurgical navigational s.
computer-controlled neurological stimulation s.
computerized bedside transfusion identification s.
computerized image analysis s.
computerized morphometric s.
Concept beachchair shoulder positioning s.
Concept Precise ACL guide s.
Concept rotator cuff repair s.
Concept self-compressing cannulated screw s.
Concept Sterling arthroscopy blade s.
Conceptus fallopian tube catheterization s.
Concept video imaging s.
Concept zone-specific cannula s.
condom catheter collecting s.
ConQuest incontinent s.
ConstaVac autoreinfusion s.
Contact SPH cups s.
contact-tip laser s.
continuous insulin delivery s. (CIDS)
continuous-wave, high-frequency Doppler ultrasound s.
continuous-wave laser s.
Continuum knee s.
Contour Genesis ultrasonic-assisted liposuction s.

Contour tilting compression mammography s.
Contrajet ERCP contrast delivery s.
Convertible trocar s.
Coombs bone biopsy s.
CooperSurgical monopolar ELSG LEEP s.
Coordinate complete revision knee s.
Corail hip s.
Cordis endovascular s.
CoreVent Implant s.
Corin hip s.
corneal topography s.
CorneaSparing LTK s.
Corometrics Medical Systems Inc. fetal monitoring s.
coronary angiography analysis s.
Coroscop C cardiac imaging s.
Cosgrove-Edwards annuloplasty s.
Cosman ICP Tele-Sensor s.
Cosman-Roberts-Wells stereotactic s.
Cotrel-Dubousset distraction s.
Cotrel-Dubousset screw-rod s.
CPD Commander combined air/fluid exchange and silicone oil delivery s.
Cragg Endopro s.
cranial osteosynthesis s.
cranial plating s.
craniomaxillofacial plating s.
CritiCore monitoring s.
Crown mattress s.
Crown recliner s.
CRS tibial torsion s.
CRW stereotactic s.
CRYOcare cryoablation s.
Cryo/Cuff knee compression dressing s.
Cryomedics electrosurgery s.
CRYO-VAC-A cryostat vacuum s.
CrystalEyes endoscopic video s.
CTDx electrostimulation s.
CT-MRI-compatible stereotactic head frame s.
C-Trak surgical guidance s.
Cuidant s.
Curix Capacity Plus film processing s.
CurvTek s.
CUSA CEM s.
Cusp-Lok cuspid traction s.
CustomCornea wavefront measurement s.
C-VEST radiation detector s.
CVIS/InterTherapy intravascular ultrasound s.
Cyberware s.
Cybex I, II+ exercise s.
Cybex 340 isokinetic rehabilitation and testing s.
Cygnet Laboratories fetal monitoring s.
Cytomax bar-guided brush cytology s.

S

system *(continued)*
Cyto-Rich cervical cytology
monolayer s.
Dall-Miles cable/crimp cerclage s.
Dall-Miles cable grip s.
Dansac irrigation s.
Dantec 12-channel Urocolor
video s.
Dantec Etude s.
Dantec Menuet s.
DAR breathing s.
DataHand s.
da Vinci surgical s.
Davol irrigation s.
DawSkin flexible protective skin s.
DCI-S automated coronary
analysis s.
Deknatel orthopedic
autotransfusion s.
DELTAmanager MedImage s.
Deltoid-Aid arm counterbalance s.
DentiCAD s.
DentiPatch lidocaine transoral
delivery s.
Dent manometry s.
Dentsply implant s.
Denver hydrocephalus shunt s.
Derma K laser s.
DermaLase laser s.
Derma 20 laser s.
DermMaster first macroabrasion s.
Desilets introducer s.
DFS 2 mattress replacement s.
Diab-A-Foot protection s.
Dialys-Aids S.
Diasonics Sonotron Vingmed CFM
800 imaging s.
dichroic filter s.
Difco ESP testing s.
Digi-Flex exercise s.
Digi Grip traction s.
Digital Add-On Bucky image
acquisition s.
Digital B s.
Digital Traumex s.
Digitrapper Mark II pH
monitoring s.
Digitron digital subtraction
imaging s.
dilator-sheath s.
DIMAQ integrated ultrasound s.
Dimension hip s.
Dinamap s.
Dingman oral retraction s.
DioLite 532 laser s.
Dioptimum s.
Director Guidewire s.
Disten-U-Flo fluid s.
Dobbhoff G/J s.
Dolphin hysteroscopic fluid
management s.
Doppler Quantum color flow s.
DORC fast freeze cryosurgical s.

Dormia extracorporeal shockwave
lithotripsy s.
DPAP interactive airway
management s.
Drake-Willock automatic delivery
DryView laser imaging s.
Dualer Plus s.
Dual-Port s.
Dual Quattrode spinal cord
stimulation s.
Dual Range Limiter s.
Dumbach mandibular
reconstruction s.
Dumon-Gilliard endoprosthesis s.
Dunlap cold compression wrap s.
Duoloid impression s.
Duovisc viscoelastic s.
DUPEL iontophoretic drug
delivery s.
Dupont distal humeral plate s.
DuPont rare earth imaging s.
Duracon PS total knee s.
Duraloc acetabular cup s.
Dur-A-Sil silicone impression s.
Durasul large diameter head s.
Duret s.
DUX s.
Dymer excimer delivery s.
Dyna-Care pressure pad s.
DynaFix external fixation s.
Dyna-Flex multilayer compression
DynaGuard LAL low-air-loss
pressure management s.
Dyna-Lok plating s.
Dynamic optical breast imaging s.
Dynamite mattress s.
Dynarad portable imaging s.
Dynasplint shoulder s.
Dyonics Dyosite office
arthroscopy s.
Dyonics IntelliJet fluid
management s.
Dyonics PS3500 drive s.
EAGLE s.
Easy Analysis s.
EasyGuide Neuro image-guided
surgery s.
Easy Introduction s.
EBI bone healing s.
E.CAM dual-head emission
imaging s.
Eccocee ultrasound s.
EccoVision acoustic rhinometry s.
EchoFlow blood velocity meter s.
Echovar Doppler s.
Eclipse infusion s.
ECTRA s.
Edentrace sleep s.
EDG s.
Edwards modular s.
e10 electrosurgery s.
Eklund breast positioning s.
Elan-E electronic motor s.
ElastaTrac home lumbar traction
Electri-Cool cold therapy s.

electroshield monitoring s.
electrotherapy s.
Elite hip s.
Ellman press-form s.
Elscint tomography s.
Embolyx liquid embolic s.
Emerald implantation s.
Emergence Profile implant s.
emergency life support s.
EnAbl thermal ablation s.
ENAC ultrasonic instrument s.
Encore ceramic hip and knee joint
  replacement s.'s
Endermologie adipose destruction s.
End-Flo laparoscopic irrigating s.
Endobag laparoscopic specimen
  retrieval s.
Endocam video camera s.
endocavitary applicator s.
Endodermologie LPG s.
Endoflex endoscopic instrument s.
EndoMed LSS laparoscopy s.
Endopath Optiview s.
Endopore dental implant s.
Endoprothetik CSL-Plus cemented-
  hip s.
EndoSaph vein harvest s.
endoscopic carpal tunnel release s.
EndoSheath endoscopy s.
Endotak lead s.
Endotek urodynamics s.
Endo Tip port s.
Endotrac blade s.
Endotrac endoscopic carpal tunnel
  release s.
EnGuard double-lead ICD s.
EnGuard pacing and defibrillation
  lead s.
ENtec surgery s.
Entree II trocar and cannula s.
Entree Plus trocar and cannula s.
Epic ophthalmic 3-in-1 laser s.
EpiLaser laser-based hair removal s.
EpiLight hair removal s.
EpiTouch Alex laser hair
  removal s.
EpiTouch ruby SilkLaser hair
  removal s.
Equinox EEG neuromonitoring s.
ErecAid vacuum s.
Ergo irrigation s.
ErgoTec vitreoretinal instrument s.
Erie s.
E-series hip s.
ESSential shaver s.
Estilux ultraviolet s.
EUB-405 ultrasound s.
EVIS 140 endoscope reprocessing s.
Evoport auditory evoked potential s.
Exact-Fit ATH hip replacement s.
Exact-Touch Saccomanno Pap smear
  collection s.
EXAKT cutting/grinding s.
EX-FI-RE external fixation s.
Exonix ultrasonic surgical s.

Explorer common bile duct
  exploration s.
Extend total hip s.
extracorporeal membrane
  oxygenation s.
eyeFix speculum s.
EyeMap EH-290 corneal
  tomography s.
EyeSys 2000 corneal topographic
  mapping s.
EZE-FIT IOL s.
E-Z-EM BioGun automated
  biopsy s.
E-Z Flap cranial flap fixation s.
E-Z Flap titanium miniplate s.
EZ-ON traction belt s.
E-Z Tac soft-tissue reattachment s.
facet screw s.
Falcon FX8000 DEEP CELL
  alternating support surface s.
F.A.S.T.1 adult intraosseous
  infusion s.
FASTak suture anchor s.
FastTake blood glucose
  monitoring s.
Feather-Lite Pouching S.
FeatherTouch SilkLaser s.
fecal containment s.
feedback s.
feedback control s.
Fenlin total shoulder s.
Ferno AquaCiser underwater
  treadmill s.
Ferno Recline-a-Bath bathing s.
Fetasonde fetal monitoring s.
FiberLase beam delivery s.
fiberoptic catheter delivery s.
fiberTome s.
Fillauer endoskeletal alignment s.
FIN s.
Finger Phantom pulse oximeter
  testing s.
Finn knee revision s.
FirstQ departure alert s.
Fischer modular stereotaxic s.
Fitnet joint testing s.
Fixateur Interne fixation s.
FlapMaker microkeratome s.
Fletcher-Suit-Delclos s.
Flexiflo gastrostomy tube enteral
  delivery s.
Flexi-Therm liquid crystal s.
F. L. Fischer modular stereotaxy s.
FlimFax teleradiology s.
Flo-Stat fluid management s.
FLOWPLUS therapeutic pneumatic
  compression s.
Flowtron DVT external pneumatic
  compression s.
Flowtron Excel DVI prophylaxis s.
FluoroPlus Roadmapper digital
  fluoroscopy s.
fluoroptic thermometry s.
"flying spot" excimer laser s.
FMA cardiovascular imaging s.

S

system *(continued)*
F-MAT screening s.
FOAMART foot impression s.
Fonar s.
Fonix 6500-CX hearing aid test s.
Foot-Station 3-D foot imaging s.
Force GSU argon-enhanced
electrosurgery s.
foreign body retrieval s.
Foundation total hip s.
Foundation total knee s.
FPS s.
fracture computer-aided surgery
(FRACAS) s.
Frag Commander ultrasonic pars
plana lensectomy s.
frameless air support therapy s.
frameless stereotaxy s.
Frank EKG lead placement s.
Frank XYZ orthogonal lead s.
Freedom leg bag collection s.
Freehand neuroprosthetic s.
FreeLock femoral fixation s.
free-standing tissue retraction
bridge s.
French Pharmacovigilance s.
Fresenius volumetric dialysate
balancing s.
FRIALITE-2 dental implant s.
F-Scan foot force and gait
analysis s.
Fuji AC2 storage phosphor
computed radiology s.
Fuji FCR9000 computed
radiology s.
Fujinon SP-501 sonoprobe s.
Galen teleradiology s.
Gambro hemofiltration s.
GastrograpH ambulatory pH
monitoring s.
Gastroscan motility s.
GDLH posterior spinal s.
GD Regainer s.
GE 9800 CT s.
GE CT Hi-Speed Advantage s.
GEL-U-SLEEP series III floatation
mattress s.
General Electric Advantx s.
GenESA closed-loop delivery s.
Genesis II total knee s.
Genotropin s.
GentleLASE laser s.
Gentle Touch colostomy/ileostomy
postoperative s.
Genucom ACL laxity analysis s.
Genucom knee flexion analysis s.
GE Senographe 2000D
mammography s.
GE Signa MR s.
GE single-axis SR-230
echoplanar s.
GFX2 coronary stent s.
Gillette double-flexure ankle joint s.

Gleeson FloVAC Hi-Flo
laparoscopic suction-irrigation s.
GliaSite radiation therapy RTS s.
Global Fx shoulder fracture s.
Global total shoulder arthroplasty
Glucocheck Pocketlab II blood
glucose s.
Glucometer DEX s.
Glucometer II home glucose
monitoring s.
GlyMed Camouflage s.
gNomos stereotactic s.
Goldenberg implant s.
Gold Series bone drilling s.
Golf exercise s.
GoodKnight 418 CPAP home-
care s.
Graf stabilization s.
Granberg cervical traction s.
Grasping Stitcher s.
Grass neurodata s.
Gravity Lumbar Traction s.
Gray revision instrument s.
Greenberg retracting s.
Greenfield vena cava filter s.
Grieshaber power injector s.
GTS great toe s.
Guardian DNA s.
Guardian two-piece ostomy s.
Guidant Heart Rhythm Technologi
Linear Ablation s.
Guidant TRIAD three-electrode
energy defibrillation s.
guided trephine s. (GTS)
Guldmann Overhead Trac s.
Gx-99 vibratory endermatherapie s
Gynecare Thermachoice uterine
balloon therapy s.
Gynecare Verascope hysteroscopy
Gyroscan HP Philips 15S whole-
body s.
HA-biointegrated dental implant s.
Haemolite autologous blood
recovery s.
Haemonetics Cell Saver s.
Haid Universal bone plate s.
Hakim valve s.
Halifax interlaminar clamp s.
Hall mandibular implant s.
Hall modular acetabular reamer s.
halo cervical traction s.
Halo CO_2 laser s.
halo retractor s.
HandiCare adult disposable pant a
pad s.
Hands Free knee retractor s.
Hariri-Heifetz microsurgical s.
Harrington rod and hook s.
Hausmann Work-Well work
hardening s.
HCMI chiropractic s.
HDI 1000, 3000, 5000
ultrasound s.
heads-up imaging s.

HeartMate implantable pneumatic left ventricular assist s.
HeartMate left ventricular assist s.
Heartport catheter s.
Heartport Port-Access s.
HeartPort PrecisionOP s.
HEARTrac I Cardiac Monitoring s.
Helios diagnostic imaging s.
Helix multihead nuclear imaging s.
HELP s.
Hematome s.
HemoCue blood glucose s.
Hemopure oxygen-based therapeutic s.
Henning s.
heparin-induced extracorporeal lipoprotein precipitation s.
HepatAssist bioartificial liver s.
Herculite XRV lab s.
Heritage hip s.
Hermes Evolution tricompartmental knee s.
Hermes total knee s.
Hermetic external ventricular drainage s.
Hermetic external ventricular and lumbar drainage s.'s
Hermetic II drainage management s.
Hessburg subpalpebral lavage s.
Hewlett-Packard 5 MHz phased-array TEE s.
Hewlett-Packard phased-array imaging s.
Hewlett-Packard Sonos 1000, 1500 ultrasound s.
Hexcel total condylar knee s.
Hex-Fix s.
Hexon illumination s.
HICOR s.
high-field s.
high-force Sundt clip s.
high-resolution brain SPECT s.
HIMAC s.
hipGRIP pelvic positioning s.
Hipokrat bimodular shoulder s.
hipRAP pelvic positioning s.
Hi-Star midfield MRI s.
Histofreezer cryosurgical s.
Hitachi EUB-405 imaging s.
Hitachi Open MRI s.
Hitachi UB 420 digital ultrasound s.
Hix-Fix fracture fixation s.
Hoek-Bowen cement removal s.
Hoffmann external fixation s.
Holter external drainage s.
Holter hydrocephalus shunt s.
Homepump infusion s.
HomMed monitoring s.
homonuclear spin s.
Hopkins angle-view 30-degree optical s.
Hopkins II optical s.
Hopkins rod lens s.
Hopkins straight-view optical s.

Horizon AutoAdjust CPAP s.
Horizon nasal CPAP s.
Hot/Ice S. III
House grading s.
Howmedica HNR s.
Howmedica pediatric osteotomy s.
Howmedica total ankle s.
Howmedica Unitrax hip fracture s.
HP SONOS 5500 ultrasound imaging s.
Humphrey ATLAS Eclipse corneal topography s.
Humphrey Mastervue corneal topography s.
Hunsaker Mon-Jet tube anesthesia s.
Hunstad tumescent anesthesia s.
Hybrid capture s.
HybridFit total hip s.
HybridFit total knee s.
Hydradjust urology s.
hydraulic capillary infusion s.
Hydra Vision ES urologic s.
Hydra Vision IV urology s.
Hydra Vision Plus urologic s.
HydroFlex irrigation s.
HydroThermAblator s.
HyperPACS s.
Hypobaric transfemoral s.
Hypobaric transtibial s.
Hysteroser contact hysteroscopy s.
HY-TEC automated allergy diagnostic s.
I&A s.
IBM Speech Server clinical reporting s.
IDIS angiography s.
ID-Micro typing s.
Igloo Heatshield s.
iiRAD DR1000C digital radiographic s.
IL 1640 blood gas/electrolyte s.
Ilizarov limb-lengthening s.
Illumina Pro Series CO_2 surgical laser s.
image analysis s.
ImageNet image digitizing s.
Image-View s.
Imatron s.
IMCOR No-Touch implant placement s.
Imexlab vascular diagnostic s.
Immediate Implant Impression s.
Immediate Response Mobile Analysis blood analysis s.
Immunomedics s.
Impact lithotriptor s.
Impact modular total hip s.
Impax PACS s.
Impingement-Free tibial guide s.
ImplaMed implant s.
Implatome dental tomography s.
IMx PSA s.
IMZ implant s.
INCA s.
Incardia valve s.

system *(continued)*
InCare pelvic floor therapy office s.
In Charge diabetes control s.
Infant Flow nasal CPAP s.
In-Fast bone screw s.
Infiniti catheter introducer s.
Infinity hip s.
InFix interbody fusion s.
InfraGuide delivery s.
Infus-a-port vascular access s.
Infuset T fluid delivery s.
InjecAid s.
Innomed arthroplasty measuring s.
Innova feminine incontinence
treatment s.
Innova home incontinence
therapy s.
Innovator Holter s.
Insall-Burstein II modular knee s.
Insight knee positioning and
alignment s.
InSIGHT manometry s.
InstaTrak s.
Instrumentation Laboratory s.
In-Tac bone anchoring s.
Integral hip s.
Integra skin replacement s.
integrated automatic stone-tissue
detection s.
integrated lead s.
integrated life support s.
Integris cardiac imaging s.
IntelliJet fluid management s.
Intensified Radiographic Imaging S.
Inteq small joint suturing s.
Interax total knee s.
Intermedics natural hip s.
International 10-20 s.
International Biomedical Mode 745-
100 microcapillary infusion s.
International compression s.
Interpore IMZ implant s.
interprobe s.
IntraArc 9963 arthroscopic power s.
IntraLuminal Safe-Steer guidewire s.
Intra-Op autotransfusion s.
intraspinal drug infusion s.
Inverter vitrectomy s.
INVOS 3100 cerebral oximeter
monitoring s.
Iontophor drug delivery s.
ipos arch support s.
IRIS OcuLight SLx indirect
ophthalmoscope delivery s.
IRMA blood gas analysis s.
Irri-Cath suction s.
irrigation bipolar s.
Irrijet DS irrigation s.
Irvine viable organ-tissue
transport s.
IS1000 gel documentation
imaging s.
Isocam scintillation imaging s.

Isocam SPECT imaging s.
Isola fixation s.
Isola spinal implant s.
Isola spinal instrumentation s.
Isolator blood culture s.
Isolex 300i stem cell selection s.
Isotechnologies B-200 back testing
and rehabilitation s.
i-STAT s.
ITI dental implant s.
Itrel II, III spinal cord
stimulation s.
IVAC needleless IV s.
JACE continuous passive motion
ankle s.
Jackson staging s.
Jay Care wheelchair seating s.
Jay seating s.
Jimmy John colonic irrigation s.
Jinotti closed suctioning s.
Jobst athrombic pump s.
Johnson & Johnson PFC Sigma
Joyce-Loebl Magiscan image
analysis s.
JS Quick-fill s.
Jurgan pin-ball s.
J-Vac closed wound drainage s.
Kaneda anterior scoliosis s.
Kaneda anterior spinal s.
Karl Storz pediatric bronchoscopy
Katena Quick Switch I/A s.
KaVo oral surgery s.
K-Centrum anterior spinous
fixation s.
Kellan capsular sparing s.
Kelley-Goerss Compass
stereotactic s.
Kelly stereotactic s.
Kendall A-V impulse s.
Kendall Ventex wound dressing s
Keratom excimer laser s.
K-Fix fixator s.
Kiethly-DAS series 500 data-
acquisition s.
Kinamed Exact-Fit ATH s.
Kin-Con isokinetic exercise s.
Kinematic II condylar and stabili
total knee s.
Kinematic II rotating-hinge knee
Kinemax modular condylar and
stabilizer total knee s.
Kinemax Plus total knee s.
Kinemetric guide s.
Kinetik great toe implant s.
King double-umbrella closure s.
Kirschner hip replacement s.
Kirschner II-C shoulder s.
Kirschner integrated shoulder s.
Kirschner Medical Dimension hip
replacement s.
Kleen-Needle s.
KLS-Martin modular
osteosynthesis s.
Knee Signature S.
Koeller illumination s.

Koenig MPJ implant and arthroplasty s.
KOH colpotomizer s.
Konan SP8000 image analysis s.
Kostuik-Harrington anterior distraction s.
Kostuik-Harrington distraction s.
Kostuik internal spine fixation s.
Kowa fluorescein s.
Kretz ultrasound s.
KTP/Nd:YAG XP surgical laser s.
KTP/532 surgical laser s.
KTP/YAG surgical laser s.
Kulzer inlay s.
laboratory automation s.
LactoSorb plating s.
LactoSorb resorbable fixation s.
LADARVision excimer laser s.
Ladd fiberoptic s.
LAGB system - Lap-Band adjustable gastric banding s.
Laitinen CT guidance s.
Laitinen stereotactic s.
Lambda Plus PDL 1, 2 laser s.
Lambotte exhaust s.
laminar flow s.
LaminOss implant s.
Lamis infusion s.
Langerman diamond knife s.
Lanier clinical reporting s.
Laparolift s.
Laparomed cholangiogram vacuum s.
laparoscopic retraction s.
Laparo Vac I&A s.
Lap-Band gastric banding s.
Lapro-Clip ligating clip s.
LaseAway ruby laser s.
laser CHRP rigid fiberscope s.
LASER I bubble s.
LaserScan LSX excimer laser s.
LCS mobile bearing knee s.
LCS total knee s.
LDD delivery s.
Lectromed urinary investigation s.
Leibinger Locking s.
Leibinger miniplate s.
Leibinger plating s.
Leibinger Profyle hand s.
Leibinger titanium mini Würzburg implant s.
Leibinger titanium Würzburg mandibular reconstruction s.
Leitz image analysis s.
Leksell Micro-Stereotactic s.
Leksell stereotactic s.
Lens Comfort ultrasound cleaning and disinfecting s.
Lens Opacities Classification S. II
Leukotrap RC storage s.
Leukotrap red cell storage s.
Level Anchorage s.
Level I normothermic irrigating s.
Liberty spinal s.
Lido Active Multijoint s.
Lidoback isokinetic dynamometry s.

Lido Passive Multijoint s.
Liebel-Flarsheim CT 9000 contrast delivery s.
Life-Air 1000 hypothermic therapy s.
Lifecore Restore wide diameter implant s.
LIFE-Lung fluorescence endoscopy s.
Lifepath AAA endovascular graft s.
LifeScan blood glucose monitoring s.
LigaSure vessel sealing s.
LINAC s.
    linear accelerator system
LINAC-based radiosurgical s.
linear accelerator s. (LINAC system)
Linear total hip s.
Link custom partial pelvis replacement s.
Link Endo-Model rotational knee s.
Link Lubinus AP hip s.
Link Lubinus SP II total hip replacement s.
Link Saddle Prosthesis Endo-Model hip replacement s.
Liposorber LA-15 s.
Liquid Embolic s.
LiteNest portable seating s.
Lithovac master suction s.
LogiCal pressure transducer s.
Lone Star retractor s.
Lorad Stereo Guide prone breast biopsy s.
Lorad Stereo Guide stereotactic breast biopsy s.
Lorenz Micro-Power dense bone drilling and cutting s.
Lorenz osteosynthesis s.
Lorenz plating s.
low-vision enhancement s.
LTK s.
Lubinus AP hip s.
Lubinus SP II anatomically adapted hip s.
Luhr maxillofacial fixation s.
Luhr microfixation s.
Luhr MRS s.
Luhr pan fixation s.
Luque II fixation s.
Luxtec fiberoptic s.
LymphoScan nuclear imaging s.
Lynco biomechanical orthotic s.
Lyra laser s.
LySonix 2000 complete ultrasonic surgical s.
LySonix Post-Operative patient s.
LySonix TTD Cannula S.
LySonix 2000 ultrasonic surgical s.
MacKool s.
Madajet XL jet-injection anesthesia s.
Madajet XL local anesthesia s.
Maestro s.
Magerl hook-plate s.

S

system *(continued)*
Magerl plate-screw s.
Magna-Site locating s.
Magnes biomagnetometer s.
Magnetic Surgery s.
Magnetom Open s.
Magnetom Vision MR s.
Magnetron MRI s.
Magnex Alpha MR s.
Magnum-Meier s.
Malcolm-Lynn radiolucent spinal retraction s.
Malcolm-Rand radiolucent headrest and retraction s.
Malis bipolar coagulating/cutting s.
Malis CMC-III electrosurgical s.
Mallinckrodt sensor s.
Mallory-Head modular calcar s.
Mammomat C3 mammography s.
Mammoscan digital imaging s.
Mammotest Plus breast biopsy s.
Mammotome biopsy s.
Manchester LDR implant s.
Maramed Miami fracture brace s.
Marex MRI s.
Marion oxygen resuscitation s.
Mark III halo s.
Mark II Sorrells hip arthroplasty retractor s.
Marlen UltraLite s.
Marquette Case-12 electrocardiographic s.
Marx bridging plate s.
Mason-Likar 12-lead EKG s.
Mastel compass-guided arcuate keratotomy s.
mattress s.
Mattrix spinal cord stimulation s.
Maturna bra s.
Mauch GaitMaster s.
Max FiberScan laser s.
Maxilift Combi patient lifting s.
maxillofacial plating s.
Maxim modular knee s.
Maxi-Myst nebulizer s.
Mayfield surgical headrest s.
MCAS modular clip application s.
McCain TMJ arthroscopic s.
McGinnis balloon s.
McGuire I&A s.
McIntyre coaxial I&A s.
Mectra I&A s.
MED^next bone dissecting s.
MEDDARS cardiac catheterization analysis s.
Medelec-Van Gogh electroencephalographic recording s.
Medex Secure s.
Medi-Duct ocular fluid management s.
Mediflex MD-7 endoscopic video s.
Medi-Ject needle free insulin injection s.
Medisorb drug delivery s.

Medi-Tech catheter s.
Mednext bone dissecting s.
Medos mechanical circulatory support s.
Medspec MR imaging s.
Medstone IRIS s.
Medstone STS lithotripsy s.
Medtronic Hemopump s.
Medtronic Interactive Tachycardia Terminating s.
Medtronic Interstim sacral nerve stimulation s.
Medtronic Micro Jewel cardiovert defibrillator s.
Medtronic Pulsor Intrasound s.
Medtronic spinal cord stimulation
Medtronics Sequestra 1000 autotransfusion s.
Medtronic Transvene endocardial lead s.
Medwatch telemetry s.
Med-Wick medication delivery s.
MEG head-based coordinate s.
Meier magnum s.
Meniscus Mender II s.
Mentor Contour Genesis ultrasonic assisted lipoplasty s.
MetaFluor s.
Metalift crown and bridge removal s.
Metasul metal-on-metal hip prosthesis s.
Metrix atrial defibrillation s.
MG II total hip s.
MG II total knee s.
MIBB breast biopsy s.
Micro-Aire facial plating s.
Micro-Aire pulse lavage s.
Micro-Aire surgical instrument s.
MicroChoice electric powered surgical s.
Micro Delta s.
microdilution s.
MicroHartzler ACS balloon catheter s.
MicroLap Gold microlaparoscopy
Microloc knee s.
MicroLux video camera s.
micromanometer catheter s.
MicroMax drill s.
Micro-Mill knee instrument s.
MicroPhor iontophoretic drug delivery s.
Micro Plus plating s.
MicroProbe integrated laser and endoscope s.
MicroShape keratome s.
MICROS infusion s.
MicroSpan minihysteroscopy s.
Microsponge delivery s.
Microstar dialysis s.
Microvasive biliary stent s.
Microvasive Ultraflex esophageal stent s.
Micro-Vent implant s.

Microvit probe s.
MIDA 1000 monitoring s.
Midas Rex instrumentation s.
Midas Rex Quick-Connect s.
Millennium CX microsurgical s.
Millennium LX microsurgical s.
Miller-Galante revision knee s.
Miller-Galante total knee s.
Milli-Q water purification s.
Minerva s.
Mini-Acutrak small-bone fixation s.
mini Hoffmann external fixation s.
MiniMed continuous glucose
  monitoring s.
mini Vidas automated
  immunoassay s.
mini Würzburg Flexplates
  craniomaxillofacial plating s.
mini Würzburg standard
  craniomaxillofacial plating s.
Mirage nasal ventilation mask s.
Mirage spinal s.
mirror optical s.
Mitek GII suture anchor s.
Mitek Vapr tissue removal s.
mitochondrial ethanol oxidase s.
Mityvac vacuum delivery s.
MKM AutoPilot stereotactic s.
MMG/O'Neil intermittent catheter s.
MMG/O'Neil sterile field urinary
  catheter s.
Mobetron electron beam s.
Mobetron intraoperative radiation
  therapy treatment s.
Modular Acetabular Revision S.
  (MARS)
Modular acetabular revision s.
modular Lenbach hip s.
modular S-ROM total hip s.
Modulus CD anesthesia s.
MOD unicompartmental knee s.
Monaldi drainage s.
Monarch IOL delivery s.
MoniTorr ICP CSF drainage and
  monitoring s.
Monotube external fixator s.
Montgomery thyroplasty implant s.
Monticelli-Spinelli circular external
  fixation s.
Moonwalker weightbearing s.
Moore hip endoprosthesis s.
MOP-Videoplan morphometric s.
Morganstern aspiration/injection s.
Moss fixation s.
Moss Miami load-sharing spinal
  implant s.
mother-baby endoscope s.
Mot-R-Pak vitrectomy s.
Mouradian humeral fixation s.
MPM I multi-parameter
  monitoring s.
Mport foldable lens placement s.
M-TEC 2000 surgical s.
Mui Scientific pressurized capillary
  infusion s.

Mulholland growth guidance s.
Mullins sheath s.
MultiDop XS s.
multileaf collimating s.
MultiLight s.
Multi Podus foot s.
MultiSPIRO s.
Myocardial Protection s.
MYOterm XP cardioplegia
  delivery s.
Natchez Mobil-Trac s.
Natural-Knee II s.
Natural Profile abutment s.
NC-stat nerve conduction s.
Nd:YAG laser s.
needle trephination s.
Neer II shoulder s.
Neer II total knee s.
Neff femorotibial nail s.
Nellcor N-400/FS s.
Nellcor Symphony blood pressure
  monitoring s.
NeoControl pelvic floor therapy s.
neodymium:yttrium-aluminum-garnet
  laser s.
NeoProbe 1000 radioisotope
  detection s.
Neosonic (P-5) SPM super powered
  mini retroprep/endo s.
Neotrend s.
NeuroCybernetic prosthesis s.
Neurogard TCD s.
Neuroguide interoperative viewing s.
NeuroLink II EEG data
  acquisition s.
Neuropak 8 s.
neuroprobe pain management s.
NeuroSector ultrasound s.
NeuroStation frameless s.
Neurostat Mark II cryoanalgesia s.
Neurotrend continuous
  multiparameter s.
Neuroview integrated visualization s.
Newport total hip orthosis s.
New Vision magnification s.
Nexerciser Plus exercise s.
NexGen complete knee s.
Nexus wheelchair seating s.
Niamtu video imaging s.
Nicolet Viking II
  electrophysiologic s.
Nidek EC-5000 refractive laser s.
Nidek MK-2000 keratome s.
Nobelpharma implant s.
NoHands foot-operated computer
  mouse s.
Nomos stereotactic s.
nonthoracotomy defibrillation lead s.
NordiCare Back Therapy s.
Norm testing and rehabilitation s.
Norwegian s.
No-Touch delivery and mounting s.
Novacor DIASYS left ventricular
  assist s.
Nova Microsonics Image Vue s.

system *(continued)*
Novapulse laser s.
NS2000 bipolar generator s.
Nu-Trake Weiss emergency
airway s.
Nuvolase 660 laser s.
Oasis sheet introducer s.
Oasis thrombectomy s.
Obtura II gutta percha s.
OCL Splint Roll Contour
splinting s.
OctreoScan s.
Oculex drug delivery s.
Ocutech Vision Enhancing s.
Ocutome II fragmentation s.
Odyssey phacoemulsification s.
OEC-Diasonics 9400 fluoroscopy C-
arm s.
OEC Mini 6600 imaging s.
OEC Series 9600 cardiac s.
Ogden plate s.
Ogden tissue reattachment mini s.
OIS image digitizing s.
Olerud PSF fixation s.
Olympus CLV-series fiberoptic s.
Olympus EVIS color computer
chip s.
Olympus GF UM3 s.
Olympus GF UM20 s.
Olympus MAJ363 FNA needle s.
Olympus OSP fluorescence
measuring s.
Olympus video urology procedure s.
Omega Plus compression hip s.
Ommaya intraventricular reservoir s.
Omnifit HA hip s.
Omnifit Plus enhanced offset
cemented hip s.
Omnifit Plus hip s.
Omni-Flow 4000 Plus medication
management s.
Omni-LapoTract support s.
Omniloc dental s.
One Action Stent Introduction S.
One Touch II hospital blood
glucose monitoring s.
OnLine ABG monitoring s.
On-Q pain management s.
Opdima digital mammography s.
open-loop insulin delivery s.
OpenPACS s.
OPERA s.
Opmilas 144 Plus laser s.
Opsis DistalCam video s.
Optetrak total knee replacement s.
optical multichannel analyzer s.
Opti-Fix total hip s.
OptiHaler drug delivery s.
OptiMax immunostaining s.
Opti-Pure s.
Opti-Qvue Mixed Venous
Saturation/CCO pulmonary artery
catheter s.
Optistar MR contrast delivery s.

OptoTrak motion-analysis s.
Oral Scan computer imaging s.
Oral Scan video imaging s.
Orascoptic acuity s.
Orfizip casting s.
OR-340 imaging s.
Orion continence s.
Orlando tibial plateau fracture
bracing s.
OrlandoTPFx bracing s.
Orth-evac autotransfusion s.
Orthodoc presurgical planning s.
Ortho-Ice Multipaks s.
Ortholoc Advantim revision knee
Ortholoc Advantim total knee s.
Orthomet Axiom total knee s.
Orthomet Perfecta total hip s.
OrthoPak bone growth stimulator
Orthotec pressurized fluid
irrigation s.
Osada XL-S30 electric handpiece
OSCAR ultrasonic bone cement
removal s.
OscilloMate 930 blood pressure
measurement s.
OSI modular table s.
Osseofix implant s.
Osseous Coagulum Trap
collecting s.
Osteobond vacuum mixing s.
osteochondral autograft transfer s.
Osteo-Clage cable s.
Osteonics Scorpio posterior crucia
retaining total knee s.
Osteonics spinal s.
OsteoView desktop hand x-ray s.
OsteoView 2000 digital imaging
Ostreg spinal marker s.
OtoScan ear aeration s.
Oulu neuronavigator s.
Ovation falloposcopy s.
oxalate s.
OxiFirst fetal monitoring s.
Oximetrix 3 s.
Oxycure topical oxygen s.
Oxydome oxygen therapy s.
oxylate dentin bonding s.
Oxy-Ultra-Lite ambulatory
oxygen s.'s
Paceart complete pacemaker
testing s.
Packard radioimmunoassay s.
PadKit sample collection s.
Palco enuretic alarm s.
PalmVue s.
Panasol II home phototherapy s.
PanoView arthroscopic s.
PapNet automated cervical
cystology s.
Pap-Perfect supply s.
Parabath paraffin heat treatment s
Paragon single-stage dental
implant s.
ParaMax ACL guide s.
paranasal sinus shaver s.

Parastep I s.
Paratrend 7 intravenous blood gas monitoring s.
Paris s.
Park-O-Tron drill s.
Parr closed-irrigation s.
Partnership s.
P.A.S. Port Fluoro-Free peripheral access s.
PASYS single-chamber cardiac pacing s.
Pathfinder microcatheter s.
Patil stereotactic s. I, II
Paulus trocar s.
PCA modular total knee s.
PCD Transvene implantable cardioverter-defibrillator s.
PDB preperitoneal distention balloon s.
PEAK anterior compression plate s.
PEAK fixation s.
PEC modular total knee s.
PEC total hip s.
Pedar in-shoe measurement s.
Pedar pressure measurement s.
pediatric circle s.
Pediatric Nutrition Surveillance S.
Pegasus Airwave pressure relief s.
Pelorus surgical s.
pelvic floor therapy s.
Pelvic Organ Prolapse-Quantified s.
PenRad mammography clinical reporting s.
Pentax-Hitachi FG32UA endosonographic s.
Percutaneous Stoller Afferent Nerve Stimulation (PerQ Sans) s.
Perfecta Interseal total hip s.
PerFixation s.
Perflex stainless steel stent and delivery system biliary s.
Performa Acoustic Imaging s.
Performa diagnostic ultrasound imaging s.
Performance modular total knee s.
Performance unicompartmental knee s.
Periotemp s.
Periotest s.
Peripheral AngioJet s.
peripheral atherectomy s.
Peritronics Medical Inc. fetal monitoring s.
Permark micropigmentation s.
permucosal implant s.
peroral pancreatoscope s.
Perspective chest imaging s.
Perspective dental imaging s.
PFC Sigma total knee s.
PFC total hip replacement s.
PF-8P peroral pancreatoscope s.
Phaco Commander phacoemulsification s.
Phacojack phaco s.

PharmChek sweat patch drug detection s.
phased-array color-flow ultrasound s.
Philips DVI 1 s.
Philips Easyguide navigation s.
Phoenix fifth ventricle s.
Phoresor II iontophoretic drug delivery s.
PhosphorImager s.
photocatalytic air filtration s.
PhotoDerm bright light delivery s.
PhotoDerm MultiLight s.
PhotoDerm VL/PL hair removal s.
PhotoGenica T laser s.
PhotoGenica T^{10} tattoo removal s.
photon-activated drug delivery s.
photonic radiosurgical s.
Photon Ocular Surgery s.
Photon Radiosurgery s.
Photopic Imaging ultrasound s.
Phototome s.
Physios CTM 01 cardiac transplant monitoring s.
Picker s.
Picket Fence fiducial localization stereotactic s.
picture archival communication s.
Picture Archiving and Communications S.
Pie Medical CAAS II analysis s.
Pie Medical ultrasound s.
Pillo-Pump alternating pressure s.
pin ball s.
Pinch Gauge and Jackson Strength Evaluation S.
pin-index safety s.
Pinnacle 3 radiation therapy planning s.
Pinn.ACL guide s.
Pinwheel s.
Pisces spinal cord stimulation s.
Placido-disk videokeratoscopy s.
PlastiCast adjustable joint cast s.
plastic endosurgical s.
Plast-O-Fit thermoplastic bandage s.
Pleur-evac autotransfusion s.
PLI-100 pico-injector pipette s.
PlumeSafe Whisper 602 smoke evacuation s.
PMT robotic fulcrumless tomographic s.
pneumohydraulic capillary infusion s.
PodoSpray nail drill s.
Polar coordinate s.
Polaroid HealthCam s.
Polarus Plus humeral fixation s.
Polarus positional humeral fixation s.
Porex drainage s.
Port-A-Cath implantable catheter s.
PortaFlo urine collection s.
PortalVision radiation oncology s.
Portex Soft-Seal cuff s.
posterior rod s.

S

system *(continued)*
Pouchkins pediatric ostomy s.
PowerGrip stent delivery s.
PowerProxi Sonic interdental
toothbrush s.
PPT insole s.
Precision hip s.
Precision Osteolock femoral
component s.
Precision QID glucose monitoring s.
Precision Strata hip s.
PreClean soak s.
Press-Fit total condylar knee s.
PressureGuard Select patient
adjustable pressure management s.
pressure transducer-monitor s.
Presto-Flash spirometry s.
Presto spirometry s.
pretarget filtration s.
Preventix modular mattress
replacement s.
Prevue s.
Price corneal transplant s.
Primbs-Circon indirect video
ophthalmoscope s.
ProAire portable rotation s.
Probe balloon-on-a dilatation s.
Procera s.
Profile mammography s.
Profile total hip s.
Profix total knee replacement s.
Profore bandage s.
programmable VariGrip II prosthetic
control s.
Prolene Hernia s.
Promise pad and pant s.
Pro-Post s.
Proscan ultrasound imaging s.
ProSeries laparoscopic laser s.
Prostalase laser s.
ProstaScint s.
Prostathermer prostatic
hyperthermia s.
ProSys Urihesive system LA and s.
Protector meniscus suturing s.
ProTime microcoagulation s.
ProTrac cruciate reconstruction s.
Providence scoliosis s.
Proxiderm wound closure s.
Pulsavac III wound debridement s.
PulseSpray pulsed infusion s.
Pump-It-Up pneumatic socket
volume management s.
Pump Vac Plus s.
punch myringotomy s.
Puno-Winter-Byrd s.
PWB transpedicular spine fixation s.
PyMaH Trimline
sphygmomanometer s.
Q-catheter catheterization
recording s.
Qlicksmart blade removal s.
Q-Plex cardio-pulmonary exercise s.
Q-prep s.

Quadracut ACL shaver s.
QuadraLase advanced surgical
fiber s.
Quadra pipetting s.
quadrature surface coil MRI s.
Quantimet 500 analyzing s.
Quantrex Sweep 650 ultrasonic
cleansing s.
Quartet s.
QuickRinse automated instrument
rinse s.
Quick-Sil silicone s.
Quimby implant s.
radiation therapy planning s.
radiofrequency needle electrode s.
radiographic image processing s.
radiographic imaging s.
RadioLucent wrist fixation s.
Radionics articulated arm s.
radionuclide carrier s.
RadNet radiology information s.
Ranawat-Burstein total hip s.
Rancho Cube s.
Rancho external fixation s.
Rasor blood pumping s.
real-time two-dimensional Doppler
flow-imaging s.
Redi-Vu teleradiology s.
Redy 2000 hemodialysis s.
Redy Sorbent dialysis s.
Reebok Slide s.
Reebok Step s.
reference coordinate s.
Refine fusion s.
Refinity Coblation s.
ReFlexion implant s.
Regulus frameless stereotactic s.
Reichert-Mundinger stereotactic s.
Reichert stereotaxy s.
Rekow s.
Relay suture delivery s.
Remac s.
Renaissance crown s.
Renaissance spirometry s.
Renatron II dialyzer reprocessing s
Replace implant s.
Replica total hip replacement s.
resorbable copolymer PGA/PLLA-
Lactosorb miniplate fixation s.
Res-Q-Vac emergency suction s.
Restoration acetabular s.
Restoration-HA hip s.
Restore ACL guide s.
Restore close tolerance dental
implant s.
Retzius s.
ReUnite resorbable orthopedic
fixation s.
Reuter suprapubic trocar and
cannula s.
Revelation hip s.
revised Salzburg lag screw s.
revised Würzburg mandibular
reconstruction s.
ReVision nail s.

RF ablation s.
rhinolaryngostroboscopy s.
Rhinoline endoscopic sinus
   surgery s.
Rhinotherm hyperthermia
   treatment s.
RiboPrinter microbial
   characterization s.
Richards fixator s.
Richards hip endoprosthesis s.
Richards modular hip s.
Richards Solcotrans orthopaedic
   drainage-reinfusion s.
Richards Solcotrans Plus drainage s.
Richard Wolf nasal epistaxis s.
rigid external distraction s.
ring-type imaging s.
r\LS red blood cell filtration s.
RLS videostroboscopy s.
Robodoc s.
Robotrac passive retraction s.
Rodenstock s.
rod-lens s.
Rod TAG suture anchor s.
Rogan teleradiology s.
Roger s.
Rogozinski screw s.
Rogozinski spinal fixation s.
Rogozinski spinal rod s.
Roho pediatric seating s.
Rolyan Reach-N-Range pulley s.
Romano surgical curved drilling s.
Romhilt-Estes point scoring s.
Rotablator s.
Rotacs s.
Rotaglide total knee s.
R-Port implantable vascular
   access s.
Rudolph breathing s.
Rumi uterine manipulation s.
Russell-Taylor femoral interlocking
   nail s.
Rx5000 cardiac pacing s.
RX Herculink 14 premounted
   stent s.
RX stent delivery s.
RZ mandibular matrix s.
Safeset blood sampling s.
Safestretch incontinence s.
SafeTrak ESP s.
Safsite IV therapy s.
Saf-T-Intima intravenous catheter
   safety s.
SalEst preterm labor test s.
SAM s.
Sanders Venturi injector s.
Sandhill esophageal motility s.
Sandman s.
SaphLITE saphenous vein s.
Sapphire premium closed wound
   drainage s.
Sarstedt s.
Save-A-Tooth tooth preserving s.
Scanmaster DX s.
scanned-slot detector s.

scanning beam digital s.
Scaphoid-Microstaple s.
scattering s.
Schmidt optics s.
Schneider-Meier magnum s.
Schwartz-Blajwas-Marcinko
   irrigation s.
Scintiview nuclear computer s.
Scintron IV nuclear computer s.
Scorpio total knee s.
Scotchcast length splinting s.
Scott chronic wound care s.
Screw-Vent implant s.
Script Stat, Inc. dispensing s.
S-D-Sorb E-Z Tac s.
S-D-Sorb suture anchor s.
Secor s.
Secure closed pressure monitoring
   and blood sampling s.
SecureStrand cervical fusion s.
Secure Yet Gentle surgical
   dressing s.
segmental spinal correction s.
Select GT blood glucose s.
selective tubal occlusion
   procedure s.
Selectron s.
Self-Cath closed catheterization s.
Sens-A-Ray digital dental
   imaging s.
SensiCath blood gas measurement s.
Sensi-Touch anesthesia delivery s.
SensoScan mammography s.
Septer closed wound drainage s.
Septi-Chek culture s.
Sequel compression s.
Sequestra 1000 blood processing s.
Sequoia Acuson s.
Sequoia echocardiography s.
Sequoia ultrasound s.
Seraton dialysis control s.
Seroma-Cath wound drainage s.
Setma hydrotherapy s.
SF-9 baculovirus-insect cell s.
Shadow-Line ACF spine retractor s.
Shape Maker s.
Sharplan sight s.
sheath and dilator s.
Sherlock bone screw
   suture/anchor s.
Sherman remote podiatric vacuum s.
Sherwood intrascopic
   suction/irrigation s.
Shiley cardioplegia s.
Shiley catheter distention s.
Shimadzu ultrasound s.
Shutt suture punch s.
SICOR cardiac catheterization
   recording s.
Side Branch Occlusion s.
Siemens somatoma plus DCT s.
Siemens Sonoline SI-400
   ultrasound s.
Sigma II hyperbaric s.
Signa Advantage s.

S

system *(continued)*
Signa GEMS MR imaging s.
Signal s.
Signature Edition infusion s.
Silberg E.U.A. s.
Silent Speaker communication s.
Silhouette spinal s.
Silhouette therapeutic massage s.
Silicon Graphics Reality Engine s.
Simal cervical stabilization s.
Simcoe I&A s.
Simmons plating s.
Simplicity adult disposable
contoured undergarment liner s.
Simpson-Robert vascular dilation s.
Simpulse irrigation s.
Simpulse lavage s.
Sinai s.
single-action pumping s.
single-incision s.
single patient s.
SinuScope s.
Sirecust 404N neonatal
monitoring s.
SiteSelect percutaneous incisional
breast biopsy s.
SITEtrac spinal surgery s.
SITE TXR diaphragmatic
microsurgical s.
SITE TXR peristaltic
microsurgical s.
SITE TXR phacoemulsification s.
SkinLaser s.
Sky-Boot stirrup s.
SKY epidural pain control s.
Skylight s.
SLS Chromos long pulse ruby
laser s.
SmartDose infusion s.
SmartKard digital Holter s.
SmartMist asthma management s.
SmartSite needleless s.
SmartSpot high-resolution digital
imaging s.
Smart System irrigation/suction s.
SmiLine abutment s.
Snuggle Warm convective
warming s.
Snugs tapeless wound care s.
Socon spinal s.
Sodas spheroidal oral drug
absorption s.
Soehendra catheter s.
Soehendra endoscopic biliary
stent s.
SoftLight laser hair removal s.
Soft & Secure 1-piece spouted
pouch s.
Soft & Secure 2-piece spouted
pouch s.
Sofwire cable s.
Solcotrans autotransfusion s.
Solcotrans closed vacuum-drainage s.
Solcotrans drainage/reinfusion s.

Solcotrans orthopaedic drainage-
refusion s.
Solcotrans Plus drainage-
reinfusion s.
Solcovac closed wound drainage
Solid Creation S.
SOLO-Surg Colo-Rectal self-retain
retractor s.
Soma Gonio s.
Soma pulley s.
Songer cable s.
sonic accelerated fracture healing
Sonicaid Vasoflow Doppler s.
Sonifer sonicating s.
SonoHeart hand-held, all digital
echocardiography s.
Sonoline Elegra ultrasound s.
Sonoline Sierra ultrasound
imaging s.
Sonoline SI-200/250 ultrasound
imaging s.
Sonomed A/B-Scan s.
Sonopsy biopsy imaging s.
Sonopsy ultrasound-guided breast
biopsy s.
Sonos imaging s.
Soprano cryoablation s.
Sorbie-Questor total elbow s.
Sorrells hip arthroplasty retractor
Sorrells Mark II hip arthroplasty
retractor s.
Souter Strathclyde total elbow s.
Sovereign Shield s.
SpaTouch PhotoEpilation s.
Spect-Align laser s.
SPECT high-resolution brain s.
Spectra 400 extended surveillance
and alert s.
SpectraScience optical biopsy s.
Spectron EF total hip s.
Spectrum lens analysis s.
Spectrum tissue repair s.
Sperm Select sperm recovery s.
SpinaLase neodymium:yytrium-
aluminum-garnet (Nd:YAG)
surgical laser s.
SpineLink s.
Spinoscope noninasive imaging s.
SpiroSense s.
Spline dental implant s.
Sportorno cementless hip
arthroplasty s.
SprayGel Adhesion Barrier s.
Square Module Seating S.
Squibb s.
Squirt wound irrigation s.
S-ROM hip replacement s.
S-ROM modular total knee s.
S-ROM proximally modular total
hip s.
Stabident s.
Stability total hip s.
Stableloc external wrist fixation s.
Stableloc II external fixator s.

Stage-1 single-stage dental implant s.
StairMaster exercise s.
STARRT falloposcopy s.
Star S2 SmoothScan excimer laser s.
Statak anchor s.
Stay-Erec s.
StealthStation image-guided s.
StealthStation image-interactive s.
Steele fiberoptic s.
steerable guide wire s.
Steffee pedicle screw-plate s.
Steffee variable spine plating s.
stent and vent s.
Step laparoscopic entry s.
StereoGuide stereotactic breast biopsy s.
Stereotaxis magnetic surgery s.
Steriking sterilization s.
Steri-Oss implant s.
Sterrad sterilization s.
stone recognition s.
stone-tissue detection s.
stone-tissue recognition s.
Storz ceiling-mounted microscope s.
Storz ear, nose and throat camera s.
Storz-Hopkins s.
Storz Millennium microsurgical s.
Straight-In surgical s.
Strata hip s.
Stratasys FDM Med Modeler s.
Stratis II MRI s.
Stryker SE3 drive s.
STS lithotripsy s.
STTOdx ophthalmic surgery s.
Sub-Vent implant s.
Sudbury s.
Sundt AVM clip s.
Sundt AVM microclip s.
Sundt suction s.
Sunrise LTK s.
Sun SPARCstation s.
Superscript preamplification s.
Superset exercise s.
Supratusion s.
Sure-Closure skin closure s.
SureScan s.
SureStart imaging s.
SureStep ankle support s.
SureTrans autotransfusion s.
Surgeons Choice stapling s.
Surg-E-Trol I/A s.
Surg-E-Trol I/A/R s.
Surgi-PEG replacement gastrostomy feeding s.
Surgitek OM-5 urodynamic s.
Sustain dental implant s.
SwimEx hydrotherapy s.
Swiss Precision cannula s.
swivel-arm s.
Symphony patient monitoring s.
Synaptic 2000 pain management s.
SynchroMed infusion s.

Synergy neurostimulation s.
Synergy posterior titanium spinal s.
Synevac vacuum curettage s.
Synthes Cervifix s.
Synthes Schuhli implant s.
Synthes Universal spinal s.
syringe-driven s.
Sysmex HS-330 robotic hematology s.
System Alloclassic hip s.
Talairach bicommissural reference s.
Talairach stereotactic s.
Talairach-Tournoux s.
Targis s.
Tarsys tilt and recline s.
Taylor Wharton 27K cryostorage s.
TCI Heartmate mechanical circulatory support s.
TD glucose monitoring s.
Tebbets EndoPlastic instrument s.
TEC atherectomy s.
Tech-Attach connection s.
Technolas 217 excimer laser s.
Technos ultrasound s.
Techstar percutaneous vascular surgery s.
Techstar XL percutaneous vascular surgery s.
TEC interface s.
TEGwire ST s.
Telefactor beehive s.
telemanipulator s.
temporolimbic s.
Tesla MRI s.
Testoderm testosterone transdermal s.
Tetrax interactive balance s.
Texas Scottish Rite Hospital screw-rod s.
ThAIRapy vest airway clearance s.
The Bodyguard emboli containment s.
The Healthy Back S.
Therabath paraffin heat therapy s.
Therabite jaw motion rehabilitation s.
Thera Cool cold therapy s.
TheraPEP positive expiratory pressure therapy s.
Thera-turn rotational s.
ThermaChoice uterine balloon therapy s.
thermal balloon s.
thermal dosimetry s.
ThermoChem-HT s.
Thermo-Flo irrigation s.
The Unfolder intraocular lens implantation s.
The Wave phacoemulsion s.
Thompson-Farley spinal retractor s.
Thompson hip endoprosthesis s.
thoracolumbosacroiliac implant s.
Thora-Klex chest drainage s.
Thoratec mechanical circulatory support s.

system *(continued)*
Thumper CPR s.
tibial torsion s.
Ti-Fit total hip s.
time-of-flight PET imaging s.
TiMesh craniofacial s.
TiMesh craniomaxillofacial plating s.
TiMesh rigid fixation bone
  plating s.
TiMesh titanium bone plating s.
tissue anchor guide s.
titanium hollow screw plate s.
titanium micro s.
TMJ Concepts patient-fitted TMJ
  prosthesis s.
TMS three-dimensional radiation
  therapy treatment planning s.
Tomey topographic modeling s.
Tomey topography s.
Tomolex tomographic s.
TomTec imaging s.
Topcon IMAGEnet digital
  imaging s.
Top Notch automated biopsy s.
topographic scanning s.
TopSS topographic scanning s.
Total O₂ s.
Total Synchrony s.
TPL-6 hip s.
Tranquility bilevel s.
transesophageal pacing s.
TransFix ACL s.
transluminal lysing s.
transtelephonic ambulatory
  monitoring s.
TraumaJet wound debridement s.
Traveler portable oxygen s.
Trex digital mammography s.
Triad SPECT imaging s.
Triage cardiac s.
Triax monotube external fixation s.
Tricomponent Coaxial s.
Tri-Motion knee s.
triple-lumen perfused catheter s.
Tri-Wedge total hip s.
trocar-cannula s.
TroGARD Finesse dilating trocar s.
TRON 3 VACI cardiac imaging s.
Tru-Close wound drainage s.
True/Fit femoral intramedullary
  rod s.
True/Flex intramedullary rod s.
True/Lok external fixator s.
True Stat s.
TruJect drug delivery s.
TruPulse CO₂ laser s.
T-TAC s.
T2 thermoablation s.
Tulip syringe s.
TurnAide therapeutic s.
Turning Board exercise s.
Turnsoft automatic turning s.
TwinMic hearing s.

Tylok high-tension cerclage
  cabling s.
UE Tech Weight Well exercise s.
Ulson fixator s.
Ultima hip replacement s.
Ultima mammography s.
Ultima OPCAB s.
Ultima total hip s.
Ultimax distal femoral
  intramedullary rod s.
Ultimax Haig II nail s.
Ultrabag s.
Ultra-Drive bone cement removal
UltraFix rotator cuff suture
  anchor s.
Ultraflex stent delivery s.
Ultra-Guard hip orthosis s.
UltraLite One-Piece convex-
  disposable s.
Ultramark ultrasound s.
UltraPACS diagnostic imaging s.
UltraPak enteral closed feeding s.
UltraPower basic drill s.
UltraPower revision drill s.
Ultrascan digital B s.
Ultraseed ultrasound-guided
  brachytherapy s.
ultrasound s.
UltraSTAR computer-based
  ultrasound reporting s.
Ultra Twin bag s.
Ultra-X external fixation s.
Ultra Y-set s.
Unica CO₂ laser s.
UniFile Imaging and Archiving s.
Uniflex nailing s.
Uni-frame patient immobilization s.
Unilink hand surgery s.
UniPlast Imaging and Archiving s.
Uni-Shunt hydrocephalus shunt s.
United Sonics J shock phaco
  fragmentor s.
Unitek I convoluted innerspring
  mattress s.
Unitrax unipolar s.
Uni-Vent Eagle portable
  ventilation s.
Universal F breathing s.
Universal Plus instrument s.
Uni-Yeast-Tek s.
Unopette s.
Up and About s.
uPACS picture archiving s.
upper collecting s.
Uro-Cup female vaginal urinary
  collection s.
Urocyte diagnostic cytometry s.
UroVive s.
USCI Probe balloon-on-a-wire
  dilatation s.
Vac-Lok patient immobilization s.
Vacupac portable vacuum s.
vacuum cassette s.
Vakutage suction s.
Valleylab CUSA CEM s.

Valleylab REM s.
Var-A-Pulse wound debridement s.
Varian brachytherapy s.
Varian MLC s.
VariCare s.
Varigrip spine fixation s.
Varis radiation oncology s.
VasoExtor lead extraction s.
VasoView balloon dissection s.
Vector II guide s.
VectorVision surgical tracking s.
venaFlow compression s.
Venodyne compression s.
Ventak PRx defibrillation s.
Ventex wound dressing s.
Ventritex TVL s.
Ventrix tunnelable ventricular
  intracranial pressure monitoring s.
VentTrak monitoring s.
Venturi-Flo valve s.
Verruca-Freeze freezing s.
Versa-Fracture femoral fixation s.
Versalok low-back fixation s.
VersaPoint s.
Versaport trocar s.
Versatrac lumbar retractor s.
VerSys hip s.
VertAlign spinal support s.
vertebral artery s.
Vertetrac ambulatory traction s.
vesicular transport s.
vessel occlusion s.
VestaBlate s.
VET-CO vacuum s.
VidaMed's TUNA s.
Vidas automated immunoassay s.
video imaging s.
view shadow projection
  microtomographic s.
Vigilance monitoring s.
Vingmed Sound CFM ultrasound s.
VircoGEN diagnostic testing s.
S. V irrigation pump
Virtuoso imaging s.
Virtuoso LX Smart CPAP s.
Virtuoso portable three-dimensional
  imaging s.
Visio-Gem color s.
Vision Sciences VSI 2000 flexible
  sigmoidoscope s.
Visitec surgical vitrectomy s.
Visulab s.
VisuPac digital s.
VISX Star S2 excimer laser s.
VISX Twenty/Twenty s.
VISX Wavefront s.
Vitatron pacing s.'s
Vitrea 3D s.
Vortex stabilization s.
VoxelView s.
Voxgram digital holography s.

VPI Non-Adhesive Colostomy s.
VPI Non-Adhesive Ileostomy s.
VPI Non-Adhesive Urostomy s.
Wagner revision hip s.
Wallaby II phototherapy s.
WarmTouch patient warming s.
Warm-Up active wound therapy s.
Wedge TAG suture anchor s.
Wheeler cyclodialysis s.
Wiktor GX Hepamed coated
  coronary artery stent s.
Wiltse pedicle screw fixation s.
Winquest tibial/femoral extraction s.
Wit portable TENS s.
Wolf aspiration/injection s.
Wolf delivery s.
Wrightlock spinal fusion s.
Würzburg maxillofacial plating s.
Xillix LIFE-GI fluorescence
  endoscopy s.
Xillix LIFE-Lung s.
XKnife stereotactic radiosurgery s.
XPS Sculpture s.
XPS Straightshot micro tissue
  resector s.
Xsensor Pressure Mapping s.
X-Sizer catheter s.
X-Trel spinal cord stimulation s.
YagLazr s.
Y-set s.
Zeiss OpMi CS-NC2 surgical
  microscope s.
Zeppelin micro-motor s.
Zeus computer-controlled robotic s.
Zeus voice-controlled robotic s.
Zimmer Anatomic hip prosthesis s.
Zimmer CPT hip s.
Zimmer cross-over instrumentation s.
Zimmer-Hall drive s.
Zimmer Pulsavac wound
  debridement s.
Zone Specific II meniscal repair s.
ZPLATE-ATL anterior spinal
  fixation s.
Zuni exercise s.
Syticon 5950 bipolar demand pacemaker
Szabo-Berci
  S.-B. endoscopic needle driver set
  S.-B. needle
  S.-B. needle driver
Sztehlo umbilical clamp
Szulc
  S. bone cutter
  S. eye magnet
  S. grommet
  S. orbital implant material
  S. vascular dilator
Szuler
  S. eustachian bougie
  S. vascular forceps
Szultz corneal forceps

T

T bandage
tonometer
  T bandage (T)
  T bar
  T clamp
  T Philips ACS-II Gyroscan
  T rotating joint
  T self-retaining drainage tube
T220L dialyzer
T-28 hip prosthesis
T2 thermoablation system
T2-weighted scan
TA
  TA II loading unit
  TA metallic staple
  TA Premium-series staple
  TA 55 stapler
TAB
  TAB acrylic
Tab
  T. grabber
Tabb
  T. crural nipper
  T. double-ended flap knife
  T. ear curette
  T. ear elevator
  T. ear knife
  T. knife pick
  T. myringoplasty knife
  T. pick knife
  T. ruler
table
  Akron tilt t.
  Albee orthopaedic fracture t.
  Allen arm surgery t.
  AlphaStar operating room t.
  American Sterilizer operating t.
  Andrews spinal surgery t.
  Back Specialist electric t.
  Back Specialist manual t.
  t. band
  Betaclassic surgical t.
  Biodex XYZ imaging t.
  Chandler t.
  chemonucleolysis t.
  Chick CLT operating t.
  Chick-Langren t.
  Chick surgical t.
  circumductor t.
  crank t.
  cutout t.
  DeLorme t.
  Diamond biomechanical t.
  Dornier Urotract cysto t.
  dual lookup t.
  Ergo style flexion t.
  Eurotech t.
  EX-OP operating t.
  EZ Lift t.
  floating t.
  fracture t.

friction-reduced segmented t.
Galaxy McManis hylo t.
Gerhardt t.
Hadlock t.
harmonic attenuation t.
Hawley t.
t. heating pad
Heidelberg-R t.
Hercules t.
Hercules drop-adjusting t.
Hill Air-Drop HA90C t.
Hill Air-Flex t.
HiLo MultiPro t.
Hixon-Oldfather prediction t.
Hydradjust IV t.
hydromassage t.
IMSI-Metripond operating room t.
intersegmental t.
Jackson imaging t.
Jackson spinal surgery t.
Kanavel t.
Leander chiropractic t.
Leander motorized flexion t.
Leander 79-Series distraction t.
lithotripsy t.
Lloyd chiropractic t.
Lloyd flexion distraction t.
Magnum 101 Plus t.
Maquet operating t.
Massage Time Pro hydromassage t.
Mayo instrument t.
McKee t.
Med-Fit cranial-sacral t.
Meridian intersegmental t.
Midland tilt t.
Multi-Lock hand operating t.
MultiPro t.
Orthostar surgical t.
over-bed t.
Paris manual therapy t.
pedestal massage t.
pivoting t.
Platinum stationary t.
Powermatic t.
PRO traction t.
Rath treatment t.
resistive exercise t.
Reuss t.
Risser cast t.
Roto Rest delta kinetic therapy
  treatment t.
Sapphire t.
Shampaine orthopaedic t.
Siemens open-heart t.
Simply Wet t.
Sister Helen Mustard ENT t.
Skytron surgical t.
slatted plinth t.
slot t.
spica t.
Stryker fracture t.
Sugita microsurgical t.

T

table *(continued)*
Surgitable hand surgery t.
Telos fracture t.
t. tie
tilt t.
Titan Apollo electric flexion t.
Titan Meridian Intersegmental
  Traction t.
Titan Nova manual flexion-extension
  multi flex t.
Topaz flexion t.
traction t.
treatment t.
Tri W-G t.
VAX-D therapy t.
table-fixed retractor
Tab-Strap knee immobilizer
TAC2 atrial caval cannula
TAC atherectomy catheter
Tach-EZ dental attachment
tachycardia-terminating pacemaker
Tachylog pacemaker
Tacit threaded anchor
tack
ACE bone screw t.
biodegradable surgical t.
Cody sacculotomy t.
Effler t.
Graftac absorbable skin t.
membrane t.
SmartTack t.
titanium retinal t.
tack-and-pin forceps
Tacoma sacral plate
Tactaid
T. hearing aid
T. I vibrotactile aid
Tacticon
T. peripheral neuropathy kit
T. peripheral neuropathy screening
  device
Tactiflex
Tactilaze
T. angioplasty laser
T. angioplasty laser catheter
tactile probe
Tactyl 1 glove
Tactylon synthetic surgical gloves
TAF175 dialyzer
TAG
tissue anchor guide
TAG instrumentation
TAG Rod II suture anchor
Tagarno
T. 3SD cineangiography projector
T. 3SD cine projector
T. 3SD cine projector for
  angiogram
Tager lever
Tahoe Surgical Instruments ligature
Takagi arthroscope
Takahashi
T. cutting forceps
T. ethmoidal forceps

T. ethmoidal punch
T. iris retractor forceps
T. nasal forceps
T. nasal punch
T. neurosurgical forceps
T. rongeur
Taka microneurosurgical sponge
Takaro clip
Takata laser
Take-apart
T.-a. forceps
T.-a. instrument
T.-a. scissors
takedown of colostomy
Take-Me-Along Personal Shocker pock
  shocker
Take-Out extractor
Talairach
T. bicommissural reference systen
T. stereotactic frame
T. stereotactic system
Talairach-Tournoux system
Talent
T. bifurcated endograft
T. stent graft
talipes hobble splint
Tallerman apparatus
Tall-ette toilet seat
Talley pump
Tamai clamp approximator
Tamarack flexure joint
tamp
CPT revision t.
interbody graft t.
Kiene bone t.
Richards t.
Robinson-Smith t.
tension band wire t.
tamper
McIntyre suture t.
tampon
Corner t.
Dührssen t.
t. forceps
Genupak t.
Merocel t.
nasal t.
Trendelenburg t.
tamponade
balloon t.
esophageal balloon t.
nasal t.
postnasal balloon t.
Silikon 1000 retinal t.
Tamsco
T. curette
T. forceps
T. periodontic scaler
T. wire-cutting scissors
Tandem
T. cardiac device
T. thin-shaft transureteroscopic
  balloon dilatation catheter
T. XL triple-lumen ERCP cannul

tandem
t. applicator
t. connector
Fleming afterloading t.
Fletcher-Suit afterloading t.
Fletcher-Suit-Delclos t.
t. and ovoid
t. scanning confocal microscope
t. stent

tangential
t. forceps
t. occlusion clamp
t. pediatric clamp
t. port

tangent screen
Tang retractor
Tanita Professional body composition analyzer
tank
Hubbard hydrotherapy t.
Imhoff t.
oxygen t.

Tanne
T. corneal cutting block
T. corneal patch
T. corneal punch

Tannenbaum stent
Tanner
T. mesher
T. mesh graft dermacarrier
T. slide

Tanner-Vandeput
T.-V. mesh dermatome

Tano
T. device
T. double-mirror peripheral vitrectomy lens
T. eraser
T. membrane scraper
T. ring

Tan spatula
tantalum
t. balloon-expandable stent
t. balloon-expandable stent with helical coil
t. gauze
t. hemostasis clip
t. mesh
t. mesh eye implant
t. "O" ring
t. plate
t. wire
t. wire monofilament suture

tantalum-178 generator
tantalum-ball marker
tantalum-wire stent
tap
t. drill
T. N' Tones
Richards bone t.
screw t.
t. water wet dressing

Tapcath esophageal electrode
tape
Aquasorb Border with Covaderm t.

Blenderm t.
t. board
Broselow t.
brow t.
Catheter-Secure t.
Cath-Secure t.
CollaTape t.
ColorZone t.
Dacron retraction t.
Deknatel wound closure t.
Delta-Lite casting t.
Dermicare hypoallergenic paper t.
Dermicel hypoallergenic cloth t.
Dermicel hypoallergenic knitted t.
Dermiclear t.
Dermiform hypoallergenic knitted t.
Dermiview hypoallergenic transparent t.
Elastikon elastic t.
foam t.
Hypafix retention t.
Hy-Tape latex-free surgical t.
instrument coding t.
Johnson & Johnson waterproof t.
lap t.
LeMaitre Glow 'N Tell t.
Leukopore t.
Leukotape P sports t.
t. marker
MaxCast fiberglass casting t.
Medipore H soft cloth surgical t.
Meditape t.
Mefix adhesive t.
Mersilene t.
Microfoam surgical t.
Micropore t.
3M matrix t.
3M Micropore surgical t.
Polyderm border with Covaderm t.
polyethylene retractor t.
Powerflex t.
Scanpor surgical t.
Scotchcast 2 casting t.
Shur-Strip wound closure t.
Sportape t.
Sta-Fix t.
Sure-Closure wound closure t.
Transpore eye t.
TSH-01 transdermal t.
umbilical t.
Vascor sterile retraction t.
Zonas porous t.

taper
collarless polished t.
funnelform t.
T. guidewire
t. hand file
laser t.
Morse t.
t. needle
t. with Zimmer shank

Tapercut
T. needle
T. suture

T

tapered
    t. blade
    t. brain spatula
    t. catheter
    t. fissure bur
    t. Micro-Vent implant
    t. needle
    t. pin
    t. reamer
    t. torque guidewire
tapered-shaft punctum plug
tapered-spring needle holder
tapered-tip
    t.-t. ear syringe
    t.-t. hydrophilic-coated push catheter
taper-jaw
    t.-j. forceps
    t.-j. rongeur
Taperloc
    T. femoral component
    T. femoral prosthesis
    T. femoral stem
Taper-Lock external hex implant
taper-point suture needle
TaperSeal hemostatic device
taping
    LowDye t.
tapper
    3-I t.
    rectangular t.
    round t.
tapping hammer
Tapscope esophageal pacing stethoscope
Tapsul pill electrode
Taq extender
TAR-200 dual-channel electronystagmograph
TARA
    TARA retropubic retractor
    TARA total hip prosthesis
Tardy osteotome
Targa+ image capture board
targeted cryoablation device
targeter
    bone screw t.
    IMP bone screw t.
targeting drill guide
Targis system
Tarlov nerve elevator
Tarnier
    T. axis-traction forceps
    T. basiotribe
    T. cephalotribe
    T. cranioclast
    T. obstetrical forceps
tarsal bar
tarsoconjunctival composite graft
Tarsys tilt and recline system
Tascon prosthetic valve
Tasserit shoulder attachment
Tassett vaginal cup bag
tattoo
    Derma-Tattoo surgical t.
tattooing needle

Tatum
    T. meatal clamp
    T. Tee intrauterine device
    T. ureteral transilluminator
Tauber
    T. ligature carrier
    T. ligature hook
    T. male urethrographic catheter
    T. needle
    T. speculum
    T. vaginal spatula
Taufic cholangiography clamp
Taut
    T. capillary drain
    T. cholangiographic catheter
    T. cystic duct catheter
    T. M55, M56, M57 catheter
    T. percutaneous introducer
    T. Safety Klip
Taveras injector
tax double needle
Taylor
    T. aspirator
    T. brain scissors
    T. Britetrac retractor
    T. catheter holder
    T. clavicle support
    T. curette
    T. dissecting forceps
    T. dural scissors
    T. fiberoptic retractor
    T. gastric balloon
    T. gastroscope
    T. halter device
    T. knife
    T. laminectomy blade
    T. percussion hammer
    T. pinwheel
    T. pulmonary dilator
    T. reflex hammer
    T. spinal frame
    T. spinal retractor
    T. spinal retractor blade
    T. spinal support apparatus
    T. spine brace
    T. splint
    T. thoracolumbosacral orthosis
    T. tissue forceps
    T. vaginal speculum
    T. Wharton 27K cryostorage syste
Taylor-Cushing dressing forceps
Taylor-Knight brace
T-bandage dressing
T-bar retractor
T-binder pressure dressing
TBird ventilator
T-buttress plate
T-C
    T-C needle holder
    T-C pin cutter
    T-C ring-handle pin and wire extractor
TC
    TC CO_2 monitor
    TC femoral stem

TC-7 adhesion barrier
TCCK unconstrained knee prosthesis
TCI Heartmate mechanical circulatory support system
TD glucose monitoring system
TDMAC heparin shunt
Teale
    T. gorget
    T. gorget lithotrite
    T. tenaculum
    T. tenaculum forceps
    T. uterine forceps
    T. vulsellum
    T. vulsellum forceps
tear
    t. duct tube
    t. strip
tear-away introducer sheath
teardrop
    t. dissector
    T. microsponge
Teare
    T. arm splint
    T. snare
TearSaver punctum plug
Tearscope
    Keeler T.
Teaser device
Tebbets
    T. EndoPlastic instrument system
    T. rhinoplasty set
    T. ribbon retractor
TEC
    TEC atherectomy device
    TEC atherectomy system
    TEC extraction catheter
    TEC interface system
    TEC liner
    TEC 2100 positioning laser
TECA-TD20 EMG machine
Tech-Attach connection system
TechMate 500 automatic immunostaining device
Techmedica
    T. implant
    T. prosthesis
technetium
    t. H2 autoanalyzer
    t. (Tc)-99m sestamibi tomographic imaging
Technicare
    T. camera
    T. Delta 2020 scanner
    T. Omega 500 CT
TechnoGel insole
Technolas 217 excimer laser system
TechnoMed
    T. C-Scan
    T. C-Scan videokeratoscope
Technos ultrasound system
Technovit acrylic resin
Techstar
    T. percutaneous closure device
    T. percutaneous vascular surgery system

    T. suturing closure device
    T. XL percutaneous vascular surgery system
Teclite fiberoptic light source
Tecmag Libra-S16 system scanner
Tecnol
    T. ankle support
    T. back support
    T. elbow support
    T. knee support
    T. wrist support
Tectonic magnet
TED
    TED antiembolism stockings
    TED hose
tedding device
Tedlar bag
Tefcat intrauterine insemination catheter
TefGen-FD guided tissue regeneration membrane
Teflo-Kapton freezing bag
Teflon
    T. block
    T. clip
    T. coating
    T. collar button
    T. ERCP cannula
    T. ERCP catheter
    T. felt
    T. glycerine-mixture injection needle
    T. glycerine-mixture syringe
    T. graft
    T. guiding catheter
    T. injection catheter
    T. injector
    T. intracardiac patch
    T. iris retractor
    T. liner
    T. mesh
    T. mesh implant
    T. mold
    T. nasobiliary drain
    T. needle catheter
    T. orbital floor implant
    T. piston
    T. plate
    T. pledget
    T. pledget suture buttress
    T. plug
    T. probe
    T. sheath
    T. sheet
    T. Silastic loop
    T. strut
    T. TFE SubLite Wall tubing
    T. tri-leaflet prosthesis
    T. woven prosthesis
Teflon-coated
    T.-c. Dacron suture
    T.-c. driver
    T.-c. guidewire
    T.-c. hollow-bore needle
Teflon-covered needle
Teflon-pledgeted suture
Teflon-tipped catheter

T

Tef-wire prosthesis
Tegaderm
    T. semipermeable occlusive dressing
Tegagel
    T. hydrogel dressing
    T. hydrogel sheet
**Tegagen HG, HI alginate wound
    dressing**
Tegam microprocessor thermometer
Tegapore contact-layer wound dressing
Tegasorb
    T. occlusive dressing
    T. ulcer dressing
Tegtmeier hand board
TEGwire
    T. balloon
    T. balloon dilatation catheter
    T. guide
    T. ST system
Tehl clamp
Tei-Shin
Tekna mechanical heart valve
Teknamed drape sheet
Tekno
    T. coagulator
    T. forceps
Tek-Pro needle
Tekscan in-shoe monitoring device
Tektronix
    T. digital oscilloscope
    T. digital phonometer
Tel-A-Fever forehead thermometer
telebinocular
TeleCaption decoder
telecentric fundus camera
Telectronics
    T. ATP implantable cardioverter-
    defibrillator
    T. Guardian ATP 4210 device
    T. Guardian ATP II ICD
    T. pacemaker
Telefactor beehive system
telemanipulator system
telemeter
    Bio-sentry t.
telemetric intracranial pressure sensor
telephone probe
telescope
    ACMI microlens Foroblique t.
    Atkins esophagoscopic t.
    Best direct forward-vision t.
    biopsy t.
    bioptic t.
    Bridge t.
    bronchoscopic t.
    Broyles t.
    Burns bridge t.
    catheterizing Foroblique t.
    convertible t.
    direct forward-vision t.
    direct-vision t.
    double-catheterizing t.
    endoscopic t.
    examining t.
    fiberoptic right-angle t.

    Foroblique bronchoscopic t.
    High-Vision surgical t.
    Holinger bronchoscopic t.
    Hopkins direct-vision t.
    Hopkins forward-oblique t.
    Hopkins lateral t.
    Hopkins nasal endoscopy t.
    Hopkins pediatric t.
    Hopkins retrospective t.
    Hopkins rigid t.
    Hopkins rod lens t.
    infant t.
    Keeler panoramic surgical t.
    Kramer direct-vision t.
    laryngeal-bronchial t.
    lateral microlens t.
    Lumina operating t.
    Lumina-SL t.
    Luxtec illuminated surgical t.
    Luxtec surgical t.
    McCarthy Foroblique operating t.
    McCarthy miniature t.
    Microlens direct-vision t.
    Microlens Foroblique t.
    Mueller t.
    nasal endoscopic t.
    Negus t.
    pediatric t.
    retrospective bronchoscopic t.
    right-angle examining t.
    Selsi sport t.
    solid-rod rigid t.
    stop collar t.
    Storz bronchoscopic t.
    Storz-Hopkins t.
    straight ahead bronchoscopic t.
    surgical t.
    Surgi-Spec t.
    transilluminating t.
    Tucker direct-vision t.
    Vest direct forward-vision t.
    Walden t.
    Zeiss binocular prism t.
telescopic view guide
telescoping
    t. brace
    t. guide
    t. plugged catheter
    t. rod
Telestill photo adapter
Teletrast gauze
Telfa
    T. adhesive pad
    T. bolster
    T. Clear nonadherent wound
    dressing
    T. gauze
    T. gauze dressing
    T. island dressing
    T. plastic film dressing
    T. Plus barrier island dressing
    T. strip
    T. 4 x 4 bandage
    T. Xtra absorbent island dressing
Telfamax ultra absorbent dressing

TeliCam intraoral camera
Teller acuity card
Telos
    T. fracture table
    T. radiographic stress device
Temco hoist
Temens curette
TEMNO biopsy needle
TE MOO mode beam laser
Tempa-DOT axillary thermometer
Tempbond dental cement
Temper
    T. foam
    T. Foam cube
    T. Foam cushion
temperature
    t. and galvanic skin response
      biofeedback device
    t. probe
temperature-sensing pacemaker
Temperlite saw blade
Temp-Kuff blood pressure cuff
template
    Bivona-Colorado t.
    Charnley t.
    dermal regeneration t.
    interimplant papillary t.
    Jacobsen t.
    Mallory-Head modular acetabular t.
    Marchac forehead t.
    Martinez universal interstitial t.
    McKissock keyhole areolar t.
    Mick prostate t.
    Moore t.
    rod t.
    Syed t.
    Syed-Neblett t.
    thermoplastic t.
    tissue expander t.
    tissue sizer t.
    total toe t.
Temple
    T. University nail
    T. University plate
Temple-Fay laminectomy retractor
Tempo denture liner
temporal
    t. bone holder
    t. electrode
temporalis
    t. sling
    t. transfer clamp
temporary
    t. pacing catheter
    t. percutaneous SCS electrode
    t. pervenous lead
    t. prosthesis
    t. skin replacement
    t. transvenous pacemaker
    t. vascular clip
    t. vessel clip
temporolimbic system
temporomandibular joint (TMJ)
TempTrac temperature monitor

Tempur-Med
    T.-M. hospital overlay
    T.-M. hospital replacement mattress
    T.-M. lumbar pad
    T.-M. O.R. table pad
    T.-M. pillow
    T.-M. seat wedge
    T.-M. stretch pad
    T.-M. wheelchair cushion
    T.-M. x-ray table pad
Tempur-Pedic
    T.-P. pressure relieving Swedish
      mattress
    T.-P. pressure relieving Swedish
      pillow
Tempur-Plus mattress
Temrex dental cement
Ten
    T. balloon
    T. system balloon catheter
tenaculum
    Abel-Aesculap-Pratt t.
    Adair breast t.
    Aesculap-Pratt t.
    Barrett uterine t.
    Braun-Schroeder single-tooth t.
    Braun uterine t.
    breast t.
    Brophy t.
    cervical t.
    Coakley t.
    Collen-Pozzi t.
    Corey t.
    Cottle single-prong t.
    double-tooth t.
    Duplay uterine t.
    Emmett cervical t.
    t. forceps
    t. holder
    t. hook
    t. hook loop
    Hulka uterine t.
    Jackson tracheal t.
    Jacobs uterine t.
    Jarcho uterine t.
    Kahn traction t.
    Kelly uterine t.
    Kennett t.
    Küstner t.
    Lahey goiter t.
    lion jaw t.
    Martin t.
    Museux t.
    nasal t.
    New t.
    Newman t.
    Potts t.
    Pozzi t.
    Pratt t.
    Revots vulsellum t.
    Ritchie cleft palate t.
    Sargis uterine t.
    Schroeder uterine t.
    single-tooth t.
    Skene uterine t.

T

tenaculum *(continued)*
Staude-Jackson uterine t.
Staude-Moore uterine t.
Staude uterine t.
straight t.
Teale t.
Thoms t.
thyroid t.
toothed t.
tracheal t.
traction t.
uterine t.
Watts t.
Weisman t.
White t.
Wylie uterine t.
tenaculum-reducing forceps
Tenador male pouch
Tena pouch
Tenax coronary stent
Tenckhoff
T. 2-cuff catheter
T. peritoneal catheter
T. renal dialysis catheter
Tender
T. subcutaneous infusion set
T. Touch extractor
T. Touch vacuum birthing cup
TenderCloud pressure pad
Tenderfoot incision-making device
Tenderlett device
Tendersorb ABD pad
TENDERWRAP Unna boot
tendon
t. carrier
t. forceps
t. gouge
t. hook
t. implant
t. knife
t. needle
t. passer
t. plate
t. prosthesis
t. stripper
t. tucker
Tutoplast anterior tibialis t.
tendon-bearing
patellar t.-b.
tendon-holding forceps
tendon-passing forceps
tendon-pulling forceps
tendon-retrieving forceps
tendon-seizing forceps
Tendril DX implantable pacing lead
Tennant
T. Anchorflex anterior chamber intraocular lens
T. Anchorflex lens implant
T. anchor lens-insertion hook
T. eye needle holder
T. intraocular lens forceps
T. iris hook
T. lens forceps

T. nuclear ball rotator
T. spatula
T. thumb-ring needle holder
T. titanium suturing forceps
T. tying forceps
Tennant-Colibri corneal forceps
Tennant-Maumenee forceps
Tennant-Troutman superior rectus forceps
Tenner lacrimal cannula
Tennessee capsular polisher
tennis
t. elbow splint
T. Racquet angiographic catheter
Ten-O-Matic TENS unit
Tenoplast elastic adhesive dressing
tenotome
Dieffenbach t.
Ljunggren-Stille t.
Ryerson t.
tenotomy
t. hook
t. scissors
TENS
transcutaneous electrical neuromuscular stimulator
TENS machine
TENS pad
TENS unit
Tensilon implant
tension
t. band wire tamp
t. clamp
t. isometer
tensioner
tension-requiring suture
Tensmax TENS unit
Tensor
T. elastic bandage roll
T. elastic dressing
Tensum coronary stent
TENS unit *(See also* unit)
Accucare TENS u.
Accu-o-Matic TENS u.
Dybex TENS u.
Electrorelaxor TENS u.
EMPI Neuropacer TENS u.
Meda 2500 TENS u.
Micro-Pulsar TENS u.
Mr. PainAway Health-Up TENS u.
Neuromod TENS u.
Neuro-Pulse TENS u.
Pulsar obstetrical two-channel TEN u.
Skylark TENS u.
Ten-O-Matic TENS u.
Tensmax TENS u.
tent
CAM t.
croup t.
Croupette child t.
hydrophilic t.
Hypan t.
KTK laminaria t.
laminaria cervical t.

mist t.
Mizutani laminaria t.
oxygen t.
Silon t.
steam t.
tentalum wire tension suture
Tenzel
    T. bipolar forceps
    T. calipers
    T. double-end periosteal elevator
Tepas retractor
Tepperwedge wedge
Teq-Trode electrode
teres knife
Terino
    T. anatomical chin implant
    T. facial implant retractor
    T. malar shell
terminal
    t. device
    t. electrode
    t. electrode adapter
    t. extensor mechanism
Ter-Pogossian cervical radium applicator
Terry
    T. astigmatome
    T. keratometer
    T. nail
    T. silicone capsular polisher
Terry-Mayo needle
Terson
    T. capsular forceps
    T. extracapsular forceps
    T. speculum
Terumo
    T. AV fistula needle
    T. dental needle
    T. dialyzer
    T. Doppler fetal heart rate monitor
    T. Glidewire
    T. hydrophilic guidewire
    T. hypodermic needle
    T. insulin syringe
    T. Radiofocus sheath
    T. SP coaxial catheter
    T. SP hydrophilic-polymer-coated
      microcatheter
    T. Steri-Cell processor
    T. Surflo intravenous catheter
    T. transducer protector
Terumo-Clirans dialyzer
Terumo/Meditech guidewire
Terumo-Radiofocus hydrophilic polymer-
    coated guidewire
Tesa S.A. hand-held electronic digital
    calipers
Tesberg esophagoscope
Tesio catheter
Tesla
    T. magnet
    T. MRI system
    T. Signa magnetic resonance imager
Tessier
    T. bone bender
    T. craniofacial instruments

T. dislodger
T. elevator
T. osteomicrotome
T. osteotome
T. spreader
Tes Tape dressing
test handle instrument
testicular implant
testing drum knife
Testoderm
    T. patch
    T. testosterone transdermal system
Testsimplets prestained slide
Test-Size orchidometer
tetrapolar esophageal catheter
Tetrax interactive balance system
Teufel cervical brace
Teurlings wrist brace
Tevdek
    T. implant
    T. pledgeted suture
    T. prosthesis
Tew
    T. cranial retractor
    T. needle
    T. spinal retractor
Texal-Muller chest binder
Texas
    T. cannula
    T. cannula tip
    T. condom catheter
    T. Goodstein sharp tip
    T. Scottish Rite Hospital
    T. Scottish Rite Hospital corkscrew
      device
    T. Scottish Rite Hospital crosslink
    T. Scottish Rite Hospital eyebolt
      spreader
    T. Scottish Rite Hospital hook
      holder
    T. Scottish Rite Hospital hook
      inserter
    T. Scottish Rite Hospital I-bolt
    T. Scottish Rite Hospital mini-
      corkscrew device
    T. Scottish Rite Hospital pedicle
      screw
    T. Scottish Rite Hospital screw-rod
      system
    T. Scottish Rite Hospital trial hook
    T. Scottish Rite Hospital (TSRH)
      instrumentation
    T. Scottish Rite Hospital wrench
Textor vasectomy clamp
TFE-coated wire guide
T-finger splint
T-Foam
    T.-F. bed pad
    T.-F. cushion
    T.-F. mattress
    T.-F. pillow
TG140 needle
T-Gel cushion
TG Osseotite single-stage procedure
    implant

T

T-grommet ventilation tube
Thackray
   T. dental forceps
   T. hip prosthesis
   T. mouthgag
Thackston retropubic bag
ThAIRapy
   T. vest
   T. vest airway clearance system
Thal-Mantel obturator
Thal-Quick chest tube
T-handle
   T.-h. bone awl
   T.-h. elevator
   T.-h. Jacob chuck
   T.-h. reamer
   T.-h. Zimmer chuck
T-handled
   T.-h. awl
   T.-h. cup curette
   T.-h. nut wrench
   T.-h. screw wrench
Tharies
   T. femoral resurfacing component
   T. hip component
   T. hip replacement prosthesis
Thatcher
   T. nail
   T. screw
The
   T. Asta-Cath female catheter guide
   T. Backstroke
   T. Beachcomber prosthetic foot
   T. Bodyguard emboli containment system
   T. Cell Sweep
   T. Corner cushion
   T. Dale tracheostomy tube holder
   T. Deluxe Button Bag
   T. Edge coated blade
   T. Feminal-female urinal
   T. Healthy Back System
   T. Heeler inflatable heel protector
   T. Hockey Stick articulating stylet
   T. Jacknobber II
   T. MMG Golden drain
   T. Original Backknobber muscle massager
   T. Original Backnobber massage tool
   T. Original Index Knobber II
   T. Original Index Knobber II massage tool
   T. Original Jacknobber massage tool
   T. Richie brace
   T. Rope stretching device
   T. Rope stretch and traction device
   T. Schneider esophageal Wallstent
   T. Sensar foldable acrylic posterior chamber intraocular lens
   T. Shark disposable biopsy forceps
   T. Side Rester cushion
   T. Travel Bath
   T. Treaser surgical instrument
   T. Trigger switch

   T. Unfolder intraocular lens implantation system
   T. Unloader brace
   T. Wave phacoemulsion system
thecoperitoneal Pudenz-Schulte shunt
Theden bandage
Theis
   T. infant rib spreader
   T. self-retaining rib retractor
   T. vein retractor
Theobald
   T. lacrimal dilator
   T. sinus probe
Thera
   T. Cane massager
   T. Cane shoulder exerciser
   T. Cool cold therapy
   T. Cool cold therapy system
Thera-Band
   T.-B. ASSIST
   T.-B. ASSIST exerciser
   T.-B. exercise ball
   T.-B. handle
   T.-B. Max band
   T.-B. strip
   T.-B. therapy band
   T.-B. therapy device
   T.-B. tubing
Therabath paraffin heat therapy syste
TheraBeads microwaveable moist heat pack
Therabite
   T. jaw exerciser
   T. jaw motion rehabilitation syste
   T. mobilizer
Thera-Boot
   T.-B. bandage
   T.-B. compression dressing
   T.-B. compression wrap
Theracloud pillow
Thera-Fit
Theraflex wrist exerciser
Theraform Selectives
Theragym ball
Ther-A-Hoop exerciser
Thera-Loop exerciser
Thera-Med cold pack
Thera-Medic shoe
Theramini 1, 2 electrotherapy stimula
TheraPEP positive expiratory pressure therapy system
therapeutic
   t. side-viewing duodenoscope
   t. splint
Therapeutica sleeping pillow
Thera-P exercise bar
Thera-Plast putty
Therap-Loop
   T.-L. door anchor
   T.-L. door handle
Thera-Pos
   T.-P. elbow orthosis
   T.-P. knee orthosis
TheraPulse pulsating air suspension b

Thera-Putty
T.-P. exercise putty
T.-P. therapy device
therapy
600 Asta frameless air support t.
t. ball
Bio t.
Burke Plus frameless air support t.
T. Carrot Finger Orthosis
Cool-Aid continuous controlled cold t.
Electri-Cool continuous controlled cold t.
Enterra t.
Facial Flex t.
GeriMend skin tear t.
Gold Probe hemostasis t.
InFerno moist heat t.
interferential t.
Kelsey unloading exercise t.
Lymphapress compression t.
MagneCore magnetic t.
magnet t.
Medtronic Activa tremor-control t.
Moxa heat t.
parachute t.
Pedi Asta frameless air support t.
Pneu-Scale frameless air support t.
ProFlo vascular compression t.
Pro-Op frameless air support t.
Pro-series frameless air support t.
Pro-Turn frameless air support t.
RT/SC 2000 frameless air support t.
Synergy frameless air support t.
Synergy Pulse frameless air support t.
Thera Cool cold t.
triple t.
VersaLight photodynamic t.
XKnife software for stereotatic radiation t.
TherArc pillow
TheraRest mattress
TheraSeed implant
Ther-A-Shapes positioner
TheraSkin wound dressing
Therasleep cervical pillow
TheraSnore
T. device
T. oral appliance
Thera-Soft hand/wrist orthosis
Therasonics lithotriptor
Therasound transducer
Thera-SR pacemaker
Theratotic
T. firm foot orthosis
T. soft foot orthosis
Theratouch 4.7 stimulator
Thera-turn rotational system
Thermacare quilt
ThermaChoice
T. catheter
T. thermal balloon ablation

T. uterine balloon
T. uterine balloon therapy system
Thermaderm epilator
Thermafil
T. plastic carrier
T. Plus obturator
Therma Jaw hot urologic forceps
thermal
t. balloon system
t. conductivity detector
t. dosimetry system
t. energy analyzer
t. knife
t. memory stent
t. plastic wrap
T. responsive non-latex nitrile surgical glove
t. space blanket
Thermalator heating unit
Thermapad pad
Thermasonic gel warmer
ThermaSplint heating bath
Thermassage
Aqua T.
ThermaStim
T. muscle warming device
T. muscule stimulator
Thermedics
T. cardiac device
T. HeartMate 10001P left anterior assist device
T. left ventricular assist device
Thermex
Direx T.
Thermex-II transurethral prostate heating device
thermistor
t. needle
nostril t.
t. probe
t. rectal thermometer
t. thermodilution catheter
Thermo
T. Cardiosystems left ventricular assist device
T. hand comforter
T. HK/Rohadur orthotic
T. HK/Tepefom orthotic
T. knee comforter
ThermoChem-HT system
thermocoagulator
Olympus CD-Z-series heat probe t.
thermocouple
Chromel-Alumel t.
copper-constantan t.
low impedance t.
Mon-a-Therm t.
needle t.
Thermocycler cycle
thermodeltameter
thermodilution
t. balloon catheter
t. cardiac output computer
t. catheter introducer kit

T

thermodilution *(continued)*
  t. pacing catheter
  t. Swan-Ganz catheter
thermoexpandable stent
ThermoFlex
  Maramed T.
  T. thermotherapy unit
Thermo-Flex suture
Thermo-Flo irrigation system
thermographic scanner
Thermograph temperature monitor
thermoluminescent
  t. dosimeter
  t. dosimeter rod
thermometer
  Acuprobe t.
  basal body t.
  Core-Check tympanic t.
  Coretemp deep tissue t.
  EZ Temp t.
  Fahrenheit flat bath t.
  FirstTemp Genius tympanic t.
  Instant Fever Tester t.
  Iso-Thermex 16-channel electronic t.
  IVAC Temp Plus II t.
  LighTouch Neonate t.
  Mon-a-Therm 6510 two-channel t.
  Ototemp 3000 t.
  Philips SensorTouch temple t.
  Quik-Temp t.
  Stik-Temp t.
  SureTemp4 oral t.
  Tegam microprocessor t.
  Tel-A-Fever forehead t.
  Tempa-DOT axillary t.
  thermistor rectal t.
  Thermoscan Pro-1 tympanic
    instant t.
  tympanic membrane t.
Thermophore
  T. bandage
  T. hot pack
  T. moist heat pad
thermoplastic
  t. splint
  t. stent
  t. template
thermopore
  Shahan t.
Thermoprep heating oven
Thermoscan Pro-1 tympanic instant
  thermometer
Thermoskin
  T. arthritic knee wrap
  T. back wrap
  T. brace
  T. heat retainer
Thermos pacemaker
Thermovac tissue pulverizer
Thero-Skin gel padding
TherOx infusion guide wire
Theurig sterilizer forceps
thick-walled Dacron-backed implant

Thiersch
  T. graft
  T. implant
  T. prosthesis
  T. skin graft knife
  T. suture
  T. wire
thigh
  t. balloon
  t. tourniquet
thigh-high antiembolic stockings
Thillaye
  T. bandage
  T. dressing
thin
  t. acupuncture needle
  t. disposable cannula
  t. film dressing
thin-layer chromatograph
ThinLine EZ bipolar cardiac pacing
  lead
Thinline uncovered orthotic
Thinlith II pacemaker
ThinPrep
  T. cytologic preparation
  T. processor
thin-shaft nasal scissors
THINSite
  T. topical wound dressing
  T. topical wound dressing with
    BioFilm hydrogel
  T. with BioFilm
thin-walled needle
thin-wall introducer catheter
thin-wire Ilizarov fixator
third generation lithotriptor
Thole
  T. goniometer
  T. pelvimeter
Thoma
  T. clamp
  T. tissue retractor
Thomas
  T. brush
  T. bur
  T. calipers
  T. cervical collar brace
  T. collar
  T. collar cervical orthosis
  T. cryoextractor
  T. cryoprobe
  T. cryoptor
  T. cryoretractor
  T. extrapolated bar graft
  T. femoral shunt
  T. fixation forceps
  T. fixator
  T. fracture frame
  T. full-ring splint
  T. heel
  T. heel orthosis
  T. hinged splint
  T. hyperextension frame
  T. I&A cannula
  T. Kapsule instruments

T. keratome
T. knee splint
T. Kodel sling
T. leg splint
T. Long-Term endotracheal tube holder
T. magnet
T. needle
T. pelvimeter
T. pessary
T. posterior splint
T. retractor
T. scissors
T. shot compression forceps
T. spatula
T. splint with Pearson attachment
T. subretinal instrument set II
T. suspension splint
T. uterine curette
T. walking brace
T. wrench
Thompson
    T. adenoid curette
    T. bronchial catheter
    T. carotid artery clamp
    T. cervical transilluminator
    T. chin support
    T. direct full-vision resectoscope
    T. dowel
    T. drape
    T. endoprosthesis
    T. evacuator
    T. femoral head prosthesis
    T. femoral neck prosthesis
    T. frontal sinus rasp
    T. hemiarthroplasty hip prosthesis
    T. hip endoprosthesis system
    T. hip prosthesis forceps
    T. hyperextension fracture frame
    T. modification of Denis Browne splint
    T. punch
    T. retractor
    T. rib shears
    T. stem rasp
Thompson-Farley spinal retractor system
Thoms
    T. pelvimeter
    T. tenaculum
    T. tissue forceps
Thoms-Allis
    T.-A. intestinal forceps
    T.-A. tissue forceps
    T.-A. vulsellum
Thomsen rib shears
Thoms-Gaylor
    T.-G. biopsy punch
    T.-G. uterine forceps
Thomson
    T. adenoidal punch
    T. lung clamp
Thomson-Walker
    T.-W. scissors
    T.-W. urethrotome
ThoraCath catheter

thoracentesis needle
thoracic
    t. artery forceps
    t. cage
    t. catheter
    t. clamp
    t. drain
    t. scissors
    t. tissue forceps
    t. trocar
thoracoabdominal (TA) 55 stapler
thoracolumbar
    t. pedicle screw
    t. spinal orthosis
    t. standing orthosis
    t. standing orthosis brace
thoracolumbosacral
    t. plate
    t. spinal orthosis
thoracolumbosacroiliac implant system
Thoracoport
    Auto Suture Soft T.
    Soft T.
    T. trocar
thoracoscope, thorascope
    Boutin t.
    Coryllos t.
    Cutler forceps t.
    Jacobaeus t.
    Jacobaeus-Unverricht t.
    Moore t.
    Sarot t.
    Storz t.
Thoracoseal drainage
thoracostomy tube
thoracotome
Thora-Drain III chest drainage
Thora-Klex
    T.-K. chest drainage system
    T.-K. chest tube
Thora-Port
    T.-P. port
thorascope (*var. of* thoracoscope)
Thoratec
    T. biventricular assist device
    T. cardiac device
    T. mechanical circulatory support system
    T. pump
    T. right ventricular assist device
Thoreau filter
Thorek
    T. gallbladder aspirator
    T. gallbladder forceps
    T. gallbladder scissors
    T. thoracic scissors
Thorek-Feldman gallbladder scissors
Thorek-Mixter gallbladder forceps
Thorlakson
    T. deep abdominal retractor
    T. lower occlusive clamp
    T. multipurpose retractor
    T. upper occlusive clamp
Thornton
    T. arcuate blade

T

Thornton *(continued)*
T. corneal marker
T. corneal press-on ruler
T. double corneal ruler
T. episcleral forceps
T. fixating ring
T. fixation forceps
T. intraocular forceps
T. iris retractor
T. K3-7991 360 degree arcuate marker
T. low-profile marker
T. malleable spatula
T. nail
T. needle
T. open-wire lid speculum
T. plate
T. T-incision diamond knife
T. tri-square blade
Thornton-Fine ring
Thornwald
T. antral drill
T. antral irrigator
T. antral perforator
T. antral trephine
Thorpe
T. calipers
T. conjunctival forceps
T. corneal forceps
T. corneoscleral forceps
T. curette
T. foreign body forceps
T. four-mirror goniolaser
T. four-mirror goniolaser lens
T. four-mirror goniolens
T. four-mirror vitreous fundus laser lens
T. gonioprism lens
T. plastic lens
T. pupillary membrane scissors
T. slit lamp
T. surgical gonioscope
Thorpe-Castroviejo
T.-C. calipers
T.-C. cataract scissors
T.-C. corneal forceps
T.-C. fixation forceps
T.-C. goniolens
T.-C. vitreous foreign body forceps
Thorpe-Westcott cataract scissors
THORP-type mandibular reconstruction plate
Thrasher
T. intraocular forceps
T. lens implant forceps
thread
BioCare t.
BioHorizon t.
polyene t.
SMIC nylon t.
t. suture
Wi-Last-Ic t.
threaded
t. cortical dowel

t. eye needle
t. guide pin
t. interbody fusion cage
t. rod
t. titanium acetabular prosthesis
threader
Allen wire t.
Borchard wire t.
cannulated wire t.
Frackelton wire t.
Hamby wire t.
t. rod holder pliers
wire t.
ThreadLoc
T. driver mount screw
T. implant
T. non-cast-to abutment
T. retaining screw
thread-locking device
three-axis gradient coil
three-bladed clamp
three-dimensional
t.-d. biocompatible scaffold
t.-d. fast spin-echo magnetic resonance imaging
t.-d. magnetic sensor
t.-d. sonic digitizer
t.-d. SPECT phantom
Three-D worker's back support
three-footed lens intraocular lens
three-head camera
three-hole
t.-h. aspiration cannula
t.-h. plate
three-legged cage heart valve
three-mirror
t.-m. contact lens
t.-m. intraocular lens
three-piece
t.-p. acrylic intraocular lens
t.-p. modified J-loop intraocular len
t.-p. silicone intraocular lens
three-point
t.-p. fixation intraocular lens
t.-p. head holder
t.-p. spreader bag
three-prong
t.-p. fork
t.-p. grasping forceps
t.-p. rake blade retractor
three-pronged
t.-p. grasper
t.-p. polyp retriever
t.-p. rake blade
three-stopcock manifold
three-turn epicardial lead
three-way
t.-w. bridge
t.-w. Foley catheter
t.-w. irrigating catheter
three-wheel walker
Threshold
T. inspiratory muscle trainer device
T. positive expiratory pressure device

Thriftcast alloy
Throat-E-Vac suction device
throat forceps
thrombectomy catheter
thrombin-soaked Gelfoam
thromboembolic
    t. disease stockings
    t. disease (TED) hose
Thrombogen absorbable hemostat
ThromboScan MRI
thrombosuction catheter
thrombus stripper
through-and-through reabsorbable suture
through-cutting forceps tip
through-the-scope (TTS)
    t.-t.-s. balloon
    t.-t.-s. bougie
    t.-t.-s. catheter probe
    t.-t.-s. dilator
    t.-t.-s. injection needle
through-the-wall mattress suture
throw-away manual dermatome blade
Thruflex
    T. balloon
    T. PTCA balloon catheter
Thrust femoral prosthesis
Thudichum nasal speculum
thulium-holmium-chromium:yttrium-
    aluminum-garnet (THC:YAG) laser
thulium-holmium:YAG laser
thumb
    t. retractor
    t. Spica bandage
    t. spica cast
    t. tissue forceps
Thumbkeeper
    Freedom T.
Thumb-Saver introducer clamp
Thumper
    T. CPR system
    T. device
ThumZ'Up functional thumb splint
Thurmond
    T. iris retractor
    T. nucleus-irrigating cannula
Thurston-Holland fragment forceps
Thymapad stimulus electrode
thymus retractor
thyroid
    t. drain
    t. forceps
    t. retractor
    t. tenaculum
Thyrx timer
Ti
    Ti alloy screw
    Ti rotor
Ti-BAC
    Ti-BAC acetabular component
    Ti-BAC II hip prosthesis
    Ti-BAC I, II acetabular cup
Tibbs
    T. arterial cannula
    T. semiautomatic suturing device

tibial
    t. aligner
    t. augmentation block
    t. bolt
    t. broach
    t. calipers
    t. collet
    t. cutter guide
    t. cutting block
    t. driver
    t. endoprosthesis
    t. fracture brace proximal support
    t. guide pin
    t. plate
    t. plateau prosthesis
    t. retractor
    t. stylus
    t. torsion system
Tickner tissue forceps
Ti/CoCr hip prosthesis
Ticonium splint
Ti-Cron suture
Ticsay transpubic needle
Tidal Wave hand-held capnograph
tie
    cable t.
    gauze neck t.
    table t.
Tieck-Halle infant nasal speculum
Tieck nasal speculum
Tiedmann rongeur
Tielle hydropolymer dressing
Tiemann
    T. bullet forceps
    T. coudé catheter
    T. nail
    T. Neoflex catheter
Tiemann-Foley catheter
Tiemann-Meals tenolysis knife
tie-on needle
tie-over
    t.-o. bolster
    t.-o. Sellotape dressing
tier
    Adson knot t.
    Harris wire t.
    knot t.
tiered-therapy
    t.-t. antiarrhythmic device
    t.-t. implantable cardioverter-
       defibrillator
Ti-Fit total hip system
tiger
    T. blade
    t. gut suture
    T. Shark forceps
tightener
    Bowen wire t.
    Charnley wire t.
    Harris wire t.
    Kirschner wire t.
    Loute wire t.
    Shiffrin bone wire t.
    Sklar wire t.

T

tightener *(continued)*
    Verner-Joseph wire t.
    wire t.
tight-to-shaft Aire-Cuf tracheostomy tube
Tiko
    T. pliable iris retractor
    T. rake retractor
    T. zonule sweeper
Tilastin hip prosthesis
Tilderquist needle holder
Tillary double-ended retractor
Tilley dressing forceps
Tilley-Henckel forceps
Tilley-Lichwitz trocar
Tillyer bifocal lens
tilt
    t. table
    T. and Turn Paragon bed
Tilt-Board
    G5 Vari-Tilt Adjustable T.-B.
tilting-disk
    t.-d. aortic valve prosthesis
    t.-d. heart valve
Tilt-In-Space wheelchair conversion
Timberlake
    T. catheter
    T. electrode
    T. evacuator
    T. irrigating tip
    T. obturator
    T. obturator electrotome
    T. obturator resectoscope
time-based counter
time-gain compensator
time-of-flight
    t.-o.-f. PET imaging system
    t.-o.-f. positron emission
       tomographic camera
timer
    Apgar t.
    Medela Apgar t.
    Medtronic automated coagulation t.
    Thyrx t.
    video t.
TiMesh
    T. bone-plate
    T. burrhole cover
    T. cranial mesh
    T. craniofacial system
    T. craniomaxillofacial plating system
    T. hardware
    T. mandibular crib
    T. orbital mesh
    T. orthognathic strap plate
    T. patient configured titanium
       craniomaxillofacial implant
    T. rigid fixation bone plating
       system
    T. screw
    T. titanium bone plating system
    T. titanium mesh
    T. titanium tray
Timeter pocket spirometer
time-to-pulse height converter

TINA monitor
tin-bullet probe
T-incision marker
Tindall scissors
tined
    t. lead pacemaker
    t. ventricular electrode
Tinel
    T. suture
    T. tapered reamer
    T. tourniquet
Tinnant gauge
tinted spectacles
Tiny-Tef ventilation tube
Tiny Tytan ventilation tube
TiOblast dental implant
tip
    ACMI cystoscopic t.
    Adson brain suction t.
    aerosol-barrier pipette t.
    Air-Shield-Vickers syringe t.
    Andrews suction t.
    Bard t.
    Batt t.
    Becker flat dissector t.
    Becker round dissector t.
    Becker twist dissector t.
    Binkhorst t.
    bipolar diathermy forceps t.
    Bruening biting t.
    buccal fat extractor t.
    Cloward cervical drill t.
    Cobra+ cannula t.
    Cobra K+ cannula t.
    Colorado electrocautery t.
    coned heparin t.
    conical inserter t.
    Cope-Saddekni catheter t.
    Cordes punch forceps t.
    Corometrics Gold Quik Connect
       Spiral electrode t.
    coronary perfusion t.
    CUSA laparoscopic t.
    custom t.
    diathermy t.
    disposable cannula t.
    double-articulated forceps t.
    Ducor t.
    eel cobra t.
    Extended Wear self-adhering urinary
       external catheter with removable
    E-Z Clean cautery t.
    Fell sucker t.
    flared ABS t.
    Flexoreamer Batt t.
    Fournier t.
    Fragmatome t.
    Frazier suction t.
    Gasparotti bevel t.
    Gess cannula t.
    Girard irrigating t.
    grasping forceps t.
    t. guard
    guillotine cutting t.
    Henke punch forceps t.

Hetter pyramid t.
Hydro-Dissection t.
Illouz modified t.
Illouz standard t.
Implantech SE-100 smoke
  aspiration t.
infraguide t.
irrigating t.
Jackson square punch t.
Japanese suction t.
Kahler double-action t.
Keeler lancet t.
Keeler micro spear t.
Keeler puncture t.
Keeler razor t.
Keeler round t.
Keeler triple-facet t.
Kelman t.
K-Flexofile Batt t.
Killian cutting forceps t.
Killian double-articulated forceps t.
Klein cannula t.
Klein 1-hole infiltrator t.
Klein multihole infiltrator t.
Krause oval punch t.
Krause punch forceps t.
Krause square-basket t.
Leasure round punch t.
Leon cobra t.
Marlow Primus t.
Mayo coronary perfusion t.
Medtronic t.
MegaDyne E-Z clean cautery t.
Mercedes t.
Micro-Probe t.
MicroTip phaco t.
Myerson biting t.
Nu-Tip disposable scissor t.
Omni laser t.
Pinto dissector t.
plumbeous zirconate titanate t.
Polaris Mansfield/Webster
  deflectable t.
pyramid Toomey t.
Quad cutting t.
Radovan tissue expander t.
Roane bullet t.
Rosenberg dissector t.
rubber acorn t.
Savary-Gilliard t.
Saverburger irrigation/aspiration t.
Scheinmann biting t.
Schuknecht suction t.
SE-100 smoke aspiration t.
Simcoe cannula t.
Simcoe interchangeable t.
Sims suction t.
SITE guillotine cutting t.
Skimmer laryngeal blade t.
Slip-Coat t.
spatula cannula t.
Spencer oval t.
Spencer triangular t.
Spencer Universal adenoid punch t.
Struyken angular punch t.

sucker t.
suction t.
Surgi-Fine reusable cannula t.
synthetic sapphire t.
Texas cannula t.
Texas Goodstein sharp t.
through-cutting forceps t.
Timberlake irrigating t.
Tischler-Morgan t.
Toledo flap dissector t.
Toledo standard dissector t.
Toledo V-dissector t.
Toomey pyramid t.
Tracer Hybrid wire guide with
  Slip-Coat t.
Trevisani cannula t.
Tricut laryngeal blade t.
TriEye t.
triport t.
tulip t.
tungsten t.
TurboSonic t.
Ultrafyn cautery t.
Unitri t.
Universal adenoid punch t.
V. Mueller cystoscopy t.
weighted t.
Yankauer tonsil suction t.

tip-deflecting
  t.-d. catheter
  t.-d. guidewire
Tip-Trol handle
tire
  t. eye implant
  implant t.
  silicone t.
  Watzke t.
tire-grooved silicone
Tischler
  T. cervical biopsy punch
  T. cervical biopsy punch forceps
Tischler-Morgan
  T.-M. biopsy punch
  T.-M. tip
  T.-M. uterine biopsy forceps
Ti-Spacer
  Cohort T.-S.
Tisseel
  T. biologic fibrogen adhesive
  T. fibrin glue
  T. surgical glue
  T. VH kit
Tissomat
Tissot spirometer
tissue
  t. anchor guide (TAG)
  t. anchor guide system
  t. culture flask
  t. desiccation needle
  t. desiccation needle electrode
  t. drain
  t. expander
  t. expander template
  t. forceps
  t. glue

T

tissue *(continued)*
t. graft press
t. lifter
t. mandrel implant material
t. morcellator
t. occlusion clamp
Ogura t.
t. plane dissector
t. press
t. protector
t. reflectance oximeter
t. retractor
t. scissors
t. sizer template
t. solder
T. Specific imaging
T. Tek-II cryostat
Tutoplast t.
tissue-engineered construct
tissue-grasping forceps
Tissue-Guard bovine pericardial patch
tissue-holding forceps
tissue-spreading forceps
tissue-wetting pak
Tis-U-Sol
Tis-U-Trap
T.-U.-T. endometrial suction
T.-U.-T. endometrial suction catheter
Tital balloon catheter
Titan
T. Apollo electric flexion table
T. endoprosthesis
T. hip cup
T. Meridian Intersegmental Traction table
T. Nova manual flexion-extension multi flex table
T. scaler
T. slow-speed handpiece
T. stent
titanate
titanium
t. alloy implant
t. alloy needle
t. aneurysm clip
t. AO plate
t. ball-cage heart valve
t. cable
t. cage
t. construct
t. elastic nail
t. fixation device
t. foil
t. half pin
t. hollow osseointegrating reconstruction plate
t. hollow-screw osseointegrating reconstruction plate
t. hollow screw plate system
t. implant material
t. mandibular staple
t. mesh
t. mesh tray
t. microconnector

t. microsurgical bipolar forceps
t. micro system
t. mini bur hole cover
t. miniplate
t. plasma sprayed dental implant
t. prosthesis
t. retinal tack
t. screw
t. spiked washer
t. urethral stent
T. VasPort port
T. Wedge electrosurgical resection device
t. wire
t. wound retractor
Titan-Mega catheter
Titmus stereo fly
Titus
T. forearm splint
T. tongue depressor
T. venoclysis needle
T. wrist splint
Tivanium
T. hip prosthesis
T. Ti-6A1-4V alloy
Tivnen tonsillar forceps
TJF-100 Olympus endoscope
TJF endoscope
TK Optimizer knee prosthesis
TL-90 stapler
TLC Baxter balloon catheter
T-lens therapeutic contact lens
TLS
TLS suction drain
TLS surgical drain
TLS surgical marker
TMJ
temporomandibular joint
TMJ acrylic
TMJ Concepts patient-fitted TMJ prosthesis system
TMJ fossa-eminence prosthesis
TMJ halter
TMJ head positioner
T-model endaural retractor
TMS-1 videokeratoscope GTS
TMS-2 videokeratoscope
TMS three-dimensional radiation therapy treatment planning system
Toad finger splint
Tobald syringe
Tobey
T. ear forceps
T. ear rongeur
Tobin anatomical malar prosthetic implant
Tobold
T. laryngeal forceps
T. laryngeal knife
T. laryngoscopic apparatus
T. tongue depressor
Tobold-Fauvel grasping forceps
Tobolsky elevator
tobramycin-impregnated PMMA implant
Tobruk splint

Tocantins bone marrow biopsy needle
tocodynamometer
   guard-ring t.
   Nihon t.
tocotonometer
Todd
   T. bur hole button
   T. cautery
   T. electrocautery
   T. eye cautery needle
   T. foreign body gouge
   T. stereotaxic guide
Todd-Wells
   T.-W. guide
   T.-W. stereotactic frame
   T.-W. stereotaxic instrument
Todt-Heyer cannula guide
ToDyeFor root canal locator
toe
   t. comb
   t. loop
   t. plate
   t. prosthesis
toedrop brace
Toennis
   T. director
   T. dissecting scissors
   T. dissector
   T. dural hook
   T. dural knife
   T. ES stand-alone constant-current
     electrical stimulator
   T. needle holder
   T. retractor
   T. tumor-grasping forceps
Toennis-Adson
   T.-A. dissector
   T.-A. dural scissors
   T.-A. forceps
Toes Protector
Tofflemire
   T. matrix band
   T. retainer
Toitu cardiovascular monitor
Tolantins bone marrow infusion catheter
Toledo
   T. dissector
   T. flap dissector tip
   T. roller
   T. standard dissector tip
   T. V-dissector cannula
   T. V-dissector tip
Tolentino
   T. prism lens
   T. ring
   T. vitrectomy lens
   T. vitreoretinal cutter
Tolman
   T. micrometer
   T. tonometer
Tomac
   T. catheter
   T. clip
   T. foam rubber traction dressing
   T. forceps

   T. goniometer
   T. knitted rubber elastic dressing
   T. vest-style holder
Tomac-Nélaton catheter
Tomas
   T. iris hook
   T. suture hook
Tomenius gastroscope
Tomey
   T. angled cannula
   T. autorefractor
   T. autotopographer
   T. G-bevel cannula
   T. retinal function analyzer
   T. standard cannula
   T. TMS-1 photokeratoscope
   T. topographic modeling system
   T. topography system
   T. trabeculectomy punch
   T. Trooper AutoLensmeter
Tommy
   T. hip bar
   T. trapeze bar
Tomolex tomographic system
Tomomatic brain scanner
tomoscanner
   Philips T-60 t.
Tompkins aspirator
TomTec
   T. cell harvester
   T. echo platform
   T. imaging system
tone-reducing ankle-foot orthosis
Tones
   Tap N' T.
tongs
   adjustable skull traction t.
   Barton-Cone t.
   Barton skull traction t.
   Böhler t.
   Cherry traction t.
   Crutchfield-Raney skull traction t.
   Crutchfield skeletal traction t.
   Edmonton extension t.
   Gardner-Wells traction t.
   Hinz t.
   Raney-Crutchfield skull t.
   Reynolds skull traction t.
   skull traction t.
   traction t.
   Trippi-Wells t.
   University of Virginia skull t.
   Vinke t.
tongue
   t. depressor
   t. forceps
   t. plate
   t. plate electrode
   t. retractor
   t. retractor blade
tongue-retaining device
Tonkaflo pump
Tonomat applanation tonometer
tonometer (T)
   Alcon t.

T

tonometer *(continued)*
    Allen-Schiotz plunger retractor t.
    applanation t.
    Bailliart t.
    Barraquer applanation t.
    Barraquer operating room t.
    Berens t.
    Carl Zeiss t.
    Challenger digital applanation t.
    Coburn t.
    CT-10 computerized t.
    Digilab t.
    Draeger t.
    Gärtner t.
    Goldmann applanation t.
    Harrington t.
    hollow visceral t.
    impression t.
    indentation t.
    Intermedics intraocular t.
    Jena-Schiotz t.
    Keeler Pulsair noncontact t.
    Krakau t.
    Linear KGT t.
    Lombart t.
    Mack t.
    MacKay-Marg t.
    Maklakoff t.
    McLean t.
    Meding tonsil enucleator t.
    Mueller electronic t.
    Musken t.
    noncontact t.
    Nuvistor electronic t.
    Pach-Pen XL t.
    Perkins applanation t.
    pneumatic t.
    pressure phosphene t.
    ProTon portable t.
    Pulsair t.
    Recklinghausen t.
    Reichert noncontact t.
    Rosner t.
    Roush t.
    Ruedemann t.
    Sauer t.
    Sauer-Storz t.
    Schiötz t.
    Sklar t.
    Sklar-Schitz jewel t.
    Sluder t.
    Sluder-Demarest t.
    Storz t.
    Storz-Schitz t.
    Tolman t.
    Tonomat applanation t.
    Tono-Pen XL t.
Tono-Pen
    Oculab T.-P.
    T.-P. XL tonometer
tonsil
    t. clamp
    t. forceps
    t. guillotine

tonsillar
    t. abscess forceps
    t. artery forceps
    t. calipers
    t. clamp
    t. coblation
    t. compressor
    t. curette
    t. dissector
    t. electrode
    t. expressor
    t. guillotine
    t. hemostatic forceps
    t. hook
    t. knife
    t. loop
    t. pillar grasping forceps
    t. pillar retractor
    t. punch
    t. punch forceps
    t. scissors
    t. screw
    t. snare
    t. snare wire
    t. sponge
    t. suction tube
    t. suture needle
    t. syringe
tonsillectome
    Ballenger-Sluder t.
    Beck-Mueller t.
    Beck-Schenck t.
    Brown t.
    Daniels hemostatic t.
    hemostatic t.
    LaForce hemostatic t.
    t. loop
    Mack lingual tonsillar t.
    Meding tonsil enucleator t.
    Moltz-Storz t.
    Myles guillotine t.
    Sauer hemostatic t.
    Sauer-Sluder t.
    Sauer-Storz t.
    Searcy t.
    Seiffert t.
    Sluder-Ballenger t.
    Sluder-Demarest t.
    Sluder-Sauer t.
    Sluder tonsillar t.
    Storz-Moltz t.
    tonsillectome t.
    Tydings t.
    Van Osdel tonsil enucleator t.
    Whiting t.
Tooke
    T. angled corneal knife
    T. angled splitter
    T. blade
    T. corneal forceps
    T. iris knife
    T. spatula
Tooke-Johnson corneal knife
tool
    AcuPressor myotherapy t.

Avenue insertion t.
Backnobber II massage t.
Gore Smoother Crucial T.
Index Knobber II massage t.
lapping t.
Lillie-Koffler t.
Magnassager massage t.
OsteoStat disposable power t.
pressure sore status t.
QuantX color quantification t.
Rolz massage t.
spud t.
The Original Backnobber massage t.
The Original Index Knobber II
    massage t.
The Original Jacknobber massage t.
Toomey
    T. bladder evacuator
    T. forceps
    T. pyramid tip
    T. surgical steel instrument set
    T. syringe
    T. syringe kit
tooth
    t. band
    t. cement
    t. guard
tooth-borne distraction device
toothbrush
    Water Pik t.
tooth-colored abutment
toothed
    t. pickups
    t. retractor
    t. tenaculum
    t. thumb forceps
    t. tissue forceps
tooth-extracting forceps
toothless forceps
Topaz
    T. CO_2 laser
    T. flexion table
Topcon
    T. aspheric lens
    T. chart projector
    T. 50IA camera
    T. IMAGEnet digital imaging
        system
    T. keratometer
    T. LM P5 digital lensometer
    T. noncontact morphometric analysis
    T. refractor
    T. RM-A2300 auto refractometer
    T. SL-45 camera
    T. SL-E series slit lamp
    T. SP-series non-contact specular
        microscope
    T. TRC-50IX ICG-capable fundus
        camera
    T. TRC-SS2 stereoscopic fundus
        camera
    T. TRC-50VT retinal camera
    T. TRC-50X retinal camera
    T. TRV-50VT fundus camera
TOP ejector punch

top-entry (open body) hook
Top-Hat supraannular aortic valve
**TopiFoam gel-backed self-adhering foam
    pad**
Top Notch automated biopsy system
topographic
    T. Modeling System-1
    t. scanning/indocyanine green
        angiography combination instrument
    t. scanning system
toposcopic catheter
Topper
    T. cannula
    T. dressing sponge
    T. mattress overlay
    T. nonadherent gauze
TopSS
    T. scanning laser ophthalmoscope
    T. topographic scanning system
Torbot
    T. cement
    T. Plastic pouch
    T. Rubber pouch
Torchia
    T. capsular forceps
    T. capsular polisher
    T. conjunctival scissors
    T. corneal knife
    T. eye speculum
    T. lens hook
    T. lens implantation forceps
    T. microbipolar forceps
    T. microcorneal scissors
    T. nucleus-aspirating cannula
    T. tissue forceps
    T. tying forceps
    T. vectis loop
Torchia-Colibri forceps
Torchia-Kuglen hook
Torchia-Vannas micro-iris scissors
**Torcon NB selective angiographic
    catheter**
toric
    crimped t.
    t. intraocular lens
Torktherm torque control catheter
torlone fixation pin
Toronto
    T. bioprosthesis
    T. Medical CPM exerciser
    T. parapodium orthosis
    T. splint
    T. SPV aortic valve
Toronto-Western catheter
TORP
    total ossicular replacement prosthesis
    TORP ossicular prosthesis
    Plastiport TORP
    Proplast TORP
    TORP strut
torpedo
    Gelfoam t.
Torpedo eye patch
Torpin
    T. automatic uterine gauze packer

T

Torpin *(continued)*
  T. obstetrical lever
  T. vectis
  T. vectis blade
  T. vectis extractor
torque
  t. attenuating diameter wire
  t. ratchet wrench
  t. vise
torque-control balloon catheter
torqued slot bracket
torque-type prosthesis
Torre Cryojet
Torres
  T. cross-action forceps
  T. needle holder
Torrington French spring needle
torsion
  t. bar splint
  t. forceps
torso phased-array coil
Toshiba
  T. biplane transesophageal transducer
  T. brain scanner
  T. echocardiograph machine
  T. electrocardiography machine
  T. ERVF 1A video floppy recorder
  T. helical CT scanner
  T. microendoprope
  T. microendoscope
  T. MR scanner
  T. Sal 38B real-time
  ultrasonography
  T. 900S helical CT scanner
  T. Sonolayer SSA250A transrectal
  ultrasonography
  T. Sonolayer SSH-140A ultrasound
  T. SSA-340A Doppler sonography
  T. TCE-M-series colonoscope
  T. video endoscope
  T. Xpress SX helical CT scanner
  T. Xvision scanner
total
  t. alloplastic TMJ reconstruction
  prosthesis
  t. contact bivalve ankle-foot orthosis
  t. contact cast
  t. gym
  T. Knee 2100 prosthetic knee
  t. ossicular prosthesis
  t. ossicular replacement prosthesis
  (TORP)
  T. O_2 system
  T. Synchrony system
  t. toe template
  t. top implant
total-body compression suit
Totallift-II lifter
totally-implantable catheter
Totco
  T. Autoclip
  T. clip
Tote-A-Neb nebulizer

Toti
  T. trephine
  T. trephine drill
Tott ring remover
TouchAmerica BodyTable
Touchlite zoom lens
Touhy-Borst connector
Touma
  T. dissector
  T. T-type grommet ventilation tu
Tourguide guiding catheter
Tournikwik tourniquet
tourniquet
  Adams modification of Bethune
  automatic t.
  t. band
  Bethune lobectomy t.
  Bethune lung t.
  Bodenstab t.
  Campbell-Boyd t.
  Carr lobectomy t.
  Conn pneumatic t.
  Conn Universal t.
  cotton-covered t.
  t. cuff
  Digikit finger t.
  Disposiquet disposable t.
  double loop t.
  Drake t.
  Dupuytren t.
  Esmarch t.
  Field t.
  forearm t.
  Fouli t.
  Gill renal t.
  Grafco t.
  Holcombe gastric t.
  horseshoe t.
  Ideal t.
  Johnson & Johnson t.
  Kidde t.
  Kidde-Robbins t.
  Linton t.
  Medi-Quet t.
  Momberg t.
  nonpneumatic t.
  Pac-Kit Army-type t.
  Petit t.
  pneumatic ankle t.
  Profex arthroscopic t.
  Quicket t.
  ratchet t.
  Robbins automatic t.
  Roberts-Nelson lobectomy t.
  Roper-Rumel t.
  Rumel-Belmont t.
  Rumel cardiovascular t.
  Rumel ratchet t.
  Samway t.
  Sebra arm t.
  Shenstone t.
  Signorini t.
  single-loop t.
  SMIC auricular t.
  t. strap

Sure-Snare t.
Surgikit Velcro t.
thigh t.
Tinel t.
Tournikwik t.
Trussdale t.
Uniquet disposable intravenous t.
Universal t.
U. S. Army t.
Velcro t.
Velket Velcro t.
Weiner t.
Wright pneumatic t.
tourniquet-eyed
    t.-e. obturator
    t.-e. ratchet stylet
Tovell tube
towel
    Charnley t.
    t. clamp
    t. clip
    DisCide disinfecting t.
    t. drape
    fat t.
    Kaycel t.
    wound t.
tower
    Concept traction t.
    T. interchangeable retractor
    Linvatec wrist arthroscopy
      traction t.
    T. muscle forceps
    T. rib retractor
    T. spinal retractor
    T. stent
Townley
    T. bone graft screw
    T. calipers
    T. implant
    T. TARA prosthesis
    T. tissue forceps
    T. total knee prosthesis
Townsend
    T. biopsy punch
    T. endocervical biopsy curette
    T. knee brace
Townsend-Gilfillan
    T.-G. plate
    T.-G. screw
toxemia curette
Toynbee
    T. curette
    T. diagnostic tube
    T. ear speculum
    T. otoscope
TPE
    T. ankle-foot orthosis
    T. biomechanical foot orthosis
T-pin handle
TPL-6 hip system
TPS-coated
    T.-c. cylinder
    T.-c. screw
TR-28 hip prosthesis

trabeculotome
    Allen-Burian t.
    Harms t.
    McPherson t.
trabeculotomy probe
Trabucco double balloon catheter
TraceHybrid wire guide
Trace hydraulic vein stripper
tracer
    T. Blood Glucose monitor
    t. catheter
    T. hybrid wire guide
    T. Hybrid wire guide with Slip-
      Coat tip
    T. ST wire
TrachCare multi-access catheter
tracheal
    t. button
    t. cannula
    t. catheter
    t. dilator
    t. forceps
    t. hook
    t. retractor
    t. safety stitch
    t. scalpel
    t. tenaculum
    t. tube
    t. tube brush
    t. tube changer
    t. tube cuff
trachelotome
    Spencer t.
tracheobronchoesophagoscope
    Haslinger t.
tracheoesophageal
    t. puncture dilator
    t. shunt
tracheopharyngeal shunt
tracheoscope
    Fearon t.
    Haslinger t.
    Jackson t.
    Storz t.
    Storz-Shapshay t.
    Tucker t.
TracheoSoft XLT tracheostomy tube
tracheostoma valve
tracheostomy
    t. button
    t. cannula
    t. hook
    Montgomery t.
    t. tube
tracheotome
    Salvatore-Maloney t.
    Sierra-Sheldon t.
tracheotomy
    t. cannula
    t. hook
    t. sponge
Trachlight
    T. lighted intubating stylet
Trach-Mist
TRACHO-FOAM adhesive disk

T

trachoma forceps
Trach-Talk device
tracker
    t. infusion catheter
    t. knee brace
    t. microcatheter
    miniBIRD position t.
    Palumbo patella t.
    patella t.
    Purkinje image t.
    t. Soft Stream side-hole
      microinfusion catheter
Tracker-18 Unibody catheter
tracker-assisted PRK laser
Trackmaster treadmill
TRACOEflex tracheostomy tube
Trac Plus catheter
traction
    Ace Trippi-Wells tong cervical t.
    Ace Universal tong cervical t.
    t. anchor
    t. apparatus
    t. bar
    t. belt
    t. bow
    Bremer halo cervical t.
    Bremer halo crown t.
    Bryant t.
    Buck t.
    cervical AOA halo t.
    C-Flex supine cervical t.
    Cotrel t.
    Crutchfield skeletal t.
    t. device
    device for transverse t.
    Dunlop elbow t.
    t. forceps
    Freiberg t.
    Frejka t.
    Georgiade visor cervical t.
    t. handle
    head halter cervical t.
    Holter t.
    Homestretch lumbar t.
    Houston halo cervical t.
    Jones suspension t.
    Kirschner skeletal t.
    Kirschner wire t.
    t. legging
    lumbosacral support pelvic t.
    McBride tripod pin t.
    Miami Acute Care cervical t.
    Miami "J" collar cervical t.
    Neufeld t.
    Perkins t.
    Philadelphia collar cervical t.
    Russell skeletal t.
    Saunders cervical HomeTrac t.
    Sayre suspension t.
    split Russell skeletal t.
    Steinmann t.
    supine C-Trax t.
    Syms t.
    t. table
    t. tenaculum
    t. tongs
    t. tongs screw
    transfer t.
    Watson-Jones t.
Tracto-Halter gait trainer
tractor
    axial t.
    banjo t.
    Blackburn skull traction t.
    Böhler t.
    Bryant t.
    Buck t.
    Dunlop t.
    Exo-Bed t.
    Exo-Static overhead t.
    Fisk t.
    Freiberg t.
    halo t.
    Hamilton pelvic traction screw t
    Handy-Buck extension t.
    Hoke-Martin t.
    Kestler ambulatory head t.
    Kirschner wire t.
    Lowsley prostatic t.
    Lowsley suprapubic t.
    Lyman-Smith t.
    Muirhead-Little pelvic rest t.
    Neufeld t.
    Orr-Buck extension t.
    Perkins split-weight t.
    prostatic t.
    Pugh t.
    Rankin prostatic t.
    Russell-Beck extension t.
    Steinmann traction t.
    Syms t.
    Trimline mobile t.
    Tupper t.
    Vinke skull t.
    Watson-Jones t.
    Wells t.
    Young prostatic t.
    Zim-Trac traction splint t.
TRAFO orthosis
tragus House hook
Trailblazer
    T. screw guide
    T. wire
trainer
    computer-aided fluency
      establishment t.
    impulse inertial exercise t.
    Monark Rehab T.
    positional feedback stimulation t.
    Posture Pump Spine T.
    Regain home EMG t.
    Sprint cross t.
    Tracto-Halter gait t.
Trake-Fit
    T.-F. endotracheal tube
    T.-F. tracheal tube holder
Trakstar balloon catheter
Tramscope 12
Tranquility
    T. Auto

T. bilevel system
T. quest CPAP
transabdominal transducer
transanal endoscopic microsurgery
transarticular screw
transaxillary needle
transbuccal trocar
transcatheter
  t. device
  t. umbrella
  t. umbrella implant material
Transcend microguidewire
transcervical tubal access catheter
transconjunctival retractor
transcranial
  t. Doppler
  t. Doppler probe
transcutaneous
  t. bilirubinometer
  t. broadband sector transducer
  t. carbon dioxide monitor
  t. cranial electrical stimulator
  t. electrical nerve stimulator
  t. electrical neuromuscular stimulator
   (TENS)
  t. extraction catheter
  t. neuromuscular electrical stimulator
  t. oxygen monitor
  t. pacemaker
TransCyte temporary skin substitute
transdermal fentanyl device
transducer
  Accuscanner t.
  Acuson linear array t.
  Acuson V5M multiplane TEE t.
  Aloka t.
  annular-array t.
  Array ultrasound t.
  ART t.
  Bentley t.
  bifocal multiplane rectal t.
  bite force t.
  Bruel & Kjaer axial t.
  bur hole t.
  catheter-borne sector t.
  Combitrans t.
  Cordis Sentron t.
  curved array t.
  Deltran disposable t.
  Diasonics t.
  Dräger MTC t.
  electromagnetic flow t.
  Elema-Siemens AB pressure t.
  endovaginal t.
  epicardial Doppler flow sector t.
  force t.
  forced displacement t.
  Gaeltec catheter-tip pressure t.
  Gould Statham pressure t.
  Hall-effect strain t.
  high-resolution linear array t.
  HP OmniPlane TEE imaging t.
  ion-specific field effect t.
  linear array t.
  linear 35-MHz t.

linear variable-differential t.
LSC 7000 curved array t.
magnetic motion t.
magnetic resonance imaging-guided
  focused ultrasound sector t.
Medex t.
microtip pressure t.
Mikro-Tip t.
Millar Mikro-Tip catheter
  pressure t.
M-mode sector t.
Nellcor Durasensor adult oxygen t.
Ocuscan 400 t.
Oxisensor oxygen t.
phased array sector t.
piezoelectric t.
piezo-resistive t.
pressure t.
puncture t.
quartz t.
rectal multiplane t.
rotatory-variable-differential t.
SensorMedics pressure t.
Siemens Endo-P endorectal t.
Sonogage System Corneo-Gage 20
  MHz center frequency t.
Sonos ultrasonographic t.
Spectramed t.
Spectranetics P23 Statham t.
Statham external t.
strain gauge t.
Therasound t.
Toshiba biplane transesophageal t.
transabdominal t.
transcutaneous broadband sector t.
transrectal multiplane 3-
  dimensional t.
TruWave pressure t.
Ultramark 8 t.
ultrasound t.
Voluson sector t.
transducer-tipped catheter
Transeal transparent wound dressing
Transelast surgical drape
transelectrical nerve stimulator
transendoscopic ultrasound
transensor
  Ommaya reservoir t.
transesophageal
  t. echocardiography probe
  t. pacing system
transfemoral endoaortic occlusion
  catheter
transfer
  t. forceps
  t. traction
TransFix ACL system
transfixion
  t. bolt
  t. screw
  t. suture
transformer
  Coolidge t.
  distribution t.
  doughnut t.

T

transformer (*continued*)
   filament t.
   high-voltage t.
   linear variable differential t.
   step-down t.
   step-up t.
transhepatic
   t. biliary stent
   t. portacaval shunt
TransiGel
   T. hydrogel-impregnated gauze
   T. woven gauze dressing
transilluminating telescope
transilluminator
   Briggs t.
   Coldite t.
   Finnoff sinus t.
   Hildreth t.
   hooded t.
   Jako t.
   Lancaster ocular t.
   National all-metric t.
   National opal-glass t.
   O'Malley-Skia t.
   rotating t.
   speculum illuminator t.
   Tatum ureteral t.
   Thompson cervical t.
   UV t.
   Welch Allyn t.
   Widner t.
transistor
   field-effect t.
   insulated gate field-effect t.
   ion-sensitive field-effect t.
   junction field-effect t.
   metal oxide semiconductor field-effect t.
   unijunction t.
transit-time flowmeter
transjugular intrahepatic portal systemic shunt
translocation needle
translucent
   t. drain tube
   t. myringotomy tube
translumbar inferior vena cava catheter
transluminal
   t. angioplasty catheter
   t. balloon
   t. endarterectomy catheter
   t. lysing system
transmandibular implant
transmission electron microscope
transmit-receive coil
transmitter
   chest-band t.
   false neurochemical t.
transmitter-receiver
   Itrel programmed t.-r.
transmural
   t. antitachycardia pacemaker
   t. electrical stimulator
transmyocardial pacing stylet

transnasal
   t. intraduodenal feeding catheter
   t. pancreaticobiliary drain
Transonic
   T. flowmeter
   T. flow probe
   T. laser Doppler perfusion monitc
transoral
   t. catheter
   t. retractor
Transorbent topical wound dressing
Transorb wound dressing
transosseous
   t. implant
   t. post
   t. suture
transosteal pin implant
transpapillary
   t. cystopancreatic stent
   t. drain
   t. endoscope
   t. endoscopic endoprosthesis
transparent
   t. adhesive film dressing
   t. drape
   t. elastic band ligating device
transpedicularly implanted anterior spinal support device
transpedicular screw
transpericardial pacemaker
Transpire wrist orthosis
transplant trephine
Transpore
   T. eye tape
   T. surgical tape dressing
Transport catheter
transpubic needle
transpupillary laser
transpyloric feeding tube
transrectal
   t. multiplane 3-dimensional transducer
   t. probe
Trans-Scan 2100 noninvasive physiological monitor
transscleral suture
transseptal
   t. cannula
   t. catheter
transsphenoidal
   t. bipolar forceps
   t. curette
   t. dissector
   t. enucleator
   t. speculum
transtelephonic
   t. ambulatory monitoring system
   t. exercise monitor
transthoracic
   t. catheter
   t. pacemaker
   t. pacing stylet
transthoracically implanted ICD
transtracheal oxygen catheter

transurethral
  t. catheter
  t. needle ablation of the prostate
    radio frequency generator
transvaginal ultrasound
Transvene
  T. nonthoracotomy implantable
    cardioverter-defibrillator
  T. tripolar electrode
Transvene-RV lead
transvenous
  t. defibrillator lead
  t. electrode
  t. pacemaker catheter
  t. ventricular demand pacemaker
transventricular dilator
transverse
  t. connector
  t. gradient coil
trap
  Allen finger t.
  Burkard spore t.
  collection t.
  Concept digit t.
  EndoDynamics suction polyp t.
  extraction t.
  filtered specimen t.
  Hirst spore t.
  in-line t.
  Kramer-Collins Spore t.
  Lukens t.
  osseous coagulum t.
  Rusch mucous t.
trapeze
  t. bar
  overhead frame t.
trapeziometacarpal joint replacement
  prosthesis
trapezium implant
trapezoid
  Superblade t.
Trapper catheter exchange device
Traquair periosteal elevator
Trattner urethrographic catheter
Traube neurological hammer
TraumaJet wound debridement system
traumatic grasping forceps
Traveler
  T. portable oxygen system
  Pulmo-Aide T.
Travenol
  T. biopsy needle
  T. heart bag
  T. infuser
  T. infusion pump
Travert needle
tray
  Bardex Lubricath sterile Foley t.
  Bard sterile infection control t.
  Bard universal Foley catheter sterile
    insertion t.
  Bard urethral catheter sterile t.
  Bucky view t.
  Curity irrigation t.
  Davol sterile irrigation t.

  Denis Browne t.
  DS-10 mobile dilator storage t.
  E-Z-EM PercuSet amniocentesis t.
  Henry instrument t.
  I-tech cannula t.
  Mayo instrument t.
  MetriTray system soaking t.
  Mobile dilator storage t.
  Monoject laceration irrigation t.
  Müller t.
  One Time sharp debridement t.
  orthodontic impression t.
  Papanicolaou smear t.
  ProTech instrument protection t.
  Russell gastrostomy t.
  TiMesh titanium t.
  titanium mesh t.
  Unimar HSG t.
  urethral intermittent catheter & t.
  Weck microsurgical t.
Treace stapes drill
treadmill
  Aquaciser underwater t.
  AquaGaiter t.
  exercise t.
  Hydrotrack underwater t.
  Jaeger LE3000 t.
  Lifestride t.
  Marquette t.
  Orbiter t.
  Q-Stress t.
  Trackmaster t.
  Tunturi Jogger-2 self-powered t.
treatment
  t. port
  t. table
Tredex
  T. bicycle
  Universal T.
tree
  BTE Assembly T.
  Finger Blocking T.
  pinch t.
  pipe t.
trefoil
  t. balloon catheter
  t. Schneider balloon
Trelat
  T. palate raspatory
  T. vaginal speculum
Trelex natural mesh
Trelles metal scleral shield
Tremble sphenoid cannula
Trendelenburg
  T. cannula
  T. tampon
Trendelenburg-Crafoord coarctation
  clamp
Trent
  T. eye retractor
  T. pick
trephine
  Arroyo t.
  Arruga eye t.
  Arruga lacrimal t.

T

trephine *(continued)*
automated t.
Bard-Parker t.
Barraquer corneal t.
Barron disposable t.
Barron epikeratophakia t.
Barron-Hessburg corneal t.
Barron radial vacuum t.
Becker skull t.
Blackburn t.
t. blade
Blakesley lacrimal t.
Boiler septal t.
Bonaccolto t.
Boston t.
Brown-Pusey corneal t.
cam-guided t.
Cardona corneal prosthesis t.
Castroviejo corneal transplant t.
chalazion t.
corneal prosthesis t.
Cross scleral t.
Damshek sternal t.
Davis t.
DeMartel t.
D'Errico skull t.
DeVilbiss skull t.
DiaPhine t.
Dimitry chalazion t.
Dimitry dacryocystorhinostomy t.
disposable t.
t. drill
Elliot corneal t.
Elschnig t.
Franceschetti corneal t.
Galt skull t.
Gradle corneal t.
Green automatic corneal t.
Greenwood spinal t.
Grieshaber calibrated corneal t.
Guyton corneal transplant t.
hand t.
hand-held t.
Hanna t.
Harris t.
Hessburg-Barron vacuum t.
Hessburg vacuum t.
Hippel t.
Horsley t.
Iliff lacrimal t.
Jentzer t.
Katena t.
Katena-Barron t.
Katzin t.
Keyes cutaneous t.
King corneal t.
lacrimal t.
Lahey Clinic skull t.
Leksell t.
Lichtenberg corneal t.
Londermann corneal t.
Lorie antral t.
t. marker
Martinez disposable corneal t.

M-brace corneal t.
Michele t.
mini t.
Moria t.
Mueller electric corneal t.
Paton see-through corneal t.
pattern t.
Paufique corneal t.
Pharmacia corneal t.
Phemister biopsy t.
Polley-Bickel t.
punch t.
razor-blade t.
Robertson corneal t.
Rochester bone t.
Schanz t.
Scheie t.
Schuknecht temporal t.
Scoville skull t.
Searcy chalazion t.
Sidney Stephenson corneal t.
sinus t.
Sisler lacrimal t.
skull t.
Stille t.
Stock eye t.
Storz chalazion t.
Storz corneal t.
Storz DiaPhine t.
Storz hair transplant t.
Surgistar corneal t.
Thornwald antral t.
Toti t.
transplant t.
Troutman tenotomy t.
Turkel t.
Von Hippel mechanical t.
Walker corneal t.
Wilder t.
Wilkins t.

Trestle prostatic bridge
Treves intestinal clamp
Trevisani
T. cannula
T. cannula tip
Trex digital mammography system
Triad
T. hydrophilic wound dressing
T. PET balloon
T. prosthesis
T. SPECT imaging system
TriaDyne bed
Triage cardiac system
trial
t. acetabular cup
t. component
t. driver
t. fracture frame
t. implant
t. prosthesis
triangle Secto dissector
Tri-angle shoulder abduction brace
triangular
t. ankle fusion frame
t. arm sling

t. bandage
t. dressing
t. encompassing clip
t. punch forceps
t. rasp
triangulated pedicle screw
triaxial semiconstrained elbow prosthesis
Triax monotube external fixation system
Tri-Beeled trapezoidal keratome
Trichodemolus epilator
Tricodur
    T. Epi compression support bandage
    T. Omos compression support
    bandage
    T. Talus compression support
    bandage
Tricomponent Coaxial system
Tri-Con component
Tricon-M
    T.-M. cruciate-sparing prosthesis
    T.-M. patellar prosthesis
Tri-Core cervical support pillow
tricuspid valve strut
Tricut
    T. blade
    T. laryngeal blade tip
Tri-Ex radiopaque triple-lumen
   extraction balloon
TriEye
    T. cannula
    T. tip
trifacet knife
tri-fin chisel
Tri-Flex auxiliary suspension belt
Tri-Float pressure reduction mattress
Tri-flow incentive spirometer
trifocal glasses
trigeminal
    t. electrode
    t. knife
    t. scissors
    t. self-retaining retractor
trigeminus cannula
trigger
    t. cannula
    Smart T.
TriggerWheel
    T. device
    T. Wand
Triguide catheter
trilaminate cushion
trileaflet prosthesis
Trilicon external breast prosthesis
Tri-Lock
    T.-L. acetabular cup
    T.-L. total hip prosthesis with
    Porocoat
Trilogy
    T. acetabular cup
    T. DC, DR, SR pulse generator
    T. DC+ pacemaker
    T. I hearing aid
    T. low-profile balloon dilatation
    catheter
    T. SR+ single-chamber pacemaker

Trilucent breast implant
Trima
    Cobe T.
Trimble suture stent
Trimedyne
    T. holmium laser
    T. Optilase 1000 device
Tri-Met apnea monitor
Trimline
    T. knee immobilizer
    T. mobile tractor
trimmer
    calcar t.
    Mallory-Head Interlok calcar t.
    Nordent margin t.
Tri-Motion knee system
Trinkle
    T. bone drill
    T. brace
    T. chuck
    T. chuck adapter
    T. screwdriver
    T. socket wrench
    T. Super-Cut twist drill
Trionix
    T. camera
    T. scanner
Trios M pacemaker
Trio-Temp X Biofil
triphasic spiral CT
Triphasix generator
triplanar
    t. protractor
    t. protractor apparatus
triplane construct
triple
    T. Care antifungal
    t. hook
    t. therapy
triple-color flow cytometry
triple-edge diamond-blade knife
triple-injection cine arthrogram
triple-lumen
    t.-l. Arrow catheter
    t.-l. balloon flotation thermistor
    catheter
    t.-l. biliary manometry catheter
    t.-l. central catheter
    t.-l. implant
    t.-l. manometry catheter
    t.-l. needle
    t.-l. perfused catheter system
    t.-l. sump drain
triple-thermistor coronary sinus catheter
tripod
    t. grasper
    t. grasping forceps
    t. intraocular lens
tri-point
    t.-p. bullet
    t.-p. K-wire sleeve
tripolar
    t. Damato curve catheter
    t. defibrillation coil electrode
    t. electrode catheter

T

tripolar *(continued)*
    t. lead
    t. w/Damato curve catheter
Tri-Port
    T.-P. hemostasis introducer sheath
      kit
    T.-P. sub-Tenon anesthesia cannula
triport tip
Trippi-Wells tongs
tri-pronged loop
tri-radial resector blade
TriStar trocar
TriStim TENS unit
Triumph VR pacemaker
Tri-Wedge total hip system
Tri W-G table
Trizol RNA extractor
TroCam
    T. endoscope
Trocam endoscopic camera
Trocan disposable CO$_2$ trocar and
  cannula
trocar, trochar
    abdominal t.
    Abelson cricothyrotomy t.
    Allen cecostomy t.
    American Heyer-Schulte-Robertson
      suprapubic t.
    AMS disposable t.
    antral t.
    Apple t.
    Arbuckle-Shea t.
    Argyle t.
    Babcock empyema t.
    BD Potain thoracic t.
    Beardsley cecostomy t.
    Birch t.
    blunt t.
    Bluntport disposable t.
    Boettcher antral t.
    Boettcher-Schnidt antral t.
    brain t.
    Bueleau empyema t.
    Bülau t.
    Cabot t.
    Campbell suprapubic t.
    Castens ascites t.
    Castens hydrocele t.
    Charlton antral t.
    Circon ACMI t.
    Coakley antral t.
    Cook urological t.
    core t.
    Core Dynamics disposable t.
    Cross needle t.
    Curschmann t.
    Davidson t.
    Dean antral t.
    Denker t.
    Dexide laparoscopic t.
    Diamond-Flex t.
    Diederich empyema t.
    Douglas antral t.
    Douglas nasal t.

    Dr. White t.
    Duchenne t.
    Duke t.
    Durham tracheotomy t.
    Emmet ovarian t.
    Endopath disposable surgical t.
    Endopath laparoscopic t.
    Endopath TriStar t.
    Endo Tip Stortz t.
    ensheathing t.
    Entree II t.
    Entree Plus t.
    Ethicon disposable t.
    Faulkner t.
    Fein antral t.
    Fleurant bladder t.
    Frazier brain-exploring t.
    Gallagher t.
    Haeggstrom antral t.
    Hargin antral t.
    Hasson laparoscopic t.
    Havlicek t.
    Hunt angiographic t.
    Hurwitz thoracic t.
    Ingram t.
    InnerDyne t.
    intercostal t.
    intestinal decompression t.
    Jako laser t.
    Jarit disposable t.
    Johannson-Stille cystotomy t.
    Judd t.
    Kidd t.
    Kido suprapubic t.
    Kolb t.
    Krause antral t.
    Kreutzmann t.
    Landau t.
    LaparoSAC t.
    laryngeal t.
    Lichtwicz abdominal t.
    Lichtwicz antral t.
    Lillie antral t.
    Livermore t.
    Marlow disposable t.
    Mayo-Ochsner t.
    Monoscopy locking t.
    Morson t.
    Myerson antral t.
    Nagashima antroscope t.
    Neal catheter t.
    t. needle
    Nelson empyema t.
    Nelson-Patterson empyema t.
    Nelson thoracic t.
    nested t.
    Ochsner gallbladder t.
    Ochsner thoracic t.
    Olympus disposable t.
    Optiview t.
    Origin t.
    Patterson empyema t.
    Patterson-Nelson empyema t.
    Pierce antral t.
    Pierce-Kyle t.

plain vesical t.
Poole t.
Potain aspirating t.
rectal t.
Reddick-Saye t.
Rica Universal t.
Richard Wolf laparoscopic t.
Roberts abdominal t.
Ruskin antral t.
Schwartz t.
Sewall antral t.
sharp t.
Singleton empyema t.
sinoscopy t.
Snyder Urevac t.
Solos disposable t.
Southey anasarca t.
Southey-Leech t.
Step laparoscopic t.
Stiwer t.
Storz disposable t.
subcostal t.
suprapubic t.
Surgiport disposable t.
Sweet antral t.
Synthes transbuccal t.
thoracic t.
Thoracoport t.
Tilley-Lichwitz t.
transbuccal t.
TriStar t.
Ueckermann-Denker t.
Uni-Shunt split t.
Universal abdominal t.
Van Alyea antral t.
Veirs t.
Visiport optical t.
Walther aspirating bladder t.
Wangensteen internal
  decompression t.
Weck disposable t.
Wiener-Pierce antral t.
Wilson amniotic t.
Wilson-Baylor amniotic t.
Wisap disposable t.
Wolf-Cottle t.
Wolf needle t.
Wright-Harloe empyema t.
Ximed disposable t.
Yankauer antral t.
trocar-cannula system
trocar-point Kirschner wire
Trocath peritoneal dialysis catheter
trochanter holder
trochanter-holding clamp
trochanteric
  t. awl
  t. bolt
  t. pin
  t. plate
  t. router
  t. wire
trochar (*var. of* trocar)
Troeltsch
  T. dressing forceps

T. ear forceps
T. ear speculum
T. eustachian catheter
TroGARD Finesse dilating trocar system
Troilius capsulotomy knife
Trokel lens
Trokel-Peyman laser lens
trolley
  Bolero lift bath t.
Trombotect tube
Tromner percussion hammer
Troncoso
  T. gonioscope
  T. gonioscopic lens implant
  T. tubular lens
TRON 3 VACI cardiac imaging system
Tronzo
  T. elevator
  T. prosthesis
troposcope
Trotter forceps
Trough gouge
trousers
  air t.
  MAST t.
  military antishock t. (MAST)
Trousseau
  T. dilating forceps
  T. esophageal bougie
  T. mouthgag
  T. tracheal dilator
Trousseau-Jackson
  T.-J. esophageal dilator
  T.-J. tracheal dilator
Troutman
  T. alpha-chymotrypsin cannula
  T. blade
  T. bladebreaker
  T. cataract extractor
  T. conjunctival scissors
  T. corneal dissector
  T. corneal forceps
  T. corneal knife
  T. corneal splitter
  T. eye implant
  T. lens loupe
  T. lens spatula
  T. mastoid chisel
  T. microsurgery forceps
  T. microsurgical scissors
  T. needle
  T. needle holder
  T. nonincisional lamellar dissector
  T. punch
  T. superior rectus forceps
  T. suture scissors
  T. tenotomy trephine
  T. tying forceps
  T. wave-edge corneal dissector
Troutman-Barraquer
  T.-B. corneal fixation forceps
  T.-B. corneal forceps
  T.-B. iris forceps
  T.-B. iris spatula

T

Troutman-Barraquer *(continued)*
T.-B. minibladebreaker
T.-B. needle holder
Troutman-Barraquer-Colibri forceps
Troutman-Castroviejo corneal section scissors
Troutman-Katzin corneal transplant scissors
Troutman-Llobera fixation forceps
Troutman-Llobera-Flieringa forceps
Troutman-Tooke corneal knife
Trowbridge
T. TerraRound foot
T. TerraRound sports limb
T. triple-speed drill
Trowbridge-Campau
T.-C. bone drill
T.-C. eye magnet
Tru-Arc blood vessel ring
Truarch wire
Tru-Area Determination wound measuring device
Tru-Canal hearing aid
Tru-Chrome band material
Tru-clip clip
Tru-Close wound drainage system
Tru-Cut
T.-C. biopsy needle
T.-C. biopsy needle holder
True
T. Blue exercise band
T. Form support stockings
T. separator
T. Sheathless catheter
T. Stat system
TrueBlue background material
True/Fit femoral intramedullary rod system
True/Flex
T. intramedullary nail
T. intramedullary rod system
True/Lok external fixator system
TrueTorque wire guide
TrueVision transvaginal probe
Tru-Fit custom molded shoe
Truflex
TruJect drug delivery system
Trulife silicone breast form
Truline forceps
Tru-Mold shoe
trumpet
t. cannula
Iowa t.
nasal t.
t. needle guide
T. Valve hydrodissector
truncated NMR probe
truncus clamp
trunnion
trunnion-bearing hip prosthesis
Trupower aspherical lens
Trupp ventricular needle
TruPro lacrimal cannula
TruPulse CO$_2$ laser system

Trush grasping forceps
Trusler-Dean scissors
Trusler infant vascular clamp
truss
Hood t.
inguinal t.
Kansas City band t.
Nu-Form t.
scrotal t.
Trussdale tourniquet
Tru-Stain acrylic powder
TruStep foot prosthesis
Tru-Support
T.-S. EW bandage
T.-S. SA bandage
Truszkowski dural dissector
Tru Taper Ethalloy needle
Tru-Trac high-pressure PTA balloon
Truvision Omni lens
TruWave pressure transducer
TruZone peak flow meter
Trylon hemostatic forceps
TSH-01 transdermal tape
T-shaped
T.-s. AO plate
T.-s. Edwards-Barbaro syringeal shunt
T.-s. forceps
T-Span tissue expander
"T" spatula
T-Spica bandage
TSRH
TSRH buttressed laminar hook
TSRH circular laminar hook
TSRH double-rod construct
TSRH hook-rod
TSRH pedicle hook
TSRH pedicle screw-laminar claw construct
T-Stick adhesive
TT-3 needle
T-TAC
T-TAC catheter
T-TAC system
TTAP-ST acetabular prosthesis
TTS
through-the-scope
TTS Aire-Cuf endotracheal tube
TTS Aire-Cuf tracheostomy tube
TTS catheter
TTS dilator
Rigiflex esophageal TTS
T-tube
bar T.-t.
T.-t. catheter
T.-t. cholangiogram
cul-de-sac irrigation T.-t.
Deaver T.-t.
T.-t. drain
French T.-t.
Goode T.-t.
Houser silicone T.-t.
Kehr T.-t.
Kelly inflatable T.-t.
lacrimal duct T.-t.

Montgomery tracheal T.-t.
polyethylene T.-t.
Pyrex T.-t.
T.-t. round suction tube
Silastic T.-t.
silicone T.-t.
T.-t. stent
vinyl T.-t.

T-type
T.-t. dental implant
T.-t. matrix band
T.-t. myringotomy tube

tub
hydrotherapy t.

tubal
t. hook
t. insufflation cannula
t. scissors

Tubbs
T. aortic dilator
T. mitral valve dilator
T. two-bladed dilator
T. valvulotome

Tubby tenotomy knife
tube
Abbott t.
Abbott-Rawson gastrointestinal
double-lumen t.
AccuMark calibrated infant
feeding t.
Activent ear t.
Adson aspirating t.
Adson brain suction t.
Adson neurosurgical suction t.
Aire-Cuf endotracheal t.
Aire-Cuf tracheostomy t.
Air-Lon laryngectomy t.
Air-Lon tracheal t.
Alesen t.
American circle nephrostomy t.
American Heyer-Schulte T-t.
Amersham J t.
Andersen mercury-weighted t.
Anderson flexible suction t.
Andrews-Pynchon suction t.
angled pleural t.
anode t.
Anthony aspirating t.
Anthony mastoid suction t.
Anthony suction t.
antifog t.
aortic sump t.
Argyle chest t.
Argyle-Dennis t.
Argyle endotracheal t.
Argyle Sentinel Seal chest t.
Armstrong beveled grommet drain t.
Armstrong beveled grommet
myringotomy t.
Armstrong ventilation t.
Armstrong V-Vent t.
Arrow t.
Asepto suction t.
aspirating t.
Aspisafe nasogastric t.

Atkins-Cannard tracheotomy t.
t. attachment device
auditory t.
Ayre t.
Baerveldt glaucoma implant t.
Baerveldt shunt t.
Baker jejunostomy t.
Baker self-sumping t.
Baldwin butterfly ventilation t.
Bard gastrostomy feeding t.
Bardic t.
Bard PEG t.
Barnes suction t.
Baron ear t.
Baron-Frazier suction t.
Baron suction t.
Baylor cardiovascular sump t.
Baylor intracardiac sump t.
Beall-Feldman-Cooley sump t.
Beardsley empyema t.
Bellocq t.
Bellucci suction t.
Bel-O-Pak suction t.
Benjamin t.
Ben-Jet t.
Bettman empyema t.
bicanalicular silicone t.
Billroth t.
Biolite ventilation t.
Biosystems feeding t.
Bivona Fome-Cuf t.
Bivona Medical Technologies
customized tracheostomy t.
Bivona sleep apnea tracheostomy t.
Bivona TTS tracheostomy t.
bladder flap t.
Blakemore esophageal t.
Blakemore nasogastric t.
Blakemore-Sengstaken t.
Blue Line cuffed endotracheal t.
blunt suction t.
bobbin myringotomy t.
Bonney uterine t.
Bouchut laryngeal t.
Bourdon t.
Bower PEG t.
Bowman t.
Brawley nasal suction t.
bronchial t.
Broncho-Cath double-lumen
endotracheal t.
bronchoscopy disposable suction t.
Bruecke t.
Bucy-Frazier suction t.
Bucy suction t.
Buie rectal suction t.
Butler tonsillar suction t.
Buyes air-vent suction t.
calibrated grasping t.
calix t.
Caluso PEG gastrostomy t.
Cantor intestinal t.
capillary t.
Carabelli endobronchial t.
Carden bronchoscopy t.

tube *(continued)*

Carden laryngoscopy t.
Carlens double-lumen endotracheal t.
Carl Zeiss myringotomy t.
Carman rectal t.
Carrel t.
Casselberry sphenoid t.
Castelli-Paparella collar button t.
cathode ray t. (CRT)
Cattell forked-type T- t.
Cattell gallbladder t.
Celestin endoesophageal t.
Celestin latex rubber t.
t. changer
Chaoul voltage x-ray t.
Charnley drain t.
Chauffin-Pratt t.
Chaussier t.
chest t.
Chevalier Jackson tracheal t.
ClearCut II with smoke eater t.
Clerf laryngectomy t.
closed-suction t.
coagulation-aspirator t.
coagulation suction t.
Coakley wash t.
Cole endotracheal t.
Cole orotracheal t.
Cole pediatric t.
Cole uncuffed endotracheal t.
collar-button t.
collecting t.
Colton empyema t.
Combitube endotracheal t.
Comfit endotracheal t.
Compat surgical feeding t.
Cone-Bucy suction t.
Cone suction t.
conical centrifuge t.
Connell breathing t.
Connell ether vapor t.
Contigen t.
continuous suction t.
Cook County Hospital tracheal suction t.
Cooley-Anthony suction t.
Cooley aortic sump t.
Cooley cardiovascular suction t.
Cooley graft suction t.
Cooley intracardiac suction t.
Cooley sump suction t.
Cooley vascular suction t.
Coolidge t.
Cope loop nephrostomy t.
corneal t.
Corpak weighted-tip, self-lubricating t.
Costen suction t.
Cottle suction t.
Coupland nasal suction t.
Crawford t.
cricothyrotomy trocar t.
Crookes-Hittorf t.
cuffed endotracheal t.

cuffed tracheostomy t.
CUI myringotomy t.
Dakin t.
Dandy suction t.
David pharyngolaryngectomy t.
Davol t.
Dawson-Yuhl suction t.
Deane t.
Dean wash t.
Deaver t.
DeBakey-Adson suction t.
DeBakey suction t.
Debove t.
Denker t.
Dennis t.
DePaul t.
Devers gall bladder t.
DeVilbiss suction t.
Devine-Millard-Frazier fiberoptic suction t.
diagnostic t.
DIC tracheostomy t.
digestive t.
digit t.
disposable Yankauer aspirating t.
disposable Yankauer suction t.
Dobbhoff gastrectomy feeding t.
Dobbhoff gastric decompression t.
Dobbhoff nasogastric feeding t.
Dobbhoff PEG t.
Doesel-Huzly bronchoscopic t.
Donaldson drain t.
Donaldson eustachian t.
Donaldson myringotomy t.
Donaldson ventilation t.
double-cannula tracheostomy t.
double-focus t.
double-lumen endobronchial t.
double-lumen suction irrigation t.
double setup endotracheal t.
doughnut tip suction t.
drain-to-wall suction t.
Dr. Bruecke aspirating t.
t. dressing
Dr. Twiss duodenal t.
dual-lumen sump nasogastric t.
Duke t.
Dundas-Grant t.
Duralite t.
Durham tracheostomy t.
Dynamic digit extensor t.
Eastman suction t.
E. Benson Hood Laboratories esophageal t.
E. Benson Hood Laboratories salivary bypass t.
EDTA-Vacutainer t.
Einhorn t.
electron multiplier t.
endobrachial double-lumen t.
endobronchial t.
endoesophageal t.
Endosoft reinforced cuffed t.
endotracheal t.
Endotrol endotracheal t.

Endo-Tube nasal jejunal feeding t.
enteroclysis t.
enterolysis t.
EntriStar feeding t.
EntriStar percutaneous endoscopic
  gastrostomy (PEG) t.
Eppendorf t.
ESKA-Buess esophageal t.
Esmarch t.
ET t.
Ethox rectal t.
eustachian t.
Ewald t.
extension t.
Fay suction t.
feeding t.
fenestrated tracheostomy t.
Ferguson-Frazier suction t.
Feuerstein drainage t.
Feuerstein split ventilation t.
fiberoptic suction t.
field emission t.
fil D'Arion silicone t.
Finsterer myringotomy split t.
Finsterer suction t.
Fitzpatrick suction t.
flanged Teflon t.
Flexiflo enteral feeding t.
Flexiflo Inverta-PEG t.
Flexiflo Sacks-Vine t.
Flexiflo Stomate low-profile
  gastrostomy t.
Flexiflo suction feeding t.
Flexiflo tap-fill enteral t.
Flexiflo Taptainer t.
Flexiflo tungsten-weighted feeding t.
Flexiflo Versa-PEG t.
flow regulated suction t.
fluffy-cuffed t.
t. foam
Fome-Cuf endotracheal t.
Fome-Cuf pediatric tracheostomy t.
Franco triflange ventilation t.
Frazier aspirating t.
Frazier brain suction t.
Frazier Britetrac nasal suction t.
Frazier-Ferguson aspirating t.
Frazier-Ferguson ear suction t.
Frazier fiberoptic suction t.
Frazier modified suction t.
Frazier nasal suction t.
Frazier-Paparella mastoid suction t.
Frazier suction t.
Frederick-Miller t.
frontal sinus wash t.
Fuller bivalve trach t.
Gabriel Tucker t.
gastric t.
gastrojejunostomy t.
Gastro-Port II feeding t.
gastrostomy feeding t.
Gavriliu gastric t.
Geiger-Müller t.
Gillquist-Stille arthroplasty suction t.
Gillquist suction t.

Glover suction t.
glutaraldehyde-tanned bovine
  collagen t.
Gomco suction t.
Goode T-t.
Goode Trim t.
Goode T-tube ventilating t.
Goodhill-Pynchon tonsillar suction t.
Gott t.
Gowen decompression t.
Grafco Martin laryngectomy t.
t. graft
graft suction t.
Great Ormond Street pediatric
  tracheostomy t.
Greiling gastroduodenal t.
grommet drain t.
grommet myringotomy t.
grommet ventilating t.
Guibor Silastic t.
Guilford-Wright suction t.
Guisez t.
Gwathmey suction t.
Haering t.
Hagan surface suction t.
Hakim t.
Haldane t.
Haldane-Priestly t.
Hardy suction t.
Har-el pharyngeal t.
Heimlich t.
Heimlich-Gavrilu gastric t.
Helsper tracheostomy vent t.
Hemagard collection t.
Hemovac suction t.
heparin-bonded Bott-type t.
Herring t.
Hi-Lo Jet tracheal t.
Holinger open-end aspirating t.
Holter t.
Hossli suction t.
hot cathode x-ray t.
Hotchkiss ear suction t.
Hough-Cadogan suction t.
House-Baron suction t.
House endolymphatic shunt t.
House-Radpour suction t.
Houser cul-de-sac irrigator t.
House-Stevenson suction t.
House suction t.
House-Urban t.
Hubbard airplane vent t.
Hugly aspirating t.
Humphrey coronary sinus-sucker
  suction t.
Hunsaker jet ventilation t.
Hymlek portable chest t.
Hyperflex tracheostomy t.
image Orthicon t.
Immergut suction t.
Immergut suction-coagulation t.
infusion t.
intracardiac suction t.
intracardiac sump t.
Isolator lysis-centrifugation t.

tube *(continued)*
Israel suction t.
Jackson aspirating t.
Jackson cane-shaped tracheal t.
Jackson cone-shaped tracheal t.
Jackson laryngectomy t.
Jackson open-end aspirating t.
Jackson-Pratt suction t.
Jackson-Rees endotracheal t.
Jackson silver tracheostomy t.
Jackson tracheal t.
Jackson velvet-eye aspirating t.
Jackson warning stop t.
Jacques gastric t.
Jako laryngeal suction t.
Jako laser aspirating t.
Jako suction t.
Jarit-Poole abdominal suction t.
Jarit-Yankauer suction t.
Javid bypass t.
jejunal feeding t.
Jesberg aspirating t.
Jiffy t.
Johnson coagulation suction t.
Johnson intestinal t.
Jones Pyrex t.
Jones tear duct t.
J-shaped t.
Jutte t.
Kangaroo silicone gastrostomy
  feeding t.
Kaslow gastrointestinal t.
Kay-Cross suction tip suction t.
Kehr gallbladder t.
Kelly t.
Keofeed feeding t.
KeyMed esophageal t.
Kidd U-t.
Killian t.
Kistner plastic tracheostomy t.
Klein ventilation t.
Knoche t.
Kos ear suction t.
Kozlowski t.
K-Tube t.
Kuhn endotracheal t.
Kurze suction t.
Lacor t.
Lahey Y-tube t.
Lanz low-pressure cuff
  endotracheal t.
Lanz tracheostomy t.
Lar-A-Jext laryngectomy t.
LaRocca nasolacrimal t.
Laryngoflex reinforced
  endotracheal t.
Laser-Shield XII wrapped
  endotracheal t.
Laser-Trach endotracheal t.
Lasertubus tracheal t.
Leiter t.
Lell tracheal t.
Lenard ray t.
Lennarson t.

Lepley-Ernst tracheal t.
Lester Jones t.
Levin-Davol t.
Levin duodenal t.
Lewis laryngectomy t.
Lezius suction t.
life-saving t.
Lindeman-Silverstein Arrow t.
Lindeman-Silverstein ventilation t.
Lindholm tracheal t.
Linton esophageal t.
Linton-Nachlas t.
Lonnecken t.
Lo-Por tracheal t.
Lord-Blakemore t.
Lore-Lawrence tracheotomy t.
Lore suction t.
L.T. Jones tear duct t.
Luer speaking t.
Luer tracheal t.
Lukens collecting t.
Lyon t.
MacKenty laryngectomy t.
Mackler intraluminal t.
Mackray short-cuffed
  endobronchial t.
Madoff suction t.
Magill Safety Clear endotracheal
Maingot gallbladder t.
Malecot nephrostomy t.
Malis-Frazier suction t.
malleable multipore suction t.
Mallinckrodt endotracheal t.
Mallinckrodt Laser-Flex t.
Martin laryngectomy t.
Martin tracheostomy t.
Mason suction t.
Massie sliding nail t.
mastoid suction t.
McGowan-Keeley t.
McMurtry-Schlesinger shunt t.
Mead Johnson t.
mediastinal t.
Medina t.
Medoc-Celestin t.
mesh myringotomy t.
Methodist vascular suction t.
Mett t.
MIC bolus gastrostomy t.
MIC gastroenteric t.
MIC jejunal t.
MIC jejunostomy t.
MIC-Key gastrostomy t.
microbore Tygon t.
Microfuge t.
Microgel surface-enhanced
  ventilation t.
microlaryngeal endotracheal t.
Micron bobbin ventilation t.
Miller-Abbott double-lumen
  intestinal t.
Miller endotracheal t.
Millin suction t.
Mill-Rose t.
Milroy-Piper suction t.

Minnesota t.
Mixter t.
modified suction t.
Molteno shunt t.
molybdenum rotating-anode x-ray t.
molybdenum target t.
Momberg t.
Montando t.
Montefiore tracheal t.
Montgomery esophageal t.
Montgomery salivary bypass t.
Montgomery T-t.
Montgomery tracheal t.
Moore t.
Morch swivel tracheostomy t.
Moretz Tiny Tytan ventilation t.
Moretz Tytan ventilation t.
Morse-Andrews suction t.
Morse-Ferguson suction t.
Morse suction t.
Mosher intubation t.
Mosher life-saving tracheal
  suction t.
Moss balloon triple-lumen
  gastrostomy t.
Moss feeding t.
Moss gastric decompression t.
Moss gastrostomy t.
Moss Mark IV t.
Moss nasal t.
Moss suction buster t.
Moss Suction Buster t.
Moulton lacrimal duct t.
Mousseau-Barbin esophageal t.
Mueller-Frazier suction t.
Mueller-Poole suction t.
Mueller-Pynchon suction t.
Mueller suction t.
Mueller-Yankauer suction t.
Muldoon t.
muscular t.
Myerson wash t.
myringotomy drain t.
Nachlas gastrointestinal t.
Nachlas-Linton t.
nasal suction t.
nasobiliary t.
nasocystic drainage t.
nasoendotracheal t.
nasoenteric feeding t.
nasogastric feeding t.
nasoileal t.
nasojejunal t.
nasotracheal t.
NCC Hi-Lo Jet endotracheal t.
nephrostomy t.
Neuber bone t.
New Luer-type speaking t.
New speaking t.
Newvicon camera t.
Newvicon vacuum chamber
  pickup t.
New York glass suction t.
NG feeding t.
Nilsson-Stille abortion suction t.

Nilsson suction t.
Nishizaki-Wakabayashi suction t.
Norton endotracheal t.
Nunez ventricular ventilation t.
Nuport PEG t.
Nyhus-Nelson gastric
  decompression t.
Nyhus-Nelson jejunal feeding t.
Nystroem abdominal suction t.
O'Beirne sphincter t.
obstructed shunt t.
Ochsner gallbladder t.
O'Dwyer t.
O'Hanlon-Poole suction t.
Olshevsky t.
Olympus One-Step Button
  gastrostomy t.
Ommaya ventricular t.
opaque myringotomy t.
open-end aspirating t.
oral endotracheal t.
oral esophageal t.
oroendotracheal t.
orogastric Ewald t.
orotracheal t.
Ossoff-Karlan laser suction t.
overcouch t.
Oxford nonkinking cuffed t.
Panda gastrostomy t.
Panda nasoenteric feeding t.
Panje t.
Paparella-Frazier suction t.
Paparella myringotomy t.
Paparella type II ventilation t.
Parker t.
Paul intestinal drainage t.
Paul-Mixter t.
pear-shaped extension t.
Pedia-Trake t.
Pee Wee low-profile gastrostomy t.
PEG t., percutaneous endoscopic
  gastrostomy tube
Penrose t.
percutaneous nephrostomy t.
Per-Lee equalizing t.
Per-Lee myringotomy t.
Per-Lee ventilation t.
Perspex t.
Pertrach percutaneous
  tracheostomy t.
pharyngotympanic t.
photoelectric multiplier t.
photomultiplier t.
pickup t.
Pierce antrum wash t.
pigtail nephrostomy t.
Pilling duralite t.
Pitot t.
Pitt talking tracheostomy t.
plastic-cuffed tracheostomy t.
pleural t.
Pleur-evac suction t.
Plumicon camera t.
Polisar-Lyons adapted tracheal t.
Polisar-Lyons tracheal t.

T

tube *(continued)*
polyethylene t.
polyvinyl chloride endotracheal t.
Ponsky-Gauderer PEG t.
Ponsky PEG t.
Poole abdominal suction t.
Poppen suction t.
Portex Blue Line tracheostomy t.
Portex Per-Fit tracheostomy t.
Portex preformed blue line
  tracheal t.
Porto-Vac suction t.
postpyloric feeding t.
preformed polyvinyl chloride
  endotracheal t.
pressure equalization t.
pressure equalizing t.
Pribram suction t.
primordial catheter t.
Proctor suction t.
Pudenz t.
Puestow-Olander gastrointestinal t.
Pynchon suction t.
Questek laser t.
Quincke t.
Quinton t.
Radius enteral feeding t.
Radpour-House suction t.
RAE endotracheal t.
RAE-Flex tracheal t.
Rand-House suction t.
Rand-Radpour suction t.
rectal t.
rectifier t.
Redivac suction t.
red rubber endotracheal t.
Rehfuss duodenal t.
Rehfuss stomach t.
Reinecke-Carroll lacrimal t.
reinforced tracheostomy t.
Replogle t.
Reuter bobbin ventilation t.
Rhoton-Merz suction t.
Rica mastoid suction t.
right-angle chest t.
Ring-McLean sump t.
Ritter suprapubic suction t.
Robertshaw t.
Robinson equalizing t.
Rochester suction t.
Rochester tracheal t.
Roller pump suction t.
Rosen suction t.
rotating anode t.
Ruschelit polyvinyl chloride
  endotracheal t.
Rusch laryngectomy t.
Rusch red rubber rectal t.
Russell suction t.
Ryle duodenal t.
Sachs suction t.
Sacks-Vine PEG t.
Safety Clear Plus endotracheal t.
Salem sump action nasogastric t.

salivary bypass t.
Samco t.
Samson-Davis infant suction t.
Sandoz balloon replacement t.
Sandoz Caluso PEG gastrostomy
Sandoz feeding/suction t.
Sandoz nasogastric feeding t.
Sandoz suction t.
Sandoz suction/feeding t.
Sapporo shunt t.
Sarns intracardiac suction t.
Saticon vacuum chamber pickup
scavenging t.
Schall laryngectomy t.
Schmiedt t.
Schuknecht suction t.
Schuler aspiration/irrigation t.
Scott-Harden t.
Scott nasal suction t.
Securat suction t.
Sengstaken-Blakemore
  esophagogastric tamponade t.
Sengstaken nasogastric t.
Sensiv endotracheal t.
separator t.
Seroma-Cath drainage t.
Seroma-Cath feeding t.
Shah myringotomy t.
Shah permanent ventilation t.
Shea-type parasol myringotomy t.
Sheehy collar-button ventilating t.
Sheehy Tytan ventilation t.
Shepard drain t.
Shepard grommet ventilation t.
Sherman suction t.
Shiley cuffless fenestrated t.
Shiley cuffless tracheostomy t.
Shiley disposable cannula low
  pressure cuffed tracheostomy t.
Shiley extra-length single cannula
  tracheostomy t.
Shiley fenestrated low pressure
  cuffed tracheostomy t.
Shiley French sump t.
Shiley laryngectomy t.
Shiley low-pressure cuffed
  tracheostomy t.
Shiley neonatal tracheostomy t.
Shiley pediatric tracheostomy t.
Shiley single cannula cuffed
  tracheostomy t.
Silastic eustachian t.
Silastic intestinal t.
Silastic sucker suction t.
Silastic tracheostomy t.
silicone t.
silicone-lubricated endotracheal t.
Silverstein permanent aeration t.
Singer-Blom t.
siphon suction t.
SMIC mastoid suction t.
Smith t.
Smokeeter t.
smoke evacuator suction t.
smoke removal t.

Snyder Hemovac suction t.
Snyder Surgivac suction t.
Snyder Urevac suction t.
Softech endotracheal t.
SoftForm t.
Soileau Tytan ventilation t.
solid-phase extraction t.
Southey capillary drainage t.
Souttar t.
speaking t.
Spetzler MicroVac suction t.
spiral-wound endotracheal t.
SS bobbin drain t.
SS bobbin myringotomy t.
Stamm gastrostomy t.
Stedman continuous suction t.
stomach t.
Stomate decompression t.
Stomate extension t.
Storz suction t.
straight chest t.
Stroud-Baron ear suction t.
suction t.
suction-coagulation t.
Suh ventilation t.
sump t.
Super PEG t.
Sustagen nasogastric t.
Swan-Ganz t.
Swenson cholangiography t.
tear duct t.
T-grommet ventilation t.
Thal-Quick chest t.
thoracostomy t.
Thora-Klex chest t.
tight-to-shaft Aire-Cuf
    tracheostomy t.
Tiny-Tef ventilation t.
Tiny Tytan ventilation t.
tonsillar suction t.
Touma T-type grommet
    ventilation t.
Tovell t.
Toynbee diagnostic t.
tracheal t.
TracheoSoft XLT tracheostomy t.
tracheostomy t.
TRACOEflex tracheostomy t.
Trake-Fit endotracheal t.
translucent drain t.
translucent myringotomy t.
transpyloric feeding t.
Trombotect t.
T self-retaining drainage t.
TTS Aire-Cuf endotracheal t.
TTS Aire-Cuf tracheostomy t.
T-tube round suction t.
T-type myringotomy t.
Tucker aspirating t.
Tucker flexible-tip t.
Tucker tracheal t.
Turkel t.
Turner-Warwick fiberoptic suction t.
Turner-Warwick illuminating
    suction t.

twist-in drain t.
twist-in myringotomy t.
tympanostomy t.
Tytan grommet ventilation t.
Tytan ventilation t.
underwater-seal suction t.
Univent endotracheal t.
urinary drainage t.
uterine t.
U-tube t.
Vacutainer vacuum t.
Valentine irrigation t.
Van Alyea antral wash t.
vascular suction t.
velvet-eye aspirating t.
Venturi bobbin myringotomy t.
Venturi collar-button myringotomy t.
Venturi grommet myringotomy t.
Venturi pediatric myringotomy t.
Vernon antral wash t.
Versatome laser fiber t.
Vidicon camera t.
Vidicon vacuum chamber pickup t.
Vinyon-N cloth t.
Vivonex gastrostomy t.
V. Mueller-Frazier suction t.
V. Mueller-Poole suction t.
Voltolini ear t.
Von Eichen antral wash t.
Vortex tracheotomy t.
Wangensteen duodenal t.
Wannagat suction t.
water-seal chest t.
Webster infusion t.
Weck coagulating suction t.
Weck suction t.
Welch Allyn suction t.
Wendl t.
Wepsic suction t.
Williams esophageal t.
Wilson-Cook nasobiliary t.
Wilson-Cook NJFT-series feeding t.
Winsburg-White bladder t.
Wolf suction t.
Woodbridge t.
woven dacron t.
Wullstein microsuction t.
Xomed endotracheal t.
Xomed straight-shank t.
Xomed Treace ventilation t.
Xomed Tytan ventilation t.
x-ray t.
Yankauer aspirating t.
Yankauer suction t.
Yasargil microsuction t.
Yasargil suction t.
Yeder suction t.
Zollner suction t.
Z-wave t.
Zyler t.

T

Tubegauz
    T. elastic net
    T. seamless tubular knitted cotton
        bandage
tubeless lithotriptor

Tube-Lok tracheotomy dressing
tube-occluding
- t.-o. clamp
- t.-o. forceps

tuberculin syringe
Tubestat lighted stylet
Tubex
- T. gauze dressing
- T. injector
- T. metal syringe

TubiFast bandage
TubiGrip
- T. dressing
- T. elastic support bandage

tubing
- t. adapter
- Argyle Penrose t.
- Bard extension t.
- t. clamp
- t. compressor
- connecting t.
- dialysate t.
- dialysis t.
- Dorsey irrigation t.
- evacuator t.
- foam t.
- t. forceps
- gel t.
- t. hand roller
- Hi Vac t.
- Intramedic PE-50 polyethylene t.
- t. introducer forceps
- Lifemed blood t.
- Nezhat irrigation t.
- Nu-Hope t.
- Ott insufflator filter t.
- Perry latex Penrose drainage t.
- polyethylene t.
- polyvinyl t.
- PVC t.
- ribbed sterile t.
- shunt t.
- Silastic t.
- Silipos mesh t.
- Simcoe connecting t.
- Sur-Fit night drainage container t.
- Surgin insufflation t.
- Teflon TFE SubLite Wall t.
- Thera-Band t.
- Tygon t.
- Y-connecting t.

Tubinger
- T. gall stone forceps
- T. self-retaining retractor

Tubipad bandage
Tubiton tubular bandage
tuboplasty surgical kit
Tubsider Kneeling Seat
tubular
- t. dressing
- t. forceps
- t. magnet
- t. plate
- t. slotted stent

Tubulitec cavity liner

Tuckables underpad
tucker
- T. anterior commissure laryngosc◦
- T. appendix clamp
- T. aspirating tube
- T. aspirating valve
- T. bead forceps
- Bishop-Black tendon t.
- Bishop-DeWitt tendon t.
- Bishop-Peter tendon t.
- Bishop tendon t.
- T. bronchoscope
- Burch-Greenwood tendon t.
- Burch tendon t.
- T. cardiospasm dilator
- Cooley cardiac t.
- Craoford-Cooley t.
- T. direct-vision telescope
- T. esophagoscope
- Fink tendon t.
- T. flexible-tip tube
- Green muscle t.
- Green strabismus t.
- T. hallux forceps
- Harrison t.
- T. hemorrhoidal ligator
- ligature t.
- McGuire tendon t.
- T. mid-lighted optic slide laryngoscope
- T. reach-and-pin forceps
- T. retrograde bougie
- Ruedemann-Todd tendon t.
- T. slotted laryngoscope
- Smith-Petersen t.
- Smuckler t.
- T. staple forceps
- T. tack and pin forceps
- tendon t.
- T. tracheal tube
- T. tracheoscope
- Twirlon ligature t.
- T. vertebrated guide
- T. vertebrated lumen finder
- Wayne t.

Tucker-Holinger laryngoscope
Tucker-Jako laryngoscope
Tucker-Levine vocal cord retractor
Tucker-Luikart blade
Tucker-McLane
- T.-M. axis-traction forceps
- T.-M. obstetrical forceps

Tucker-McLane-Luikart forceps
Tucker-McLean forceps
Tudor-Edwards
- T.-E. bone-cutting forceps
- T.-E. costotome
- T.-E. rib shears
- T.-E. rib spreader

Tufcote epilation probe
Tuffier
- T. abdominal retractor
- T. abdominal spatula
- T. arterial forceps

T. rib retractor
T. rib spreader
Tuffier-Raney laminectomy retractor
Tuffnell bandage
Tuf Nex neck exerciser
Tuf-Skin tape adherent
Tuke bone saw
Tulevech lacrimal cannula
Tuli heel cup
tulip
    t. pedicle screw
    t. probe
    t. sheath
    T. syringe system
    t. tip
tulle gras dressing
Tumble
    T. Forms feeder
    T. Forms roll
tumbling E cube
Tum-E-Vac
    T.-E.-V. gastric lavage
    T.-E.-V. gastric lavage kit
tumor
    t. forceps
    t. probe
    t. screw
tumor-grasping forceps
tumor-replacement endoprosthesis
tunable
    t. dye laser
    t. notch filter
tungsten
    t. anode
    t. carbide bur
    t. eye shield
    t. microdissection needle
    t. microelectrode
    t. tip
tungsten-halogen lamp
tuning fork
tunnel
    t. drill guide
    t. graft
tunnelable ventricular ICP catheter
tunneled eye implant
tunneler
    Cooley cardiac t.
    CPI t.
    Crafoord t.
    Crawford-Cooley t.
    Davol t.
    DeBakey femoral bypass t.
    DeBakey vascular t.
    Diethrich-Jackson femoral graft t.
    Dosick t.
    Hallman t.
    Jackson t.
    Kelly-Wick vascular t.
    Noon AV fistular t.
    Noon modified vascular access t.
    Oregon t.
    Scanlan vascular t.
    vascular access t.
tunnel-type implant material

Tunstal connector
Tunturi
    T. EL400 bicycle ergometer
    T. hand exerciser
    T. Jogger-2 self-powered treadmill
Tuohy
    T. catheter
    T. lumbar aortography needle
    T. spinal needle
Tuohy-Borst
    T.-B. adapter
    T.-B. connector
Tupman osteotomy plate
Tupper
    T. hand-holder
    T. hand-holder and retractor
    T. tractor
turbinate
    t. electrode
    t. forceps
    t. scissors
turbinectomy scissors
Turbo-Inhaler
    Spinhaler T.-I.
Turbo-Jet dental bur
TurboSonic tip
TurboStaltic pump
Turbuhaler inhaler
Turchik instrument holder
TUR-Cue photometer
Turek spinous process spreader
Turkel
    T. bone biopsy trephine set
    T. liver biopsy needle
    T. prostatic punch
    T. sternal needle
    T. trephine
    T. tube
turkey-claw clamp
TurnAide therapeutic system
turnbuckle
    t. ankle brace
    t. distractor
    t. elbow splint
    t. functional position splint
    Giannestras t.
    t. knee brace
    t. wrist orthosis
Turnbull
    T. adhesion forceps
    T. applicator
    T. cannula
    T. nail nipper
Turn-Easy transfer aid
turner
    t. biopsy needle
    t. cord elevator
    t. cystoscopic fulgurating electrode
    t. dilator
    t. periosteal elevator
    t. pin
    t. prosthesis
    rotating t.
    t. spinal gouge
Turner-Babcock tissue forceps

T

Turner-Doyen retractor
Turner-Warwick
    T.-W. adult retractor ring
    T.-W. bladder neck spreader
    T.-W. blade
    T.-W. diathermy scissors
    T.-W. fiberoptic suction tube
    T.-W. illuminating suction tube
    T.-W. malleable spoon
    T.-W. needle holder
    T.-W. pediatric perineal retractor ring
    T.-W. posterior urethral retractor
    T.-W. post-urethroplasty review speculum
    T.-W. prostate retractor
    T.-W. stone forceps
    T.-W. urethral staff
    T.-W. urethroplasty needle
Turner-Warwick-Adson forceps
Turning Board exercise system
turn-Q-plus
    microAir t.-Q.-p.
Turnsoft automatic turning system
turnstile casting stand
Turrell
    T. rectal biopsy forceps
    T. sigmoidoscope
    T. specimen forceps
Turrell-Wittner rectal biopsy forceps
Turtle chart
Turvy internal screw fixation
tutoFix cortical pin
Tutoplast
    T. anterior tibialis tendon
    T. auditory ossicle
    T. bone
    T. Dura
    T. fascia lata
    T. processed allograft
    T. tissue
Tuttle
    T. dressing forceps
    T. obstetrical forceps
    T. proctoscope
    T. sigmoidoscope
    T. thoracic forceps
    T. thumb forceps
    T. tissue forceps
Tuttle-Singley thoracic forceps
Tuwave galvanic stimulator/TENS unit
Twardon grommet
Twee alternating cut-off compressor stockings
Tweedy canaliculus knife
tweezers
    Arti-holder t.
    Dumont t.
    jeweler's t.
    Kaprelian easy-access t.
    Laser T.
    soldering t.
twill dressing
twin
    t. edgewise bracket

    T. Flash scanner
    T. Jet nebulizer
    t. knife
twin-beam CT
twin-coil dialyzer
TwinMic hearing system
twin-pattern chisel
Twirlon ligature tucker
Twisk
    T. forceps
    T. microscissors
    T. needle holder
    T. scissors
twist
    t. drill
    t. drill catheter
    t. fixation hook
twisted
    t. cotton nonabsorbable surgical suture material
    t. cotton suture
    t. dermal suture
    t. linen suture
    t. silk suture
    t. virgin silk suture
    t. wire snare loop
twister
    Batzdorf cervical wire t.
    Baumgarten wire t.
    cerclage wire t.
    Cooley-Baumgarten wire t.
    Corwin wire t.
    Miltex wire t.
    Ochsner wire t.
    orthotic coiled spring t.
    Richards wire t.
    Vital-Cooley-Baumgarten wire t.
    Vital-Cooley wire t.
    Vital wire t.
    wire t.
twist-in
    t.-i. drain tube
    t.-i. drain tube inserter
    t.-i. myringotomy tube
Twist-Lock drill guard
Twist-Mate ligator
Twist MTX implant
two-angled polypropylene loop
two-arm goniometer
two-bladed dilator
two-by-two strung sponge
two-hole
    t.-h. miniplate
    t.-h. plate
two-microphone acoustical rhinometer
two-point discriminator
two-pronged
    t.-p. dural hook
    t.-p. stem finger prosthesis
two-prong rake retractor
Tworek
    T. bone marrow-aspirating needle
    T. screw guide
    T. transorbital leukotome
    T. Universal gouge

two-stage Sarns cannula
two-stream irrigating forceps
two-toothed forceps
two-turn epicardial lead
two-wavelength near-infrared spectroscope
two-way
    t.-w. cataract-aspirating cannula
    t.-w. catheter
    t.-w. syringe
    t.-w. towel clip
two-wing Malecot drain
Tycos
    T. gauge
    T. manometer
    T. pressure infusion line
Tycron suture
Tydings
    T. automatic ratchet snare
    T. tonsillar clamp
    T. tonsillar forceps
    T. tonsillar knife
    T. tonsillar snare
    T. tonsillectome
Tydings-Lakeside tonsillar forceps
Tygon
    T. catheter
    T. esophageal prosthesis
    T. tubing
    T. tubing circuit
tying forceps
Tyler-Gigli saw
Tyler spiral Gigli saw
Tylok
    T. cerclage
    T. high-tension cerclage cabling
    system
tympanic membrane thermometer

tympanomastoid suture
tympanometer
    diagnostic t.
    MicroTymp2 hand-held t.
    Welch Allyn MicroTymp
      impedance t.
tympanoplasty
    t. forceps
    t. knife
tympanoscope
    Hopkins t.
    ulcer marker Quinton t.
tympanostomy tube
tympanum
    t. perforator
    t. perforator handle
Typhoon
    T. cutter blade
    T. microdebrider blade
Tyrer nerve root retractor
Tyrrell
    T. clamp
    T. foreign body forceps
    T. hook retractor
    T. iris hook
    T. skin hook
    T. tympanic membrane hook
Tyrrell-Gray suture
Tyshak
    T. balloon
    T. balloon valvuloplasty catheter
T-Y stent
Tytan
    T. grommet ventilation tube
    T. tube inserter
    T. ventilation tube

T

U.

U. S. Army bone chisel
U. S. Army double-ended retractor
U. S. Army gauze scissors
U. S. Army gouge
U. S. Army osteotome
U. S. Army tourniquet
U. S. Army umbilical scissors
U-1100 UV-Vis spectrophotometer
UAM
UAM Osteon bur adapter
UAM universal fixation driver
UC
UC strip
UC strip catheter tubing fastener
UCAC diagnostic catheter
UCBL prosthesis
U-channel stripping dural substitute
UCI prosthesis
Uckermann cotton applicator
UCLA
UCLA CAPP TD hook
UCLA functional long leg brace
UCOheal orthotic
UCOlite orthotic
Uebe applicator
Ueckermann-Denker trocar
UE Tech Weight Well exercise system
Uffenorde bone curette
UG-70 stapler
UGI endoscope
Ulanday double cannula
Ulbrich wart curette
ulcer
u. dressing
u. marker Quinton tympanoscope
Uldall
U. subclavian hemodialysis cannula
U. subclavian hemodialysis catheter
Ullrich
U. bone-holding forceps
U. dressing forceps
U. drill guard
U. drill guard drill
U. fistula knife
U. self-retaining laminectomy
retractor
U. tubing clamp
U. uterine knife
U. vaginal speculum
Ullrich-Aesculap forceps
Ullrich-St.
U.-S. Gallen forceps
U.-S. Gallen self-retaining retractor
ulnar
u. rasp
u. ruler
Ulrich bone-holding clamp
Ulson fixator system
Ultec Pro alginate hydrocolloid dressing
Ultex
U. lens

U. lens implant
U. Thin extra thin hydrocolloid
dressing
Ultigard underpad
Ultima
U. Bloc bite block
U. C femoral component
U. hip replacement system
U. mammography system
U. OPCAB system
U. 2000 photocoagulator
U. total hip system
Ultimate
U. knee
U. quilted comply underpad
Ultimax
U. distal femoral intramedullary rod
system
U. Haig II nail system
Ultra
U. Cover transducer cover
U. Dream Ride car bed
U. Duet Colostomy
U. Duet Colostomy irrigating sleeve
U. Duet Urostomy
U. Low resistance voice prosthesis
U. mag lens
U. pacemaker
U. Stim silver electrode
U. Twin bag system
U. ultrasonic aspirator
U. view SP slit lamp lens
U. Voice speech aid
U. Y-set system
Ultrabag system
Ultrabrace orthosis
Ultra-Care heel/elbow protector
Ultracast alloy
UltraCision
U. harmonic laparoscopic cutting
shears
U. ultrasonic knife
**UltraCon rigid gas permeable contact
lens**
Ultra-Core biopsy needle
Ultracor prosthetic valve
Ultracranio T
Ultra-Cut
U.-C. Cobb curette
U.-C. Cobb spinal gouge
U.-C. Cobb spinal instrument
U.-C. Hoke osteotome
U.-C. Smith-Petersen osteotome
Ultra-Drive bone cement removal system
UltraEase ultrasound pad
UltraEdge keratome blade
ultrafast
u. CT scanner
u. magnetic resonance imaging
u. MRI
Ultrafera wound dressing
ultrafiltration membrane

U

UltraFine erbium laser
Ultra-Fit brief
UltraFix
  U. anchor
  U. MicroMite anchor suture
  U. rotator cuff suture anchor
    system
Ultraflex
  U. ankle dorsiflexion dynamic splint
  U. esophageal prosthesis
  U. Microvasive stent
  U. nitinol expandable esophageal
    stent
  U. self-adhering male external
    catheter
  U. self-expanding stent
  U. stent delivery system
UltraFoam seating cushion
UltraForm therapeutic mattress
Ultrafuse catheter
Ultrafyn cautery tip
Ultra-Guard hip orthosis system
Ultra-Image A-scan scanner
Ultraject
  U. contrast media syringe
  U. prefilled syringe
UltraLine
  U. laser
  Lasersonic ACMI U.
UltraLite
  U. flow-directed microcatheter
  U. One-Piece convex-disposable
    system
Ultramark
  U. 9 echocardiograph
  U. scanner
  U. 8 transducer
  U. 4 ultrasound
  U. ultrasound system
Ultramatic Rx Master Phoroptor
  refractor
Ultramer catheter
Ultra-Neb nebulizer
UltraPACS diagnostic imaging system
UltraPak enteral closed feeding system
UltraPower
  U. basic drill system
  U. bur guard
  U. revision drill system
UltraPulse
  U. CO$_2$ laser
  U. surgical laser
Ultrascan digital B system
Ultrascope obstetrical Doppler
Ultraseed ultrasound-guided
  brachytherapy system
Ultra-Select nitinol PTCA guidewire
UltraShaper keratome
Ultra-Sil cannula
UltraSling glenohumeral joint sling
ultrasmall-shafted balloon
ultrasonic
  u. aspirating device
  u. biomicroscope
  u. bone-cutting instrument

  u. cataract removal lancet
  u. cataract-removal lancet needle
  u. cleaner basket
  u. dissector
  u. electrode
  u. flow director
  u. harmonic scalpel
  u. lithotriptor
  u. micrometer
  u. nebulizer
  u. probe
  u. scaler
  u. stone crusher
  u. tactile sensor
ultrasonically activated scalpel
ultrasonogram
  A-scan u.
  B-scan u.
  gray-scale u.
ultrasonography
  contact B-scan u.
  Doppler u.
  endoscopic u.
  endoscopic color Doppler u.
  intraportal endovascular u.
  Siemens Sonoline u.
  Toshiba Sal 38B real-time u.
  Toshiba Sonolayer SSA250A
    transrectal u.
ultrasonometer
  Achilles+ u.
  QUS-2 calcaneal u.
ultrasonoscope
  Acuson XP-10, -128 u.
  Bronson u.
ultrasound
  Acuson u.
  ADR Ultramark 4 u.
  Advantage u.
  AI 5200 diagnostic u.
  Alcon Digital B 2000 u.
  Aloka linear u.
  Aloka OB/GYN u.
  Aloka sector u.
  Ansaldo AU560 u.
  Aspen digital u.
  ATL/ADR Ultramark 4/9 HDI u.
  ATL real-time u.
  ATL Ultramark-series u.
  Axisonic II u.
  BladderManager u.
  BladderScan u.
  u. bone analyzer
  Bruel & Kjaer u.
  u. catheter probe
  catheter probe u.
  color Doppler u.
  colorvascular Doppler u.
  CooperVision u.
  Diasonics u.
  Doppler pulsed u.
  duplex u.
  Dynatron 150 u.
  Eccocee u.
  EchoEye u.

Elscint ESI-3000 u.
endoanal u.
EndoSound endoscopic u.
General Electric Model RT-3200 u.
GE RT 3200 Advantage II u.
HDI u.
Hewlett-Packard 2500 Sonos u.
Hitachi u.
u. inhaler
Interspec XL u.
Intertherapy intravascular u.
intraductal u.
intraluminal u.
Intrascan u.
Irex Exemplar u.
LeFort urethral u.
u. monitor
Netra intravascular u.
NeuroSector u.
Olympus EUS-20 endoscopic u.
OR 340 Intraoperative u.
u. pad
Performa u.
Pie Medical u.
power Doppler u.
PowerVision u.
pulsed Doppler u.
Rich-Mar 510 external u.
RT Advantage u.
Shimadzu cardiac u.
Shimadzu IIQ u.
Shimadzu SDU-400 u.
Siemens SI 400 u.
Siemens Sonoline Elegra u.
Siemens Sonoline Prima u.
SieScape u.
Sonicator portable u.
Sonoline Prima u.
Sonos 5500 cardiovascular u.
Spectra-Diasonics u.
u. stethoscope
Synergy u.
u. system
Toshiba Sonolayer SSH-140A u.
u. transducer
transendoscopic u.
transvaginal u.
Ultramark 4 u.
vaginal probe u.
Vingmed System Five u.
UltraSTAR computer-based ultrasound reporting system
ultrastiff wire
Ultrata
    U. capsulorhexis forceps
Ultra-Thin
    U.-T. balloon
ultra-thin
    u.-t. pancreatoscope
    u.-t. surgical blade
Ultratome
    U. double-lumen sphincterotome
    Microvasive U.
    U. XL triple-lumen sphincterotome

Ultratone electrical transcutaneous neuromuscular stimulator
ultraviolet
    u. detector
    u. light
    u. light-polymerized resin
    u. radiation (UVR)
ultraviolet-blocking intraocular lens
Ultra-vue amniocentesis needle
Ultra-X external fixation system
Ultrec
    U. cylinder
    U. Plus penile prosthesis
Ultroid coagulator
ULT-Svi calibrated end-tidal gas analyzer
umbilical
    u. clip
    u. cord clamp
    u. scissors
    u. tape
    u. tape drain
    u. tape suture
    u. venous catheter
umbiliclamp
    u. clamp
    SurgiMed u.
Umbili Clip
Umbilicutter clamp
umbrella
    Bard clamshell septal u.
    Bard PDA u.
    Clamshell septal u.
    u. dissector
    u. filter
    PDA u.
    U. punctum plug
    Rashkind u.
    u. retractor
    transcatheter u.
umbrella-type prosthesis
UMI
    UMI amniocentesis kit
    UMI catheter
    UMI Cath-Seal sheath
    UMI needle
    UMI transseptal Cath-Seal catheter introducer
U-Mid-O$_2$ Jet set
unabsorbable suture
uncoated mesh stent
unconstrained prosthesis
undergarment
    Attends beltless u.
    Dignity Plus briefmates beltless u.
    First Quality belted u.
    MaxiCare adult disposable u.
    Protection Plus belted u.
    Safe & Dry u.
    strap on u.
underpad
    Attends u.
    Birdseye quilted u.
    Brethables air-permeable u.
    Canadian Ibex quilted u.

U

underpad *(continued)*
Chamois u.
Comfort Quilt u.
Dignity Plus u.
Dri-flo u.
Excel Plus u.
Excel quilted u.
First Quality high performance and nighttime u.
Harmonie u.
Macima reusable u.
MaxiCare disposable u.
MaxiFlo breathable disposable u.
Med-I-Pad u.
Night Preservers u.
PatientGuard u.
Pinnacle reusable u.
Polylite quilted u.
PrimeTime disposable u.
Protection Plus disposable u.
Provide u.
reusable and washable u.
Safe & Dry u.
Sahara super absorbent reusable u.
Senepads u.
Sofnit Birdseye reusable u.
Sofnit 300 reusable u.
Spectra quilted u.
SureCare/Medical disposable u.
Tuckables u.
Ultigard u.
Ultimate quilted comply u.
underwater
u. Bovie
u. diathermy
u. electrode
underwater-seal suction tube
undyed suture
unfilled resin
uniaxial strain gauge
unibevel chisel
Unica CO₂ laser system
Unicare breast pump
Unicath all-purpose catheter
Unicat knife
unicompartmental knee implant
unicondylar prosthesis
UniFile Imaging and Archiving system
Uni-Flate 1000 penile prosthesis
Uniflex
U. calibrated step drill
U. distal targeting awl
U. dressing
U. drill bushing
U. intramedullary nail
U. nailing system
Uni-frame patient immobilization system
Uni-Gard
U.-G. piggyback connector
U.-G. Quik Cath
Unigraft knife
unijunction transistor
Unilab Surgibone surgical implant

unilateral
u. bar
u. calcaneal brace
u. removable partial denture
Unilink
U. anastomotic device
U. hand surgery system
Unilith pacemaker
Unimar
U. Cervex-Brush
U. HSG tray
U. J-needle
U. Pipelle curette
UniMax 2000 laser micromanipulator
union
u. broach retention drill
u. broach retention pin
Unipass endocardial pacing lead
uniplanar intraocular lens
Uniplane rocker
UniPlast Imaging and Archiving system
unipolar
u. atrial pacemaker
u. atrioventricular pacemaker
u. cautery
u. cutting loop
u. glass electrode
u. J-tined passive-fixation lead
u. sequential pacemaker
UniPort hemostasis introducer sheath k
UniPuls electrostimulation instrument
Uniquet disposable intravenous tourniquet
UniShaper single-use keratome
Uni-Shunt
U.-S. abdominal slip clip
U.-S. catheter passer
U.-S. cranial anchoring clip
U.-S. hydrocephalus shunt system
U.-S. right-angle clip
U.-S. split trocar
U.-S. with elliptical reservoir
U.-S. with reservoir introducer
Unistat bilirubinometer
Uni-sump drain
Unis Universal guide
unit
Acu-Ray x-ray u.
AdvanTeq II TENS u.
Alcon cryosurgical u.
Alcon Phaco-Emulsifier phacoemulsification u.
Amoils cryosurgical u.
Amoils-Keeler cryo u.
Arrow-Trerotola rotator drive u.
Atmolit suction u.
Autocon electrosurgical u.
Autoflex II continuous passive motion u.
Back Bubble gravity traction u.
Baird Electric System 5000 Power Plus electrosurgical u.
Bair Hugger patient heating u.
Bart abdominoperipheral angiography u.

BCD Plus cardioplegic u.
BICAP u.
BiLAP bipolar cautery u.
BioMed TENS u.
Biosound 2000 II ultrasound u.
BiPAP u.
bipolar electrosurgical u.
Birtcher Hyfrecator electrosurgical u.
Bovie electrocautery u.
Bovie electrosurgical u.
Bovie retinal detachment u.
Buck Universal convoluted
  traction u.
Burdick microwave diathermy
  electrosurgical u.
Cadwell 5200A somatosensory
  evoked potential u.
Cal-20 central dialysate
  preparation u.
calf compression u.
C-arm fluoroscopy u.
C-arm portable x-ray u.
Cavitron cautery u.
Cavitron phacoemulsification u.
Celay milling u.
Centry 2 cps dialysis u.
Century bicarbonate dialysis
  control u.
Cilco ultrasound u.
Clinitron Elexis air fluidized
  therapy u.
Clinitron II air fluidized therapy u.
Clinitron uplift air fluidized
  therapy u.
Collins Eagle I spirometry u.
Conmed Aspen Excalibur-Plus
  electrosurgical u.
Contimed II measuring u.
CoolPac hands-free u.
CooperVision I&A u.
cryosurgical u.
CSV Bovie electrosurgical u.
Cybex Trunk Extension Flexion u.
DeVilbiss I&A u.
Diasonics DRF ultrasound u.
diathermy u.
Discover Cryo-Therapy u.
DualStim TENS u.
DynaLator ultrasound u.
Dynasplint knee extension u.
Dystrophile exercise u.
ECG triggering u.
Eclipse TENS u.
Econo 90 traction u.
EEA disposable loading u.
Efica CC dynamic air therapy u.
EIE MiniEndo piezoelectric
  ultrasonic u.
Elan electrosurgical u.
ElastaTrac home lumbar traction u.
electricator electrosurgical u.
electrosurgical u. (ESU)
EMI u.
Empac-Cavitron I&A u.

enhanced external
  counterpulsation u.
EXAKT cutting/grinding u.
Exo-Bed traction u.
Exo-Overhead traction u.
Flexicair eclipse low-air-loss
  therapy u.
Flowtron DVT prophylactic deep
  venous thrombosis u.
Fox I&A u.
FracSure u.
Freedom dental u.
FreeDop portable Doppler u.
Frigitronics cryosurgical u.
Gass I&A u.
Gaymar Thermacare warming u.
G5 Fleximatic massage/percussion u.
GIA II loading u.
Gibson I&A u.
Girard ultrasonic u.
Hampton electrosurgical u.
Heliodent dental x-ray u.
Hewlett-Packard ultrasound u.
Hounsfield u.
Hyde irrigator & aspirator u.
Hydrocollator heating u.
Iceman continuous cold therapy u.
image-processing u.
inhalation breath u.
Intermedics phaco I & A u.
intrapleural sealed drainage u.
Irvine I&A u.
JACE hand continuous passive
  motion u.
JACE-STIM electrotherapy u.
kallikrein-inhibiting u.
Keeler cryophake u.
Keeler cryosurgical u.
Kelman-Cavitron I&A u.
Kelman cryosurgical u.
Kelman I&A u.
Kelman phacoemulsification u.
KeyMed u.
King-Armstrong u.
Kreiselman resuscitation u.
Kry-Med cryopexy u.
laminar air flow u.
Leksell stereotactic gamma u.
L-F Uniflex diathermy
  electrosurgical u.
linear accelerator u.
Lithostar lithotripsy u.
Living Air XL-15 u.
LIZ-88 ablation u.
low-grade suction u.
Lumix dental x-ray u.
Magnatherm pulsed therapy high-
  frequency u.
Magnatherm SSP electromagnetic
  therapy u.
Magnetrode cervical u.
Malis electrocoagulation u.
Maxima II TENS u.
Mayfield radiolucent base u.
McKesson suction bottle u.

U

U. eye shield
U. F breathing system
U. Fitstep
U. forceps
U. gastroscope
U. goniometer
U. head holder
U. hex screwdriver
U. joint device
U. Kerrison rongeur
U. laminectomy set
U. Mack lamp
U. malleable valvulotome
U. nasal instrument handle
U. nasal saw
U. nasal saw blade
U. pelvic traction belt
U. Plus instrument system
U. prosthesis
U. radial component
U. reducer cap
U. retractor
U. screwdriver
U. sheath
U. slit lamp
U. speculum
U. speculum holder
U. stent
U. straight-tube stylet
U. support splint
U. swivel
U. T-adapter
U. tourniquet
U. Tredex
U. two-speed hand drill
U. vaginal probe
U. wire clamp
U. wire scissors

Uni-Versatil sling
University
U. of Akron artificial heart
U. of British Columbia brace
U. of California Biomechanics
Laboratory heel cup
U. of Florida linear accelerator
U. of Illinois biopsy needle
U. of Illinois marrow needle
U. of Illinois sternal puncture
needle
U. of Iowa cotton applicator
U. of Kansas corneal forceps
U. of Kansas hook
U. of Kansas spatula
U. of Michigan gonioscope
U. of Michigan Mixter thoracic
forceps
U. of Virginia skull tongs
Univision low-vision microscopic lens
Uniweave catheter
Uni-Yeast-Tek system
Unna
U. boot
U. boot bandage
U. boot dressing
U. comedo extractor

Unna-Flex
U.-F. compression dressing
U.-F. compression wrap
U.-F. elastic Unna boot
U.-F. paste bandage
U.-F. Plus dressing
U.-F. PLUS Venous ulcer
convenience pack
U.-F. Plus venous ulcer kit
Unopette
U. pipette
U. system
unsegmented bar
unstented pulmonary homograft heart
valve
unzipper
Katzen flap u.
Up and About system
uPACS picture archiving system
up-angled curette
up-angle hook
upbiting
u. biopsy forceps
u. cup forceps
u. peapod
up-cupped forceps
upcurved basket forceps
Updegraff
U. cleft palate needle
U. staphylorrhaphy needle
updraft nebulizer
UPLIFT
Carter-Thomason UPLIFT
UPO-16 stapler
upper
u. body dressing
u. cervical spine anterior construct
u. cervical spine posterior construct
u. collecting system
u. esophagoscope
u. extremity myoelectric prosthesis
U. Hands self-retaining retractor
u. lateral scissors
U. 7 model head halter
u. occlusive clamp
upper-lateral exposing retractor
Uppsala gall duct forceps
upturned forceps
upward bent forceps
upward-cutting triangular knife
Urban
U. microscope
U. microsurgery closed-circuit color
TV camera
U. retractor
U. Walkers
Urbanski strut guide
Urbantschitsch
U. eustachian bougie
U. nasal forceps
Ureflex ureteral catheter
Uresil
U. biliary catheter
U. embolectomy thrombectomy
catheter

U

Uresil *(continued)*
- U. irrigation catheter
- U. occlusion balloon catheter
- U. radiopaque silicone-band vessel loops
- U. Vascu-Flo carotid shunt

ureteral
- u. basket stone dislodger
- u. brush biopsy kit
- u. catheter forceps
- u. catheter obturator
- u. clamp
- u. dilatation catheter
- u. implant
- u. isolation forceps
- u. meatotomy electrode
- u. occlusion catheter
- u. stent
- u. stone basket
- u. stone dilator
- u. stone extractor
- u. stone forceps
- u. stone retriever
- u. stylet
- u. visualization instrument

ureteric retrieval net
ureteropyeloscope
- Karl Storz flexible u.

ureterorenoscope procedure sheath
ureteroscope
- Applied Medical mini u.
- Circon ACMI MR-series u.
- flexible u.
- Gautier u.
- Micro-6 u.
- Olympus URF type P2 flexible u.
- PanoView rod-lens u.
- stiletto u.
- Storz 27022 SK u.
- Wolf rigid u.

ureterotome
- Campbell u.
- Korth u.
- optical u.
- Otis u.

urethane
- Poron cellular u.

urethral
- u. barrier device
- u. candle
- u. catheter
- u. female dilator
- u. instillation cannula
- u. intermittent catheter & tray
- u. male dilator
- u. meatus dilator
- u. sound
- u. staff

urethrographic
- u. cannula
- u. cannula clamp
- u. catheter

urethroplasty needle
urethro-profilometer

urethroscope
- Albarran u.
- Judd u.
- Lowsley u.
- Microlens u.

urethrotome
- u. blade
- bougie u.
- Hertel bougie u.
- Huffman-Huber infant u.
- infant u.
- Keitzer infant u.
- Kirkheim-Storz u.
- Maisonneuve u.
- Otis u.
- Riba u.
- Sachs u.
- Storz u.
- Storz-Kirkheim u.
- Thomson-Walker u.

Uri-Aid
Urias pressure splint
Uribe orbital implant
Uridome catheter
Uri-Drain
- U.-D. leg bag
- U.-D. male incontinence device

Uridrop catheter
Urihesive
- U. expandable adhesive
- U. moldable adhesive strip

urinal
- condom u.
- Feminal u.
- Millie female u.
- The Feminal-female u.

urinary
- u. catheter
- u. control urethral insert
- u. drainage bag and urine meter
- u. drainage tube
- u. incontinence clamp
- u. incontinence prosthesis
- u. leg bag
- u. night drainage bottle

urine
- u. collection device

Urisheath
- Conveen self-sealing U.

Uri-Two petri dish
Uro-Bond II brush-on silicone adhesive
Urocam video camera
Urocare
- U. Foley catheter
- U. latex reusable leg bag

Uro-Cath molded latex male external catheter
UroCoil self-expanding stent
Uro-Con Texas style male external catheter
Uro-Cup female vaginal urinary collection system
UroCystom unit
Urocyte diagnostic cytometry system
urodynamic catheter

Jroflo cystometer
*roflowmeter, uroflometer
   Dantec Urodyn u.
   Drake u.
   Etude cystometer u.
   Synectics-Dantec Flo-Lab II u.
Jrofoam-1, -2 adhesive foam strip for
  male external catheter
JroGold laser
Jro-Guide stent
JROLAB Janus II
Jrolase
   U. CO$_2$ laser
   U. neodymium:YAG laser fiber
*urological
   u. catheter
   u. soaking basin
Uroloop
   U. electrode
   U. instrument
UroLume
   U. endourethral Wallstent prosthesis
   U. urethral stent
   U. Wallstent
UroMax II high-pressure balloon
  catheter
Uro-Safe vinyl disposable leg bag
Uro-San Plus external catheter
Uroseal valve
Urosheath incontinence device
UroSnare cystoscopic tumor snare
Urosoft stent
Urospiral urethral stent
Urostomy
   Ultra Duet U.
Urovac bladder evacuator
UroVive system
Urowave
Urquhart periosteal elevator
Urrets-Zavalia
   U.-Z. depressor
   U.-Z. localizer
   U.-Z. probe
   U.-Z. retinal surgical lens
Urschel-Leksell rongeur
Urschel rongeur
URYS 800 nerve stimulator
USA
   USA Elite System GYN rotating
     continuous-flow resectoscope
   USA plaster spreader
   USA retractor
   USA Series Distortion Free Hydro
     laparoscope
USCI
   USCI Bard catheter
   USCI bifurcated Vasculour II
     prosthesis
   USCI cannula
   USCI Finesse guiding catheter
   USCI Goetz bipolar electrode
   USCI guiding catheter
   USCI Hyperflex guidewire
   USCI introducer

   USCI Mini-Profile balloon dilatation
     catheter
   USCI NBIH bipolar electrode
   USCI pacing electrode
   USCI PET balloon
   USCI Positrol coronary catheter
   USCI probe
   USCI Probe balloon-on-a-wire
     dilatation system
   USCI Sauvage EXS side-limb
     prosthesis
   USCI shunt
   USCI Vario permanent pacemaker
USCI-DeBakey vascular prosthesis
U-shaped
   U.-s. cannula
   U.-s. forceps
   U.-s. retractor
U-sheet
   impervious U.-s.
Usher
   U. Marlex mesh dressing
   U. Marlex mesh implant
   U. Marlex mesh implant material
   U. Marlex mesh prosthesis
Uslenghi drill guide
U-splint splint
Ussing chamber
US 1005 uroflow meter
U-sutures
   Cooley U.-s.
Utah
   U. arm electronic prosthesis
   U. artificial arm
   U. total artificial heart
UTAS 2000 electroretinography
  instrument
uterine
   u. artery forceps
   u. aspirator
   u. biopsy curette
   u. biopsy punch
   u. biopsy punch forceps
   u. clamp
   u. cornual access catheter
   u. dilator
   u. elevator
   u. evacuator
   u. Explora Curette endometrial
     sampling device
   u. injector
   u. irrigating curette
   u. manipulator
   u. needle
   u. ostial access catheter
   u. polyp forceps
   u. probe
   u. scissors
   u. scoop
   u. self-retaining cannula
   u. sound
   u. specimen forceps
   u. suction curette
   u. tenaculum
   u. tenaculum forceps

U

uterine *(continued)*
  u. tube
  u. vacuum aspirating curette
  u. vacuum cannula
  u. vulsellum forceps
uterine-dressing forceps
uterine-elevating forceps
uterine-grasping forceps
uterine-holding forceps
uterine-manipulating forceps
uterine-packing forceps
Uterobrush endometrial sample collector
utility
  u. bandage scissors
  u. forceps
  u. shears
Utrata
  U. capsulorhexis forceps
  U. foldable lens cutter

U-tube
  U.-t. drain
  U.-t. stent
  U.-t. tube
U-type dental implant
UV
  UV blocking filter
  UV transilluminator
uvea-fixated intraocular lens
uvea-supported intraocular lens
Uvex lens
UV-Flash ultraviolet germicidal excha
  device
Uviolite lamp
UVR
  ultraviolet radiation
UVR-absorbing intraocular lens
uvular retractor
U X-Acto gouge

V.

V. Mueller amputating saw
V. Mueller aortic clamp
V. Mueller auricular appendage clamp
V. Mueller-Balfour abdominal retractor
V. Mueller biopsy forceps
V. Mueller blunt hook
V. Mueller bone-cutting forceps
V. Mueller bulldog clamp
V. Mueller cross-action bulldog clamp
V. Mueller curved operating scissors
V. Mueller cystoscopy tip
V. Mueller diamond rasp
V. Mueller embolectomy catheter
V. Mueller fiberoptic retractor
V. Mueller-Frazier suction tube
V. Mueller-Gigli saw
V. Mueller-LaForce adenotome
V. Mueller laser Backhaus towel forceps
V. Mueller laser Crile micro-arterial forceps
V. Mueller laser micro-Allis forceps
V. Mueller laser Rhoton microforceps
V. Mueller laser Rhoton microneedle holder
V. Mueller laser Rhoton microscissors
V. Mueller laser Rhoton microtying forceps
V. Mueller laser Singley tissue forceps
V. Mueller laser tubal scissors
V. Mueller mastoid curette
V. Mueller myringotomy blade
V. Mueller nonperforating towel forceps
V. Mueller operating scissors
V. Mueller paracervical nerve block needle
V. Mueller-Poole suction tube
V. Mueller pudendal nerve block needle
V. Mueller ruler
V. Mueller ruler calipers
V. Mueller screwdriver
V. Mueller Tip-Trol handle
V. Mueller TUR drape
V. Mueller tying forceps
V. Mueller Universal handle
V. Mueller vascular loop
V. Mueller vena cava clamp
V. Mueller-Vital laser Babcock forceps
V. Mueller-Vital laser Heaney needle holder
V. Mueller-Vital laser Julian needle holder
V. Mueller-Vital laser Mayo dissecting scissors
V. Mueller-Vital laser Potts-Smith forceps

V1 halo ring
V33W high-density endocavity probe
Vabra
  V. assembly
  V. cannula
  V. catheter
  V. cervical aspirator
  V. suction curette
Vac
  Sani V.
Vacher self-retaining retractor
Vac-Lok
  V.-L. immobilization cushion
  V.-L. patient immobilization system
Vac-Pac positioner
Vac-Pak Pad
Vactro
  V. perilimbal suction
  V. perilimbal suction apparatus
Vacuconstrictor erection device
Vaculance
  Microlet V.
Vacupac portable vacuum system
Vac-U-Port
  Bemis V.-U.-P.
Vacurette
  Berkeley V.
  V. catheter
  V. suction curette
Vacutainer
  V. drain
  V. holder
  V. needle
  V. vacuum tube
Vacu-tome
  Barker V.-t.
  V.-t. knife
Vacutron suction regulator
vacuum
  v. apparatus
  v. aspiration catheter
  v. aspirator
  v. assisted closure dressing
  v. cassette system
  v. constriction device
  v. curette
  v. drain
  v. entrapment device
  ErecAid v.
  v. erection device
  v. extraction device
  v. fixation ring
  v. intrauterine cannula
  v. intrauterine probe
  MacroVac v.
  v. pillow

881

vacuum *(continued)*
Quiet-Vac v.
Rainbow v.
v. retractor
v. tube voltmeter
v. tumescence-constrictor device
v. uterine cannula
vacuum-assisted
v.-a. closure
v.-a. closure device
vacuuming needle
vacuum-operated viscous restraint
VAD
vascular access device
venous access device
ventricular assist device
HeartSaver VAD
V.A.D.
Covaderm plus V.A.D.
Vaduz hand
vaginal
v. aluminum electrode
v. bag
v. candle
v. contraceptive film
v. cuff clamp
v. cylinder
v. dilator
v. hysterectomy forceps
v. laser measuring rod
v. probe ultrasound
v. prolapse prosthesis
v. retractor
v. spatula
v. speculum
v. speculum loop
v. stent
Vaginard metal speculum
vaginometer
vaginoscope
Huffman-Huber infant v.
Huffman infant v.
vagotometer
Burge v.
vagotomy
v. retractor
v. stripper
Vail
V. lid everter
V. lid retractor
Vairox high-compression vascular
stockings
Vaiser-Cibis muscle retractor
Vaiser sponge
Vakutage
V. curette
V. suction system
Valdoni clamp
Valentine
V. irrigation tube
V. irrigator
V. splint
valgus bar
Validyne manometer

Valin
V. forceps
V. hemilaminectomy self-retaining
retractor
Valle hysteroscope
Valleylab
V. ball electrode
V. cautery
V. CUSA CEM system
V. electrocautery
V. Force IC electrosurgical
generator
V. laparoscopic instrument
V. loop electrode
V. pencil
V. REM system
Valliex uterine probe
Valls prosthesis
Valtrac
V. absorbable biofragmentable
anastomosis ring
V. anastomosis device
V. BAR
ValueWalker brace
valve
Abrams-Lucas flap heart v.
Accu-Flo pressure v.
Ahmed glaucoma artificial v.
Ambu-E v.
Angell-Shiley bioprosthetic heart v
Angell-Shiley xenograft prosthetic
Angiocor prosthetic v.
antisiphon v.
aortic bioprosthetic v.
apicoaortic conduit heart v.
apicoaortic shunt heart v.
Argyle anti-reflux v.
Argyle-Salem sump anti-reflux v.
ball-occluder v.
Baxter mechanical v.
Beall disk heart v.
Beall mitral v.
Beall-Surgitool ball-cage
prosthetic v.
Beall-Surgitool disk prosthetic v.
Benchekroun ileal v.
Beverly referential v.
Bianchi v.
Bicarbon Sorin v.
Bicer-val mitral heart v.
Bicer-val prosthetic v.
bileaflet tilting-disk prosthetic v.
Biocor porcine stented aortic v.
Biocor porcine stented mitral v.
Biocor prosthetic v.
Biocor stentless porcine aortic v.
biological tissue v.
bioprosthetic heart v.
Bio-Vascular prosthetic v.
Björk-Shiley mitral v.
Björk-Shiley Monostrut v.
Blom-Singer v.
bovine heart v.
bovine pericardial v.
Braunwald-Cutter ball prosthetic v.

Braunwald heart v.
bulb and thumb screw v.
Capetown aortic prosthetic v.
CarboMedics bileaflet prosthetic
  heart v.
CarboMedics "Top-Hat" supra-
  annular v.
Carpentier-Edwards bioprosthetic v.
Carpentier-Edwards mitral
  annuloplasty v.
Carpentier-Edwards pericardial v.
Carpentier-Edwards porcine supra-
  annular v.
Carpentier pericardial v.
Carpentier ring heart v.
Codman Hakim programmable v.
Codman-Medos programmable v.
convexoconcave heart v.
Cooley-Bloodwell-Cutter v.
Cooley-Cutter disk prosthetic v.
Coratomic prosthetic v.
Cordis-Hakim v.
Cross-Jones disk prosthetic v.
CRx v.
CryoLife-O'Brien v.
cryopreserved homograft v.
Cutter-Smeloff mitral v.
DeBakey heart v.
DeBakey prosthetic v.
DeBakey-Surgitool prosthetic v.
Delrin disk heart v.
Delta v.
Denver v.
Diamond v.
diastolic fluttering aortic v.
v. dilator
double spring ball v.
Dua antireflux v.
dual-chamber flushing v.
Duostat rotating hemostatic v.
Duraflow heart v.
Duromedics bileaflet mitral v.
eccentric monocuspid tilting-disk
  prosthetic v.
Edmark mitral v.
Edwards-Duromedics bileaflet
  heart v.
Edwards seamless heart v.
Emiks heart v.
expiratory v.
fascia lata heart v.
Fink v.
flexible cardiac v.
floating disk heart v.
flushing v.
four-legged cage heart v.
Freestyle v.
Frumin v.
GateWay Y-adapter rotating
  hemostatic v.
Georgia v.
glutaraldehyde-tanned bovine
  heart v.
glutaraldehyde-tanned porcine
  heart v.

Gott butterfly heart v.
Guangzhou GD-1 prosthetic v.
Hakim high-pressure v.
Hakim precision v.
Hall-Kaster heart v.
Hall prosthetic heart v.
Hammersmith heart v.
Hancock bioprosthetic heart v.
Hancock heterograft heart v.
Hancock modified orifice v.
Hancock porcine v.
Hans Rudolph three-way v.
Harken ball heart v.
Harken prosthetic v.
Harken-Starr v.
Hasner v.
heart v.
Heidbrink expiratory spill v.
Heimlich chest drainage v.
Heimlich heart v.
Heimlich Vygon pneumothorax v.
Hemex prosthetic v.
Heyer-Pudenz v.
Heyer-Schulte v.
v. holder
hollow Silastic disk heart v.
Holter elliptical v.
Holter-Hausner v.
Holter high-pressure v.
Holter medium-pressure v.
Holter mini-elliptical v.
Holter straight v.
Hufnagel-Kay heart v.
Hufnagel prosthetic v.
Intact xenograft v.
Ionescu-Shiley artificial cardiac v.
Ionescu-Shiley pericardial v.
Ionescu tri-leaflet v.
I-S artificial cardiac v.
Jatene arterial switch v.
Jatene-Macchi prosthetic v.
Kay-Shiley heart v.
Kay-Suzuki heart v.
Krupin-Denver eye v.
Lanz pressure regulating v.
v. leaflet excision scissors
lens mitral heart v.
LeVeen v.
Lewis-Leigh positive-pressure
  nonrebreathing v.
Lifemed heterologous heart v.
Liks Russian disk rotation heart v.
Lillehei-Kaster pivoting-disk
  prosthetic v.
Liotta-BioImplant LPB prosthetic v.
Lopez enteral v.
low-profile mitral heart v.
Magovern-Cromie ball-cage
  prosthetic v.
Magovern heart v.
Malteno glaucoma artificial v.
Medos v.
Medos-Hakim v.
Medtronic-Hall monocuspid tilting-
  disk v.

V

valve *(continued)*
Medtronic-Hall prosthetic heart v.
Medtronic Hancock II tissue v.
Medtronic prosthetic v.
Mishler dual-chamber v.
Mishler flushing v.
Mitamura fine ceramic heart v.
Mitroflow pericardial prosthetic v.
Monostrut Bjödork-Shiley v.
Monostrut heart v.
Montgomery speaking v.
Mosaic v.
multipurpose v.
Nezhat-Dorsey trumpet v.
nonrebreathing v.
Novus hydrocephalic v.
Novus mini v.
Omnicarbon prosthetic heart v.
Omniscience tilting-disk v.
On-X-mechanical bi-leaflet prosthetic
    heart v.
Orbis-Sigma cerebrospinal fluid
    shunt v.
v. outflow strut
Passy-Muir tracheostomy speaking v.
Peep v.
Pemco prosthetic v.
Phoenix ancillary v.
Phoenix cruciform v.
polyethylene seat heart v.
pop-off v.
porcine heart v.
programmable v.
prosthetic heart v.
Provox tracheoesophageal
    speaking v.
PS Medical Flow Control v.
Pudenz flushing v.
Puig Massana-Shiley annuloplasty v.
pulmonary autograft v.
Pyrolyte ball-cage heart v.
Quick Drain v.
Ross pulmonary porcine v.
rotating hemostatic v.
Rudolph one-way respiratory v.
Safsite v.
Sanders v.
Shiley convexoconcave heart v.
Shiley low-pressure cuffed
    tracheostomy tube with pressure
    relief v.
Shiley monostrut heart v.
Shiley Phonate speaking v.
silicone ball heart v.
silicone disk heart v.
Singer-Blom v.
Smeloff-Cutter ball-cage
    prosthetic v.
Smeloff heart v.
SmokEvac trumpet v.
Sophy mini programmable
    pressure v.
Sorin prosthetic v.
Spitz-Holter v.

Spivack v.
Starr ball heart v.
Starr-Edwards ball-cage v.
Starr-Edwards cloth-covered metal
    ball heart v.
Starr-Edwards heart v.
Starr-Edwards prosthetic aortic
Starr-Edwards prosthetic mitral
Starr-Edwards Silastic v.
Starr-Edwards silicone rubber
    ball v.
Stellite ball-cage heart v.
Stellite ring material of
    prosthetic v.
stented bioprosthetic v.
stented homografts heart v.
stentless porcine aortic v.
stent-mounted allograft v.
stent-mounted heterograft v.
Stephen-Slater v.
St. Jude bileaflet prosthetic v.
St. Jude Medical bileaflet tilting
    disk aortic v.
St. Jude Medical BioImplant v
Tascon prosthetic v.
Tekna mechanical heart v.
three-legged cage heart v.
tilting-disk heart v.
titanium ball-cage heart v.
Top-Hat supraannular aortic v.
Toronto SPV aortic v.
tracheostoma v.
Tucker aspirating v.
Ultracor prosthetic v.
unstented pulmonary homograft
    heart v.
Uroseal v.
Vascor porcine prosthetic v.
Wada-Cutter heart v.
Wessex prosthetic v.
X-Cell v.
Xenomedica prosthetic v.
Xenotech prosthetic v.
valved voice prosthesis
valve-ended catheter
valvotome
    expanding v.
    spade-shaped v.
valvuloplasty balloon catheter
valvulotome, valvutome
    angioscopic v.
    antegrade v.
    Bakst v.
    bread knife v.
    Brock v.
    Carmody v.
    Chalnot v.
    Derra v.
    Dogliotti v.
    Dubost v.
    expandable LeMaitre v.
    Gerbode mitral v.
    Gohrbrand v.
    Hall v.
    Harken v.

Himmelstein pulmonary v.
Intramed angioscopic v.
Leather antegrade v.
Leather retrograde v.
Longmire v.
Longmire-Mueller curved v.
Malm-Himmelstein pulmonary v.
Mills v.
Neider v.
Potts expansile v.
Potts-Riker v.
retrograde v.
Samuels v.
Sellor v.
Tubbs v.
Universal malleable v.
VA magnetic orbital implant
van
v. Alyea antral cannula
v. Alyea antral trocar
v. Alyea antral wash tube
v. Alyea frontal sinus cannula
v. Alyea sphenoid cannula
v. Aman pigtail catheter
v. Buren bone-holding forceps
v. Buren canvas roll sound
v. Buren catheter
v. Buren catheter guide
v. Buren dilating sound
v. Buren dilator
v. Buren sequestrum forceps
v. Buren urethral sound
v. de Graaf generator
v. Der Pas hysteroscope
v. Doren uterine biopsy punch
  forceps
v. Hove bag
v. Loonen operating keratoscope
v. Osdel guillotine
v. Osdel irrigating cannula
v. Osdel tonsil enucleator
  tonsillectome
v. Rosen splint
v. Ruben forceps
v. Slyke apparatus
v. Sonnenberg gallbladder catheter
v. Sonnenberg sump catheter
v. Sonnenberg sump drain
v. Sonnenberg-Wittich catheter
v. Struyken nasal forceps
v. Struyken nasal punch
v. Tassel pigtail catheter
Vancaillie uterine cannula
Vance
V. percutaneous Malecot
  nephrostomy catheter
V. prostatic aspiration cannula
Vance-Kish urethral illuminated catheter
Vancenase Pockethaler
Vanderbilt
V. arterial forceps
V. deep-vessel forceps
V. University hemostatic forceps
V. University vessel forceps
V. vessel clamp

Vander Pool sterilizer forceps
Vanghetti limb prosthesis
Vanguard endograft
VanishPoint syringe
Vannas
V. abscess knife
V. capsulotomy scissors
V. corneal scissors
V. fixation forceps
V. iridocapsulotomy scissors
Vantage
V. ophthalmoscope
V. Performance monitor
V. tube-occluding forceps
Vantec
V. dilator
V. grasping forceps
V. loop retriever
V. occlusion balloon catheter
V. stone basket
V. ureteral balloon dilatation
  catheter
V. urinary stent
Vantos vacuum extractor
VAPC dorsiflexion assist orthosis
Vaper Vac II
VAPORbar instrument
vaporizer
cool mist v. (CMV)
Cool-vapor v.
Dench v.
draw-over v.
flow-over v.
Fluotec v.
Goldman v.
Israel Benzedrine v.
Maxi-Myst v.
Muraco v.
Ohmeda Sevotec 5 v.
Penlon v.
vaporizing rust inhibitor
VAPORloop instrument
vapor-permeable dressing
VaporTome resection electrode
VaporTrode
V. roller electrode
VAPR coagulation and cautery device
Var-A-Pulse wound debridement system
Varco
V. dissecting clamp
V. gallbladder clamp
V. gallbladder forceps
V. thoracic forceps
variable
v. axis knee
v. flow insufflator
v. rate pacemaker
v. spinal plating
variable-focus scope
Variable Spot Dermastat
Varian
V. accelerator
V. Assoc. Cary 118C
  spectrophotometer

V

Varian *(continued)*
V. Associates 11.7-T, 51-mm bore spectrometer
V. brachytherapy system
V. CT scanner
V. LINAC
V. MLC system
V. model 3600 gas chromatograph
V. NMR spectrometer
Vari-Angle
V.-A. clip
V.-A. McFadden clip applier
V.-A. temporary clip approximator
Vari bladebreaker
VariCare system
Varick elastic dressing
Varicoscreen
Vari-Duct hip and knee orthosis
Varidyne drain
Variflex catheter
Vari-Flex prosthetic foot
Varigray
V. implant
V. lens
Varigrip spine fixation system
Variject needle
Varilux
V. Infinity lens
V. lens implant
V. Plus lens
Varimic 900 microscope
Vari-Mix II amalgamator
Vari/Moist wound dressing
Varioligator kit
Varis radiation oncology system
Vari-Stim
V.-S. III hand-held nerve stimulator
V.-S. unit
VariTone
Varivas
V. loop graft
V. R vein graft
Vari-Zone variable density convoluted mattress overlay
vas
v. clamp
v. hook
v. isolation forceps
Vasamedics PR-434 implantable prism laser probe
Vas-Cath Opti-Plast peripheral angioplasty catheter
Vasceze vascular access flush device
Vasconcelos-Barretto clamp
Vasco-Posada orbital retractor
Vascor
V. porcine prosthetic valve
V. sterile retraction tape
VascuClamp
V. minibulldog vessel clamp
V. vascular clamp
VascuCoil peripheral vascular stent
Vascu-Guard peripheral vascular patch

vascular
v. access catheter
v. access device (VAD)
v. access flush device
v. access tunneler
v. clip
v. clip applier
v. dilator
v. dissector
v. graft clamp
v. hemostatic device
v. loop
v. needle holder
v. scissors
v. sealing device
v. sheath
v. silk suture
v. spring retractor
v. suction tube
v. tissue forceps
VascuPatch
Shelhigh No React V.
Vascushunt carotid balloon shunt
Vascutech circular blade
Vascutek
V. gelseal vascular graft
V. knitted vascular graft
V. vascular prosthesis
V. woven vascular graft
vasectomy forceps
Vaseline
V. gauze dressing
V. wick dressing
Vaso-Cath peritoneal dialysis catheter
vasocillator
v. fracture appliance
v. fracture frame
VasoExtor lead extraction system
VasoSeal vascular hemostasis device
vasovasostomy clamp
VasoView balloon dissection system
Vasport access port
Vastack needle
Vasx
Neuro V.
Vauban speculum
Vaughan
V. abscess knife
V. periosteotome
Vaughn sterilizer forceps
Vaxcel catheter
VAX-D therapy table
VBH
VBH head holder
V-blade plate
VC2 atrial caval cannula
vectis
Anis irrigating v.
anterior chamber irrigating v.
v. blade
v. cesarean forceps
cul-de-sac irrigating v.
Drews-Knolle reverse irrigating v.
irrigating/aspirating v.
Knolle-Pearce v.

Look irrigating v.
v. loop
Peczon I&A v.
Pierce I&A v.
Pierce irrigating v.
plastic disposable irrigating v.
Sheets irrigating v.
Snellen v.
Torpin v.
Vector
V. II guide system
V. large-lumen guiding catheter
VectorVision surgical tracking system
VectorX large-lumen guiding catheter
Vedder loop
Veeder tip snare
Veenema-Gusberg
V.-G. prostatic biopsy cup
V.-G. prostatic biopsy needle
V.-G. prostatic punch
Veenema retropubic self-retaining retractor
Vehmehren costotome
Veidenheimer resection clamp
veil
Conformant 2 nonadherent transparent wound v.
vein
deep dorsal v.
v. dilator
v. graft cannula
v. graft ring marker
v. graft stenting stent
v. hook retractor
v. stripper
vein-coated stent
Veingard dressing
VEINLASE captured-pulse laser
Veirs
V. canaliculus rod
V. cannula
V. dacryocystorhinostomy set
V. needle
V. trocar
Velcro
V. extenders splint
V. fastener dressing
V. tourniquet
Velex woven Dacron vascular graft
Veley headrest
Velket Velcro tourniquet
velocimeter
Doppler laser v.
FloMap v.
laser Doppler v.
optical Doppler v.
Velocity stent
velolaryngeal endoscope
velour collar graft
Velpeau
V. bandage
V. cast
V. shoulder immobilizer
V. sling
V. sling dressing

V. snare
V. stockinette
V. wrap
velum
Baker v.
velvet-eye aspirating tube
vena
v. cava clamp
v. cava clip
v. cava forceps
v. caval cannula
V. Tech dual vena cava filter
V. Tech-LGM vena cava filter
Venable
V. bone plate
V. screw
Venable-Stuck
V.-S. fracture pin
V.-S. nail
Venaflo needle
venaFlow compression system
Venaport catheter
veneer retention wire
Venflon
V. cannula
V. needle
Veni-Gard stabilization dressing
venipuncture needle
Vennes pancreatic dilation set
venoclysis cannula
Venodyne
V. boot
V. compression system
V. pneumatic compressive device
Venofit medical compression stockings
Venoflex medical compression stockings
Venoflow PTFE graft
venoscope
Landry vein light v.
venous
v. access device (VAD)
v. access port
v. cannula
v. irrigation catheter
v. needle
v. plethysmograph
v. pressure gradient support stockings
v. thrombectomy catheter
v. Y-adapter
v. Y connector
Ventak
V. AICD pacemaker
V. ECD pacemaker
V. Mini II AICD
V. Mini III implantable defibrillator
V. Prizm implantable defibrillator
V. PRx defibrillation system
V. PRx pacemaker
Ventana
V. 320 automated immunostainer
V. Immuno-automated machine
VentCheck monitor
vented-electric HeartMate LVAD

Ventex
V. dressing
V. wound dressing system
Ventifoam traction dressing
ventilated
v. incontinence pad
v. mask
ventilation
v. adapter
v. tube inserter
ventilator (*See also* respirator)
Aequitron v.
Amadeus v.
Amsterdam v.
Avian transport v.
BABYbird II v.
Babyflex v.
Bear adult-volume v.
Bear 1, 2 adult-volume v.
Bear Cub infant v.
Bennett pressure-cycled v.
Bio-Med MVP-10 pediatric v.
Bird MK VIII pressure-cycled v.
Bird pressure-cycled v.
Bird 8400STi v.
blow-by v.
Bourns-Bear I v.
Bourns LS104-150 infant v.
Breeze infant v.
CPAP v.
Critical Care v.
cuirass v.
Dräger v.
Emerson postoperative v.
Hamilton v.
Healthdyne v.
high-frequency jet v.
high-frequency oscillation v.
High Frequency Oscillatory v.
HVF v.
ICV-10 v.
Infant Star high-frequency
  500/950 v.
Infrasonics v.
IVAC v.
Lifecare v.
Max v.
mechanical v.
MicroVent v.
Monaghan 300 v.
Morch v.
MVV v.
nebulization v.
Newport v.
Ohio critical care v.
Peep v.
Pneumotron v.
pneuPAC v.
Porta-Lung noninvasive
  extrathoracic v.
pressure v.
pressure-cycled v.
v. pressure manometer
pressure-preset v.
Pulmo-Aide v.

Puritan-Bennett v.
Searle volume v.
Sechrist infant v.
Sechrist neonatal v.
Servo v.
Siemens-Elema Servo 900C v.
Siemens Servo v.
Smart Trigger Bear 1000 v.
Star v.
TBird v.
Venturi v.
Veolar v.
Vickers Neovent v.
VIP Bird neonatal v.
Vix infant v.
volume-limited v.
Wave v.
Yung percutaneous mastoid v.
Venti mask
venting
v. aortic Bengash needle
v. catheter
Vent-O-Vac aspirator
Ventra catheter
Ventricor pacemaker
ventricular
v. arrhythmia monitor
v. asynchronous pacemaker
v. cannula
v. catheter
v. catheter introducer
v. demand-inhibited pacemaker
v. demand pacemaker
v. demand pulse generator
v. demand-triggered pacemaker
v. needle
v. sump
ventricular-suppressed pacemaker
ventricular-triggered pacemaker
ventriculogram retractor
ventriculography catheter
ventriculoperitoneal shunt
ventriculoscope
four-channel Aesculap v.
rigid v.
ventriculosubarachnoid (VS)
Ventritex
V. Augstrom MD implantable
  cardioverter-defibrillator
V. Cadence device
V. Cadence ICD
V. Cadence implantable cardioverte
  defibrillator
V. Contour
V. generator
V. TVL system
Ventrix tunnelable ventricular
intracranial pressure monitoring
system
ventroposterolateral (VPL)
VentTrak monitoring system
Ventura spreader
Venture sponge
Ventureyra ventricular catheter

Venturi
  V. apparatus
  V. aspiration vitrectomy device
  V. bobbin myringotomy tube
  V. collar-button myringotomy tube
  V. grommet myringotomy tube
  V. insufflator
  V. mask
  V. meter
  V. pediatric myringotomy tube
  V. spirometer
  V. ventilation adapter
  V. ventilator
Venturi-Flo valve system
Veolar ventilator
Vera bond alloy
Vera-Lift
Veratex cotton roll
Verbatim balloon catheter
Verbrugge
  V. bone clamp
  V. bone-holding clamp
  V. bone-holding forceps
  V. needle
  V. retractor
Verbrugge-Mueller bone lever
Verbrugge-Souttar craniotome
Veress
  V. laparoscopic cannula
  V. peritoneum cannula
  V. pneumoperitoneum needle
  V. spring-loaded laparoscopic needle
Veress-Frangenheim needle
Verhoeff
  V. capsular forceps
  V. capsule forceps
  V. cataract forceps
  V. dissecting scissors
  V. lens expressor
  V. suture
Veriflex guidewire
Verifuse ambulatory infusion pump
Verlow brace
Vermont spinal fixator
Verner
  V. speculum
  V. stripper
Verner-Joel cutter
Verner-Joseph
  V.-J. scissors
  V.-J. wire tightener
Verner-Kalinowski speculum
Verner-Smith monitor
Vernier calipers
Vernon
  V. antral wash tube
  V. David sigmoidoscope
  V. wire cutter
  V. wire-cutting scissors
Vernon-David
  V.-D. proctoscope
  V.-D. rectal speculum
Verruca-Freeze freezing system
VersaClimber exercise machine
Versadopp Doppler probe

Versaflex steerable catheter
Versaflow pump
Versa-Fracture femoral fixation system
Versa-Fx femoral device
VersaLight
  V. laser
  Lübke-Berci V.
  V. photodynamic therapy
Versalok
  V. low-back fixation device
  V. low-back fixation system
Versalon all purpose sponge
Versa-PEG gastrostomy kit
VersaPoint
  V. system
Versaport trocar system
VersaPulse
  V. holmium laser
  V. Select laser
Versatack stapler
Versatome
  V. laser fiber
  V. laser fiber tube
Versatrac lumbar retractor system
Versatrax
  V. cardiac pacemaker
  V. II pacemaker
Verse-Webster clamp
Versi-Splint carry bag
VerSys hip system
VertaBrace brace
VertAlign spinal support system
vertebral
  v. artery system
  v. body impactor
vertebrated
  v. catheter
  v. probe
Vertetrac ambulatory traction system
Vertex camera
vertical
  v. forceps
  v. ring curette
  v. self-retaining bone retractor
vertometer
Vesely nail
Vesely-Street nail
Vesica
  V. percutaneous bladder neck suspension kit
  V. Sling Kit
vesical retractor
vesicoamniotic shunt
vesicular transport system
Vess chair
vessel
  v. band
  v. clamp
  v. clip
  v. dilator
  v. forceps
  v. knife
  v. loop
  v. occlusion system

vessel *(continued)*
    v. punch
    v. retractor
vessel-occluding clamp
vessel-sizing catheter
VEST
    V. ambulatory ventricular function monitor
vest
    Breast V.
    Bremer AirFlo thoracic stabilization v.
    Bremer halo v.
    Circumpress gynecomastia v.
    V. direct forward-vision telescope
    E-Z-On v.
    halo v.
    Little cargo v.
    Mark VII cooling v.
    Standard E-Z-On V.
    ThAIRapy v.
    weighted v.
VestaBlate
    V. system
    V. system balloon device
vestibular clamp
Vestibulator positioning tumble forms
VET-CO vacuum system
Vezien abdominal scissors
VG slit lamp
VIA arterial blood gas and chemistry monitor
Viadrape drape
Viasorb occlusive film dressing
Viboch iliac graft retractor
Vibram rockerbottom shoe
Vibrant D, P soundbridge
Vibrasonic hearing instrument
vibrating scissors
vibrator
    Magic Wand v.
Vibrodilator probe
Vibro-Graver
    Burgess V.-G.
vibrometer
Vic
    V. hair transplant knife
    V. Vallis running hair knife
Vicat needle
Vick-Blanchard hemorrhoidal forceps
Vickerall round ringed forceps
Vickers
    V. isolator
    V. M85a microdensitometer
    V. needle holder
    V. Neovent ventilator
    V. ring-tip forceps
    V. Treonic hemoheater
Vico angled manipulator
Vicor pacemaker
Vicryl
    V. pop-off suture
    V. Rapide suture
    V. SH suture

Victor-Bonney forceps
Victoreen dosimeter
Victorian collar dressing
Victory alloy
Vidal-Ardrey modified Hoffman device
Vidal device
Vidal-Hoffman fixator frame
VidaMed's TUNA system
Vidar scanner
Vidas automated immunoassay system
Vidaurri
    V. cannula
    V. irrigator
video
    v. densitometer
    v. disk
    v. display camera
    v. duodenoscope
    v. endoscope
    v. imaging system
    v. monitor
    v. otoscope
    v. processor
    v. push enteroscope
    v. recorder
    v. specular microscope
    v. timer
videocolonoscope
    EVE Fujinon v.
videoduodenoscope
    Fujinon ED7-XU2 v.
    Fujinon 310XU v.
videoelectroscope
    Fujinon CEG-FP-series v.
    Fujinon EG7-series v.
videoendoscope, video endoscope
    double-channel v.
    fiberoptic v.
    Olympus GIF-series v.
    Olympus GIF-series double-channel therapeutic v.
    Olympus GIF-SQ-series v.
    Olympus GIF-T-series v.
    Olympus GIX-XQ-series v.
    Pentax EG-series v.
videogastroscope
    Pentax EG-2900 v.
videoHydrolaparoscope
videohydrothoracoscope
    Circon v.
videohydrothorascope
    Circon v.
videokeratoscope
    computer-assisted v.
    EyeSys v.
    PAR-C-Scan v.
    TechnoMed C-Scan v.
    TMS-2 v.
videolaparoscope
videoscope
    Cabot Medical Corporation v.
videosigmoidoscope
videostrobe

idicon
V. camera tube
V. vacuum chamber pickup tube
i-Drape
V.-D. bowel bag
V.-D. drape
V.-D. dressing
ienna
V. Britetrac nasal speculum
V. wire suture
iers
V. erysiphake
V. needle
ieth-Mueller horopter
iew shadow projection
microtomographic system
iewSite video monitor
igger-5 eye forceps
igiFoam dressing
igilance monitoring system
igilon
V. drain
V. gel dressing
V. primary wound dressing
igor DDDR pacemaker
igorimeter
Martin V.
iking
V. cannula
V. II nerve monitoring device
V. needle
ilex cannulated screw
illalta retractor
illard button
illasenor-Navarro fixation ring
illasensor ultrasonic pachymeter
imentin filament
Vim needle
Vim-Silverman
V.-S. biopsy needle
V.-S. needle
Vimule pessary
Vingmed
V. Sound CFM ultrasound system
V. System Five ultrasound
Vinke
V. retractor
V. skull tractor
V. tongs
vinyl
v. gloves
v. T-tube
Vinyon-N cloth tube
Vioform gauze dressing
Viomedex surgical marking pen
VIP Bird neonatal ventilator
Viper PTA catheter
Virag injector
ViraType probe
Virchow
V. brain knife
V. cartilage knife
V. chisel
V. skin graft knife

VircoGEN diagnostic testing system
Virden rectal catheter
Viresolve ultrafiltration membrane
virgin
V. hip screw
v. silk suture
Virginia needle
Viro Glove
Viro-Tec suture
virtual
v. labor monitor
v. reality head-mounted display
v. reality simulator
v. retinal display
Virtuoso
V. imaging system
V. LX Smart CPAP system
V. portable three-dimensional
imaging system
Virtus
V. splinter clamp
V. splinter forceps
viscera-holding forceps
visceral forceps
viscera retainer
Viscoadherent Occucoat viscoelastic
Viscoat viscoelastic
viscoelastic
Cilco v.
CooperVision v.
sodium hyaluronate v.
Viscoadherent Occucoat v.
Viscoat v.
Viscoflow angled cannula
Viscoheel
V. K, N orthosis
V. K, N prosthesis
V. SofSpot orthosis
V. SofSpot prosthesis
Viscolens lens
viscometer
Brookfield v.
Viscopaste PB7 gauze dressing
Viscoped insole
Viscospot heel cushion
vise
allograft bone v.
Benda finger v.
v. forceps
Gam-Mer v.
pin v.
Starrett pin v.
torque v.
vise-grip pliers
Visi-Black surgical needle
Visicath
V. endoscope
V. viewing catheter
Visidex II blood glucose testing strip
Visi-Drape
V.-D. Elite ophthalmic drape
V.-D. Mini Aperture drape
V.-D. Mini Incise drape
Visiflex drape

VISI-FLOW
  V.-F. irrigation starter set
  V.-F. stoma cone
Visijet hydrokeratome
Visilex polypropylene mesh
Visiline disposable sigmoidoscope
Visio-Gem color system
Vision
  V. camera
  V. Epic wheelchair
  V. MRI scanner
  V. PTCA catheter
  V. Sciences VSI 2000 flexible
    sigmoidoscope system
  V. System EndoSheath
  V. Tech lens
  V. Ten V-scan scanner
Visiport
  V. optical trocar
  V. port
Visi-Spear eye sponge
Visitec
  V. angled lens hook
  V. anterior chamber cannula
  V. aspiration unit
  V. capsule polisher curette
  V. circular knife
  V. Company lens
  V. corneal shield
  V. corneal suture manipulating hook
  V. cortex extractor
  V. crescent knife
  V. double-cutting cystitome
  V. double iris hook
  V. EdgeAhead phaco slit knife
  V. I&A cannula
  V. intraocular lens dialer
  V. iris retractor
  V. lens pusher
  V. nucleus removal loop
  V. retrobulbar needle
  V. RK zone marker
  V. stiletto knife
  V. straight lens hook
  V. surgical vitrectomy system
  V. syringe
  V. vico manipulator
  V. vitrectomy unit
Visi-Tube catheter
Vismark surgical skin marker
Visometer
  Lotman V.
visor
  Georgiade v.
Vista
  V. American Health Tesla MRI
    scanner
  V. disposable skin stapler
  V. pacemaker
Vistaflex balloon expandable, platinum alloy biliary stent
Vistech wall chart
Vistec x-ray detectable sponge

Vistnes
  V. applier bar
  V. rubber band
visual
  v. acuiometer
  v. acuity
  v. endoscopically controlled las
  v. hemostatic forceps
  v. obturator
Visual-Tech machine
Visuflo wand
Visulab system
Visulas
  V. argon C laser
  V. Nd:YAG laser
  V. YAG C laser
visuometer
VisuPac digital system
visuscope ophthalmoscope
VISX
  VISX 2020 excimer laser
  VISX Star S2 excimer laser s
  VISX Twenty/Twenty system
  VISX Wavefront system
Vitacrilic
VitaCuff
  V. cuff
  V. dressing
  V. infection control device
  V. tissue-interface barrier
Vitadur-N porcelain powder
Vita-Gel acrylic
Vitagraft
  V. arteriovenous shunt
  V. vascular graft
Vital
  V. French-eye needle holder
  V. general tissue forceps
  V. intestinal forceps
  V. lung-grasping forceps
  V. microsurgery needle holder
  V. microvascular needle holder
  V. needle holder forceps
  V. neurosurgical needle holder
  V. operating scissors
  V. skin stapler
  V. wire-cutting scissors
  V. wire twister
Vitalab
  V. Flexor clinical chemistry
    analyzer
  V. ViVa clinical chemistry ana
Vital-Adson tissue forceps
Vital-Babcock tissue forceps
Vital-Baumgartner needle holder
Vital-Castroviejo eye needle holder
Vital-Cooley
  V.-C. French-eye needle holder
  V.-C. general tissue holder
  V.-C. intracardiac needle holder
  V.-C. microvascular needle hold
  V.-C. neurosurgical needle hold
  V.-C. operating scissors
  V.-C. wire-cutting scissors
  V.-C. wire twister

Vital-Cooley-Baumgarten wire twister
Vitalcor
    V. cardioplegia infusion cannula
    V. venous return catheter
Vital-Cottle dorsal angled scissors
Vital-Crile-Wood needle holder
Vital-Cushing tissue forceps
Vital-DeBakey cardiovascular needle
  holder
Vital-Derf eye needle holder
Vital-Duval intestinal forceps
Vital-Evans pelvic tissue forceps
Vital-Finochietto needle holder
Vital-Fomon angular scissors
Vital-Halsey eye-needle holder
Vital-Heaney needle holder
Vital-Jacobson spring-handled needle
  holder
Vital-Julian needle holder
Vital-Kalt eye needle holder
Vital-Knapp
    V.-K. iris scissors
    V.-K. strabismus scissors
Vitallium
    V. allow cobalt-chrome prosthesis
    V. alloy
    V. clip
    V. cup
    V. device
    V. drill
    V. Elliott knee plate
    V. eye implant
    V. Hicks radius plate
    V. implant material
    V. mesh component
    V. miniplate
    V. Moore self-locking prosthesis
    V. nail
    V. screw
    V. Wainwright blade plate
    V. Walldius mechanical knee plate
Vital-Masson needle holder
Vital-Mayo dissecting scissors
Vital-Mayo-Hegar needle holder
Vital-Metzenbaum
    V.-M. dissecting scissors
    V.-M. scissors
Vital-Mills vascular needle holder
Vital-Neivert needle holder
Vital-Nelson dissecting scissors
Vital-New Orleans needle holder
Vitalock
    V. cluster acetabular component
    V. solid-back acetabular component
    V. talon acetabular component
Vitalograph spirometer
Vital-Olsen-Hegar needle holder
Vital-Potts-Smith forceps
Vital-Rochester needle holder
Vital-Ryder needle holder
Vital-Sarot needle holder
Vital-Stratte needle holder
Vital-Wangensteen
    V.-W. needle holder
    V.-W. tissue forceps

Vital-Webster needle holder
Vita-Stat automatic device
Vitatrax II pacemaker
Vitatron
    V. Diamond ICD
    V. Diamond II pacemaker
    V. Diamond pacemaker
    V. E catheter
    V. pacing systems
Vitax female catheter
Vit Commander vitreous cutter
Vitesse
    V. Cos laser catheter
    V. E-II coronary catheter
Vitox femoral head
Vitrasert
    V. intraocular implant
Vitrathene jacket
Vitrea 3D system
vitrectomy sponge
vitrector
    Alcon v.
    catheter v.
    Cilco v.
    CooperVision v.
    Frigitronics v.
    Kaufman v.
    Kaufman II v.
    Machemer VISC v.
    mechanical v.
    Microvit v.
    ocutome v.
    O'Malley v.
    Peeler-Cutter v.
    Peyman v.
    v. probe
    Storz Premiere Microvit v.
vitreophage
    Kaufman v.
vitreoretinal infusion cutter
vitreous
    v. infusion suction cutter
    v. pencil
    v. strand scissors
    v. sweep spatula
    v. transplant needle
vitreous-aspirating
    v.-a. cannula
    v.-a. needle
vitreous-grasping forceps
ViVa binocular infrared vision analyzer
Vivalith-10 pacemaker
Vivalith II pulse generator
Vivant ultrasonic scaler
Vivatron pacemaker
Vivonex
    V. gastrostomy tube
    V. jejunostomy catheter
Vivosil
    V. implant
    V. prosthesis
Vix infant ventilator
V-lance
    V.-l. blade

V-lance *(continued)*
    V.-l. eye knife
    V.-l. Sharpoint
V-Lok disposable blood pressure cuff
Vmax series
V-medullary nail
VoCoM thyroplasty implant
Voda catheter
Vogel-Bale-Hohner head holder
Vogelfanger-Beattie stapler
Vogelfanger blood vessel stapler
Vogel infant adenoid curette
Vogler hysterectomy forceps
Vogt-Barraquer corneal needle
Vogt toothed capsular forceps
voice
    v. button
    v. intensity controller
    v. prosthesis sizer
voiding cystourethrogram
Volk
    V. conoid implant
    V. conoid lens
    V. high-resolution aspherical lens
    V. Minus (-) noncontact adapter
    V. panretinal lens
    V. Plus (+) noncontact adapter
    V. QuadrAspheric fundal lens
    V. retinal scale adapter
    V. SuperField aspherical lens
    V. SuperPupil NC lens
    V. Super Quad 160 pan retinal lens
    V. Ultra Field aspherical lens adapter
    V. yellow filter adapter
Volkmann
    V. bone curette
    V. bone hook
    V. finger retractor
    V. hand retractor
    V. oval curette
    V. pocket retractor
    V. rake retractor
    V. scoop
    V. splint
    V. spoon
    V. vas hook
Voller curette
voltmeter
    digital v.
    electronic v.
    vacuum tube v.
Voltolini
    V. ear tube
    V. nasal speculum
Voltz wrist joint prosthesis
volume-limited ventilator
volumeter
    Dräger v.
    foot v.
    hand v.
volumetric infusion pump
Volurex incentive spirometer

Voluson sector transducer
Volutrol control apparatus
volvulus
    gastric v.
vomerine gouge
vomer septal forceps
von
    v. Andel biliary dilation catheter
    v. Eichen antral cannula
    v. Eichen antral wash tube
    v. Graefe cautery
    v. Graefe cystitome
    v. Graefe electrocautery
    v. Graefe fixation forceps
    v. Graefe iris forceps
    v. Graefe knife needle
    v. Graefe muscle hook
    v. Graefe strabismus hook
    v. Graefe tissue forceps
    v. Hippel mechanical trephine
    v. Lackum surcingle
    v. Lackum transection shift jack
    v. Langenbeck periosteal elevator
    v. Mandach capsule fragment forceps
    v. Mandach clot forceps
    v. Petz apparatus
    v. Petz clip
    v. Petz forceps
    v. Petz intestinal clamp
    v. Rosen splint
    v. Saal medullary pin
    v. Seemen rongeur
    v. Szulec hook
Voorhees
    V. bag
    V. needle
Voris intervertebral disk rongeur
Voris-Oldberg intervertebral disk forceps
Vorse
    V. tube-occluding clamp
    V. tube-occluding forceps
Vorse-Webster
    V.-W. forceps
    V.-W. tube-occluding clamp
Vortex
    V. Clear-Flow port
    V. router
    V. stabilization system
    V. tracheotomy tube
VORTX vascular occlusion coil
VoxelView system
Voxgram digital holography system
Voyager Aortic IntraClusion device
VPI
    Coloscreen VPI
    VPI Non-Adhesive Colostomy system
    VPI nonadhesive condom catheter
    VPI Non-Adhesive Ileostomy system
    VPI Non-Adhesive Urostomy system
    VPI stone basket
    VPI urinary leg bag
VPI-Ambrose resectoscope forceps

VPI-Jacobellis microhematuria catheter
set
VPL
    ventroposterolateral
      VPL thalamic electrode
VS
    ventriculosubarachnoid
      VS femoral stem
      VS shunt
VSI 2000 sigmoidoscope
V-slit lamp
V-type intertrochanteric plate
vulcanite
    v. bur
    v. chisel
vulsellum
    Bland v.
    cervical v.
    v. clamp
    Donald v.
    Fenton bulldog v.
    v. forceps

    Henrotin v.
    Jacobs v.
    Kelly v.
    MGH v.
    Schroeder v.
    Seyand v.
    Skene v.
    Teale v.
    Thoms-Allis v.
Vu-Max vaginal speculum
VVD mode pacemaker
VVI
    VVI bipolar Programalith pacemaker
    VVI single-chamber pacemaker
VVI/AAI pacemaker
VVIR single-chamber rate-adaptive
    pacemaker
VVT pacemaker
Vygantas-Wilder retinal drainage probe
Vygon Nutricath S catheter
Vynacron resin
Vynagel dental resin

W.
W. D. Johnson epicardial retractor
W. W. Walker appliance
WACH
wedge adjustable cushioned heel
WACH shoe
Wachsberger bur
Wachtenfeldt
W. butterfly clip
W. clip-applying forceps
W. suture clip
W. wound clip
Wachtenfeldt-Stille retractor
Wackenheim clivus canal line
Wacker Sil-Gel 604 silicone cement
Wada-Cutter heart valve
Wada hingeless heart valve prosthesis
Wadia elevator
Wadsworth
W. lid clamp
W. lid forceps
W. scissors
Wadsworth-Todd
W.-T. electrocautery
W.-T. eye cautery
wafer
BCNU-impregnated polymer w.
carmustine w.
Coloplast w.
Curagel w.
Gliadel w.
polyanhydride biodegradable
polymer w.
Stomahesive sterile w.
wax bite w.
Waffle
W. seating cushion
Wagener hook
Wagner
W. antral punch
W. apparatus
W. bone lever
W. knife
W. laryngeal brush
W. leg-lengthening distraction device
W. resurface prosthesis
W. revision hip system
W. rongeur
Wainstock eye suturing forceps
waist belt
Wakeling fetal heart monitor
Walb knife
Waldeau fixation forceps
Walden-Aufricht nasal retractor
Waldenberg apparatus
Waldenstrom laryngeal forceps
Walden telescope
Waldeyer
W. forceps
W. ring
Waldmar link

Wales
W. rectal bougie
W. rectal dilator
walker
w. articulator
w. aspirator
ATO w.
Body Armor short leg w.
CAM W.
Castaway leg w.
w. cautery
w. coagulating electrode
w. coagulator
Comfy w.
w. corneal scissors
w. corneal trephine
Delta w.
DH pressure relief w.
EasyStep pressure relief w.
Equalizer air w.
w. forceps
front-wheeled w.
w. gallbladder retractor
Guardian w.
hemiambulator w.
w. hollow quill pin
w. lid everter
w. lid retractor
Low Profile w.
Lumex w.
w. magnet
Merry W.
Moon W.
Nextep Contour lower-leg w.
Nextep Silhouette lower-leg w.
obese w.
ORLAU swivel w.
pneumatic w.
ProROM w.
w. ring curette
Rollator Nova w.
w. ruptured-disk curette
Sabel cast w.
w. scleral ruler
short leg w.
w. submucous elevator
w. suction tonsillar dissector
Sure-Gait folding w.
three-wheel w.
w. tonsillar needle
Urban W.'s
w. ureteral meatotomy electrode
Walker-Apple scissors
Walker-Atkinson scissors
Walker-Lee sclerotome
walking
w. brace
w. heel
w. heel cast
w. pole
Walk-'n-tone exerciser
Wallaby II phototherapy system

Wallace
W. cesarean forceps
W. Flexihub central venous pressure cannula
W. pipette
Wallace-Maloney knife
Wallach
W. Bio-Tool sterilizer
W. cryosurgical pain blocker
W. cryosurgical pencil
W. Endocell device
W. Endocell endometrial cell sampler
W. freezer cryosurgical device
W. LL100 cryosurgical Cryogun
W. minifreezer cryosurgical instrument
W. pencil cryosurgical device
W. ZoomStar colposcope
Wallach-Papette disposable cervical cell collector
Walldius Vitallium mechanical knee prosthesis
Wallgraft endoprosthesis
Wallich
W. abortion scoop
W. curette
W. placental scoop
Wallner interstitial prostate implanter
Wallstent
W. biliary endoprosthesis
W. delivery device
W. esophageal prosthesis
Schneider Magic W.
W. spring-loaded stent
The Schneider esophageal W.
UroLume W.
Wal-Pil-O neck pillow
Walrus
W. Advancit catheter
W. Angioflus catheter
Walser
W. corneoscleral punch
W. matrix
Walsh
W. dermal curette
W. footplate chisel
W. hook
W. hook-type dermal curette
W. pressure ring
W. tissue forceps
Walsham
W. nasal forceps
W. septal forceps
W. septal straightener
W. septum-straightening forceps
Walter
W. corneal spud
W. nasal retractor
W. Reed implant
W. splinter forceps
Walter-Deaver retractor
Waltham-Street bougie
Walther
W. aspirating bladder trocar

W. female catheter
W. kidney pedicle clamp
W. pedicle clamp
W. tissue forceps
W. urethral dilator
W. urethral sound
Walther-Crenshaw meatal clamp
Walton
W. comedo extractor
W. corneoscleral punch
W. curette
W. ear knife
W. foreign body gouge
W. meniscal clamp
W. meniscal forceps
W. rib shears
W. rongeur
W. round gauge spud
W. scissors
Walton-Allis tissue forceps
Walton-Liston forceps
Walton-Ruskin rongeur
Walton-Schubert
W.-S. punch
W.-S. uterine biopsy forceps
waltzing areolar lifter
Walzl hysterectomy forceps
wand
Acc ESS W.
Arthrocare thermal w.
CLO Cool W.
CollagENT w.
Connor straight nonirrigating w.
Elekta viewing w.
flexible w.
Hummingbird w.
Powell w.
programmer w.
ReFlex w.
TriggerWheel W.
Visuflo w.
wandering atrial pacemaker
Wang
W. applicator
W. lens
W. needle
Wang-Binford edge detector
Wangensteen
W. anastomosis clamp
W. apparatus
W. awl
W. deep ligature carrier
W. dissector
W. drain
W. dressing
W. duodenal tube
W. gastric-crushing anastomotic clamp
W. internal decompression trocar
W. intestinal forceps
W. intestinal needle
W. needle holder
W. patent ductus clamp
W. retractor
W. suction

W. suction unit
W. tissue forceps
W. tissue inverter
Wangensteen-Vital needle holder
Wannagat
    W. injection needle
    W. suction tube
Wappler
    W. bridge
    W. cold cautery
    W. cystoscope with microlens optics
    W. electrode
    W. microlens cystourethroscope
    W. pneumotome
    W. polypectomy snare
    W. resectoscope with microlens
      optics
Warburg apparatus
Ward
    W. French-eye needle
    W. French needle
    W. nasal chisel
    W. nasal osteotome
    W. periosteal elevator
Ward-Lempert lens loop
Ware cancer cell collector
Warm
    W. 'n Form lumbosacral corset
    W. Springs brace
    W. Springs crutch
warmer
    Alton Dean blood/fluid w.
    Bair Hugger forced-air w.
    Echowarm gel w.
    fluid w.
    gel w.
    high-capacity fluid w.
    HOTLINE blood and fluid w.
    hypothermia oxygen w.
    Kreiselman infant w.
    Ohio w.
    Omni infant heel w.
    radiant heat w.
    Thermasonic gel w.
Warm'N'Form insert
WarmTouch patient warming system
Warm-Up active wound therapy system
Warne penile sheath
Warren-Mack rotating drill
Warren-Wilder retriever
Warsaw hip prosthesis
Wartenberg
    W. neurological hammer
    W. pinwheel
Warthen
    W. forceps
    W. spur crusher
    W. spur-crushing clamp
Warwick James elevator
Was-Catheter catheter
washer
    barbed plastic w.
    biconcave w.
    connector with lock w.
    contoured w.

    w. crimper
    female w.
    Gravlee jet w.
    w. holder
    male w.
    narrow w.
    Olympus Europe ETD automated
      endoscope w.
    plate-spacer w.
    rotation-stop w.
    Salzburg biconcave w.
    spiked w.
    Synthes ligament w.
    titanium spiked w.
    wide w.
WasherLoc implant
washing catheter
washout cannula
Wasko common duct probe
wasp-waist laryngoscope
Watanabe
    W. apparatus
    W. arthroscope
    W. catheter
    W. pin
    W. pin holder
watchmaker forceps
Watco 2001 knee immobilizer
water
    w. bed
    w. bottle
    w. cushion lithotriptor
    w. dressing
    w. gauge
    W. Pik irrigator
    W. Pik toothbrush
    w. probe
    w. scalpel
Waterfield needle
water-filled balloon sheath
water-infusion esophageal manometry
  catheter
Waterman
    W. folding bronchoscope
    W. rib contractor
    W. sump drain
water-perfused catheter
Waterpillow
    Mediflow W.
Waters
    W. M-440 fixed wavelength
      detector
    W. muscle stimulator
water-seal
    w.-s. chest tube
    w.-s. drain
water-sealed spirometer
water-trap drain
Watson
    W. capsule
    W. duckbill forceps
    W. heart value holder
    W. skin graft knife
    W. speculum
    W. tonsil-seizing forceps

W

Watson-Cheyne dry dissector
Watson-Jones
    W.-J. bone gouge
    W.-J. bone lever
    W.-J. dressing
    W.-J. elevator
    W.-J. frame
    W.-J. guide pin
    W.-J. nail
    W.-J. traction
    W.-J. tractor
Watson-Williams
    W.-W. conchotome
    W.-W. ethmoidal punch
    W.-W. ethmoid-biting forceps
    W.-W. intervertebral disk rongeur
    W.-W. nasal forceps
    W.-W. needle
    W.-W. polyp forceps
    W.-W. sinus rasp
Watts
    W. locking clamp
    W. tenaculum
Watzke
    W. band
    W. cuff
    W. forceps
    W. silicone sleeve
    W. tire
Waugh
    W. dissection forceps
    W. dressing forceps
    W. prosthesis
    W. tissue forceps
Waugh-Brophy forceps
wave
    w. guide catheter
    W. ventilator
wave-edge knife
wave-tooth forceps
wax
    Aluwax impression w.
    w. bite wafer
    Bite wafer denture bite w.
    bone w.
    w. bougie
    Carver dental w.
    w. curette
    dental w.
    Flex-E-Z w.
    Flexo w.
    Godiva w.
    Horsley bone w.
    Kwik w.
    Parafil w.
    PD dental w.
    Peck inlay w.
    Plastodent w.
    Swissedent w.
    Sylver-Wax dental w.
wax-removing spatula
Wayfarer prosthesis
Wayne
    W. tucker
    W. U-crimper

WD2 welding device
wearable
    w. cardioverter-defibrillator device
    w. speech processor
Weary
    W. brain spatula
    W. nerve hook
    W. nerve root retractor
Weaveknit vascular prosthesis
Weaver
    W. chalazion clamp
    W. chalazion curette
    W. chalazion forceps
    W. sinus probe
    W. trocar introducer
Webb
    W. bolt nail
    W. cannula
    W. interchangable vein stripper
    W. pin
    W. retractor
    W. stove bolt
Webb-Balfour self-retaining abdominal
retractor
Weber
    W. aortic clamp
    W. canaliculus knife
    W. colonic insufflator
    W. hip implant
    W. iris knife
    W. lens scoop
    W. Permalock
    W. rectal catheter
    W. tissue scissors
    W. winged catheter
Weber-Elschnig
    W.-E. lens
    W.-E. lens loop
Web needle holder
Webril
    W. bandage
    W. dressing
web-spacer
    C-bar w.-s.
Webster
    W. abdominal retractor
    W. coronary sinus catheter
    W. infusion cannula
    W. infusion tube
    W. needle holder
    W. orthogonal electrode catheter
    W. ruler
    W. skin graft knife
Webster-Halsey needle holder
Webster-Kleinert needle holder
Webster-Vital needle holder
Weck
    W. astigmatism ruler
    W. clamp
    W. clip applier
    W. coagulating suction tube
    W. dermatome
    W. disposable cannula
    W. disposable trocar
    W. electrosurgery pencil

W. endoscopic suture punch
W. eye shield
W. Hemoclip clip
W. high-flow laparator
W. hysterectomy forceps
W. iris scissors
W. knife
W. microscope
W. microsurgical tray
W. rectal biopsy forceps
W. shears
W. sponge
W. suction tube
W. suture-removal scissors
W. suture scissors
W. towel forceps
W. uterine biopsy forceps
W. wire-cutting scissors
Weck-cel
    W.-c. dressing
    W.-c. implant
    W.-c. microsponge
    W.-c. surgical spear sponge
Weck-Edna nonperforating towel clamp
Weck-Harms forceps
Weck-Prep
    W.-P. blade
    W.-P. orderly razor
Weck-Spencer suture scissors
Wedeen wire passer
Weder
    W. dissector
    W. retractor
Weder-Solenberger
    W.-S. pillar retractor
    W.-S. tonsillar retractor
wedge
    w. adjustable cushioned heel
    (WACH)
    w. adjustable cushioned heel shoe
    ball w.
    bumper w.
    C. B. T. bumper w.
    disconnect w.
    Duo-Cline contoured bed w.
    w. electrosurgical resection device
    w. filter
    Good 'N Bed w.
    inner heel w.
    Kaltenborn-Evjenth Concept Wedge
    mobilization w.
    knee w.
    Livingston peribulbar w.
    medial heel w.
    medial heel-and-sole w.
    medial sole w.
    Medline w.
    Medpor biomaterial w.
    membrane delamination w.
    Positex knee w.
    w. pressure balloon catheter
    w. resection clamp
    roof w.
    Saunders mobilization w.
    self-adhering varus/valgus w.

w. TAG suture anchor system
Tempur-Med seat w.
Tepperwedge w.
wedge-line needle
wedge-shaped support
Weeks
    W. eye forceps
    W. eye speculum
    W. needle
Weerda
    W. distending operating
    laryngoscope
    W. endoscope
    W. laparoscope
Wegenke stent exchange accessory
Wehbe arm holder
Wehmer cephalometer
Wehrs incus prosthesis
Weider tongue depressor
Weiger-Zollner forceps
weight
    ankle w.
    w. boot
    EyeClose external eyelid w.
    Femina vaginal w.
    FemTone vaginal w.
    gold w.
weight-activated locking knee
weightbearing brace
weighted
    w. glove
    w. posterior retractor
    w. tip
    w. vaginal speculum
    w. vest
weight-relieving orthosis
Weil
    W. ear forceps
    W. ethmoidal forceps
    W. implant
    W. lacrimal cannula
    W. pelvic sling
    W. pelvic snare
    W. pituitary rongeur
Weil-Blakesley
    W.-B. conchotome
    W.-B. ethmoidal forceps
    W.-B. rongeur
Weil-modified Swanson implant
Weimert epistaxis packing
Weinberg
    W. blade
    W. "Joe's hoe" double-ended
    retractor
    W. rib spreader
    W. vagotomy retractor
Weiner
    W. cannula
    W. speculum
    W. tourniquet
    W. uterine biopsy forceps
Weingartner
    W. ear forceps
    W. rongeur

W

Weinstein
    W. horizontal retractor
    W. intestinal retractor
Weis chalazion forceps
Weise jack screw
Weisenbach sterile forceps holder
Weisman
    W. cannula
    W. ear curette
    W. forceps
    W. tenaculum
Weisman-Graves open-sided vaginal speculum
Weiss
    W. forceps
    W. gold dilator
    W. needle
    W. speculum
    W. spring
Weissbarth vaginal speculum
Weitlaner
    W. brain retractor
    W. hinged retractor
    W. microsurgery retractor
    W. self-retaining retractor
Welch
    W. Allyn anal biopsy forceps
    W. Allyn anoscope
    W. Allyn disposable sigmoidoscope
    W. Allyn dual-purpose otoscope
    W. Allyn fiberoptic sigmoidoscope
    W. Allyn flexible sigmoidoscope
    W. Allyn halogen penlight
    W. Allyn hook
    W. Allyn illuminated speculum
    W. Allyn KleenSpec fiberoptic disposable sigmoidoscope
    W. Allyn KleenSpec vaginal speculum
    W. Allyn laryngoscope
    W. Allyn laryngoscope blade
    W. Allyn MicroTymp impedance tympanometer
    W. Allyn operating otoscope
    W. Allyn ophthalmoscope
    W. Allyn pocket scope
    W. Allyn proctoscope
    W. Allyn rectal probe
    W. Allyn single fiber illumination headlight
    W. Allyn standard retinoscope
    W. Allyn streak retinoscope
    W. Allyn suction tube
    W. Allyn transilluminator
    W. Allyn video colonoscope
    W. Allyn video endoscope
Weldon miniature bulldog clamp
Wellaminski antral perforator
Weller
    W. cartilage forceps
    W. cartilage scissors
    W. meniscal forceps
    W. total hip joint prosthesis

Wellington
    W. Hospital vaginal retractor
    W. Hospital vaginal speculum
well-leg
    w.-l. holder
    w.-l. support
Wells
    W. enucleation scoop
    W. enucleation spoon
    W. forceps
    W. irrigator
    W. Johnson cannula
    W. pedicle clamp
    W. scleral suture pick
    W. stereotaxic apparatus
    W. tractor
Wellwood-Ferguson introducer
Welsh
    W. cortex extractor
    W. cortex-stripper cannula
    W. flat olive-tipped
    W. flat olive-tipped double cannu
    W. iris retractor
    W. olive-tipped needle
    W. ophthalmic forceps
    W. pupil-spreader forceps
    W. rubber bulb erysiphake
    W. Silastic erysiphake
Wendl tube
Wenger slotted plate
Wepsic
    W. fiberoptic cautery
    W. suction tube
Werb
    W. angled stricturotome
    W. right-angle probe
    W. scissors
Wergeland
    W. double cannula
    W. double needle
Wertheim
    W. deep surgery scissors
    W. hysterectomy forceps
    W. kidney pedicle clamp
    W. needle holder
    W. splint
    W. uterine forceps
    W. vaginal forceps
Wertheim-Cullen
    W.-C. compression forceps
    W.-C. hysterectomy forceps
    W.-C. kidney pedicle clamp
    W.-C. kidney pedicle forceps
Wertheim-Navratil
    W.-N. forceps
    W.-N. needle
Wertheim-Reverdin pedicle clamp
Weser dental hinge
Wesley-Jessen lens
Wesolowski
    W. bypass graft
    W. Teflon graft
    W. vascular prosthesis
Wessex prosthetic valve

Wesson
- W. mouthgag
- W. perineal self-retaining retractor
- W. vaginal retractor

West
- W. blunt dissector
- W. blunt elevator
- W. bone gouge
- W. hand dissector
- W. lacrimal cannula
- W. lacrimal chisel
- W. nasal chisel
- W. nasal-dressing forceps
- W. nasal gouge
- W. plastic dissector
- W. Shur cartilage clamp

West-Beck
- W.-B. periosteotome
- W.-B. spoon curette

Westco Neurostat-Mark II
Westcott
- W. biopsy needle
- W. conjunctival scissors
- W. double-end scissors
- W. micro scissors
- W. spring-action scissors
- W. stitch scissors
- W. tenotomy scissors
- W. utility scissors

Westcott-Scheie scissors
Wester
- W. meniscal clamp
- W. meniscectomy scissors

Westerman-Jansen needle
Westermark-Stille forceps
Westermark uterine dressing forceps
Western external urinary catheter
Westfield-style
- W.-s. acromioclavicular immobilizer
- W.-s. envelope sling

Westmacott dressing forceps
Weston rectal snare
Westphal
- W. gall duct forceps
- W. hemostatic forceps

wet
- w. bandage
- w. cup
- w. dressing

wet-field
- w.-f. cautery
- w.-f. coagulator
- w.-f. electrocautery

wet-to-dry dressing
Weve electrode
Wexler
- W. abdominal retractor
- W. catheter
- W. deep-spreader blade abdominal retractor
- W. large-frame abdominal retractor
- W. lateral side-blade abdominal retractor
- W. malleable-blade abdominal retractor

- W. self-retaining retractor
- W. Universal joint abdominal retractor
- W. vaginal retractor
- W. X-P large abdominal retractor

Wexler-Balfour retractor
Wexler-Bantam retractor
Wextran sponge
whalebone
- w. eustachian probe
- w. filiform bougie
- w. filiform catheter

Wheaton
- W. brace
- W. Pavlik harness
- W. tissue homogenizer

wheel
- w. bur
- Carborundum grinding w.
- Excell polishing w.
- pin w.
- shoulder w.

wheelchair
- Action Jr. w.
- Amigo mechanical w.
- Applause Super-Hemi w.
- W. Buddy
- w. cushion
- Epic w.
- HiRider motorized lift w.
- Hoveround HVR 100 power control programmable w.
- Invacare w.
- Jay J2 w.
- Kid-Kart w.
- Kusch'kin Ace w.
- Lumex lightweight w.
- Lumex Tilt-in-Space reclining w.
- manual w.
- Nitro w.
- w. pad
- power w.
- Quickie Carbon w.
- Quickie EX w.
- Quickie GP w.
- Quickie GPS w.
- Quickie GP Swing-Away w.
- Quickie GPV w.
- Quickie Kidz w.
- Quickie Recliner w.
- Quickie Ti w.
- self-propelling w.
- Skil-Care reclining w.
- Slam'r w.
- Spirea adjustable foldable w.
- Vision Epic w.
- 4XP Tilt System w.
- Zippie 2 w.
- Zippie P500 w.

Wheeler
- W. blade
- W. cyclodialysis spatula
- W. cyclodialysis system
- W. cystitome
- W. discission knife

Wheeler *(continued)*
W. graft
W. iris knife
W. iris spatula
W. malleable-shape knife
W. plaque forceps
W. prosthesis
W. spherical eye implant
W. vessel forceps
whip
W. appliance
w. bougie
Whip-Mix articulator
whirlpool
whirlybird
Hough w.
w. needle
w. probe
w. stapes excavator
whisker
slotted w.
whisk-packets dressing
whistle
Bárány noise apparatus w.
Galton ear w.
peak flow w.
w. stent
Whistler bougie
Whistle-Stop wireless aversive stimulator
whistle-tip
w.-t. drain
w.-t. Foley catheter
w.-t. ureteral catheter
Whitacre spinal needle
Whitcomb-Kerrison
W.-K. laminectomy punch
W.-K. rongeur
white
W. bone chisel
w. braided silk suture
W. clamp
W. foam pessary
W. glaucoma pump shunt
W. mallet
w. nylon suture
W. Plume absorbent gauze
W. scissors
W. screwdriver
W. tenaculum
W. tonsillar forceps
w. twisted suture
Whitehall Glacier Pack
Whitehead-Jennings mouthgag
Whitehead mouthgag
White-Lillie
W.-L. retractor
W.-L. tonsillar forceps
White-Oslay prostatic forceps
White-Proud uvular retractor
Whiteside prosthesis
White-Smith forceps
Whiting
W. mastoid curette

W. mastoid rongeur
W. tonsillectome
Whitman
W. arch support
W. fracture appliance
W. fracture frame
W. plate
Whitmore bag
Whitney
W. single-use plastic curette
W. superior rectus forceps
Whittle spud
Whitver penile clamp
whole-body
w.-b. counter
w.-b. digital scanner
Wholey
W. balloon occlusion catheter
W. Hi-torque modified-J guidewir
W. wire
Wholey-Edwards catheter
Whylie uterine dilator
Wiberg
W. fracture staple
W. fracture stapler
W. raspatory
Wichman retractor
wick
Bone-Dri femoral surgical w.
W. catheter
w. dressing
gauze w.
Glaucoma W.
Pope w.
Silastic w.
Staar glaucoma w.
wicking glue patch
Wickman uterine forceps
Wideband urinary catheter
wide-base quad cane
wide-field eyepiece
wide-seal diaphragm
wide washer
Widex hearing aid
Widner transilluminator
Wiechel scissors
Wiechel-Stille bile duct scissors
Wieder
W. dental retractor
W. pillar retractor
W. tonsillar dissector
Wieder-Solenberger pillar retractor
Wiegerinck culdocentesis puncture set
Wiener
W. antral rasp
W. corneal hook
W. eye needle
W. eye speculum
W. hysterectomy forceps
W. keratome
W. MRI filter
W. nasal rasp
W. scleral hook
W. suture hook
W. Universal frontal sinus rasp

Wiener-Pierce
   W.-P. antral rasp
   W.-P. antral trocar
Wies chalazion forceps
Wiet
   W. graft-measuring instrument
   W. otologic cup forceps
   W. otologic scissors
   W. retractor
Wigand endoscopic instrument
Wigderson ribbon retractor
Wigmore plaster saw
Wikco ankle machine
Wikström
   W. arterial forceps
   W. gallbladder clamp
Wikström-Stilgust clamp
Wiktor
   W. balloon-expandable coronary
   stent
   W. GX coronary stent
   W. GX Hepamed coated coronary
   artery stent system
Wi-Last-Ic thread
Wild
   W. laser
   W. lens
   W. M 690 microscope
   W. operating microscope
Wildcat wire
Wilde
   W. ear forceps
   W. ear polyp snare
   W. ethmoidal exenteration forceps
   W. ethmoidal punch
   W. intervertebral disk forceps
   W. intervertebral disk rongeur
   W. laminectomy forceps
   W. nasal-cutting forceps
   W. nasal-dressing forceps
   W. nasal punch
   W. nasal snare
   W. septal forceps
Wilde-Blakesley
   W.-B. ethmoidal forceps
   W.-B. scissors
Wilde-Bruening
   W.-B. ear snare
   W.-B. nasal snare
Wilder
   W. band spreader
   W. cystitome
   W. cystitome knife
   W. dilating forceps
   W. foreign body hook
   W. lacrimal dilator
   W. lens hook
   W. lens loop
   W. lens scoop
   W. loupe
   W. pick
   W. scleral depressor
   W. scleral self-retaining retractor
   W. trephine
Wilde-Troeltsch forceps

Wildgen-Reck metal locator magnet
Wildhirt laparoscope
Wiles prosthesis
Wilgnath alloy
Wilkadium alloy
Wilke
   W. boot
   W. boot brace
   W. boot prosthesis
Wilkerson
   W. choanal bur
   W. intraocular lens-insertion forceps
Wilkes self-retaining retractor
Wilkinson
   W. abdominal retractor
   W. ring-frame abdominal retractor
   W. self-retaining abdominal retractor
Wilkinson-Deaver blade abdominal
   retractor
Wilkins trephine
Wilkoro alloy
Willauer
   W. intrathoracic forceps
   W. raspatory
   W. scissors
Willauer-Allis
   W.-A. thoracic forceps
   W.-A. tissue forceps
Willauer-Deaver retractor
Willauer-Gibbon periosteal elevator
Willett
   W. clamp
   W. placental forceps
   W. placenta previa forceps
   W. scalp flap forceps
William
   W. Dixon Cratex point
   W. Harvey arterial blood filter
   W. Harvey cardiotomy reservoir
William-House suction-irrigator
Williams
   W. back brace
   W. cardiac device
   W. cartilage knife
   W. clamp
   W. craniotome
   W. cystoscopic needle
   W. diskectomy forceps
   W. esophageal tube
   W. eye speculum
   W. gastrointestinal forceps
   W. interlocking Y nail
   W. internal pelvimeter
   W. intestinal forceps
   W. lacrimal dilator
   W. lacrimal probe
   W. L-R guiding catheter
   W. microclip
   W. microlumbar retractor
   W. orthosis
   W. perforator
   W. rod
   W. rod self-retaining retractor
   W. screwdriver
   W. splinter forceps

Williams *(continued)*
W. tissue forceps
W. tonsillar electrode
W. Uni-Quad leg holder
W. uterine forceps
W. varices injection overtube
W. vessel-holding forceps
Williamsburg forceps
Williamson biopsy needle
Williamson-Noble scissors
Williams-Watson ethmoidal punch
Williger
W. bone curette
W. ear curette
W. elevator
W. hammer
W. raspatory
Willock respiratory jacket
Wills
W. eye lacrimal retractor
W. Hospital eye cautery
W. Hospital ophthalmic forceps
W. spoon with spatula
W. utility forceps
Wilman clamp
Wilmer
W. chisel
W. conjunctival scissors
W. cryosurgical iris retractor
W. iris forceps
W. iris retractor
W. iris scissors
W. refractor
Wilmer-Bagley
W.-B. iris expressor
W.-B. lens expressor
W.-B. retractor
Wilmer-Converse conjunctival scissors
Wilmington plastic jacket
Wilson
W. amniotic trocar
W. awl
W. Bimetric arch
W. bolt
W. clamp
W. fracture appliance
W. intraocular scissors
W. retractor
W. rib spreader
W. spinal frame
W. spinal fusion plate
W. vein stripper
W. vitreous foreign body forceps
Wilson-Baylor amniotic trocar
Wilson-Cook
W.-C. bronchoscope biopsy forceps
W.-C. Carey capsule set
W.-C. coagulation electrode
W.-C. colonoscope biopsy forceps
W.-C. cytology brush
W.-C. dilating balloon
W.-C. double-channel sphincterotome
W.-C. eight-wire basket stone extractor

W.-C. electrode needle
W.-C. endoprosthesis
W.-C. ERCP Cottontome
W.-C. esophageal balloon prosthes
W.-C. esophageal Z-stent
W.-C. feeding tube kit
W.-C. fine-needle-aspiration cathet
W.-C. French stent
W.-C. gastric balloon
W.-C. gastroscope biopsy forceps
W.-C. grasping forceps
W.-C. hot biopsy forceps
W.-C. low-profile esophageal prosthesis set
W.-C. minibasket
W.-C. ministent retriever
W.-C. nasobiliary tube
W.-C. NJFT-series feeding tube
W.-C. papillotome
W.-C. plastic prosthesis
W.-C. polypectomy snare
W.-C. prosthesis repositioner
W.-C. Protector guidewire
W.-C. retrieval forceps
W.-C. Saaed six shooter
W.-C. standard wire guide
W.-C. stone basket
W.-C. Tracer guidewire
W.-C. tripod retrieval forceps
W.-C. wire-guided sphincterotome
Wilson-Kirbe speculum
Wilson-Mayo stand
Wiltberger spinous process spreader
Wiltek papillotome
Wil-Tex alloy
Wilton-Webster
W.-W. coronary sinus thermodilutio catheter
W.-W. thermodilution flow and pacing catheter
Wiltse
W. iliac retractor
W. pedicle screw fixation system
W. system cross-bracing
W. system double-rod construct
W. system H construct
W. system single-rod construct
W. system spinal rod
Wiltse-Bankart retractor
Wiltse-Gelpi self-retaining retractor
WinABP ambulatory blood pressure monitor
Wincor enucleation scissors
Windmill suction evacuation unit
window
w. clip
w. rasp
w. rasp marker
windowed
w. esophageal balloon
Winer catheter
wing
w. clip
w. suture

inged
  w. catheter
  w. retractor blade
  w. steel needle

Wingfield fracture frame

Winkelmann circumcision clamp

Winquest tibial/femoral extraction system

Winsburg-White
  W.-W. bladder tube
  W.-W. retractor

Winston
  W. cervical clamp
  W. SD catheter

Winter
  W. arch bar
  W. elevator
  W. facial fracture appliance
  W. Helping Hand
  W. ovum forceps
  W. placental forceps
  W. shunt
  W. splint

Winter-Nassauer placental forceps

Winternitz sound

wipe
  Alkare adhesive remover w.
  Allkare protective barrier w.
  Kimwipes w.
  Microclens w.
  Remove adhesive remover w.
  Sani-Cloth HB disposable w.
  Sani-Cloth Plus germicidal
    disposable w.

wire (*See also* guidewire, guidewire)
  ACS microglide w.
  Amplatz torque w.
  Ancrofil clasp w.
  w. appliance
  atrial pacing w.
  auger w.
  Australian orthodontic w.
  Australian Special Plus w.
  Babcock stainless steel suture w.
  Baron suction tube-cleaning w.
  bayonet-point w.
  beaded cerclage w.
  Bentson exchange straight guide w.
  Bentson floppy-tip guide w.
  Bentson-type Glidewire guide w.
  Birtcher Hyfrecator cautery w.
  w. bivalve vaginal speculum
  bone fixation w.
  braided w.
  brass w.
  Brooker w.
  Bunnell pull-out w.
  central core w.
  cerclage w.
  cesium-137 w.
  Charnley trochanter w.
  circumdential w.
  Coffin transpalatal w.
  coiled spiral pusher w.
  Commander PTCA w.
  Compere fixation w.

Conceptus Robust guide w.
control w.
Cope w.
Cordis Stabilizer marker w.
Cragg Convertible w.
Cragg FX w.
Cragg infusion w.
crenulated tantalum w.
w. crimper
Crozat orthodontic w.
curved J-exchange w.
w. cutter
Dall-Miles cerclage w.
delivery w.
Dentaflex w.
diathermy w.
double keyhole loop w.
w. drill
w. driver
Drummond w.
ear snare w.
eel w.
endocardial w.
Eve-Neivert tonsillar w.
E wildcat orthodontic w.
extra-stiff Amplatz w.
w. fixation bolt
FlowWire Doppler guide w.
Force w.
w. frame spectacles
Geenan Endotorque w.
Gigli spiral saw w.
Gilmer w.
Glidewire Gold surgical guide w.
Guidant guide w.
guide w., guidewire
w. guide
Hahnenkratt orthodontic w.
Hancock temporary cardiac
  pacing w.
high-torque w.
Hi-Per Flex exchange w.
House piston w.
HPC guide w.
hydrophilic-coated guide w.
intermaxillary w.
interosseous w.
intracoronary Doppler flow w.
intravascular Doppler-tipped
  guide w.
Isola w.
Isotac pilot w.
Ivy w.
J-w.
Jagwire w.
Jarabak arch w.
J exchange w.
Johnson canaliculus w.
K w.
Katzen infusion w.
Killip w.
Kirschner w. (K wire, K-wire)
Kirschner boring w.
K wire
K-wire

wire *(continued)*
    w. lid speculum
    ligature tie w.
    lingual w.
    Linx extension w.
    w. loop
    w. loop stapes dilator
    Lunderquist coat hanger w.
    Luque cerclage w.
    Luque sublaminar w.
    magnet w.
    w. mandrin
    Markley orthodontic w.
    Medi-Tech w.
    w. mesh eye implant
    monofilament snare w.
    Monorail guide w.
    Mullan w.
    Mustang steerable guide w.
    nasal snare w.
    needle-knife w.
    Neivert-Eves tonsillar w.
    nitinol shape-memory alloy w.
    olive w.
    outrigger w.
    over-tying w.
    pacing w.
    w. passer
    Pathfinder w.
    PD orthodontic w.
    piston w.
    platinum w.
    Prima laser guide w.
    w. probe
    w. prosthesis-crimping forceps
    prosthesis smooth w.
    protector plus w.
    Puestow guide w.
    pusher w.
    Quadcat w.
    QuickSilver hydrophilic-coated
      guide w.
    RadiMedical fiberoptic pressure-
      monitoring w.
    rectal cautery w.
    rectangular w.
    Remaloy w.
    Remanium w.
    Respond w.
    Roadrunner w.
    Rotablator w.
    Rotafloppy w.
    round chuck-end Kirschner w.
    Sadowsky hook w.
    Sage w.
    w. saw
    Scimed-Choice floppy w.
    w. scissors
    Seldinger retrograde w.
    w. side blade
    Silk guide w.
    Simcoe anterior chamber
      retaining w.
    Sippy esophageal dilator pusher w.

    smooth transfixion w.
    snare w.
    w. snare
    space-age w.
    spinous process w.
    w. splint
    square w.
    stainless steel w.
    w. stapes prosthesis
    Sterling-Spring orthodontic w.
    Stertzer-Myler extension w.
    stiffening w.
    Storz twisted snare w.
    w. stylet
    w. stylet catheter
    sublaminar w.
    suture w.
    tantalum w.
    TherOx infusion guide w.
    Thiersch w.
    w. threader
    w. tightener
    titanium w.
    tonsillar snare w.
    torque attenuating diameter w.
    Tracer ST w.
    Trailblazer w.
    trocar-point Kirschner w.
    trochanteric w.
    Truarch w.
    w. twister
    ultrastiff w.
    veneer retention w.
    Wholey w.
    Wildcat w.
    Wironit clasp w.
    Wirotom clasp w.
    Wizdom guide w.
    Zimaloy beaded suture w.
    w. Zytor suture
wire-closure forceps
wire-crimping forceps
wire-cutting suture scissors
wire-fat ear prosthesis
wire-fixation buckle
wire-guided
    w.-g. hydrostatic balloon
    w.-g. metal spiral retrieval dev
    w.-g. oval intracostal dilator
    w.-g. papillotome
    w.-g. polyvinyl bougie
    w.-g. sphincterotome
wire-loop
    w.-l. keratoscope
    w.-l. strut
wire-mesh self-expandable stent
wire-passing
    w.-p. awl
    w.-p. bur
wire-pulling forceps
wire-tightening clamp
wire-twisting forceps
wiring retractor
Wironit clasp wire
Wirosol investment material

Wirotom clasp wire
Wirovest investment material
Wirthlin splenorenal shunt clamp
Wisap
    W. diagnostic laparoscope
    W. disposable cannula
    W. disposable trocar
    W. insufflator
    W. operating laparoscope
Wisconsin
    W. laryngoscope
    W. laryngoscope blade
Wise
    W. dilator
    W. iridotomy laser lens
    W. orbital retractor
    W. sphincterotomy laser lens
Wis-Foregger laryngoscope
Wishard ureteral catheter
Wis-Hipple laryngoscope
Wissinger
    W. rod
    W. set
Wister
    W. forceps holder
    W. nipper
    W. vascular clamp
Withers tendon passer
Wit portable TENS system
Witt dental light
Wittmoser optical arm
Wittner
    W. cervical biopsy punch
    W. uterine biopsy forceps
Witzel
    W. enterostomy catheter
    W. gastrostomy
Wixson hip positioner
Wizard
    W. cardiac device
    W. disposable inflation device
    W. gamma counter
    W. microdebrider
Wizdom guide wire
Woakes nasal saw
Wolf
    W. antral needle
    W. arthroscope
    W. aspiration/injection system
    W. biopsy forceps
    W. biting-basket forceps
    W. cataract delivery forceps
    W. curved-basket forceps
    W. delivery system
    W. dermal curette
    W. disposable cannula
    W. drain
    W. drainage cannula
    W. endoscope
    W. eye forceps
    W. graft
    W. hemostatic bag
    W. implant
    W. insufflation laparoscope
    W. lithotrite

    W. Loktite mouthgag
    W. meniscal retractor
    W. needle trocar
    W. nephrostomy catheter
    W. photolaparoscope
    W. Piezolith 2300 lithotripsy device
    W. prosthesis
    W. return-flow cannula
    W. rigid panendoscope
    W. rigid ureteroscope
    W. suction tube
    W. uterine cuff forceps
Wolf-Castroviejo needle holder
Wolf-Cottle trocar
Wölfe-Böhler
    W.-B. cast breaker
    W.-B. cast remover
    W.-B. plaster cast spreader
Wölfe-Krause
    W.-K. graft
    W.-K. implant
Wolfe loop electrode
Wolferman drill
wolffian drain
Wolf-Henning gastroscope
Wolf-Knittlingen gastroscope
Wolf-Post rhinoscope
Wolfram needle electrode
Wolf-Schindler gastroscope
Wolfson
    W. forceps
    W. gallbladder retractor
    W. intestinal clamp
    W. spur crusher
    W. spur-crushing clamp
Wolf-Yoon
    W.-Y. applicator
    W.-Y. ring
Wollaston doublet
Wolvek
    W. fixation device
    W. sternal approximation fixation
    W. sternal approximator
Women's Tradition brace
WonderBrace Convertible
Wong-Staal scissors
Wood
    W. aortography needle
    W. bulldog clamp
    W. colonic kit
    W. glasses
    W. lamp
    W. light
    w. roll dressing
    W. screw
    w. tongue blade
    w. tongue depressor
Woodbridge tube
Wooden Wobble balance ball
Woodruff
    W. screw
    W. screwdriver
    W. spatula knife
    W. ureteropyelographic catheter

Woodson
- W. dental periosteal elevator
- W. double-ended dissector
- W. dural separator
- W. obstetrical spoon
- W. packer
- W. plug
- W. probe
- W. spatula

Woods Surgitek bra

Woodward
- W. antral rasp
- W. forceps
- W. retractor
- W. sound
- W. thoracic artery forceps

Woodward-Potts intestinal forceps
Woolley tibia punch
Wool'n Gel seating cushion
Wooten eye needle
Worcester
- W. City Hospital speculum
- W. instrument holder

Word Bartholin gland catheter
Work-Bruening diagnostic head
world standard Olsen bipolar cable
Worrall
- W. deep retractor
- W. headband

Worst
- W. corneal bur
- W. corneal contact glasses
- W. double-ended pigtail probe
- W. gonioprism contact lens
- W. lobster-claw lens
- W. Medallion lens
- W. needle
- W. probe

Wort antral retractor
Worth
- W. advancement forceps
- W. amblyoscope
- W. chisel
- W. cystitome
- W. muscle forceps
- W. strabismus forceps

wound
- w. clip
- w. drain
- w. drainage collector
- w. drainage reservoir
- w. dressing
- w. forceps
- w. towel

wound-clip forceps
Wound-Evac kit
Woun'Dres natural collagen hydrogel wound dressing
WoundSpan Bridge II dressing
woven
- w. cotton gauze
- w. Dacron catheter
- w. dacron tube
- w. Dacron tube graft

- w. elastic bandage
- w. silk catheter

woven-tube vascular graft prosthesis
Wozniak Sur-Lok chuck
wrap
- Ace w.
- ArtAssist w.
- bias w.
- Biocell w.
- BodyIce w.
- braceRAP w.
- CircPlus w.
- Circulon w.
- Coban w.
- Coflex w.
- digit w.
- Dura-Kold reusable compression ice w.
- Dura-Soft soft-compression reusable ice or heat w.
- Dyna-Flex w.
- DynaWraps w.
- Elasto-Gel hot/cold w.
- Elasto-Gel shoulder therapy w.
- Elasto-Link joint w.
- Electro-Link joint w.
- Fabco w.
- FLEX-WRAP self-adherent w.
- Ice Wedge hot/cold therapy w.
- iodophor-impregnated adhesive w.
- kastRAP w.
- Kerlix w.
- kneeRAP w.
- Kold W.
- loop-over w.
- magnetic w.
- 3M Coban LF self-adherent w.
- Nylatex w.
- Ocu-Guard ophthalmic w.
- Primer compression w.
- shoulderRAP w.
- Stimprene w.
- super w.
- SurePress compression w.
- Thera-Boot compression w.
- thermal plastic w.
- Thermoskin arthritic knee w.
- Thermoskin back w.
- Unna-Flex compression w.
- Velpeau w.
- Zipzoc compression w.

wraparound
- w. dressing
- w. inactive electrode

Wratten 6B filter
wrench
- Barton w.
- beaded pin w.
- Canakis w.
- Cloward spanner w.
- DynaTorq w.
- Hagie w.
- Halifax w.
- Harrington flat w.
- hexagonal w.

hex socket w.
Kurlander orthopaedic w.
Richmond subarachnoid w.
Santa Casa w.
slotted w.
socket w.
spanner w.
spinal slip w.
Stader w.
Stille w.
Texas Scottish Rite Hospital w.
T-handled nut w.
T-handled screw w.
Thomas w.
torque ratchet w.
Trinkle socket w.

Wright
W. Care-TENS device
W. fascia needle
W. knee plate
W. knee prosthesis
W. nasal snare
W. ophthalmic needle
W. peak flow meter
W. peak flowmeter
W. pneumatic tourniquet
W. ptosis needle
W. respirometer
W. tonsillar snare
W. Universal brace
Wright-Crawford needle
Wright-Guilford
W.-G. curette
W.-G. cutting block
W.-G. double-edged knife
W.-G. drum elevator
W.-G. elevator knife
W.-G. fenestrometer
W.-G. flap knife
W.-G. footplate pick
W.-G. incudostapedial knife
W.-G. middle ear instrument
W.-G. roller knife
W.-G. stapes pick
W.-G. wire cutter
Wright-Harloe empyema trocar
Wrightlock spinal fusion system
Wright-Rubin
W.-R. forceps
W.-R. forceps guard
Wrigley forceps
Wristaleve support
wristband
Sea-Band acupressure w.
wrist-driven prehension orthosis

Wristlet
Freedom USA W.
Wrist Restore brace
W-shaped ileoneobladder
W-shape forceps
Wullen stone dislodger
Wullstein
W. chuck adapter
W. contra-angle handpiece
W. diamond bur
W. double-edged knife
W. drill
W. ear forceps
W. ear scissors
W. high-speed bur
W. microsuction tube
W. ototympanoscope otoscope
W. ring curette
W. self-retaining ear retractor
W. transplant spatula
W. tympanoplasty forceps
Wullstein-House forceps
Wullstein-Paparella forceps
Wullstein-Weitlaner self-retaining retractor
Wunderer modification activator
Wurd catheter
Wurmuth spatula
Wurth
W. spur crusher
W. vein stripper
Würzburg
W. maxillofacial plating system
W. plate
Wurzelheber dental elevator
Wutzler scissors
Wyler subdural strip electrode
Wylie
W. carotid artery clamp
W. drain
W. endarterectomy set
W. endarterectomy stripper
W. hypogastric clamp
W. "J" clamp
W. lumbar bulldog clamp
W. renal vein retractor
W. spatula
W. splanchnic retractor
W. stem pessary
W. tenaculum forceps
W. uterine dilator
W. uterine forceps
W. uterine tenaculum
Wylie-Post rhinoscope
Wynne-Evans tonsillar dissector

W

X-Acto utility knife
Xanar
    X. 20 Ambulase CO_2 laser
    X. laser adapter
    X. laser bronchoscope
X-Cel dental x-ray unit
X-Cell valve
XeCl
    XeCl excimer laser
Xemex pulmonary artery catheter
XenoDerm graft
xenograft
    bovine pericardial heart valve x.
    Carpentier-Edwards x.
    Ionescu-Shiley pericardial x.
Xenomedica prosthetic valve
xenon
    x. arc
    x. arc coagulator
    x. arc photocoagulator
    x. cold light fountain
    x. lamp
    x. light source
xenon-chloride excimer laser
Xenophor femoral prosthesis
Xenotech prosthetic valve
Xercise
    X. band
    X. tube resistive device
Xeroflo dressing
Xeroform
    X. dressing
    X. gauze
Xertube
Xillix
    X. LIFE-GI fluorescence endoscopy
    system
    X. LIFE-Lung system
Ximatron simulator
Ximed
    X. disposable cannula
    X. disposable trocar
Xi-scan
    X.-S. fluoroscope
    Linde X.-S.
XKnife
    X. knife
    X. software for stereotatic radiation
    therapy
    X. stereotactic radiosurgery system
XL
    XL illuminator
    Jung Autostainer XL

XL-11 Ranfac percutaneous
    cholangiographic catheter
X-long cement forceps
Xoman drill
Xomed
    X. Audiant bone conductor
    X. Doyle nasal airway splint
    X. dual-chamber balloon
    X. endotracheal tube
    X. intraoral artificial larynx
    X. Kartush tympanic membrane
    patcher
    X. micro-oscillating saw
    X. rectal probe
    X. Silastic splint
    X. sinus irrigation kit
    X. sinus-secretion collector
    X. skimmer shaver
    X. straight-shank tube
    X. Treace ventilation tube
    X. Tytan ventilation tube
Xomed-Treace nerve integrity monitor
XO-soft-sole orthotic
XP
    X. peritympanic hearing instrument
    X. Xcelerator ultrasound enhancer
Xpeedior catheter
Xpress/SW helical CT scanner
Xpress/SX helical CT scanner
XPS
    XPS Sculpture system
    XPS Straightshot micro tissue
    resector system
    XPS Striaghtshot micro tissue
    resector
XQ video instrument
x-ray
    x.-r. calipers
    x.-r. detectable laparotomy sponge
    x.-r. generator
    x.-r. overlay
    x.-r. spectrometer
    x.-r. tomographic microscope
    x.-r. tube
Xsensor Pressure Mapping system
X-Sizer catheter system
X-tend back protector
X-TEND-O knee flexer
X-Trel spinal cord stimulation system
X-Trode electrode catheter
Xyrel pacemaker

Y-adapter
YAG
yttrium-aluminum-garnet
YAG laser
Yaghouti LASIK Polisher
YagLazr system
Yale
Y. brace
Y. Luer-Lok needle
Y. Luer-Lok syringe
Yalon intraocular lens
Yamagishi stapler
Yamanda knife
Yang needle
Yankauer
Y. antral punch
Y. antral trocar
Y. aspirating tube
Y. bronchoscope
Y. ear curette
Y. esophagoscope
Y. ethmoidal forceps
Y. eustachian catheter
Y. hook
Y. laryngoscope
Y. ligature passer
Y. middle meatus cannula
Y. nasopharyngeal speculum
Y. punch
Y. salpingeal curette
Y. salpingeal probe
Y. scissors
Y. septal needle
Y. suction
Y. suction tube
Y. suture needle
Y. tonsil suction tip
Yankauer-Little forceps
Yannuzzi fundus laser lens
Yarmo morcellizer
Yasargil
Y. aneurysm clip-applier
Y. angled forceps
Y. applying forceps
Y. arachnoid knife
Y. arterial forceps
Y. bayonet needle holder
Y. bayonet scissors
Y. bipolar forceps
Y. carotid clamp
Y. clip applier
Y. clip-applying forceps
Y. cross-legged clip
Y. curette
Y. dissector
Y. flat serrated ring forceps
Y. ligature carrier
Y. microclip
Y. microdissector
Y. microforceps
Y. microneedle holder
Y. microraspatory

Y. microscissors
Y. microsuction tube
Y. microvascular bayonet scissors
Y. microvessel clip-applying forceps
Y. neurosurgical bipolar forceps
Y. raspatory
Y. retractor
Y. scoop
Y. spring hook
Y. straight forceps
Y. suction tube
Y. tissue lifter
Yasargil-Aesculap
Y.-A. instrument
Y.-A. spring clip
Yasargil-Leyla brain retractor
Yashica Dental Eye II camera
Yazujian cataract bur
Y-bandage dressing
Y-bone plate
Y B Sore cushion
Y-connecting tubing
Yeates drain
Yeder suction tube
Yellen circumcision clamp
Yellow
Y. Springs Instrument Co., Inc. (YSI)
Y. Springs probe
yellow-eyed dilating bougie
yellow-tip aspirator
Yeoman
Y. biopsy punch
Y. probe
Y. proctoscope
Y. sigmoidoscope
Y. uterine biopsy forceps
Y. uterine forceps
Yeoman-Wittner rectal forceps
Yield nonadherent gauze dressing
Y-jaws
Y-Knot device
Yoon-ring applicator
Yoon tubal sterilization ring
Yoshida
Y. dental x-ray unit
Y. tonsillar dissector
Youens lens
Youlten nasal inspiratory peak flow meter
Young
Y. anterior prostatic retractor
Y. bifid retractor
Y. bladder retractor
Y. boomerang needle holder
Y. bulb retractor
Y. cystoscope
Y. cystoscopic rongeur
Y. intestinal forceps
Y. lateral prostatic retractor
Y. ligature carrier
Y. lobe forceps

Young *(continued)*
  Y. needle holder
  Y. pediatric rectal dilator
  Y. prostatectomy forceps
  Y. prostatic enucleator
  Y. prostatic forceps
  Y. prostatic retractor
  Y. prostatic tractor
  Y. renal pedicle clamp
  Y. rubber dam fracture frame
  Y. tongue forceps
  Y. urological dissector
  Y. uterine forceps
  Y. vaginal dilator
Younge
  Y. endometrial curette
  Y. irrigator
  Y. uterine curette
  Y. uterine forceps
Younge-Kevorkian forceps
Young-Hryntschak boomerang needle holder
Young-Millin boomerang needle holder

Younken double-lumen drain
Yours Truly asymmetrical external breast form
Y-port connector
Y-set system
YSI
  Yellow Springs Instrument Co., Inc.
    YSI Foley probe
    YSI neonatal temperature probe
Y-trough catheter
yttrium-aluminum-garnet (YAG)
  y.-a.-g. laser (YAG laser)
Y-tube
  Lahey Y.-t.
Yuan screw
Yucca wood splint
Yu-Holtgrewe
  Y.-H. malleable blade
  Y.-H. prostatic retractor
Yund
  Y. acetabular skid
  Y. ligamentum teres knife
Yung percutaneous mastoid ventilator

Ziegler *(continued)*
  Z. lacrimal dilator
  Z. lacrimal probe
  Z. needle probe
  Z. wash bottle
Ziegler-Furness clamp
Zielke
  Z. bifid hook
  Z. curette
  Z. derotator bar
  Z. pedicular instrumentation
  Z. rod
  Z. scoliosis gouge
  Z. screw
zigzag stent
Zilkie device
Zimalate twist drill
Zimaloy
  Z. beaded suture wire
  Z. cobalt-chromium-molybdenum
   alloy
  Z. epiphyseal staple
  Z. femoral head prosthesis
Zimberg esophageal hiatal retractor
Zimcode traction frame
Zim-Flux dressing
Zimfoam
  Z. head halter
  Z. pad
  Z. pad and patient positioner
  Z. pin
  Z. splint
Zimmer
  Z. airplane splint
  Z. Anatomic hip prosthesis system
  Z. antiembolism stockings
  Z. arthroscope
  Z. bone cement
  Z. bur
  Z. cartilage clamp
  Z. Centralign Precoat hip prosthesis
  Z. clavicular cross splint
  Z. clip
  Z. CPT hip system
  Z. cross-over instrumentation system
  Z. dermatome
  Z. extractor
  Z. fracture frame
  Z. Gigli-saw blade
  Z. goniometer
  Z. hand drill
  Z. head halter
  Z. low-viscosity adhesive
  Z. Orthair ream driver
  Z. pin
  Z. protractor
  Z. Pulsavac wound debridement
   system
  Z. saw
  Z. screw
  Z. screwdriver
  Z. shoulder prosthesis
  Z. skin graft mesher
  Z. snare

  Z. suction irrigator
  Z. telescoping nail
  Z. tibial bolt
  Z. tibial nail cap
  Z. tibial prosthesis
  Z. Universal drill
Zimmer-Hall drive system
Zimmer-Hoen forceps
Zimmer-Hudson shank
Zimmer-Kirschner hand drill
Zimmer-Schlesinger forceps
Zimmon
  Z. biliary stent
  Z. catheter
  Z. endoscopic biliary stent set
  Z. endoscopic pancreatic stent set
  Z. esophagogastric balloon
   tamponade set
  Z. papillotome
  Z. sphincterotome
Zimocel dressing
Zim-Trac
  Z.-T. traction splint
  Z.-T. traction splint tractor
Zim-Zip rib belt splint
zinc
  z. ball electrode
  z. oxide bandage
Zinco
  Z. Gunslinger II shoulder
   immobilizer
  Z. Hyperex thoracolumbar brace
Zinnanti
  Z. clamp
  Z. uterine manipulator/injector
  Z. Z-clamp
Zinn endoillumination infusion cannula
zipper
  Z. anti-disconnect device
  Z. Medical hypoallergenic
   tracheostomy tube neck band
  Z. Medical tracheostomy tube
   neckband
  z. ring
Zippie
  Z. P500 wheelchair
  Z. 2 wheelchair
Zipser
  Z. meatal clamp
  Z. meatal dilator
  Z. penile clamp
Zipster rib guillotine
Zipzoc
  Z. compression wrap
  Z. stocking compression dressing
  Z. stockings
Ziramic
  Z. femoral head
  Z. femoral head prosthesis
Zirconia
  Z. orthopaedic prosthesis
  Z. orthopaedic prosthetic head
Ziskie operating laparoscope
Ziski iris clip intraocular lens
Zitron pacemaker

M-1 colonoscope
-Med balloon catheter
murkiewicz
    Z. brain clip
    Z. clip applier
obec sponge dressing
oeffle soft intraocular lens
oellner
    Z. hook
    Z. needle
    Z. raspatory
    Z. scissors
oladex implant
oll
    Z. NTP noninvasive pacemaker
    Z. PD1200 external defibrillator
ollinger
    Z. leg holder
    Z. multipurpose tissue forceps
    Z. splint
ollinger-Gilmore vein stripper
ollner suction tube
onas
    Z. porous adhesive tape dressing
    Z. porous tape
Zone Specific II meniscal repair system
onule
    z. separator
    z. stripper
Zoomscope colposcope
Zoroc resin plaster dressing
Zower speculum
ZPLATE-ATL anterior spinal fixation
    system
Z-plate plate
Z-Sampler endometrial suction curette
Z-Scissors hysterectomy scissors
Z-stent
    covered Z.-s.
    modified Z.-s.
    Wilson-Cook esophageal Z.-s.
Zucker
    Z. cardiac catheter
    Z. multipurpose bipolar catheter
    Z. splint

Zucker-Myler cardiac device
Zuelzer
    Z. awl
    Z. hook plate
Zuker bipolar pacing electrode
Zuma coronary guiding catheter
ZUMI uterine manipulator
Zund-Burguet apparatus
Zuni
    Z. exercise system
    Z. gym
    Z. harness
Zurich dilatation catheter
Zutt clamp
Zwanck radium pessary
Z-wave tube
Zweifel
    Z. angiotribe
    Z. appendectomy clamp
    Z. needle holder
    Z. pressure clamp
Zweifel-DeLee cranioclast
Zweymuller-Alloclassic prosthesis
Zweymuller hip prosthesis
Zyderm collagen implant
zygoma
    z. elevator
    z. hook
Zyler
    Z. head halter
    Z. tube
Zylik
    Z. cannula
    Z. microclip
    Z. ophthalmoendoscope
Zylik-Joseph hook
Zylik-Michaels
    Z.-M. retractor
    Z.-M. scissors
    Z.-M. speculum
Zyoptix laser
Zyplast implant
Zyranox femoral head
Zywiec electrode

Appendix 1
Common Manufacturers & Websites

Editor's Note: Mergers, acquisitions, and new entrants in the medical and scientific equipment industry contribute to this collection. In the "Website" column below, "na" indicates that website addresses were not available when this edition went to print.

Manufacturer	Website
Abbey Home Healthcare	www.ecatcorp.com
Abbott Laboratories	www.abbott.com
ABCO Dealers, Inc.	www.goetzedental.com/abco.html
Access Surgical International, Inc.	www.biopsys.com
Accurate Surgical & Scientific Instrument Corp.	na
Accuscope	www.accuscope.com
Achilles USA	www.achillesusa.com
ACI Medical	www.acimedical.com
Ackrad Laboratories, Inc.	www.ackrad.com
Acme United Corporation, Medical Division	www.acmeunited.com
ACMI Circon	www.circon.com
ACS (Applied Cardiac Systems)	www.acsholter.com
Action Products, Inc.	www.actionproducts.com
Acuson, Inc.	www.acuson.com
Adenna, Inc.	www.adenna.com
Advanced Neuromodulation Systems	www.ans-medical.com
AdvantaJet	www.advantajet.com
Aesculap, Inc.	wwww.aesculap.de
Alcon Surgical, Inc.	www.alconlabs.com
Aldrich Chemical Company	www.sigma-aldrich.com/aldrich/
Alimed, Inc.	www.alimed.com
Allegiance Healthcare Corp.	www.allegiance.net
Allied Healthcare	www.alliedhpi.com
Alltech Associates, Inc.	www.alltechweb.com
Aloka Company, LTD.	www.aloka.co.jp.
AMAC Inc./Immunotech, Inc.	www.immunotech.com
American Endoscopy/Amersham Corp.	www.amersham.co.uk/
American Type Culture Collection	www.atcc.org
American Optical Corporation	www.americanopticaleyewear.com
Amersham Corporation	www.amersham.co.uk/
Apple Medical Corporation	www.applemed.com
Applied Cardiac Systems, Inc. (ACS)	www.acsholter.com
Applied Imaging Corp.	www.cytovision.com

Manufacturer	Website
Arrow International, Inc.	www.arrowintl.com
Arzco Medical Systems, Inc.	www.arzco.com
Astra U.S.A., Inc.	www.astra.com
Atlas Surgical	www.sahaj.com
AUTO SUTURE	www.clubcoelio.com/autosuture.htm (French)
AVECOR Cardiovascular, Inc.	www.clubcoelio.com/autosuture.htm
AVL Medical Instruments	www.avlmed.com
Bard, Inc., C. R.	www.crbard.com
Baxter Healthcare Corporation	www.baxter.com
Bayer Diagnostics	www.bayerdiag.com
BBL Microbiology Systems/ Becton Dickinson	www.bd.com
Beckman Coulter, Inc. (Beckman Instruments)	www.beckman.com
Becton Dickinson and Company	www.bd.com
Beere Precision Medical Instruments, Inc.	www.beeremedical.com
Beltone Electronics Corporation	www.beltone.com
Bennett X-Ray Corporation	www.bennettx-ray.com
Bergen Brunswig Corp.	www.bergenbrunswig.com
BioChem Pharma	www.biochem-pharma.com
Biodex Medical Systems, Inc.	www.biodex.com
Bio-Logic Systems, Corp.	www.blsc.com
Bio-Lok International, Inc.	www.biolok.com
Bio-Med Devices, Inc.	www.biomeddevices.com
Bio-Medicus, Inc.	www.medtronic.com
Bio-Rad Laboratories Ltd.	www.bio-rad.com
Bioject, Inc.	www.bioject.com
Biomet, Inc.	www.biomet.com
Biosound, Inc.	www.biosound.com
Bird & Cronin Medical	www.birdcronin.com
Bird Life Design	www.trianim.com
Birtcher Medical Systems, Inc.	na
Bivona Medical Technologies	www.bivona.com
Bledsoe Brace Systems	www.bledsoebrace.com
Boehm Surgical Instrument Corporation	na
Boehringer Mannheim Corporation	www.boehringer-mannheim.com
Boekel Scientific	www.boekelsci.com
Bollinger Healthcare Products	na
Boston Scientific Corporation	www.bsci.com
Braintree Scientific, Inc.	www.braintreesci.com

Manufacturer	Website
Brasseler USA/Komer Medical	www.brasselerusa.com
Braun Medical Inc.	www.bbraunusa.com
Breas	www.breas.com
Bristol-Myers Co./Mead Johnson & Company	www.bms.com
	www.meadjohnson.com
Bristol-Myers Squibb Pharmaceutical	www.bms.com
Bruel & Kjaer Instruments, Inc.	www.bk.dk
Bruker Instruments	www.bruker.com
Burroughs Wellcome Co.	www.glaxowellcome.com
C.B. Fleet Co., Inc.	www.cbfleet.com
Cabot Medical Corporation	na
Cameron-Miller, Inc.	na
Canon USA, Inc.	www.usacanon.com
Carbomedics, Inc.	www.carbomedics.com
Cardiovascular Imaging Systems (CVIS)	www.bsci.com
Cardio-Vascular Innovations, Inc.	www.mmm.com/cardiovascular
	www.cvico.com
Cardiovascular Systems/3M Health Care	na
Carolina Medical, Inc.	www.caromed.com
Carrington Laboratories, Inc.	www.carringtonlabs.com
Cavitron CO_2 Laser Systems/Cooper Life Sciences, Inc.	na
Cavitron Surgical Systems, Inc./ Valleylab, Inc.	www.valleylab.com
Cavitron/Syntel Division/Alcon Surgical	www.alconlabs.com
Cell Robotics	www.cellrobotics.com
Cetylite Industries, Inc.	www.cetylite.com
Chiron Corporation	www.chiron.com
Cho-Pat, Inc.	www.cho-pat.com
Ciba Corning Diagnostics Corporation	na
Ciba Vision Corporation	www.cibavision.com
Cilco/Alcon Surgical	www.cilco.com
	www.alconlabs.com
Cincinnati Surgical Company	www.cincinnatisurgical.com
Circon Corporation	www.circoncorp.com
Circon ACMI	www.circoncorp.com/company/ co-divisions.html#acmi
Clarus Medical Systems, Inc.	www.clarusmedical.com
Clinimed, Inc.	www.clinimed.com
Clinipad Corporation	na
Cliniex Medical Corporation	www.clinitex.fr (French)

Manufacturer	Website
COBE Laboratories, Inc. (Gambro BCT)	www.cobebct.com
Codman & Shurtleff, Inc.	www.codmanjnj.com
Coherent, Inc.	www.cohr.com
Color Max Technologies	www.color-vision.com
Conmed	www.conmed.com
Cook Incorporated	www.cookgroup.com
Cook Urological, Inc.	www.cookgroup.com/cook-urological.htm
CooperSurgical, Inc.	www.coopercos.com
CooperVision, Inc.	www.coopervision.com
Cordis Corporation (Johnson & Johnson ultimate parent)	www.cordis.lu
Core Dynamics, Inc.	www.core-dynamics.com
Corometrics Medical System, Inc.	http://www.icem.com/award/1999/ design_html/417. htm
Corpak, Inc.	www.bldmedical.com
Coulter Corporation	www.coulter.com
Craft de Pak	http://users.erols.com/craftdepak
C. R. Bard, Inc.	www.crbard.com
Critikon, Inc.	www.dinamap.com
Cryomedics, Inc./Cabot Medical Corp.	www.circoncorp.com
Custom Ultrasonics, Inc.	www.customultrasonics.com
CVIS (Cardivascular Imaging Systems)/ InterTherapy, Inc.	www.cvico.com
Dainabot Company (Japan)	na
DAKO Corp.	www.dakousa.com
Datascope Corp.	www.datascope.com
Datex-Ohmeda	www.ohmeda.com
Davol, Inc.	www.davol.com
Denison Orthopedic Appliance Corp.	www.cddenison.com
Dentsply International, Inc.	www.dentsply.com
Denver Biomaterials, Inc.	www.denverbio.com
DePuy Orthopaedics, Inc.	www.depuy.com
DeRoyal Industries. Inc.	www.deroyal.com
Diasonics	www.diasonics.com (GE Medical)
Dicon	www.dicon.com
Doran Instruments, Inc.	www.diagnosysllc.com
Dornier Medical Systems, Inc.	www.dornier.com
Dow Medical	www.dow.com
Draeger, Inc. Critical Care Systems	www.draeger.com
Du Pont Company	www.dupont.com
Dyna-Med	www.dynamed.com
Dynacor	www.dynacor.com (French)

Manufacturer	Website
Dynorthotics, Inc.	na
Dyonics, Inc./Smith & Nephew Dyonics, Inc.	www.smithnephew.at
E-Z-EM, Inc.	www.ezem.com
EBI Medical Systems, Inc./Biomet, Inc.	www.biomet.com www.ebimedical.com
Eli Lilly	www.lilly.com
Elmed, Inc.	www.elmed.com
Elscint. Inc.	www.elscint.co.il
Endo Direct. Inc.	www.heartport.com
Erie Scientific Co.	www.eriesci.com
Ethicon Endo-Surgery	www.eesonline.com
Euro-Med/CooperSurgical	www.euromed.nl
Everest Medical Corp.	www.everestmedical.com
FCS Laboratories, Inc.	na
Fenwal Electronics, Inc.	www.fenwal.com
Fibra-Sonics, Inc.	www.fibrasonics.com
Fillauer Inc.	na
Fischer Imaging Corporation	www.fischerimaging.com
Fisher Scientific Co.	www.fisher.co.uk
Flents Products Co., Inc.	na
Flexiflo	na
FlexMedics Corp.	na
Flowtronics, Inc.	www.techexpo.com
Freeman Manufacturing Company	www.freemanmfg.com
Fresenius USA, Inc.	www.fmcna.com
Fujinon, Inc.	www.fuginon.co.jp
Gambro BCT (formerly COBE BCT)	www.cobebct.com
Geiger Instrument Corp.	www.geigerinst.com
GE Medical Systems	www.gemedicals.com
General Electric CGR USA	www.ge.com
GIBCO Laboratories/Life Technologies, Inc.	www.lifetech.com
Glaxo, Inc.	www.glaxowellcome.com
Global Medi-Tex, Inc.	www.globalmeditek.com
Gomco/Allied Health Care Products, Inc.	www.alliedhpi.com
Gore & Associates, Inc., W. L. (Gore-Tex)	www.gore.com
Gould Instrument Systems, Inc.	www.gould.co.uk
Graham-Field, Inc.	www.grahamfield.com
Grass Instrument Co.	www.aesnet.org/VEC/grass/grass.htm

Manufacturer	Website
Greenwald Surgical Co., Inc.	na
Grieshaber & Company, Inc.	na
Guidant Corp.	www.guidant.com
Healthdyne Technologies	na
Hemocue, Inc.	www.hemocue.se
Hemostatix Corp.	www.inductothermindustries.com
HemoTec, Inc.	na
Heraeus Lasersonics, Inc./ Heraeus Surgical, Inc.	www.laserscope.com
Hewlett-Packard Co.	www.hp.com
HGM Medical Laser Systems, Inc.	www.hgmmedical.com
Hitachi Denshi America, Ltd.	www.hdal.com
Hitachi Instruments, Inc.	www.hii.hitachi.com
Hoefer Scientific Instruments	na
Hoffman-La Roche, Inc./Roche Diagnostic Systems, Inc.	www.roche.com
Hoffman-Nagel Medical Systems, Inc.	na
Hollister, Inc.	www.hollister.com
Hologic, Inc.	www.hologic.com
Howmedica, Inc.	www.osteonics.com
Hu-Friedy Manufacturing Co., Inc.	www.hu-friedy.com
Hybritech (USA)	www.coulter.com
Hyclone Laboratories, Inc.	www.hyclone.com
Hydro-Med, Inc.	www.hydromed.com
Imex Medical Systems, Inc. (now Nicolet Vascular, Inc.)	www.nicoletvascular.com
Immunotech Corp.	www.immunotech.com
Inamed Corp.	www.inamed.com
Incstar Corp.	www.diasorin.com
Infimed, Inc.	www.infimed.com
Infrasonics, Inc.	na
Intermedics Inc.	www.intermedics.com
International Biomedical, Inc.	www.interbio.com
Interventional Therapeutics Corp. (ITC)	na
Interzeag Inc. USA	www.interzeag.haag-streit.com (German)
Invacare Corporation	www.invacare.com
Iolab Corp.	na
Iovision, Inc.	www.iovision.com
IPAS	www.ipaas.org
Isotec Corporation	www.isotec.de
IVAC Corporation (IVAC Medical)	www.ivac.com

Manufacturer	Website
ralon, Inc. (Ivalon Surgical Products)	www.pactmed.com/products/ivalon
rit Instruments	www.jarit.com
ly Medical Ltd. (now Rehab Designs, Inc.)	www.rehabdesigns.com
ohnson & Johnson	www.johnsonandjohnson.com
app Surgical Instrument, Inc.	www.kappsurgical.com
atena Products, Inc.	www.katena.com
endall Co.	www.kendallhq.com
err Corporation	www.kerrdental.com
eymed, Inc.	www.keymedinc.com
inamed, Inc.	www.kinamed.com
irschner Medical Corp.	na
irwan Surgical Products, Inc.	www.kirwans.com
leen Test Products Co. (Meridian Industries)	www.meridiancompanies.com
MI, Inc.	www.kmiinc.com
odak Company	www.kodak.com
onigsberg Instruments, Inc.	na
ontron Instruments, Inc.	www.kontronmedical.com (French)
owa Optimed, Inc.	www.optimedtech.com
T Medical, Inc.	na
urzweil Applied Intelligence, Inc.	www.kurzweiltech.com www.voicerecognition.com
& M Instruments, Inc.	na
abconco Corp.	www.labconco.com
aparomed Corp.	na
arkotex Company	www.larkotex.com
aser Photonics, Inc.	www.lpg.man.ac.uk
aserscope	www.laserscope.com
awton USA Surgical Instruments	na
DB Enterprises, Ltd.	www.lab-enterprises.com
eibinger L.P.	www.leibinger.de (German)
eisegang Medical, Inc.	www.leisegang.com
eisure Lift	www.leisurelift.com
enox Hill Brace Co., Inc.	www.lenoxhill.com
ife Medical Technologies, Inc. (Life Medical Equipment)	www.lifemedicalequipment.com
ife Support Products, Inc. (Allied Healthcare)	www.alliedhpi.com
ife-Tech, Inc.	www.life-tech.com
ink America, Inc.	www.linkorthopedics.com
invatec Corporation	www.linvatec.com

Manufacturer	Website
LKB Diagnostics, Inc./Wallace, Inc.	www.wallac.fi
LKC Technologies, Inc.	www.lkc.com
Lone Star Medical Products	www.lsmp.com
Lorenz Surgical, Walter	www.lorenzsurgical.com
Lukens Medical Corp.	www.cepz.com/lukens
Lumex	www.lumex.com
Lumiscope Company, Inc.	www.lumiscope.net
Luther Medical Products, Inc.	www.opitsourcebook.com/luther_medical.html
Luxar Corp.	na
Luxtec Corp.	www.luxtec.com
Machida, Inc.	www.machidascope.com
Mallinckrodt Medical, Inc.	www.mallinckrodt.com
Mansfield/Boston Scientific Corp.	www.bsci.com
Maramed Orthopedic Systems	www.maramed.com
Marlow Surgical Technologies, Inc.	www.marlow-surgical.com
Marquette Electronics Inc., (USA)	www.gemedicals.com
Maxxim Medical	www.maxximmedical.com
Medical Graphics Corporation	www.mbbnet.umn.edu
Medical Devices International	www.cprmicroshield.com
Medical Innovations Corporation	www.aedi.com
M.E. Meditek Co., Ltd.	www.devicelink.com
Meditron Devices, Inc.	www.s-und-s.de/pages-NEU-eng/UB3/filtration/UB3-body-meditron.html
Medix Biotech, Inc.	www.genzyme.com/bin/gensrch.pl
Medline Industries, Inc.	www.medline.com
Medrad, Inc.	www.medrad.com
Medtronic Heart Valves, Inc.	www.medtronic.com
Medtronic, Inc.	www.medtronic.com
MegaDyne Medical Products, Inc.	www.megadyne.net
Mennen Medical Corp.	www.mennenmedical.com
Mentor Corp.	www.mentorcorp.com
Meridian Industries	www.meridiancompanies.com
Merlyn Pharmaceuticals	www.inc.com/users/merlyn.html
Merocel Corporation	www.xomed.com/specialtybrochures/sinus.asp
Micro-Aire Surgical Instruments, Inc.	www.microaire.com
Micro-Bio-Logics	www.microbiologics.com
Micromedics, Inc.	www.micromedics-usa.com
Microtek Medical, Inc.	www.microtekmed.com
Microvasive/Boston Scientific Corp.	www.bsci.com
Midas Rex Pneumatic Tools	www.midasrexlp.com

Manufacturer	Website
Midmark Corporation	www.midmark.com
Miles, Inc., Diagnostics Division	http://guide.labanimal.com/company/237.html
Milex Products, Inc.	www.milexproducts.com
Mill-Rose Laboratories, Inc.	www.mrlabsinc.com
Millar Instruments, Inc.	www.millarinstruments.com
Miltex Instrument Co., Inc.	www-miltex.com
Minntech Corporation	www.minntech.com
	www.mbbnet.umn.edu/company_folder/mnn.html
Mityvac/Neward Enterprises, Inc.	www.mityvac.com
MMI, Inc.	www.mmicompanies.com
Moss Tubes, Inc.	www.mosstubeinc.com
Narco Bio-Systems, Inc.	www.int-bio.com/narcobio.htm
Natvar Company (now Plastron)	www.plastron.com
Nautilus	www.nautilus.com
NDL Products	www.ndlwest.com
Nellcor, Inc. (formerly Akcess Med-Prods., Inc.)	www.mallinckrodt.com
Neostar Medical Technologies, Inc.	na
Nevco International, Inc.	na
New Life Systems, Inc.	na
Ney Company, J. M.	www.jmney.com
Nichols Institute	www.nicholsdiag.com
Nicolet Vascular	www.nicoletvascular.com
Nihon Kohden (America), Inc.	www.nkusa.com
Nikon Inc., Instrument Group	www.nikonusa.com/products/industrial
Nomos Corporation	www.nomos.com
Nordic Track	www.nordictrak.com
Nova Biomedical Corporation	www.nova.ch
Nova Ortho-Med, Inc.	www.novaortho-med.com
Novartis	www.novartis.com
Novo Industri A/S	www.novo.dk
Nuaire, Inc.	www.nuaire.com
Nalge Nunc International	www.nalgenunc.com
Oculus of America/Insight Instruments, Inc.	www.insightinstruments.com
OEM Medical	www.bigskylaser.com
Ohio Medical Instrument Co., Inc.	www.ohiomed.com
Ohmeda (Datex-Ohmeda)	www.ohmeda.com
Olympus America, Inc.	www.olympus.com
Onyx Medical Corp.	www.onyxmedical.com

Manufacturer	Website
Optima Worldwide, Ltd.	www.optimacompany.com
Orion Medical Products, Inc.	www.orimed.com
Ormco Corp.	www.ormco.com
Orthoband Company, Inc.	www.prlink.com/orth.html
Ortho-Care, Inc.	na
Ortho Diagnostic Systems, Inc.	www.pslgroup.com
Orthomedics, Inc.	na
Ortho Med, Inc.	www.novaortho-med.com
Orthopedic Systems, Inc.	na
OrthroTex	www.medix.de/orthomed/orthotex.htm
Osada Electric Co., Inc.	www.osadausa.com
Osteotech, Inc.	www.osteotech.com
Ote Biomedica	www.modulusa.net
Oto-Med, Inc.	www.otomed.com
Ovamed Corporation	na
Oxboro Medical, Inc.	www.oxboromedical.com
Padgett Instruments, Inc.	www.padgettinst.com
Palco Laboratories	www.palcolabs.com
Pall Biomedical Products Company	www.pall.com
Pall Gelman Laboratory	www.pall.com/gelman/
Palumbo Orthopaedics	www.brace4u.com/palumbo/
Paramedical Distributors	na
Pascal Company, Inc.	www.pascaldental.com
Peace Medical (Global Medi-Tek, Inc.)	www.globalmeditek.com
Pentax Precision Instrument Corp.	www.pentaxmedical.com
Perma-Type Co., Inc.	na
Perkin-Elmer Corp., Nelson Analytical	www.perkin-elmer.com www.galactic.com/instruments/nelson-analytical.htm
Philips Medical Systems North America	www.medical.philips.com
Phillips & Jones (U.S.A.), Inc.	na
Phoenix Biomedical Corp.	www.shunt.com/biomedical/
Physitemp Instruments, Inc.	www.physitemp.com
Picker International Inc., Health Care	www.picker.com
Pie Medical USA	www.piemedical.com
Pilling-Rusch	na
Pilling Weck, Inc.	www.pillingweck.com
Pioneer Medical, Inc.	www.pioneermed.com
Plastron	www.plastron.com
PLC Medical Systems	www.plcmed.com
PML Microbiologicals	www.pmlmicro.com

Manufacturer	Website
PMT Corp.	www.pmtcorp.com
Polaroid Corp. Medical Products	www.polaroid-oem.com/medical.htm
Polaron Instruments, Inc./Bio-Rad, Microscience Division	www.bio-rad.com
Pollenex	www.rivco.com/products/pollenex/ pollenexmain.htm
Poly Scientific R&D Corp.	www.polyrnd.com
Poly Vac, Inc.	www.polyvac.com
Popper & Sons, Inc.	www.popperandsons.com
Portlyn Medical Products	na
Pozzi Dental Products	www.americantooth.com/pozzi.htm
Precision Medical, Inc.	www.beeremedical.com
Premier Dental Products Co.	www.premusa.com
Proctor & Gamble	www.pg.com
Profex Medical Products	na
Propper Manufacturing Co., Inc.	www.proppermfg.com
Puritan Bennett Corp. (Nellcor Puritan Bennett)	www.cpapman.com
PyMaH Corp. (Acquired by 3M in 1996)	www.3m.com
Quest Medical, Inc. (Advanced Neuromodulation Systems)	na
Quinton Instrument Co.	www.ihf.co.uk
Ramvac Corporation	www.ramvac.com
Ranfac Corporation	www.ranfac.thomasrejiolo.com
Redfield Corporation	na
Rehab Designs, Inc. (formerly Jay Medical Ltd.)	www.rehabdesigns.com
Rehabilicare	www.rehabilicare.com
Rica Surgical Products	na
Ricca Chemical Company	www.riccachemical.com
RJL Systems, Inc.	www.rjlsystems.com
Roche Diagnostic Systems, Inc.	www.roche.ch
Rocky Mountain/Orthodontics	www.rmortho.com
Roho, Inc.	www.rohoinc.com
Ross Laboratories/Ross Products Division	www.rosslaboratories.com www.ross.com
Rusch, Inc.	http://ruschinc.com/rusch.shtml
Rush-Berivon, Inc.	www.netdoor.com/com/berivon
S&K Reagents, Inc.	na
Sammons Inc. (Fred Sammons, Inc.)	na
Sanderson-Macleod, Inc.	www.smbrushes.com

Manufacturer

Website

Manufacturer	Website
Sandhill Scientific, Inc.	www.carsengroup.com/sandhill
Sandoz Pharmaceutical Corporation (now Novartis)	www.novartis.com
Sargent-Welch Scientific Co.	www.sargentwelch.com
Sarns, 3M Health Care	www.jtp.com/applied/sarns.htm
Scanlan International, Inc.	www.scanlangroup.com
Schering-Plough Corporation	www.schering-plough.com
Schlueter Instruments, Corp.	www.iscpubs.com/bg/us/manu/ manu1978.html
Schneider (USA), Inc. (Boston Scientific subsidiary)	http://www.bsci.com/index.html
Schott Fibre Optics, Inc.	www.schott.co.uk
Schuco	www.schuco.co.uk
SciMed Life Systems (Boston Scientific)	*www.bsci.com/divisions/scimedTech. html*
Searle & Co., G.D./Buchler Instruments (Labconco)	www.searle.com www.labconco.com
Sechrist Industries, Inc.	www.sechristind.com
Seitz Corporation	www.seitzcorp.com
SensorMedics Corp.	www.sensormedics.com
Shandon Lipshaw, Inc.	www.shandon.com
Sharpe Endosurgical Corp.	na
Sharplan Lasers, Inc.	www.escmed.com
Sharpoint/Surgical Specialties Corp.	www.sharpoint.com
Sherwood Medical Company	www.sherwood.de
Shimadzu Precision Instr. Inc./ Med. Systems	www.shimadzu.com
Shippert Medical Technologies Corp.	www.shippertmedical.com
Siemens Corporation	www.siemens.com
Siemens Elema	www.siemens.fi
Sigma Diagnostics	www.sigma-aldrich.com
Sil-Med Corporation	www.silmed.com
Silipos	www.silipos.com
Sklar Instrument Company	www.sklarcorp.com
SMI	www.smi.de
Smith & Nephew	www.smith-nephew.com
SmithKline Beecham	www.sb.com
Snowden-Pencer	www.snowdenpencer.com
Sodem Systems	www.sodem.ch/
Sofamer Danek Group	www.sofamerdanek.com
Sola Optical USA Inc./ Sola Ophthalmics	www.sola.com

Manufacturer	Website
Sontec Instruments, Inc.	www.sontecinstruments.com
Sony Electronics, Inc., Medical Systems	www.sony.com
Sony	www.ultrasoundsales.com
Sony	www.medelex.com
Sony	www.avsupply.com/sonymed.htm
SpaceLabs Medical, Inc.	www.spacelabs.com
Sparta Surgical Corp.	www.pillingweck.com/sparta.html
Spectrum Surgical Instruments Co.	www.spectrumsurgical.com
Spencer Technologies	www.spencertechnologies.com
Star Guide Corp.	www.starguide.com
Stephens Instruments, Inc.	www.stephensinst.com
St. Jude Medical Co.	www.sjm.com
Stortz Instrument Company	www.elmed.com
Strato/Infusaid	na
Stryker Corp., Medical Division	www.strykercorp.com
Stubbs C., Inc., Frank	www.inmax.com/homecare/fs/fs.html
Sulzer Carbomedics, Inc.	www.carbomedics.com
Sumitomo Electric USA	www.sci.co.jp
Sun-Med, Inc.	www.sunmedica.com
Surgical Instrument Co. of America	na
Surgical Instrument Manufacturers, Inc.	na
Surgical Specialties Instrument Co., Inc.	na
Surgidyne, Inc.	na
Surgilase, Inc.	www.laserengineering.com
Surgitek	www.circoncorp.com
Surgitex Int'l. Corp. of America (Color Max Technologies)	www.colormaxtech.com
Sutter Corp.	www.sutter.com
Sybron Corp.	www.sybron.com
Synectic Engineering, Inc.	www.synectic. net
Tartan Orthopedics, Ltd.	na
Taut, Inc.	www.taut.com
Tava Surgical Instruments	www.tava.com
Telectronics Pacing Systems, Inc.	na
Teledyne, Inc.	www.waterpik.com
Terumo Cardiovascular Systems	www.terumo-us.com
Texas Medical Products, Inc.	www.surgimedics.com
Thomas Scientific	http://thomassci.com
Tidi Products Inc., National	www.bantahealthcare.com
Toolmex Corporation	www.toolmex-polmach.co.uk
TomTec	www.tomtec.de
Topcon America Corporation	www.topcon.co.jp

Manufacturer	Website
Toshiba America Medical Systems	www.toshiba.com
Trimedyne, Inc.	www.trimedyne.com
Truform Orthotics & Prosthetics	www.truform-otc.com
Tulip Company, The	www.tulipmedical.com
Tuzik Corporation	na
Tyco International	www.tycoint.com
Unisurge, Inc.	na
United Instrument Corp.	na
United States Catheter & Instrument Co./Bard Inc. (USCI)	www.crbard.com
United States Surgical Corp. (see AUTO SUTURE)	
Urocare Products, Inc.	www.urocare.com
U.S. Clinical Products, Inc.	na
U.S. Endoscopy Group	www.usendoscopy.com
U.S. Orthotics, Inc.	na
USCI (United States Catheter and Instrument Co./Bard, Inc.)	www.crbard.com
Vacumed	www.vacumed.com
Valley Forge Scientific Corp.	www.vfsc.com
Valleylab, Inc.	www.valleylab.com
Varian	www.varian.com
Vasamedics	www.vasamedics.com
Velcro USA, Inc.	www.velcro.com
Ventritex	www.cardion.cz/ventritex.htm
Veratex Corporation	www.veratex.com
Vicon Industries, Inc.	www.vicon-cctv.com
Victoreen, Inc.	www.victoreen.com
Vingmed U.S.A.	www.vingmed.se
Vision Sciences	www.visionscience.com
Visitec Company	www.visitec.com
Vistec, Inc.	www.vistec.net
Visx, Inc.	www.visx.com
Vital Signs, Inc.	www.vital-signs.com
Volk Optical	www.volk.com
Vygon Corp.	www.vygonusa.com
Wampole Laboratories	www.wampolelabs.com
W.J. Medical Instruments, Inc.	na
Weck & Co., Inc., Edward	www.weckclosure.com
Weck Instruments	www.teleflex.com
	www.pilling-wecksurgical.com